Also available...

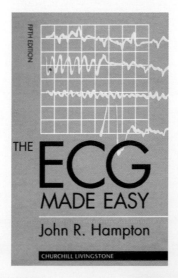

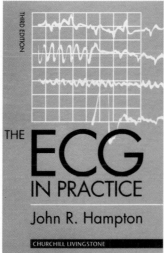

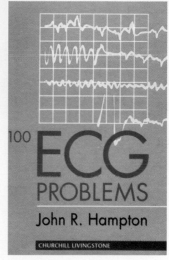

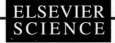

Cardiac Nursing

For Churchill Livingstone:

Senior Commissioning Editor: Ninette Premdas
Project Development Editor: Dinah Thom
Project Manager: Jane Dingwall
Design Direction: George Ajayi

Cardiac Nursing

A Comprehensive Guide

Edited by

Richard Hatchett RN MSc BA(Hons) CertH/Promotion

Principal Lecturer, Faculty of Health, South Bank University, London, Visiting Lecturer, St Batholomew School of Nursing and Midwifery, City University, London, UK

David R Thompson RN MA BSc MBA PhD FRCN FESC

Professor of Nursing, University of York, York, UK

Foreword by

Sarah Mullally RGN BSc(Hons) MSc

Chief Nursing Officer, Department of Health, England

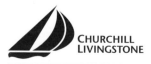

CHURCHILL
LIVINGSTONE

EDINBURGH LONDON NEW YORK PHILADELPHIA ST LOUIS SYDNEY TORONTO 2002

CHURCHILL LIVINGSTONE
An imprint of Elsevier Science Limited

First published 2002
Reprinted 2002

ISBN 0 443 06346 X

British Library Cataloguing in Publication Data
A catalogue record for this book is available from the British Library

Library of Congress Cataloging in Publication Data
A catalog record for this book is available from the Library of Congress

Note
Medical knowledge is constantly changing. As new information becomes available, changes in treatment, procedures, equipment and the use of drugs become necessary. The editors, contributors and the publishers have taken care to ensure that the information given in this text is accurate and up to date. However, readers are strongly advised to confirm that the information, especially with regard to drug usage, complies with the latest legislation and standards of practice.

 your source for books, journals and multimedia in the health sciences

www.elsevierhealth.com

The publisher's policy is to use **paper manufactured from sustainable forests**

Printed in China

Contents

There is a colour plate section between pages 226 and 227.

Contributors

Maree Barnett RN BSc(Hons) DipMngt
Senior Nurse Cardiac Services, Barts and the London
NHS Trust, Cardiac Directorate, London, UK

Claire Bennett RN DipN
Clinical Specialist in Vascular Intervention, Guidant
Corporation, Basingstoke, UK

Frances Blackburn RN BA(Hons)
Senior Sister Cardiology, Coronary Care Unit,
Freeman Hospital, The Newcastle upon Tyne
Hospitals NHS Trust, Newcastle upon Tyne, UK

Beverley Bookless RN RM MBA
Project Manager, National Service Framework –
Coronary Heart Disease, NHS
Executive Northern and Yorkshire, Durham
University Science Park, Durham, UK

Glen Brice RN BSc(Hons)
Research Nurse, Department of Cardiological
Sciences, St George's Hospital Medical School,
London, UK

Angela Bygrave RN BSc(Hons)
Former Arrhythmia Nurse Specialist, Department of
Cardiological Sciences, St George's Hospital Medical
School, London; Currently: Cardiology Unit, The
John Radcliffe Hospital, The Oxford Radcliffe NHS
Trust, Oxford, UK

Carol Cox RN MSc BSc(Hons) MAEd PG DipEd PhD
Professor, Advanced Clinical Practice, St
Bartholomew School of Nursing and Midwifery,
City University, London, UK

Wendy Cox RN BSc(Hons)
Former Sister, Transplant Unit, Harefield Hospital,
The Royal Brompton and Harefield NHS Trust,
London, UK

Nigel Cross HNC
Chief Perfusionist, Theatres, The Great Ormond
Street Hospital for Children NHS Trust, London, UK

Lianne Daniels RN DipN
Sister, Coronary Care Unit, University Hospital of
Wales and Llandough Hospital NHS Trust, Cardiff,
UK

Moira Durbridge RN BSc
Head of Nursing, Cardiorespiratory Directorate,
University Hospitals of Leicester NHS Trust,
Leicester, UK

Lynda Filer RN MSc BSc(Hons) PGCE(A)
Lecturer in Applied Biological Sciences, St
Bartholomew School of Nursing and Midwifery,
City University, London, UK

Sarah Fisher RN MSc BSc
Assistant Director of Nursing, University College
London Hospitals NHS Trust, London, UK

Mary Gould RN MSc BSc(Hons)
Nurse Specialist, Heart Failure, Department of
Cardiological Sciences, St George's Hospital Medical
School, London, UK

Fiona Halstead RN DipN
Cardiology Manager, Barts and the London NHS
Trust, Cardiac Directorate, London, UK

Mary Ibbotson RN BSc(Hons)
Former Cardiothoracic Research Sister, Cardiothoracic
Department, Barts and the London NHS Trust,
Cardiac Directorate, London, UK

Jayne James RN CertEd MSc
Senior Lecturer, Faculty of Social Care, University of
the West of England, Bristol, UK

Stuart Jones RN
Cardiothoracic Liaison Charge Nurse, Cardiothoracic
Liaison Office, Manchester Royal Infirmary, Central
Manchester and Manchester Children's University
Hospitals NHS Trust, Manchester, UK

Grace Lindsay RN MN BSc(Hons) RM PhD
Lecturer, Nursing and Midwifery School, University
of Glasgow, Glasgow, UK

Sue Mason RN MA
Practice Development Nurse, The Glenfield Hospital,
University Hospitals of Leicester NHS Trust,
Leicester, UK

Barbara Novak RN RSCN RNT RM MSc BEd(Hons)
Lecturer in Applied Biological Sciences,
St Bartholomew School of Nursing and Midwifery,
City University, London, UK

Ann O'Donoghue RN
Cardiomyopathy Nurse Specialist, Department of
Cardiological Sciences, St George's Hospital Medical
School, London, UK

Ann-Marie Openshaw RN BSc
Senior Nurse Cardiac Services, Barts and the London
NHS Trust, Cardiac Directorate, London, UK

Tom Quinn RN MPhil FESC
Honorary Visiting Fellow, Department of Health
Studies, University of York, York, UK

Jillian Riley RN BA(Hons) RM MSc
Senior Lecturer, Thames Valley University,
Department of Education, Royal Brompton and
Harefield NHS Trust, London, UK

Catherine Rimmer RN DipCommunityHealthStudies
Cardiothoracic Liaison Nurse, Cardiothoracic Liaison
Office, Manchester Royal Infirmary, Central
Manchester and Manchester Children's University
Hospitals NHS Trust, Manchester, UK

Graham Rumbold RN MSc BA NDN RNT CHNT
Co-ordinator, International Affairs and CPD, Centre
for Health Care Education, University College
Northampton, UK

Prashant Sanghani MSc MRPharmS BPharm
Senior Directorate Pharmacist, Medical and
Emergency, Barts and the London NHS Trust,
London, UK

Myrna Scott RN MSc BSc(Hons)
Critical Care Nursing Team Research Fellow,
St Batholomew School of Nursing and Midwifery,
City University, London, UK

Helen Stokes RN PhD
Visiting Professor, Faculty of Health Sciences,
University of Ottawa, Ottawa, Canada

Adelaide Tunstill RN RSCN BA(Hons)
Grown Up Congenital Heart Nurse Specialist, GUCH
Unit, The Middlesex Hospital, University College
London Hospitals NHS Trust, London, UK

Brian Turner MSc DCR(R)
Superintendent Radiographer, X-Ray Department,
Barts and the London NHS Trust, London, UK

Gill Walsh RN FETC DMS
Theatre Manager, The Heart Hospital, London, UK

Rosemary Webster RN BSc(Hons)
Clinical Nurse Specialist, Coronary Care Unit, The
Leicester General Hospital, University Hospitals of
Leicester NHS Trust, Leicester, UK

Stephen Wilson BSc
Senior Chief Cardiac Technician, Formerly Barts and
the London NHS Trust, Cardiac Directorate, London;
Currently: Treliske Hospital, Truro, UK

Jane Young RN MBA
Senior Sister, Coronary Care Unit, University
Hospital of Wales and Llandough Hospital NHS
Trust, Cardiff, UK

Foreword

Cardiac care is rapidly developing, with a huge evidence base to support many interventions to reduce suffering and speed recovery. But there is also evidence to suggest that uptake of 'proven' therapies for people with heart disease is uneven. There is clearly much to be done to spread good clinical and working practice to benefit all patients, wherever they may be.

The substantial, and ever growing, evidence base for cardiac care covers the whole spectrum of activity from prevention through to improvements in primary care, emergency care, specialized care and rehabilitation. This 'patient pathway' is recognized in current Government policies in England aimed at reducing the high death rates from coronary heart disease (CHD) in particular.

The White Paper *Saving Lives: Our Healthier Nation* (DoH 1999a) sets out the challenge: a 40% reduction in premature deaths from circulatory diseases by 2010. The *National Service Framework for CHD* (CHD NSF) (DoH 2000) published in March 2000, sets out the blueprint for how this will be achieved, providing for the first time clear national standards, service models and monitoring mechanisms to ensure progress across the country. The National Institute for Clinical Excellence has already published guidelines on the use of treatments for heart patients and will continue to appraise new evidence as it becomes available.

The NHS Plan sets out how the NHS will develop to provide people with a service that is built around the needs of the patient: a health service fit for the 21st century. It also sets out plans to make the NHS a better place in which to work. The NHS Plan prioritizes cardiac care through, for example, a commitment to more rapid assessment of suspected angina, shorter waiting times for cardiac surgery, faster treatment for people who suffer a heart attack, and an expansion in cardiac rehabilitation services. The first ever national survey of CHD patients' experiences, published in 2000, gives an insight into the things that matter to patients and presents challenges to nurses and other health workers to address physical comfort and dignity, communication and information-giving in particular.

Successful implementation of the NHS Plan and the CHD NSF is dependent on a skilled, informed, professional nursing workforce for its successful delivery. The evidence base for effective nurse-led interventions in primary, emergency and specialist care continues to grow. In both hospital and community settings, nurses are demonstrating their contribution, in collaboration with medical, paramedical and other colleagues, to improving patients' experience. The CHD Partnership Programme, established with the NSF, is working on 60 projects in 10 local cardiac networks to redesign services for patients. Nurses are key players in each network.

The NHS Plan gave me the opportunity to identify 10 key roles for nurses, setting out ways in which nurses can improve patient care by being able to order diagnostic tests, make and receive referrals, admit and discharge patients within agreed protocols, manage patient caseloads, run clinics, prescribe treatments, carry out resuscitation procedures, perform minor surgery, perform triage, and take the lead in the way local health services are organized and run. In cardiac care, there are great opportunities for nurses to test out and develop these roles, in line with the frameworks outlined in *Making a Difference* (DoH 1999b) and the United Kingdom Central Council's *Code of Professional Conduct and Scope of Professional Practice* (UKCC 1992).

This comprehensive new textbook will make an important contribution to preparing nurses to improve the patients' experience of health care. It is written by an impressive team of authors, all of whom can justly consider themselves experts in their field, bringing a wealth of experience in caring for patients with heart disease, supporting families, and researching better ways of providing care.

The first edition is published at an ideal time to influence the delivery of the Government's priorities for improving heart health. It will play an important part in developing the knowledge base essential for nurses embarking on a career in cardiac care in a range of settings. It will provide a useful source of reference for more experienced nurses who are committed to keeping up to date with contemporary practice. It will stimulate many to explore further the evidence base on which their current practice is founded.

2001   Sarah Mullally

REFERENCES

Department of Health 1999a Saving lives: our healthier nation. Stationery Office, London
Department of Health 1999b Making a difference: strengthening the nursing, midwifery and health visiting contribution to health and healthcare. Department of Health, London

Department of Health 2000 National Service Framework for Coronary Heart Disease. Department of Health, London
United Kingdom Central Council 1992 Code of professional conduct and scope of professional practice. UKCC, London

Preface

Expanding horizons

So often we hear that cardiac nursing is changing more now than ever before. It remains a view inextricably linked to even further technological advances. But is this the whole story and what does this mean to the hospital or community nurse? Is nursing care provision really altering beyond merely learning further aftercare of new treatments? This book is a 3-year project which is a testimony to the changes in cardiac nursing that are occurring from within the profession and from much more than technology. Change is occurring from a variety of angles that clearly impact not only on health-care provision on the wider scale but down to the grass roots of individual practice.

The National Service Framework for Coronary Heart Disease has now been published, with its emphasis on standardizing the high quality of care we want all patients with cardiac disease to receive. As Stuart Jones and Catherine Rimmer discuss, cardiac liaison teams and nurse-led clinics are emerging to facilitate seamless care and to fill the gap in monitoring and maintaining optimum health in those living with chronic cardiac disease. They also offer that valued element of care, the opportunity to enhance communication and explanation to our patients and carers. Myrna Scott explores the concept of critical/integrated care pathways as a method for providing auditable care to a more uniform standard. It will be of continued interest to note how nursing, among other disciplines, adapts the pathways to incorporate areas such as individual assessment and aims to more fully record the process of achieving set outcomes.

It is important to ourselves and the contributors that this book is not about nurses and nursing responding to a medical model. Disease processes, which all nurses need to understand, are explored in detail by expert colleagues in these areas. Yet surrounding these are patient management issues, detail of fast tracking and surgery without bypass. This extends to the wider scope of cardiac health promotion, rehabilitation and initiatives such as nurse-led thrombolysis programmes and the need to meet the requirements of young people with congenital heart defects. For certain of our patients, we now know that there is a growing need to utilize and learn from the skills of palliative care colleagues. We have asked our contributors to excel themselves, providing all those whose interest is cardiac nursing care with sound rationale, the debates for varying forms of care and a rich source of references to explore further.

Cardiac nursing remains exciting. It is exhausting, it is changing and, in an era of nurse shortages and long waiting times for patients, offers the chance to provide innovation in breaking traditional boundaries and to work with related disciplines in providing enhanced and competent care. We both come from a cardiac nursing background but our differing interests, together with the excellent contributors from all over the United Kingdom, will offer a challenging and stimulating book to enhance cardiac nursing as we move into the 21st century. We sincerely thank all those involved in this book.

London and York 2001

Richard Hatchett
David Thompson

Acknowledgements

The editors and publishers sincerely thank all the health professionals and colleagues who gave their time, including permission to reproduce illustrations, in the preparation of this book: John Albarran, Maureen Aruede, Carol Bavin, Darren Bull, Megan Burrows, Simon Croom-Hollingsworth, Dr Anne Child, Andy Cox, Dot Crowe, Jane Curle, Justine Davie, Professor Michael Davies, Rory Farrelly, Lynda Filer, Margaret Findley, Jane Gallagher, Emma Gardner, Gill Glennon, Alison Harvey, Hilary Hollis, Dr Siân Hughes, Corinne Leck, Belinda Linden, Abid Mahboob, Joy MacDonald, Professor William McKenna, Helene Metcalfe, Celeste Morison, Corinna Petre, Professor Chris Price, Jill Riley, Di Robertshaw, Desiree Robson, Dr Mary Sheppard, Mark Stevens, Cath Taylor, Lee Thorogood, Caroline Westgate, Mark Whitbread

and all the reviewers whose signatures we saw but whose faces we didn't.

Epidemiology, health promotion and living with heart disease

SECTION CONTENTS

This section explores the sociolgical and human impact of heart disease. Epidemiology is explored in relation to important factors such as gender, ethnicity and geographic region. The theory behind the varying concepts of health is presented. This aims to assist the practitioner in understanding how this concept may vary between differing patients and clients and inform nursing care. Models of health promotion and their contribution to cardiac nursing care are evaluated, while the role and value of cardiac rehabilitation and the necessity for a structured approach are explored in detail.

1

The sociological and human impact of coronary heart disease

Richard Hatchett
David Thompson

Cardiovascular disease is at present the United Kingdom's biggest killer. This general term encompasses circulatory disorders including cerebrovascular accidents (CVAs or strokes) and coronary heart disease, with over 250 000 deaths a year attributed to this overall cause (British Heart Foundation (BHF) 2000). Coronary heart disease (CHD) itself, which can be defined as the gradual narrowing of the arteries supplying blood to the heart, inevitably demonstrates lower figures yet it remains the most common cause of death in the UK, accounting for approximately one in four deaths in men and one in five in women. This ultimately is a figure in excess of 135 000 deaths per year (BHF 2000). In reading and interpreting demographic studies, it is important to note that various terminology is used with regard to classifying conditions. An additional term used in the latter part of this chapter is ischaemic heart disease, because this is the term used in those particular reports. The term tends to pertain to CHD, which produces symptoms of ischaemia and excludes the general circulatory disorders that cardiovascular disease encompasses.

This opening chapter aims to provide an overview of the trends in heart disease incidence, highlighting age-related, regional, gender and ethnic differences. The reports highlighting inequalities in health across social class will also be discussed. It must always be remembered that CHD is a progressive, degenerative disease. Medicine, through pharmacological measures and revascularization techniques, can alleviate many of the symptoms, reducing the incidence of sudden death, but once present, CHD will limit the quality of life and result in premature death.

GENERAL TRENDS FOR CORONARY HEART DISEASE IN THE UK

In comparison with the rest of the world, the UK still has one of the highest death rates for CHD. However, these figures have in recent years been superseded by rapidly rising numbers in the countries of Eastern and Central Europe, where much political and sociological unrest has been experienced. Within the UK a north–south divide does seem to exist. You are more likely to die of CHD in Scotland, the north of England and Northern Ireland than in Wales and the south of England.

CHD and general disease statistics can take some time to correlate and process, so they will never reflect the exact moment. However, the trend or movement of figures can also provide valuable information regarding disease processes and their occurrence. In studying Figure 1.1, it can be noted that the premature death rate for men living in the north of England is over 50% higher than in the counties of East Anglia and nearly 90% higher for women. Within Wales, the north of England and Scotland the highest mortality rates tend to concentrate in urban areas (BHF 1999). Other recent figures indicate that the premature death rate from CHD for men living in Scotland is over 60% higher than in East Anglia and over 70% higher for women (BHF 2000).

When health trends are examined from the early 20th into the 21st century, a changing pattern can be seen, with a move from infectious disease and high infant mortality to an era of chronic, incurable diseases. The latter include respiratory disorders, diabetes, HIV infection and of course cardiovascular disease. In 1997 average life expectancy at birth in the UK was approaching 75 years for males and 80 for females. This was compared with just over 50 years for men and 54 for women in 1911. The 1998-based population projections indicated that in 2021 the life expectancy at age 60 years will be a further 22 years, compared with 18.8 in 1997 (Social Trends Dataset 2000). Improvements, notably in public health, sanitation and the success of vaccination programmes, have produced a marked decrease in infant mortality, with only two occasions in the last 50 years when the figure increased from one year to the next. It is interesting to note that although medicine has played its part it is the public health measures that have impacted to a far

greater degree on the general decline of infectious diseases (Fig. 1.2).

Improvements in the health of people generally have inevitably led to an older and ageing population and this has impacted on health-care provision through the occurrence of the aforementioned incurable and chronic diseases. Although the picture now appears to show sicker people living longer, it is important to remember that health is a wide and in many ways a highly personal term. In the mid 1990s evidence from the General Household Survey showed that about 60% of all people over the age of 65 suffered from some form of chronic illness or disability, rising to 70% for those over 75 years (Sidell 1995). Yet, when asked in the same survey to rate their quality of health, less than 25% rated it as poor (Sidell 1997). Coronary heart disease itself has been declining since the 1970s but still remains at a worryingly high level (Fig. 1.3).

Figure 1.3 illustrates that deaths from CHD have not fallen to the same degree amongst the various age groups. The figures have fallen fastest in the younger age groups, with a 40% fall in death rates in men aged 35–44 in the 10 years between 1986 and 1996. However, in women, this decline in the same age group over the same years has been only 17% (BHF 2000).

THE RISK FACTORS

Figures for 1996 demonstrated that, in England, 28% of men and 27% of women still smoked. This figure relates to 28% of adults aged 16 years and over (Department of Health (DoH) 1998). The figures have been declining substantially since 1976 but there is evidence that the level of decline has slowed and may indeed have reversed (DoH 1998). The prevalence of cigarette smoking is higher in manual than non-manual socio-economic groups. In 1996 13% of children aged 11–15 regularly smoked cigarettes – 11% of boys and 15% of girls. Although more men smoke than women, there is now a narrowing in the gap between the sexes. Within the various ethnic groups males from the Bangladeshi and Caribbean communities show particularly high smoking rates: 49% and 42% respectively (BHF 2000).

In 1990 the Department of Health began a series of health surveys for England. Each year these have chosen one or a small group of specific topics. The early surveys concentrated on cardiovascular disease and this was again covered in the 1998 report (DoH 1999a). Interviews were held with 19 654 persons representing households across England; 15 908 were aged 16 and over and 3746 were aged 2–15. The households, as opposed to institutions, were drawn from a random

The term 'age standardized' is not uncommon in research reports. The aim of standardization is to allow more precise comparison of two or more crude rates, i.e. collected figures, by eliminating the effect of factors such as the differences in age structure between two or more populations or groups. If you have an unduly high number of elderly people in a group death rates will inevitably be higher, even without the presence of a disease process. Nurses who are keen to understand demographics in more detail should purchase a good overview text such as Newell (1994).

MEN AGED 35–74

	1978	1979	1980	1981	1982	1983	1984	1985	1986	1987	1988	1989	1990	1991	1992	1993	1994	1995	1996	1997
United Kingdom	578	537	521	507	497	502	490	488	470	453	434	407	393	379	364	357	325		292	295
England	523	515	501	486	473	481	471	468	449	433	414	388	377	363	349	341	311	298	281	260
North	613	610	594	572	562	576	576	562	539	531	517	490	468	454	448	422	378	366	337	324
Yorkshire and Humberside	603	582	559	558	545	541	532	534	528	499	490	450	438	410	395	379	345	325	310	290
North West	612	601	583	578	575	572	564	578	538	512	514	474	460	429	413	417	376	359	338	319
East Midlands	535	510	502	491	490	493	475	463	445	436	427	404	384	377	351	342	303	295	281	259
West Midlands	519	508	500	501	498	495	493	496	480	468	436	427	416	382	371	370	323	322	303	284
East Anglia	462	430	432	407	385	390	420	366	382	368	335	318	305	312	290	283	275	333	240	211
South East	464	463	450	431	421	430	410	411	335	375	349	325	319	317	303	297	275	240	250	228
South West	489	500	474	442	434	431	428	416	418	390	368	343	332	317	306	296	279	265	243	225
Wales	629	584	582	534	533	560	518	539	501	489	467	443	427	403	379	390	348	262	318	293
Scotland	656	653	616	621	606	617	595	591	581	565	538	518	481	468	458	453	408	340	371	347
Northern Ireland	653	666	658	630	571	596	598	592	602	541	562	505	483	440	437	413	380		338	323

WOMEN AGED 35–74

	1978	1979	1980	1981	1982	1983	1984	1985	1986	1987	1988	1989	1990	1991	1992	1993	1994	1995	1996	1997
United Kingdom	202	179	174	171	171	172	172	173	167	162	156	150	145	141	134	131	120		104	98
England	171	168	163	161	160	162	162	162	158	153	146	141	137	133	127	123	142	107	99	92
North	235	235	217	215	220	212	222	223	210	222	209	209	196	186	176	172	164	141	134	130
Yorkshire and Humberside	205	209	192	203	196	202	205	203	189	190	183	167	173	162	155	142	130	125	116	112
North West	220	209	210	206	205	210	210	211	205	196	194	188	178	168	167	161	148	136	129	116
East Midlands	170	179	165	158	161	161	171	164	167	155	151	148	141	136	127	130	108	111	99	95
West Midlands	177	167	167	161	167	166	175	172	167	165	161	158	146	139	134	136	118	116	110	103
East Anglia	145	136	134	120	124	122	127	126	123	115	104	101	100	106	94	97	87	110	76	70
South East	139	137	134	133	131	135	130	130	127	122	114	108	107	109	104	100	94	91	81	75
South West	147	142	136	135	126	134	137	133	133	120	112	113	113	110	97	94	90	83	77	70
Wales	195	199	204	178	134	183	187	186	182	177	166	162	154	144	142	142	131	120	112	108
Scotland	256	245	241	242	245	236	228	241	220	226	219	212	201	195	182	180	160		140	136
Northern Ireland	233	246	228	233	226	219	204	222	207	200	209	187	177	164	168	162	153		127	115

ICD codes 410–414, age standardized using the European Standard Population.

Sources: *Office for Population Censuses and Surveys (1994) Mortality Statistics 1992, DHS series. HMSO: London and previous editions;*
World Health Organization (1994) World Health Statistics Annual 1993. WHO: Geneva;
World Health Organization (1997) http://www.who.ch/;
The Office for National Statistics, personal communication (1993–1997 figures).

Figure 1.1 Age-standardized UK death rates from CHD per 100 000 population by standard region, 1978–97. (Reproduced with permission from the British Heart Foundation Statistics Database 1999.)

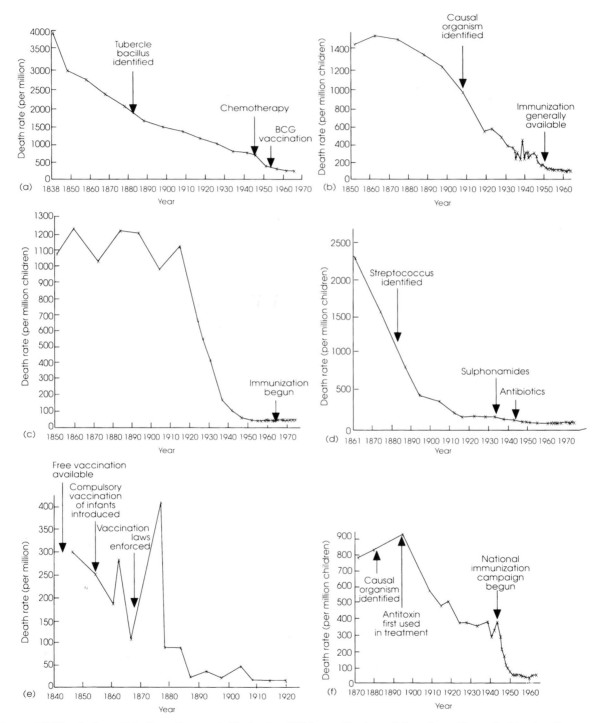

Figure 1.2 The decline of infectious diseases in England and Wales and implementation of specific medical treatment.
a: Respiratory tuberculosis. b: Whooping cough: death rates of children under 15. c: Measles: death rates of children under 15.
d: Scarlet fever: death rates of children under 15. e: Smallpox: death rates. f: Diphtheria: death rates of children under 15.
(Reproduced with permission from McKeown & Lowe 1974.)

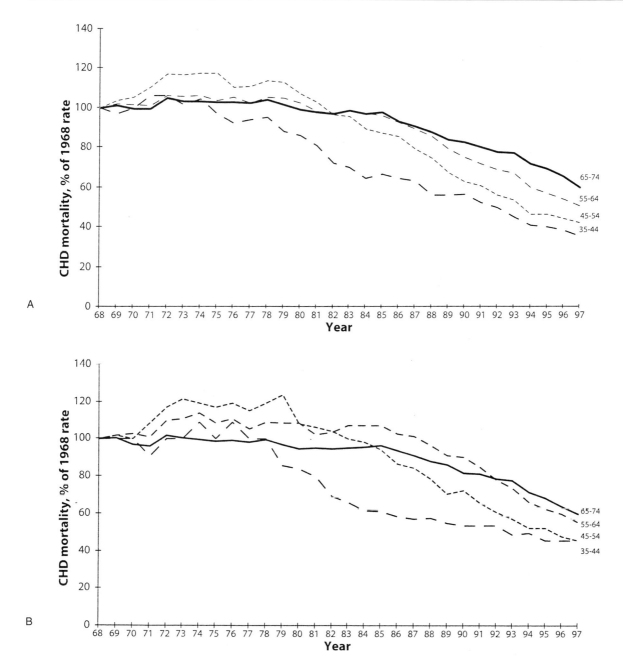

Figure 1.3 Age-specific UK death rates from CHD, 1968–97, plotted as a percentage of the rate in 1968. A: Men. B: Women. (Reproduced with permission from the British Heart Foundation Statistics Database 1999.)

sample of 13 680 address sectors in the postal code address file; 720 postcode sectors were selected and 19 addresses were selected within each sector.

In addition to interviews, blood samples were taken to analyse six variants including total cholesterol, high-density lipoprotein (HDL) cholesterol (known to be a protective factor for heart disease), haemoglobin and fibrinogen (a clotting agent – raised levels can contribute to cardiovascular disease and stroke). The nicotine metabolite cotinine, which is present in saliva following smoking, was also analysed. The survey reinforced the generally accepted figures of smoking prevalence, with 28% of men and 27% of women reporting smoking cigarettes. It was highest in those aged 16–24 (41% of men and 38% of women), declining with increasing age to 9% in men aged 75 years and over and 10% in women of the same age group. The 1998 survey also showed the well-documented social class gradient in cigarette smoking. The age-standardized prevalence in men in social class I was 18%, rising to 42% in social class V. Corresponding figures in women were 14% and 37% (DoH 1999a).

In all social classes in the survey fat consumption was higher in men than women, the mean fat source being 34.0 for men and 28.3 for women. There was a clear social class gradient in age-standardized high fat intake in both sexes. In men this increased from 19% in social class I to 38% in social class V; the corresponding figures in women were 19% and 17%. Slightly over one-third (35%) of men stated that they added salt to food without tasting it first. Men over 55 years were more likely to do this. The proportion of women adding salt without tasting food first was lower, at 24% (DoH 1999a). Fibre intake was assessed from fruit and vegetable, breakfast cereal and bread consumption. Again, there was a strong social class gradient in the prevalence of low fibre intake, increasing steadily in both men and women from social class I (45%, 47%) to social class V (59%, 68%).

Exercise is known to both increase a sense of well-being and reduce the incidence of CHD. It is difficult to gain figures as easily as other risk factors for CHD. However, levels of physical activity are low in the United Kingdom, with only 37% of men and 25% of women meeting the activity guidelines suggested by the government (30 minutes of moderate intensity exercise on 5 or more days of the week, e.g. brisk walking, cycling or climbing stairs) (BHF 2000). In terms of activity to lower the risk of CHD, the exercise has to be regular and aerobic. The latter involves using the large muscle groups in the arms, legs and back steadily and rhythmically so that the breathing and heart rate are significantly increased (BHF 2000). The health survey for England (DoH 1999a) noted that 42% of men had participated in some sports or exercise in the past 4 weeks, of at least 15 minutes' duration. The participation of women in sports and exercise was lower, at 36%. Twenty-two percent of men were classified as at least moderately active, compared with women at 12%. The survey summarized participation in physical activity into various groups. Group 3 was seen as a level that fulfilled the current recommended activity guidelines. Men were far more likely to be classified in group 3 than women, 37% compared to 25% (DoH 1999a).

In terms of body mass, the health survey for England (DoH 1999a) demonstrated that the mean body mass index (BMI) was 26.5 kg/m^2 in men and 26.4 kg/m^2 in women. Overall, obesity (a BMI >30 kg/m^2) was more prevalent in women (21.2%) than in men (17.3%). Notably, what may be termed morbid obesity (a BMI > 40 kg/m^2) was 30% higher in men than women. The BMI and prevalence of obesity have continued to increase in both sexes since 1994 (DoH 1999a).

Raised blood pressure remains of concern as a risk factor for CHD. This is notably because it appears that the condition is often undiagnosed, while the practitioner's technique for recording the pressure can often be improved (see Chapter 5). In England, the mean systolic blood pressure for ages 16–24 years is 128.4 mmHg, rising to 150.3 mmHg at age 75 and over. In women the figures are 120.1 and 155.4 mmHg respectively (DoH 1999a). There appears to have been a general tendency for the mean systolic pressure to decrease between 1994 and 1998, with the change greater amongst women than men. The mean diastolic pressure ranges from 62.7 mmHg at ages 16–24 in men and 78.7 mmHg at age 75 and over. For women the figures are 63.6 mmHg and 76.9 mmHg (DoH 1999a).

The survey provided a new definition for high blood pressure with a systolic reading of ≥140 mmHg and diastolic ≥90 mmHg. The prevalence of high blood pressure increased from 16% in men aged 16–24 years to 72.8% in the age group 75 years and over. For women the figures were 4.2% and 77.6% for the same age groups. Treatment for hypertension was examined. This was calculated by the proportion defined as hypertensive in the survey and receiving antihypertensive medication. The treatment rate was 61% in men and 68% in women (DoH 1999a). Very little variation was found in the prevalence of high blood pressure between social classes in this particular survey.

The mean blood cholesterol level for men in the UK is about 6.2 mmol/l and for women about 6.1 mmol/l. Approximately 37% of men and 34% of women aged 35–64 years have blood cholesterol levels above 6.5 mmol/l (BHF 1999). The pattern of rising cholesterol between the sexes is interesting. In women, the mean cholesterol level does appear to rise with age but flattens off above the age of 75 years. In men it increases more rapidly with age and from 25 to about 50 years is higher than women's. After that it levels off, while women's mean cholesterol continues to increase, becoming substantially higher than men's from age 60 years (DoH 1999a).

Women are noted as having higher levels of HDL cholesterol, which is a protective factor against CHD, when compared to men (1.6 mmol/l compared to 1.3 mmol/l). Mean HDL cholesterol appears the same for all age groups in men, while for women it did seem to fluctuate between 1.5 mmol/l and 1.6 mmol/l in the health survey for England (DoH 1999a). Total cholesterol levels show little social class variation in either sex, although mean HDL cholesterol appears lower for women in manual as opposed to non-manual classes (DoH 1999a).

MORBIDITY

The health survey for England examined the prevalence of cardiovascular disease (CVD) and ischaemic heart disease and the incidence of angina and myocardial infarction (heart attack). The prevalence of ischaemic heart disease (defined as angina or heart attack) was 7.1% in men and 4.6% in women. It was almost three times as high among those aged 55–64 (13.6% in men and 6.3% in women) as amongst those aged 45–54 (4.3% in men and 1.8% in women).

Overall, 5.3% of men reported having ever had angina and 3.2% reported having it currently. Among women the corresponding figures were 3.9% and 2.5%. In both sexes the prevalence increased with age, from being almost negligible under the age of 35 years to almost 1 in 5 in those aged 75 and over. Again overall, 4.2% of men reported ever having had a heart attack and 0.6% reported having it in the last 12 months. Amongst the women in the survey, the prevalence was less than half that in men. Age did increase the prevalence and in those men aged 65 years and over, more than 10% had had a heart attack. One-tenth of these were in the last 12 months (DoH 1999a).

The age-standardized prevalence of any CVD condition (including high blood pressure) was generally higher in manual than non-manual social classes in both sexes. In men, prevalence was lowest in social class I (professional workers) (28.6%) and highest in social class V (unskilled manual workers) (38.2%). However, the gradient was not consistent. In women the prevalence of CVD increased steadily from social class I (31.8%) to social class IV (39.7%), then decreased to 36.6% in social class V (DoH 1999a). From the various sources of morbidity data available, it can be estimated that approximately 270 000 people have a myocardial infarction each year in the UK (BHF 2000). More recent figures reveal that an estimated 1.3 million people in the UK have survived a myocardial infarction, of whom 850 000 are men (BHF 2001). More than 2 million people suffer from angina and 760 000 people are living with chronic heart failure (BHF 2001). The World Health Organization MONICA (Monitoring Trends and Determinants in Cardiovascular Disease) project from the early 1980s monitored trends over 10 years in coronary heart disease across 37 populations in 21 countries (Tunstall-Pedoe et al 1999). Deaths as a result of causes such as coronary heart disease, acute myocardial infarction and risk factors in men and women aged 35–64 years were monitored. The study demonstrated that cities such as Glasgow and Belfast still maintained some of the highest figures for myocardial infarction in the world, with 823 age-standardized events per 100 000 for men and 256 for women in Glasgow while 781 events per 100 000 men and 197 for women occurred in Belfast (Tunstall-Pedoe et al 1994). In comparison, the figures for men in Catalonia, Spain, were 187 events per 100 000 and only 30 for women. Overall, Beijing in China appeared in the study as the lowest, with 76 events per 100 000 for men and 37 events for women.

WOMEN AND CORONARY HEART DISEASE

There are clear differences in the occurrence of CHD in women. In what may be termed premature death, before the age of 75 years, 16% can be attributed to coronary heart disease in women, compared to 26% in men. However, the mortality figure for women from heart and circulatory disease is still twice as high as for cancer (BHF 2000). The difference in the figures between men and women in the earlier years is not least because of factors such as premenopausal hormone protection. Once beyond the menopause, women catch up in the coronary heart disease figures very quickly. By the age of 65 cardiovascular disease is equally common in men and women (Jackson 1994). It should be noted that when death occurs in females under 65 years from myocardial infarction, one quarter are under the age of 45 (Jackson 1994).

In the 1990s an increasing awareness grew that coronary heart disease research had primarily focused upon white, middle-aged men. Particular groups, such as women, were noted as presenting differently and having specific needs in terms of treatment and care (Jackson 1994). Women have been noted as having a higher mortality following myocardial infarction, with a higher operative risk at the time of coronary artery bypass grafting (double that of men) and angioplasty (Jackson 1994). This may in part be due to the more advanced nature of the presenting CHD and factors such as smaller coronary arteries. Clarke et al (1994) presented work that suggested that in terms of treatment, women did not receive the same as men following a myocardial infarction. They took longer to reach hospital, but this may have reflected a lack of awareness of the possibility of infarction. Women tended to have more severe infarcts and were older at presentation. They were therefore more likely to have severe CHD, which increases mortality (Clarke et al 1994).

INEQUALITIES IN HEALTH

Inequalities in health have been noted for many years. This can be linked to an increasing social awareness which led to the commencement of slum clearance and improved sanitation in the 19th century. However, it took the publication of the *Black Report* in 1980 to demonstrate the continuing scale of health inequalities related to social class. The report concluded that the poor health experiences of lower occupational groups applied at all stages of life. The report stated that if the mortality rates of occupational social class I (professional workers and members of their families) had applied to classes IV and V (partly skilled and unskilled manual workers and members of their families) during 1970–2, 74 000 lives under 75 years would not have been lost (Townsend et al 1992). This estimate included nearly 10 000 children and 32 000 men aged between 15 and 64 years.

The controversial report put the emphasis for reducing the inequalities outside the scope of the National Health Service. Social and economic factors such as income, the type of work, the environment, education and housing were seen as affecting health and all favoured the wealthier or, as the report described them, 'the better off'. The *Black Report* was controversial to the new Conservative government in the 1980s and its 37 recommendations were unheeded. These had included recommendations for rapidly phasing out all advertising and sales promotion of tobacco products, the further provision of non-smoking areas in public places, an increase in the level of child benefits to 5.5% of the average gross male industrial earnings and a non-means tested scheme for free milk for mothers with preschool and school children. The emphasis was to lie initially with couples with their first infant child and infant children in large families.

Patrick Jenkin, the then Secretary of State, made it clear 'that the additional expenditure on the scale which would result from the report's recommendations – the amount involved would be upward of two billion pounds a year – is quite unrealistic in present or any foreseeable economic circumstances, quite apart from any judgement that may be formed of the effectiveness of such expenditure in dealing with the problems identified' (Townsend et al 1992, p. 4). Inequalities in health were noted as widening throughout the rest of the century, in reports such as *The health divide* in 1987, updated again in 1992 (Townsend et al 1992).

At the close of the 20th century several reports reiterated concerns about persistent inequalities in health. These included the 1998 *Independent Inquiry into Inequalities in Health Report* (Stationery Office 1998) and the White Paper *Saving lives: our healthier nation* in 1999 (DoH 1999b). The former report was subsequently criticized for not presenting a costing for its 39 recommendations. It was welcomed by some but still produced more of a non-hierarchical 'shopping list' with no particular emphasis, together with a lack of specific strategy to aid implementation (Davey Smith et al 1998).

The Labour government re-emphasized its concerns with the launch in July 1999 of the aforementioned White Paper *Saving lives: our healthier nation* (DoH 1999b). This highlighted that the projected life expectancy at birth of a baby boy was still about 5 years less in social classes IV and V than in social classes I and II. The figures were 70 and 75 years respectively. It also reiterated that social class inequalities in death rates as judged by the gradient between highest and lowest social classes appeared to have been increasing over the previous 40 years. The White Paper addressed health issues such as mental health, cancer and accidents. Chapter 6 focused upon coronary heart disease and outlined an aim to reduce the death rates from this cause and stroke-related diseases (cerebrovascular accident: CVA) in people under 75 years, by at least two-fifths by the year 2110.

This was estimated to save some 200 000 lives in total. The variety of approaches included the proposal of up to £50 million for a smoking cessation public education campaign and the particular targeting of health action zones, areas known to be particularly socially deprived. In June 1999 regulations were published with the intention of moving towards banning tobacco advertising, an original recommendation of the *Black Report*. For those with established heart disease easier access to and more equity in services provided throughout the country were seen as a priority. This led to the setting up of a task force to produce a National Service Framework (NSF) for Coronary Heart Disease which set national standards and defined service models for health provision, disease prevention, diagnosis, treatment, rehabilitation and care (DoH 2000). On its publication in April 2000, a task force accountable to the Chief Medical Officer assisted health-care professionals and organizations in achieving the targets outlined in the White Paper.

ETHNIC POPULATIONS AND CORONARY HEART DISEASE

Throughout the 1980s increased evidence emerged regarding the health inequalities for various ethnic groups within the United Kingdom. *The health divide* (1987), unlike the preceding *Black Report* in 1980, discussed the issue in relative detail. A high mortality caused by ischaemic heart disease was found in immigrants from the Indian subcontinent, while what was termed a 'strikingly high' mortality was noted in immigrants from the Caribbean and Africa from hypertension and stroke (Townsend et al 1992, p. 258).

Immigrant groups with raised mortality in the early 1970s showed little improvement over the decade and mortality from ischaemic heart disease increased amongst Indians by 6% in men and 13% in women (Townsend et al 1992). Currently, the figures remain poor, particularly for those from the Indian subcontinent. The statistics released in 2000 still show that together, South Asians living in the UK (Indians, Bangladeshis, Pakistanis and Sri Lankans) have a higher premature death rate from CHD than average. The rate is 46% higher in men and 51% higher in women (BHF 2000). The reasons may be complex but it is important to remember also that the causes of CHD are often multifactorial. Ethnic minorities settling in Britain may experience poverty, poor housing and employment difficulties, all of which can correlate with poor health. Learning how to access medical services and basic rights may be difficult, particularly if English is not a first language.

The difference in death rates between South Asians and the rest of the population is widening. This is partly due to the fact that the death rate from CHD is not declining as fast in this group as in the general population. Wild & McKeigue (1997), in reviewing census data from 1971 and 1991, noted that the standardized mortality ratios (SMR) for ischaemic heart disease fell by 29% for men and by 17% for women. Caribbean immigrants showed a steeper decline of 38% for men and 40% for women, while South Asian immigrants showed a shallower decline of 20% for men and only 7% for women. The report highlighted that high SMR figures for ischaemic heart disease and cerebrovascular disease in South Asian men and women are consistent with rates in this group worldwide. They appear associated with an increased prevalence of central obesity and insulin resistance (McKeigue et al 1989).

It was not clear why Afro-Caribbean people, in whom the prevalences of diabetes and hypertension were high, had relatively low rates of ischaemic heart disease. A genetic factor may play a part. The high incidence of death from stroke in African and Caribbean populations is still a concern. For West Africans the rate is nearly three times higher than the general population and 81% higher for women. In Caribbeans it is 68% higher for men and 57% for women (BHF 2000).

CARDIAC INTERVENTIONS

The numbers of interventions for CHD occurring in Britain provide further detail on morbidity, by offering a suggestion of the severity of heart disease in individuals. It is important at this point to realize that there has been concern in more recent years regarding variations in the use of cardiac services within specific areas, particularly amongst the social classes and in areas of social deprivation (Ben-Shlomo & Chaturvedi 1995, HMSO 1993, Payne & Saul 1997). The use of services has not always appeared commensurate with need, when symptoms of conditions such as angina are linked to the coronary artery revascularization techniques available (Payne & Saul 1997). However, such findings have not always been conclusive. Ben-Shlomo & Chaturvedi (1995), in examining the North East Thames Regional Health Authority, concluded that inequities may have existed in the provision of coronary artery bypass grafting (CABG) operations for men in the region. However, the ratio of CABG operations to ischaemic heart disease mortality by deprivation was relatively constant in women, suggesting equitable provision. Kee et al (1993), examining access to coronary catheterisation or angiography in acute hospitals across Northern Ireland, noted that there was no significant difference in invasive investigation rates for heart disease in areas of varying deprivation or affluence. The reports do, however, suggest a clear need to monitor such demographics and access to service, to ensure greater equity.

The number of CABG operations has increased steadily since the late 1970s. In 1996–7 a total of 22 160 CABG operations were performed in the United Kingdom, while only 2653 occurred in 1978 (BHF 1999). A total of over 28 000 CABG operations now occur each year (BHF 2000). The British Cardiovascular Intervention Society (De Belder 1997) provides details of percutaneous coronary interventions (PCIs). The number of centres performing these in 1997 was 58: 45 NHS and 13 private hospitals. This was a growth of five centres (four NHS and one private) since 1996. All the centres reported performing diagnostic cardiac catheterisation. Another 32 centres performed diagnostic but not intervention procedures. One NHS and two private hospitals provided no data but from the remaining 55 centres, a total of 22 902 coronary interventions were reported for the year 1997; 20 885 were performed in NHS hospitals. This compares to a total of 20 511 reported in 1996, an annual increase of 11.7%. In the NHS centres, the mean number of adult catheter sessions per week was 16.1 in 1996 (nine in the private hospitals) and 15.7 in 1997

(9.5 in the private hospitals). The mean annual number of adult diagnostic angiograms per centre in 1996 was 2087 (909 in the private hospitals) and 2547 in 1997 (734 in the private hospitals). The mean annual number of adult intervention procedures per centre was 460 in 1996 (137 in the private hospitals) and 475 in 1997 (183 in the private hospitals). The society had previously reported a growth in stent procedures and this continued in 1997, with 60% of all cases being treated with this modality (data from 47 centres; De Belder 1997).

CHD costs the UK health-care system approximately £1600 million a year. However, in addition, CHD costs the UK economy about £8500 million because of days lost due to death, illness and informal care of people with the disease (BHF 2000). Thus, the costs of CHD, both human and economic, are substantial.

Two more recent key national initiatives have emphasized the role that nurses play in combating cardiovascular disease. The first, a national nursing strategy for England (DoH 1999c), emphasizes the need for nurses to extend their roles and make better use of their knowledge and skills. It highlights evidence supporting the development of nurse-led initiatives in risk assessment, cardiac rehabilitation and secondary prevention.

The second, the aforementioned National Service Framework for Coronary Heart Disease, a blueprint for tackling heart disease and improving cardiac services in England (DoH 2000), is a radical and far-reaching programme designed to transform prevention, diagnosis and treatment. It sets out a 10-year programme designed to achieve a target of cutting CHD and stroke by 40% by 2010. It sets 12 standards for the prevention, diagnosis and treatment (including rehabilitation) of CHD, describes service models and explains how the standards can be delivered and how progress will be monitored. The introduction of this framework was part of the government's strategy to improve the quality of services by setting standards. As the Framework points out (DoH 2000, section 1.13), the evidence shows:

- rates of CHD vary according to social circumstances, gender and ethnicity
- differences across the social spectrum have been growing
- many people are not receiving or acting on advice and help that could stop them developing CHD in the first place
- many people with CHD are not receiving treatment of proven effectiveness
- there are unjustifiable variations in quality and access to some CHD services.

The NSF continues (section 1.15) that its aim is to:

- specify interventions that are known to be effective
- identify models of care that deliver those interventions reliably
- provide the means to implement improved systems of care
- develop audit tools and performance indicators to help ensure services are being delivered to an acceptable standard
- indicate milestones and goals by which the NHS can monitor progress towards delivery
- identify gaps in knowledge or standards to inform the research and other agendas
- institute a system for receiving and updating the contents of the NHS in line with developments.

Thus, the effect of the NSF will be to reduce undesirable variations and inconsistencies in service delivery access, improve overall quality of care and thereby improve the overall health of the population. Northern Ireland and Wales do not have frameworks but are working to reduce CHD. In Scotland a CHD taskforce was set up in 1998.

By April 2001 the health service was required to have introduced smoking cessation clinics, producing quantitive data no older than 12 months regarding this implementation by April 2002. 100 rapid access chest-pain clinics have to be in place by April 2002. The 'call to needle' time for thrombolysis is required to be 30 minutes for 75% of eligible patients by April 2002 and 20 minutes by April 2003. Nurses will continue to play a key role, particularly in running 'cardiac prevention clinics', providing 'outreach' follow-up and leading 'heart failure clinics', in addition to their usual contribution to prevention, management and rehabilitation.

In conclusion, statistics and trends in coronary heart disease can provide general information regarding both how the disease is declining and how effective social and medical measures may be. Regional variations offer a correlation with factors which may be linked to lifestyle and the environment. The papers emerging following the *Black Report* (1980) have notably focused upon these latter issues. Variations between ethnic groups can assist health-care professionals and those involved in broader social planning and health promotion to target and monitor groups more likely to succumb to heart disease. The issue of women and CHD has allowed us to reflect whether we have been addressing care and treatment issues based upon research amongst groups that are not homogeneous.

REFERENCES

Ben Shlomo Y, Chaturvedi N 1995 Assessing equity in access to health care provision in the UK: does where you live affect your chances of getting a coronary artery bypass graft? Journal of Epidemiological and Community Health 49(2): 200–204

British Heart Foundation 1999 The British Heart Foundation coronary heart disease statistics. British Heart Foundation Statistics Database, London

British Heart Foundation 2000 The British Heart Foundation coronary heart disease statistics database: annual compendium. British Heart Foundation, London

British Heart Foundation 2001 Coronary heart disease statistics: morbidity supplement 2001. British Heart Foundation, London

Clarke KW, Gray D, Keating NA, Hampton JR 1994 Do women with acute myocardial infarction receive the same treatment as men? British Medical Journal 309: 563–566

Davey Smith G, Morris JN, Shaw M 1998 The Independent Inquiry into Inequalities in Health is welcome, but its recommendations are too cautious and vague (editorial). British Medical Journal 317: 1465–1466

De Belder M 1997 Cardiac intervention procedures in the United Kingdom 1997. Council of the British Cardiovascular Intervention Society, London

Department of Health 1998 Statistics on smoking: England 1976 to 1996. Bulletin 1998/25. Department of Health, London

Department of Health 1999a Health survey for England: cardiovascular disease 1998. Stationery Office, London

Department of Health 1999b Saving lives: our healthier nation. Department of Health, London

Department of Health 1999c Making a difference: strengthening the nursing, midwifery and health visiting contribution to health and healthcare. Department of Health, London

Department of Health 2000 National Service Framework for Coronary Heart Disease. Department of Health, London

HMSO 1993 Clinical standards advisory group. Coronary artery bypass grafting and coronary angiography: access to and availability of specialist services. HMSO, London

Jackson G 1994 Coronary artery disease and women (editorial). British Medical Journal 309: 555–557

Kee F, Gaffney B, Currie S, O'Reilly D 1993 Access to coronary catheterisation: fair shares for all? British Medical Journal 307(6915): 1305–1307

McKeigue PM, Miller GJ, Marmot MG 1989 Coronary heart disease in South Asians: a review. Journal of Clinical Epidemiology 42: 597–609

McKeown T, Lowe CR 1974 An introduction to social medicine. Blackwell Science, Oxford

Newell C 1994 Methods and models in demography. John Wiley, Chichester

Payne N, Saul C 1997 Variations in use of cardiology services in a health authority: comparison of coronary artery revascularisation rates with prevalence of angina and coronary mortality. British Medical Journal 314: 257–261

Sidell M 1995 Health in old age: myth, mystery and management. Open University Press, Buckingham

Sidell M 1997 Older people's health: applying Antonovsky's salutogenic paradigm. In: Sidell M, Jones L, Katz J, Peberdy A (eds) Debates and dilemma in promoting health. Open University and Macmillan, Basingstoke, pp. 9–15

Social Trends Dataset 2000 Expectation of life at selected ages by gender, 1911–2021 (selected years). National Statistics Information and Library Service, London

Stationery Office 1998 Independent Inquiry into Inequalities in Health. Stationery Office, London

Townsend P, Davidson N, Whitehead M 1992 Inequalities in health: The Black Report and The Health Divide. Penguin Books, Harmondsworth

Tunstall-Pedoe H, Kuulasmaa K, Amouyel P, Arveiler D, Rajakangas AM, Pajak A 1994 Myocardial infarction and coronary deaths in the World Health Organization MONICA project. Registration procedures, event rates, and case fatality rates in 38 populations from 21 countries in four continents. Circulation 90(1): 583–612

Tunstall-Pedoe H, Kuulasmaa K, Mahonen M, Tolonen H, Ruokokoski E, Amouyel P 1999 Contribution of trends of survival and coronary-event rates to changes in coronary heart disease mortality: 10-year results from 37 WHO MONICA project populations. Monitoring trends and determinants in cardiovascular disease. Lancet 353: 1547–1557

Wild S, McKeigue P 1997 Cross sectional analysis of mortality by country of birth in England and Wales 1970–92. British Medical Journal 314: 705

2

Health promotion and its application in coronary heart disease

Grace Lindsay

This chapter examines health as a concept from different perspectives, taking into account theoretical definitions, lay viewpoints and health-related quality of life. Theories relating to health beliefs, locus of control, social support and behavioural change will be examined in general and specifically, where they may be helpful to the understanding of health behaviours in the cardiac patient or client. Contemporary, wider definitions of health promotion, its objectives, focus and individual components will be discussed and limitations to the medical model of health highlighted. Examples of interventions based on theoretical perspectives of behavioural change will be used to highlight their application to clinical practice within cardiac nursing.

HEALTH AS A CONCEPT

There is a general consensus that health is a multidimensional phenomenon. It is not merely the absence of an identifiable disease but a positive state of well-being and a reserve of overall health determined in large part by individual constitution (Blaxter 1985, Herzlich 1973, Pill & Stott 1982). Although health is generally viewed as a positive entity to be desired, individuals may also recognize that high levels of health can co-exist in the presence of serious or long-term illness (Blaxter 1990). This may be seen as a paradox, in that individuals are perfectly capable of admitting to serious illness and yet claiming to be healthy while on the other hand, there are those who report low levels of health but who have no discoverable pathology. This indicates a growing consensus that individuals have important knowledge of their own health state (Tuckett et al 1985) and therefore this view should be carefully recorded and monitored. This in turn has fuelled the search for better subjective measures of health.

DEFINITION OF HEALTH

The World Health Organization (WHO) definition of health has embodied a multifaceted view with distinct components through which optimal levels of health can exist, with or without the presence of disease. Health has been described as 'the state of complete physical, mental and social well-being and not merely the absence of disease or infirmity' (WHO 1977). This definition was widely endorsed but is now relatively dated and has been criticized for several reasons. It described 'health' as a 'state' which implied that it was a fixed and static entity and was viewed as a utopian ideal with few direct applications to individuals or populations in practice. However, it was considered an advance at that time because it introduced a multidimensional view of health and moved away from the disease model. One of its important concepts was related to the possibility of high levels of health in the presence of disease. More recently, the WHO has explored a variety of newer definitions of health including 'a resource for living'.

ILL HEALTH AND DISEASE

The 'disease-based' view of ill health is based on the premise that poor health is a function of an abnormality and the term 'disease' therefore has been used in a limited and scientific manner (Field 1976). Illness, conversely, refers to a person's subjective experience of 'ill health' indicated by reported symptoms and personal accounts, such as pain, distress or discomfort. Furthermore, objectively defined 'disease' does not bear a simple causal relationship with subjectively reported experience of illness. As MacIntyre (1986b) noted, screening studies of random cross-sections of the population have shown that very few people are without some abnormalities that can be defined as 'disease', even though many of the affected individuals are unaware of the disorders.

In a similar manner to the perspective of illness, the term 'well-being' can also be viewed as a subjective view of a health state. In the Oxford Health Lifestyle Survey (Wright et al 1992), of those reporting long-term chronic illness, only 28% reported that their health was fair or poor on a scale of excellent, good, through to fair and poor. This highlights the complexities of assessing health where individuals are very well aware of the diseased state and yet rate their overall health as good. It would suggest that there is a complex meaning that people attach to this term 'health'. Many studies support the view that health should be regarded as a multidimensional concept; that is, not only the absence of disease but a positive state of well-being and a reserve of overall health determined in large part by individual constitution (Blaxter 1985, Herzlich 1973, Pill & Stott 1982).

HEALTH WITHIN ILLNESS

Dunn (1973) defined health as 'an integrated method of functioning ... orientated towards maximizing the potential of which the individual is capable'. Others have described it as 'the adaptive potential of the individual' (Dubos 1965), 'harmony with self and environment' (Neuman 1990) and conformity to social norms (Parsons 1972). These viewpoints consider health status to include subjective dimensions that relate uniquely to the individual. Neuman (1990) proposed that health should be viewed as a continuum representing the degree of client wellness existing at any point in time. The energy level of wellness was considered to range from its maximum value at optimal health to zero (total energy depletion) at death. This theoretical perspective of health could be considered to provide the basis for quantitative measurement of different levels of health.

Pender (1989) supported the need for a new approach to understanding health that combined both objective and subjective health perspectives. This approach excluded the possibility of physical and behavioural dimensions of health being viewed as separate or in opposition to experiential aspects of health. As a result, a unitary view was proposed (Neuman 1990, Newman 1986) where health is the positive state to be desired and illness or disease is the negative state to be avoided. Therefore a polarized view of health was generated where the positive state, identified with optimal health, was diametrically opposite to the negative state, identified with disease (Pender 1989). The 'either/or' dichotomy that was thereby created precluded the existence of high levels of health in the presence of disability or disease. As such it does not explain the complex and varied nature of health status in the context of disease or in its absence.

There has not been general support for the latter polarized view of health. Moch (1989) proposed that there are many positive health states in the presence of illness. She justified this stance on the basis that the experience of illness has been credited with many rewarding attributes such as 'stimulating personal transformation', a 'means of learning about oneself' and the 'opportunity to reflect on the meaningfulness of life' (Moos 1982).

In a qualitative study, the experience of feeling healthy for people living with a chronic illness and/or disability was explored in a group of eight individuals using an interpretative phenomenological approach (Lindsey 1996). The essential attributes that were identified by the participants were: honouring the self; seeking and connecting with others; creating opportunities; celebrating life; transcending the self; and acquiring a state of grace (Lindsey 1996). These positive experiences were not documented by previous work that examined the impact of chronic illness. Factors such as a loss of self-identity and strained and problematic relationships with others have been reported (Charmaz 1997). A process of adaptation in order to cope has been identified by others and described as similar to grief (Matson 1977). These differing perspectives of health within illness may be a result of the focus of the research question. The different accounts that were given could be explained by simply changing the emphasis of the area of enquiry from that of 'health' to that of 'illness'.

HEALTH FROM A LAY PERSPECTIVE

Medical knowledge rests upon the concept of disease, whereas the lay perspective of health affected by illness has been described as being rooted in the experience of illness, either personally or through others (Williams & Wood 1986). Lay beliefs about illness are many and varied and do not simply mirror medical science. Although this may imply that they lack any scientific and valid basis, they have been shown to be logical, consistent and coherent, providing narrative reconstructions of the relationship between illness, health and health-related behaviours (Williams & Popay 1996). Lay perspectives have been shown to bring together different aspects of the person's experience of the onset, course and effects of their illness in an attempt to make sense of this in causal terms (Blaxter 1983). While the biological basis may be considered to shape and set limits on human experience, the recognition that 'it may tell us little about the social meaning and significance ascribed to such knowledge' has been cited as its major limitation in terms of understanding health (McIntyre 1986a).

Perceptions of health have been shown to change over the course of life, although there are some common elements. These include the ability to function, energy and vitality, psychosocial well-being and the understanding and recognition that high levels of health can be present despite a major illness (Blaxter 1990). The world of everyday life can therefore be viewed as the total sphere of an individual's experiences, being circumscribed by the objects of living and encompassing what is seen to be true or real to each individual.

Lay perspectives of health and well-being in patients with coronary heart disease

A qualitative study interviewed 12 women and 13 men at around 2 weeks and 5 months following their myocardial infarction (heart attack) (Wiles 1998). Although at initial interview, information provided by health professionals about recovery was central to people's understanding about the nature of heart attack and their future risk, this was not maintained. As they came to terms with the shock of the event, contradictory accounts of cause and recovery with evidence from lay epidemiology tended to emerge. It was concluded that the failure of health-care professionals to recognize the random nature of the occurrence of heart attack, its severity and level of recovery fuelled people's reluctance to take on board the lifestyle messages as rational action to take to prevent another heart attack.

In a study examining the health and well-being of 215 patients awaiting coronary artery bypass grafts (CABG), a thematic analysis of responses to enquiry about perceptions of health and well-being was undertaken (Lindsay et al 2000). In general, the comments relating to health covered a broad range of issues relating to many dimensions. The all-pervading effect of heart disease on health was summarized by one subject who said that it 'affects every facet of life and the thought of having an operation ... makes me so anxious even to think about it'. The key issues relating to their health experience were captured within two main themes that emerged from analysis of the memos collected during the structured interview: dependency and impending doom. Dependency was the most common theme to emerge and on more detailed examination, three subthemes were identified within the dependency theme: dependency on functional status, dependency on others and dependency on medication.

Dependency on functional capability was the most frequently raised issue by patients in the study and different strategies in dealing with its limitations were described. Many patients reported that they were not free to make choices about even very basic everyday activities such as visiting a friend or doing housework: 'I have to think and plan what I am doing in advance'. This planning took the form of making an assessment of their health in terms of the level of cardiac symptoms and general tiredness at a particular moment, because their capacity to cope with activity varied considerably and was unpredictable far in advance. Some patients found it difficult to express in broad terms a view of their health and well-being because of the changeability as highlighted in the following comments: 'How I feel is variable', 'I have good days and bad days'. Some patients described a sense of their activity being driven by their symptoms or lack of them. They employed a strategy of undertaking activities a little at a time and continually reviewed how they felt as captured in this statement: 'I have to pace myself, hills a big problem'. High levels of functional disability were reported by many patients: 'Can only walk about 50 yards before pain starts'. A dependency on walking routes that were relatively flat with no steps or stairs was highlighted: 'I avoid hills and inclines like the plague'.

Forward planning was reported by the majority of subjects; an example of one comment was that the subject 'never tackled unknown areas on foot'. Detailed planning of journeys where walking would be involved was reported: 'Frightened to go too far a distance walking and can't get back, get very uptight', with one man reporting that in stark contrast to his previous disinterest in shops, when he was planning to walk anywhere he would make sure that the route passed by shops, so that he had an 'excuse to stop' or what he considered to be a legitimate reason for stopping to relieve chest pain and breathlessness. He reported feeling embarrassed at having to stop which was made worse if he was in open spaces.

Others reported a high degree of reliance on glyceryl trinitrate (GTN) spray for angina symptoms as reported by one man: 'I have to take a spray before I do anything, even washing and shaving'. Not only was a high degree of dependency reported but also the issue of the need for forward planning where medication was undertaken in advance of activity in order to minimize worsening of symptoms or initiating chest pain. This led again to advance planning to ensure that when this cardiac medication was needed it would be close to hand.

Dependency on others to take care of their usual responsibilities within the family setting was mentioned: 'My daughter is having her first baby, don't know how I can plan to help; I depend on my husband and daughter to keep things going'. In this case the patient had the additional concern of not being able to participate in supporting her daughter at a very important and special time in both their lives. Another level of dependency described by a small number of the patients was related to adherence to medical advice: 'As long as I do what doctor says, I'll be OK', in a broader sense than solely relating to medication. Responsibility for their health and well-being was devolved to their doctor with a sense of lack of any personal control or influence over their health status.

These accounts are provided by patients who were awaiting coronary surgery with moderate to severe angina and breathlessness. However, although these perspectives are not necessarily generalizable to all patients with CHD they do provide some insights into the impact of the disease on general health and well-being. In addition, they highlight strategies employed by patients in order to cope with the limitations imposed by their symptoms.

HEALTH-RELATED QUALITY OF LIFE

A single comprehensive view of health has been considered widely to include a dimension of quality. Calman defined quality of life as 'the extent to which a person's hopes and ambitions are matched and fulfilled by experience' (Calman 1984). Quality of life, as it has been traditionally viewed, embodies broader issues related to agencies and experience outside the domain of health (Farquhar 1995, Meeberg 1993). In addition to health, quality of life encompasses many other factors such as job satisfaction, family relations, standard of living, neighbourhood type and so forth. The term 'health-related quality of life' has been introduced to help focus on factors that are more directly attributed to health and health service activity.

In essence, the meaning of 'quality of life' still remains a matter of debate. There are no agreed definitions upon which to guide health-care practice or research. Quality of life can be viewed from two broad conceptual bases. The first is that of a subjective interpretation of views and events (Bergner 1985, Campbell et al 1976, McDowell & Newell 1987) and the second takes the view that quality of life can be reduced into functional component parts that can be used in health outcome measurement (Aaronson 1988, Jenkins et al 1990, Stewart & Ware 1992). In the literature terms such as health status, functional status, well-being and life satisfaction are sometimes used interchangeably with quality of life (Spitzer 1987). There is general agreement that quality of life is a multidimensional concept (Jenkins et al 1990, McDowell & Newell 1987) that can be useful as a measure of changes in health status as a result of health-care interventions. Some authors believe that quality of life remains a fashionable idea rather than a rigorously defined concept in the health sciences (Harrison et al 1996, McDowell & Newell 1987). Harrison et al (1996) described 'quality of life' in the context of assessment of health outcome as a person's 'conception of their health status and aspects of their life considered important in relation to their expectations of normal living'. This view encompasses the notions of a subjective evaluation of one's life against what is normal, an acknowledgement of expectations against natural capacity and meeting personal goals by narrowing the gap between one's expectations and one's achievements.

For the purposes of outcome measurement, the operational definitions are usually more restrictive and situation specific (Waltz et al 1991). In the case of health-related quality of life, the domains important to the study population and the health intervention under investigation are most commonly used as the focus for quality of life. Many available therapies offer similar morbidity and mortality outcomes but different effects on quality of life. Bypass surgery is cited as one such therapy.

Health status and quality of life in individuals with CHD

Coronary heart disease (CHD) affects different individuals in different ways. In some it may have no apparent effect. In others it may cause death preceded or not by symptoms and in a third group, it may cause incapacity due to angina. In the search for objectivity we often try to quantify the degree of incapacity due to angina with treadmill or bicycle exercise tests (Cowley 1995). Even when these tests are continued to their maximum workload, there is no indication that this correlates well with the incapacity experienced during daily life. More subjective assessment and accounts are necessary in order to improve understanding of the full impact of disease on an individual's lifestyle.

In a study comparing the symptoms and well-being following myocardial infarction (MI) in men and women, agreement was seen with previous studies, whereby female patients were older and sicker, they more often had angina, congestive heart failure and hypertension (Kitler 1992). In terms of symptomatic differences, these ranged from more pronounced symptoms to psychological complaints. This indicated that women had more difficulty in adapting after a MI. Another study examining survivors of a MI at 5 years showed that women had significantly poorer health-related quality of life in terms of fatigue, sleep disturbances, emotional complaints, mobility, pain and social isolation (Wiklund et al 1989).

Women are more likely to seek medical care when symptoms emerge (Verbrugge & Wingard 1987) compared with men and also have higher overall rates of physical illness, disability days, physicians' visits and drug use (Verbrugge 1989). Women claimed that their health status interfered to a greater extent with house-work and social life than in men. This may be due to the fact that the responsibility for household and social chores in most families still lies almost entirely on the woman in the family. Nevertheless, after an MI, home and daily activity priorities tend to prevail. This may be one reason why women do not utilize cardiac rehabilitation programmes as often as men (Conn et al 1991, Hamilton 1990).

The quality of life of people suffering from CHD was evaluated in a study that included 100 patients who had undergone CABG surgery, 100 angioplasty and 80 medically treated patients (Lukkarinen & Hentinen 1997). The New York Heart Association (NYHA) classification, which is a measure of grades of functional status, was used as a quality of life assessment. Almost two-thirds of the patients (65%) were graded as having class 3 or 4 severity of symptoms, which meant that they had chest pain upon slight exercise or at rest. The health-related quality of life across the six dimensions of health as measured by the Nottingham Health Profile (McEwen 1993) was significantly poorer in a group of CHD patients than in an age- and gender-matched general population sample. The differences were most obvious on the dimensions of energy, pain, emotional reaction, sleep and physical exercise. Social isolation correlated with age, employment, financial status, mood, smoking and physical exercise. The authors concluded that CHD appears to handicap the person's entire life and to interfere with their basic daily activities, preventing physical mobility and sleep, causing a decline of energy. This arouses the inevitable emotional reactions of fear and depression, resulting in an overall feeling of illness. The authors found that the Nottingham Health Profile was well suited to measuring the quality of life of CHD patients. It provided an accurate view of the subfactors in different patient groups, although it did not yield profound information on an individual's subjective quality of life.

A large study using the SF-36 questionnaire, a generic health-related quality of life tool, to evaluate the benefits of the addition of a glyceryl trinitrate (GTN) patch to their usual treatment in 4400 patients with stable angina showed more positive results over a 6-month period (Charlier et al 1997). The study objectives were to prospectively record the number of anginal attacks, the need for rescue medication (sublingual nitrates) and SF-36 scores following the addition of the GTN transdermal patch in patients with stable angina. The design was open, non-comparative and prospective. The SF-36 scores ranged from 36.25 to 55.49 at baseline to 46.16 to 79.77 at 6 months. A maximum possible score of 100 indicates the highest healthy state, with a minimum score of 0 indicating the worst health state. The scores were correlated with a statistically significant reduction in both frequency of angina attacks (3.38 per week vs 0.86 per week, p<0.001) and use of rescue medication (2.5 tablets/day vs 0.67 tablets/day, p<0.001).

The authors acknowledge the potential for bias inherent in open studies without a randomized control group, together with a well-established placebo effect of the introduction of new therapy in the management of angina pectoris, which may produce favourable influence on subjective assessments of health status. However, all eight domains of the health status profile clearly improved significantly during the study and correlated with positive changes in clinical presentation. The SF-36 instrument was therefore able to detect changes in health status with changes in clinical status for patients with stable angina pectoris.

SOCIO-ECONOMIC DEPRIVATION

The impact of socio-economic circumstances on health is highlighted by the existence of large differences in health and disease experience across socio-economic groups. This is a fact that will be highlighted throughout this book. The relationship between increased risk of ill health and disease with lower socio-economic status has been recognized for hundreds of years (Smith et al 1995). Depending on the classification used, twofold, threefold and fourfold differences in mortality have been reported in the UK (Davey-Smith et al 1990, Goldblatt 1990, Morris & Carstairs 1991). Socio-economic-related gradients in health have been explained in terms of their association with both social position and with different material circumstances such as bad housing, poor diet, inadequate heating, unemployment and poverty (Wilkinson 1997).

Furthermore, psychosocial effects of adverse social position have been implicated in the generation of health inequalities through an increased exposure to risk of chronic mental and emotional stress, together with the related coping strategies of cigarette smoking and alcohol excess. These associations were also outlined in the *Black Report* (Townsend et al 1992), initially published in 1980 and now considered synonymous with the relationship between socio-economic deprivation and ill health. It was concluded that smoking, diet and other behavioural factors interact with biological effects to contribute to, but not fully explain, health inequalities.

An individual's biological development takes place within a social context. This structures their life chances so that advantages and disadvantages tend to cluster cross-sectionally and accumulate longitudinally (Bartley et al 1997). Examples of these relationships have been documented in many areas of achievement and in health status. In particular, children of less affluent families are more likely to fail at school (Essen & Wedge 1992), to find work in the more disadvantaged areas of the workplace and to experience unemployment earlier in their working lives (Ashton et al 1987). In addition, less affluent families are more likely to give birth to babies of lower birth weight, a factor which has been linked to socio-economic disadvantage in childhood and adolescence (Bartley et al 1994). Other studies of low birth weight have linked this early disadvantage to an increased incidence of both cardiovascular risk factors (Blane et al 1996) and chronic disease in middle age. This effect has been attributed to early biological programming of important homeostatic physiological functions (Barker 1992).

The effect of socio-economic group on the incidence, management and survival after MI and coronary death was analysed using a community coronary event register (Morrison et al 1997). CHD events increased with age for both genders and were greater in men than women at all ages. The event rate increased 1.7-fold in men and 2.4-fold in women from the least to the most deprived socio-economic group (as defined by lowest quartile) (Morris & Carstairs 1991). The proportion of individuals treated in hospital (66%) decreased with age, was greater in women than men and decreased in both sexes with increasing deprivation category. The study concluded that higher socio-economic deprivation group increased an individual's likelihood of a CHD event but decreased the chance of hospital admission. The likelihood of death following acute MI was higher in individuals from lower socio-economic groups.

Morris & Carstairs' deprivation scores (Morris & Carstairs 1991) have been developed as a measure of socio-economic deprivation based on postcode of geographical area of residence. An updated version using 1991 census data had been used in this study (McLoone 1994). Use of postcode has been reported to be more accurate than occupational classification when discriminating between socio-economically deprived groups. This is because of high unemployment rates in sectors of the community (Tunstall-Pedoe et al 1996). The information was routinely available on both death certificates and hospital discharge data. It has been criticized because it does not relate to characteristics of the individual or personal circumstances but to geographical area. However, postcodes have been shown to be useful in describing variation over a wide range of mortality, morbidity and other health-related population measurements (Morris & Carstairs 1991, Watt 1993, Woodward 1996).

HEALTH LOCUS OF CONTROL

Locus of control beliefs have been described as whether an individual uses internal or external attributions to explain events and actions related to their own health (Wallston et al 1976). The health locus of control (HLOC) model (Wallston et al 1976) has therefore been developed to measure the extent to which individuals believe that their health is influenced either by their own behaviour (internal locus of control) or by external forces (external locus of control). The latter may be luck, chance or other powerful forces beyond the person's direct control. The concept has been derived from social learning theory (Rotter 1954) which states that behaviour is a function of expectancy beliefs and the value that is placed on certain outcomes. Future behaviours, in a broad range of activities, are considered to be determined by socialization experiences. Internal locus of control beliefs have been related in a positive way to health practices and general well-being with the converse being true for external locus of control. However, these relationships have not been confirmed universally in studies that have assessed and evaluated measures of locus of control and health behaviour intentions (Wallston et al 1976). The HLOC construct has been applied in a wide range of behaviours. Some studies have documented a positive relationship between internal HLOC beliefs and indices of preventive health practices (Duffy 1988, Weiss & Larsen 1990).

In a follow-up study of 110 patients with established CHD, who had been admitted to hospital with exacerbation of symptoms, locus of control assessment and mastery of stress estimations were made using validated self-completed questionnaires (Younger et al 1995). Mastery of stress has been described as a process through which stressful or difficult situations are overcome. This is through the development of new capabilities, changing the environment and/or re-organizing the self to re-establish meaning and purpose to life (Younger 1991). Approximately 25% of the sample were noted to have participated in the outpatient cardiac rehabilitation programme. Results showed that there were no differences in estimates of locus of control or mastery skills between attendees and non-attendees. However, internal HLOC was significantly and positively associated with a higher mastery score and with positive changes in health behaviours. These findings add support to the hypothesis that those who may be termed 'health-internals' make more attempts to control their environment and lifestyle. A similar

finding was reported in a small study examining the effect of HLOC on compliance to smoking cessation one month following CABG. It showed that those who believe that they are in control of their health were found to be more compliant with smoking cessation than those who believed that their health is the result of chance or is controlled by others (Galindo-Ciocon 1989). By contrast, other studies have failed to establish such a relationship (Steptoe et al 1994).

HLOC remains of debatable use to health-care professionals in terms of predicting behaviour changes and in the evaluation of determinants of health-care outcomes. However, developments to incorporate HLOC assessment into a more general theory of health behaviour are being investigated in which the three concepts of the health value, self-efficacy and locus of control are combined (Wallston 1992). The theory suggests that self-efficacy predicts health behaviour when the individual values their health and has an internal health locus of control. This interpretation remains to be tested although the author believes that self-efficacy is one of the most powerful predictors of health behaviour because it outlines a role for health locus of control as a more peripheral predictor of health behaviour. It also has the potential for improving our understanding of health behaviour.

Interpretation of the impact of HLOC on health behaviour is made more difficult because of the confounding effect of social class. This is because beliefs about illness have been linked to socio-economic class (Pill & Stott 1982). In their study examining factors that individuals thought were causative agents for ill health, Pill & Stott (1982) noted that home-owners were more likely to view a variety of diseases, such as CHD and cancer, to be caused in part by aspects of individual behaviour. This included diet, mental attitude to work and lifestyle habits. This contrasted with the beliefs of those who rented their homes from the local authority (Pill & Stott 1982). The authors interpreted home ownership as part of a cluster of social attitudes that emphasized the individual's control over life as opposed to notions of fatalism. The authors concluded that specific social and material conditions within socio-economic categories need to be considered in order to understand attitudes to health.

More than 10 years later, a large survey of approximately 1026 men and 1700 women aged between 20 and 45 years examined factors related to preventive health behaviour. It again confirmed a strong relationship with social class (Pill et al 1995), which existed in men and women. The particular factors related to social class were identified as education, tenure, residential overcrowding index and salience of lifestyle.

In conclusion, preventive health behaviour has been strongly linked to social class status and therefore an examination of the relationship between health locus of control and health practices should take into account the possible confounding effects of social class.

SOCIAL SUPPORT

Social support has been defined in the literature as the 'assistance and protection given to others', especially by individuals to individuals (Shumaker & Bronwell 1984). An additional earlier definition described 'shielding people from the adverse effects of life stresses' (Cobb 1976). Several conceptual definitions have been proposed and many different measurement instruments have been developed (O'Reilly 1988). The form that support and protection may take can range from specific objective interventions such as financial aid to less tangible acts of caring and emotional support achieved through the sharing of issues and concerns. The main sources of social support have been shown to be associated with the availability of a spouse or confidant, close ties with friends and the nearness of relatives (Brandt & Weinert 1981). The key areas through which social support has positive health benefits have been related to its ability to enhance personal competence, health maintenance behaviours, especially coping behaviours such as perceived control, positive affect, sense of stability, recognition of self-worth, decreased anxiety and depression, and psychological well-being (Langford 1997).

Many positive consequences of social support have been described with several large epidemiological studies documenting extension to life in people who are socially integrated (Berkman 1995, House et al 1988). Increased risk of total mortality has been reported in socially isolated individuals (Kaplan et al 1988, Orth-Gomer & Johnson 1987). In a 4-year prospective study of adult males aged 42–77 years, social networks were assessed at baseline and correlated with total mortality, incidence of cardiovascular disease and cerebrovascular accident (Kawachi et al 1996). Socially isolated men were at increased risk of cardiovascular mortality (age-adjusted relative risk 1.09; 95% CI 1.07, 3.37) compared to men with the highest level of social networks.

In a study examining the role of social support and long-term recovery after CABG surgery, different aspects of social support were examined (King et al 1992). The five areas of social support that were included were: support in appraisal, self-esteem, sense of belonging, closeness and tangible sense of social support. Utilizing an interpersonal support evaluation list (Cohn & Hoberman 1983) to measure social support, the study demonstrated that the perceived availability of social support was related to outcome for patients and their spouses up to one year following CABG surgery. The results indicated that there was a differential influence in the five types of social support examined. In addition, perception of the availability of esteem support was the only type of support that consistently accounted for the unique share of the relationship between social support and outcomes. Esteem support was associated more strongly with positive emotional outcome and this may be because it is most strongly associated with close relationships and is received at minimal social cost.

In summary, the literature acknowledges the difficulties in measuring social support although, using a variety of assessment approaches, it has clearly demonstrated a positive relationship between high levels of social support and improved health status.

HEALTH PROMOTION
Definitions

Health promotion has been defined as 'the organised application of educational, social and environmental resources enabling individuals to adopt and maintain behaviours that reduce risk of disease and enhance wellness' (Petosa 1986).

Others have defined the concept as 'the process of enabling people to increase control over the determinants of health and thereby improve their health' (WHO 1986). However, it should be remembered that just as health itself means different things to different people, the concept of health promotion may equally be interpreted widely, with different emphases placed on its individual components. In practice, the term 'health promotion', used alone or in combination with disease prevention, embraces a wide variety of perspectives from preventing premature death to legislative and physical measures to improve health. This is in addition to the promotion of individuals' responsibility for the maintenance of healthy ways of living and mobilizing the support of communities as part of health improvement programmes.

Health promotion in practice

In the last 20 years there have been major developments in preventive medicine. This has been fuelled by an increasing acceptance in medical and political circles that the common chronic diseases of middle and later life constitute the principal health issues of industrialized societies. This movement has become characterized by the emergence of a clear policy agenda based on the management of mass behaviour change. These developments have brought to the fore the concept of lifestyle, a loose aggregation of behaviours and conditions encompassing body size, shape, diet, exercise and the use of drugs, both legal and illegal. Improving the lifestyle of the population soon became the major challenge deemed necessary to improve the health of the population.

The concept of empowerment is central to the philosophy and practice of health promotion. In one sense it parallels the concept of health, in that it can be said to be both a desirable end in itself and a means to an end. Empowerment of individuals and communities acts instrumentally to facilitate healthy decision making. It has to do with the relationship between individuals and their environment where the relationship is recognized to be reciprocal. At the micro level empowerment is also a key health promotion goal. For instance, as part of a planned contract of behaviour modification, people might learn how to avoid environmental circumstances which trigger their consumption of tobacco or alcohol. They might acquire skills in resisting social pressure and receive clear examples of how the rhetoric of empowerment can be operationalized and translated into specific educational objectives. Self-empowerment concepts include beliefs about control, e.g. perceived locus of control and self-efficacy beliefs, values such as self-esteem and a variety of specific social and personal skills which might be encapsulated in the term 'health and life skills' (Sidell & Peberdy 1987).

Models of health promotion

A widely accepted model of health promotion is that described by Downie et al (2000) (Fig. 2.1) which describes three overlapping spheres of activity: health education (such as lifeskills work with adolescents), health protection (for example, a smoking-free workplace) and health prevention (an example being a cervical screening programme). The model is essentially a description of the main strategies that may be employed to improve health and their inter-relationship. It can be used in practice to map out all possible options that may be available affecting large initiatives and individual patient care. However, it does not take into account the social and environmental context which has been shown to be a major determinant of health.

Beattie's (1991) model suggests that there are four paradigms for health promotion which are generated

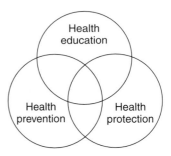

Figure 2.1 A model of health promotion. (Adapted from Downie et al 2000.)

from two dimensions of activity: the style and focus of the intervention (Fig. 2.2). The 'style' dimension ranges from authoritative (top down and expert led) to negotiated (bottom up, supporting individual autonomy). The 'focus' dimension relates to the target group, ranging from the individual to the collective group. On the basis of these dimensions four strategies for health promotion are described as follows.

- Health persuasion, describing interventions that are focused on the individual and are led by professionals.
- Legislative action covers activities that are professionally led and directed to community population groups. An example of this approach is that of health-care professionals lobbying for better access to exercise facilities in areas of high socio-economic deprivation.
- Personal counselling describes interventions that are client led and focus on personal development, with the health promotion action focused on facilitation rather than directive. An example of this approach could be that of one-to-one stress counselling by a cardiac rehabilitation nurse, whereby specific strategies to deal with stress are individualized and negotiated with the client.
- Community development describes interventions through which community groups are supported in taking action to improve their environment. An example of this approach would be supporting and encouraging individuals to form action groups to lobby for improved local employment opportunities.

HEALTH BELIEFS

Theories describing health-related behavioural change are based on the premise that if an individual has sufficient information and understands the relationship between an activity and its effect on health, this will in

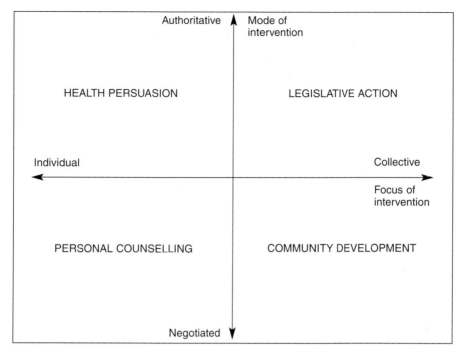

Figure 2.2 Strategies of health promotion. (Reproduced with permission from Beattie 1991.)

turn influence behaviour. The health belief model (Becker 1974) (Fig. 2.3) is probably the best known theoretical model highlighting the function of belief in health-care decision making. It has been used to predict protective health behaviour such as screening or vaccination uptake and compliance with medical advice.

The model suggests that whether or not a patient changes their behaviour will be influenced by an evaluation of both the feasibility of making changes and the benefits likely to be gained against the actual costs. According to this theory, an individual must believe that they are capable of carrying out the intended behaviour.

For behavioural changes to take place, the model suggests that an individual should feel:

- there is an incentive to make change
- threatened by their current behaviour
- change would have few adverse consequences
- competent to carry out the changes.

Central to this is the degree to which individuals perceive themselves to be susceptible to a particular illness or injury and how serious they consider the consequences. An individual's perception and assessment of risk is therefore important and is likely to be influenced by their previous personal experience,

ability to change the situation and a general feeling that illness or danger has drastic consequences. However, in many situations there may be an unrealistic expectation that it won't happen to them. It has been suggested that people need to have some kind of cue to take action to change their behaviour. The issue needs to become relevant to them and this may be the result of appreciating the adverse effects of their own lifestyle or being closely involved in the illness of others.

The degree to which individuals, following a major cardiac event, complied with diet, activity, medication, stress reduction and smoking cessation was examined in relation to two concepts of the health belief model: perceived benefits and perceived barriers (Kison 1992). Results showed that those who perceived more benefits than barriers to medical check-ups were more compliant. However, the highest degree of compliance was with medications and the lowest in modifying responses to stress. The subgroup of patients who had undergone CABG were least likely to stop smoking. Perhaps this latter finding was related to a perceived cure as a result of the procedure and therefore removal of the threat from heart disease. In addition, individuals from higher socio-economic groups were more likely to perceive benefits than barriers from undergoing

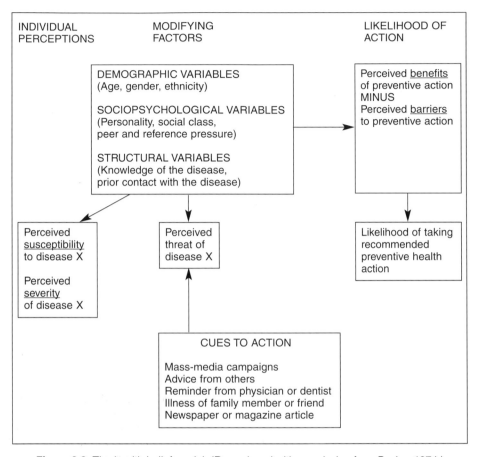

Figure 2.3 The health belief model. (Reproduced with permission from Becker 1974.)

health check-ups. This may provide some insight into possible underlying reasons for the higher levels of ill health related to lower socio-economic groups.

BEHAVIOURAL CHANGE THEORY

Motivation to change adverse aspects of one's lifestyle has been described within the context of the stages of change model (Prochaska & DiClemente 1984) (Fig. 2.4). This approach evaluates an individual's readiness to make changes and bases interventions on that assessment, i.e. those who were willing to make changes were helped to do so, whereas those who were resistant to change were given general advice and information. Individuals who are receptive to making changes are encouraged to evaluate the positive and negative aspects of their lifestyle and, through endorsement of the positive aspects, supported in making changes to more healthy behaviours.

The implementation of this approach to facilitating lifestyle changes was shown to be effective when used in the management of patients on the waiting list for CABG (McHugh et al 2001). During the waiting time of approximately one year, patients randomized to a care programme managed by a cardiac specialist nurse in partnership with the practice nurse improved several aspects of lifestyle-associated CHD risk factors. The intervention was based on a shared care programme of family-centred health education and counselling sessions according to individual need. These sessions were carried out monthly alternating between the patients' own homes and the general practice setting. Patient-held records were used as a communication tool and an aid to motivating behavioural change. Sessions consisted of:

- assessment of an individual's readiness to make change
- tailored counselling and lifestyle advice

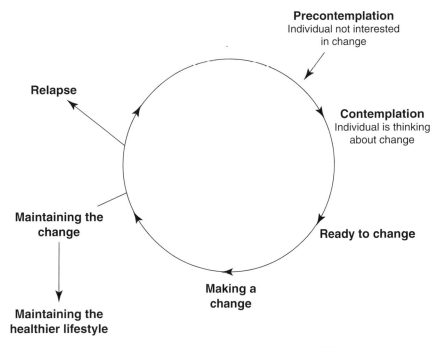

Figure 2.4 The stages of change model (after Prochaska & DiClemente 1984).

- information and advice re CABG surgery
- family support
- measurement and monitoring of CHD risk factors
- back-up telephone advice.

Greater improvement in smoking cessation was achieved in the intervention group compared to the control group. Similarly, numbers of patients who were overweight were improved, with moderate obesity reduced by 54% in the intervention group but at the same time increasing by 71% in the usual care group. There was a 30% decrease in the proportion of patients with total plasma cholesterol levels greater than 5.2 mmol (p=0.003).

The study concluded that nurse counselling based on the behavioural change model was effective at facilitating positive changes to health-related lifestyle habits for patients during the year-long wait for CABG surgery. Positive results were also achieved in a larger randomized controlled study conducted in primary care of nearly 900 men and women with one or more modifiable risk factors (Steptoe et al 1999). The inter-

vention group used brief behavioural counselling on the basis of the stages of change model. This was implemented by appropriately trained practice nurses to reduce smoking and dietary fat intake and to increase physical activity. Favourable differences were recorded in dietary fat intake, the taking of regular exercise and the number of cigarettes smoked per day, although there was no difference in smoking cessation rates or body mass index.

CONCLUSION

This chapter has provided an overview of theoretical perspectives of health, health promotion and models that have been proposed to explain and predict an individual's health behaviour pattern. Examples have been used to demonstrate their application to practice, highlighting their strengths and weakness. Behavioural counselling based on the stages of change model is currently showing the most promise for motivating and facilitating healthy lifestyle behaviour changes when used to guide practice.

REFERENCES

Aaronson NK 1988 Quality of life: what is it? How should it be measured? Oncology 2: 69–74

Ashton DN, Maguire MJ, Spilsbury M 1987 Labour market segmentation and the structure of the youth labour market. In: Brown P, Ashton DN (eds) Education, unemployment and labour markets. Falmer Press, London, pp. 160–178

Barker DJP 1992 Fetal and infant origins of adult disease. BMJ Books, London

Bartley M, Power C, Blane D, Davey-Smith G, Shipley M 1994 Birthweight and later socioeconomic disadvantage: evidence from the 1958 British cohort study. British Medical Journal 309: 1475–1478

Bartley M, Blane D, Montgomery S 1997 Health and the life course: why safety nets matter. British Medical Journal: 314: 1194–1196

Beattie A 1991 Knowledge and control in health promotion: a test case for social policy and social theory. In: Gabe J, Calnan M, Bury M (eds) The sociology of the health service. Routledge, London, pp. 162–202

Becker MH (ed) 1974 The health belief model and personal health behaviour. Slack, Thorofare, New Jersey

Bergner M 1985 Measurement of health status. Medical Care 23: 696–704

Berkman LF 1995 The role of social relations in health promotion. Psychosomatic Research 57(3): 245–254

Blane DB, Hart CL, Davey-Smith G, Gillis CR, Hole DJ, Hawthorne VM 1996 The association of cardiovascular disease risk factors with socioeconomic position during childhood and during adulthood. British Medical Journal 313: 1434–1438

Blaxter M 1983 The causes of disease. Women talking. Social Science and Medicine 17(2): 59–69

Blaxter M 1985 Self definition of health status and consulting rates in primary care. Quarterly Journal of Social Affairs 1: 131–171

Blaxter M 1990 Health and lifestyles. Routledge, London

Brandt PA, Weinert C 1981 The PRQ: a social support measure. Nursing Research 30(5): 277–280

Calman KC 1984 Quality of life in cancer patients – an hypothesis. Journal of Medical Ethics 10: 124–127

Campbell A, Converse PE, Rodgers WL 1976 The quality of American life. Russell Sage Foundation, New York

Charlier L, Dutrannois J, Kaufman L 1997 The SF-36 questionnaire: a convenient way to assess quality of life in angina pectoris patients. Acta Cardiologica 3: 247–260

Charmaz K 1997 Loss of self: a fundamental form of suffering in the chronically ill. Sociology of Health and Illness 5(2): 168–198

Cobb S 1976 Social support as a moderator of life stress. Psychosomatic Medicine 38(5): 300–313

Cohn S, Hoberman HM 1983 Positive events and social supports as buffers of life change stress. Journal of Applied Social Psychology 13: 99–125

Conn VS, Taylor SG, Abele F 1991 Myocardial infarction survivors: age and gender differences in physical health, psychological state and regimen adherence. Journal of Advanced Nursing 16: 1026–1034

Cowley AJ 1995 The clinical impact of coronary artery disease: are subjective measures of health status more relevant than laboratory-assessed exercise tolerance? European Heart Journal 16: 1461–1462

Davey-Smith G, Shipley M, Rose G 1990 Magnitude and causes of socioeconomic differentials in mortality: further evidence from the Whitehall Study. Journal of Epidemiology and Community Health 44: 265–270

Downie RS, Tannahill C, Tannahill A 2000 Health promotion: models and values, 2nd edn. Oxford University Press, Oxford

Dubos R 1965 Man adapting. Yale University Press, New Haven, Connecticut

Duffy ME 1988 Determinants of health promotion in mid-life women. Nursing Research 37: 358–362

Dunn HL 1973 High level wellness. Beatty, Arlington, Virginia

Essen J, Wedge P 1992 Continuities in childhood disadvantage. Heinemann Educational, London

Farquhar M 1995 Definitions of quality of life: a taxonomy. Journal of Advanced Nursing 22: 502–508

Field D 1976 The social definition of illness. In: Tuckett D (ed) An introduction to medical sociology. Tavistock, London, pp. 334–365

Galindo-Ciocon DJ 1989 Smoking behavior, health beliefs and locus of control of patients who have had open heart surgery. PhD thesis, University of Miami

Goldblatt P 1990 Mortality and alternative social classifications. In: Goldblatt P (ed) Longitudinal study 1971–1981: mortality and social organisation. HMSO, London

Hamilton GA 1990 Recovery from acute myocardial infarction in women. Cardiology 77 (suppl 2): 58–70

Harrison MB, Juniper EF, Mitchell-DiCenso A 1996 Quality of life as an outcome measure in nursing research. 'May you have a long and healthy life.' Canadian Journal of Nursing Research 28(3): 49–68

Herzlich C 1973 Health and illness. Academic Press, London

House JS, Landis KR, Umberson D 1988 Social relationships and health. Science 241: 540–545

Jenkins CD, Jono RT, Stanton BA, Stroup-Benham CA 1990 The measurement of health related quality of life: major dimensions identified by factor analysis. Social Science and Medicine 31(8): 925–931

Kaplan GA, Salonen JT, Cohen RD, Brand RJ, Syme SL, Puska P 1988 Social connections and mortality from all causes and from cardiovascular disease: prospective evidence from Eastern Finland. American Journal of Epidemiology 128: 370–380

Kawachi I, Colditz GA, Ascherio A et al 1996 A prospective study of social networks in relation to total mortality and cardiovascular disease in men in the USA. Journal of Epidemiology and Community Health 50: 245–251

King KB, Porter LA, Norsen LH, Reis HT 1992 Patient perceptions of quality of life after coronary artery surgery: was it worth it? Research in Nursing and Health 15(5): 327–334

Kison C 1992 Health belief and compliance of cardiac patients. Applied Nursing Research 5(4): 181–185

Kitler ME 1992 Differences in men and women in coronary artery disease, systemic hypertension and their treatment. American Journal of Cardiology 70: 1077–1080

Langford CPH 1997 Social support: a conceptual analysis. Journal of Advanced Nursing 25: 95–100

Lindsay GM, Smith LN, Hanlon P, Wheatley DJ 2000 Coronary artery disease patients' perceptions of their health and expectations of benefit following coronary artery bypass grafting. Journal of Advanced Nursing 32(6): 1412–1421

Lindsey E 1996 Health within illness: experiences of chronically ill/disabled people. Journal of Advanced Nursing 24: 465–472

Lukkarinen H, Hentinen M 1997 Assessment of quality of life with the Nottingham Health Profile among patients with coronary heart disease. Journal of Advanced Nursing 26: 73–84

Matson RR 1977 Adjustment to multiple sclerosis: an exploratory study. Social Science and Medicine 11: 245–250

McDowell I, Newell C 1987 Measuring health: a guide to rating scales and questionnaires. Oxford University Press, New York

McEwen J 1993 The Nottingham Health Profile: a measure of perceived health. In: Walker SR, Rosser RM (eds) Quality of life: key issues in the 1990s. Kluwer Academic, London, pp. 111–130

McHugh F, Lindsay GM, Hanlon P et al 2001 Nurse-led shared care for patients on the waiting list for coronary artery bypass surgery: a randomised controlled trial. Heart (in press).

McIntyre S 1986a Health and illness. In: Burgess RG (ed) Key variables in social investigation. Routledge, London

McIntyre S 1986b Health and illness. In: Burgess RG (ed) Key variables in social investigation. Routledge, London, pp. 99–122

McLoone P 1994 Carstairs scores for Scottish postcode sectors from the 1991 census. Public Health Research Unit, Glasgow

Meeberg GA 1993 Quality of life: a concept analysis. Journal of Advanced Nursing 18: 32–38

Moch SD 1989 Health within illness: conceptual evolution and practice possibilities. Advanced Nursing Science 11(4): 23–31

Moos R 1982 Coping with acute health crisis. In: Miller T, Green C, Meagher R (eds) Coping with life crisis: an integrated approach. Plenum Books, New York

Morris R, Carstairs V 1991 Which deprivation? A comparison of selected deprivation indexes. Journal of Public Health Medicine 13: 318–326

Morrison C, Woodward M, Leslie W, Tunstall-Pedoe H 1997 Effect of socioeconomic group on incidence of, management of, and survival after myocardial infarction and coronary death: analysis of community coronary event register. British Medical Journal 314: 541–546

Neuman BM 1990 Health as a continuum based on the Neuman systems model. Nursing Science Quarterly 3(3): 129–135

Newman MA 1986 Health as expanding consciousness. CV Mosby, St Louis

O'Reilly P 1988 Methodological issues in social support and social network research. Social Science and Medicine 26: 863–873

Orth-Gomer K, Johnson J 1987 Social network interaction and mortality. A six year follow-up study of a random sample of the Swedish population. Journal of Chronic Disease 40: 949–958

Parsons T 1972 Definitions of health and illness in the light of American values and social structure. In: Jaco E, Gartley E (eds) Patients, physicians and illness: a sourcebook in behavioural science and health. Collier-Macmillan, London, pp. 97–117.

Pender NJ 1989 Expressing health through lifestyle patterns. Nursing Science Quarterly 3(1): 115–122

Petosa R 1986 Emerging trends in adolescent health promotion. Health Values 10(3): 22–28.

Pill R, Stott NCH 1982 Concept of illness causation and responsibility: some preliminary data from a sample of working class mothers. Social Science and Medicine 16: 43–52

Pill R, Peters TJ, Robling MR 1995 Social class and preventive health behaviour: a British example. Journal of Epidemiology and Community Health 49(1): 28–32

Prochaska JO, DiClemente CC 1984 The transtheoretical approach: crossing traditional foundations of change. Don Jones, Irwin, Homewood, Illinois

Rotter JB 1954 Social learning and clinical psychology. Prentice-Hall, Englewood Cliffs, New Jersey

Shumaker SA, Bronwell A 1984 Towards a theory of social support: closing conceptual gaps. Journal of Social Issues 40(4): 11–33

Sidell M, Peberdy A (eds) 1987 Debates and dilemmas in promoting health: a reader. Open University/Macmillan, Basingstoke

Smith GD, Carroll D, Rankin S, Rowan D 1995 Socioeconomic differentials in mortality: evidence from Glasgow graveyards. British Medical Journal 305: 1554–1557

Spitzer WO 1987 State of science 1986: quality of life and functional status as target variables for research. Journal of Chronic Diseases 40: 465–471

Steptoe A, Wardle J, Vinck J, Tuomisto M, Holte A, Wickstrom L 1994 Personality and attitudinal correlates of health and unhealthy lifestyles in young adults. Psychology and Health 9: 331–343

Steptoe A, Doherty S, Rink E, Kerry S, Kendrick T, Hilton S 1999 Behavioural counselling in general practice for the promotion of healthy behaviour among adults at increased risk of coronary heart disease: randomised trial. British Medical Journal 319: 943–948

Stewart AL, Ware JE 1992 Measuring functioning and wellbeing: the medical outcomes study. Duke University Press, London

Townsend P, Davidson N, Whitehead M 1992 Inequalities in health: the Black Report and the Health Divide. Penguin Books, Harmondsworth

Tuckett D, Boulton M, Olson C, Williams A 1985 Meetings between experts. Tavistock, London

Tunstall-Pedoe H, Morrison C, Woodward M, Fitzpatrick B, Watt G 1996 Sex differences in myocardial infarction and coronary deaths in the Scottish MONICA population of Glasgow 1985–91. Circulation 93: 1981–1992

Verbrugge LM 1989 The twain meet. Empirical explanations of sex differences in health and mortality. Journal of Health and Social Behaviour 30: 282–304

Verbrugge LM, Wingard DC 1987 Sex differentials in health and mortality. Women and Health 12: 103–145

Wallston BS, Wallston KA, Kaplan GD, Maides SA 1976 Development and validation of the Health Locus of Control (HLC) Scale. Journal of Consulting and Clinical Psychology 44: 580–585

Wallston KA 1992 Hocus-pocus, the focus isn't strictly on locus: Rotter's social learning theory modified for health. Cognitive Therapy and Research 16: 183–199

Waltz CF, Strickland OL, Lenz ER 1991 Operationalizing nursing concepts. In: Measurement in nursing research, 2nd edn. FA Davis, Philadelphia, pp. 27–59

Watt GCM 1993 Differences in expectation of life between Glasgow and Edinburgh. Implications for health care policy in Scotland. Health Bulletin 51: 407–417

Weiss GL, Larsen DL 1990 Health value, health locus of control and the prediction of health protective behaviors. Social Behavior and Personality 18: 121–136

WHO 1977 Manual for the international statistical classifications of diseases, injuries and causes of death. World Health Organization, Geneva

WHO 1986 Ottawa charter for health promotion. Journal of Health Promotion 1: 1–4

Wiklund I, Herlitz J, Hjalmarson A 1989 Quality of life five years after myocardial infarction. European Heart Journal 10: 464–472

Wiles R 1998 Patients' perceptions of their heart attack and recovery: the influence of epidemiological 'evidence' and personal experience. Social Science and Medicine 46: 1477–1486

Wilkinson RG 1997 Health inequalities: relative or absolute material standards? British Medical Journal 314: 591–595

Williams G, Popay J 1996 Lay knowledge and the privilege of experience. In: Gabe J, Kelleher D, Williams G (eds) Challenging medicine. Routledge, London, pp. 118–139

Williams G, Wood PHN 1986 Common-sense beliefs about illness: a mediating role for the doctor. Lancet II: 1435–1437

Woodward M 1996 Small area statistics as markers for personal social status in the Scottish Heart Health Study. Journal of Epidemiology and Community Health 50: 570–576

Wright LD, Harwood A, Coulter A 1992 Health and lifestyles in the Oxford region. Health Services Research Unit, Oxford

Younger J 1991 A theory of mastery. Advances in Nursing Science 14(1): 76–89

Younger J, Marsh KJ, Grap MJ 1995 The relationship of health locus of control and cardiac rehabilitation to mastery of illness-related stress. Journal of Advanced Nursing 22: 294–299

3

Cardiac rehabilitation

Helen Stokes
David Thompson

This chapter aims to provide an overview of the key issues in cardiac rehabilitation. It is regarded as a progression from the previous chapter, which explored the concept of health promotion.

REHABILITATION

Cardiac disease is a chronic health condition, which may also present with acute events. Chronic illness has been defined as 'an altered health state not cured by surgery or short-term medication' (Morrow & Oglesby 1996). In addition to a long-term timescale, the implications of chronic ill health potentially include uncertainty of outcomes, loss of or change in functional capacity, lifestyle changes, social isolation and economic consequences. Rehabilitation may be perceived as a means of restoring best possible capacity across a broad spectrum, including physical, psychological and socio-economic functions. The ultimate goal of rehabilitation is often described as helping the patient to achieve independence, but the meaning of independence is open to interpretation. As Banja (1988, p. 382) points out, 'independence is a situation wherein an individual is capable of and is encouraged to determine his or her best interests, and then can assume available measures in society to secure the satisfaction of those interests'. In other words, the individual should be helped to make their own decisions and to put those decisions into action, using whatever personal, professional or social support is required to do so.

This philosophy is supported by the World Health Organization in its *International classification of impairments, activities and participation* (ICIDH-2) (WHO 1997). The ICIDH-2 attempts to categorize what the consequences of a particular health condition may be; that is, the extent to which a health condition impacts on the individual by causing an impairment of function, a limitation of activity or a restriction of participation. The ICIDH-2 is envisaged as a tool to provide a common language for assessment and communication not only amongst patients themselves and healthcare professionals but also in social security, insurance, education, labour, legislation and other sectors.

Definition of cardiac rehabilitation

Cardiac rehabilitation is defined by the WHO (1993) as 'The sum of activities required to influence favourably the underlying cause of the disease, as well as to ensure the patients the best possible physical, mental and social conditions so that they may, by their own efforts, preserve, or resume when lost, as normal a place as possible in the life of the community. Rehabilitation cannot be regarded as an isolated form of therapy, but must be integrated with the whole treatment, of which it forms only one facet' (p. 5). This is, of course, an all-embracing definition but it is endorsed by countries in Europe and beyond.

It is important to appreciate that cardiac rehabilitation is a relatively recent intervention and has developed from older and more unidimensional concepts of exercise-based rehabilitation, which had evolved in response to treatment regimens involving prolonged bedrest. In essence, cardiac rehabilitation services are comprehensive programmes involving education, exercise, counselling and behaviour modification designed to limit the deleterious physiological and psychological consequences of heart disease, reduce the risk of death or recurrence of the cardiac event and enhance the psychosocial and vocational state of patients. The national standard for cardiac rehabilitation, contained within the National Service Framework (NSF) for Coronary Heart Disease (Department of Health (DoH) 2000) states that: 'National Health Service (NHS) Trusts should put in place agreed protocols/systems of care so that, prior to leaving hospital, people admitted to hospital suffering from coronary heart disease have been invited to participate in a multidisciplinary programme of secondary prevention and cardiac rehabilitation. The aim of the programme will be to reduce their risk of subsequent cardiac problems and to promote their return to a full and normal life'.

It can be seen that cardiac rehabilitation is a multidisciplinary and multifaceted activity that requires a range of skills to bring together medical treatment, education, sexual and vocational counselling, risk factor modification and secondary prevention. It should be regarded as an integral part of cardiac care, throughout both acute and community settings. Nurses have been at the forefront in establishing and co-ordinating programmes; they are ideally placed to

deliver the service in both primary and secondary care, as they have continuous contact with the patient and family/carers at all stages of recovery, as well as frequent contact with other health and social care professionals.

Ideally, the cardiac rehabilitation process should start at, or even before, the time of hospital admission, continue through the hospital stay and hand over seamlessly to rehabilitation and aftercare in the community. A flexible approach to the later stages of rehabilitation is essential, with the outcomes, particularly in respect of physical activity, smoking cessation and dietary modification, being more important than rigid adherence to set procedures.

HISTORICAL PERSPECTIVE

Reference is frequently made to the observations of William Heberden in 1777 regarding the regular efforts of one of his patients in sawing wood and the subsequent improvement in his (presumed) angina. However, cardiac rehabilitation did not really begin to develop until the mid-20th century. Harrison (1944) commented on 'The abuse of rest as a therapeutic measure for patients with cardiovascular disease' at a symposium of the American Medical Association. Further work in the United States during the 1950s by Levine & Lown (1952) demonstrated the benefits of early mobilization of cardiac patients, at least by allowing them to sit in a chair rather than keeping them on constant bedrest. The 1960s saw the development of coronary care units for cardiac patients, which led to specialization in both cardiology and cardiac nursing.

Despite these developments, it was not until the late 1970s that cardiac rehabilitation programmes began to appear in the United Kingdom (UK). A handful of programmes were set up at this time and these mainly explored the benefits of increased physical activity as opposed to the mere early mobilization of inpatients (Bethell et al 1983, Carson et al 1982). Relatively little increase in activity was seen until the late 1980s when a joint initiative was developed, between the Chest, Heart and Stroke Association and the British Heart Foundation. The initiative was designed to provide funding to 'pump-prime' cardiac rehabilitation programmes and was a significant factor in enabling the majority of UK programmes to begin. By this time, there was a growing awareness of the need for cardiac rehabilitation to encompass more than increased physical activity, as the impact of psychosocial and socioeconomic factors on the individual was recognized.

The early 1990s saw an explosion in the number of programmes commencing, with over half of the existing programmes starting during that period (BACR 1998). Due to the growing interest in this field, other initiatives developed accordingly: the British Association for Cardiac Rehabilitation (BACR) was launched in 1992, as was the Heart Manual (Lewin et al 1992); the National Health Service Executive funded a national survey (Thompson et al 1997a); the first edition of the BACR Guidelines was published (Coats et al 1995); and guidelines and audit standards were developed (Stokes et al 1998, Thompson et al 1996a,b, 1997b).

EVIDENCE FOR EFFECTIVENESS

Though it is increasingly being recognized as an important part of comprehensive cardiac care, there remains some scepticism regarding the effectiveness of cardiac rehabilitation and some ignorance of its potential (Thompson & Bowman 1997). Yet, there is now available strong evidence attesting to the benefit of cardiac rehabilitation (Dinnes et al 1999, NHS Centre for Reviews and Dissemination 1998, Wenger et al 1995). These benefits include:

- improvements in exercise tolerance
- improvement in symptoms
- improvement in blood lipid levels
- reduction in cigarette smoking
- improvements in psychosocial well-being
- reduction of stress.

A recent Effective Health Care bulletin concluded that cardiac rehabilitation can promote recovery, enable patients to achieve and maintain better health and reduce the risk of death in people who have heart disease. It also concluded that a combination of exercise and psychological and educational interventions appears to be the most effective form of cardiac rehabilitation (NHS Centre for Reviews and Dissemination 1998). Because cardiac rehabilitation is often a multifaceted intervention, it can be difficult to ascertain whether benefits, if they accrue, are due to a single component or a combination of components. It may be that some interaction of factors is responsible; in other words, the whole of the intervention is more than the sum of the parts.

COST AND COST EFFECTIVENESS

At present little is known about the economic aspects of cardiac rehabilitation. Hence, there is an urgent need to assemble information on the cost and cost effectiveness of such services. To date, the only full cost-effectiveness study of cardiac rehabilitation in the United States of America found no gain in effectiveness (Oldridge et al 1993).

A study of the cost of cardiac rehabilitation services in England and Wales (Gray et al 1997) used workload and resource data returned to calculate cost per centre, per patient and per session. Annual staffing costs for each cardiac rehabilitation centre were in the range of £10 000–62 000, with a mean of just under £33 000 (median £32 000). Mean cost per patient completing the rehabilitation programme was £370 (median £223) and mean cost per patient per session was £47 (median £26). There was substantial intercentre variation in costs. Costs for each patient were closely related to patient throughput and hours of contact time.

Clearly cardiac rehabilitation is not a homogeneous service and there is a range of factors that influence the costs and cost effectiveness of the process, including scale of the programme, location, components, intensity of the process, the patient population and adherence.

GUIDELINES, STANDARDS AND AUDIT

Clinical guidelines are aids to, not substitutes for, clinical judgement and are powerful tools for helping to put research evidence into practice and as such are an important part of any clinical effectiveness initiative (Thompson & Kitson 1999). Cardiac rehabilitation guidelines have been available in the United States for some years and are updated regularly (AACVPR 1999). UK national guidelines have been developed with the aim of ensuring that cardiac rehabilitation is offered to all who are likely to benefit, based on an individual assessment of need, and followed by a later menu of options. It should be accompanied by audit and individual monitoring of patient progress.

The national standards identify interventions that should be offered at each stage of the rehabilitation process as including: comprehensive assessment of physical, psychological and social risk and needs, a written individual plan, lifestyle advice, psychological interventions, use of effective medications, the involvement of carers, access to cardiac support groups, and long term follow-up. Other interventions may include health promotion and vocational advice, structured exercise sessions, or referral to specialist services as appropriate. The stated goal of the NSF is that: 'more than 85% of people discharged from hospital with a primary diagnosis of acute myocardial infarction or after coronary revascularisation are offered cardiac rehabilitation; and that 1 year after discharge at least 50% of people are non-smokers, exercise regularly and have a body mass index (BMI) <30 kg/m² (DoH 2000). These data should be less than 12 months old; therefore audit and individual monitoring of patient progress needs to be an integral part of the service. Models of care need to be developed in order to systematically identify those who would benefit from these services, assess their needs and risks, provide, document and review service delivery, integrate cardiac care and evaluate the quality of the service.

CLIENT GROUPS

The national guidelines advocate that cardiac rehabilitation services should be available not only to those post-myocardial infarction or post-coronary artery bypass surgery but also those with heart failure, valvular heart disease, angina and hypertension (Thompson et al 1996b). Despite these recommendations, the majority of cardiac rehabilitation programmes are still only available to a minority of patients who are likely to benefit. Most centres tend to restrict access to young, male, white patients who have suffered a (usually first, uncomplicated) myocardial infarction (Lewin et al 1998; Thompson et al 1997a). At present, comparatively little is known about the needs and experiences of women, elderly and physically disabled people and low income and ethnic groups. They are rarely offered rehabilitation or, when they are, frequently fail to take up services. In addition, very little is known about the effects of cardiac rehabilitation on patients with heart failure or angina or those who have undergone heart transplantation. This is surprising when one considers the prevalence of a disease such as heart failure and the costs, both human and economic, that it can incur (Bowman et al 1998a).

LOCATION OF REHABILITATION SERVICES

There is a need to offer a range of cardiac rehabilitation programmes that will widen entry for patients. Though traditionally, cardiac rehabilitation has tended to be a hospital-based service, there is a strong case for an expansion of community-based programmes, which have been shown to be effective, may be more acceptable to consumers and are in line with government policy on shifting care from secondary to primary settings in the UK. The development of community- and home-based programmes could widen access to older people and others who might find hospital-based programmes unsuitable or inconvenient (Bowman et al 1998b).

Placing cardiac rehabilitation in the community should ensure greater awareness of the individual needs of the person and his or her family. Community-based rehabilitation can address the importance of the social and environmental context of the person's life in the rehabilitation process.

Hildingh & Fridlund (1992) provide an illustration of a client-led service in Sweden. A large number of self-help groups for older people who have experienced a myocardial infarction have been set up with the support of nurses and a national patient association. In the UK, the British Heart Foundation has facilitated the formation of a network of patient support groups, co-ordinated by regional advisors. These groups have regular meetings, together with a variety of other activities, including exercise groups in some areas.

PHASES OF REHABILITATION

A systematic and structured framework for the provision of cardiac rehabilitation services is a useful way of providing the appropriate service at the right time and in the right place. Many programmes use a framework consisting of four phases.

- Phase 1: inpatient stay (variable). This includes explanation of the disease, the prognosis and a positive approach to recovery, early mobilization and discharge planning.
- Phase 2: immediate post-discharge period (up to 6 weeks). This includes further investigations, liaison with community-based health-care professionals, assessment and health education as appropriate.
- Phase 3: intermediate post-discharge period (commonly 6–12 weeks, may be longer). This includes rehabilitation interventions, such as a tailored/supervised exercise programme, psychosocial interventions such as a stress management programme and vocational evaluation or retraining.
- Phase 4: long-term maintenance period (indefinite). This includes chronic disease management: monitoring of secondary prevention, maintenance of lifestyle changes.

For information on programme management, administration and funding, the reader is referred to Chapters 2 and 4 of the BACR *Guidelines on cardiac rehabilitation* (Coats et al 1995).

PROCESS OF REHABILITATION

The process of rehabilitation, as described above, should contain the following elements (Thompson et al 1996b).

- Element 1: the process of explanation and understanding. This includes medical diagnosis and management, nursing practice and teamwork.
- Element 2: specific rehabilitation interventions. These include individually tailored secondary prevention, exercise training and psychological support.
- Element 3: the process of re-adaptation. This includes education for, and adaptation to, long-term lifestyle changes.

It should be emphasized that the phases and the elements contained within them should be flexible and tailored to suit the individual needs of the patient and his or her partner and family. This means that the timing and location of sessions need to be flexible and the length of participation in a programme should be variable in order to cater for the wide range of clients. In order to tailor the services, comprehensive assessment of the individual's needs is essential.

RISK STRATIFICATION

Risk stratification is the assessment of future risk to an individual, traditionally viewed according to their clinical status. This is broadening to take into account functional and behavioural aspects as well; for example, a patient post-myocardial infarction could have a low *clinical* risk but if they continue to smoke heavily then their *behaviour* is increasing their future risk. Risk stratification is normally considered in three categories: low, moderate and high (see Box 3.1)

Box 3.1 Stratification for risk of event (not specific solely to exercise) (reprinted by permission from AACVPR 1999)

Lowest risk
- No significant LV dysfunction (EF >50%)

- No resting or exercise-induced complex dysrhythmias

- Uncomplicated MI; CABG; angioplasty, atherectomy or stent:
  - absence of CHF or signs/symptoms indicating post-event ischaemia

- Normal haemodynamics with exercise or recovery

- Asymptomatic including absence of angina with exertion or recovery

- Functional capacity ≥7.0 METs*

- Absence of clinical depression

Lowest risk classification is assumed when each of the risk factors in the category is present.

Moderate risk
- Moderately impaired LV function (EF = 40–49%)

- Signs/symptoms including angina at moderate levels of exercise (5–6.9 METs) or in recovery

Moderate risk is assumed for patients who do not meet the classification of either highest risk or lowest risk.

Highest risk
- Decreased LV function (EF <40%)

- Survivor of cardiac arrest or sudden death

- Complex ventricular dysrhythmia at rest or with exercise

- MI or cardiac surgery complicated by cardiogenic shock, CHF and/or signs/symptoms of post-procedure ischaemia

- Abnormal haemodynamics with exercise (especially flat or decreasing systolic blood pressure or chronotropic incompetence with increasing workload)

- Signs/symptoms including angina pectoris at low levels of exercise (<5.0 METs) or in recovery

- Functional capacity <5.0 METs*

- Clinically significant depression

Highest risk classification is assumed with the presence of any one of the risk factors included in this category.

---

*NOTE: If measured functional capacity is not available, this variable is not considered in the risk stratification process. CABG = coronary artery bypass grafting, CHF = congestive heart failure, EF = ejection fraction, LV = left ventricular, MET = metabolic equivalent value, MI = myocardial infarction

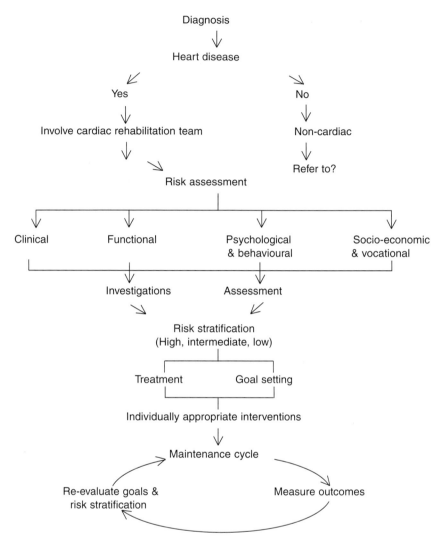

Figure 3.1 Patient pathway through cardiac rehabilitation services.

ASSESSMENT

Assessment in cardiac rehabilitation may be divided into the following areas, each of which will be discussed: clinical, functional, psychological and behavioural, social and vocational. These may be illustrated in a pathway as shown in Figure 3.1.

Clinical assessment

Clinical assessment, leading to diagnosis and management of the specific conditions for the client groups outlined above, is covered in the various chapters in this book. Assessment of clinical risk status may include graded exercise testing. This may also be performed as part of a functional assessment – see below.

Functional assessment

Having assessed the level of cardiac damage, the impact of this on the daily life of the individual should be considered. If a graded exercise test has been completed, then the metabolic equivalent unit (MET) value achieved at the maximum point of the test can be used to assess the individual's ability to carry out activities of daily living, which may be personal, sexual, social, recreational or vocational (see Table 3.1) (1 MET = 3.5 ml O_2 consumed per kilogram body weight per minute).

Table 3.1 Metabolic equivalent values for activities of daily living (ADLs), household tasks, recreational activities and vocational activities (adapted from Pashkow & Dafoe 1999)

	Energy requirements (METs)	
	Min	Max
ADLs		
Dressing	2	3
Sexual intercourse	3	5
Showering	3	4
Bathing	2	3
Walking 2 mph	2	3
Walking 4 mph	5	6
Household tasks		
Carrying 20–44 lbs	4	5
Carrying 18 lbs upstairs	7	8
Cooking (standing)	2	3
Vacuuming	2.9	3.6
General housework	3	4
Light gardening	2	4
Pushing power mower	3	5
Washing car	6	7
Recreational activities		
Bowling	2	4
Cycling 5 mph	2	3
Cycling 10 mph	5	6
Ballroom dancing	4	5
Golf carrying clubs	4	5
Running 12 min/mile	8	9
Tennis singles	4	9
Swimming slow	4	5
Swimming crawl	9	10
Swimming breaststroke	8	9
Vocational activities		
Assembly-line work	3	5
Bricklaying	3	4
Desk work	1.5	2
Handyman	5	6
Painting	4	5
Trucking	3	4

Cardiac rehabilitation is a multidisciplinary activity and it may be necessary to involve the skills of a physiotherapist or an occupational therapist (especially where there may be other pathology involved such as osteo-arthritis), to help in assessing functional capacity and in discharge planning.

Psychological assessment

Psychological assessment should include the measurement of factors such as anxiety, depression and quality of life. It may also cover factors such as aggression, anger and hostility. Stress is a term that carries with it many misconceptions and individual interpretations may vary considerably. The concept of stress may be defined as including biochemical, physiological,

behavioural and psychological changes. Stressors are the external factors that cause a response, which may be harmful (distress) or beneficial (eustress) (Ogden 1996, p. 201).

Quality of life

Health-related quality of life measures include generic instruments, which address multiple aspects of quality of life across a range of different patient or illness groups, and disease-specific instruments, which comprise content specific to the disease in question and thus are more clinically sensitive and potentially more responsive in detecting change. An example of the former includes the Medical Outcomes Study Short-Form 36-item (SF-36) Health Survey (Jenkinson et al 1993) while the latter includes the Quality of Life after Myocardial Infarction (QLMI) questionnaire (Oldridge et al 1991). Each of these measures has its particular strengths and weaknesses and there is some merit in combining both types in the assessment of quality of life.

Other assessment tools include:

- Hospital Anxiety and Depression (HAD) Scale
- State-Trait Anxiety Inventory (STAI)
- Zung Self-Rating Depression Scale
- Profile of Mood States (POMS).

The advantages of these tools are that they are relatively brief and have been used with a cardiac population. A review of quality of life measurement scales and their application may be found in Bowling (1997) and Spilker (1996).

There has been a rapid and significant growth in the measurement of quality of life as an indicator of health outcome. In the management and care (including rehabilitation) of the patient with coronary heart disease there is an increasing awareness that the assessment of physical outcomes alone is not sufficient and as a consequence, assessment of well-being and health-related quality of life is considered to be important (Thompson et al 1998).

Cardiac rehabilitation aims to prolong life, relieve symptoms and improve function in patients and it is imperative that well-validated and appropriate measures of outcome are utilized to assess the impact on functioning and well-being. Measurement of quality of life is important in evaluating the efficacy of interventions, including cardiac rehabilitation (McGee 1996).

Despite the widespread use of the phrase, there is vagueness and little agreement as to the precise definition of quality of life, though health, defined as physical, social and mental well-being, is an important aspect. As a consequence, health-related quality of life measures have evolved in order to assess the impact of treatment on those patients with recognized medical conditions. Such measures provide an assessment of the patient's experience of his or her health problems in areas such as physical function, emotional function, social function, role performance, pain and fatigue.

Behavioural assessment

Assessment of behavioural risk will include assessment of both risk factors and health beliefs and behaviours. Health behaviours may be positive (for example, seeking health information, leading a healthy life style) or negative (for example, ignoring health advice, smoking, avoiding healthy activities) (Kasl & Cobb 1966, Matarazzo 1984). There are a variety of theories relating to health behaviours and health beliefs; for a description and overview, see Ogden (1996), Chapters 2 and 3.

Social assessment

Social support has been defined by Wills (1985) as:

- esteem support – where other people increase one's self-esteem
- informational support – where other people are available for advice
- social companionship – support through activities
- instrumental support – involves physical help.

It has been suggested that increased social support may be linked to decreased mortality (Berkman & Syme 1979) and to well-being (Waltz 1986). This effect on health may be linked to stress, in that lack of social support acts as a stressor or that social support acts as a buffer between the individual and the stressor. Socio-economic deprivation is associated with both an increased risk of developing myocardial infarction (MI) and a poorer prognosis afterwards (Pell et al 1996). A comprehensive assessment of social networks on admission is therefore essential to discharge planning. This may be an issue of asking the right questions, or it may include involving other agencies as part of a more formal assessment of social circumstances, including financial assessment or socio-economic status.

Vocational assessment

Factors which influence return to work may include lower socio-economic status and depression immediately following an MI (Abbott & Berry 1991), as well as place of residence, age, education, perceived job stress and clinical complications during hospitalization (Maeland & Havik 1986). Failure to return to work is affected by a number of individual factors and is not necessarily related to the severity of the clinical condition. An occupational health assessment may be needed and retraining possibilities explored. A graded exercise test to evaluate the individual's functional capacity and the use of MET values in relation to vocational activities is recommended (see Table 3.1).

INTERVENTIONS

The process of cardiac rehabilitation may be perceived as starting from the earliest possible opportunity after diagnosis. The following interventions progress through the various phases outlined earlier.

Mobilization

Early mobilization in hospital is recommended, both to avoid the complications of bedrest and to encourage a positive approach to recovery. Nursing observation of the individual's capacity to perform activities of daily living is important, as part of the assessment process and discharge planning.

Risk factor management

Identification of risk factors will divide into modifiable and non-modifiable factors. Involvement of partners and family members in any health education process may be helpful in reinforcing important messages and facilitating changes in lifestyle.

Health education

Acknowledging the principles of adult learning will help the nurse to assess and plan appropriate health education interventions. A range of information suited to different learning capacities and needs is important. Adult learning principles have been identified in the AACVPR Guidelines (1999) as follows.

- Readiness is achieved when the learner is physically stable, has adequate energy, is emotionally stable and is aware of the problem or need to learn.
- Adults learn only if and when they are ready to learn.
- Adults prefer to be self-directed, participate in decision making relative to their health and treatment and be actively involved in the learning process.
- Adults use their cumulative experience as a learning resource.

- Adults learn by problem solving and learn best in the immediate time frame.

The ability to absorb and retain information will vary according to the individual and the time frame.

Psychosocial interventions

These may include specific sessions on stress management or a broader programme such as behaviour modification. The principles of behaviour modification include setting appropriate and achievable goals, with feedback and positive reinforcement. These principles are used in cognitive behavioural therapy, which is based upon the links between feelings, thoughts and behaviours. Behaviour modification may be used to address a specific risk factor issue, such as smoking cessation, or broader issues such as anxiety and depression. A stress management programme may include the identification of individual stressors and methods of coping with these. For further information, see also Chapter 6 in the BACR *Guidelines for cardiac rehabilitation* (Coats et al 1995).

Physical activity

Cardiac rehabilitation is frequently associated with a programme of supervised exercise. The principle of rehabilitation should be perceived more broadly than this, as a means of improving physical function and being able to achieve activities of daily living and recreational and vocational activities as appropriate. Depending on individual risk stratification, physical activity may be supervised or unsupervised or a mixture of both. The aim should be to improve cardiovascular function as well as general fitness. Targets may vary from aiming at, for example, 10–15 minutes of daily activity to three or four sessions of 30–40 minutes per week of cardiovascular exercise, regulated by a percentage (between 60% and 80%) of maximum heart rate.

AUDIT AND EVALUATION

Historically, cardiac rehabilitation in the UK has suffered from a lack of common audit data (Horgan et al 1992, Thompson et al 1997b). An audit tool has been developed alongside the national guidelines and piloted in three centres; the tool is composed of three elements: individual patient data, summarized patient data and data relating to the facility or service provision (Thompson et al 1997b,c). It should be emphasized that audit is a cyclical activity and that information gathering is only the first step in the process. It is important to evaluate the data obtained in order to improve clinical practice and service provision. This emphasizes the importance of collecting data that relate not only to the patients but also to all aspects of the service.

Local audit initiatives are increasing and in an attempt to co-ordinate the data collected, the British Heart Foundation (BHF) is developing a computerized audit package which will be widely available after piloting.

RESEARCH ISSUES

It is clear that further research is required to identify the optimal method of delivering cardiac rehabilitation. It will be important to compare the clinical and cost effectiveness of, for instance, home-based and community-based services with hospital-based programmes. It will also be important to ascertain the optimal mix of components and the frequency and duration of the programme. Finally, research is needed to ascertain the reasons for the low uptake of services by elderly people, women and ethnic groups and to devise and test strategies to improve this uptake.

CONCLUSION

Cardiac rehabilitation is a multifaceted, multidisciplinary activity that has developed rapidly over the past two decades in the UK. The National Service Framework for Coronary Heart Disease (DoH 2000) should be helpful in improving the quality and consistency of services in terms of prevention and treatment, including rehabilitation. Individual assessment, careful formulation of treatment, effective delivery and systematic evaluation will help to ensure that cardiac rehabilitation is improved (Thompson & De Bono 1999).

REFERENCES

Abbott J, Berry N 1991 Return to work during the year following first myocardial infarction. British Journal of Clinical Psychology 30: 268–270

American Association of Cardiovascular and Pulmonary Rehabilitation (AACVPR) 1999 Guidelines for cardiac rehabilitation and secondary prevention. Human Kinetics, Champaign, Illinois

Banja JD 1988 Independence and rehabilitation: a philosophic perspective. Archives of Physical Medicine and Rehabilitation 69: 381–382

Berkman LF, Syme SL 1979 Social networks, lost resistance and mortality: a nine year follow up study of Alameda County residents. American Journal of Epidemiology 109: 186–204

Bethell HJN, Larvan A, Turner SC 1983 Coronary rehabilitation in the community. Journal of the Royal College of General Practitioners 33: 285–291

Bowling A 1997 Measuring health: a review of quality of life measurement scales. Open University Press, Buckingham

Bowman GS, Thompson DR, Lewin RJP 1998a Why are patients with heart failure not routinely offered cardiac rehabilitation? Coronary Health Care 2: 187–192

Bowman GS, Bryar RM, Thompson DR 1998b Is the place for cardiac rehabilitation in the community? Social Sciences in Health 4: 243–254

British Association for Cardiac Rehabilitation 1998 Database. Unpublished

Carson P, Phillips R, Lloyd M et al 1982 Exercise after myocardial infarction: a controlled trial. Journal of the Royal College of Physicians of London 16: 147–151

Coats AJS, McGee HM, Stokes HC, Thompson DR 1995 BACR guidelines for cardiac rehabilitation. Blackwell Science, Oxford

Department of Health 2000 National Service Framework for Coronary Heart Disease. Deparment of Health, London

Dinnes J, Kleijnen J, Leitner M, Thompson DR 1999 Cardiac rehabilitation. Quality in Health Care 8: 65–71

Gray AM, Bowman GS, Thompson DR 1997 The cost of cardiac rehabilitation services in England and Wales. Journal of the Royal College of Physicians of London 31: 57–61

Harrison TR 1944 Abuse of rest as a therapeutic measure for patients with cardiovascular disease. Journal of the American Medical Association 125: 1075–1077

Hildingh C, Fridlund B 1992 Supporting elderly coronary patients in self-help groups with a guidebook: a nurse intervention for public health. Journal of Clinical Nursing 1: 259–264

Horgan J, Bethell H, Carson P et al 1992 Working party report on cardiac rehabilitation. British Heart Journal 67: 412–418

Jenkinson C, Wright L, Coulter A 1993 Quality of life measurement in health care. A review of measures and population norms for the UK SF-36. Health Services Research Unit, Oxford

Kasl SV, Cobb S 1966 Health behaviour, illness behaviour and sick role behaviour. II. Sick role behaviour. In: Ogden J (ed) Health psychology: a textbook. Open University Press, Buckingham

Levine SA, Lown B 1952 Armchair treatment of acute coronary thrombosis. Journal of the American Medical Association 14: 1365–1369

Lewin B, Robertson IH, Cay EL, Irving JB, Campbell M 1992 Effects of self-help post-myocardial-infarction rehabilitation on psychological adjustment and use of health services. Lancet 339: 1036–1040

Lewin RJP, Ingleton R, Newens A, Thompson DR 1998 Adherence to cardiac rehabilitation guidelines: a survey of rehabilitation programmes in the United Kingdom. British Medical Journal 316: 1354–1355

Maeland JG, Havik OE 1986 Return to work after a myocardial infarction: the influence of background factors, work characteristics and illness severity. Scandinavian Journal of Social Medicine 14: 183–195

Matarazzo JD 1984 Behavioural health: a 1990s challenge for the health sciences professions. In: Matarazzo JD, Miller NE, Weiss SM, Herd JA (eds) Behavioural health: a handbook of health enhancement and disease prevention. John Wiley, New York

McGee HM 1996 Can the measurement of quality of life contribute to evaluation in cardiac rehabilitation services? Journal of Cardiovascular Risk 3: 148–153

Morrow EJ, Oglesby FM 1996 Acute and chronic illness: similarities, differences and challenges. Orthopedic Nursing 15: 47–51

NHS Centre for Reviews and Dissemination 1998 Cardiac rehabilitation. Effective Health Care 4(4): 1–12

Ogden J 1996 Health psychology: a textbook. Open University Press, Buckingham

Oldridge N, Guyatt G, Jones N, Crowe J, Singer J 1991 Effects on quality of life with comprehensive cardiac rehabilitation after acute myocardial infarction. American Journal of Cardiology 74: 1240–1244

Oldridge N, Furlong W, Feeny D et al 1993 Economic evaluation of cardiac rehabilitation soon after acute myocardial infarction. American Journal of Cardiology 72: 154–161

Pashkow FJ, Dafoe WA 1999 Clinical cardiac rehabilitation: a cardiologist's guide, 2nd edn. Williams and Wilkins, Baltimore

Pell J, Pell A, Morrison C, Blatchford O, Dargie H 1996 Retrospective study of influence of deprivation on uptake of cardiac rehabilitation. British Medical Journal 313: 267–268

Spilker B (ed) 1996 Quality of life and pharmacoeconomics in clinical trials. Lippincott Raven, Philadelphia

Stokes HC, Thompson DR, Seers K 1998 The implementation of multiprofessional guidelines for cardiac rehabilitation: a pilot study. Coronary Health Care 2: 60–71

Thompson DR, Bowman GS 1997 Evidence for the effectiveness of cardiac rehabilitation. Clinical Effectiveness in Nursing 1: 64–75

Thompson DR, De Bono DP 1999 How valuable is cardiac rehabilitation and who should get it? Heart 82: 545–546

Thompson DR, Kitson AL 1999 Development of multi-professional guidelines for cardiac rehabilitation: a survey based approach. In: Hutchinson A, Baker R (eds) Making use of guidelines in clinical practice. Radcliffe Medical Press, Oxford.

Thompson DR, Bowman GS, De Bono DP, Hopkins A 1996a The development and testing of a cardiac rehabilitation audit tool. Journal of the Royal College of Physicians of London 31: 317–320

Thompson DR, Bowman GS, Kitson AL, De Bono DP, Hopkins A 1996b Cardiac rehabilitation: guidelines and audit standards. Heart 75: 89–93

Thompson DR, Bowman GS, Kitson AL, De Bono DP, Hopkins A 1997a Cardiac rehabilitation services in England and Wales: a national survey. International Journal of Cardiology 59: 299–304

Thompson DR, Bowman GS, De Bono DP, Hopkins A 1997b Cardiac rehabilitation: guidelines and audit standards. Royal College of Physicians, London

Thompson DR, Bowman GS, De Bono DP, Hopkins A 1997c The development and testing of a cardiac rehabilitation audit tool. Journal of the Royal College of Physicians 31: 317–320

Thompson DR, Meadows K, Lewin RJP 1998 Measuring quality of life in patients with coronary heart disease. European Heart Journal 19: 693–695

Waltz M 1986 Marital context and post-infarction quality of life: is it social support or something more? Social Science and Medicine 22: 791–805

Wenger NK, Froelicher ES, Smith LK et al 1995 Cardiac rehabilitation. Clinical practice guideline No. 17. Agency for Health Care Policy and Research and National Heart, Lung, and Blood Institute, Rockville, Maryland

Wills TA 1985 Supportive functions of interpersonal relationships. In: Cohen S, Syme SE (eds) Social support and health. Academic Press, Orlando, Florida

World Health Organization 1993 Needs and action priorities in cardiac rehabilitation and secondary prevention in patients with CHD. WHO Regional Office for Europe, Copenhagen

World Health Organization 1997 International classification of impairments, activities and participation. Beta-1 draft for field trials June 1997. World Health Organization, Geneva

FURTHER READING

American College of Sports Medicine 2000 Guidelines for exercise testing and prescription, 6th edn. Williams and Wilkins, Baltimore

Bowling A 1997 Measuring health: a review of quality of life measurement scales. Open University Press, Buckingham

Coats AJS, McGee HM, Stokes HC, Thompson DR 1995 BACR guidelines for cardiac rehabilitation. Blackwell Science, Oxford

Jones D, West R 1995 Cardiac rehabilitation. BMJ Books, London

Julian D, Wenger N 1997 Women and heart disease. Martin Dunitz, London

Pollock M, Schmidt D 1995 Heart disease and rehabilitation, 3rd edn. Human Kinetics, Champaign, Illinois

Wenger NK, Froelicher ES, Smith LK et al 1995 Cardiac rehabilitation. Clinical practice guideline No. 17. Agency for Health Care Policy and Research and National Heart, Lung, and Blood Institute, Rockville, Maryland

Cardiac structure and function

This section explores the structure and function of the cardiovascular system. The altered physiology which is a hallmark of many cardiac conditions dictates nursing care. This section therefore discusses the anatomy and physiology of the cardiac system in preparation for the disease processes and conditions discussed throughout the text. The emphasis is placed upon the application of biological principles to cardiac nursing care.

4

The applied anatomy and physiology of the cardiovascular system

Barbara Novak
Lynda Filer
Richard Hatchett

The biological sciences provide the underpinning for cardiac nursing care. As coronary heart disease progresses, the failing heart has a unique ability to initiate a variety of compensatory mechanisms to assist and maintain tissue perfusion. However, it is frequently such mechanisms that result in a cycle of worsening heart failure for the patient. Much of non-surgical treatment consists of breaking and manipulating these biological and essentially physiological mechanisms. To understand the variety of treatments and associated nursing care currently implemented, there is a clear need for a knowledge of the heart's structure, function and its ability to adapt to failure. In addition, in an era of chronic heart disease, patients themselves are being empowered to understand their own illness and aim for greater medication compliance and lifestyle changes. This requires a nursing team with a confident and competent knowledge base regarding the anatomy and physiology of the cardiovascular system. Finally, the emergence of specialties within cardiac care, such as the angiography nurse and those caring for adults with congenital cardiac abnormalities, indicates the need for a practitioner with a comprehensive understanding of specific and particular anatomical areas.

This chapter explores in detail the structure of the heart and its normal function in preparation for the adaptive mechanisms examined within this text, as part of the development of disease. The reader is encouraged to review all areas of cardiac anatomy and physiology but this chapter provides an overview of the major areas of relevance related to nursing care.

The cardiovascular system is a sophisticated transport mechanism capable of delivering the required metabolic substrates to tissue and cells. This is in addition to facilitating the removal of undesirable byproducts from various organs, for elimination from the body. The blood vessels in this dynamic circulatory network provide the pathways for distributing and collecting the bloodborne substrates. However, the blood can only perform its many complex roles if it circulates continually and in a pulsatile fashion through the pulmonary and systemic vascular compartments linking the external environment to the tissues and cells. The heart itself generates the required energy for moving the blood through the closed but selectively permeable circulatory network.

The shaping of the cardiovascular system in preparation for its complex function takes place in early embryonic life. To this end the formation of the cardiovascular system begins in the first 3 weeks of pregnancy with the establishment of a single heart tube, which gradually evolves into the four-chambered heart. As part of its gradual development and shaping the heart is connected to the systemic and pulmonary vessels. This makes the cardiovascular system fit for its future dual function in terms of maintenance of the pulmonary and systemic circulations.

THE ANATOMY OF THE ADULT HEART

The normal position and shape of the heart

The normal human heart is cone shaped and located in the mediastinum, one-third to the right of the sternum and the remaining two-thirds to the left. This is clearly apparent on the normal anteroposterior (AP) chest X-ray. Unusually, the top of the heart is referred to as the base and the pointed lower section as the apex. The base of the heart lies in an oblique position behind the sternum and its apex lies to the left, in the fifth intercostal space in the mid-clavicular line. The normal position of the heart ensures maximal protection from the thoracic cavity and particularly the lungs and diaphragm.

The adult heart is about the size of the person's fist and varies in weight from 230 to 340 g, a weight which is achieved between the ages of 17 and 20 years of age (Gabella 1995). Considering that mammalian life depends on the continual pumping action of this organ, it is somewhat awesome to realize that it weighs less than 1 lb. Functionally, the heart may be considered as a hollow fibromuscular organ consisting of two highly specific pumps (a left and a right), each of which includes a set of valves. These guide the continuous flow of blood to the pulmonary and the systemic circulations (Fig. 4.1).

The pathway of blood through the heart

Deoxygenated blood returns to the right side of the heart from the body via the inferior and superior vena cavae. The blood enters the right atrium, then passes through the tricuspid valve to the right ventricle. From here it passes through the pulmonary artery to the lungs. In the lungs oxygenation occurs and the blood flows back to the left side of the heart to be pumped around the body. The circuit to and from the lungs is referred to as the **pulmonary circuit**.

Oxygenated blood returns to the left side of the heart via the pulmonary veins into the left atrium. From there it passes into the left ventricle via the mitral (bicuspid) valve. The term 'mitral' is used clinically, whilst the term 'bicuspid' is seen in physiology texts. The oxygenated blood then passes from the left ventricle to the body via the aorta. The circuit supplying blood to the body (other than the lungs) is referred to as the **systemic circuit**.

Each side of the heart consists of an upper chamber, the atrium, and a lower chamber, the ventricle. Thus the heart consists of four chamber (see Fig. 4.2). The right and left sides of the heart are divided by a partition known as the septum. Although the fibromuscular framework and conduction tissue of these pumps are structurally interwoven, each pump is physiologically independent but always capable of contributing to the pulmonary and systemic circulations. The division of the heart into four chambers produces characteristic external boundaries, which frequently present as deep grooves containing prominent structures such as coronary vessels. An example of such anatomical cardiac demarcations is the atrioventricular groove, which separates the atria from the ventricles and embodies the main trunks of the coronary arteries. Similarly, the interventricular groove corresponds to the interventricular septum, which divides the two ventricular chambers.

The chambers and valves of the heart

The atria

The atria are thin-walled muscular chambers that form the most anterior aspect of the heart (Gabella 1995). A fibromuscular septum separates the two atria, forming the distinctive right and left atrium. This septum features a fairly central fibrous oval depression known as the **fossa ovalis**. According to Gabella (1995), approximately 33% of normal adult hearts have a small slit in the upper margins of the fossa ovalis, a phenomenon which is generally asymptomatic but may be detected in expectant mothers and in later life.

Gabella (1995) divides the atrial myocardium into a superficial and a deep layer. The superficial layer spans over and encircles both atria, inserting into the

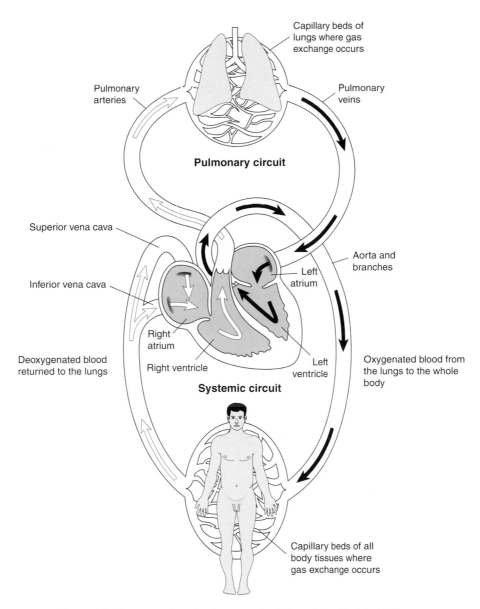

Figure 4.1 The systemic and pulmonary circulations (after Marieb 1998).

annulus fibrosus. By contrast, the deep layer is independent for each atrial chamber, its fibres run at right angles to the superficial muscle fibres and make up the major muscle mass of the atria. However, the arrangement of both fibres is such that they form distinctive muscular loops, which encircle the vessel inlets to the atria.

The function of the atria is to serve as storage reservoirs for blood returning to the heart from the systemic and pulmonary circulations. This function is particularly significant during ventricular systole when the forward flow of blood is stopped by the competent closure of the atrioventricular valves. In these circumstances the returning blood collects in and distends the atrial cavities. However, the atria can also be compared to the venous network in that they are collapsible when partially filled. This phenomenon may be attributed to the relative thinness of the atrial myocardium. The advantage of this relative compliance is that both chambers will adapt to the volume

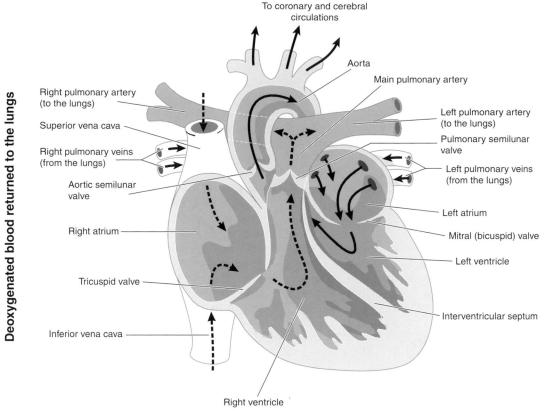

Figure 4.2 Internal structure of the heart.

they hold, distending when they are full or overfilled and reducing in size when venous return is compromised. In addition, there are flap-like protrusions, attached to each atrial chamber. These are known as **auricles** and contribute to the expelled atrial volume. As the left atrium, in addition to being smaller, is less distensible, the venous return from the lungs will invariably maintain a slightly higher left atrial pressure than that of the right. Finally, the insides of the atrial walls are not smooth but have ridges of muscle called **pectinate muscles**.

Atrioventricular (AV) valves

The tricuspid valve is the largest valvular orifice in the adult heart and is situated between the right atrium and the right ventricle. A ring of collagen and fibrous tissue acts as the base for the attachments of the three cusps or leaflets (flaps), which make up this valve. The three cusps are separated by commissures, which are tethered by fan-shaped **chordae tendinae** of varying length and thickness. The chordae tendinae insert into the anterior and septal papillary muscle.

The mitral (bicuspid) valve guards the inlet to the left ventricle from the left atrium. This valve is fixed to an annulus or a ring of fibrocollagenous tissue. The consistency of this tissue seems important as it allows for major changes in the shape of annulus and valve during the different stages of the cardiac cycle. In other words, the compliance of this tissue ensures optimal efficiency in valve function. The valve itself is formed by two extensive leaflets, which are joined by commissures. These leaflets are also tethered by chordae tendinae, attached to papillary muscles emerging from the ventricular walls.

The cusps or leaflets of the AV valves hang loosely into the ventricles when the valves are in their open state. This allows blood to flow from the atria to the ventricles. The increase in pressure that occurs when the ventricles contract causes the blood to push up against the cusps, allowing them to come together and close. This prevents the flow of blood travelling back from the ventricles to the atria in a retrograde fashion. Valvular disease and incompetence is not an uncommon occurrence seen in cardiac nursing care. The details and specific management are explored in detail in Chapter 13.

The ventricles

The function of the ventricles is to maintain the circulation via their pumping action. The two chambers are divided by the interventricular septum. An intact septum ensures that the two separate but integrated circulations are maintained. The right ventricle pumps deoxygenated blood through the pulmonary circulation, whilst the left ventricle pumps oxygenated blood through the systemic circulation. If the septum is damaged, either congenitally or as the result of an infarct, there is a mixing of the blood between the two ventricles. If the shunt is predominantly from the higher pressure left ventricle through to the right ventricle, there will be inadequate oxygenation of the blood. Shunts can also flow in the other direction. More detail regarding these defects is explained in Chapter 12.

The right ventricle extends from the tricuspid valve almost to the apex itself. In comparison to the left ventricle, it is much smaller and with thinner walls, reflecting its role of pumping blood to the pulmonary circulation, as opposed to the entire body. The left ventricle is larger, more powerful and has additional electrical pathways (**fascicles**). This highlights its role as a powerful systemic pump, maintaining tissue oxygenation. In both ventricles the muscle fibres follow a distinctive spiral path. The fibres sweep from the base of the heart to the apex, forming a 360° clockwise rotation. This spiral arrangement ensures that when the ventricles contract, blood is propelled into the respective outflow tracts, the aorta and the pulmonary artery.

The semilunar valves (Fig. 4.3)

The pulmonary valve lies between the right ventricle and the pulmonary artery. This is generally considered as a semilunar valve, which consists of three cusps that are joined to each other by commissures. The aortic valve guards the left ventricular outflow tract. This is also a three-cusp, semilunar valve with a similar structure to the pulmonary valve. However, it is stronger in construction due to the higher pressure generated by the left side of the heart. The leaflets of the aortic valve are attached to the annulus, which forms part of the **aortic sinuses of Valsalva**. This structure creates a well-defined complete circumferential tubular area, consisting largely of non-contractile collagenous tissue. This creates an ideal and structurally stable arrangement for the coronary arteries that open near the upper part of the sinus.

The semilunar valves open and close in a particular fashion. As the ventricles contract, interventricular pressure rises above the pressure in the aorta and the pulmonary trunk. This pumps blood out of the ventricles into the blood vessels, pushing the valves open and forcing the cusps against the walls. When the pressure in the ventricles falls below that of the major vessels, blood will begin to flow backwards, fill the cusps and shut the valve.

As the ventricles contract and intraventricular pressure rises, blood is pushed up against the semilunar valves, forcing them open

As the ventricles relax and intraventricular pressure falls, blood flows back from the arteries, filling the cusps of the semilunar valves and forcing them to close

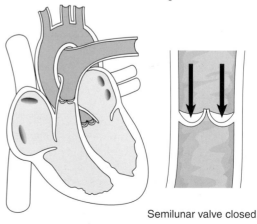

Aorta

Pulmonary artery

A

Semilunar valve open

B

Semilunar valve closed

Figure 4.3 The semilunar valves (after Marieb 1998).

The layers of the heart

The walls of the heart consist of three anatomically distinct layers: the outer protective pericardium, a middle layer known as the myocardium, or the muscle of the heart, and the inner layer known as the endocardium which lines the chambers of the heart (Fig. 4.4).

The pericardium

The pericardium is the outermost layer of the heart. It forms a firm fibrous sac within which the heart is suspended by its attachments to the aorta and the pulmonary artery. This mechanism seems a physiological necessity that fixes the base but leaves the apex of the heart relatively free. This phenomenon seems important to ventricular function, especially as the dimensions of the ventricles change during contraction, moving the apex forward and thus allowing it to strike against the left side of the chest wall in the area of the fifth intercostal space.

The role of the pericardium is to provide physical protection for the heart against mechanical force. It consists of two components, the fibrous and the serous pericardium. The **fibrous** pericardium consists of mesothelium, a compact collagenous fibrous tissue, which encloses the heart and merges with the **tunica adventitia** of the major vessels. The **serous** pericardium, on the other hand, is a double-layered membrane consisting of flat secretory epithelium, connective tissue and some adipose tissue. The quantities of the adipose tissue are related to the general body fat. The innermost layer of the serous pericardium, the

epicardium, is fused to the surface of the myocardium, thereby forming the **visceral** pericardium.

Conversely, the outer layer of the serous pericardium is fused with the inner aspect of the fibrous pericardium and now forms the **parietal** pericardium. The two layers of the serous pericardium are joined at the juncture of the great vessels with the heart, forming a small fluid-filled cavity – the pericardial cavity (see Fig. 4.4).

The pericardium receives its blood supply from arteries derived from the internal thoracic and musculophrenic arterial network and the descending thoracic aorta. The pericardial venous drainage is returned to the internal thoracic veins. The pericardial nerve supply is derived from branches of the vagus nerve, the phrenic nerves and the sympathetic trunk. Disruptions to the pericardium can cause medical emergencies such as cardiac tamponade which occurs when fluid collects, through trauma, malignancy or following surgery, within the pericardial cavity. This can constrict the heart's pumping action. Conversely, pericarditis can occur due to an alteration in the serous fluid. This causes a roughening of the membranous surfaces and results in the classic 'pericardial rub' heard on auscultation (see Chapter 16).

The myocardium

The myocardium, the middle layer, forms the bulk of the heart. It is composed primarily of cardiac muscle cells (**myocytes**). Others include the autorhythmic cells with their propensity to generate electrical impulses devoid of external stimuli. It is the layer that generates the cardiac pumping action. When relating

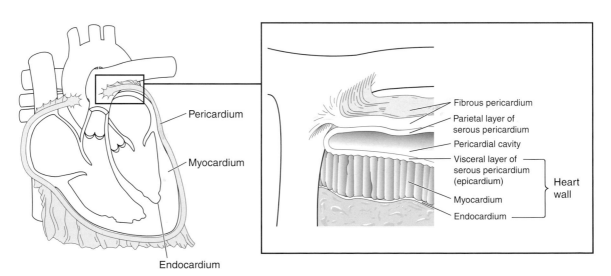

Figure 4.4 The layers of the heart (after Marieb 1998).

the anatomical features of the heart to its function as a pump, it is helpful to focus first upon the fibrous zone. This forms the cardiac skeleton into which insert myocardial fibres and the annulus of the heart valves. The interposition of the fibrous skeleton between the atria and the ventricles also prevents myocardial continuity between these two chambers. Consequently, the atrial myocardium is confined to the atrial chambers and the ventricular myocardium is confined to ventricular chambers. The myocardium is important within cardiac nursing care, primarily due to the serious conditions of myocardial ischaemia and infarction (see Chapter 9). More detail regarding this area and the cardiac myocytes themselves will be discussed later.

The endocardium

This is the inner layer lining the heart and is composed of squamous epithelium. Along with the vascular endothelium, it is regarded as one continuous sheet (Li et al 1993). Significantly, the vascular endothelium is known to be the source of numerous chemical mediators, including nitric oxide (NO), previously identified as endothelium-derived relaxing factor, and endothelin, that are involved in vasoregulation. Nitric oxide is a vasodilator, while endothelin is a powerful vasoconstrictor.

It has been proposed that, when stretched, the endocardium releases an endothelin-type mediator known as endocardin. This could increase the length and duration of contraction (Brutsaert & Andries 1992). This could be considered to be a 'safety mechanism', in that a dilated, failing ventricle has the ability to release endocardin to strengthen the force of contraction, thus autoregulating an inotropic stimulus.

Infective endocarditis (IE) occurs when microorganisms colonize the endocardial surface of the heart and valves, causing local tissue destruction. It remains a debilitating and in many cases a life-threatening disease. Chapter 14 explores the condition in depth.

The coronary blood vessels

Figure 4.5 provides a useful diagrammatic representation of the coronary circulation. The development of specialist roles within cardiac nursing, such as the angiography nurse, has led to the need for a clear overview of the coronary circulation and, importantly, which areas of the myocardium the various blood vessels serve. The right and left coronary arteries are the first vessels to arise from the anterior and left posterior sinuses of the ascending aorta. The opening orifices of these arteries are generally found above the aortic cusp margins. The two arteries form an oblique crown by way of anastomoses in the atrioventricular sulcus. In encircling the heart along the atrioventricular groove, the coronary arteries form a distinctive ring that gives off branches supplying the atria and ventricles.

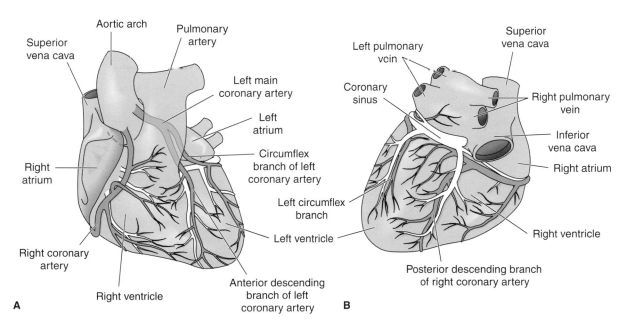

Figure 4.5 The adult coronary artery circulation. A: Anterior view. B: Inferior-posterior view.

The right half of this ring, which is formed by the **right coronary artery**, gives off a short penetrating artery which supplies the atrioventricular node. Correspondingly, the left half of the ring is formed by the **left coronary artery**, which divides to deliver oxygenated blood to both ventricles. However, according to West (1990), in 90% of human subjects the right coronary artery is the dominant larger vessel that traverses down the groove between the right atrium and the right ventricle, giving rise to branches that supply both chambers. This artery then turns toward the apex as it reaches the posterior aspect of the heart. At this point the artery becomes the **posterior descending branch** which supplies the lower aspect of the left ventricle.

The left coronary artery is a short vessel, which divides into an anterior descending branch (LAD) and a circumflex branch (CX). The LAD branch supplies the interventricular septum and the anterior surface of the left ventricle. The circumflex artery supplies the lateral aspect and part of the posterior aspect of the left ventricle. Whilst this is a common distribution there are many variations in coronary artery anatomy and in some subjects the left coronary artery may be the dominant vessel. In such circumstances, the right coronary artery (RCA) is very small and the circumflex supplies the inferior wall of the left ventricle. The pattern of coronary artery distribution is of course critically important, as any alteration in the coronary blood flow may result in changes in the blood supply to specific areas of the heart.

As the heart is an aerobic (requiring oxygen), constantly active organ, an efficient coronary circulation must provide a rich blood supply to the myocardium. For this reason a rich network of capillaries passes through the myocardium, creating a relatively short diffusion distance between the myocytes and their energy-producing mitochondria. Mitochondria, which occupy a large proportion of each myocyte, are often described as the powerhouse of the cell, producing the energy (such as adenosine triphosphate ATP) that the cells need to survive and function (Opie 1998). It is for this reason that some degree of arterial anastomosis may occur in the mature heart in conditions of myocardial hypoxia and coronary artery disease. These may be anastomoses between two branches of the same coronary artery or connections of branches of the RCA with branches of the left. The functional importance of this collateral circulation is debated. It is unclear if it protects the heart or represents more severe ischaemia (McCance & Richardson 1994).

The cardiac veins, which collect the venous blood returning from the heart itself, consist of numerous venous tributaries and a coronary sinus. The anterior cardiac veins drain the anterior region of the right ventricle (see Fig. 4.6). The large majority of cardiac veins drain into the wide **coronary sinus**, which is about 2 or 3 cm long, lying posterior to the coronary sulcus between the left atrium and the left ventricle. The coronary sinus opens into the right atrium between the orifice of the inferior vena cava and the atrioventricular annulus. An endocardial fold, known as the semilunar valve of the coronary sinus, guards its opening.

The great cardiac vein begins at the apex of the heart and ascends in the anterior interventricular sulcus en route to the coronary sulcus, turning to the left as it eventually enters the coronary sinus. A range of smaller cardiac veins, which receive deoxygenated blood from specific regions of the heart, thus support the work of the great cardiac vein. These smaller vessels can be identified in Figure 4.6.

Lymph drainage of the heart

A substantial lymphatic network supports the heart. In this context fine thin-walled lymphatic vessels are distributed throughout the myocardium, forming a plexus immediately below the endocardial surface. The lymph channels follow the path of the conductive tissue. The bundle branches and the atrial surfaces of the tricuspid and mitral valves have a particularly extensive lymph vessel supply. A single large channel carries the lymph to a pretracheal node near the arch of the aorta.

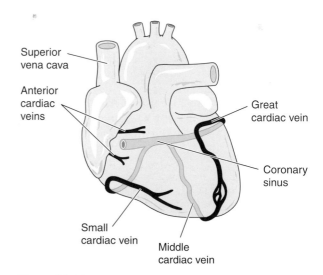

Figure 4.6 The coronary venous circulation (after Marieb 1998).

The innervation of the heart

The heart receives its nerve supply from the sympathetic and parasympathetic branches of the autonomic nervous system. Branches of the afferent and efferent fibres of the vagus and phrenic nerves and the thoracic and cervical cardiac nerves convey impulses to the cardiac plexus. Silver (1991) defines the cardiac plexus as a group of nerve ganglia positioned between the aortic arch and the bifurcation of the trachea. Further networks of nerve ganglia are found in the subendocardium of the right atrium, the interatrial septum and the epicardium near the roots of the aorta and the pulmonary artery. Branches of the sympathetic and the parasympathetic nervous system also supply the sinoatrial (SA) and AV nodes. However, the sympathetic and parasympathetic nerves of the cardiac plexus only serve to modulate myocardial performance, they do not participate in the propagation of the action potentials through the myocardium.

The myocardial architecture

The myocardium is predominantly composed of cardiac muscle, which makes up the greater proportion of the muscular walls of the heart. The myocardial cells can be classified into two main types. The most important of these are the myocytes, which are elongated force-generating cells (Fig. 4.7). The second type, which are in the minority, are those with autorhythmic properties. These form a specialized electrical pathway (the conduction pathway) that will be discussed later in this chapter.

The myocytes are embedded in a matrix of connective tissue and surrounded by a rich network of blood vessels, capillaries, lymph vessels and nerves. They are cylindrical in shape but branch freely. The myocytes vary in size, depending on their atrial or ventricular origin. However, they are small. Atrial myocytes are less than 10 μm in diameter and about 20 μm in length, whilst ventricular myocytes are 10–20 μm in diameter and 50–100 μm long (Levick 1995, Opie 1998).

The branching myocytes are attached to each other at junctions known as **intercalated discs** (Fig. 4.8). These discs contain desmosomes and gap junctions. The function of desmosomes is to anchor the adjacent cells together, possibly by a proteoglycan glue (Levick 1995), to prevent them separating during muscle contraction. Gap junctions (or nexus) allow the movement of ions from one cell to another via connexons, which are protein particles with a central channel that spans the gap. This direct movement of ions from one cell to

Sarcomere (a segment of a myofibril)

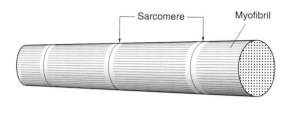

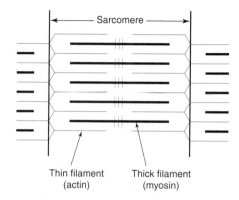

Figure 4.7 Microscopic anatomy of a myocyte (after Marieb 1998).

another ensures that the entire myocardium behaves as one unit and this is referred to as a **functional syncytium**. In ischaemia, gap junctions become progressively uncoupled which alters the ease with which ions move from one cell to another. It has been proposed that a result of this uncoupling is the poor conduction seen during myocardial ischaemia and recorded on the electrocardiogram (ECG) (Levick 1995).

The myocytes contain mitochondria, whose function is to produce energy for the cells, in the form of adenosine triphosphate (ATP). ATP is an organic molecule that stores and releases chemical energy for use within cells (Marieb 1998). Therefore cardiac muscle cells that are constantly working need a large amount of energy and thus large mitochondria. The myocytes also contain organelles called **sarcoplasmic reticulum** whose function is to store calcium ions. The surface of the cell consists of a membranous structure known as the **sarcolemma** (cell membrane). The cell membrane protrudes down into the cell, forming a set of transverse tubules (T-tubules) whose function is to rapidly transmit the external electrical stimulus inside the cell.

The cardiac muscle cells are filled with cross-striated myofibrils, which are similar to those in skeletal

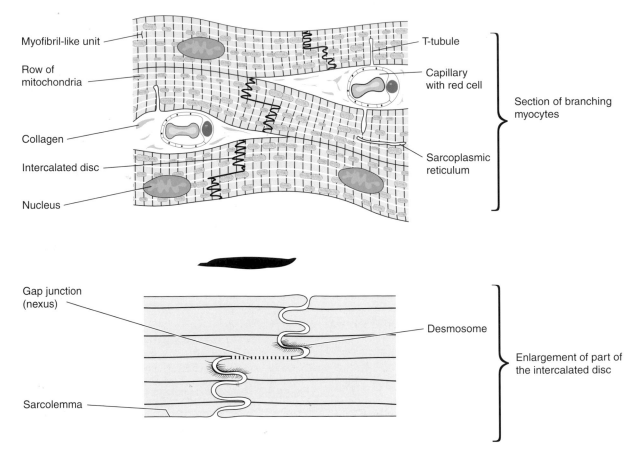

Myofibril-like unit

Row of mitochondria

Collagen

Intercalated disc

Nucleus

T-tubule

Capillary with red cell

Section of branching myocytes

Sarcoplasmic reticulum

Gap junction (nexus)

Desmosome

Enlargement of part of the intercalated disc

Sarcolemma

Figure 4.8 The intercalated discs.

muscle. They are composed of smaller units known as **sarcomeres** (the contractile units).

The sarcomere

Within the sarcomere are two types of protein filament (**myofilaments**) that are arranged in such a way that when there is a muscle contraction, they partially slide over each other to cause shortening, known as the sliding filament theory (see Fig. 4.7). The two types of protein filament are known as the thick and the thin filaments. The former is composed of the protein myosin. The myosin molecules are made up of two globular heads and a rod-like region, consisting of a neck and tail, which provide stability to the molecule. The globular head contains active sites that hydrolyse ATP and interact, forming bridges, with designated sites of the actin molecule.

The thin filament, although predominantly made of actin, contains two other types of protein, tropomyosin and troponin. These filaments are functionally involved in tension generation and muscle contraction. The tropomyosin filaments are positioned in the grooves of the actin helix. Attached to the tropomyosin, at intervals of 40 nm, are the troponin complexes, consisting of three distinguishable proteins known as troponin-T, troponin-C and troponin-I. Collectively the troponin tropomyosin molecules are responsible for the regulation of actin–myosin function.

The above principles offer some clarification of the sliding filament hypothesis, which is a major contributor to the current understanding of muscle contraction. The theory implies that although a muscle shortens during contraction, the length of both the thick and thin filaments remains constant and unchanged. Indeed, the shortening events are best described in terms of the thin filaments being pulled into the lattice of the thick filaments. Each contraction therefore depends on the thin filaments being pulled towards the centre of the sarcomere. Thus the degree of contraction is limited by the length of the sarcomere. Starling's Law of the heart states that, within physiological limits, the greater the degree of stretch, the greater the force of contraction. The term 'physiological limit' refers to the sarcomere; if stretched too far then some of the bridges between the myosin and actin become detached and will reduce the force of contraction.

The cardiac nurse needs to have an increased knowledge of the myocardial architecture to fully understand advances made in cardiology. Examples include the discovery that some forms of hypertrophic cardiomyopathy are due to new mutations in parts of myosin filaments (Watkins et al 1992) and the identification of cardiac troponins as highly sensitive and specific markers for diagnosing myocardial infarction (Plebani & Zaninotto 1999).

The conduction pathway

A knowledge of the conduction system, together with the associated recordings of the electrocardiogram (ECG), is essential for the cardiac nurse. Nurses working within acute units need to understand how conduction abnormalities will manifest and the subsequent appropriate treatments. The management of cardiopulmonary resuscitation by nursing and medical staff against printed algorithms is one example.

The autorhythmic cells within the myocardium, in health, function in a specific order, known as the con-

duction pathway: first the sino-atrial (SA) node, then the atrioventricular (AV) node or junction, then the bundle of His, left and right bundle branches and the Purkinje fibres (Fig. 4.9).

The cardiac 'pacemaker' or SA node initiates each cardiac cycle. Its anatomic location at the junction of the embryonic sinus venosus and the right atrium proper appears to be ideally suited to its function, ensuring that the atria are depolarized first. A plaque of subepicardial fat frequently covers this node, which makes it visible to the naked eye. The node has its own large central artery, which takes its origin from either the right or the circumflex coronary artery. The structural features of this node include some slender cells, which are confined to the nodal centre surrounding the nodal artery. These cells are arranged somewhat more irregularly on the external surfaces and are considered as the specialized pacemakers of the heart. They initiate the wave of electrical depolarization that is eventually propagated through the entire myocardium. They make functional contact with each other and the adjacent transitional myocytes, which are smaller than the contractile myocytes. Katz (1992) suggests that these transitional cells establish a zone, which forms a junction between the SA node and the surrounding myocardium.

The AV node is located in the muscular part of the AV septum. Its interior aspect enters a central fibrous body forming the atrioventricular bundle, also known as the **bundle of His**. This node consists of irregular

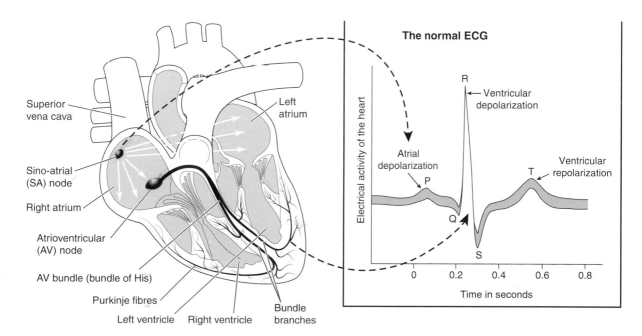

Figure 4.9 The internal conduction system of the heart and associated ECG trace.

collagenous reticulum which enmeshes the myocytes, forming a compact and a transitional zone. The transitional zone is thought to be responsible for the delays in the cardiac impulse. However, the myocardial discontinuity must permit the bundle of His to penetrate the central fibrous body and establish a bridge of excitable tissue between the atria and the ventricles. This anatomical feature is of considerable physiological significance as it provides the only acceptable pathway for the conducting system between atria and ventricles. Generally the AV node receives its blood supply from a tributary of the RCA, although in a small percentage of people this may be from the left circumflex artery. The blood supply to the SA and AV nodes and other components of the conduction pathway is of great relevance to the cardiac nurse. This knowledge will assist in predicting conduction problems in association with blockages to the coronary arteries (see Chapter 9).

The bundle of His is the direct extension of the AV node. It branches on the upper surface of the muscular interventricular septum, forming a right and a left bundle branch. The blood supply to the bundle of His and the first few millimetres of the bundle branches is via the tributory of the RCA that supplies the AV node and also from branches of the left anterior descending artery.

The **right and left bundle branches** are similar in structure. However, the left bundle branch consists of two sets of fibres, termed anterior and posterior fascicles, whilst the right bundle is a single cord-like structure. The right bundle branch is embedded in the myocardium and subendocardium, radiating towards the apex of the right ventricle and reaching the anterior papillary muscles. It then forms fine subendocardial conduction pathways, which supply the remainder of the right ventricular wall. The left bundle branch forms a framework down the smooth left ventricular septum, which eventually give rise to a rich subendocardial network, which first surrounds the papillary muscles and then the remaining part of the left ventricle. The bundle branches are supplied by branches of the left anterior descending artery.

The smallest structures of the conduction system are the **Purkinje fibres** which are large pale cells containing more glycogen and fewer contractile filaments than the cells of the contractile myocardium (Katz 1992). Contact between the Purkinje fibres and the contractile myocardium is best established in the subendocardial regions. This arrangement permits the papillary muscles to contract first. This is followed by a wave of excitation and the ensuing contraction then travels from the apex to the ventricular outflow tract. As the Purkinje network is subendocardial, myocardial excitation and contraction proceed from the endocardium to the epicardium. The spread of the excitation is rapid but not instantaneous. A short delay allows different parts of the right and left ventricles to receive their impulse at slightly different times.

The functional relationship of the conduction pathway to the heart as a whole allows us to appreciate how failure in the conduction system may not necessarily block myocardial contractility, but the function of the heart as a pump will become poorly co-ordinated. Importantly, as slower conduction and alterations in rhythm occur, a 'new' dominant pacemaker may arise from focal spontaneous myogenic activity in the contractile myocytes or distal part of the conduction system. Arrhythmias, particularly tachycardias, occur when an irritable focus predominates, becoming for that period of time the pacemaker of the heart.

Although the autonomic nervous system influences various functions of the heart, including the frequency and vigour of each contraction, cardiac function is not entirely dependent on neural stimulation and control. This is because **automaticity** and **rhythmicity** are physiological phenomena intrinsic to the myocardium and its conduction system. The heart will continue to beat even when denervated. Therefore, providing the coronary blood vessels are perfused, rhythmic myocardial contraction will continue. The transplanted heart is a clear example of this.

ELECTROPHYSIOLOGY

Action potential Changes that occur in the cell membrane, allowing the inward and outward flow of ions during depolarization and repolarization.

Depolarization The moment when the interior of the cardiac cell is maximally charged with positive ions.

Repolarization The process of restoration of a cell to its normal resting membrane polarity following depolarization.

As highlighted previously, autorhythmicity of the heart is masterminded by the SA node, which is commonly regarded as the master pacemaker. The SA node depolarizes spontaneously 65–85 times a minute. Due to the dominance and magnitude of action potentials initiated within the node, the electrical stimuli spread rapidly but in an orderly fashion, throughout the myocardium.

One of the features of the pacemaker cells is that they do not require external stimuli to depolarize. Indeed, the pacemaker cells are perceived to have an unstable resting potential, which allows them to depolarize continually. This is turn generates a threshold, which permits the firing of the dominant rhythmic action potentials, which spread throughout the heart initiating the characteristic ECG recording depicted in Figure 4.9.

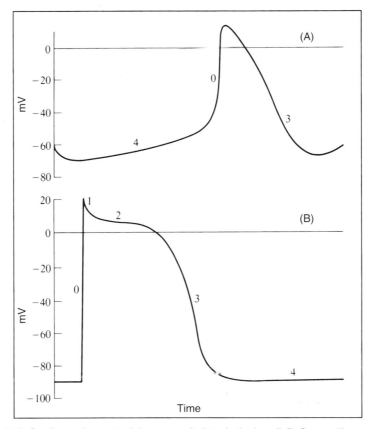

Figure 4.10 Cardiac action potential sources. A: Autorhythmic cell. B: Contractile myocyte.

Overview of the action potential

The action potential of the autorhythmic cells (Fig. 4.10A)

The autorhythmic cells do not depend on an extrinsic (external) nerve supply as the stimulus as they have an intrinsic ability to depolarize. The precise mechanism of how this occurs is unclear. However, the belief is that the autorhythmic cells have a reduced membrane permeability to potassium (K^+). Yet, sodium (Na^+) permeability is unchanged and it continues to diffuse into the cell at a slow rate. As the interior of the cell becomes less negative, gates along the cell open and allow sodium in at a rapid rate. The membrane interior thus becomes less and less negative and slowly more positive. Ultimately, when a certain threshold is reached, fast calcium channels open, allowing an explosive and fast entry (influx) of calcium into the cell from the extracellular space. Therefore, in autorhythmic cells an influx of calcium, rather than sodium, produces the rising phase in the action potential and rapidly reverses the membrane potential, creating an electrical impulse (Marieb 1998).

The falling phase of the action potential, **repolarization**, reflects an increased potassium (K^+) permeability and its efflux (exit) from the cell. Once repolarization is complete, the potassium ion channels are inactivated and the membrane permeability to K^+ is reduced. Then the whole process of depolarization begins again.

Autorhythmicity of the heart has been described as spontaneous diastolic depolarization and is initiated in the SA node (Katz 1992). Each action potential thus generated by the SA node will set up the propagated wave of depolarization that initiates the systole in all regions of the heart. However, the action potentials of the SA node are small with a slow upstroke, which suggests that the sodium ion channels in these cells may not be fully functioning (Katz 1992). It could also be argued that the absence of an inward sodium current is partly due to the high resting potential enjoyed by the SA node. As a high resting potential will inactivate sodium ion channels, it must be assumed that the upstroke of the action potentials generated within the SA node is largely due to an influx of calcium ions.

Spontaneous pacemaker activity exists in all regions of the AV node (Katz 1992). However, this node appears to be under the control of the autonomic nervous system. As in the SA node, the characteristic slow AV node depolarization reflects the absence of functional sodium ion channels. A slow inward calcium current primarily causes the spontaneous diastolic depolarization. Control of this current by neurotransmitters such as adrenaline (epinephrine) from the sympathetic fibres and acetylcholine from the parasympathetic plays a critical role in regulating the slow conduction velocity. However, slow conduction in the AV node is also due to the small nodal cell size and the relatively small number of gap junctions, which are responsible for a high internal resistance. By contrast, the cells of the remaining part of the conduction system pathway have action potentials that are long and of large magnitude. This ensures that impulses do not re-enter the Purkinje system after they have activated the ventricles.

In addition to the SA and AV nodes, many other regions of the heart have the capacity to generate characteristic action potentials. These are specific for their specialized electrophysiological role. However, two dominant action potentials may be noted with respect to the heart: the **fast response** action potentials that occur in the atrial and ventricular myocytes and Purkinje fibres; and the **slow response** action potentials which occur in the SA and AV nodes.

The physiological relationship between the electrical events of the action potential and the actual mechanical contraction of the muscle is detailed later. Katz (1992) argues that rapid depolarization precedes the development of muscle force and the completion of depolarization generally coincides with peak force or contraction. Of course, the duration and magnitude of the action potential will influence the duration of the muscle contraction. On the other hand an unacceptable increase in the number of action potentials in a given time will result in a decrease in the time committed to each impulse and, of course, a corresponding decrease in the mechanical contraction of the muscle.

The action potential in the autorhythmic cells can be summarized in the following phases:

- phase 0 representing depolarization
- phase 3 representing repolarization
- phase 4 representing the 'resting potential'. However, as this can be regarded as unstable, it is not truly a resting potential.

The action potential of the contractile myocytes (Fig. 4.10B)

Although the ionic basis of the action potential in myocytes continues to be investigated, the assumption is that any abrupt changes in the resting membrane

potential will result in a propagation of an action potential (Katz 1992, West 1990). This assumption gives rise to a belief that the rapid myocyte depolarization or excitation (phase 0) may be almost exclusively attributed to a sudden increase in sodium influx. The influx of the sodium ions diminishes the transmembrane potential and this increases the influx of sodium ions further, causing the membrane potential to become positive. The sodium channels then close and the membrane potential begins to fall (phase 1). This is due to a short period when chloride ions re-enter the cell. However, it is at this point that there is a sustained inward current of calcium ions. This prolongs the action potential for a brief period of time (200–400 ms) and prevents the myocyte from rapidly repolarizing. This is the plateau phase (phase 2).

In phase 3, repolarization, the cell membrane returns to its resting potential of about −90 mv. The falling phase of the action potential reflects an increased potassium (K^+) permeability and its efflux (exit) from the cell. Once repolarization is complete, the potassium channels are inactivated and phase 4 or the resting state is reached. The inside of the cell is once again negative due to the K^+ leakage. An excess of sodium remains in the cell, because the membrane is much less permeable to this ion. The sodium–potassium pump is then activated, pumping sodium out of the cell and moving potassium inside. According to Katz (1992), at phase 3 of the action potential, some of the gates of the sodium ion channels open and as the channels recover from their inactivation, sodium influx resumes and the myocyte begins to respond again but rather weakly initially.

The action potential in the contractile myocytes can be summarized in the following phases:

- an upstroke (phase 0) representing depolarization
- a brief partial repolarization (phase 1)
- a plateau (phase 2)
- a gradual but progressive repolarization (phase 3)
- a resting potential (phase 4).

During the plateau period, the myocyte is said to enter its effective refractory period. The benefit of this mechanism is considerable as the refractory period prevents **tetanic contraction** (a sustained muscle contraction) of the myocardium.

Excitation–contraction coupling

As indicated earlier, co-ordinated myocardial contractility is initiated by the rhythmic discharge of action potentials that spread across the myocardium. However, the mechanisms involved in the excitation

Box 4.1 Summary of the events of contraction

The action potential is generated speedily to the myofibrils via the T-tubules. There is an influx of calcium into the myocardial cytoplasm and also liberation of calcium from the sarcoplasmic reticulum (the intracellular calcium stores). The calcium ions bind to troponin, causing a change in conformation and freeing tropomysin from its position, which is blocking the binding sites on actin. Contraction can then occur because the myosin can form crossbridges with the actin, pulling the actin filament inwards. Actin–myosin detachment is dependent on the binding of magnesium and ATP to the ATPase site of the myosin head region. The ATP is hydrolysed, leaving the myosin head energized. During repolarization, calcium ions are removed; some are pumped into the sarcoplasmic reticulum and some become extracellular. This then re-instates the tropomyosin blockage and relaxation of the muscle occurs.

and contraction of the myocardium overlap considerably in time. Consequently, the ending of an action potential coincides with the beginning of myocardial relaxation. This characteristic relationship seems entirely appropriate to the pump action of the heart. An important event of the excitation–contraction coupling is the influx of calcium into the myocytes during the action potential which prolongs both the action potential and the refractory period (Schmidt & Thews 1987).

The co-ordination of cardiac activity

The rhythmic action potentials that drive the heart as a pump originate in a group of pacemaker cells in the SA node and spread rapidly but sequentially through the atria and then the ventricles, depolarizing them to contract. This mechanism ensures that the human (adult) heart pumps ceaselessly at about 70–80 cycles per minute, maintaining a constant perfusion of the pulmonary and systemic tissue. However, as the entire cardiovascular system enjoys a certain capacity for adaptability, the heart rate and stroke volume (the amount of blood ejected in one heart beat) fluctuate in accordance with the prevailing physiological demands of the individual.

The principal events of a cardiac cycle are complex and dependent on precise timing of the many mechanical operations. Neural influences are important contributors in that they adapt the intrinsic cardiac rhythm to functional demands made on the cardiovascular system by the whole of the body.

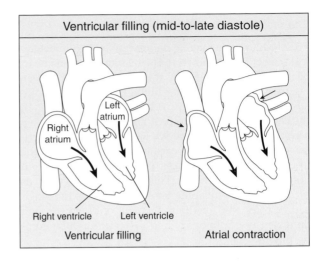

Ventricular filling (mid-to-late diastole)

Left atrium

Right atrium

Right ventricle   Left ventricle

Ventricular filling   Atrial contraction

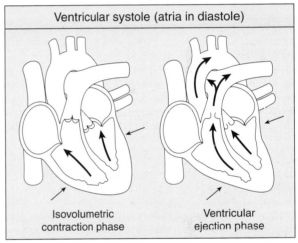

Ventricular systole (atria in diastole)

Isovolumetric contraction phase   Ventricular ejection phase

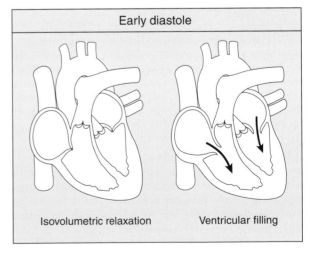

Early diastole

Isovolumetric relaxation   Ventricular filling

Figure 4.11 The mechanical events of the cardiac cycle (after Marieb 1998).

The mechanical events of the cardiac cycle

The cardiac cycle may be defined in terms of mechanical events that occur from the beginning of one heart beat to the beginning of the next, as illustrated in Figure 4.11. As the resting human heart rate is maintained at approximately 70 beats/min the phases of the cardiac cycle need to be accomplished in less than a second (about 0.8 seconds). Furthermore, the electrical activation of the myocardium must ensure that the four chambers of the heart contract sequentially but not entirely in synchrony. This allows the atria to act as primer pumps whilst the ventricles provide the major source of power for the movement of blood through the extensive pulmonary and systemic vascular compartments.

The cardiac cycle is characterized by a series of pressure changes within the heart that result in blood flowing from high to low pressure areas. Healthy cardiac valves prevent blood from flowing in the wrong direction. The cardiac cycle, due to its continuous nature, can be described from different starting points. This description will start when the ventricles are relaxing, in diastole. The terms 'diastole' and 'systole', by convention, refer to the state of the ventricle. When they are used for the atria, this will be specifically stated.

Mid to late ventricular diastole. The pressures are low in the heart and the blood passively returns to the atria and to the ventricles through the open AV valves. About 70–80% of ventricular filling occurs by this route. The semilunar valves are closed because the pressure in the major vessels (the pulmonary artery and aorta) is greater than in the ventricles and this prevents backflow of blood.

There is then depolarization, that spreads throughout the atria (the P wave on the ECG) and atrial contraction (systole) follows, forcing the remaining 20–30% of blood into the ventricles. Atrial contraction is normally slightly asynchronous as the right atrium contraction occurs ahead of the left atrium by approximately 0.02 seconds but this has no significant effect on cardiac output. The atria then relax for the rest of the cycle.

Ventricular systole. As the atria relax, the ventricles depolarize (the QRS complex on the ECG). There is then ventricular contraction (systole) which causes an increase in the pressure within the ventricles. As the pressure starts to rise, the AV valves close. So at this stage in the cycle, all four valves are closed and the volume of blood in the ventricles is constant. This is known as **isovolumetric contraction**. As the ventricle continues to contract the rapidly rising pressure

exceeds the pressure in the major vessels and the semilunar valves open. This occurs when the left ventricular pressure rises slightly above 80 mmHg and the right ventricular pressure slightly above 27–30 mmHg. This marks the onset of the ejection phase.

During the ejection phase the pressures in the left ventricle and the aorta briefly rise to a maximum of about 120 mmHg. At this point the systolic and diastolic pressures in the right ventricle and the pulmonary artery are thought to be approximately 25–8 mmHg.

Early ventricular diastole. There is then repolarization of the ventricles (T wave on the ECG) and as a consequence the ventricles then relax (diastole). The pressure then drops in these chambers, allowing the raised aortic and pulmonary artery pressures to push blood back towards the ventricles, a process that snaps the aortic and pulmonary valves into a closed position (the dicrotic notch on the arterial pressure trace marks this event; see Chapter 5). So once again the ventricles are closed chambers and this is known as **isovolumetric relaxation**. During the period of ventricular activity, the atria have been filling. Eventually the pressure in the ventricles will be lower than that in the atria and so the AV valves will open, allowing blood to flow through into the ventricles.

Each cardiac cycle is about 0.8 seconds, although this will depend on heart rate. Atrial systole takes 0.1 seconds, ventricular systole takes 0.3 seconds so for 0.4 seconds the heart is totally relaxed. An increase in heart rate will decrease the resting period (the diastolic time), which has implications as the coronary arteries fill during diastole and therefore any reduction in filling time may impair the blood supply to the myocardium.

Atrial function. The function of the atria may be normally represented by characteristic pressure curves and haemodynamic recordings identify three major pressure elevations (Fig. 4.12).

● An 'a' wave which is initiated by atrial contraction. In the healthy adult, the right atrial pressure may rise to 5 or 6 mmHg during systole and the left atrial pressure may rise to approximately 7 or 8 mmHg.

● A 'c' wave which is initiated by the beginning of ventricular contraction. Guyton & Hall (1996) attribute this positive wave to the slight backflow of blood towards the AV valves and a corresponding backward bulging of these valves into the atria as the ventricles begin to contract and the ventricular pressure rises.

● A 'v' wave, which arises as a consequence of the slow return of venous blood to the atria while the AV

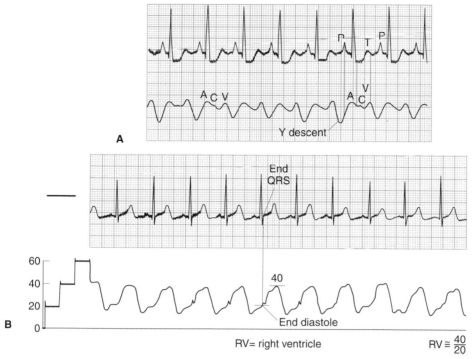

Figure 4.12 ECG correlation with the component parts of the atrial (A) and ventricular (B) pressure waveforms. (Reproduced with permission from Ahrens 1992).

valves are closed during ventricular contraction. Characteristically the 'v' wave appears towards the end of ventricular contraction and disappears as the ventricles relax and the AV valves open, allowing the accumulated atrial blood to flow rapidly into the respective ventricles, causing the 'v' wave to disappear again.

The significance of the end-diastolic, end-systolic volume and stroke volume

The period of diastole normally allows the ventricles to increase their volume to about 110–125 ml each and this is known as the **end-diastolic (filling) volume** or **preload**. The preload is defined as the volume of blood that stretches the muscles of the ventricular chambers prior to contraction. During systole, in a resting individual, the ventricles eject approximately 70 ml of blood; this is known as the **stroke volume output**. The remaining volume in each ventricle, about 40–55 ml, is known as the **end-systolic volume**. There is, however, considerable variation in the volume of blood ejected during each systole. This variation is largely influenced by the activity of the individual person; for example, when the heart con-

tracts more forcefully during exercise, the end-systolic volume can fall to as little as 10–20 ml. Conversely, when large quantities of blood are returned to the ventricles during diastole, the end-diastolic volume may increase to 150–250 ml. Therefore, by increasing the end-diastolic volume and decreasing the end-systolic volume, the stroke volume output will be increased significantly and may even double at times of high metabolic demand.

Another physiological variable of considerable clinical importance is the **ejection fraction**, a concept which defines the ratio of stroke volume to end-diastolic volume. Essentially the ejection fraction describes the stroke volume as a percentage of the ventricular end-diastolic volume, normally approximately 50–65%. However, when evaluating ventricular function it has to be remembered that the ejection fraction is a measure of pump function rather than contractility, as it is influenced by a number of haemodynamic variables. These include the preload, afterload and the heart rate. The **afterload** is the resistance against which the left ventricle must eject its volume of blood during systole. The blood present in the vascular compartment and the blood vessel walls themselves generate this resistance. The ejection fraction can, however, distinguish between two major types of heart failure. For example, in circumstances of impaired myocardial contractility, the ejection fraction is low. Conversely, in circumstances where ventricular relaxation is impaired, for example in some presentations of hypertrophic cardiomyopathy, the ejection fraction may increase.

NORMAL HEART SOUNDS

An understanding of the sequence of electrical and mechanical events that occur in the right and left sides of the heart is central to the appreciation of the timing of heart sounds and murmurs. Auscultation with the aid of a stethoscope is one of the best established methods used to distinguish between the different sounds of the heart. When listening to a normal heart, one hears sounds generally described as 'lub ... dub ... lub ... dub'. The 'lub', also known as the first sound, is associated with the closure of the AV valves at the onset of systole. The 'dub' gives rise to the second heart sound and is associated with the closure of the semilunar valves at the end of systole.

The first heart sound

West (1990) argues that the first heart sound is attributed to vibrations caused by the taut AV valves immediately following their closure. These vibrations are enhanced by sounds generated by the blood, the walls of the heart and of course the major vessels around the heart. Contraction of the ventricles causes sudden backflow of blood against the closed tricuspid and mitral valves, causing them to bulge towards the atria. The elastic nature of these valves then redirects the blood back into the ventricles. This causes a turbulence in the blood and establishes the characteristic vibrations, which travel through the adjacent tissue to the chest wall. The duration of the first heart sound averages 0.14 seconds (Guyton 1991).

The second heart sound

The second heart sound is attributed to the sudden closure of the aortic and pulmonary valves. As these valves close they bulge towards the ventricles. However, as the elastic tissue of these valves recoils the blood is moved back into the arteries, which causes characteristic vibrations that are then transmitted to the chest wall.

The duration of the second heart sound averages 0.11 seconds. The shorter sound is attributed to the extra tautness of the semilunar valves, which gives rise to a

shorter vibration period in comparison to the vibrations of the AV valves. However, the second heart sound normally has a higher (pitch) frequency than the first heart sound. The rationale for this can again be found in the greater tautness of the semilunar valves in comparison to the AV valves and the greater elasticity of the arteries in comparison to the looser ventricular chambers.

The third heart sound

Occasionally a third sound is heard in middle diastole. The cause of this sound is attributed to the oscillation of blood between the walls of the ventricles, which is initiated by the entry of blood from the atria. The reason for this sound appearing in mid-diastole is presumably that in the early part of diastole the heart is not filled sufficiently to generate tension in the ventricles, which is essential for the rumbling reverberation characteristic of the third sound. The frequency (pitch) of this sound is normally very low, making it difficult to hear on auscultation.

The fourth heart sound

This sound is frequently referred to as the atrial sound because it occurs as the atria contract. The main contributor to this sound is the flowing of blood into the ventricles, which initiates the characteristic low-frequency vibrations. Due to its low frequency, this sound can almost never be heard on auscultation.

THE REGULATION OF THE PUMPING HEART

As indicated earlier the heart is a highly adaptive organ. Its activities are regulated in accordance with the activities and metabolic needs of the body as a whole. The two most responsive mechanisms that regulate the 'pumping' of the heart are:

● the intrinsic cardiac regulation, which augments the pumping action of the heart in direct response to changes in the volume of the blood flowing into the heart
● the autonomic nervous system.

Intrinsic regulation of the mechanical activities of the heart

The pumping activity of the heart and the amount of blood pumped each minute are determined by the rate of blood flow into the heart. This is generally known as the venous return, which may vary in volume depending on the physical demands made on the body. In the systemic circulation the venous return consists of deoxygenated blood being returned to the right atrium and thus the right ventricle. By contrast, the pulmonary venous circulation consists of oxygenated blood being returned through the pulmonary veins to the left atrium and left ventricle. The heart then automatically pumps the oxygenated blood into the aorta and the deoxygenated blood into the pulmonary artery (see Fig. 4.1).

The intrinsic capacity of the heart to adapt to changing volumes of returning blood is referred to as the **Frank–Starling mechanism** (Starling's Law) of the heart. Starling's Law of the heart is based simply on the notion that a greater stretch of the myocardial fibres during filling will generate a greater subsequent force of contraction, resulting in larger volumes of blood being pumped by the ventricles. The basis of this law may be outlined as follows. The additional volume of blood returning to the heart causes the myocardial fibres to stretch to a greater length. This in turn stimulates the myocardium to contract with increased force as actin and myosin filaments are brought to a nearly optimal degree of interdigitation required for force generation. However, Guyton & Hall (1996) draw attention to a further point which implies that stretching the right atrial wall as a consequence of greater venous return raises the heart rate by 10–20%. Of course, this will also increase the amount of blood pumped each minute, although its contribution is not as great as that of the Frank–Starling mechanism.

Control of the heart function by the autonomic nervous system

The effectiveness and efficiency of the pumping action of the heart are controlled by parts of the sympathetic and parasympathetic (vagus) nerves, which supply the heart abundantly. Under normal physiological conditions, the sympathetic nerve fibres to the heart discharge continuously at a slow rate that maintains cardiac pumping at about 30% (Katz 1992) above that which would occur with no sympathetic stimulation. Consequently when the activity of the sympathetic nervous system is depressed, a reduction in the heart rate and force of ventricular contraction becomes evident. This eventually contributes to a significant reduction in cardiac output. Conversely, the parasympathetic (vagal) stimulation can induce significant bradycardia. This may be demonstrated clinically by any 'vagal manoeuvre'. This is a purposeful stimulation of the vagus nerve, perhaps carotid sinus massage under the jaw or asking the patient to breathe out against a closed epiglottis (the Valsalva manoeuvre).

This is used to slow an excessive tachycardia that may be compromising the haemodynamic status and, if successful, avoids the use of drug therapy. However, under physiological conditions the heart will resume beating normally again within a short period of time.

In some circumstances strong vagal stimulation will also decrease the force of myocardial contraction by 20–30%. However, this has a relatively small impact, which is attributed to the limitations of the vagal fibre distribution, being predominantly in the atria. As vagal fibre distribution to the ventricles is limited any impact on the force of ventricular pumping is also limited. Nevertheless, a significant reduction in the heart rate combined with the moderate decrease in myocardial contractility will have a considerable impact on ventricular pumping and so cardiac output.

Finally, sympathetic nerve stimulation may increase cardiac output by more than 100%. Indeed, the general consequences of sympathetic stimulation are:

- raised (adult) heart rate to 200 beats per minute
- increases in the force of myocardial contractility
- raised ventricular ejection pressure
- raised cardiac output.

In view of the above, it must be argued that neural stimulation augments the heart rate and the contractile force of the myocardium. Under physiological conditions, the heart rate determines the cardiac output, although there are important limitations to this. For instance, when the heart rate rises above the critical point, the force of myocardial contractility decreases. Guyton & Hall (1996) suggest that this phenomenon may be attributed to the myocardial overuse of metabolic substrates. In addition, in such circumstances, the period of diastole is significantly reduced so that ventricular filling is compromised and stroke volume reduced. However, the reduction in the stroke volume may be just one of the physiological adaptations manifested by the heart in clinically significant tachycardia.

THE CARDIAC OUTPUT AND DISTRIBUTION OF BLOOD

The cardiac output (CO) may be defined as the volume of blood ejected by each ventricle per unit of time. This is usually measured in litres per minute and can be calculated as follows:

Heart rate (HR) × stroke volume (SV) = cardiac output (CO).

In the resting individual the cardiac output generally amounts to approximately 5 l/min, e.g. normal heart rate 70 beats/min × stroke volume 70 ml = 4900 ml/min = 4.9 l/min. Slight normal variations do exist and this is particularly evident in the different values noted for females (4.6 l/min) and males (5.6 l/min). However, for all individuals the cardiac output can be increased to many times this value by an increased heart rate and a greater stroke volume. Conversely, bradycardia and reductions in the effective circulating blood volume and stroke volume may significantly reduce the cardiac output.

It may therefore be concluded that cardiac output is the most critical factor that must be taken into consideration when evaluating a patient's cardiovascular function. However, cardiac output is not a fixed entity sustained only by myocardial contractility and the amount of blood volume present in the circulation. In reality, the cardiac output is determined principally by the sum of various factors that control local and regional blood flow throughout the body. The sum of this local blood flow forms the venous return to the heart.

Although the individual's cardiac output is largely dependent on intrinsic cardiac factors, such as the heart rate and myocardial contractility, other factors also play an important role. The two major factors identified are the venous return and the peripheral resistance.

The venous return

Blood returning to the heart via the systemic and pulmonary veins is generally known as the venous return: the sum of all the local blood flow from the individual segments of the peripheral circulation. It follows, therefore, that the cardiac output is the sum of all the blood flow regulations. Local and regional blood flow is almost always responsive to the variations of tissue metabolism. Consequently, when local tissue oxygen consumption increases the volume of blood flow is augmented in proportion to that tissue metabolism. The advantage of such fine local adaptation is that blood flow increases in response to greater metabolic activities. This ensures that the appropriate substrates are delivered to the relevant area and the waste products are removed.

Peripheral resistance

One of the important factors that could affect the cardiac output is the physical resistance offered by the peripheral blood vessels. This phenomenon may be detailed as follows. Under physiological conditions and normal arterial pressure, the long-term cardiac output is reciprocal to the changes in the peripheral resistance. This implies that as peripheral resistance increases, the cardiac output falls. Conversely, as peripheral resistance decreases, the cardiac output rises. However, there are limitations to the amount of

blood that the heart can pump. These limitations are best expressed in the form of cardiac output curves. The systemic vascular resistance (SVR) can be measured clinically with a pulmonary artery (PA) catheter. It is frequently regarded as the afterload, as it is a resistance offered to the ejecting left ventricle by the arterial system. The usual range is 770–1500 dynes/sec/cm^{-5}. More details regarding cardiac output and systemic vascular resistance can be found in Chapter 18.

The vascular system (Fig. 4.13)

Essential to the function of the cardiovascular system is the circulating blood volume, which is propelled in a pulsatile, continuous fashion through the body. The lumen of all blood vessels is lined by endothelium, which usually consists of a single layer of flat cells. The endothelium occupies an important location, being situated between blood and tissues. It has now been discovered that the vascular endothelium not only has an important role in regulating cardiovascular homeostasis in health but also contributes to the pathophysiology of cardiovascular disease (Rubanyi 1993). The endothelium has the ability to respond to changes, whether physical, chemical or humoral, by the production of biologically active mediators that influence the control of the vascular diameter, e.g. prostacyclin, nitric oxide (NO) and endothelin. The endothelium also mediates haemostasis, cell proliferation and inflammatory mechanisms in the cell wall. Damage to the endothelium disrupts its normal functions and results in endothelial dysfunction. Endothelial dysfunction is an important area of research as it is a key feature of atherosclerosis, the most common cause of coronary artery disease, and seems to play a role in myocardial ischaemia and infarction.

In addition, all blood vessels, with the exception of the capillary network, are made up of varying amounts of elastic and collagen fibres as well as smooth muscle fibres. The elastic fibres, particularly in the tunica intima (the inner layer composed of endothelium), form a relatively dense network and can easily be stretched to many times their original length. These fibres exert a certain degree of tension, which opposes the tendency of the blood pressure to stretch the lumen of the vessels, without the use of any energy. Conversely, in the tunica media (the middle layer) and tunica adventitia (the outer layer), the collagen fibres form a network that offers a great deal more resistance to stretch than the elastic fibres. The spindle-shaped smooth muscle cells are connected to one another as well as to the elastin and collagen fibres. Their chief function is to provide active tension in the

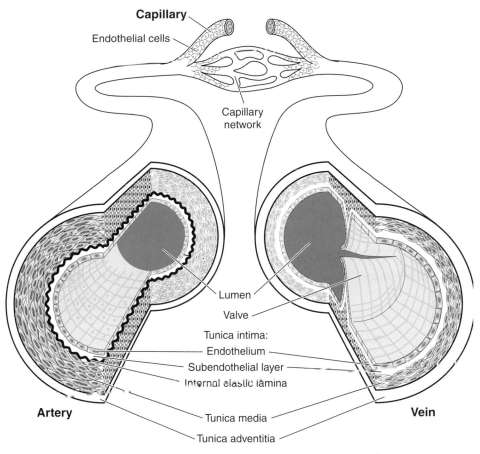

Figure 4.13 The structure of arteries, veins and capillaries (after Marieb 1998).

vessel wall (**myogenic vascular tone**) and to regulate the size of the lumen in response to the tendency of the blood pressure to stretch it. Autonomic nerve fibres innervate the smooth muscle in the blood vessels.

Although the vascular compartment is generally divided into the pulmonary and systemic units, from a functional point of view the blood vessels can be classified into elastic vessels, resistance vessels, sphincter vessels, capillaries and capacitance vessels or veins. Whilst all these vessels are important to the efficient function of the cardiovascular system, the resistance vessels appear to make the greatest contribution in the regulation of the volume of blood flow, within each vascular bed. The aorta and its dominant arterial branches account for about 19% of the total resistance to blood flow. The contribution of the terminal arteries and arterioles amounts to just under 50%. That is, vessels only a few millimeters long, due to their small capacity, generate half of the resistance to blood flow.

However, resistance in capillaries is also considerable, amounting to approximately 25% of the total resistance. The venous compartment offers a fairly small resistance to blood flow, averaging 4% for venules with the remaining larger veins contributing only about 3%.

Venules and veins largely determine the post-capillary resistance. Venules are tiny vessels formed when capillaries unite. As they return blood to the heart from the capillary beds, they join together to form larger veins. Significantly, veins also serve as the capacitance or reservoir vessels, in that their distensibility allows them to hold or pass on large quantities of blood without marked effect on other parameters of the circulation. Furthermore, some veins have anatomical characteristics that make them particularly capacious storage areas. This applies in particular to the venous network in the liver, the splanchnic region and the subpapillary plexus of the skin. Together these vessels can hold more than 1000 ml of blood for release as required. However, the pulmonary vessels too can be used for short-term storage or mobilization of fairly large amounts of blood, by altering venous return or augmenting the left ventricular volume output.

The term **systemic vascular resistance** (SVR) is used to define the overall resistance of the systemic circulation; that is, the resistance of all the vascular beds together. Together the SVR and the cardiac output determine the blood pressure.

Blood pressure

The pressure differences between the various vascular regions make the flow of blood possible because in response to the pulsatile ejection of blood from the left ventricle, blood flows from high-pressure regions to lower pressure regions. The evolving pressure gradient provides the force that overcomes the resistance to the flow of blood. Resistance to flow may vary depending on the differences in the blood vessels and the viscosity of the blood.

The pressures in the vascular compartment, that is the arterial and venous blood pressures, are equivalent to the force per unit area exerted by the blood on the walls of the vessels. Clinically, however, blood pressure implies the arterial pressure in the systemic circulation. Under normal circumstances the blood pressure fluctuates with each heart beat between a maximum value known as the **systolic pressure**, which occurs during systole, and a minimum value referred to as the **diastolic pressure**, attributed to the diastole of the cardiac cycle. The difference between the systolic and diastolic pressure values is known as the **pulse pressure**. However, the clinically significant blood pressure in critical care areas is the **mean arterial pressure** (MAP). This is the decisive pressure that reflects the blood flow through the body (see Chapter 5). Although mean arterial pressures are not used in some cardiac areas, it is important that the nurse has some understanding of the term as these figures appear on the automatic blood pressure recording machines.

The intrinsic regulation of the vascular system ensures that the entire body receives adequate amounts of blood at rest and during various changing physical circumstances. This must involve:

- the maintenance of a minimum blood flow to all organs
- the optimal regulation of cardiac activity and blood pressure
- the redistribution of blood to active organs when required, at the expense of the resting organs.

The regulation of blood flow, systemic vascular resistance and blood pressure are achieved predominantly by alterations in the diameter of the blood vessels. Local effects, neural activity and hormonal signals influence the state of tension (tone) of the smooth muscle of the blood vessels. At rest, most blood vessels are in an intermediate state of tension and this is known as the **resting tone**. The primary purpose of local control of circulation is to autoregulate the local blood flow and ensure its constancy in the face of constantly changing blood pressure. Furthermore, blood flow must be carefully adjusted in line with the metabolic needs of a specific organ or tissue. The autoregulation may be of myogenic origin (smooth muscle of the vessels) or of metabolic origin such as through oxygen deficiency or a rise in local tissue metabolites. Both mechanisms will induce vasodilatation, which will contribute towards the solution of the problem. Branches of the sympathetic nervous system mediate neural control of the blood vessels, principally the arterioles. In this fashion, postganglionic transmission involves α-1-receptors, the stimulation of which leads to vasoconstriction, and β-2-receptors, the stimulation of which results in vasodilatation.

The arterial blood pressure needs to be maintained within an appropriate physiological range but be able to fluctuate to meet the demands of everyday living. There are three main regulatory mechanisms that assist in blood pressure control. The immediate or short-term mechanism involves the autonomic nervous system. The medium-term control is regulated via a hormonal mechanism whilst the long-term control is, perhaps surprisingly, under the influence of the renal system.

Neural control

Pressure receptors (baroreceptors) are found in the aortic arch in the thorax and carotid sinuses which are situated in the neck. These are strategically placed to monitor any pressure changes in the blood supply to the body (via the aortic arch) and to the brain (via the carotid sinuses). They then transmit afferent impulses to the cardiovascular control centre in the medulla, part of the brainstem. The primary function in this instance is to stabilize the blood pressure. For example, an acute rise in blood pressure will initiate an increase in the firing of afferent impulses. This mechanism will in turn activate the parasympathetic nervous system, thus setting off a reflex response via the vagus nerve. This reduces cardiac activity. In addition, the sympathetic nerve pathway initiates vasodilatation and gives rise to a decrease in systemic vascular resistance. These two responses bring about a lowering of the elevated blood pressure.

Conversely, a drop in blood pressure will be detected by the baroreceptors and sympathetic cardiac and vasoconstrictor nerve activity will be increased, accompanied by a decreased parasympathetic activity. This will result in an increase in heart rate and stroke volume and cause arteriolar and venous vasoconstriction. This then gives rise to an increased cardiac output and systemic vascular resistance. This mechanism elevates the blood pressure to a physiologically desirable value.

Hormonal control

As the cardiac output lowers, catecholamines are released from the chromaffin cells of the adrenal medulla. Adrenaline (epinephrine) and noradrenaline (norepinephrine) are the primary catecholamines. The latter has a more specific action on the peripheral vessel α-adrenergic receptors, raising the systemic vascular resistance and therefore the blood pressure. Adrenaline has a wider range of effects including stimulating the β-1-adrenergic receptors to increase the heart rate and myocardial contractility. The general stimulatory actions will therefore raise the heart rate to increase the cardiac output and promote arterial and venous constriction. In specific areas, the constrictive action in the renal vasculature promotes excessive sodium and water retention. The arterial constriction will raise the systemic vascular resistance and hence the blood pressure and tissue perfusion. Venous constriction will cause a natural augmenting of Starling's Law of the heart, by shunting blood into the right side of the heart to raise the preload and increase the cardiac output. The above responses are similar to those of the sympathetic nervous system but they are longer lasting.

Renal control

The kidneys control blood pressure in two ways, directly and indirectly. Renal physiology is complex and so this section is only a brief overview, introducing the reader to the kidneys' effect on the cardiovascular system.

The direct mechanism involves altering blood volume. When blood pressure or volume rises, the kidneys respond by producing more urine. This reduces volume and therefore blood pressure and is the principle for the administration of diuretics in hypertension. On the other hand, if blood pressure or volume drops, water is conserved. This increases volume and therefore blood pressure. Although antidiuretic hormone (ADH), which is released from the posterior pituitary gland but produced by the hypothalamus, stimulates the kidneys to save water, this tends to play

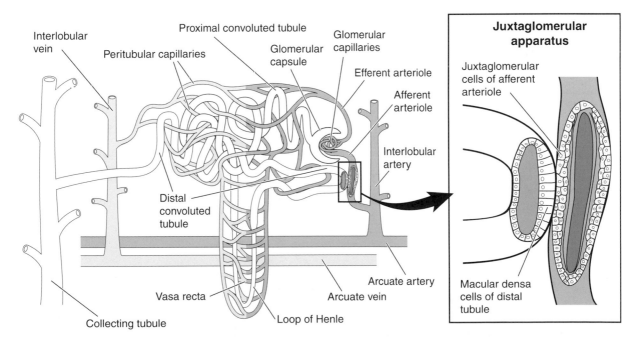

Figure 4.14 The anatomy of a nephron (after Marieb 1998).

a more prominent role in blood pressure regulation when there is a large reduction in blood volume. At this stage, ADH also causes vasoconstriction.

The indirect mechanism occurs when there is a reduction in the blood supply to the kidneys. The juxtaglomerular apparatus (JGA) is an area where the distal tubules and afferent arterioles of the kidney lie in close proximity. The afferent arterioles feed blood into the glomerular capsule, part of the nephron that ultimately creates urine. The distal convoluted tubule is the lower part of this nephron coiled back to come into contact with the afferent arteriole vessel (Fig. 4.14). The response to a reduction in blood pressure, volume or osmolarity is complex but ultimately results in the release of renin from the juxtaglomerular cells of the JGA. This commences what is known as the renin–angiotensin–aldosterone mechanism.

Renin acts to convert circulating angiotensinogen to angiotensin I. This is then converted, notably in the lining of the lungs, to angiotensin II which is a potent vasoconstrictor, raising the systemic vascular resistance, and causing the blood pressure to rise. In addi-

tion, it stimulates the adrenal cortex to release aldosterone which causes the renal tubules to reclaim sodium from the filtrate. Osmotically water follows sodium and hence the intravascular blood volume rises to induce an elevation in the blood pressure (Marieb 1998). Additionally, the preload will rise, augmenting Starling's Law of the heart and hence increasing the cardiac output. Treatments such as the diuretics reduce this excessive fluid retention, while the angiotensin-converting enzyme inhibitors are used as long-term therapy to block this chronic effect.

CONCLUSION

This chapter has discussed the anatomy and physiology of the cardiovascular system and aims to assist the reader in applying biological concepts to cardiac nursing practice. Throughout this text the knowledge will provide a useful underpinning not only to normal functioning but also to understanding the compensatory mechanisms that the cardiovascular system is capable of demonstrating in varying disease processes.

REFERENCES

Ahrens TS 1992 Haemodynamic waveform recognition. WB Saunders, Philadelphia

Brutsaert DL, Andries LJ 1992 The endocardial endothelium. American Journal of Physiology 263: H985–H1002

Gabella G 1995 Cardiovascular system. In: Bannister L (ed) Gray's anatomy. Churchill Livingstone, New York, pp. 1454–1605

Guyton A 1991 Textbook of medical physiology. WB Saunders, Philadelphia, pp. 97–271

Guyton A, Hall J 1996 Textbook of medical physiology. WB Saunders, Philadelphia, pp. 107–293

Katz A 1992 Physiology of the heart. Raven Press, New York

Levick JR 1995 An introduction to cardiovascular physiology, 2nd edn. Butterworth Heinemann, Oxford

Li K, Rouleau JL, Calderone A et al 1993 Endocardial function in pacing-induced heart failure in the dog. Journal of Molecular and Cellular Cardiology 25: 529–540

Marieb EN 1998 Human anatomy and physiology, 4th edn. Benjamin/Cummings, Menlo Park, California

McCance KL, Richardson SJ 1994 Structure and function of the cardiovascular and lymphatic systems. In: McCance

KL, Huether SE (eds) Pathophysiology: the biologic basis for disease in adults and children, 2nd edn. CV Mosby, St Louis, pp. 943–999

Opie LH 1998 Heart: physiology, from cell to circulation. Lippincott-Raven, Philadelphia

Plebani M, Zaninotto M 1999 Cardiac markers: present and future. International Journal of Clinical and Laboratory Research 29(2): 56–63

Rubanyi GM 1993 The role of endothelium in cardiovascular homeostasis and diseases. Journal of Cardiovascular Pharmacology 22 (suppl 4): S1–S14

Schmidt R, Thews G 1987 Human physiology. Springer-Verlag, Berlin

Silver M 1991 Cardiovascular pathology, vol. 1. Churchill Livingstone, Edinburgh

Watkins H, Thierfelder L, Hwang D-S et al 1992 Sporadic hypertrophic cardiomyopathy due to de novo myosin mutations. Journal of Clinical Investigation 90: 1666–1671

West J 1990 Physiological basis of medical practice. Williams and Wilkins, Baltimore

FURTHER READING

Berridge M, Bootman M, Lipp P 1998 Calcium: a life and death signal. Nature 395: 645–648

Brutsaert DL 1989 The endocardium. Annual Review of Physiology 51: 263–273

Haber E 1995 Molecular cardiovascular medicine. Scientific American Inc, New York

Holden A 1998 A last wave from the dying heart. Nature 392(6671): 20–21

Marieb EN 2001 Human anatomy and physiology, 5th edn. Benjamin/Cummings, Menlo Park, California

Thorogood P 1997 Embryos, genes and birth defects. John Wiley, Chichester

Clinical assessment

This section explores in detail the important issue of skilled and accurate clinical assessment of the cardiac patient or client. The more complex monitoring devices are explored, but the emphasis is placed upon a sound knowledge of physical assessment and the presenting physiological signs, before such devices and techniques are used. Subsequent chapters will build upon the principles presented in this section.

5

Clinical observation and monitoring devices

Richard Hatchett

This chapter explores the variety and range of monitoring devices available for assessing the cardiac patient's clinical status. These include the non-invasive methods such as accurately recording the blood pressure and the more invasive devices such as the central venous and pulmonary artery catheters. In more recent years, there has been concern about the overzealous use of these more invasive monitoring devices (Paladichuk 1998, Taylor et al 1997). Arguments have centred around the cost and risk of infection, with line insertion only being justified if the data gained are used to improve, rather than merely confirm, the patient's condition. Research continues on the actual patient outcomes achieved when using these more complex devices.

The management of hypertension is also addressed within this chapter. The emphasis is placed on the non-pharmacological methods for lowering a chronically elevated blood pressure. The estimation of the coronary heart disease (CHD) risk together with recording blood pressures is now considered a vital part of the overall management of hypertension. The various societies' guidelines currently available are invaluable in both offering evidence-based practice and enabling the standardization of service delivery.

In considering monitoring devices, several important factors need to be highlighted at this early point. It is important to remember that there is a patient at the end of our monitoring devices. The equipment may make us appear clinically impressive but can be very frightening to the patient. An explanation and reassurance to both patient and family or carers, particularly if more equipment is added or alarms are sounding, are always needed. The normal range for many of the measured parameters within this chapter is wide, notably the central venous pressure (CVP) and data gained from the pulmonary artery (PA) catheter. This emphasizes the need to take measurements at regular intervals and observe the trend patterns. Single measurements are useful but will only demonstrate readings that are outside the normal range. Regular recordings will demonstrate a movement towards the higher or lower limit even before that point is reached. Interventions can then be applied before grossly abnormal readings are encountered.

It is also important not to consider readings in isolation but to consider the patient's presenting clinical condition and what his/her normal cardiac status might be. Many of our patients live with cardiac disease and to expect, for example, their usual CVP to be anything other than slightly elevated might be wishful thinking. Working clinically with experienced staff is where such skills are gained and this chapter will guide you in that direction. Finally, as highlighted above, you need to ask why you are gaining the data. This prevents you from blindly recording observations without using them and encourages a good team discussion with nursing and medical colleagues. The rationale for observations may be a concern that the patient's condition has shown signs of deterioration or that there is a likelihood this may occur. You may also be using the monitoring devices to manipulate the haemodynamics and improve tissue perfusion, as described in Chapter 18.

NON-INVASIVE MONITORING

It is always important to emphasize the value of the non-invasive monitoring devices. Frequently there is little need for a PA catheter to confirm that a patient's cardiac condition is deteriorating. Community colleagues have been achieving this for years. An early sign may include the cardiac patient who is becoming increasingly breathless at rest, indicating the inability to effectively pump blood forward from the lungs, resulting in pulmonary oedema. He or she may be gaining weight each day through fluid retention. The colour and temperature of the skin is another highly useful guide to a rapidly worsening cardiac condition. As the cardiac system fails, neurogenic stimulation and catecholamine release causes peripheral vessels to constrict to maintain the blood pressure and tissue perfusion. As a consequence the skin becomes pale and clammy, often before a notable drop in blood pressure.

Following cardiac surgery nursing staff frequently measure the core-to-toe temperature. A temperature probe is placed usually in the axilla and another in the centre of the foot. As the patient warms following surgery the central temperature and then the peripheral temperature rise. If the two measurements begin to drift apart, this is a sign that the skin is cooling and, in the presence of an unchanging environmental temperature, could indicate a drop in cardiac output as the peripheral vessels constrict (Hill & Summers 1994).

Weighing the patient daily, usually before breakfast and in the same or similar clothing, offers a valuable assessment of deterioration or amelioration of the cardiac condition. Retention of fluid is a problem for all patients with long-term cardiac failure and this can lead to extra work for the heart and exacerbation of the condition. As described in Chapter 4, when the heart fails aldosterone actively encourages the retention of sodium and water to maintain the blood pressure and stretch the myocardium. This should subsequently increase the cardiac output. In addition, poorly perfused and functioning kidneys, together with failing myocardial contractility, will lead to the patient gaining in weight due to an increased fluid load.

The fluid balance chart, which records over a 24-hour period oral and intravenous intake minus urinary and gastrointestinal output, is useful as an additional way of assessing the degree of fluid retention. In severe cases of heart failure a restriction on fluid input may be prescribed and this can be achieved through using the chart. However, the charts are problematic in any patient other than those restricted to intravenous fluids and with a urinary catheter and measuring urometer. Patients tend to miscalculate exactly how much they have had to drink and if a bed pan is not used it is impossible to accurately measure how much urine was passed. Daily weights offer a more accurate assessment of fluid retention.

However, fluid balance charts should never be discarded, as they provide detailed information that a general weight cannot. For example, if the patient is losing weight daily but their fluid input has markedly reduced or they are vomiting, then pharmacological treatment alone cannot be wholly responsible for the weight reduction. The urinary response to diuretic therapy can also be assessed, particularly if the time and dose of the drug are recorded on the fluid balance chart.

In addition to the fluid balance, the measured urinary output remains one of the most important monitored signs in acute cardiac nursing. Every adult patient should pass a minimum of 0.5 ml of urine per kg of body weight per hour (1 ml/kg/hour in children). This means that a 90 kg man or woman should pass at least 45 ml of urine per hour. Frequently 30 ml an hour is quoted but this is rather imprecise for the variety of differing patient weights encountered.

Urinary output is much more than an assessment of renal function. As the cardiac system fails, organ oxygen perfusion is prioritized and blood is actively shunted to the areas considered to be in most need, the vital or life-sustaining organs of heart, brain and lungs. The kidneys, and now we also know the gut (Ball 1994), have blood actively shunted away through the compensatory mechanisms maintaining tissue perfusion.

As blood to the kidneys is reduced, the glomerular filtration rate slows and urine production drops. If the patient is passing at least 0.5 ml/kg/hour without an artificially enforced diuresis, then the vital organs must be adequately if not optimally served with oxygen, as they receive the priority blood supply first. When there is no urinary output due to a compromised cardiac system, there is no way of knowing how near or far the vital organs are from an adequate blood supply for their functioning needs. This is the reason, regardless of blood pressure, that the doctor will frequently ask what the urinary output is for the patient in acute cardiac failure.

Cardiac nurses are increasingly moving into the domain of auscultating the heart and breath sounds, particularly with the emergence of study courses in physical assessment. Chapter 4 describes the various heart sounds and recognizing them is a skill that requires listening to both the normal and abnormal and then undergoing a period of clinical supervision. For practising this skill, a variety of tapes are now available and placing the stethoscope over the loud-speaker can assist in mimicking the sounds heard. Breath sounds are highly useful, particularly in the intensive care environment, for assessing patients following cardiac surgery for signs of consolidation, the correct placement of the endotracheal tube and general restriction and wheezing of the airways. Cox & McGrath (1999) provide a useful guide for assessing breath sounds and augment this with a need to observe the rate, rhythm and quality of breathing as well as the configuration of the thorax, before even using the stethoscope. The use of palpation, using the hands to sense the sounds and feel of the chest, is a part of the overall assessment.

BLOOD PRESSURE

In cardiac nursing the blood pressure (BP) appears in two management guises. In the acute units there is frequently the need for regular recordings, often with the use of an indwelling arterial line, due to haemodynamic instability. Community colleagues and staff within clinics frequently monitor the BP to aid the management of essential hypertension, a clear risk factor for coronary heart disease. Essential hypertension is the term used where there is no identifiable cause, for example renal failure, for the chronically elevated blood pressure and is the most common form of the disease. BP is frequently measured and moni-

tored with non-invasive devices and raises the issue of accuracy in both clinical and patient-initiated recordings.

The incidence of coronary events, such as myocardial infarction together with conditions such as stroke and retinal changes, clearly increases with raised BP (Gueyffier et al 1997). Hypertension has been termed 'the silent killer' and the need to take steps to correct this condition cannot be overemphasized. National and international surveys continue to reveal underdiagnosis of hypertension (Ramsay et al 1999), with only approximately 25% of UK patients with high blood pressure having their condition adequately controlled (MacGregror & Kaplan 1998, p. 62). A variety of factors contribute to this poor figure, including a lack of routine monitoring, poor patient compliance and a reduced understanding of the risks associated with hypertension.

In addition to the variety of complications highlighted above, others such as left ventricular hypertrophy are not uncommon, with between 10% and 40% of patients with mild hypertension developing this condition (Vann Jones et al 1998). Such ventricular enlargement is a chronic response to an increasing afterload imposed on the heart by a gradually increasing arterial pressure and peripheral resistance. It does, however, more commonly occur with BP in excess of 160/95 mmHg (Vann Jones et al 1998).

Microvascular aneurysms, renal failure and the acceleration of atherosclerosis are further recognized complications of hypertension. The exact mechanism of the latter is unclear but may involve the higher pressure leading to abnormalities in endothelial function. Changes in arterial compliance and turbulent blood flow appear to facilitate lipid transport into atheromatous lesions. With BP reduction, this progression is reduced (MacGregor & Kaplan 1998, p. 14). Prior to the introduction of antihypertensive drugs, patients with a diastolic pressure between 130 and 150 mmHg had only a 40% 2-year survival. Death usually occurred with stroke, myocardial infarction, heart or renal failure (O'Brien et al 1995, p. 37).

The factors creating and influencing the blood pressure are described in Section 2 of this book. Blood pressure is the force per unit area exerted on the walls of a blood vessel by its contained blood (Marieb 1998, p. 699). It is influenced by blood flow, which is the volume of blood flowing through a vessel, and the peripheral resistance. The blood pressure is always measured in millimetres of mercury (mmHg), traditionally by the use of a sphygmomanometer and inflatable cuff. However, due to the toxic nature of mercury, this substance is slowly being removed in blood pressure and other devices such as thermometers throughout the world. Devices are available which do not use mercury to measure the blood pressure but there is a need to assess what testing has occurred to ensure their accuracy.

Direct (invasive) measurement of the blood pressure

Direct techniques utilize an indwelling arterial line, which is transduced to a monitor. This provides a pressure waveform and continually records numerical values of the BP. The arterial lines designed for this direct technique are usually inserted into the radial artery and are used in critically ill patients where there is a need for continual BP monitoring. This may occur after cardiac surgery or where acute cardiac failure has occurred, with the BP maintained at a persistently low level.

The primary indications for an indwelling arterial line are therefore:

- to provide continual monitoring in a labile or persistently low/elevated reading, which is compromising haemodynamic stability
- to allow a persistently low BP to be monitored, where the traditional auscultation technique may not detect the pressure
- to monitor the immediate effects of treatments, such as inotropic therapy
- to gain regular arterial blood gas samples for oxygen, carbon dioxide and acid–base analysis.

Figure 5.1 illustrates the insertion technique and monitoring system used with an arterial line. The radial artery is frequently used but the brachial, dorsalis pedis and femoral arteries are other, rare, sites of cannulation. An experienced physician, anaesthetist, technician or occasionally nurse will insert the line and attach it to a water manometer set, which in turn is attached to a fluid-filled pressure bag. This usually contains heparin to prevent the arterial line attracting clot formation and providing inaccurate recordings. It is important to highlight that adequate skin cleaning is vital to prevent the risk of intravascular device-related septicaemia. The choice of cleaning agent has traditionally been divided between chlorhexidine, iodine or alcohol-based solutions. Maki et al's work (1991) supported the view that chlorhexidine-based solutions are probably the best for cutaneous disinfection in terms of reduced incidence of catheter-related infections, with devices such as arterial and central lines.

Arteries contain blood at high pressure and to attach the line to a normal intravenous giving set would result in blood tracking quickly back up to the infusion bag. The pressure bag and transducer prevent this occurring and allow a slow trickle of fluid, usually 3 ml per hour if the pressure bag is inflated to 300 mmHg, to keep the arterial line clear. In insertion, a small cannula, perhaps of 20 g or 22 g size, is used.

The issue of whether the flush bag should contain heparin has raised interest since the mid-1980s, when the routine heparin flushing of peripheral lines was found to be essentially unnecessary (Jowett et al 1985, Taylor et al 1989). With regard to arterial lines, provided that a high pressure of approximately 300 mmHg is maintained on the flush bag, it appears that line patency can be maintained for up to 7 days with saline alone (Gamby & Bennett 1995). However, differing research and discussion are likely to produce varying protocols within cardiac units. When a single flush device is used on two lines such as arterial and CVP and one is switched off, perhaps being flushed with saline only occasionally, clots will form around this cannula tip. Evidence regarding the choice of flush frequency or solution has at present proved difficult to gain due to differing variables used within contrasting research papers (Clifton et al 1991, Hook et al 1985, Leighton 1994).

Before arterial cannula placement, the Allen's test was previously recommended but is now considered inappropriate. In this test the two arteries, the ulnar and radial, would be compressed in the wrist and the patient would make a repeated tight fist to squeeze blood from the hand. Once the hand was pale, the ulnar artery was released and a flush of colour should have occurred within 5–10 seconds. This would indicate that the ulnar artery would provide an adequate blood supply when the radial artery was cannulated (Darovic & Franklin 1999). However, ischaemia does not seem to correlate to a positive test or, indeed, negative results exclude ischaemic complications (Hinds & Watson 1996).

Arterial lines remain useful, therefore, for continuous BP monitoring. Changes can be noted quickly whereas a non-invasive method, even with an automatic inflating cuff attached to a monitor, cannot record the BP frequently enough. Arterial lines will also sense the BP at low levels, where with auscultation the nurse's ears cannot. Such lines are also useful in obtaining arterial blood samples for blood gas analysis, without the need for repeatedly inserting a needle into an artery (arterial stab).

The characteristic arterial trace is seen in Figure 5.2. The undulating pattern of the arterial trace

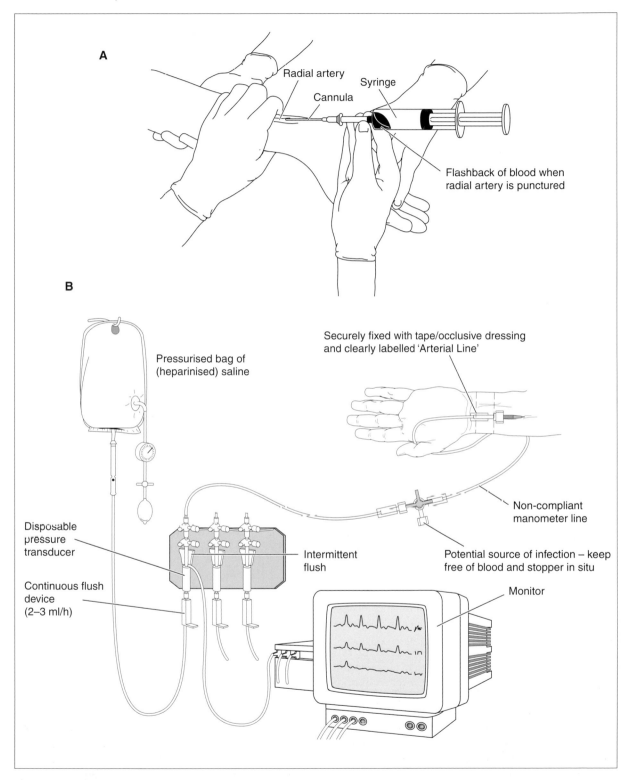

Figure 5.1 Insertion technique (A) and monitoring system (B) for an indwelling arterial cannula.

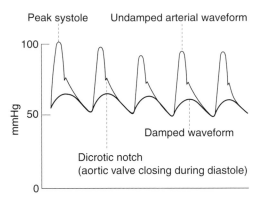

Peak systole   Undamped arterial waveform

Damped waveform

Dicrotic notch
(aortic valve closing during diastole)

Figure 5.2 A normal and damped arterial pressure trace.

demonstrates systole, diastole and a slight hump on the downward stroke. This is the dicrotic notch indicating the aortic valve closing. As with all monitored pressures, it is important to ensure the monitor is recording a baseline of zero when the port on the transducer is open to air and is at the level of the right atrium (re zeroing). This ensures that the waveform recorded above this zero mark is an accurate reflection of arterial pressure. All monitors for recording haemodynamic waveforms have the facility to zero pressure to atmospheric air (see Central Venous Pressure Monitoring below).

The monitor senses the pressure from the arterial line through a fluid-filled manometer line. The actual interface of fluid lines and electrical cable is at the transducer. Occasionally a bubble of air can become trapped in the small transducer plate, perhaps during the priming of the line from the pressurized flush bag. This will result in a damped trace and an inaccurate arterial line pressure reading (Fig. 5.2). The experienced nurse or technician can remove the bubble with a syringe or by disconnecting to allow the air to exit. If the arterial line becomes pushed against the arterial wall or, with time, blood is clotting around the cannula tip, the same effect may be seen. It is vital that nursing and medical staff recognize a damped trace to ensure treatment decisions are based on accurate recordings.

Invasive arterial monitoring, when correctly calibrated, is regarded as more accurate than auscultation. The indirect and direct methods can present a discrepancy in measurement which can vary from 12 mmHg (difference between mean of direct and indirect measurements; Asiain et al 1990) to 25 mmHg (Pickering 1991). It is important when taking care of a patient to record a non-invasive blood pressure and compare this to the arterial line trace.

The arterial line is another source of infection and hands should be washed and gloves worn to protect yourself and the patient. Gloves must be changed between patients. The line must be labelled clearly, usually written in red on tape attached near to the line's entry. Primarily, this prevents drugs being administered into this line and acute ischaemia of the limb occurring. The arm and occasionally femoral area where the line is inserted should be kept exposed, so that disconnection and the potential large loss of blood are noted immediately. Signs of ischaemia in the limb from arterial line placement, notably digital ischaemia of fingers, are rare but the nurse needs to observe for this so that the decision to remove the cannula can be made. Note also if the insertion site becomes inflamed or exudes any discharge, indicating possible infection. This again is an indication for removal.

The need for accuracy in indirect (non-invasive) BP recordings

The use of the mercury sphygmomanometer is slowly disappearing throughout the world, due to the known hazards of this substance. However it is valuable to reflect that what had become an apparently simple task is rarely performed with the necessary care although its results clearly affect treatment planning. Sphygmomanometry itself has undergone no substantial technological improvement in nearly 100 years. Literature demonstrates that there often appears to be little reference to extraneous variables which will affect the reading or, indeed, practitioners updating or reviewing their technique (Feher et al 1992, Kennedy & Curzio 1996, Torrance & Serginson 1996). Torrance & Serginson (1996), in observing 54 student nurses nearing the end of their common foundation programme (18 months into the course) measuring the BP with a sphygmomanometer, discovered a variety of factors which could alter the readings. In 44% of the observations the arm was above or below the heart level, only 5% of the students obtained an estimate of the systolic pressure through palpation and none inquired about extraneous variables such as recent coffee consumption or smoking.

The British Hypertension Society and the Nurses Hypertension Association guidelines require the correct size cuff to be wrapped around the arm (Box 5.1). This is inflated until the mercury column in the sphygmomanometer rises to 30 mmHg above the estimated systolic pressure (Box 5.2). This will have been estimated by palpating the brachial or radial artery pulsation and inflating the cuff until the pulsation disappears. Such a measure prevents unnecessary inflation of the cuff to a high level.

When taking the BP reading, a stethoscope is placed over the pulsating area of the brachial artery and is used to auscultate the characteristic sounds. Once the cuff is inflated the valve is used to carefully release the air, so that the column of mercury slowly lowers at a rate of 2–3 mmHg per second. This occurs until a repetitive clear, tapping sound is heard for two consecutive beats; this is the systolic or upper pressure. The diastolic pressure is noted when the repetitive sounds disappear (phase 5). If the tapping does not disappear on auscultation, diastolic pressure is estimated when the sound muffles (phase 4) (O'Brien & Davison 1994). However, the muffling of sounds should not be taken as the diastolic pressure, unless sound continues to a very low level (MacGregor & Kaplan 1998). The sounds heard are referred to as the Korotkoff sound technique, after the Russian surgeon who modified sphygmomanometry in 1905.

The issue of using the correct cuff size is highlighted as an important source of error in a large number of papers (Croft & Cruickshank 1990, Maxwell 1982). The bladder (the inflatable section inside the material cuff) must be at least 80% of the arm circumference. If the person has a large arm and too short a bladder is used, the BP will be overestimated (O'Brien et al 1995). Similarly, if the arm is raised above heart level when reading the blood pressure, the reading will be underestimated and if below the heart, there will be overestimation. Box 5.1 provides the correct size of cuff for various arm circumferences.

Changing practice habits or behaviour, particularly if they are not perceived as being at fault, is difficult. The Treating Hypertension in North Yorkshire through Clinical Effectiveness (THINYCE) project implemented, on a large scale, a three-stage approach to improve hypertension management in local GP practices (Maskrey 1999). Local educational events demonstrated the correct technique for BP recording and again illustrated how poor those in the practices were at measuring blood pressures accurately. As a second stage, independent checks of the maintenance and condition of sphygmomanometers were offered, again showing the poor functioning of much of the equipment. 109 machines were checked, with only one practice emerging with most of their sphygmomanometers in good working condition. It is a frequent finding that sphygmomanometers are simply not serviced. The final stage of the project involved an audit programme, with nine practices who cared for a total population of 73 000 people. Findings illustrated that over 90% of patients identified as hypertensive had been reviewed in the preceding 12 months. The project steering group set the audit standard for BP control at 160/96 mmHg or less and this was achieved in 60% of patients (Maskrey 1999).

Box 5.2 highlights the recommended procedure for recording the BP with a sphygmomanometer and stethoscope, as well as the factors influencing the accuracy of the reading. Many of these are of value whether a sphygmomanometer is used or the newer alternative devices, which remove the use of mercury.

Figure 5.3 illustrates the correct method for recording the blood pressure with a sphygmomanometer and auscultation technique.

'White coat' hypertension is the term used for BP readings which tend to be higher when taken in a clinical setting, usually by a doctor. The occurrence has been noted for some time, with the claim that 20% of patients diagnosed with mild hypertension may have the increase confined purely to the doctor's surgery (Pickering 1968, 1994). Interestingly, there is evidence that nurses do tend to record lower BP readings in the same patient when compared to medical colleagues (Pickering 1994). Those who are correctly diagnosed with this condition may not require antihypertensive drugs and, indeed, have a good prognosis in terms of complications of hypertension (Verdecchia et al 1994). It is important not to dismissively label 'white coat'

Box 5.1 Correct cuff sizes (after the British Hypertension Society (BHS) and the Nurses Hypertension Association 1997)			
	Cuff width (cm)	*Cuff length (cm)*	*Arm circumference (cm)*
Normal	12.0–13.0	23	Up to 33
Alternative adult	12.5–13.0	35	Up to 42
Children	7.5–9.0	22.5–23.5	Up to 26
Infants	4.0–6.0	11.5–18.0	Up to 17
Larger bladders for arms >42 cm circumference may be required.			

Box 5.2 Blood pressure measurement: techniques based on the British Hypertension Society and the Nurses Hypertension Association (1997), Ramsay et al (1999) and Feather (2001)

- Explain the procedure to the patient.
- Position patient lying, standing or sitting with arm supported (on a pillow).
- Ensure patient rests calmly for at least 3 minutes before taking reading (1 minute if standing).
- Apply appropriately sized cuff; if arm circumference exceeds 33 cm, a large cuff must be used.
- Place centre of the bladder over the brachial artery.
- Do not inflate over clothing.
- Ensure lower edge of the bladder is above antecubital fossa.
- Ensure tubing leaves from the top of the cuff, to avoid interfering with auscultation.
- Position the sphygmomanometer at eye level, to accurately read meniscus.
- The patient's arm must be at their heart level, not above or below.
- Estimate systolic blood pressure by palpating the brachial or radial artery and inflating cuff until pulsation stops, noting measurement on sphygmomanometer.
- When listening with stethoscope allow column of mercury to drop at 2–3 mm/s. Measure systolic (first sound) and diastolic (sound disappearing) to nearest 2 mmHg.
- With no disappearance of sound, diastolic pressure is the muffling of sound.

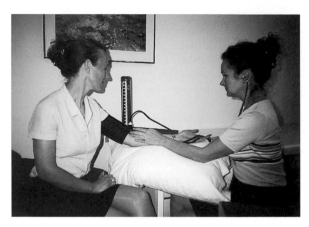

Figure 5.3 Recording the blood pressure with a sphygmomanometer and stethoscope (auscultation). Note that both the patient and practice nurse are seated comfortably, the correct size cuff is positioned above the antecubital fossa and the arm is well supported. (The sphygmomanometer is at eye level and the level of the heart.) The principles can be applied to non-mercury and digital devices.

hypertensive patients as normal, as there is some evidence that this phenomenon is an early manifestation of haemodynamic disturbance that may manifest later as sustained hypertension (O'Brien et al 1995, p. 32).

Such an occurrence has led to the increasing use of ambulatory blood pressure monitoring devices (ABPM), where the blood pressure is recorded intermittently, usually every 30 minutes, outside the clinical setting. The use of the device has offered the opportunity for recordings to more directly correlate to the individual's everyday living. The machine normally performs this task automatically, with the cuff worn continually for a period of time, often 24 hours. Its use is generally confined to the above patients and predominantly to those with borderline hypertension; this has been defined as a surgery or clinic pressure of 140/90–160/100 mmHg by Prasad & Isles (1996). In addition, patients who complain of hypotensive symptoms, such as dizziness, while receiving drug treatment may benefit from this monitoring device. This would follow an assessment of the standing

blood pressure in the clinic, to assess for postural hypertension.

The advantages of the ambulatory device are that it provides a whole series of readings during everyday life and avoids observer error and bias. It does have disadvantages in that the equipment is expensive and the patient must understand why the device is being used and how it will affect their everyday life. They will need to stop and hold the arm still as the cuff inflates and records. It can interfere with sleep as it automatically inflates. It should be taken off for bathing but must be replaced. Heavy manual work should be avoided due to its delicate workings (Prasad & Isles 1996). In addition, the individual should be able to keep a diary of events so that interpretation has a relevance to everyday living.

Initially, it is advisable to record the BP in the other arm to assess the accuracy of the device. If there is a discrepancy of over 10 mmHg, then the device is swapped to the other arm to assess if the difference is due to the recorder or the arm. The importance of an appropriately sized cuff must again be emphasized to ensure as accurate a recording as possible is made each time. Many ambulatory devices are available but those validated by the British Hypertension Society (BHS) are know to be accurate in their recordings (Prasad & Isles 1996).

Nursing staff play a vital role in assessing whether the patient will be able to cope with the device as it regularly inflates or whether they will be compelled to remove it. Increasingly in nurse-led clinics, nurses themselves will be involved in deciding whether the device is a viable option in the management of the patient's hypertension. Importantly, there is also the issue of how much teaching time can and will need to be allotted to explain and review the device with the patient. Normal ranges for ambulatory readings based on age and sex are available to chart a person's position within blood pressure centiles (O'Brien et al 1995, p. 30).

As highlighted, it is important to note that many countries are banning the use of mercury devices in health care due to concerns regarding its toxic properties, the potential risk of spillages and the risk involved in servicing mercury devices. The problem is finding a suitable and accurate alternative (O'Brien 2000). There are a large number of machines of the automatic variety and ambulatory devices for recording the BP over a period of time currently available. The former provides a cuff and a digital reading of the blood pressure, dispensing with the need for auscultation via a stethoscope. The issue with all these devices is their reliability and accuracy in recordings and concerns have been raised in the past (O'Brien et al 1990). However, the BHS and the Association for the Advancement of Medical Instrumentation offer an information service which includes those devices considered to be accurate to their high standards. The BHS is currently based in the Blood Pressure Unit of St George's Hospital Medical School in South London.

Management issues in hypertension

Defining high blood pressure is problematic, not least because in the given population the spread of diastolic pressures assumes a bell shape, creating a blurring of normotensive and hypertensive patients (O'Brien et al 1995, p. 37). The perceived risk to the patient of the presenting findings, together with subsequent treatment, will be influenced by a variety of factors. These will include the patient's age and risk factors such as smoking and family medical history. This has led to a rather pragmatic definition, whereby hypertension is the level above which treatment trials have shown that lowering the blood pressure is beneficial (MacGregor & Kaplan 1998, p. 10). There has been debate regarding which is the more important in hypertension management, the systolic or diastolic pressure. In fact, both are important risk factors for cardiovascular disease and

should be considered in planning management. However, current practice, at the time of going to press, indicates that the systolic blood pressure should be regarded as the more important (Ramsay et al 1999).

Figure 5.4 illustrates the current joint British recommendations regarding the management of blood pressure. There are different guidelines available but these have been created by four societies, including the BHS and the Cardiac Society, consulting together and producing a pragmatic approach. The emphasis is placed on health promotion and lifestyle changes for all patients, together with the initial need to estimate the overall coronary heart disease risk for the individual. The coronary heart disease risk is defined as the likelihood of non-fatal myocardial infarction and coronary death. It is estimated in individuals who have not developed symptomatic CHD or other major atherosclerotic disease. The 10-year risk of developing CHD is estimated by choosing a graph relating to whether the individual is male or female, a smoker or non-smoker and whether they are diabetic. Within the graph the risk is estimated according to the systolic blood pressure (vertical axis) and the ratio of total cholesterol to high density lipoprotein (HDL) cholesterol (horizontal axis). The latter is a protective factor in CHD. The point on the graph will relate to one of three CHD risk levels: <15% over the next 10 years, 15–30% and >30% over the same time period. The estimated risk will influence the treatment thresholds in hypertension (Wood et al 1998) (see Fig. 5.4).

Non-pharmacological measures

Box 5.3 highlights the many factors that have been shown to influence the management of hypertension. It is difficult to prioritize order but in considering non-pharmacological measures to control the blood pressure, a factor such as a low potassium intake is of less importance than discussing with the patient the issues of controlling obesity, salt intake and inactivity.

All patients with hypertension or with a strong family history of the condition should be offered non-pharmacological advice and support. Weight loss is correlated with a reduction in BP and appears the most effective of all non-pharmacological measures used to treat hypertension (Carretero & Oparil 2000). Weight reduction of as little as 10 lb reduces the blood pressure in a large proportion of overweight hypertensive patients. In addition, there is a beneficial effect on associated CHD risk factors such as diabetes, hyperlipidaemia and left ventricular hypertrophy (Carretero & Oparil 2000). Support and encouragement to lose

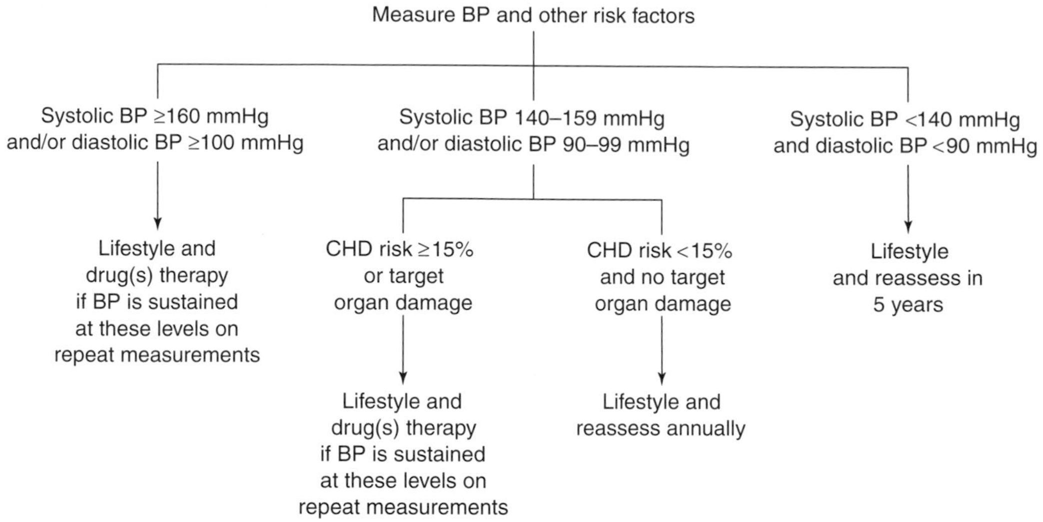

Measure BP and other risk factors

Systolic BP ≥160 mmHg
and/or diastolic BP ≥100 mmHg

Systolic BP 140–159 mmHg
and/or diastolic BP 90–99 mmHg

Systolic BP <140 mmHg
and diastolic BP <90 mmHg

Lifestyle and
drug(s) therapy
if BP is sustained
at these levels on
repeat measurements

CHD risk ≥15%
or target
organ damage

CHD risk <15%
and no target
organ damage

Lifestyle
and reassess in
5 years

Lifestyle and
drug(s) therapy
if BP is sustained
at these levels on
repeat measurements

Lifestyle and
reassess annually

Figure 5.4 Joint British recommendations on the prevention of coronary heart disease in clinical practice: management of blood pressure (from Wood et al 1998; reproduced with kind permission of Professor PN Durrington).

Box 5.3 Factors which can precipitate essential hypertension

- Obesity
- Inactivity
- High salt intake
- Family history of hypertension
- Diabetes
- High alcohol intake
- Low potassium intake

---

weight and maintain this through the variety of support groups and methods available should be undertaken.

Increased physical activity, and not necessarily of a strenuous variety, is known to reduce blood pressure in both normotensive and hypertensive individuals (Carretero & Oparil 2000). Moderate activity may lower the systolic blood pressure by 4–8 mmHg (Puddey & Cox 1995). At least 30 minutes of moderately intense physical activity, such as brisk walking, swimming or bicycling, is recommended at least three times per week and preferably once a day (Carretero & Oparil 2000).

Reducing salt intake for all cardiac patients is recommended because in Britain general consumption within the population remains high. Salt intake is recognized as one of the most important determinants of

BP differences both between and within populations (Elliot et al 1996). If a reduction in intake from the current UK level of 10 g per day to 5 g is undertaken, there is a decrease of 1.0–1.5 litres in extracellular volume, with a corresponding weight loss of 1.0–1.5 kg (Antonios & MacGregor 1996). This relatively moderate move can be as effective in managing hypertension as single drug treatment (MaGregor & Kaplan 1998, p. 40). Certainly controlled trials in reducing salt intake to 3, 6 and 12 g/day demonstrated raised and lowered BP measurements within the separate groups (MacGregor et al 1989).

The advent of the fridge has reduced the need for heavily salted, preserved foods but 70–80% of a patient's salt intake may still come from processed food (MacGregor & Kaplan 1998, p. 42). Processed meats, ready-made meals, soups and many instant foods are particularly noted for their higher salt content (MacGregor & Kaplan 1998, p. 43), which is used as a cheap method to make relatively unpalatable foods, such as meat products, more edible. Furthermore, the higher the salt content, the more water can be added, increasing weight at little cost. The investment connection between soft drink companies and snack foods with a high salt intake is significant, because salt and thirst are of course linked.

Labelling of food for salt content is confusing. Salt may appear as 'sodium', which will contain other chemicals such as sodium bicarbonate and not sodium chloride alone. Generally a sodium content of less than 0.2 g/100 g is advocated. If you examine the tinned and processed foods in your own cupboard for the salt content against this recommended figure, this will demonstrate the high level of salt added during food processing.

In practical terms this indicates that advising patients not to add salt at table and to cooking is strongly recommended, due to its clear beneficial effect. However, it can have a limited impact if discussion regarding the high salt content in processed foods is not undertaken. Initially, when undertaking a lower salt diet, food will taste bland but taste receptors do adjust, making the former higher salt intake inedible after 3 or 4 weeks (MacGregor & Kaplan 1998).

The link between a high alcohol intake and elevated blood pressure has been consistent (Carretero & Oparil 2000). The effects do increase with age and do not appear to be linked to particular beverages. Studies demonstrate that BP falls 4–5 mmHg in days to weeks with abstinence from alcohol (Beilin et al 1996). However, it is known that moderate alcohol consumption does reduce overall CHD risk in the general population (McConnell et al 1997). Intake should be reduced to moderate levels. This is 1 oz alcohol per day for most men and half that in women and small men (Carretero & Oparil 2000). This equates to 3–4 units of alcohol per day for men and 2–3 units per day for women. The patient will need to be provided with information regarding the amount of alcohol within each type of drink, because blind figures will mean nothing if effective management is to be attempted.

The link between potassium levels and blood pressure has been known for some time (Geleijnse et al 1994, Knaw & Thom 1982). Raising potassium levels does lower blood pressure but advice is restricted to encouraging a healthy diet with an increased consumption of fruit and vegetables, rather than administering potassium supplements (Carretero & Oparil 2000).

Drug treatment

This chapter focuses primarily on monitoring devices, while Chapter 19 specifically addresses antihypertensive drug management. The important issues are, however, outlined in this section. In terms of thresholds for treatment, the third working party for the British Hypertension Society reported in 1999 and the reader is referred to this more detailed document and discussion (Ramsay et al 1999). However, Figure 5.4 provides perhaps a simpler and more pragmatic approach to the threshold for treatment interventions. The emphasis in management is still placed initially on lifestyle changes and on estimating the CHD risk to the patient.

Monotherapy for hypertension usually commences with a low-dose thiazide diuretic, unless there are contra-indications (Ramsay et al 1999). However, the majority of hypertensive people will require combined therapy to achieve optimal BP control. At least one-third will require three or more drugs (Ramsay et al 1999). In management the first drug may be substituted for an alternative drug if the hypertension is mild and uncomplicated but the response to the drug is small.

The major classes of drugs tend to have additive effects on BP. This can produce a better BP response with fewer of the side-effects linked to the individual drugs. Combination therapies will include a diuretic and β-blocker, diuretic with angiotensin-converting enzyme (ACE) inhibitor, β-blocker with calcium antagonist and a calcium antagonist with ACE inhibitor. There is no longer a clear guide or set prescribing sequence across all hypertensive patients. There are indications for using specific drugs in specific patient groups but also compelling contra-indications. The choice of drug will depend on the relative indications and contra-indications in the individual patient (Ramsay et al 1999). The BHS guidelines should be checked before adjusting or prescribing is undertaken. This will include management advice for drug therapy in varying groups such as the elderly, those with renal disease and ethnic groups. The latter is of interest, with evidence that black subjects are more responsive to diuretic and calcium antagonists (Materson et al 1994), while limited data in British South Asians appear to show a drug response in hypertension similar to white Europeans.

Multidisciplinary planning

As has been highlighted, essential hypertension is a chronic condition and requires regular but accurate monitoring. The use of the sphygmomanometer technique appears misleadingly simple but is rarely performed competently. A high standard of care with all blood pressure devices is required to obtain accurate and reproducible readings, because significant treatment decisions are based on the results (Mann 1999).

The issue of hypertension lends itself to multidisciplinary planning for effective management and encourages the utilization of nursing in the form of appropriately trained practice nurses in the community and nurse-led clinics in the hospital setting. Once

---

Box 5.4. The primary care issues in hypertension

- Hypertensive patients may feel asymptomatic and can experience difficulties in understanding why treatment is necessary. Careful discussion and accurate recordings on more than one occasion should therefore be normal practice before initiating treatment, unless the reading is grossly abnormal.
- Inaccuracies in recording the blood pressure have been well documented. Equipment needs to be regularly serviced and calibrated, with continued staff education to standardize best practice within clinics and units.
- In considering the use of automatic blood pressure recording devices, it is prudent to utilize those that have been validated by the British Hypertension Society as accurate and reliable.
- When ambulatory or home blood pressure devices are used, the patient needs to demonstrate clear understanding of the rationale for this method of recording and show clearly that they can use the device. It is advisable for the individual to maintain a diary of events to correlate activity with measurements.
- Non-pharmacological measures clearly have a place in the management of hypertension. The risk factors outlined in Box 5.3 should be considered and non-pharmacological advice offered to all hypertensive patients. Giving advice regarding risk factors to non-hypertensive patients is always prudent practice.
- The management of hypertension has been augmented by the release of evidence-based practice guidelines. These should always be utilized as the basis of good practice to maintain standards and uniformity of practice within units and clinics.
- Estimating the coronary heart disease (CHD) risk factor is a useful approach in assisting with lifestyle changes. It is now also used in considering the threshold for antihypertensive treatment.

Box 5.5 Mean arterial pressure calculation

$$MAP = diastolic + \frac{(systolic - diastolic)}{3}$$

If the blood pressure were 130/50 mmHg:

$$MAP = 50 + \frac{(130 - 50)}{3}$$
$$= 50 + \frac{80}{3}$$
$$= 50 + 27$$
$$MAP = 77 \text{ mmHg}$$

---

professional barriers to management are reduced, nurses can offer the opportunity of greater patient contact time to monitor the blood pressure, explore non-pharmacological measures with the patient and, within agreed protocols, adjust treatment to optimize hypertension control. Multidisciplinary discussion within the practice and adherence to national or local guidelines can again increase the efficacy of the service offered to hypertensive patients.

THE MEAN ARTERIAL PRESSURE

The mean arterial pressure (MAP) is increasingly used in addition to the blood pressure within acute cardiac units. The MAP offers the average pressure through the whole cardiac cycle and takes account of both variations in the diastolic and systolic pressures and the amount of time each takes within the cardiac cycle. There are several ways to calculate the MAP, although it frequently appears as the whole number in brackets below the systolic and diastolic readings on the monitor. It can be calculated, especially if the blood pressure is recorded without a manometer line and monitor, as shown in Box 5.5.

The normal range is approximately 60–80 mmHg. The calculation cannot be gained by adding the systolic and diastolic pressures together and dividing by two, because diastole is longer in the cardiac cycle than systole.

PULSE OXIMETRY

Pulse oximetry has been one of the greatest advances in monitoring in recent years. The device, which consists of a finger, toe or ear probe, connects to a portable unit or to the cardiac monitor (Fig. 5.5). Pulse oximetry measures the oxygen saturation of haemoglobin at the arterial tissue level; the normal range is 94–98% (Hill & Summers 1994, p. 117). The great advantage of the device is that it is both non-invasive and easy to apply. The pulse rate and a plethysmographic waveform of the pulse are also displayed.

The system functions by alternately emitting two light beams, via a light-emitting diode (LED), at red and infrared frequencies on one side of the finger or ear. The beam frequencies are 660 nm and 940 nm respectively, while on the other side of the diode is a sensitive photodetector (Al-Shaikh & Stacey 1995, p. 90). The two light sources are absorbed to different degrees by oxyhaemoglobin (oxygen-saturated haemoglobin) and deoxyhaemoglobin. The intensity of the light reaching the photodetector is converted into an electrical signal. Absorption due to static structures such as tissues and venous blood is subtracted from the beat-to-beat variation of arterial saturation (Gwinnutt 1996, p. 138). The technique offers an

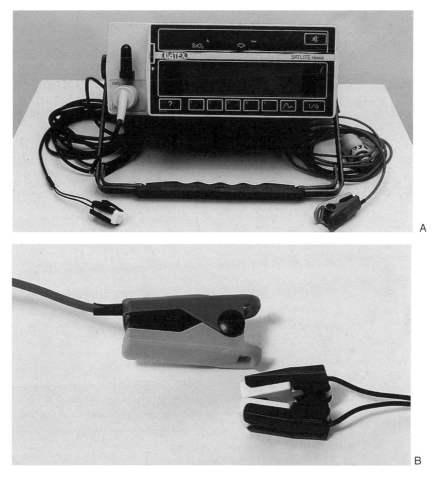

Figure 5.5 A: The pulse oximeter and probes. B: Finger (top) and ear (bottom) probes. (Reproduced with permission from Al-Shaikh & Stacey 1995.)

accuracy of ± 2%, over the range of 70–100% saturation (Hill & Summers 1994).

The device is useful both in ensuring that the patient's oxygen saturation is satisfactory and in reducing the need for frequent arterial blood gas analysis. However, the device does not provide any information on the PaO_2 or $PaCO_2$ levels within the blood or the acid–base balance (see Chapter 7 for analysis of arterial blood gases). In addition, the effort that the patient may be expending to produce good oxygenation saturations is not provided by the device. The patient may be tachypnoeic with a high level of inspired oxygen or be in no respiratory distress at all. As with all monitoring devices, pulse oximetry should be used as part of an overall patient assessment and not merely accepted at face value.

Sources of error in pulse oximetry

Cases have been recorded where the device provides information that appears inaccurate in view of the patient's presenting condition (Ralston et al 1991, Webb et al 1991). This has been particularly noteworthy in paediatrics. Poets et al (1993) noted an oximetry probe that had become detached from a premature baby's foot yet still provided a pulsatile signal and saturations of 98–99%. It became apparent that the readings disappeared when the room lights were switched off. Patients who have cold extremities, such as with poor circulation or hypothermia, create problems for the pulse oximeter and may result in non-detection of oxygen saturation.

As the device works by detecting light absorption by the oxygen-carrying haemoglobin, it is unable to distinguish between normal and abnormal haemoglobins. In patients with carbon monoxide poisoning, where this lethal gas replaces oxygen carried within the haemoglobin, creating carboxyhaemoglobin, a reading may still be gained indicating satisfactory oxygen saturation despite acute desaturation. Drugs which produce dysfunctional haemoglobins such as methaemoglobinaemia, which contains oxidized or ferric iron, are another source of error. Coloured nail varnish can produce inaccuracies but skin pigmentation does not affect the reading (Al-Shaikh & Stacey 1995, p. 91).

THE CHEST X-RAY

Interpretation of the chest X-ray is becoming a skill increasingly required by the acute cardiac nurse. As with the ECG, a systematic approach to interpretation can yield useful information with regard to caring for the patient, anticipating complications and instigating appropriate treatment. As a starting point it is useful to invest in a good text such as Corne et al (1997) or establish seminars, usually with the unit radiographer or physiotherapist, to acquire a working knowledge. Physiotherapy texts such as Smith & Ball (1998) may also provide valuable information. Skill in interpretation comes with supervised practice. Attempts to photocopy articles tends to produce poor-quality X-rays for learning purposes.

The main areas within the chest X-ray that can be identified for nursing work are:

- position of lines such as central venous pressure, PA catheter and nasogastric tubes, together with correct placement of the endotracheal (ET) tube
- the heart size
- areas of lobar consolidation and collapse
- the position and identification of artificial valves
- calcification of areas such as the aorta
- abnormalities of the lung fields, such as the development of pulmonary oedema.

The X-ray is basically shadows caused by a form of light energy cast on a film. Areas that are very dense, such as bone or alveolar consolidation, absorb the X-rays and appear as white on the film. Areas with reduced density, such as air in the lungs, do not absorb the beam and appear dark.

In examining the chest X-ray, the first step involves identifying from the film the correct patient's name and required date. A suitable light box should be used, rather than holding the X-ray up to the light or by a window. The film should be assessed from a distance of approximately 4 feet (1.2 m) and also close up to ensure all detail is seen (Corne et al 1997).

The practice of ascertaining if the patient has had a chest X-ray before admission is recommended. This is frequently the case with elective surgery and allows this X-ray to be placed alongside the most recent film, for comparison of any changes. The issue of pre-admission X-rays is important, because such films will have been taken in the radiography department, rather than at the bed area and will be of a superior quality. Chest X-rays utilize a beam that will be either anteroposterior (AP) or postero-anterior (PA). When taken in the radiography department, this will be PA. The beam enters from behind the patient who is standing and taking a good inspiration to allow a clear representation of the structures. The chest will be against the X-ray plate in front.

There are several advantages in utilizing the PA technique. The film will produce a much truer representation of the heart size, as it is directly against the plate. Emergency X-rays, such as the portable X-rays taken in coronary care and the acute units, are usually AP. The plate is behind the patient and the beam enters from the front. The patient may not be able to take a clear breath to allow all the structures to be clearly seen and may not be positioned optimally when in bed or a chair. Organs such as the heart will appear larger because they are at a distance from the film and cast a larger shadow. Exposure is also set manually and therefore may be inconsistent (Juniper & Garrard 1997). In reality, comparison of PA and AP films can be extremely difficult.

All films should be labelled as either PA or AP; if unlabelled (and all should be labelled) it is regarded as a PA, this being the standard format (Corne et al 1997, p. 8). The film will also be marked erect or supine. This is important as factors such as the thin line of a fluid level will disappear if the patient is lying flat (supine). This position may also obscure radiological findings such as pleural effusion and pneumothorax (Juniper & Garrard 1997).

Figure 5.6 shows a normal chest X-ray illustrating the various structures that may be seen. Figure 5.7 offers a diagrammatic representation.

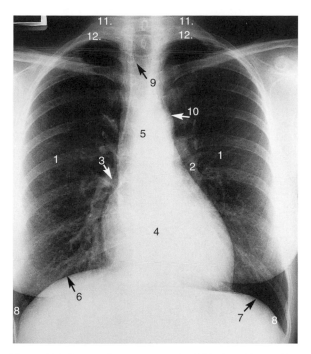

Figure 5.6 A normal postero-anterior (PA) chest X-ray with associated structures. (Adapted from Corne et al 1997.) 1. Lung fields. These should be of equal transradiancy, with no field whiter or darker than the other. 2&3. The hila. The left hilum (2) should be higher than the right (3). 4. The heart shadow. The maximum diameter should be half of the maximum thoracic diameter. Note that two-thirds of the heart are to the left of centre and one-third to the right. 5. The mediastinum. This should be clear; some blurring may occur where the heart meets the diaphragm. 6&7. Right and left diaphragms. The right should be higher than the left. The difference should be less than 3 cm. 8. The costophrenic angles. These should be sharp to the corners. 9. The trachea overlying the vertebrae and passing between the two clavicles. 10. The aortic knuckle. 11&12. The first and second ribs.

A systematic approach to basic chest X-ray interpretation

1. Check the name of the patient and date of the chest X-ray.

2. Establish whether the film is PA or AP and erect or supine.

3. Utilize a light box source and place the X-ray as if it were the patient's left or right, not the reader's. A marker on the film 'L' or 'R' will demonstrate this. The film is viewed as if you are looking at the patient in front of you.

4. Establish if the patient is positioned in line with the film. The patient may be rotated slightly which will distort the image. To assess this, note the inner (medial) ends of the clavicles and ensure that the vertebrae lie between the two ends (9). If one clavicle is nearer than the other to the spinous process, the lung on that side will appear whiter.

5. Note if the exposure (penetration) of the film is correct. To assess this, observe the lower part of the cardiac shadow (4). The vertebrae of the spinal column should only just be visible. If they are very clear, the film is overpenetrated and if they cannot be seen at all, the film is underpenetrated and the lung fields will appear falsely white (Corne et al 1997). Note this particularly if comparing various chest X-rays from the patient.

6. Note bilaterally each of the 12 ribs, both anteriorly and posteriorly. Descriptions of chest findings are often related to the rib number where the abnormality is located. The anterior end of the first rib is located just below the medial end of the clavicle (Kelly-Heidenthal & O'Connor 1994). Numbers 11 and 12 on Figure 5.6 identify the first and second ribs.

7. Note the heart size (4). The maximum width (transverse diameter) should be less than 15.5 cm in men and less than 14.5 cm in women. The usual method is to assess the cardiothoracic ratio, that is the widest part of the heart in comparison to the maximum width of the thoracic diameter. The widest point of the heart should have a ratio of less than 0.5, just under half of the widest part of the thoracic diameter (Desai & Chan 1992). It is normal for two-thirds of the heart to be to the left of the film and a third to the right.

8. Observe the two hemidiaphragms (6,7). The right is always higher than the left, which is pushed down by the heart, but the difference should not exceed 3 cm. The outline should be smooth.

9. The costophrenic angles at the bottom edges of the lung fields can be seen at 8. These should be clear and pointed. Obliteration of these can mean that the bases of the lungs are consolidated and full lung expansion is poor.

10. The hila (meaning the indentation in an organ) are on the right and left of the heart shadow (2,3). The left hilum is higher than the right and both should be concave in shape and not altered in density. The difference in height between the two is up to 1.5 cm but never less (Desai & Chan 1992).

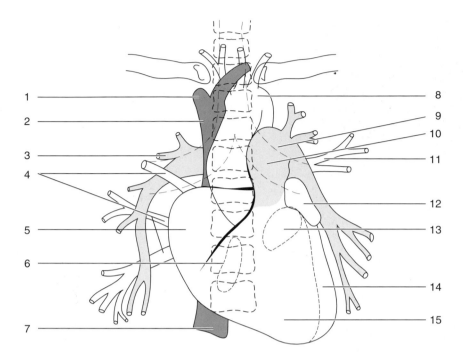

1. Right innominate vein
2. Superior vena cava
3. Right main branch of the pulmonary artery
4. Upper and lower lobe veins
5. Right atrium
6. Tricuspid valve
7. Inferior vena cava

8. Arch of the aorta
9. Left main branch of the pulmonary artery
10. Main pulmonary artery
11. Left upper lobe vein
12. Appendage of the left atrium
13. Mitral valve
14. Left ventricle
15. Right ventricle

Figure 5.7 Diagrammatic representation of the normal anatomical landmarks of the chest X-ray. (Reproduced with permission from Gedgaudas et al 1985.)

11. The chambers of the heart can be identified in Figure 5.7. Above the right atrium are the superior vena cava and hilum. The left ventricle is found to the left of the sternum and this rests on the diaphragm. Above the left ventricle is the left atrium and above these, the pulmonary artery and aortic knuckle (Kelly-Heidenthal & O'Connor 1994). The latter can be seen at 10 in Figure 5.6).

12. The correct positioning of lines will produce characteristic X-ray images (Fig. 5.8).

13. To identify pleural effusion, consolidation and collapse on the chest X-ray requires supervised practice. A pleural effusion occurs as an area of whiteness (Fig. 5.9A). To differentiate, collapse will tend to cause mediastinal shift towards the white lung field, while consolidation usually causes more heterogeneous shadowing, typically with an air bronchogram (Corne et al 1997). Collapse will also produce an area of white lung on the chest X-ray. Lateral X-rays are commonly ordered with collapse as they assist in confirming the diagnosis. Collapse can be caused by a misplaced endotracheal tube if, for example, it has entered the right main bronchus, preventing left lung expansion. Airway obstruction, such as a large plug of mucus, and also carcinomas and bronchial trauma are other causes (Smith & Ball 1998). An entire lung can collapse or just a lobe (Fig. 5.9B).

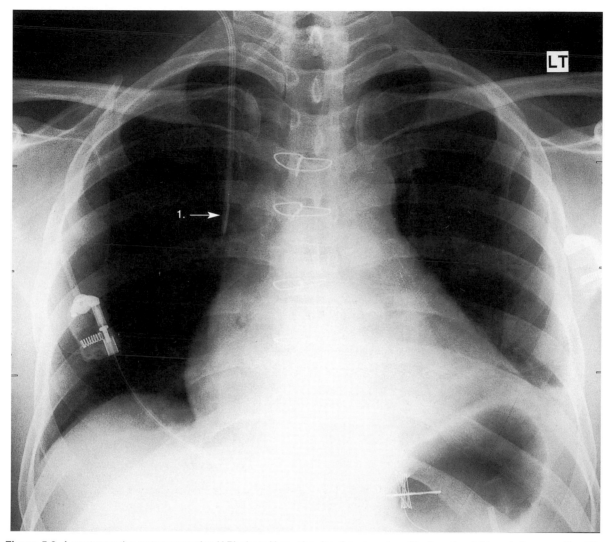

Figure 5.8 A postoperative anteroposterior (AP) chest X-ray showing the correct positioning of a right central venous line (1).

There is a loss of volume in the affected area, so that landmarks on the X-ray become distorted. Comparison of old films are very useful to highlight the presenting distortions; for example, the heart will deviate to the side of the collapse. The horizontal fissure, which divides the right upper lobe from the middle lobe and which extends from the middle of the hilum to the sixth rib, will pull up with right upper lobe collapse and down with right lower lobe collapse (Corne et al 1997). Unfortunately the horizontal fissure is not easy to see but appears as a fine hair-like line. The heart border will appear blurred next to the collapsed lung. Again, with upper lobe collapse, the trachea will deviate towards the collapsed area.

Consolidation is the filling of the alveoli with oedema fluid, blood, pus or cells (Fig. 5.9C). Many disease processes can cause consolidation, including pneumonia and acute respiratory distress syndrome (ARDS). Consolidation characteristically produces fluffy (white) pulmonary opacities (Smith & Ball 1998). When the alveoli are filled with little or no involvement of the airways, darker tube-like markings filled with air will occur amongst the opaque areas. This is the aforementioned air bronchogram. Further factors that differentiate consolidation from collapse include a shadowing that is not uniform and without a clearly demarcated border. Fluid will sink, so that the area of consolidation will appear more dense as your eye travels down (Corne et al 1997).

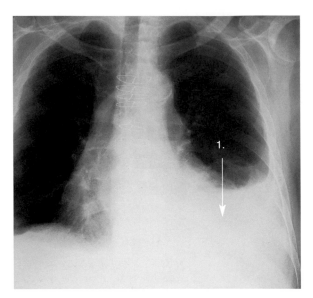

Figure 5.9 A: A chest X-ray primarily showing a pleural effusion at the left base (1). A smaller one is at the right base. Consolidation tends to produce more heterogenous shadowing, typically with the presence of an air bronchogram (Corne et al 1997). In a pleural effusion the upper border is generally concave as fluid collects with a meniscus.

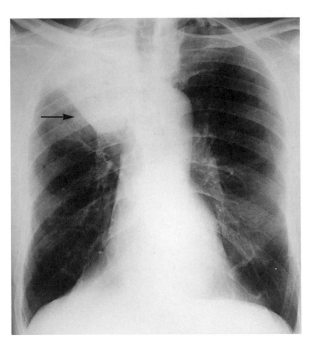

Figure 5.9 C: A chest X-ray of consolidation. This can be hard to diagnose. The arrow indicates the presence of an air bronchogram, created from the smaller airways retaining air and making them dark. The patient's previous X-rays are always useful: if the consolidation shadowing is not present, then fibrosis, which is usually a chronic condition, can generally be excluded. Consolidation is also likely to produce a pyrexia.

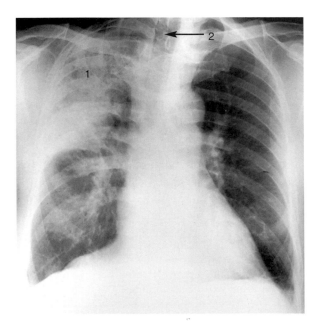

Figure 5.9 B: Right upper lobe collapse. There is a whiteness in the upper zone of the right lung (1) and the trachea is deviated to the right (2). The ribs over the area of whiteness are closer together than is normal. The horizontal fissure is elevated.

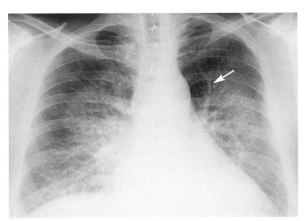

Figure 5.9 D: Pulmonary oedema from left ventricular failure. The white arrow indicates the prominent and dilated upper lobe blood vessels. The heart is also enlarged. (B, C, D reproduced with permission from Corne et al 1997.)

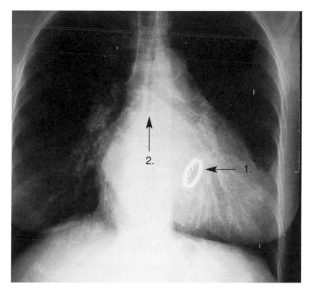

Figure 5.9 E: Artificial valve. This chest X-ray shows clearly an artificial mitral valve (1). Note also that the heart is enlarged. The X-ray also shows the bifurcation of the trachea into its two main branches (2).

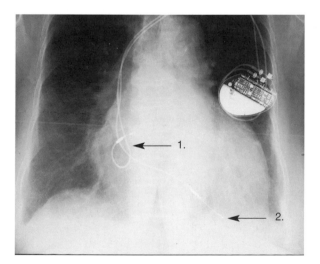

Figure 5.9 F: A permanent pacing system with atrial (1) and ventricular (2) pacing wires.

14. Cardiogenic pulmonary oedema (Fig. 5.9D) is sometimes indistinguishable from a non-cardiogenic cause, e.g. ARDS. However, in the latter the heart size may be normal while in the former it may be enlarged

due to progressive heart failure. It is important to remember the problem of estimating heart size in an AP film. The shadowing across the lungs in pulmonary oedema presents with Kerley B lines, horizontal white lines near the peripheries of the lungs, usually seen near to the costophrenic angles. For the experienced eye, upper lobe blood vessels should be narrower than those in the lower lobes in the erect film. If the vessels are the same size as in the lower lobe, this may indicate heart failure as lower vessels constrict due to alveolar hypoxia (Corne et al 1997). Fig. 9E and F provide further examples of the use of the chest X-ray in cardiac nursing care.

THE CENTRAL VENOUS PRESSURE

Measurement of the central venous pressure (CVP) is used to estimate the fluid status of the patient. Primarily this is to assess the relative state of hyper- or hypovolaemia. The word 'relative' is used here, as the patient may be unable to effectively pump their existing fluid volume without there having been any additional infusion. This is the presentation in acute heart failure (cardiogenic shock). The CVP will be elevated and may require manipulation with the use of diuretics, nitrates if the blood pressure is not too low and possibly inotropic therapy. Manipulating haemodynamics is an important skill for the acute cardiac nurse and is dealt with more fully in Chapter 18.

It is possible to estimate the venous pressure through non-invasive methods. The external jugular veins are visualized, usually with the patient supine with the bed's backrest at 30°. In this position the top of the venous column is just above the superior border of the mid clavicle. It is difficult to identify and often requires pressure from the forefinger over the site. This allows the vein to fill from above and to distend to the level of the jaw. On removing the finger the vein collapses and the visible fluid top falls to its previous level (Darovic & Franklin 1999). Generally as CVP rises, so does the top of the venous column above the mid clavicle. In severe heart failure distension may be seen to the level of the jaw.

The CVP catheter is an invasive but relatively simple means of measuring the fluid status of the patient. In this role it is highly valuable but offers very little information on the functioning of the left side of the heart, which delivers oxygenated blood to the tissues. The CVP is a manometer line introduced under sterile conditions, often at the bedside and usually into a central neck vein. This is frequently the internal jugular or subclavian vein (Hatchett & Robinson 2000).

The patient is laid flat, the skin is anaesthetized and towels are draped over the area. Chlorhexidine 0.5% is the recommended solution for cleaning the skin. The bed is often tipped slightly head down to engorge the neck veins for placement and to reduce the catastrophic effects of air entering the great veins during insertion. Lying flat can be distressing for the patient, particularly if breathless, and reassurance is of paramount importance. The patient will be required to lie still with the head turned away from the insertion site. Sedation can be used if the patient is unable to lie still but is frequently contra-indicated due to the haemodynamic status.

Once the catheter is introduced by the physician, blood is withdrawn to avoid introducing air and the line is flushed and attached to a transducer to visualize the pressure trace on a monitor. Alternatively it may be attached to a water manometer on an infusion stand (Fig. 5.10).

Both methods require the equipment to be 'zeroed' before measurements are taken. This means both devices take atmospheric pressure as zero or the starting point from which to measure the central venous pressure. This requires the transducer table to be at the level of the right atrium, achieved with the use of a

spirit level (Fig. 5.10A). A three-way tap attached to the water-filled manometer line on the transducer table is opened to air. A button on the monitor is pressed which records this atmospheric pressure as a zero point. The three-way tap is then closed so that the monitor can measure the pressure of fluid transmitted along the manometer line from the central veins. It then provides an accurate numerical value of the CVP. Occasionally a transducer table may not be used and the three-way tap is attached with tape under the patient's arm at the level of the right atrium. This is often seen when the patient returns from theatre.

Alternatively, without a monitor, the bottom of the vertical section of the manometer line is regarded as zero (Fig. 5.10B). This is in line with the right atrium, again achieved with a spirit level. Normally the device is attached to a fluid bag which both acts as an intravenous hydration fluid and keeps the central line patent. For the CVP reading, the vertical manometer line running against a tape measure is gently filled with fluid via a three-way tap, from the infusion bag. The three-way tap is then turned so that the fluid from the vertical tubing drips slowly into the central vein. When it reaches a resistance, that is the back pressure of circulating blood, the infusion stops. The top of the

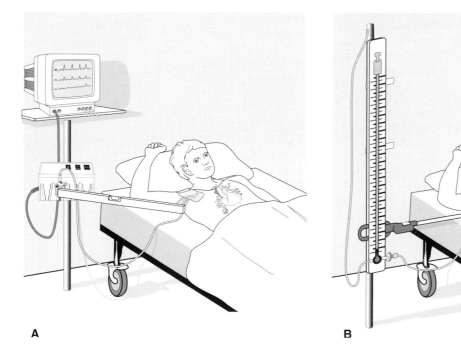

A   **B**

Figure 5.10 Measuring the central venous pressure (CVP). A: Transducer table to a monitor. B: Via a manometer set and infusion stand. Note in B that the base of the spirit level is the point from which zero is measured, as this is the level of the right atrium.

fluid in the vertical column is then read against the tape measure (the nurse must bend down so that the meniscus is at eye level). This is regarded as the CVP. After reading, the three-way tap is then turned so that the infusion bag can continue infusing into the line.

The normal range of the CVP is wide, approximately 3–11 cmH$_2$O if being transduced via a water manometer on an infusion stand or 0–8 mmHg if transduced to a monitor (see Fig. 5.10) (Darovic & Franklin 1999). Each of these ranges applies to a CVP device zeroed at mid axilla. Any monitored trace or rise of water in the manometer column on an infusion stand above this zero point is regarded as the CVP figure. To find this zero point a spirit level is used to align the transducer table with the centre of the underarm, mid axilla (Fig. 5.10). It may be useful to put a small pen mark here to ensure the same mid-axilla point is used for each measurement. Fluoroscopic imaging has ascertained that the mid-chest point is a more accurate reflection of the placement of the left ventricle than zeroing to the sternum (Lambert et al 1989, p. 283).

As the CVP is a *direct* measurement of the venous pressure, it is one of the earliest parameters to alter if there are changes in the fluid status. A rising pulse rate is a *compensatory* mechanism in response to such alteration and assists in maintaining the cardiac output. Except in the most extreme loss of fluid volume, the blood pressure may be maintained for some time as peripheral vessels constrict. The CVP is therefore also useful in identifying covert bleeding, such as internal haemorrhage following trauma or surgery.

Within cardiac nursing one of the major roles of the CVP is in the skill of manipulating haemodynamics. Here, measured parameters are altered with intravenous fluids, inotropes and occasionally left ventricular assist devices. The aim is to maximize oxygen delivery to aid organ functioning and recovery. Cardiac patients, due to their presenting fluid status and pre-existing cardiac function, will require differing amount of intravenous colloids and crystalloids to enhance the cardiac output. Administering too much fluid could worsen the cardiac condition, leading to reduced contractility and pulmonary oedema. The CVP can therefore be used to guide the filling process to the best effect. The use of the CVP in this respect, together with all the other aspects of utilizing monitoring devices to manipulate haemodynamics, is discussed in Chapter 18.

The CVP is essentially measuring the pressure in the venous system. If the patient is losing fluid and becoming dehydrated or hypovolaemic then the haemostatic pressure in the venous system drops and the CVP reading is low. If the patient for some reason is retaining fluid, such as in cardiac failure, where the heart is having difficulty pumping blood forward, then the CVP will rise. From the wide normal range it can be seen that patients exist with a variety of normal CVPs. This is why, as with all monitoring, regular observations and assessing the trend of movement is so important.

The CVP measurement is influenced by several factors which need to be considered when assessing the reading. Box 5.6 highlights the main factors that should be considered.

The venous tone reflects the degree of constriction of the vessels which return blood to the right side of the heart and from where the CVP is measured. If these vessels are unduly constricted, such as with hypovolaemia or hypothermia, blood will be shunted into the central circulation, elevating the CVP. The reading gained may not be a true reflection of the circulating volume.

The venous return simply signifies that the amount of blood returning to the right side of the heart will influence the measurement gained from the central venous circulation.

A variety of factors may alter and decrease the right ventricular compliance. Patients with pre-existing heart failure will often have a stiffer ventricle. Hypertrophy, myocardial fibrosis and ischaemia can all lead to a decrease in compliance. This reduced ability of the ventricles to distend means that the CVP can be higher than expected for the circulating blood volume (Darovic & Franklin 1999).

The effects of breathing will cause the CVP to rise and fall. This respiratory 'swing' can be seen with the gently rising and falling meniscus when the CVP is measured from a water-filled manometer on an infusion stand. Correspondingly the tracing on the monitor can also be seen to swing with each breath. This effect is normal but accentuated when the patient is dehydrated. At this point the great veins have limited blood volume and this reduced rigidity means they can easily be compressed by changes in the intrathoracic pressure throughout the respiratory cycle.

Box 5.6 Factors influencing the central venous pressure

- Venous tone
- Venous return
- Right ventricular compliance
- Intrathoracic pressure, notably with continuous positive airway pressure (CPAP) therapy and mechanical ventilation

When the patient is mechanically ventilated the positive pressure is transmitted to the great veins, elevating the CVP. The effect is enhanced with positive end expiratory pressure (PEEP). This occurs when the ventilator is set to prevent all of the gas leaving the chest at the end of each breath and is measured in cmH_2O. The aim is to aid gaseous exchange throughout the whole respiratory cycle and prevent alveolar collapse. However, particularly at higher levels, it can impede venous return and raise the CVP disproportionally to the circulating volume.

The CVP is therefore a sensitive measurement of the patient's fluid status. It is useful in administering intravenous fluids in a safe manner appropriate to the patient's needs, particularly with cardiac patients who require adequate filling pressures but who may develop pulmonary oedema very quickly. Covert haemorrhage will be sensed by the CVP at an earlier stage than other measured parameters. In reading a CVP several factors should be considered. The equipment should be correctly zeroed so that the zero point, either at the base of the water manometer on the infusion stand or on the transducer table, is at the level of the right atrium. Serial measurements are important. The normal range is wide and unless the reading is outside this range, it will be impossible to note a CVP that is gradually rising or falling. It is important to consider the four factors in Box 5.6 which can create a reading that is disproportional to the circulating volume. It should be remembered that when reading the CVP, the line should be flushed and no other drugs or infusions should be in progress. In addition, as the CVP line will need occasional flushing, infusing drugs in the same line can result in a bolus of the drug entering the patient.

THE PULMONARY ARTERY CATHETER

The pulmonary artery (PA) catheter was first described in 1970 by Swan and colleagues (Swan et al 1970), hence its more popular title, the Swan–Ganz catheter. The advantage of this device is that it offers data on the functioning of the left side of the heart and hence the chambers that provide oxygenated blood. The PA catheter is basically a long manometer line which is introduced in much the same way as the CVP line, into a central vein. This is usually the internal jugular or subclavian vein. Insertion is performed at the bedside with the patient lying flat and under sterile conditions. The skin around the neck area is sterilized with a solution, usually chlorhexidine based, anaesthetized and towels are draped over the area.

As with insertion of the CVP catheter, the head of the bed is often tipped downwards. Prior to the device being inserted a monitor and pressure transducer should be prepared and connected to the line. This allows the various pressures of the chambers to be noted as the catheter enters. It is these pressure tracings that tell the physician when the catheter has reached the pulmonary artery (Fig. 5.11).

On the end of the PA catheter is a tiny balloon which is inflated with approximately 1.5 ml of air as the catheter is introduced. This allows the tip to become buoyant and the catheter to float with the blood flow through the chambers of the heart. The catheter enters the right atrium, crosses the tricuspid valve into the right ventricle before being swept with the blood flow out into the pulmonary artery. This artery carries deoxygenated blood to the lungs and quickly splits into smaller and smaller tributaries. Eventually the catheter cannot be passed any further and becomes wedged in the pulmonary artery. At this point the pressure tracing alters to a classic occluded or 'wedged' tracing (see Fig. 5.11). The line is then secured to the patient's skin, the little balloon is deflated and the catheter is in place.

As the catheter is passed through the chambers of the right side of the heart it is not uncommon to notice ventricular ectopics and occasionally runs of ventricular tachycardia on the ECG. This usually subsides once the catheter is in place. However, for some patients it can be a persistent problem indicating early removal of the device.

When specific measurements are not being taken, the balloon must be deflated and the syringe which initiates this always has a Luer lock device to prevent accidental inflation. As the PA catheter sits in the pulmonary artery, if the balloon did become inflated, blood flow from the right ventricle through to the lungs would be impeded, leading to a pulmonary infarct. The pressure tracing from the pulmonary artery is always monitored to allow the classic sign that the balloon is inflated or that the tip has advanced further forwards and occluded the artery to be quickly noted and the catheter pulled back.

Box 5.7 illustrates the variety of data and the normal values obtained from the PA catheter. Of note are the cardiac output, cardiac index and the systemic vascular resistance (SVR). The cardiac output is the amount of blood ejected by the left ventricle in 1 minute to oxygenate the tissues. In health this is approximately 4–8 l/min. This can be calculated by what is termed the thermodilution technique. A known volume and temperature of crystalloid, usually cold but no longer chilled, is injected at speed and emerges at an early port in the PA catheter. This is usually in the right atrium. The contracting heart moves this cooled blood forward to a temperature probe at the catheter tip. The

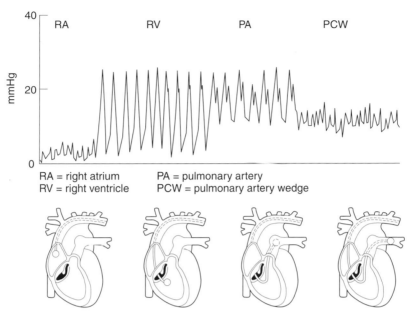

Figure 5.11 The placement and pressure tracings from the PA catheter. (Originally published in Stokes P, Jowett N 1985 Intensive Care Nursing 1: 3–12.)

Box 5.7 Values gained from the PA catheter (after Darovic 1995, Darovic & Franklin 1999)

- PA pressure 15–30/6–12 mmHg
- CVP 3–8 mmHg
- Pulmonary artery occlusion pressure (PAOP or 'wedge') 4–12 mmHg
- Cardiac output (resting) 4–8 l/min
- Cardiac index (resting) 2.5–4.2 l/min m²
- Systemic vascular resistance (SVR) 770–1500 dynes/sec/cm⁻⁵
- Systemic vascular resistance index (SVRI) 1680–2580 dynes/sec/cm⁻⁵/m²
- Mixed venous saturation (SvO_2) 65–75%

---

speed and degree of temperature change noted indicates the strength of contractility and hence a numerical cardiac output can be calculated and displayed on the monitor. Technology has now allowed PA catheters to offer continuous cardiac output readings through the use of thermal filaments which emit pulsating energy, warming the blood and utilizing the same thermodilution principle. The cardiac index is the cardiac output related to each metre squared of body surface area. This allows comparison between patients of varying body sizes. In health this value is approximately 2.5–4.2 l/min/m². The SVR is the resistance offered by the arterial and venous systems to the ejecting left ventricle. It is essentially the measurement of the afterload (see Chapter 18). It has a wide range of

770–1500 dynes/sec/cm⁻⁵. The systemic vascular resistance index (SVRI) is again the SVR related to each metre squared of body surface area, the range being 1680–2580 dynes/sec/cm⁻⁵/m².

It is an important measurement because, as mentioned throughout this book, when the patient experiences a compromised cardiac system, the body initiates a variety of often overzealous compensatory mechanisms to maintain tissue perfusion. Neurogenic and catecholamine release will cause active vessel constriction which may result in a normal or near normal blood pressure in the presence of a poor cardiac output. Therefore a measurement of the SVR or SVRI allows the team to note how far the body is compensating to maintain the blood pressure and, with the other clinical measurements such as cardiac output, how effective tissue perfusion actually is.

The value of monitoring the mixed venous saturation

The mixed venous saturation, commonly written as the SvO_2, is recorded by the PA catheter from a sensor in the pulmonary artery. The reading represents the oxygen saturation of the blood returning to the right side of the heart via the inferior and superior vena cavae. The normal range is 65–75%, while the arterial oxygen saturation (SaO_2), which indicates oxygenated blood being delivered to the tissues, is 95–98% (Baxter

1996, p. 3). As the SvO_2 is still a relatively high saturation, there is an oxygen reserve that may ultimately be utilized in times of increasing tissue demand.

The amount of oxygen consumed by the tissues every minute is often written as the VO_2. It is calculated by subtracting the amount of oxygen returning to the right side of the heart from the amount delivered to the tissues. Normally, at rest, the VO_2 is 200–290 ml O_2/min. The index, related to varying body sizes, is 115–160 ml O_2/min/m^2 (Darovic & Franklin 1999).

As with all measurements within cardiac work, the SvO_2 must be read in conjunction with other presenting signs and with an understanding of the factors influencing the supply and demand of oxygen at the tissue level. Chapter 4 highlighted many of the factors involved in maintaining this delicate balance, including the ability of the pulmonary system to diffuse an adequate amount of oxygen into the bloodstream, the affinity of haemoglobin for oxygen and the ability of the cardiac system to maintain an adequate flow and pressure of blood to meet the changing oxygen demands of the tissues. Such factors are crucial as the body is unable to maintain a store of oxygen.

More complex but important factors include the ability of haemoglobin to maintain a greater affinity and carrying capacity for oxygen in areas of plentiful supply, such as in the alveolar areas of the lungs, but to have a weaker bond where surrounding oxygen levels are lower, such as in the body's tissue areas.

Figure 5.12, the infamous oxyhaemoglobin dissociation curve, demonstrates haemoglobin's affinity for

oxygen at varying partial pressures of oxygen (PaO_2). Note that the curve flattens when the PaO_2 is high, demonstrating the greater binding of haemoglobin and oxygen, but in the areas of low PaO_2, a steep curve occurs, the bond is weaker and oxygen readily dissociates from the haemoglobin. This may be at tissue level. Certain factors alter the curve, moving it to the right or left of its normal plotting. In times of increased body temperature, elevated blood carbon dioxide levels and when an acidosis occurs, the curve shifts to the right. At this point the bond between the haemoglobin and oxygen is weaker for any given PaO_2. This can be useful because highly active tissues, such as occur during exercise, become hot. The weaker bond thus makes an easier dissociation of oxygen from the haemoglobin into the tissues. Conversely when the patient is hypothermic or there is an increased pH of the blood indicating a move towards an alkalotic state, the bond between haemoglobin and oxygen is strengthened.

A falling SvO_2 measurement below the normal range indicates that the tissues are extracting a greater amount of oxygen from the reserve than would be expected. Either the above factors which maintain an adequate oxygen supply are not sufficient or the tissues are demanding an unusually high degree of oxygen.

Normally when there is a need to increase the supply of oxygen to the tissues, an increase in cardiac output is the primary mechanism (Baxter 1996, p. 9). Increased oxygen extraction, indicated by a falling SvO_2, is very much a last line of defence. At this point therapeutic interventions such as intravenous colloids, inotropes or left ventricular assist devices may be considered if the cardiac system alone cannot maintain adequate tissue oxygen delivery.

Box 5.8 demonstrates the variety of factors that may result in either a high or low SvO_2. It is important to remember that the SvO_2 represents the very end point of the balance of oxygen delivery and consumption at the tissue level.

Obviously the monitoring of the SvO_2 is reserved for the acute situation, where the cardiac system is compromised. The *trends* of SvO_2 can act as an early warning system that the usual compensatory mechanisms for maintaining tissue oxygenation are not functioning sufficiently and that therapeutic interventions may be necessary. It is also important to look at the points where the SvO_2 may have dipped before returning to a normal range. At these points the demand for oxygen was too high for the compensatory mechanisms to maintain the supply. Nursing action can then be modified when the cause has been found.

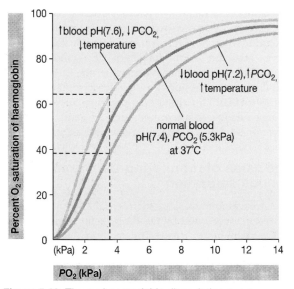

Figure 5.12 The oxyhaemoglobin dissociation curve.

Box 5.8 The factors influencing high and low SvO_2 measurements

High SvO_2
- Increased oxygen delivery
  - A high FiO_2 (fraction of inspired oxygen)
- Reduced oxygen demand
  - Anaesthesia
  - Paralysing agents
  - Sepsis, hypothermia

Low SvO_2
- Increased oxygen demand
  - Shivering, pain, hyperthermia, seizures
- Poor delivery of oxygen
- Reduced SaO_2 (arterial oxygen saturation)
  - Hypoxia, suctioning
- Low cardiac output
  - Cardiogenic shock, hypovolaemia
- A lowered haemoglobin
  - Anaemia, haemorrhage

A drop in SvO_2 may be precipitated by suctioning of the endotracheal tube, which both reduces oxygen supply and can agitate the patient. Further patient reassurance, reducing the incidence of suctioning and pre-oxygenating may assist in eliminating dangerous drops in the SvO_2 reading. In cardiac surgery, shivering following surgery markedly increases the demand for oxygen which may temporarily not be met, causing the SvO_2 to drop.

It will be clear throughout this book that what appears to be an adequate cardiac output or blood pressure in acute cardiac units does not necessarily mean the tissues are receiving adequate oxygenation. The SvO_2 is a useful parameter in this respect, in individualizing haemodynamic parameters to patient needs. If the blood pressure drops but the SvO_2 remains within the normal range, then it is likely that therapeutic intervention may not be required. If, however, the blood pressure drops with a concomitant drop in SvO_2, therapy may be needed to support the cardiac system (Baxter 1996, p. 21).

THE TRANSOESOPHAGEAL DOPPLER TECHNIQUE FOR MEASURING THE CARDIAC OUTPUT

This technique offers an alternative method to ascertain continuous cardiac output measurements. Although it does involve a transducer passed into the oesophagus, it does not breach the skin and is therefore primarily non-invasive. From within the oesophagus, the transducer's angled head emits ultrasound waves across the descending aorta (Batson 1994). Moving red blood cells reflect back the ultrasound waves to the transducer, where the velocity of the blood flow is calculated. The frequency of the reflected wave is essentially the same during diastole as the red blood cells are static. In systole the cells move away from the transducer and therefore reflect back a lower signal, rather like the changing sound of a fire engine siren travelling ahead (Batson 1994). The faster the red cells move away, the lower the reflected ultrasound. The cardiac output can be estimated to an accuracy of approximately 80–90% with this technique (Adam & Osborne 1997, p. 100). It may also be helpful in establishing whether invasive measurements are likely to be of value to a patient (Hayes 1997, p. 169). A lack of familiarity with the approach, together with the cost of equipment, has restricted this form of cardiac output measurement to a few specialist centres in Britain.

CONCLUSION

As this chapter closes it is also worth mentioning the electronic patient record or paperless form of charting. Already many acute units receive laboratory results via a computerized system but some units are advancing further. Computer programs and electronic interfaces between medical devices now make it possible to collect, integrate, archive and review all parameters gathered from medical equipment such as patient monitors, ventilators, syringe pumps and even urinary catheters. This information can then be viewed and even queried on a screen either at the patient's bedside or in a nearby office via a number of clinicians at one time, accessed via a password for security. Each password has individual access rights, enabling some clinicians to prescribe and/or validate information whilst others may have access rights to view data only. Each time the system is accessed an audit trail will be set up enabling every entry to be tracked: your personal password becomes your signature.

The method by which this information is displayed on the screen is dependent on the program. Some patient data management systems (PDMS) or clinical information systems (CIS), as they are known, allow the hospital to display the information in a similar format to their paper chart, displaying trended information for haemodynamics and fluids, so important in managing a cardiac patient. All patient data are stored on the local hard disk at the bedside and simultaneously mirrored onto a second workstation within the unit for back-up purposes.

The benefit of a CIS becomes apparent when one realizes that at least 30–50% of a nurse's time is spent charting at the beside. This time could be used for other activities that may improve patient outcome, change clinical practice and make the best use of limited resources. Some systems also perform automated intake/output, haemodynamic and ventilation calculations, send off pharmacy requests and prompt staff when something needs to be done for the patient.

With all forms of change there are valid concerns, many of which can be alleviated by familiarization. However, one of the primary concerns is the training and supporting of staff who will inevitably vary in their information technology experience. Fortunately many companies are now addressing this concern and employ staff whose responsibility it is to train and educate users. However, packages vary and this is still a relatively new concept and should be a consideration for any unit looking at purchasing a system. As the recording of observations and their interpretation are crucial activities in any cardiac unit, a dedicated hospital team should be established for this purpose. Accurate planning and implementation can be the only pathway to success.

Among the positive aspects of a CIS are the ability to have information automatically recorded before and during emergency situations; drug orders being 100% legible and standardized (thereby reducing the risk of errors) and having the ability to analyse information for research purposes. Some systems can also identify an apparently incorrect prescription and warn the prescriber (who can over-ride the warning or confirm the dose). On the negative side, as health-care workers, we must decide how safe we feel if all information is not available in a paper format. Also the cost/benefit equation should be carefully considered. However, overall, the advantages of a CIS should prevail over any negative aspects and enable staff to benefit from what the technology can offer.

In conclusion, this chapter has highlighted both the variety of monitoring devices available to the cardiac nurse and the need to use them in unison as a source of holistic information. Through assessing the whole picture and by considering the underlying patient condition, a more accurate understanding of the appropriate nursing and medical care required is gained. Students may initially learn through the provision of what Benner has referred to as 'context-free rules', focusing upon the normal parameters and ranges without situational experience (Benner 1984, pp. 20–21), but it is through clinical experience and supervised practice that these norms can be honed more appropriately to the individual patient. Chapter 18 takes the monitoring devices further, by utilizing the data they provide to manipulate the haemodynamics of the patient and augment the cardiac output.

Case study 5.1

Mr Hayes, a 75-year-old man, returns from theatre to the intensive care unit (ICU) following coronary artery bypass grafting (CABG). There were complications in theatre and Mr Hayes remained in surgery for longer than was expected. Consequently, his body temperature has dropped to 33.5°C and a pulmonary artery (PA) catheter is in place. The following measurements are taken by the intensive care team.
- Heart rate: 130 bpm
- Blood pressure: 95/60 mmHg
- Skin: cool, pale and clammy
- Core temperature: 33.5°C
- Peripheral temperature: 30°C
- Urinary output: 150 ml/h at present
- CVP: 8 mmHg (via PA catheter)
- Cardiac output: 3.5 l/min
- SVR: 1900 dynes/sec/cm^{-5}
- PA occlusion pressure: 20 mmHg
- SvO$_2$: 55%

This case demonstrates the need to look holistically at all the findings and link them to the known history. Initially, if you look at the urine output it is very high. This would indicate good tissue perfusion, if the rule of 0.5 ml/kg/h were applied. However, a knowledge of cardiac surgery would indicate that this man has been administered a large dose of diuretics in theatre to aid removal of the cardiopulmonary bypass (CPB) support and to encourage his own circulation to support tissue perfusion. The central venous pressure (CVP) appears within a normal range but the patient is very cold, so one of the four factors affecting this reading comes into play, with an excessively constricted venous system (venous tone) elevating the reading.

If the nurse accepted the measured CVP and did not begin gentle intravenous colloid filling, the peripheral vessels would eventually dilate as the patient warmed and the haemodynamic pressures would rapidly fall. Such a decompensation would be highly dangerous in view of the compromised cardiac function and the need to keep the new coronary grafts patent.

The PA catheter reveals a low cardiac output and a high occlusion pressure. This indicates that the myocardial contractility is poor and tissue perfusion will not be good. This is further supported by the falling mixed venous saturation (SvO$_2$), indicating that the body is now drawing from the oxygen reserve which would normally be returned to the lungs via the venous system. The peripheral constriction demonstrated in the high SVR is still maintaining a relatively good blood pressure.

It is likely at this stage that intravenous fluids would be administered to elevate the CVP and augment cardiac output and to prevent the aforementioned predicted peripheral dilatation. A positive inotrope may also be considered in view of the poor cardiac contractility. Chapter 18 highlights the variety of methods utilized in manipulating haemodynamics to increase tissue oxygen perfusion.

REFERENCES

Adam SK, Osborne S 1997 Critical care nursing: science and practice. Oxford Medical Publications, Oxford

Al-Shaikh B, Stacey S 1995 Essentials of anaesthetic equipment. Churchill Livingstone, Edinburgh

Antonios TFT, MacGregor GA 1996 Salt – more adverse effects. Lancet 348: 250–251

Asiain MC, Montes Y, Costa-Ramos ML, Imizcoz P 1990 Blood pressure measurement: an evaluation of direct and indirect methods. Intensive Care Nursing 6: 111–117

Ball C 1994 Intestinal barrier failure and the development of the systemic inflammatory response syndrome. Intensive and Critical Care Nursing 10(4): 252–256

Batson S 1994 Measuring cardiac output. Nursing Times 90: 37–63

Baxter 1996 Understanding continuous mixed venous oxygen saturation (SvO2) monitoring with the Swan–Ganz oximetry TD system, 2nd edn. Cardiovascular Group, Edwards Critical Care Division, Berkshire

Beilin LJ, Puddey IB, Burke V 1996 Alcohol and hypertension: kill or cure? Journal of Human Hypertension 10 (suppl 2): S1–S5

Benner P 1984 From novice to expert: excellence and power in clinical nursing practice. Addison-Wesley, California

British Hypertension Society and the Nurses Hypertension Association 1997 Blood pressure measurement. Recommended techniques. British Hypertension Society, St George's Hospital, London

Carretero OA, Oparil S 2000 Essential hypertension part II: treatment. Circulation 101: 446–453

Clifton D, Kelly HJ, Record KE, Thompson JR 1991 Comparison of normal saline and heparin saline for the maintenance of arterial catheter patency. Heart and Lung 20(2): 115–118

Corne J, Carroll M, Brown I, Delany D 1997 Chest X-ray made easy. Churchill Livingstone, Edinburgh

Cox CL, McGrath A 1999 Respiratory assessment in critical care units. Intensive and Critical Care Nursing 15: 226–234

Croft PR, Cruickshank JK 1990 Blood pressure measurement in adults: large cuffs for all? Journal of Epidemiological and Community Health 44(2): 170–173

Darovic GO 1995 Hemodynamic monitoring: invasive and noninvasive clinical application. WB Saunders, Philadelphia

Darovic GO, Franklin CM 1999 Handbook of hemodynamic monitoring. WB Saunders, Philadelphia

Desai S, Chan O 1992 Interpretation of a normal chest X-ray. Nursing Standard 4(7): 38–39

Elliot P, Stamler J, Nichols R et al 1996 Intersalt revisited: further analysis of 24 hour sodium excretion and blood pressure within and across populations. British Medical Journal 312: 1249–1253

Feather C 2001 Blood pressure measurement. Nursing Times 97(4): 33–34

Feher M, Harris-St John K, Lant A 1992 Blood pressure measurement by junior hospital doctors – a gap in medical education? Health Trends 24(2): 59–61

Gamby A, Bennett J 1995 A feasibility study of the use of non-heparinised 0.9% sodium chloride for transduced arterial and venous lines. Intensive and Critical Care Nursing 11: 148–150

Gedgaudas E, Moller JH, Castaneda-Zuniga MD et al 1985 Cardiovascular radiology. WB Saunders, Philadelphia

Geleijnse JM, Witteman JCM, Bak AAA, Den Breeijen JH, Grobbee DE 1994 Reduction in blood pressure with a low sodium, high potassium, high magnesium salt in older subjects with mild to moderate hypertension. British Medical Journal 309: 436–440

Gueyffier F, Boutitie F, Boissel JP et al 1997 Effect of antihypertensive drug treatment on cardiovascular outcomes in women and men: a meta-analysis of individual patient data from randomized, controlled trials. Annals of Internal Medicine 126: 761–767

Gwinnutt CL 1996 Clinical anaesthesia. Blackwell Science, Oxford

Hatchett R, Robinson T 2000 Central venous catheterisation 1. Nursing Times 96(11): 53–54

Hayes B 1997 Non-invasive cardiovascular monitoring. BMJ Books, London

Hill DW, Summers R 1994 Medical technology – a nursing perspective. Chapman and Hall, London

Hinds CJ, Watson D 1996 Intensive care: a concise textbook, 2nd edn. WB Saunders, London

Hook M, Reuling J, O'Brien Norris S, Leonard MR 1985 Comparison of the patency of arterial lines maintained with heparinised and non-heparinised infusions. Heart and Lung 16(6): 693–699

Jowett NI, Stephens JM, Thompson DR, Sutton TR 1985 Do indwelling cannulae on coronary care units need a heparin flush? Intensive Care Nursing 2: 16–19

Juniper MC, Garrard CS 1997 The chest X-ray in intensive care. Care of the Critically Ill 13(5): 198–200

Kelly-Heidenthal P, O'Connor M 1994 Nursing assessment of portable AP chest X-rays. Dimensions of Critical Care Nursing 13(3): 127–132

Kennedy S, Curzio J 1996 Blood pressure points. Practice Nurse 11(1): 25, 27–29

Knaw KT, Thom S 1982 Randomised double-blind cross-over trial of potassium on blood-pressure in normal subjects. Lancet 11: 1127–1129

Lambert CR, Pepine CJ, Nichols WW 1989 Pressure measurement. In: Pepine CJ, Hill JA, Lambert CR (eds) Diagnostic and therapeutic cardiac catheterisation. Williams and Wilkins, Baltimore, p. 283

Leighton H 1994 Maintaining the patency of transduced arterial and venous lines using 0.9% sodium chloride. Intensive and Critical Care Nursing 10: 23–25

MacGregor GA, Kaplan NM 1998 Hypertension. Health Press, Oxford

MacGregor GA, Sagnella GA, Markandu ND, Singer DRJ, Cappuccio FP 1989 Double blind study of three sodium intakes and long-term effects of sodium restriction in essential hypertension. Lancet 2: 1244–1247

Maki DG, Ringer M, Alvarado CJ 1991 Prospective randomised trial of povidone-iodine, alcohol, and chlorhexidine for prevention of infection associated with central venous and arterial catheters. Lancet 338(8763): 339–343

Mann R 1999 Blood pressure – when to treat? Or 'the appliance of science'. Cardiology 2(4): 10–11

Marieb E 1998 Human anatomy and physiology, 4th edn. Benjamin/Cummings, Menlo Park, California

Maskrey N 1999 Has the rule of halves in hypertension been replaced by the rules of (almost) two-thirds and (almost) three-quarters? Cardiology 2(4): 12–13

Materson BJ, Reda J, Cushman WC 1994 For the Department of Veterans Affairs Cooperative Study Group on Antihypertensive Agents. Single drug therapy for hypertension in men. A comparison of six antihypertensive agents with placebo. New England Journal of Medicine 328: 914–921

Maxwell MH 1982 Error in blood pressure measurement due to incorrect cuff size in obese patients. Lancet 11: 33–36

McConnell MV, Vavouranakis I, Wu LL, Vaughan DE, Ridker DM 1997 Effects of a single daily alcoholic beverage on lipid and hemodynamic markers of cardiovascular risk. American Journal of Cardiology 80(9): 1226–1228

O'Brien ET 2000 Replacing the mercury sphygmomanometer. British Medical Journal 320: 815–816

O'Brien ET, Davison M 1994 Blood pressure measurement: rational and ritual actions. British Journal of Nursing 3(8): 393–396

O'Brien ET, Mee F, Atkins N, O'Malley K 1990 Inaccuracies of seven popular sphygmomanometers for home-measurement of blood pressure. Journal of Hypertension 8: 621–634

O'Brien ET, Beevers DG, Marshall HJ 1995 ABC of hypertension, 3rd edn. BMJ Books, London

Paladichuk A 1998 Interview: life-saver or money waster? The PA catheter goes under the microscope. Critical Care Nurse 18(1): 88–93

Pickering GW 1968 High blood pressure. Churchill Livingstone, London

Pickering TG 1991 Ambulatory monitoring and blood pressure variability. Science Press, London

Pickering TG 1994 Blood pressure measurement and detection of hypertension. Lancet 11: 31–35

Poets CF, Seindenberg J, Von Der Hardt H 1993 Failure of pulse oximeter to detect sensor detachment. Lancet 341: 244

Prasad N, Isles C 1996 Ambulatory blood pressure monitoring: a guide for general practitioners. British Medical Journal 313: 1535–1541

Puddey IB, Cox K 1995 Exercise lowers blood pressure – sometimes or did Pheidippides have hypertension? Journal of Hypertension 13: 1229–1233

Ralston AC, Webb RK, Runciman WB 1991 Potential errors in pulse oximetry: 1 pulse oximeter evaluation. Anaesthesia 46: 202–206

Ramsay LE, Williams B, Johnston GD et al 1999 Guidelines for management of hypertension: report of the Third Working Party of the British Hypertension Society. Journal of Human Hypertension 13(9): 569–592

Smith M, Ball V 1998 Cardiovascular/respiratory physiotherapy. CV Mosby, Philadelphia

Swan HJC, Ganz W, Forrester J et al 1970 Catheterisation of the heart in man with the use of a flow-directed balloon-tipped catheter. New England Journal of Medicine 283: 447–451

Taylor N, Hutchinson E, Milliken W, Larson E 1989 Comparison of normal versus heparinised saline flushing infusion devices. Journal of Nursing Quality Assurance 3(4): 49–55

Taylor RW, Ahrens T, Beilin Y et al 1997 Pulmonary artery catheter consensus conference. Consensus statement. Critical Care Medicine 25: 910–925

Torrance C, Serginson E 1996 An observational study of student nurses' measurement of arterial blood pressure by sphygmomanometer and auscultation. Nurse Education Today 16: 282–286

Vann Jones J, Patel KCR, Dalton GR, Levi AJ 1998 Hypertension and the heart. Cardiology News 2(2): 6–11

Verdecchia P, Porcellati C, Schillaci G et al 1994 Ambulatory blood pressure: an independent predictor of prognosis in essential hypertension. Hypertension 24(6): 793–801

Webb RK, Ralston AC, Runciman WB 1991 Potential errors in pulse oximetry: II effects of changes in saturation and signal quality. Anaesthesia 46: 207–212

Wood D, Durrington P, Poulter N, McInnes G, Rees A, Wray R 1998 Joint British recommendations on prevention of coronary heart disease in clinical practice: management of blood pressure. Heart 80 (suppl 2): S1–S29

6

The ECG: its role and practical application

Jillian Riley

The electrocardiogram or ECG depicts the electrical activity of the heart. It is following this electrical excitation that the mechanical events of contraction, relaxation and the cardiac cycle occur. By placing electrodes at various sites on the surface of the body, the depolarization and repolarization of the myocardial cells can be detected from different angles. These electrodes are known as 'leads' and make up the ECG. By presenting information on myocardial cell activity in different parts of the heart, the ECG is able to contribute to patient assessment. It can be used therefore to inform or refute diagnoses, predict consequences, alert to a deteriorating condition or adverse haemodynamic event and enable practitioners to be proactive in their patient care and management.

In the early 1900s, Einthoven attached electrodes to the right and left arms and to the left leg, to record the heart's electrical activity. These were bipolar leads; they had both negative and positive poles and recorded the difference between the electrical potential at the poles. They provided three views of the electrical activity of the heart and form what has become known as the Einthoven triangle (leads I, II and III). However, this left a gap in our knowledge of the electrical activity of the heart in the angles between these points so by 1932, Frank Wilson devised a method for recording these views and the additional limb leads of aVR, aVF and aVL were developed (Wagner & Marriott 1994). These latter leads are unipolar with only a positive lead and so amplify the signal from one point. When using an electrocardiograph to record them, the signal is automatically augmented by 50% over the actual voltage, thereby enhancing the waveform. These same leads are used today as the six standard limb leads and record the electrical activity of the heart on a frontal plane (Fig. 6.1).

Today the ECG is recorded using 12 leads: the six standard limb leads and six precordial leads, the latter also being unipolar leads. These precordial leads are termed V1–V6 and are positioned around the chest

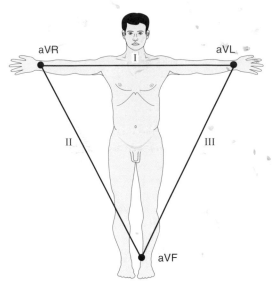

Figure 6.1 Einthoven's triangle depicting the six standard limb lead positions.

wall. They complete the cardiac assessment by presenting a view of the heart's electrical activity on a horizontal plane.

Although Figure 6.2 indicates the traditional precordial lead placement used in Britain, alternative

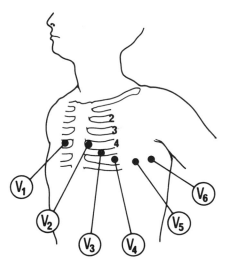

Figure 6.2 The leads are carefully placed at intervals around the chest wall V1 – 4th intercostal space, right sternal margin. V2 – 4th intercostal space, left sternal margin. V3 – midway between V2 and V4. V4 – 5th intercostal space, mid-clavicular line. V5 – midway between V4 and V6. V6 – 5th intercostal space on mid-axillary line. (Reproduced with permission from Hampton JR 1997 The ECG Made Easy 5E. Churchill Livingstone, Edinburgh.)

positions may sometimes be used. For example, right chest leads may be used if a right ventricular myocardial infarction or hypertrophy is suspected. Leads may also be placed around the posterior thoracic wall, where they are useful to confirm a diagnosis of a posterior wall myocardial infarction (Wagner & Marriott 1994).

By using the six standard limb leads and six precordial leads, the electrical activity at various surfaces of the heart can be interpreted. This is invaluable, for example, in diagnosing the area where a myocardial infarction has taken place. The areas are summarized as follows.

- Leads V1–V2 = right ventricle
- Leads V3–V4 = anterior wall of the left ventricle
- Leads V5–V6 = anterior and lateral walls of the left ventricle
- Leads II, III, aVF = inferior surface of the heart
- Leads I, aVL, V5–V6 = lateral surface of the heart
- Lead aVR = atria

RECORDING THE ECG

Most ECG bedside monitors use bipolar leads, with only one view of the heart recorded at any one time. The three leads are positive, negative and ground/earth. This latter lead removes any interference from other electrical impulses, such as nearby electrical equipment. Frequently the lead II position is chosen, recording a more positive R-wave and a clear view of the P-wave. Although useful for bedside monitoring this does not present a complete picture of the heart's electrical activity so it may be necessary, in situations where the patient is experiencing severe chest pain or as an assessment tool, to record a 12-lead ECG. Consistent and accurate placement of the electrodes is essential as each lead reflects a different view of the electrical activity of the heart.

The best position for limb leads is at the distal portion of the arms and legs but for continuous tracings this position will produce too much artefact through muscle movement and so the leads are placed on the torso. To help reduce muscle tremor the 12-lead recording should be taken with the patient in the supine position, whenever this can be tolerated. As skin is a poor conductor of electricity, it should be prepared carefully to reduce its resistance. Today adhesive electrodes are used, pre-prepared with an electrode jelly to enhance contact with the skin and the transference of the impulses. Substances that may prevent adhesiveness of the electrode or create impedance, such as dressings, should be removed and abra-

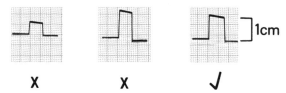

X   X   √

Figure 6.3 Calibration of the ECG machine where 1 mV = two large squares. Poor calibration may affect the magnitude and width of the complexes. (Reproduced with permission from Hampton JR 1997 The ECG Made Easy 5E. Churchill Livingstone, Edinburgh.)

sion may be necessary to remove rough skin cells. (Natural skin oils should not be removed with alcohol, contrary to popular practice.) Poor contact may result, causing the iso-electric line (the baseline or the part of the ECG where no electrical activity is occurring) to wander, making ECG interpretation difficult and possibly inaccurate.

NB: Impedance caused by a large thorax or large muscle mass around the thoracic cage will affect the amplitude of the ECG tracing. Attention to positioning of the patient and electrodes is therefore important.

The electrocardiograph should be standardized and typically two large squares are used to represent 1 millivolt (mV). Nowadays the electrocardiograph will produce a calibration mark at the end of each line. This should be assessed, as the stylus should produce a clean upstroke to the calibration mark of two large squares (Fig. 6.3).

The paper is marked out in squares and the paper speed is generally 25 mm/s. The thin lines are spaced 1 mm apart, representing 0.04 s on the horizontal axis and 0.1 mV on the vertical axis. As five fine squares make a large square, each large square represents 0.2 s and 0.5 mV respectively (Fig. 6.4). This enables the waveform to be analysed more accurately for rate, regularity and amplitude.

INTERPRETING THE ELECTRICAL ACTIVITY

When resting, the myocardial cell is negatively charged and the ECG recording will show a straight

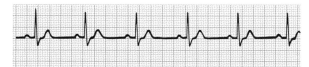

Figure 6.4 ECG paper is divided into millimetre squares, with five squares making one large square. The horizontal axis measures time with one small square representing 0.04 s. The vertical axis measures amplitude in mm. (Reproduced with permission from Hampton JR 1997 The ECG Made Easy 5E. Churchill Livingstone, Edinburgh.)

line called the **iso-electric line**. It is not until the cell is stimulated and sodium ions, primarily, rush into the cell that it becomes positively charged (depolarization) and the electrical activity causes a waveform. The ECG detects the wave of electrical activity that travels towards the positive pole of the lead and produces a positive or upright deflection in that lead. If the electrical activity travels away from the positive pole, it will produce a negative deflection. When all cells are depolarized there is no electrical charge moving towards the electrode and the ECG returns to the iso-electric line. Following this there is a wave of repolarization as the cell returns to its resting membrane potential and is negatively charged (Fig. 6.5). This wave of electrical activity is termed the **action potential** of the cell and is described in full in Chapter 4.

- An electrical current that travels towards a lead will produce a positive (upward) deflection.
- An electrical current that travels away from the lead will produce a negative (downward) deflection.
- An electrical current that travels perpendicular to the lead will produce a biphasic deflection.

From Chapter 4 you will recall that the wave of depolarization passes from the sino-atrial (SA) or sinus node to the atrioventricular (AV) node. This is shown on the ECG as the P-wave.

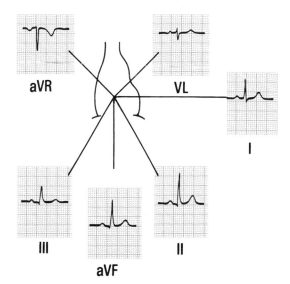

Figure 6.5 As the mean vector travels in an inferior and leftwards direction through the atria it will show as a positive waveform in leads I, II and aVF. In aVR the vector travels away from it, shown by a negative waveform. (Reproduced with permission from Hampton JR 1997 The ECG Made Easy 5E. Churchill Livingstone, Edinburgh.)

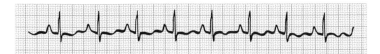

Figure 6.6 Enlargement of the right atria will result in a wide P-wave. The shape is referred to as **P-pulmonale** and is frequently associated with high pulmonary artery pressures from pulmonary disease, congenital heart defects or disease of the pulmonary or tricuspid valves. (Reproduced with permission from Hampton JR 1997 The ECG in Practice 3E. Churchill Livingstone, Edinburgh.)

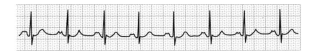

Figure 6.7 Enlargement of the left atria will result in a double-peaked P-wave. This shape is referred to as **P-mitrale** and is frequently associated with high left ventricular pressures, caused by mitral valve disease.

How the impulse is conducted through the atria is a subject of some controversy. It is generally considered that there are three internodal tracts passing through the atria: the anterior, middle and posterior internodal pathways. These are considered to be small bundles of fibres that exist where the ends of the SA node fibres fuse with the atrial muscle fibres and enable the rapid propagation of the action potential and therefore of the wave of contraction (Guyton & Hall 1996). However, although this is the traditionally taught theory, there appears to be no histological evidence for it (Moorman & Lamers 1999, Thompson 1983) and it must be concluded that conduction passes through atrial tissue from the SA to the AV node.

The P-wave is usually a rounded dome-shaped deflection. However, as the initial portion of the P-wave represents right atrial contraction and the middle portion left atrial contraction, any abnormality of the atria will alter the shape. It is during this P-wave that the AV node is stimulated (Figs 6.6 and 6.7).

Following the P-wave, the atria contract (atrial systole). For complete filling of the ventricles this must be complete prior to ventricular contraction. Within the cardiac cycle this is referred to as the 'atrial kick' when approximately one-third of ventricular filling occurs, accounting for about 25 ml of blood in the adult. The AV node delays impulse conduction and hence contraction of the ventricles. This not only protects the ventricles from abnormal, chaotic or rapid impulses but also enables a more complete filling of the ventricle. By applying the Frank–Starling Law of cardiac contractility (see Chapter 4), you can see that by allowing time for ventricular filling, the stroke volume increases the myocardial fibre length, which in turn increases the tension and therefore the force of ventricular contraction. This therefore contributes to cardiac output.

The importance of the interval between the P-wave and ventricular contraction (the P–R interval) is clear. A P–R interval long enough for complete ventricular filling will enhance cardiac output. A reduced P–R interval will decrease cardiac output. Following the P–R interval, atrial repolarization takes place but is obscured by the QRS complex.

Initial depolarization of the ventricles is from left to right through the septum, while through the ventricular wall the current passes from the endocardial surface outwards. As the left ventricle has more muscle mass than the right it exerts a greater influence on the ECG. This is depicted by the QRS complex (Fig. 6.8). The breadth of this complex describes the length of time for electrical activity to depolarize the ventricular cells. If widened, it may indicate abnormal conduction through the ventricles.

The S–T segment follows the QRS complex and represents the end of ventricular depolarization and the start of repolarization, also referred to as the refractory period, during which coronary artery perfusion takes place. This should be an iso-electric (flat) line gently curving towards the T-wave (Fig. 6.8).

S–T segment abnormalities, predominantly elevation or depression of the S–T segment, are referred to in Chapter 9 with reference to the identification of myocardial ischaemia, injury or infarction.

The final wave of the ECG is the T-wave, representing repolarization of the ventricles. The Q–T interval, measured from the beginning of ventricular depolarization to the end of repolarization (Q-wave → end of T-wave) represents ventricular ejection. It has an inverse relationship to the heart rate and varies with

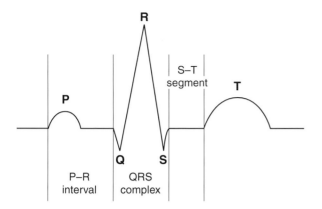

Figure 6.8 The ECG complex.

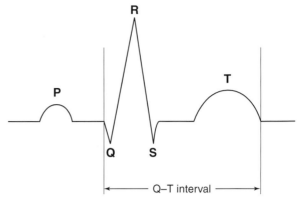

Figure 6.9 The Q–T interval represents depolarization and repolarization of the ventricles and ranges from 0.3–0.4 s.

age and gender. Hence the QTc is sometimes recorded, which is the Q–T interval corrected for a heart rate of 60 beats per minute (bpm) (Fig. 6.9).

To summarize these points:

- normal P–R interval = 0.12–0.2 s (3–5 small squares)
- Q-wave = first large negative deflection after the P-wave = 0.04–0.12 s (three small squares)
- R-wave – first positive deflection <13 mm amplitude (height from the iso-electric line) around 0.3–0.4 s
- S-wave = first large negative deflection following the positive upright deflection.

When referring to the QRS complex, lower or upper case letters are used to describe the relative size. The term q-wave will be used when the deflection is small, while Q-wave will be used to describe a large deflection.

THE CARDIAC AXIS

Six views of the electrical activity of the heart are possible by using the standard limb leads and the hexaxial reference system is frequently used to describe this plane (Fig. 6.10). With only 30° angles of unknown electrical activity between each lead, it enables a reasonably accurate assessment of the axis of the heart.

The mean electrical activity through the ventricles is used to determine the axis of the heart. Through the ventricles the vectors swing progressively towards the left due to the increased electrical activity of the larger left ventricle. The mean vector (mean electrical activity) travels towards the left and downwards and so towards the positive pole of lead II. Matching this to

the hexaxial reference system, we can see that the normal axis is around +60°.

- Normal axis = 0 to +90°.
- Left axis = 0 to –90°.
- Right axis = +90 to +180°.

Recalling how the wave of electrical activity affects the waveform, we are able to determine the direction of the mean flow of current. Therefore when assessing the six standard limb leads, the lead with the greatest deflection indicates the greatest mean vectors in that plane. Hence if the mean vectors travel towards lead II, it will have the largest positive deflection on the ECG. If the mean vectors travel away from a lead, it will produce a large negative deflection. As the electrical current travelling perpendicular to a lead produces a biphasic wave, that can also be added to our equation. Hence the principles for axis determination are as follows.

- Step 1. Examine the six standard leads to identify the lead that is most positive, most negative and biphasic.
- Step 2. Look at the lead perpendicular to the biphasic lead.
- Step 3. If the deflection in the lead you are now looking at is positive, then this shows the direction of the axis. If it is negative, then the opposite pole is the direction of the axis.

See Case studies 6.1 and 6.2.

Where a myocardial infarction results in a large portion of ventricular mass becoming dysfunctional then the cardiac axis will shift away from this area. Hence a large infarct of the inferior wall may result in LAD, while an extensive lateral infarct may lead to RAD.

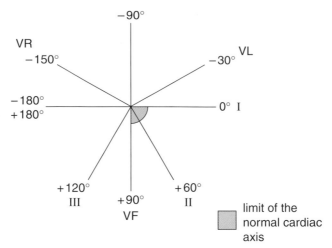

Figure 6.10 The hexaxial reference system. (Reproduced with permission from Hampton JR 1997 The ECG Made Easy 5E. Churchill Livingstone, Edinburgh.)

INTERPRETING THE HEART RATE

We can add to our knowledge of the waveform by assessing the heart rate. Using the squares of the recording paper, we can calculate this as:

- one large square = 0.2 s
- 300 large squares = 1 min.

Clearly we cannot count the number of waveforms in 300 squares so an easier option is to count the number of large squares between two complexes and divide this into 300.

Hence:
three large squares = 100 bpm
four large squares = 75 bpm
six large squares = 50 bpm.

Box 6.1 Causes of axis deviation

Causes of left axis deviation (LAD)
- Emphysema
- Cardiomyopathy
- Left bundle branch block
- Mechanical shifts due to factors such as expiration, pregnancy, ascites

Causes of right axis deviation (RAD)
- Respiratory disorders with right ventricular hypertrophy
- Right bundle branch block
- Congenital heart abnormalities with dominant right-sided heart chambers

---

This method only provides a guide and will not help assess the heart rate in the presence of a very irregular rhythm.

Rhythm interpretation

Analysis of cardiac rhythms requires an assessment of the ECG. Hence the principles of arrhythmia recognition require an assessment of the following.

- Rates: of the P-wave and QRS complex
- P-wave: shape, size and regularity
- P–R interval: length
- QRS: shape, size and regularity
- S–T segment
- Determine the cardiac axis.

12-lead ECG interpretation

Using the principles already discussed, it is possible to analyse a 12-lead ECG and Figure 6.11 shows the standard format. When reviewing a 12-lead ECG it is often easiest to start by looking at lead II.

The P-wave is a small dome-shaped deflection and so indicates normal conduction through the atria. The P–R interval = 0.2 s (five small squares) and is within normal parameters, indicating normal conduction through the AV node. The Q-wave = 0.08 s (two small squares) and is within normal parameters, indicating normal conduction through the ventricles.

A P-wave precedes each QRS complex so each beat initiated in the atria is conducted through to the ventricles. From this assessment it is possible to determine that there is normal conduction through the heart. The heart rate can be estimated. As there are 2.5 large squares between each QRS complex a heart rate of around 120 bpm can be estimated. It can be concluded, therefore, that the ECG demonstrates a sinus tachycardia.

However, when applying these same principles to the 12-lead ECG in Figure 6.12 it is possible to see that in leads II, III and aVF, the S–T segment is elevated to 2 mm (two small squares), above the iso-electric line. As these leads assess the electrical activity of the inferior surface of the heart it is possible to suggest that electrical activity in the ventricular cells of the inferior surface of the heart is abnormal. The reason for the elevated S–T segment is unclear although it has been suggested that the loss of resting membrane potential of damaged cells causes the iso-electric line to be depressed, resulting in a falsely elevated S–T segment (Wagner & Marriott 1994). As these changes are seen in three contiguous leads, they are suggestive of an inferior wall myocardial infarction. This diagnosis should be confirmed by the clinical assessment of the patient.

The 12 leads provide a picture of the electrical activity at various points. As electrical activity travels towards a lead, an upright deflection will be produced on the ECG. When reviewing Figure 6.11 it is clear that lead II shows a positive deflection to the QRS complex and therefore suggests that electrical activity is moving towards this lead. However, by reviewing the principles of determining the cardiac axis, lead I shows the largest positive deflection and so it may be assumed that the mean vectors are travelling towards this lead. This can be confirmed through using all the steps for cardiac axis determination.

- Step 1. Lead I is most positive, aVR is most negative, aVF is biphasic.
- Step 2. The lead perpendicular to the biphasic lead is lead I.
- Step 3. The deflection in lead I is positive. The direction of the axis is towards this lead. From the hexaxial reference system the angle is determined at 0° (a normal axis). A 12-lead ECG, with a normal cardiac axis, should always demonstrate a negative deflection in lead aVR.

The six precordial leads continue to enhance the picture of electrical activity through the ventricular wall. Electrical activity through the ventricles travels from the endocardial surface towards the epicardial surface. Hence, where the ventricular muscle wall is thickest, the deflection of the QRS complex will produce the largest positive deflection in these precordial leads. As V1–V2 are positioned to look at the electrical activity of the right ventricle, in health the smaller muscle mass, the deflection will be downwards as most of the electrical activity moves away from these leads. Lead V3 is positioned to assess the electrical activity of the septum, where electrical activity neither travels directly away from nor towards this lead; hence the deflection should be biphasic. Leads V4–V6 travel progressively around the left side of the thorax and therefore indicate the electrical activity of the left ventricle and should all produce upright, positive deflections.

As lead V5 is positioned around the area of thickest muscle, this should have the largest positive deflection. This picture of the QRS complex in the precordial leads can be seen in Figure 6.11 and demonstrates what is termed **R-wave progression**. This is useful for assessing the thickness of the ventricular walls and also the activity of the muscle. Therefore, for example, if there is death to an area of tissue in the left ventricle, the R-wave assessing this area of muscle would not demonstrate the expected deflection and the R-wave progression would be abnormal.

ARRHYTHMIA FORMATION

There are two major causes for arrhythmia formation: altered automaticity and the re-entrant phenomenon.

Altered automaticity

Again, from Chapter 4, you will recall the principles of cardiac cell automaticity and the threshold potential for rhythm initiation of –60 mV (see Figure 4.10A). Therefore the cells can spontaneously depolarize at this voltage. Pacemaker cells (such as the SA node) have a steep slope to phase 4 of the action potential. If this is altered then the principle of automaticity will be affected. The slope of phase 4 is steep in the following situations, leading to enhanced automaticity: hypoxia, hypokalaemia, hyperthermia and sympathetic nervous system stimulation. It is decreased in hyperkalaemia, hypothermia and parasympathetic nervous system stimulation.

Excitability is the property of responding to a stimulus. In a refractory state, the cell is not able to respond to the stimulus because the cell voltage is not sufficiently negative. During the latter phases of repolarization (the lower slope of the T-wave), the cell may be stimulated, leading to what is referred to as the R-on-T phenomenon.

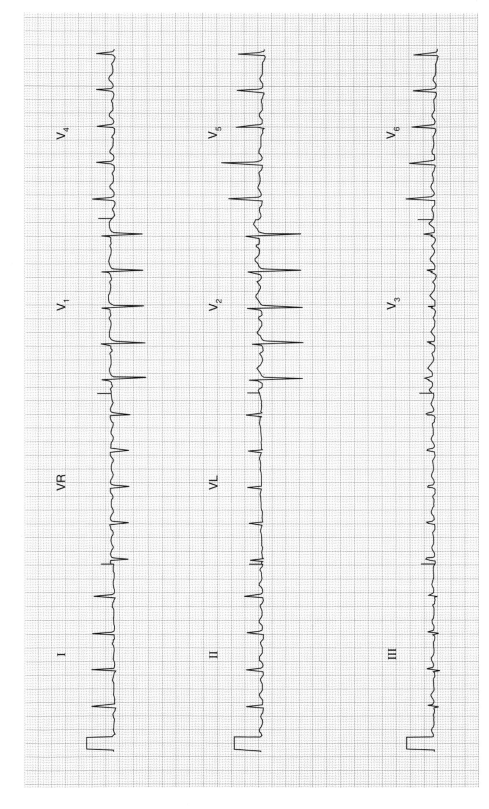

Figure 6.11 12-lead ECG demonstrating a sinus tachycardia. (Reproduced with permission from Hampton JR 1997 The ECG Made Easy 5E. Churchill Livingstone, Edinburgh.)

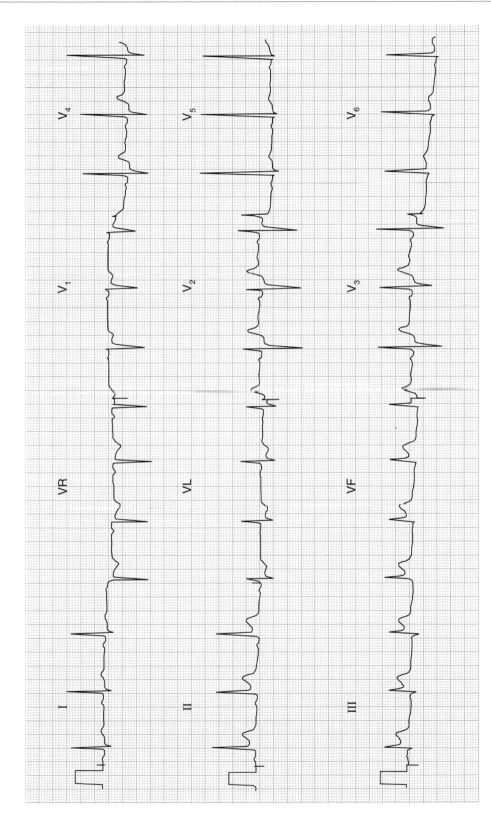

Figure 6.12 12-lead ECG demonstrating an inferior wall myocardial infarction. (Reproduced with permission from Hampton JR 1997 The ECG Made Easy 5E. Churchill Livingstone, Edinburgh.)

Re-entrant phenomenon

This may occur in areas of the heart where conduction is slowed. The impulse is conducted through the healthy cells, followed by the cells with slowed conduction. Re-entry occurs when this conduction is slow enough to allow previously stimulated cells to pass their refractory stage and hence be able to propagate the impulse again. If the impulse travels down the re-entry circuit once only then a single abnormal beat will result. However, the re-entry circuit may be repeated, leading to a more sustained rhythm such as a tachycardia. If this circuit is in a small portion of the heart such as the atria, then it is termed a micro re-entry circuit; if it bypasses the AV node and involves ventricular tissue, it is termed macro re-entry.

Sinus rhythms

The SA node is the pacemaker of the heart. This means that in health it is the over-riding rate setter. As such, the SA node has the property of spontaneous depolarization at a rate of 60–100 bpm. This is controlled by the sympathetic and parasympathetic nervous system to a rate of approximately 70 bpm. As sinus rhythm (Fig. 6.13) represents the normal rhythm of the heart the criteria referred to in the explanation of the normal waveform should be present. Normally the SA node has the steepest slope to phase 4 of the action potential and so depolarizes earlier than the other cardiac cells. This explains why in health it is the pacemaker of the heart, initiating the heart beat.

Sinus bradycardia

Sinus bradycardia (Fig. 6.14) occurs when the SA node takes longer to depolarize than usual. In other words, the slope of phase 4 of the action potential is decreased and the cell takes longer to reach its threshold potential. The rhythm has all the criteria for normal sinus rhythm but at a rate below 60 bpm.

As the heart rate is a component of cardiac output (cardiac output (in litres per minute) = heart rate × stroke volume), a sinus bradycardia may lead to a decreased cardiac output, although generally it is well tolerated. A fall in cardiac output may occur where coronary heart disease (CHD) has led to poor ventricular function and the heart is unable to increase its stroke volume as a compensatory mechanism. A bradycardia may also reduce coronary artery perfusion. For a fuller explanation of cardiac output and stroke volume, refer to Chapter 4.

The slope of phase 4 and hence automaticity are reduced in cells distal to the SA node as they are not normally the pacemaker cells of the heart. However, if the sinus rate falls below the intrinsic rate of subsidiary pacemaker cells, the cardiac rhythm may originate as an escape rhythm. For example, if the SA node rate falls, then the cells in an area with the next highest rate of automaticity (atrial tissue or AV node area) may take over this role.

Box 6.2 Primary causes of sinus bradycardia

- Stimulation of the vagus nerve through, for example:
  - carotid sinus massage
  - vasovagal attacks
  - vomiting
  - β-blockers
- Hyperkalaemia
- SA node disease or ischaemia
- Myocardial infarction affecting the blood supply to the SA node

---

Sinus tachycardia

Sinus tachycardia (Fig. 6.15) results in a normal sinus beat but at a rate greater than 100 bpm. In order to depolarize at this faster rate, the slope of phase 4 of the action potential is increased so the threshold is reached more quickly. Due to the action of the AV node, the rate rarely exceeds 150 bpm in adults.

As the diastolic time, enabling coronary artery perfusion and ventricular filling, is reduced at heart rates above 130 bpm, a sinus tachycardia may result in a fall in cardiac output, together with a reduced myocardial blood supply. Sinus tachycardia also increases myocardial work and may extend the size of a myocardial infarction (MI). Following a MI, sinus tachycardia may indicate poor left ventricular function and is therefore associated with a poor prognosis in the initial period. In conjunction with mitral stenosis, a tachycardia will

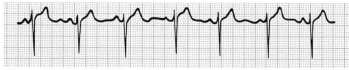

Figure 6.13 Sinus rhythm. (Reproduced with permission from Hampton JR 1997 The ECG Made Easy 5E. Churchill Livingstone, Edinburgh.)

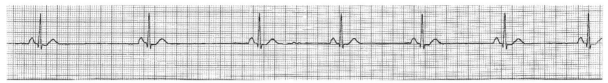

Figure 6.14 Sinus bradycardia. (Reproduced with permission from Hampton JR 1997 100 ECG Problems. Churchill Livingstone, Edinburgh.)

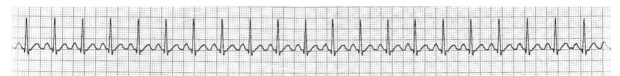

Figure 6.15 Sinus tachycardia. (Reproduced with permission from Hampton JR 1997 The ECG Made Easy 5E. Churchill Livingstone, Edinburgh.)

further decrease ventricular filling, leading to an increased chance of pulmonary oedema developing.

Sinus arrhythmia

Sinus arrhythmia (Fig. 6.16) occurs when there is a cyclic variation to the sinus rhythm. Commonly this occurs in response to changes in vagal nerve stimulation associated with changes in intrathoracic pressure. Therefore at the end of inspiration the SA node speeds up a little and slows down at the end of expiration. It is associated with health and found more frequently in young adults. If the cyclical pattern is not associated with respiration then sinus arrhythmia may indicate SA node disease.

Box 6.3 Primary causes of sinus tachycardia

- Stimulation of the sympathetic nervous system through, for example:
  pain
  anxiety
  stress
  hyperthyroidism
  isoprenaline or adrenaline administration
  physiological response to hypotension
  hypovolaemia
- Compensation for low stroke volume such as in left ventricular failure, where an increase in heart rate will help to raise the overall cardiac output

---

Atrial rhythms

Due to the property of automaticity within cardiac cells, the atrial cells may initiate the impulse and take over the SA node function as the heart's pacemaker. This may be due to changes in the resting membrane potential caused by increased levels of catecholamines, stretched atrial fibres (as in left atrial enlargement) or drug therapy. The consequent unco-ordinated activity may lead to a fall in cardiac output.

Atrial fibrillation

Atrial fibrillation (AF) (Fig. 6.17) is probably one of the more commonly recognized arrhythmias and is frequently found in the elderly (Kern 1998). Although it may occur in paroxysms, it is likely to become a chronic, established rhythm if left untreated, or to become unresponsive to treatment, for a period greater than 3 weeks.

In atrial fibrillation the atria fire at a chaotic and disorganized rate from several foci with multiple micro

---

Box 6.4 Primary causes of sinus arrhythmia

- Normal if related to respiration
- Inferior myocardial infarction if not related to respiration

---

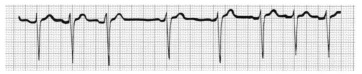

Figure 6.16 Sinus arrhythmia. (Reproduced with permission from Hampton JR 1997 The ECG in Practice 3E. Churchill Livingstone, Edinburgh.)

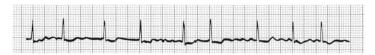

Figure 6.17 Atrial fibrillation. (Reproduced with permission from Hampton JR 1997 The ECG in Practice 3E. Churchill Livingstone, Edinburgh.)

re-entry circuits forming throughout the atria. As a result there is an irregular ventricular response leading to the classic ECG waveform of an irregular heart rate with no definable P-waves. Fibrillatory waves are seen on the ECG as a wavy line, with the ventricular response indicated by an irregularly spaced QRS complex. The ventricular response is normal and the QRS complex has a normal shape and size. Occasionally the atrial beat is conducted to the AV node and bundle branches when they are still refractory (phase 3 of the action potential), leading to aberrant conduction and an abnormal shape to the QRS complex.

Transient AF may frequently occur following cardiac surgery (Sideris et al 1994). This may be for a number of reasons, ranging from cellular disorders, ischaemia and electrolyte imbalance to acute stretch of left atrial tissue caused by sudden increases in afterload or preload. Clinically, atrial emptying is reduced, leading to reduced ventricular filling and cardiac output. Some patients may notice symptoms only when exercising, when they are more susceptible to the reduced cardiac output. The reduced atrial emptying becomes most noticeable when AF is associated with mitral stenosis, when it may worsen pulmonary congestion.

Atrial fibrillation is diagnosed on an ECG but may be suspected when there is a pulse deficit between the apex and radial counts or the patient complains of the symptoms of poor cardiac output. The risk of a cerebrovascular event is increased in patients with AF due to the formation of atrial thrombi in the fibrillating atria. This risk of embolism is greatest during the first year from onset and the use of an anticoagulant in patients with AF is now recommended. Unfortunately for some patients, atrial fibrillation is only diagnosed once they have suffered a cerebrovascular accident (CVA).

Atrial flutter

Here a micro re-entry circuit originates in an abnormal focus within the atria and conducts in a pathway around the atrial tissue in the region of the vena cavae and tricuspid ring. The atria may depolarize at a rate of 300 bpm but are blocked by the AV node, usually to a regular, slower ventricular rate. This results in fast flutter waves (with a saw tooth appearance; Fig. 6.18), representing atrial contraction which is blocked in a regular pattern. Consequently there may be four flutter waves to every ventricular beat. This would be termed a 4:1 block. The rate of block by the AV node is constant but could be 2:1, 3:1, 4:1, etc., depending on the rate of atrial beats.

As the atria do not contract well and blood stasis occurs, thrombus formation within the atria may occur but is less common than in AF. This is due to the stronger and more regular atrial contraction that occurs.

Premature atrial contraction (PAC) or atrial extrasystole/ectopic

PACs may precede the onset of AF or supraventricular (narrow complex) tachycardia (SVT). The stimulus is initiated from irritable atrial cells due to the myocardial cells' intrinsic property of automaticity. The pathway is abnormal, resulting in an abnormal and premature P-wave. If the ventricles are fully repolarized then the premature P-wave will be followed by a normal QRS complex (Fig. 6.19). However, if the bundle branches are not fully repolarized, a

---

Box 6.5 Primary causes of atrial fibrillation

- Left atrial enlargement (acute/chronic)
- Ischaemia/hypoxia
- Coronary heart disease
- Heart failure
- Valvular disease, notably mitral stenosis
- Thyrotoxicosis
- Alcoholism

Box 6.6 Primary causes of atrial flutter

Coronary heart disease
- Right atrial enlargement
- Heart failure
- Chronic pulmonary disease
- Thyrotoxicosis

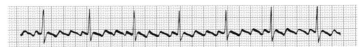

Figure 6.18 Atrial flutter with 3:1 block, i.e. there are three flutter waves to every ventricular conducted beat. (Reproduced with permission from Hampton JR 1997 The ECG in Practice 3E. Churchill Livingstone, Edinburgh.)

wide QRS complex will follow, indicating aberrant conduction through the bundles and ventricular cells. Occasionally the premature atrial contraction will occur so early that all the cells are in their refractory period. The impulse cannot be propagated and no QRS complex will following the P-wave.

As PACs may be rapid, the importance of the AV node in slowing conduction to the ventricles is clear. If not inhibited, a tachycardia could develop, dramatically reducing the cardiac output.

Paroxysmal atrial tachycardia (PAT)

Atrial tachycardia is a rapid rhythm occurring at a rate of 150–200 bpm. The origin may be an abnormal focus or a re-entry circuit. When the rhythm abruptly starts and stops it is termed paroxysmal (Fig. 6.20). As the AV node functions to slow ventricular response, not all these impulses are necessarily conducted, leading to a paroxysmal atrial tachycardia with block. As the rhythm is regular with co-ordinated atrial and ventricular activity, the effect upon cardiac output is less severe than in atrial fibrillation, where the reduced cardiac output is due to the unco-ordinated activity between the two chambers.

Supraventricular tachycardia (SVT) or narrow complex tachycardia

This term is used for any tachycardic rhythm originating from a focus above the ventricles, but where the exact origin is uncertain. Therefore it may be seen as an umbrella term for atrial flutter, atrial tachycardia or junctional tachycardia where the focus is situated within the junctional tissue of the AV node. As a tachycardia the rate is greater than 100 bpm and may be as fast as 280 bpm. The P-wave is unclear or not present, indicating an uncertain origin for the arrhythmia. The QRS complex may be normal if the ventricular cells can conduct the rhythm or, as is more commonly seen, is narrow (Fig. 6.21).

However, if the impulse passing through the AV node is early and meets the bundle of His when it is refractory, then it will be conducted with a wide QRS complex indicative of aberrant conduction. As the right bundle has a longer refractory period than the left, the aberrant beat is generally conducted with a right bundle branch block (RBBB) pattern. In practice, it may be difficult to differentiate between SVT with aberrant conduction and ventricular ectopic beats and it may be necessary to rely upon clinical signs.

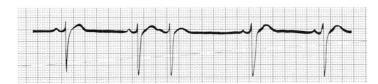

Figure 6.19 Premature atrial contraction or atrial extrasystole/ectopic. The atrial beat is seen early, followed by a normally conducted ventricular beat. (Reproduced with permission from Hampton JR 1997 The ECG in Practice 3E. Churchill Livingstone, Edinburgh.)

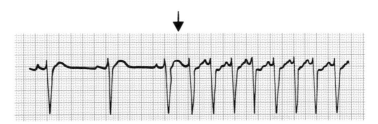

Figure 6.20 Paroxysmal atrial tachycardia. (Reproduced with permission from Hampton JR 1997 The ECG Made Easy 5E. Churchill Livingstone, Edinburgh.)

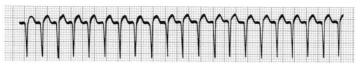

Figure 6.21 Supraventricular tachycardia. (Reproduced with permission from Hampton JR 1997 The ECG in Practice 3E. Churchill Livingstone, Edinburgh.)

As it is a fast rate, the cardiac output can be reduced. The patient may complain of cool fingers and palpitations.

Box 6.7 Primary causes for premature atrial tachycardia or supraventricular tachycardia

- Caffeine intake
- Alcohol
- Nicotine
- Stress (psychological/physiological)

Ventricular arrhythmias

These originate from cells in the ventricular muscle mass or the Purkinje fibres and are considered the most dangerous and potentially life threatening. Due to their effect upon ventricular contraction, they can severely reduce cardiac output.

Box 6.8 Primary causes for premature ventricular contractions

- Myocardial ischaemia
- Hypoxia
- Heart failure
- Increased catecholamines, e.g. due to stress, anxiety
- Alcohol, nicotine, caffeine

Premature ventricular contraction (PVC), ventricular extrasystoles/ventricular ectopic beats (VE)

Due to early depolarization of the ventricular cells, the impulse is conducted abnormally through the ventricles, leading to a QRS complex with a broad and bizarre shape. If the PVCs occur in groups of three or more they are referred to as salvoes. It is only when they become more frequent than around 10/min, if there are multiple sites of origin (multifocal) or they occur in salvoes that they may become dangerous. PVCs are probably one of the most common arrhythmias but in the absence of coronary heart disease are usually benign; however, they may lead to sudden death.

Typically the beat is early and has a wide and abnormal QRS complex without evidence of any prior atrial contraction (Fig. 6.22). If it occurs close to the preceding T-wave it may precipitate ventricular tachycardia (VT) or ventricular fibrillation (VF). When the stimulation for depolarization occurs just after the relative refractory period (or the downstroke of the T-wave) the impulse may be propagated prematurely. This is termed the R-on-T phenomenon. It is very likely that this will precipitate VF.

Ventricular tachycardia (VT)

This is either caused by rapid firing from ectopic foci or macro re-entry circuits and results in rapid impulse propagation within the ventricles. Consequently the causes are the same as those for PVCs. Due to the speed of the rhythm, the reduction in cardiac output is even more severe and may rapidly lead to unconsciousness (Fig. 6.23).

Ventricular fibrillation (VF)

Here there is a rapid, fibrillatory waveform originating in the ventricles, leading to ineffective emptying. Without adequate ventricular contraction, there will be no pulse or cardiac output and without immediate attention, it will become a fatal arrhythmia. It can progress from a coarse to a very fine tracing. The latter is less likely to be terminated by defibrillation and therefore necessitates treatment at the earliest opportunity (Fig. 6.24).

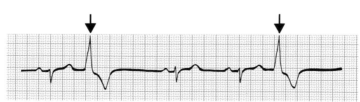

Figure 6.22 Premature ventricular contractions. (Reproduced with permission from Hampton JR 1997 The ECG in Practice 3E. Churchill Livingstone, Edinburgh.)

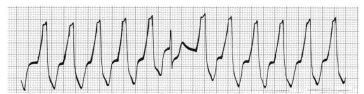

Figure 6.23 Ventricular tachycardia. (Reproduced with permission from Hampton JR 1997 The ECG in Practice 3E. Churchill Livingstone, Edinburgh.)

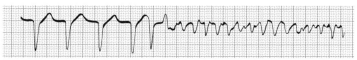

Figure 6.24 Ventricular fibrillation (developing from VT). (Reproduced with permission from Hampton JR 1997 The ECG in Practice 3E. Churchill Livingstone, Edinburgh.)

ATRIOVENTRICULAR CONDUCTION ABNORMALITIES

First-degree AV block

Here the impulse is delayed in the AV node longer than normal and so is seen on the ECG as a P–R interval >0.2 s. All impulses are conducted so there is a P-wave preceding every QRS complex which has a normal configuration, indicating normal conduction through the ventricles. Frequently an asymptomatic arrhythmia, it may precede more severe forms of heart block (Fig. 6.25).

Second-degree heart block

Type I (Wenckebach)

Here the delay in conduction by the AV node progressively worsens over consecutive beats. The P–R interval lengthens until a P-wave is finally not conducted and the sequence starts again (Fig. 6.26).

Type II

This is seen as an intermittent block to the atrial impulse by the AV node and may occur in a pattern of 2:1, 3:1. As there is a consistent pattern of a non-conducted P-wave, it indicates a worse condition than the heart blocks previously discussed (Fig. 6.27).

Third-degree heart block (complete heart block)

Here there is no conduction of the atrial beats to the ventricles. The atria beat at around 60 bpm (under the influence of the SA node) and the ventricles beat at their own intrinsic rate of around 40 bpm. There is complete disassociation between the atria and ventricles and the consequences to the patient are clear. Cardiac output falls with the loss of atrial filling. If this happens gradually, as with fibrosis associated with old age, the normal compensatory mechanisms for reduced cardiac output may maintain homeostasis. It

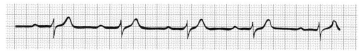

Figure 6.25 First-degree heart block. P–R interval is lengthened to 0.32 s (eight small squares). (Reproduced with permission from Hampton JR 1997 The ECG in Practice 3E. Churchill Livingstone, Edinburgh.)

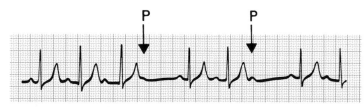

Figure 6.26 Second-degree heart block; Wenckebach. The P–R interval gradually lengthens until a P-wave is not conducted (arrowed) and the sequence starts again. (Reproduced with permission from Hampton JR 1997 The ECG in Practice 3E. Churchill Livingstone, Edinburgh.)

P

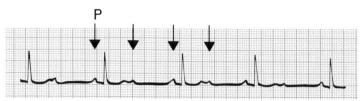

Figure 6.27 Second-degree heart block; 2:1 block where every other P-wave is conducted to the ventricles. (Reproduced with permission from Hampton JR 1997 The ECG in Practice 3E. Churchill Livingstone, Edinburgh.)

Box 6.9 Primary causes of heart blocks

- Coronary heart disease
- Degenerative disease such as fibrosis, ageing
- Infarction of the conduction pathways, e.g. anterior MI
- Inferior MI – usually reversible ischaemia of the AV node
- Valvular heart disease, especially aortic disease
- Acute rheumatic fever
- Atrial septal defect (ASD)
- Surgical heart block
- Dilated cardiomyopathy
- Connective tissue disorders: systemic lupus erythematosus (SLE), sarcoidosis, amyloidosis

---

is only when the cardiac output is not compensated for or the disturbance is sudden (for example, following a MI) that rapid treatment may be necessary. The presence of Stokes–Adams attacks (syncope resulting from a sudden and temporary cessation of cardiac activity of possibly only a few seconds) may indicate third-degree heart block (Fig. 6.28).

THE BUNDLE BRANCHES

Conduction disturbance of the bundles is referred to as bundle branch block and is usually of the right or left bundle. Although the left bundle branch divides into the anterior and posterior fascicles, recognition of left anterior/superior hemiblock is beyond the scope of this text. If either of the right or left bundles is blocked, conduction through the ventricles will be delayed, resulting in a broad QRS complex. Recognition of

which bundle is affected is made through assessing the precordial leads looking at the right and left ventricles – leads V1 and V6 respectively.

Right bundle branch block (RBBB)

As the septum normally depolarizes from left to right resulting in the r-wave in the V1 lead and small septal q-wave in V6, this will be unchanged in the presence of RBBB. The excitation then travels through the left branch to depolarize the left ventricle as normal. However, depolarization of the right ventricle is delayed, leading to a broad QRS complex and a second R-wave (termed R1) in V1 and an S-wave in V6. Hence the QRS >0.12 s and there is a subsequent rSR pattern in V1 (Fig. 6.29).

Left bundle branch block (LBBB)

Here the normal left-to-right depolarization of the septum cannot take place and consequently it depolarizes from right to left. This results in a Q-wave in V1 and R-wave in V6. The right ventricle is then depolarized before the left but due to its smaller muscle mass, exerts less influence on the ECG and causes a small R-wave in V1 and an S-wave in V6. Depolarization of the left ventricle occurs following this, leading to the wide ventricular complex and QRS pattern in V1 and the RSR pattern best seen in V6. This latter configuration is commonly referred to as 'rabbit ears' (Fig. 6.30).

As the initial part of the QRS complex is abnormal, once the diagnosis of LBBB is made, no further

P

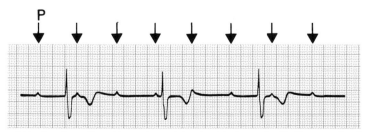

Figure 6.28 Complete heart block, where the atria and ventricles beat independently. Note on the rhythm strip normal P-waves (marked with an arrow) are blocked and hence totally dissociated to the ventricular escape beats. The latter will maintain some form of cardiac output. (Reproduced with permission from Hampton JR 1997 The ECG Made Easy 5E. Churchill Livingstone, Edinburgh.)

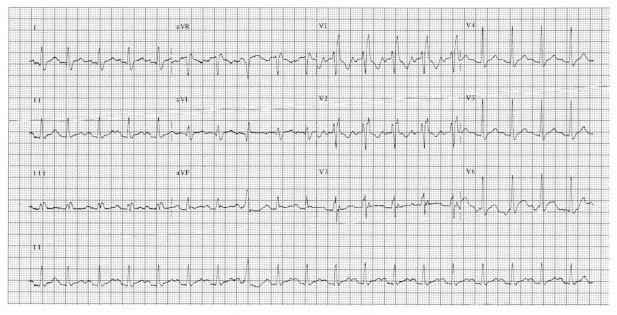

Figure 6.29 Right bundle branch block. Note the rSR pattern in V1 particularly.

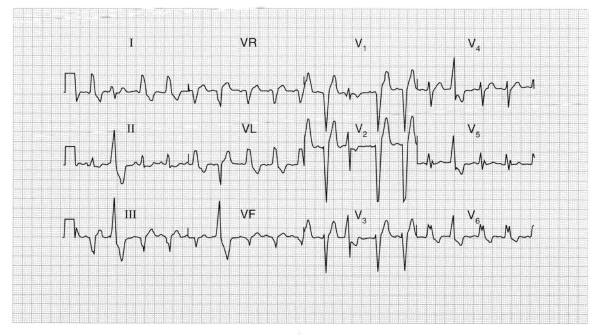

Figure 6.30 Left bundle branch block. Note the presence of ventricular ectopics (extrasystoles) and the M shape ('rabbit ears') notably in V6. (Reproduced with permission from Hampton JR 1997 100 ECG Problems. Churchill Livingstone, Edinburgh.)

Table 6.1 Treatment guide for common cardiac arrhythmias

Rhythm	Treatment
Sinus bradycardia	If symptomatic: atropine 0.5–1 mg (intravenously)
	Occasionally a pacemaker may be necessary
Sinus tachycardia	Treat the cause (usually asymptomatic)
Sinus arrhythmia	No treatment necessary
Atrial fibrillation	Drug therapy such as digoxin or amiodarone
Atrial flutter	Synchronized cardioversion
Premature atrial contractions (PAC)/	Drug therapy such as digoxin or amiodarone
atrial ectopics	Synchronized cardioversion
	Usually no treatment is necessary
Paroxysmal atrial tachycardia	Drug therapy such as digoxin, amiodarone
	Synchronized cardioversion
Supraventricular (narrow complex) tachycardia	Carotid sinus massage/Valsalva manoeuvre
	Drug therapy: adenosine 6 mg (increased in progressive doses if necessary to 12 mg) or verapamil 5–10 mg (intravenously)
Premature ventricular contractions (PVC)/	Check serum potassium levels and correct hypokalaemia if present
ventricular ectopics	Lidocaine (lignocaine) may be used if the PVCs are problematic
Ventricular tachycardia	If pulseless: defibrillation
	If haemodynamically unstable: synchronized cardioversion
	If haemodynamically stable: drug therapy such as lidocaine (lignocaine) 1 mg/kg (intravenously) or synchronized cardioversion
Ventricular fibrillation	Defibrillation
First-degree heart block	Usually no treatment needed
Second-degree heart block	Type I: atropine to increase rate may be considered
	Type II: pacemaker
Complete heart block	Pacemaker usually considered

NB: Synchronized cardioversion refers to the use of defibrillator paddles to terminate an arrhythmia by using an electrical impulse (usually of around 100–200 joules) to rapidly depolarize the heart. It is timed to avoid the T-wave of the ECG and hence the refractory period of the cardiac cycle. Cardioverting at this point could induce ventricular fibrillation.

Box 6.10 Primary causes of bundle branch blocks

Right
- Pulmonary embolism
- Chronic right ventricular strain as in chronic lung disease, pulmonary valve disease, pulmonary hypertension or congenital heart disease
- Coronary heart disease

Left
- Coronary heart disease
- Disease/ischaemia of conduction tissue
- Left ventricular hypertrophy
- Cardiomyopathy

---

diagnostic process can be undertaken using the QRS complex.

Intermittent bundle branch block is a form of aberrant conduction. The bundle (usually the right) is still refractory, leading to re-entry. This usually occurs when the heart rate increases. If the right ventricle enlarges, the right bundle branch has longer to travel and may well show on the ECG as RBBB. As the left bundle branch divides into the two fascicles, enlargement of the left ventricle may not lead to LBBB but to incomplete LBBB and show a wide QRS complex with increased amplitude.

CONCLUSION

This chapter has reviewed how the ECG is formed and recorded for clinical assessment. A huge amount of data regarding the functioning of the heart's electrical activity can be gained from the ECG and interpretation is a matter of understanding the principles, together with practice through analysing examples, preferably within the clinical setting.

The ECG can highlight existing abnormalities, prewarn regarding the potential for a worsening cardiac conduction and is invaluable in guiding treatment in cardiac emergencies where cardiac output is lost. The learning materials available to maintain competence in ECG interpretation are now extensive and the advancement of computer technology allows a huge choice of learning resources to be accessed.

THE PRINCIPLES OF 12-LEAD ECG INTERPRETATION

Case Study 6.1

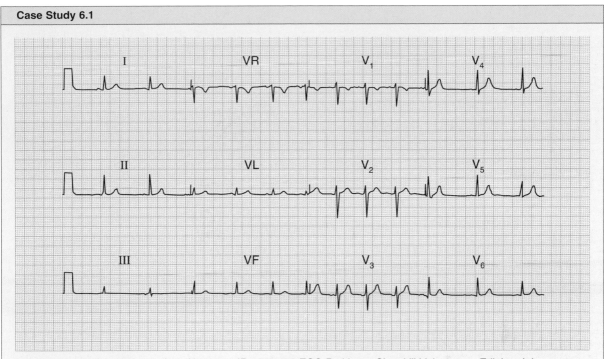

(Reproduced with permission from Hampton JR 1997 100 ECG Problems. Churchill Livingstone, Edinburgh.)

This ECG was recorded on a young man who was fit and healthy. Using the principles described previously, we can start to analyse the recording.
- Rate: P-wave and QRS complex. The P-wave is slightly irregular with roughly five large squares from the beginning of one P-wave to the beginning of the next. By dividing 5 into 300 we can determine that the heart rate = 60 bpm There is one QRS complex to each P-wave, indicating that each beat is conducted through the ventricles.
- P-wave: shape, size and regularity. The duration of the P-wave is two small squares (0.08 s) and dome shaped. This indicates a normal pattern of conduction through both the left and right atria. The P-wave is small but present.
- P–R interval: length = 4 small squares (0.16 s). The P–R interval is within normal limits, suggesting normal atrial emptying.
- QRS: shape, size and regularity. The shape and size of the QRS are normal. The width of the QRS complex is one small square, so conduction through the ventricle is normal. The QRS complex has a slight irregularity to it in time, with some complexes further apart than others.

- S–T segment: This follows the QRS complex and is on the iso-electric line.
- Determine the cardiac axis.

Step 1
Lead II is the most positive lead.
Lead aVR is the most negative lead.
Lead III is the biphasic lead.

Step 2
Lead aVR lies perpendicular to lead III.

Step 3
Lead aVR is negative. Hence the mean electrical vectors travel away from this lead.

The cardiac axis is in the region of 30° and so is within the limits for a normal cardiac axis.

Conclusion
The ECG is normal, indicating normal sinus rhythm. The slight irregularity to the timing of the complexes varies with inspiration and expiration and is termed sinus arrhythmia. This can be normal in young adults.

Case Study 6.2

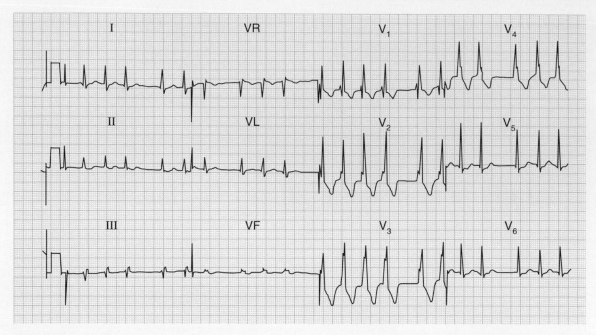

(Reproduced with permission from Hampton JR 1997 100 ECG Problems. Churchill Livingstone, Edinburgh.)

This ECG was recorded from a 60-year-old man. Using the principles of ECG interpretation, we can start to analyse the recording.

- Rate: P-wave and QRS complex. It is difficult to determine any P-waves. A QRS complex is evident but appears irregularly spaced. It is therefore not possible to determine the heart rate using the principles previously discussed. There are approximately two large squares between each QRS complex, so an estimate of the heart rate can be made in the region of 150 bpm. The ventricles are therefore beating at a fast rate, allowing little time for coronary artery perfusion.
- P-wave: shape, size and regularity. The P-waves are not clearly defined and have to be assumed to be absent. The rhythm therefore indicates that the atria are not contracting as one unit and that the cardiac output will consequently be reduced.
- P–R interval: length – indeterminate.
- QRS: shape, size and regularity. The width of the QRS complex is one small square in the six standard leads. However, the shape of the complex is abnormal in the precordial leads, indicating abnormal conduction through the ventricles. Further analysis of these changes indicates a QRS complex of three small squares (0.12 s) which is the wider limit of normal. However, there is a second R-wave in lead V1. From this RSR pattern in lead V1, right bundle branch block can be concluded.

- S–T segment: This follows the QRS complex and is on the iso-electric line.
- Determine the cardiac axis.

Step 1
Lead I is the most positive lead.
Lead aVR is the most negative lead.
Lead aVF is the biphasic lead.

Step 2
Lead I is perpendicular to aVF.

Step 3
Lead I is positive therefore the mean electrical vectors travel towards the positive pole of this lead. The cardiac axis is 0 and is therefore normal.

Conclusion
The ECG has the appearance of atrial fibrillation with right bundle branch block. On examination, the man would be likely to demonstrate the clinical symptoms of a reduced cardiac output such as cool extremities. The atrial fibrillation will result in loss of atrial filling, decreasing the cardiac output. The fast rate is likely to lead to the man complaining of palpitations. The presence of atrial fibrillation and right bundle branch block may indicate that this patient has coronary heart disease.

REFERENCES

Guyton AC, Hall JE 1996 Textbook of medical physiology, 9th edn. WB Saunders, Philadelphia

Kern L 1998 Management of postoperative atrial fibrillation. Journal of Cardiovascular Nursing 12(3): 57–77

Moorman A, Lamers W 1999 Development of the conduction system of the vertebrate heart. In: Harvey RP, Rosenthal N (eds) Heart development. Academic Press, San Diego, pp. 195–207

Sideris D, Toumanidis S, Theodorakis M 1994 Some observations on the mechanisms of pressure related atrial fibrillation. European Heart Journal 15(11): 1585–1589

Thompson D 1983 Specialized internodal pathways. International Journal of Cardiology 4(3): 393–396

Wagner GS 1994 Marriott's practical electrocardiography, 9th edn. Lippincott Williams and Wilkins, Baltimore

7

Interpreting arterial blood gases

Richard Hatchett

The interpretation of arterial blood samples for partial pressure of oxygen, carbon dioxide and acid–base balance is a common requirement of the cardiac nurse, particularly those working in the acute unit areas. The process will utilize samples obtained from either an indwelling arterial line or an arterial 'stab' where a pre-heparinized syringe with a needle is used to access the artery through the skin. In examining the acid–base balance of the body, it is important to remember that all enzyme reactions require an optimal level of pH, that is a maintenance of the delicate balance of acidity and alkalinity, to function adequately. Hinds & Watson (1996) describe a 'metabolic chaos' that may ensue if this balance is not maintained. In this state some reactions proceed faster than they should, while others slow down. Severe metabolic acidosis can cause cerebral and myocardial depression, while the respiratory centre is stimulated initially but subsequently becomes depressed as the acidosis becomes more severe (Hinds & Watson 1996). Conversely, a marked metabolic alkalosis may combine with an associated hypokalaemia (low serum potassium) to depress cardiac function. The body naturally tends towards an acidic state as our metabolic processes tend to produce hydrogen ions (H^+). There is a need therefore for a reactionary system to address this, to maintain the body in a relatively constant state of acid–base balance. When analysing arterial blood samples, this is referred to as the compensatory mechanisms.

pH

The acidity or alkalinity of the blood is measured in pH units. The pH scale runs from 0 to 14 and is logarithmic. Therefore a change of 1 in the pH value means a 10-fold change in hydrogen ion concentration. The pH value of a solution is the negative logarithm of the hydrogen ion concentration in moles per litre (Marieb 2001). A solution is neutral at pH 7. At this point the number of free hydrogen ions equals the number of hydroxyl ions, the latter being dissociated from alkaline hydroxides. Solutions lower than pH 7 are acidic and those higher are alkaline. As highlighted, a pH of 6 has 10 times the number of hydrogen ions as pH 7.

BUFFERS

Within acid–base balance the terms buffers or buffering systems and bases are often discussed. A **buffer** is a substance with the ability to bind and release hydrogen ions (Adam & Osborne 1997). Examples are proteins and other molecules such as phosphoric acid and its salts and haemoglobin. Therefore, the buffering system, as a first line of defence, allows hydrogen ions to be transported from their site of production to the site of excretion with a minimal alteration in the blood pH itself. A **base** is an alkaline substance and an acceptor of hydrogen ions (H^+), for example bicarbonate (Alspach 1998). Below is the example for bicarbonate (HCO_3^-) combining with free hydrogen ions (H^+) to produce weaker carbonic acid (H_2CO_3), which in turn produces carbon dioxide (CO_2 excreted through the lungs) and water (H_2O). This is an example of an effective and rapid buffering system to maintain the acid–base balance in the body.

$$H^+ + HCO_3^- \rightleftharpoons H_2CO_3 \rightleftharpoons CO_2 + H_2O$$

Note that the equation moves in two directions. It therefore effectively buffers the altering pH in a variety of situations. For example, if more carbon dioxide builds up within the patient, such as in respiratory depression, the equation moves to the left and consequently more hydrogen ions (H^+) are produced, increasing the acidity of the blood. Yet if more hydrogen ions are produced, the equation will ultimately move back to the right, with free hydrogen ions being buffered by the bicarbonate base.

Interpretation of arterial blood gases, as with so many other skills, is a matter of understanding the underlying physiology and dedicated practice. This chapter reviews in a pragmatic form the principles of arterial blood gas analysis but does not explore in depth the complete physiology of gaseous exchange and acid–base balance.

OBTAINING AN ARTERIAL BLOOD SAMPLE

It is worth reviewing and emphasizing here the importance of a sterile technique in obtaining an arterial blood sample from an arterial line before exploring the analysis. Chapter 5 discussed the use and placement of an indwelling arterial line in greater depth. Before the sample is obtained the practitioner must wear well-fitting gloves, usually latex, to prevent spillage of blood onto the hands and to reduce crossinfection.

The *Marsden manual of clinical nursing procedures* (Mallett & Dougherty 2000) provides a clear overview of the procedure. The arterial line will have a three-way tap, which ideally should be within 5–10 inches of the arterial line to reduce the need to draw a large amount of infusion fluid from the line to access the blood. Approximately 5 ml of blood are withdrawn with a syringe attached to the port or until the line is clear of infusion fluid. The three-way tap is then turned diagonally to prevent blood leaking out of the port and to close off the infusion fluid from the pressurized bag.

Another syringe, this time pre-heparinized, is attached to obtain the sample. It is usual now to find pre-heparinized syringes on acute units. These contain approximately 60 units of heparin for a 1 ml sample. If the latter are not available, heparin solution of 1000 units per ml can be used and flushed through the syringe. No more than 0.1 ml should remain in the syringe, before drawing about 2 ml of blood into the barrel. It is important not to draw too much heparin into a syringe to prevent overdilution of the sample and, conversely, to avoid a tiny drop of heparin with a large volume of blood. Once the sample is obtained the three-way tap is closed off to the port so that the infusion can be flushed manually via the actuator to clear the line of blood. Mallett & Dougherty (2000) emphasize cleaning the port with a swab of chlorhexidine in 70% alcohol to remove accumulated blood both before obtaining the sample and after, as the cap is replaced.

The arterial sample must be processed immediately to allow an accurate analysis of blood. All air must be expelled from the syringe and a plastic bung placed over the end. This prevents accidental spillage but also seals the blood from atmospheric air, contact with which may affect the accuracy of the reading. Air bubbles will equilibrate with those in the blood, lower the PCO_2 and usually raise the PO_2 of the sample (Hinds & Watson 1996). All new clinical staff are advised to seek assistance from colleagues familiar in using the particular blood gas machine, to ensure the correct procedure is followed for analysis.

An ongoing debate for all health-care personnel is whether data regarding the patient's temperature should be introduced into the machine as the sample is processed. This is commonly called 'temperature correcting' the pH, PCO_2 and PO_2 values. This is based on the observation that large differences in the blood gas values are present when the patient is profoundly hyper- or hypothermic (Shapiro 1995).

There is still no conclusive evidence that we should be temperature correcting samples. Shapiro believes that we do not yet fully understand the complexities of the effects of patient temperature changes on metabolism, vascular function and respiration. Therefore the conclusion at this time remains that corrected and uncorrected blood gas values are of uncertain utility in patients with significant deviations in body temperature. Certainly there appears no clear clinical advantage to using values other than 37°C. Interpretation of the corrected values will also deviate from the familiar guidelines for processing samples at this standard temperature. Of course, it is worth the clinical team discussing these issues, so that all staff are adhering to standard practice. A more ominous scenario would be temperature-corrected values being used alongside other non-corrected measurements. The debate is set to continue until further physiological data and clinical evidence become available.

PARAMETERS

Box 7.1 highlights what each of the parameters from the arterial blood gas analysis indicates.

The analysis printout will also often provide other details such as the serum potassium level (3.5–4.8 mmol/l), haemoglobin (Hb) level (adult men 12–17 g/100 ml and adult women 11–17 g/100 ml) and the oxygen saturation of haemoglobin (approximately 95%).

INTERPRETING THE ARTERIAL BLOOD GAS MEASUREMENT

The first step is to have a basic understanding of the presenting condition of the patient. The blood gas results are merely measured parameters and will require interpretation and understanding of what may be occurring. Relating the results to the patient is of vital, as well as logical importance.

The blood gas results will inform you whether the following are occurring.

- A respiratory acidosis or alkalosis.
- A metabolic acidosis or alkalosis.
- A combined (mixed) metabolic and respiratory acidosis or alkalosis.
- Whether the body has initiated any compensatory mechanisms to correct the above.

An acidosis or alkalosis of respiratory origin indicates that the body is having difficulty eliminating carbon dioxide and carbonic acid is accumulating (**respiratory acidosis**). In cardiac patients a more common cause of

---

Box 7.1 Arterial blood gas analysis: interpretation of parameters

pH units 7.35–7.45
The pH measures the level of free hydrogen ions (H$^+$) in the blood sample. An accumulation of free hydrogen ions results in an acidosis (an acid blood). A depletion causes an alkalosis (the blood is alkalotic). An acidosis results in lowering of the measured pH while an alkalosis results in a figure above the normal range.

PaCO$_2$ 5–6 kPa or 38–42 mmHg
Commonly written just as PCO$_2$, this measures the arterial carbon dioxide pressure in the blood. Carbon dioxide is in itself not acidotic but with water it produces acidic carbonic acid (H$_2$CO$_3$).

PaO$_2$ 10–13 kPa or 80–100 mmHg
Commonly written as PO$_2$, this measures the arterial oxygen pressure in the blood.

HCO$_3^-$ (actual) 24 mmol/l (range 22–26 mmol/l)
This is the measure of the serum bicarbonate concentration in the blood. Bicarbonate is an alkaline solution and can act as a buffer or a base. A base has the property of combining with free hydrogen ions (H$^+$) and thus reducing the effects of accumulated metabolic acids in the blood. Bicarbonate's measured decrease therefore indicates the presence of a metabolic acid in the blood.

The **standard bicarbonate** is used to assess the contribution of metabolic factors, while disregarding changes due to alteration in PaCO$_2$. The standard bicarbonate is therefore the amount of bicarbonate that would be present in a particular blood sample if the PaCO$_2$ were 5.3 kPa (40 mmHg), the temperature was 37°C and the blood was fully oxygenated at sea level (Hinds & Watson 1996).

B/excess + to –2.5 mmol/l
The base excess was best described by Neutze et al (1982, p. 16): `The amount by which the plasma bicarbonate ion concentration is decreased is called the *base deficit*, which is an assessment of the number of hydrogen ions that have reacted in this way. In most laboratories a base deficit is reported as a negative *base excess*'. Alternatively Hinds & Watson (1996, p. 115) define the base deficit as `a convenient number for calculating the amount of sodium bicarbonate required to correct a metabolic acidosis. It is calculated as the amount of base that needs to be added to or subtracted from each litre of extracellular fluid to return the pH to a value of 7.4 at a PCO$_2$ of 5.3 kPa at 37°C'.

NB: 1 mmHg = 0.133 kPa

---

respiratory acidosis is the administration of too much analgesia which has depressed the respiratory centre and reduced the rate of breathing. The inappropriate use of opiates is an example. The respiratory system fails to excrete sufficient carbon dioxide and a respiratory acidosis results.

Conversely, elimination of carbon dioxide via the respiratory system may be too excessive (**respiratory alkalosis**). The latter occurs in hyperventilation, for example during panic attacks or through mechanical ventilation, where the respiratory rate is set too high.

An acidosis or alkalosis of metabolic origin results from an imbalance in acids that are not respiratory in origin. In the cardiac patient, it may be due to poor tissue perfusion resulting in an accumulation of lactic acid, which results from anaerobic metabolism. Other causes of acid accumulation include renal failure, diabetic ketoacidosis and the ingestion of toxins, perhaps chemical or drugs.

Alkalosis is rare but may be due to excessive vomiting, overzealous nasogastric aspiration with non-return of the aspirate or iatrogenic causes such as the overadministration of sodium bicarbonate. The latter is rare now, particularly with its cautionary use in cardiac arrest situations. Depletion of the extracellular fluid volume and a reduction of total body potassium levels are both important precipitating factors of metabolic alkalosis. Contraction of the extracellular compartment causes increased sodium reabsorption by the kidneys in exchange for the acidic hydrogen ions (H^+). Similarly, potassium depletion causes the kidneys to retain potassium in exchange for the hydrogen ions (Hinds & Watson 1996).

pH

Firstly look at the pH. This will indicate whether there is a presenting acidosis <7.36 or an alkalosis >7.42.

Cause

Secondly, try to ascertain the cause. If it is respiratory in origin, the PCO_2 will have altered and may be higher or lower than usual. If it is higher then carbon dioxide in the form of carbonic acid is accumulating. If it is lowered, it could indicate overventilation as the primary cause. However, this is rare and a lowered carbon dioxide level usually indicates a compensatory mechanism by the body in response to high levels of a metabolic acid.

If the PCO_2 is normal, look for a metabolic cause. This will be indicated in the HCO_3^- (bicarbonate) and the base excess. Although the results will record directly the carbon dioxide level, there is no direct measurement of the metabolic acids that may be accumulating. The results indicate their presence by the degree to which bicarbonate levels have dropped in an attempt to buffer (or mop up) the metabolic acid. Therefore a lowering bicarbonate and a corresponding

	pH	CO_2	Bicarb.
Respiratory acidosis	↓	↑	Normal Compensation ↑
Respiratory alkalosis	↑	↓	Normal Compensation ↓
Metabolic acidosis	↓	Normal Compensation ↓	↓
Metabolic alkalosis	↑	Normal Compensation ↑	↑

Figure 7.1 Primary causes of acid–base imbalance.

move of the base excess into a negative figure indicates the presence of a metabolic acid (see Fig. 7.1).

Compensatory mechanisms

Finally, ascertain if the primary cause of the acidosis or alkalosis has initiated any compensatory mechanism. Although there are several mechanisms within the body, the blood gas results indicate the predominant ones. As highlighted above, the carbon dioxide level will drop to compensate for a metabolic acidosis. This means the body is having difficulty eliminating the metabolic acid, which stimulates the respiratory centre and results in hyperventilation. This reduces carbonic acid levels and lowers the overall acid accumulation.

The pH will then tend towards normal, depending on how successful the compensation is. This can be seen to good effect in the diabetic ketoacidotic patient who demonstrates heavy (Kussmaul's) respirations. The change in PCO_2 exhibits a linear correlation with the change in HCO_3^-. The equation predicting the respiratory response to a metabolic acidosis is known as Winter's formula (Hornick 1999). This calculation functions for PCO_2 levels measured in mmHg.

$$\text{Expected } PCO_2 = (1.5 \times HCO_3^-) + (8 \pm 2)$$

If the serum HCO_3^- is measured at 12 mmol/l, then the PCO_2 should be 24–28 mmHg. If it falls outside this range, then an additional respiratory disturbance must be occurring concurrently (Hornick 1999).

In the presence of a respiratory acidosis the renal system will reduce the excretion of bicarbonate to act as a buffer to carbonic acid. Thus, a rise in bicarbonate in the presence of a respiratory acidosis will move the pH towards normal. This is best seen in chronic respiratory disorders such as chronic obstructive pulmonary disease (COPD).

It is important to remember that the compensatory mechanism initiated by the respiratory centre may occur almost immediately, while those involving the bicarbonate levels can take several hours to occur.

CASE STUDIES

Case study 7.1

pH 7.24
PCO_2 7.4 kPa
PO_2 9 kPa
HCO_3^- 23 mmol/l
B/excess −1.5 mmol/l
O_2 sat 93%

pH 7.24 ↓
PCO_2 7.4 ↑
PO_2 9 ↓
HCO_3^- 23 (−)
B/excess − 1.5 (−)
O_2 sat 93% (−)

In this example, it is clear that the patient is acidotic as the pH is below the lower end of normal (7.36). In utilizing the second step of looking for a cause, an elevated PCO_2 can be seen, indicating an accumulation of carbon dioxide, as carbonic acid in solution. Thirdly, in ascertaining a compensatory mechanism, the bicarbonate is seen as normal. If this were a patient with a chronic respiratory disorder, for example, compensation would be seen and the pH would be near or in the normal range.

In assessing this patient, it was noted that he was extremely sleepy, having complained of excessive pain following cardiac surgery. A large amount of opiates had been administered which had depressed the respiratory function. The use of a patient-controlled analgesic device (PCA) may have been more appropriate, if the patient had been able to use this, to provide a more even level of pain control. The partial pressure of oxygen (PO_2) is also lowered.

Result: uncompensated respiratory acidosis due to opiate use.

Case study 7.2

pH 7.31
PCO_2 4.1 kPa
PO_2 12.4 kPa
HCO_3^- 17 mmol/l
B/excess −8 mmol/l
O_2 sat 95%

pH 7.31 ↓
PCO_2 4.1 ↓
PO_2 12.4 (−)
HCO_3^- 17 ↓
B/excess −8 ↓
O_2 sat 95% (−)

This patient was admitted to the coronary care unit in left ventricular failure. He was breathless and had a lowered blood pressure. The results indicate an acidosis with the pH lower than the beginning of the normal range. In looking for the cause, the PCO_2 is noted as slightly low and can probably be accounted for by the breathlessness. It could not therefore possibly account for the excess acid.

In examining the HCO_3^-, it can be seen that a metabolic acid is present as the bicarbonate level has lowered. The base excess in response has also moved into a negative figure. Any compensation for a metabolic acid would come from the respiratory centre and it is fortunate that the PCO_2 has lowered, as this will have moved the pH towards a more normal level. The patient probably has poor tissue perfusion producing an accumulation of acid, notably lactic acid. Two types of lactic acid production exist: type A and type B. Type A is more common and is due to inadequate tissue perfusion, cellular hypoxia and anaerobic glycolysis (Hinds & Watson 1996, p. 118). Type B occurs in the absence of tissue hypoxia. This may be with, for example, diabetic ketoacidosis, severe liver disease, methanol poisoning or ethanol ingestion.

Result: (partially) compensated metabolic acidosis.

Case study 7.3

pH 7.50
PCO_2 5.8 kPa
PO_2 12.3 kPa
HCO_3^- 33 mmol/l
B/excess +7 mmol/l
O_2 sat 95%

pH 7.50 ↑
PCO_2 5.8 (−)
PO_2 12.3 (−)
HCO_3^- 33 ↑
B/excess +7 ↑
O_2 sat 95% (−)

On the cardiac ward this patient had developed gastro-intestinal problems and had been vomiting all day, despite attempts to rectify this. A nasogastric (NG) tube was passed to empty the stomach but the aspirate was thrown away. The pH indicates an alkalosis, because it is above the upper limit of the normal range (7.42).

Case study 7.3 *continued*

In looking for the cause, the PCO_2 is normal. The bicarbonate level, however, is high. This could have resulted from an overinfusion of sodium bicarbonate but you would be aware from the patient history that this had not occurred. What has happened is that excessive vomiting and NG aspiration has altered the acid–base balance in favour of reduced acid, allowing the level of bicarbonate to dominate, resulting in a metabolic alkalosis.

The compensation for this would be a reduced respiratory rate to allow levels of carbonic acid to rise. In reality, an effective slowing in respirations is never a noted compensatory mechanism. In this situation it is rare to encounter a PCO_2 >6.5 kPa (Hinds & Watson 1996, p. 118).

Result: uncompensated metabolic alkalosis.

Case study 7.4

pH 7.20
PCO_2 7.2 kPa
PO_2 8.3 kPa
HCO_3^- 17 mmol/l
B/excess −8 mmol/l
O_2 sat 87%

pH 7.20 ↓
PCO_2 7.2 ↑
PO_2 8.3 ↓
HCO_3^- 17 ↓
B/excess −8 ↓
O_2 sat 87% ↓

This patient was discovered in cardiac arrest in the bathroom of the cardiac ward. It took up to a minute to pull the patient to safety and into an area where effective basic life support could commence. It remained difficult in this confined area.

The pH demonstrates a clear acidotic state. In examining the cause, the PCO_2 can be seen to be elevated, indicating a possible poor ventilatory technique from those initiating basic life support. This level of carbon dioxide dissociated in the blood as carbonic acid will certainly add to the altered pH. In addition, the HCO_3^- has dropped, together with the base excess becoming grossly negative, indicating the additional accumulation of metabolic acid(s). It is impossible therefore to note any compensatory action.

The PO_2 and oxygen saturation indicate poor oxygenation of the patient. The overall blood gas result indicates that basic life support may not be as efficient as it could be.

Result: combined (mixed) respiratory and metabolic acidosis.

Case study 7.5

pH 7.36
PCO_2 7.9 kPa
PO_2 7.8 kPa
HCO_3^- 32 mmol/l
B/excess +7 mmol/l
O_2 sat 86%

pH 7.36 (−)
PCO_2 7.9 ↑
PO_2 7.8 ↓
HCO_3^- 32 ↑
B/excess +7 ↑
O_2 sat 86% ↓

This patient was admitted to the CCU with a diagnosis of myocardial infarction (MI). On admission it was noted that he was having difficulty in breathing, using all his accessory muscles and leaning forward in the bed. His face and lips appeared a dusky colour.

The arterial blood gas indicates a normal pH, although at the low end of the range. However, further examination shows that the PCO_2 is outside the

normal range, being elevated. This would normally produce a respiratory acidosis and a lowering of the pH value yet this is not occurring, so some form of compensatory mechanism must be in place.

Analysis of the bicarbonate indicates an elevated level, together with a base excess in the positive figures. This compensatory mechanism, which is moving the pH to the normal range, would normally take some time to occur, indicating the presence of a chronic respiratory condition. This man has been a smoker all his life and has developed quite severe chronic obstructive pulmonary disease (COPD), in addition to the MI he is now experiencing. Oxygen administration must be kept to a low percentage, due to his respiratory drive now being initiated by low levels of oxygen (the hypoxic drive).

Result: fully compensated respiratory acidosis. Note the term 'fully compensated' is used. When a compensatory mechanism is in place but is not fully effective, it is termed 'partially compensated'.

THE ANION GAP

The anion gap can best be described as the difference between the positively charged cation electrolytes in the blood (chiefly sodium) and the negatively charged anions (chiefly chloride and bicarbonate). The significance of the anion gap is that it increases in the presence of organic acids. It therefore simplifies the possible causes of a metabolic acidosis.

In theory there should be no anion gap (Hatchett 1993). The sum of the serum cations should equal the sum of the anions. However, in reality they do not evenly balance, due to the presence of small amounts of anions that are unaccounted for.

The normal anion gap is therefore ≤ 12 mEq/1 (Hornick 1999). An anion metabolic acidosis produces an anion gap <12 mEq/1. It is calculated as follows.

$$(Na^+ + K^+) - (Cl^- + HCO_3^-) = \text{the anion gap}$$

The anion gap is increased by three factors (Hatchett 1993):

- decreased unmeasured cations
- increased unmeasured anions
- a miscalculation of the sodium, bicarbonate and chloride levels.

As highlighted, it is commonly the increase in organic acids (unmeasured anions) that increases the gap. This can occur with renal failure or ketoacidosis, as in the case of a hyperglycaemic diabetic patient. Drugs capable of increasing the anion gap include salicylates, methanol, paraldehyde and ethylene glycol (the latter is antifreeze, a not uncommon alcohol substitute in vagrant alcoholics).

This chapter has offered the cardiac nurse a pragmatic approach to the analysis of arterial blood samples. It is necessary to relate the recorded results to the patient's underlying condition and to grasp the relationship between the various recorded values in order to understand the compensatory mechanisms that can occur. Calculations such as the anion gap can assist in narrowing down the causes of a metabolic acidosis, when this is not clearly known.

REFERENCES

Adam SK, Osborne S 1997 Critical care nursing: science and practice. Oxford Medical Publications, Oxford
Alspach JG 1998 Core curriculum for critical care nursing. American Association of Critical-Care Nurses. WB Saunders, Philadelphia
Hatchett R 1993 A severe and fatal case of ethylene glycol poisoning. Intensive and Critical Care Nursing 9: 183–190
Hinds CJ, Watson D 1996 Intensive care: a concise textbook. WB Saunders, London
Hornick DB 1999 An approach to the analysis of arterial blood gases and acid–base disorders. Department of Internal Medicine, University of Iowa College of Medicine, US. Website: http://www.int-med.uiowa.edu/education/abg.htm
Mallett J, Dougherty L 2000 The Royal Marsden Hospital: manual of clinical nursing procedures, 5th edn. Blackwell Science, Oxford
Marieb EN 2001 Human anatomy and physiology, 5th edn. Benjamin/Cummings, Menlo Park, California
Neutze JM, Möller CT, Harris EA, Horsburgh MP, Wilson MD 1982 Intensive care of the heart and lungs, 3rd edn. Blackwell Science, Oxford.
Shapiro BA 1995 Temperature correction of blood gas values. Respiratory Care Clinics of North America 1(1): 69–76

FURTHER READING

Williams AJ 1998 ABC of oxygen: assessing and interpreting arterial blood gases and acid–base balance. British Medical Journal 317: 1213–1216

8

Diagnostic procedures

Fiona Halstead
Brian Turner
Stephen Wilson

In considering any medical consultation, whether in the general practitioner (GP) surgery, in a cardiac out-patient clinic or indeed a hospital casualty department, the assessment will comprise the same important considerations when attempting to identify a potential cardiac problem.

- Can a positive assumption of a real problem be made?
- What are the differential diagnoses under consideration?
- What is likely to be the underlying pathology and probable causes and risk factors?
- What is the likely degree of severity of the condition?

The answers to the above questions are based on two major points of reference:

1. the accepted templates for normality and abnormality of patient presentation that have developed through experience over time
2. the medical interpretation of each individual presentation as determined by the experience and knowledge of the diagnostician.

Thereafter consideration of two further issues can be made.

- Is confirmation of the preliminary diagnosis indicated and how is this to be achieved?
- What course(s) of action need to be taken to treat the problem?

Utilizing the above principles, this chapter explores the variety of diagnostic procedures available to those involved in treating and managing cardiac clinical conditions. The information will be useful to nurses involved in explaining the plethora of investigations that may be undertaken, allowing patients to make informed decisions regarding their managed care. Reassurance and explanation regarding each step of the various procedures will not only reduce anxiety for patient and carers but may aid compliance if there is an understanding of what is happening. Nursing staff have always worked with the medical and technical teams involved in the procedures, ensuring a safe environment and assisting in gaining appropriate data to make as accurate a diagnosis as possible.

ELEMENTS OF THE DIAGNOSTIC ROUTE

'The due appreciation of the patient's sensations is essential to a knowledge of the condition of the heart.' (Sir James MacKenzie MD 1916, p. 48)

This statement still remains at the centre of diagnostic procedures, however complex they have now become. At the disposal of each initial consultation process are two principal sources of information.

- Patient history: skilfully gleaned from a series of pointed questions, the subsequent answers and direct observations of the presenting patient.
- Clinical information: derived from the pre-existing physical signs and appearance of the patient, together with findings of direct clinical examination.

Typically any assessment or consultation takes place within 15–30 minutes and during this short period the information that will form the basis for subsequent management must be drawn from the patient. Although attempts have been made to formalize the clinical evaluation process by construction of data sheets and even computerized methods, direct personal assessment has still proved irreplaceable. However, some degrees of standardization have been adopted – for example, the New York Heart Association (NYHA) classification for the level of heart failure disability.

The nature of the complaint must be established as precisely as possible to aid the direction of the ensuing examination. Typically the presentations of cardiac disease may include, but would not be limited to:

- dyspnoea
- precordial (and/or radiating) chest pain
- palpitations
- syncope (a transient loss of consciousness, due to a reduced cerebral blood flow), presyncope or dizziness
- haemoptysis
- cyanosis
- oedema
- embolic event with a possible cardiac implication
- other more general features such as fatigue, fever, a temperature, cough.

A patient history is carefully elucidated with the use of questioning to ascertain full previous medical history (including medication history), occupational history and an assessment of the patient's social and personality profile. Through this an assessment of the predisposing cardiac risk factors (such as age, family history, smoking, diet, obesity, alcohol intake, psychosocial status, physical activity status, etc.) is made, together with some insight into the patient's comprehension, reaction and perspective on the future.

A clinical examination for physical signs of cardiac abnormality is conducted to complete the initial evaluation process. This will include, but again is not limited to:

- assessment of height and weight
- observation of features of the general appearance, specifically including the eyes, mouth, skin, abdomen and extremities
- palpation to examine the characteristics of the arterial and venous pulse
- auscultation to assess the nature of the heart sounds.

The examination process should observe the holistic picture with consideration given to concomitant or multisystem disorders. Generally speaking, a successful diagnosis can be made from a comprehensive patient history and a well-conducted physical examination in approximately 90% of cases. Thereafter, once a preliminary diagnosis has been decided upon, the third element of the diagnostic route, namely selective 'laboratory-based' testing, may be indicated to confirm the suspected condition and validate the degree of severity. In addition to diagnostic information, detailed subsequent testing may also reveal information of important prognostic value.

Today's cardiologists have a comprehensive battery of tests at their disposal, ranging from the simple electrocardiogram (ECG) or chest X-ray (CXR) through to the high technology areas of magnetic resonance imaging (MRI) and cardiac angiography. However, irrespective of the degree of complexity, fundamental to the process is the use of suitably qualified and trained personnel to both perform the tests and similarly to interpret and report on the results obtained.

Selective laboratory testing is usually designed to examine a single feature, or a combination of associated features, in order to demonstrate the likely existence of an abnormality. This is, however, not an infallible exercise, especially where information is inferred rather than directly observed or may be more anatomical than functional in nature. Furthermore, both false-positive and false-negative results may exist

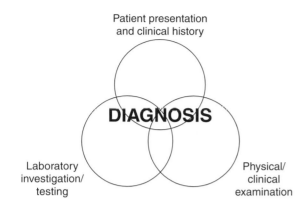

Patient presentation
and clinical history

DIAGNOSIS

Laboratory
investigation/
testing

Physical/
clinical
examination

Figure 8.1 Methods by which cardiovascular abnormalities can be identified.

alongside the reality of true positives and true negatives. As much as possible, these inaccuracies are limited by the refinements of test design and equipment, the fullness to which a test is applied and the interpretive skill applied to the result obtained. It should be remembered that testing may only demonstrate the probability of disease and brief mention should therefore be given to a few statistical terms and considerations of the 'meaningfulness' of a given test.

Two useful measures are **sensitivity** and **specificity**, both of which confer some degree of confidence to the test result, albeit in a converse manner. These are defined by the following equations (where TP = true positives, TN = true negatives, FP = false positives and FN = false negatives):

Sensitivity = true positive result/total tested *with the condition* × 100%, i.e. TP/TP + FN
Specificity = true negative result/total tested *without the condition* × 100%, i.e. TN/TN + FP.

In any patient population sensitivity and specificity will both show their highest values (ideally 100%) where there is a clear boundary for what constitutes a normal and an abnormal test result; that is, one is assured of a high TP count together with an acceptably low FP count. Implicit in this concept is the expectation that both sensitivity and specificity will be improved as the severity of the pre-existing disease state increases. Thus, testing multivessel coronary artery disease (CAD) should reveal higher specificity and sensitivity values than testing single-vessel disease; similarly, testing severe aortic stenosis should enable greater confidence levels in the results than those obtained for the mild disease state.

However, regardless of the disease state, both sensitivity and specificity will be seen to show additional variance in accordance with the particular circum-

stances of a given test. For example, if the definition of positivity is widened then an inverse relationship develops with sensitivity increasing but specificity decreasing (and vice versa). This serves to emphasize the need not only for accuracy but also for uniformity, continuity and standardization in test application.

Once a result has been obtained, whether positive or negative, further validation of the 'meaningfulness' of the test may be gained from its **predictive value** (PV). Predictive value is represented by the following equations:

PV of a positive result, i.e. the test result positively reflects the diagnosis
= true positive results/total tested for condition × 100%
= TP/TP + FP

whereas,

PV of a negative result, i.e. the test result does not reflect the diagnosis
= true negative results/total tested for condition × 100%
= TN/TP + FP.

This measure of 'accuracy' will also show some inherent variation according to a fundamental statistical principle known as Bayes theorem. This states that the predictive accuracy of any test is directly related to the prevalence of the disease or condition within the population under study. In general, patient populations must show inherent variation and consequently PV cannot be derived merely from sensitivity and specificity values.

When a test with a certain sensitivity and specificity is applied to a population with a low prevalence of disease, the calculated PVs will differ from those containing a high prevalence of disease. This statistical concept can be used to illustrate, for example, why routine screening programmes (high true-negative counts) also produce higher false-positive counts when compared to a symptomatic population undertaking a similar test.

In addition to considering single populations such as a symptomatic group, the Bayesian concept introduces the relevance of considering the additive results of different selective tests, together with specific aspects of patient profiling. Profiling may include factors such as age, sex, ethnic origin, concurrent risk factors and so forth that act to redefine the population under consideration and enhance predictive accuracy. For example, a combination of positive test A + positive test B + risk factor C significantly enhances the overall predictive accuracy of a subsequent test result (and hence final diagnosis) beyond that provided by a single factor alone.

> *Note: Of necessity this section represents an oversimplification of the statistical viewpoint by which results can be judged. The concepts can be very complex and although the same principles apply to considerations of routine testing, they tend to be more a feature of research work, trial design and the subsequent manner in which such results are processed and interpreted.*

Once additional testing is indicated, further considerations become integral to the developing clinical process. The physician should inform the patient of the tests that are necessary, including a brief description together with any inherent risks, however small, and gain consent if necessary. Nursing advocacy may be indicated to enhance or supplement the medical input and deal with other important aspects of overall patient care. For example, a patient may require a more detailed description of the test and need the opportunity to voice more individual concerns such as likely time frames, the availability of results, family and home support issues, etc. Additional factors that the nurse may therefore need to consider include evaluation of the patient's psychological and social status, a knowledge of sources of patient education (helplines, pre-admission clinics, discharge planning and so forth), together with a discussion of future needs: lifestyle planning, rehabilitation programmes, etc. Ultimately, the test results need to be carefully explained and again a combination of medical and nursing advocacy may be required to ensure that the patient fully comprehends the significance of the result and its implications.

CLINICAL TESTS

A wide and comprehensive battery of tests are available to investigate the many different aspects of heart disease. For the purposes of this chapter these can be categorized as either cardiological or radiological (diagnostic imaging) procedures, although some commonality may exist. Acknowledgements must also be given to those other hospital services that may be integral to obtaining a full diagnosis, most notable amongst which would be the services of the pathology unit.

The aforementioned degree of commonality may exist between certain cardiological and radiological tests whereby different methods are capable of producing information of a similar nature and often with a similar diagnostic accuracy. The test protocol is therefore selected according to medical preference,

any special circumstances of the particular patient plus considerations of the following.

- Time constraints such as prioritization due to the severity of the condition, waiting lists, etc.
- Risks, complications or indeed contra-indications to certain test modalities.
- Facilities available: the specialist nature of some tests may require referral to a specialist centre.
- Cost; for example, widespread population screening may be the ideal in certain situations but is rarely a cost- or resource-effective option.

From the medical and especially the patient perspective, all tests may be further categorized as being of an invasive or non-invasive nature. Although most procedures can hold some fears for the patient, generally they will be less amenable to tests involving the small but nevertheless inherent risk of complications associated with procedures of a genuinely invasive nature.

The majority of these procedures are of long standing, with detailed descriptions found in many excellent publications (see Further Reading). Constraints dictate that the remainder of this chapter is concerned only with a brief description of the salient features of each procedure, with some mention given to current/future developments.

CARDIOLOGICAL PROCEDURES
Non-invasive

The electrocardiograph

The fundamental mechanisms that generate the electrocardiogram (ECG) commence at a biochemical/cellular level and proceed as an electrophysiological event ultimately to be detected, amplified and printed as an impression on a paper trace for interpretation. Within the clinical evaluation process, the ECG represents a fundamental diagnostic tool as *the* first-line means of assessing potential cardiac problems and is integral to the majority of cardiac clinical evaluations.

An ECG is quick, painless and easy to perform. Tracings can be produced in single or multichannel lead formats. The diagnostic potential generally increases with the number of leads recorded. Conventionally, a standard 12-lead ECG recording covering the main regional aspects of the heart is nominally required. Other lead configurations have been developed such as the XYZ orthogonal system, although nowadays this is mainly confined to specialist and research use.

Each individual 12-lead ECG recording contains a wealth of potentially useful information to the trained eye. Moreover, this information can be further supplemented by continuous 'rhythm strip' recordings or serial recordings from a particular patient, to provide information of a progressive or evolving nature.

The ECG provides information on everything from heart rate to rhythm, from intracardiac electrical conduction defects to the degree of muscle hypertrophy and may indicate valvular dysfunction. Not least, a potential insight into both the chronic and acute ischaemic status of the myocardium can be obtained. Moreover, the diagnostic value of the ECG exceeds that of simply highlighting the current state of affairs, by acting as a pointer to implicate other associated symptoms and lesions. As examples, pathological Q-waves are indicative of previous myocardial infarction, while a combination of a short P–R interval and a pre-excited QRS complex indicates accessory pathway conduction (overt Wolff–Parkinson–White syndrome). Long Q–T intervals and associated T-wave morphologies are suggestive of a possible substrate for ventricular tachycardia (torsade de pointes) and bradycardia, or evidence of a high-grade heart block revealing a possible mechanism for syncopal episodes.

As a development of the standard ECG, the **signal-averaged ECG** (SAECG) is a more specialist tool principally utilized by the electrophysiologist for prognostic purposes. It is based on the rationale that muscle fibres at the border of infarcted territory produce local small electrical activity, termed late potentials, occurring after those of normal myocardial activation. Using surface ECG electrodes (typically the three XYZ orthogonal bipolar leads), a series of several hundred complexes are recorded, electrically processed and filtered to cancel out random noise. This averaging technique produces a single clean composite vector ECG trace, designed to reveal the presence of late potentials that represent a potential substrate region for re-entrant excitation and consequent ventricular arrhythmias. Although exhibiting varying sensitivity as a specific test for a ventricular tachycardia (VT) substrate, a positive SAECG is regarded as being of high prognostic value for the potential occurrence of VT when considered in addition to other known risk factors, such as an established infarct, reduced left ventricular function or complex ectopy. Thus the SAECG represents an important tool in investigations concerning sudden cardiac death, a topic of much current research and investigation.

In the quest for additional 'hidden' information contained within the ECG, certain other features of electrocardiography are currently under evaluation as potential markers for pathological associations and possessing a certain prognostic value. These markers include:

- QT dispersion (i.e. distribution of the QT duration) as an indicator of electrical instability and a propensity for arrhythmic events
- heart rate variability (i.e. beat-to-beat variation in R–R interval) as an independent predictor of cardiac mortality in patients following myocardial infarction
- signal-averaged P-wave (to assess prolongation of the filtered P-wave) as an indicator of vulnerability to atrial fibrillation from global atrial conduction delays
- T-wave alternans (beat-to-beat alternation of the morphology, amplitude and polarity of the T-wave) as an indicator for sudden cardiac death in the setting of ventricular tachycardia.

Holter (ambulatory) monitoring/event recording. It is apparent that the standard 12-lead ECG has a major limitation in that any single recording represents only a snapshot of cardiac activity in the history of the patient. Unfortunately ECG abnormalities are not always quite so obliging as to manifest themselves during the few seconds it takes to generate a 12-lead recording. Hence, principally to assist in the diagnosis of symptom-related bradyarrhythmias and tachyarrhythmias (but equally, at times, to demonstrate the absence of ECG abnormalities during symptomatic episodes), systems were pioneered in the late 1950s by Holter. These were able to record a continuous ECG over a prolonged period of time. Technological developments in Holter monitoring made over the years have been many and varied and many systems are currently commercially available (see below).

The advances made in anti-arrhythmic pharmacology have also enhanced the value of ambulatory monitoring as a relatively inexpensive and accessible tool for the cardiologist. However, with regard to the intended use of these devices, all fall within a few simple categories according to:

- the expected frequency and severity of symptoms
- the required duration of recording (short or long term)
- the degree of patient compliance required.

Fundamentally all recordings are best supplemented with some form of direct patient feedback, either verbal or as a written diary. This allows an ECG abnormality to be linked to patient activity at the time. This may, for example, be sleeping, running for a bus and so forth.

As in many other areas, the current state of advancement in ambulatory monitoring owes much to the advent of digital technology. In addition to a reduction

---

Box 8.1 Types of ambulatory ECG devices

1. 24 (or 48) hour single/dual-channel ECG Holter. These short-term recording devices utilize a continuous 24-hour recording ability to standard audio cassette via direct ECG electrode attachment. To identify relevant points on the recording these devices usually incorporate some form of event marker, activated by the patient at the time of symptoms. The inherent time constraints imposed by the recording method indicate the use of this system for relatively frequent symptoms.

2. For less frequent symptomatic episodes, devices were developed whereby recordings could be initiated by the patient at the onset of symptoms. For convenience, some such devices possess integral electrodes as metal contact plates on the unit to pick up an ECG when pressed against the chest wall. They therefore avoid direct, permanent attachment of ECG electrodes. By utilizing a loop magnetic strip, the recording capacity of such devices was initially somewhat limited compared to the continuous tape system above. However, the development of solid-state recording media in the current generation of devices has significantly increased recording capacity. To facilitate data transfer to the cardiology unit and enable an instantaneous analysis, these units often utilize a transtelephonic link capacity to download recorded information directly via a standard telephone line, enabling an instant response capability. Patient compliance for this type of system is obviously paramount and therefore may not be appropriate for certain elderly patients. Additionally, by virtue of the fact that recording is totally reliant on

patient activation, asymptomatic arrhythmias will be missed.

3. For a similar indication but for specific use where symptoms are severe enough to preclude a warning or debilitate/disable the patient from initiating an immediate recording, the retrospective recorder was developed. Such units necessitate continual attachment via ECG electrodes but possess a retrospective recording ability (via a continual loop mechanism). This is activated by the patient on recovery from a symptomatic episode such as post dizziness, syncope, profound chest pain, etc.

4. The implantable loop recorder represents a refinement of the retrospective recorder. It is a relatively new concept in ambulatory ECG monitoring utilizing aspects of permanent pacemaker technology. As a significantly more costly option at this time but with a power source lasting some 18–24 months, use of this device is limited to the specific indication of particularly infrequent but very severe symptoms such as otherwise unexplained syncope in the young patient. The device is implanted subcutaneously in a pectoral location and possesses the ability to monitor an ECG directly via internal surface contact. Recordings are automatically triggered from programmed upper and lower heart rate limits or may also be patient activated retrospectively (by means of an external telemetry unit) and stored in the device memory. This information can subsequently be downloaded whilst the device is still implanted, using a telemetry link to an appropriate programming unit.

---

in overall device size, other notable features include arrhythmia detection algorithms for automatic initiation of recordings, the use of smart cards (digital media) for data recording and PC/Internet interfacing for the transfer, management and storage of information. Furthermore, as information is digitally processed, additional elements have been introduced into the analytical processes to enable automatic assessments of ECG features, such as heart rate variability and frequency of ectopy.

Ambulatory blood pressure (BP)

These monitoring devices may be considered in a similar way to ambulatory ECG monitoring and utilize auscultation to measure patient blood pressure at timed intervals. This can be used to investigate postural or circadian fluctuation and evaluate the effects of drug treatment. Additional investigative adjuncts may also be integral features of modern units; for example, supplementary information can be gleaned on arterial distensibility in relation to blood pressure.

Exercise tolerance testing (ETT)

Also known as stress testing or exercise testing. This basic extension to 12-lead electrocardiography is utilized to observe the changing nature of the ECG when the heart and cardiovascular system are exposed to increasing aerobic stress. Not all patients are suitable for exercise testing and although not definitive, the following is a list of conditions generally considered as contra-indications to testing.

- Severe aortic stenosis
- Left mainstem coronary disease
- Unstable angina
- High-grade cardiac failure
- Recent myocardial infarction (MI) (within 5 days)
- Hypertension (systolic >220 mmHg, diastolic >120 mmHg)
- Hypotension (systolic <90 mmHg)
- Second- or third-degree heart block
- Recent embolism
- Acute infectious disease
- Acute myocarditis

In addition to the above listing, it must be remembered that there are inherent risks to exercising any cardiac patient and full resuscitation facilities are mandatory to any ETT protocol. The patient is connected to a full 12-lead ECG (with the limb leads modified to the Mason and Liker torso configuration to avoid limb movement artefact). They are continually monitored, together with periodic measurement of the blood pressure during exercise on a treadmill (or cycle ergometer). The exercise regime follows a standardized time/speed/gradient workload protocol (typically Bruce or modified Bruce). The intention of the protocol is to provide both a diagnosis and some quantification of the result. Each test would normally continue to a point where one or more of the following endpoint criteria has been reached. It is acknowledged that different centres may have slightly different termination markers.

- Patient non-compliance (i.e. refuses to continue)
- Patient confused or cyanotic
- Development of pronounced dyspnoea/fatigue/ faintness/vertigo/unsteadiness
- Development of significant retrosternal chest pain or substernal discomfort
- Development of hypertension (systolic >230 mmHg)
- Development of hypotension or a drop in BP during exercise >10 mmHg
- Development of horizontal ST depression ≥2 mm 40–80 ms post J point with accompanying symptoms that are indicative of myocardial ischaemia
- Development of planar ST depression 3 mm 40–80 ms post J point without accompanying symptoms
- Development of arrhythmias (supraventricular (narrow complex) tachycardia (SVT) or ventricular tachycardia (VT)) or frequent multifocal ventricular ectopics
- Attainment/tolerance of submaximal heart rate (representing 85% of maximal heart rate, where maximal heart rate is 220 bpm minus age for a male and 210 beats per minute (bpm) minus age for a female) unless a symptom limited test has been requested

Certain predictable changes to the ECG under stress are considered normal. These include a shortening of the P–R and Q–T intervals, together with more subtle and largely ignorable changes to the P, QRS and T-waves components and the ST segment. However, other more marked morphological changes may indicate the presence of a pathological substrate. In the setting of coronary heart disease, which is the main

indication for exercise testing, the principal function of the test is to assess:

- symptom-related aerobic/exercise capacity
- chronotropic competence (increase in heart rate) and BP response to exercise
- the incidence of exercise-induced arrhythmias/ectopy and the corresponding patient tolerance
- ischaemic status from an evaluation of the ST segmental movement.

All these factors are equally relevant to testing both before and after medical/pharmacological intervention. However, ETT should not be considered as confined to the investigation of coronary heart disease alone and it has a certain role in the evaluation of other disease states. For example, the cardiomyopathies have various direct associations with rate-related left bundle branch block (LBBB), ventricular ectopy, other arrhythmias and atrioventricular (AV) block. Similarly, the effort-induced symptoms of valvular heart disease require full evaluation with regard to an appropriate management strategy. In addition, other patients considered at risk of sudden cardiac death may undergo ETT as part of their work-up to full electrophysiological study (EPS). In the latter case, should internal cardioverter-defibrillator (ICD) device therapy be indicated, exercise testing may play a role in assessing the anti-arrhythmic medication regimen and aid post implant device programming.

Exercise tolerance testing is one clinical area in which the sensitivity and specificity of testing can demonstrate particular inherent variation. Results are dependent on factors such as age, sex and ethnic origin, the extent of the underlying cardiac condition, current medication regimen, the fullness of the test applied and the criteria set for a positive result. Consequently, both false negatives and false positives are not infrequent findings and the predictive value of any result should be carefully considered.

Tilt testing

This is a diagnostic tool developed principally to investigate the propensity to develop vasopressor (or vasovagal) syncope. This is a syndrome in which a spectrum of underlying mechanisms and aetiologies exist that may be cardiac or neurological such as panic, fright, pain, carotid sinus hypersensitivity, micturition, etc. Normally, when an upright posture is assumed, lower body blood pooling acts to reduce arterial pressure. This initiates an initial increase in sympathetic tone, with a corresponding increase in heart rate (HR), BP and levels of circulating catecholamines. This is

mediated via the carotid sinus/aortic arch barorecep-
tor input to the medullary vasopressor region of the
brain-stem. In the abnormal subject this reflex is over-
ridden with suppression of sympathetic tone and
vagal tone over-riding. The consequences are vasodilatation, blood pooling in the lower body, reduced
cardiac filling/cardiac output, bradycardia and possibly presyncope or syncope.

The tilt test protocol involves strapping the patient
to a special table which is then tilted to a head-up
position (60–85° off horizontal) for a period of
40–60 minutes whilst continuously monitoring the HR
and BP response. Time is no predictor of outcome in
tilt testing and overt symptoms of sudden (or more
gradual) bradycardia and hypotension may manifest
at any point. Normality can usually be restored simply
by lowering the patient back to a supine position;
however, as with exercise testing, full resuscitation
facilities are mandatory. A positive result may be categorized according to HR and BP response as:

- type I (mixed response)
- type IIA (cardio-inhibitory)
- type IIB (cardio-inhibitory)
l type III (pure vasodepressor).

It is important to note that the main component of the
vasodepressor syndrome is vasodilatation (rather than
bradycardia), hence only a small percentage of
patients exhibiting syncope or presyncope would
obviously benefit from subsequent dual-chamber
pacing therapy. The diagnostic and prognostic value of
tilt testing is somewhat uncertain. There is a positive
test sensitivity ranging from 30% to 70% for patients
presenting with syncope of unknown origin and a
specificity in the order of 90% (Fogoros 1999).
However, tilt testing continues to represent a useful
tool in patients presenting with syncope of unknown
origin where other non-invasive testing has proven
inconclusive and it remains a useful precursor to full
electrophysiological testing in some patients.

Transthoracic echocardiography (TTE)

This first appeared as a medical tool in the mid 1950s
and as a true non-invasive procedure has dramatically revolutionized diagnostic cardiology. Even
though ultrasound technology has a 50-year history, it
continues to evolve to meet the increasing demands of
cardiology.

Utilizing the principles of sonar (similar to that used
by bats and dolphins), cardiac ultrasound uses sound
waves in the 2–7 MHz band, transmitted from a transducer source. Such ultrasound signals are capable of
penetrating the body where they undergo differential
reflection at tissue interfaces, such as pericardium, heart
wall, blood pools, valves, etc. The same transducer
receives back the reflected waves and these signals are
processed based on timing and intensity characteristics.
The received signals can display the underlying
anatomy in various formats or modalities, each offering
specific qualitative or quantitative information and contributing to the overall diagnostic picture.

The common modes currently in use are termed M-
mode, 2D mode, spectral Doppler and colour flow
Doppler. Visually the most recognizable of these is 2D
(two-dimensional) echocardiography whereby a
picture image is formed by a fan of 'echo' pulses creating a sector that illustrates a sectional cut of the heart.
This picture provides direct anatomical and structural
information about the myocardium, heart valves and
associated structures. The image is continually
updated throughout the cardiac cycle thus illustrating
the relative movements and relationships of the
various heart structures during systole and diastole.
Other echo modalities are used to supplement this
information and help quantify direct observations
made from the 2D mode. For example, measurements
of muscle wall thickness and cavity dimensions are
obtained from M-mode studies, measurements of
blood flow velocity with secondary derivations of
valve area and pressure gradients from spectral
Doppler and qualitative assessment of regurgitant
valve jets from colour-encoded Doppler signals.

To a large degree image quality is dependent on the
ultrasound frequency emitted from the selected transducer. The lower frequencies offer better depth penetration but less resolution and vice versa. The
diagnostic value of TTE is currently somewhat dependent on a reasonable degree of 'echogenicity' on the
part of the patient as certain body tissues, notably
bone and lung (air), represent a poor transmission
medium for ultrasound waves. TTE images are thus
reliant on a good echo 'window' through which the
heart can be 'visualized' from an external chest position, i.e. avoiding rib and lung tissue.

The indications for echocardiography remain widespread but may be summarized as shown in Box 8.2.

As a means of directly observing cardiac anatomy,
2D echocardiography (supplemented by anecdotal
information from other echo modalities) is able to
demonstrate both high sensitivity and specificity for
certain conditions or abnormalities. These include
assessment of left ventricular (LV) function, structural
valve lesions (such as a calcified aortic valve or mitral
valve prolapse) and the presence of a LV thrombus.
However, the shortcomings of TTE should also be

Box 8.2 Primary indications for echocardiography

- Evaluation of murmurs and valve morphology for structural and functional abnormalities. Disease aetiology. Identification and quantification of lesions. Detection of associated abnormalities such as a postinfarct ventricular septal defect (VSD) or mitral regurgitation due to papillary muscle rupture and a flail mitral valve, the presence of intracavity thrombus or a pericardial effusion.
- Ischaemic heart disease (IHD) especially where the ECG is non-diagnostic for regional wall information. As a future development in the postinfarct setting, echocardiography may act as a means to differentiate myocardial scar tissue and help assess ischaemia as transient or chronic in nature.
- Cardiomyopathies – dilated, hypertrophic, restrictive, diastolic dysfunction.
- Constrictive pericarditis, effusions, cardiac tamponade.
- Masses/tumours (intra- and extracardiac).
- Associated vasculature such as aortic aneurysm, aortic dissection.
- General 'screening' for structural abnormalities in the context of syncope or arrhythmias.
- Congenital abnormalities.

acknowledged, with both ultrasound-generated artefact and unfavourable patient 'echogenicity' being potentially problematical to each investigation. Accordingly the value of TTE for certain other indications becomes lessened, for example when required to demonstrate the presence of vegetations in suspected infective endocarditis. Similarly, the overall diagnostic value of TTE is compromised in 'non-echogenic' patients where a poor echo 'window' may exist, for example in those of large build, those suffering chronic obstructive pulmonary disease (COPD) or those in the immediate postcardiac operative period (due to factors such as oedema and swelling).

In some cases where evaluation of regional and global cardiac function is not facilitated by true exercise testing, for example ischaemic changes masked by co-existing LBBB or limitations due to respiratory or mobility issues, alternative methods have been sought to mimic exercise. Stress echocardiography is an investigation increasingly adopted that utilizes pharmacological stress agents to increase myocardial contractility and heart rate. Intravenous introduction of inotropes such as dobutamine and dipyridamole enables echocardiographic assessment of 'exercising' myocardium, not only to evaluate regional and global wall movement in ischaemic heart disease (IHD) but also to 'unmask' apparently stunned or dormant myocardium as potentially viable muscle that may respond to revascularization techniques.

Echocardiography continues to evolve and has been notably aided by the progression of digital technology. This has enabled advances not only in directions that establish newer echocardiography modalities such as 3D reconstruction imaging, but also those designed to enhance image quality and border definition. This becomes especially pertinent to the non-echogenic subjects where factors such as obesity, chronic lung disease and prior thoracic surgery may well limit images of real diagnostic value. Development of harmonic imaging techniques (both tissue and contrast orientated) that boost the received signal frequencies for better resolution and colour enhancement (colour kinesis) has already assisted the assessment and quantification of regional myocardial wall movement, contractility and also stunned myocardium viability. Border definition is a key feature of the development of contrast echocardiography. This technique utilizes agents introduced into the venous blood that are capable of traversing the transpulmonary circuit and are designed specifically to aid delineation of the blood–tissue interface within the left heart, aiding assessment of regional wall motion.

Other specialist ultrasound uses in the cardiac context include visualization of the coronary vasculature from enhanced blood flow imaging, intravascular ultrasound (IVUS), currently in widespread use but only able to examine the proximal segment of the arterial tree, and intracavity echocardiography (ICE). The latter two techniques are also mentioned later in the invasive cardiology section on cardiac catheterisation.

Transoesophageal echocardiography (TOE). This represents a development of the transthoracic specialty that is not encumbered by the same issues of patient echogenicity. Essentially, TOE represents a semi-invasive test type as the ultrasound transducer, mounted on a flexible endoscope and commonly with multiplane steerability, is passed orally down the oesophagus to lie directly adjacent to the posterior aspect of the heart. In this way tissue penetration becomes less of an issue, enabling use of higher frequency (better resolution) ultrasound transducers, affording excellent image resolution and clarity. The technique can be performed with or without sedation, depending on operator experience and preference, but ultimately patient compliance is the issue. The procedure therefore requires nursing support, especially when sedation is utilized, with a potential need for extended patient care including pulse oximetry, oral suction, oxygen administration and subsequent aftercare.

> **Box 8.3** Common indications for transoesophageal echocardiography (TOE)
>
> - Dysfunction of a mechanical mitral prosthesis
> - Endocarditis
> - Transient ischaemic attack (TIA) or cerebral infarct
> - Aortic dissection
> - Poor TTE images
> - Intra-operative assessment of aortic or mitral valve repairs
> - Intra-operative assessment of myomectomy procedures (for hypertrophic cardiomyopathy)
> - Assessment of suitability for balloon mitral valvuloplasty/valvotomy, mitral valve repair
> - Visualization of the left atrial appendage for the presence of thrombus (prior to DC cardioversion)

Pacemakers and internal cardioverter-defibrillators

Although occurring essentially in a post-therapy setting, permanent pacemaker (PPM) and internal cardioverter defibrillator (ICD) clinical follow-up nevertheless merits inclusion in this section as such procedures can aid the ongoing evaluation and optimization of treatment. Ostensibly guided by patient symptoms and feedback, such clinical assessments are further enhanced by the considerable advances made in the diagnostic capabilities of implantable devices, notably of the dual-chamber variety. These capabilities include such features as heart rate and AV delay histograms to monitor chronotropic response and measure proportions of intrinsic (sensed) and paced activity, high atrial and ventricular rate counters to monitor tachyarrhythmias together with recordings of intracardiac electrograms (EGMs) to aid their identification, plus measures to monitor pacemaker response to such arrhythmias.

The programmable parameters available to address persistent postimplant symptoms extend far beyond the standby pacing rate. 'Physiological' (variable) rate-responsive devices have programmable upper rates and sensors with programmable activation thresholds and sensitivities that automatically adjust to the level of patient activity. Many dual-chamber devices also possess sophisticated algorithms to activate 'mode switch' responses to avoid ventricular tracking of atrial tachycardias and most units have mechanisms to eliminate the potential for pacemaker-induced/mediated tachycardias (PMTs).

Implantable atrial devices, originally designed to detect and provide overdrive pacing therapy in the setting of medically unresponsive poorly tolerated SVTs, are little used of late. This is largely due to the advances made in ablation therapy. However, the development of dual-chamber ICDs, coupled with research into the management of atrial fibrillation utilizing implantable devices, has revitalized interest in this area. Dual-chamber defibrillation devices that can evaluate both ventricular and atrial arrhythmias are increasingly available with algorithms (based on criteria such as tachycardia onset and stability, EGM morphology and atrial/ventricular signal relationship) to discriminate SVT from VT and thereby avoid delivery of inappropriate shocks for 'benign' arrhythmias. Such devices may also offer advanced pacing modalities overtly intended to suppress atrial arrhythmias. If unsuccessful, however, their capabilities, including accurate tachycardia definition, allow delivery of appropriate therapies including overdrive pacing for SVT and, if appropriate, DC cardioversion for episodes of paroxysmal atrial fibrillation (PAF) together with the 'standard' protective therapies for ventricular arrhythmias (see Chapter 25).

Invasive

Cardiac catheterisation

What is cardiac catheterisation? Cardiac catheterisation, also known as coronary angiography, is an invasive procedure used to make a medical diagnosis or otherwise confirm a diagnosis that has been indicated from non-invasive tests. This is achieved by introducing a catheter into a peripheral vein or artery, which is then advanced under X-ray guidance (fluoroscopy) to the heart and coronary arteries for detailed contrast imaging, measurement of haemodynamic pressure data and blood sampling.

Under fluoroscopic (X-ray) imaging contrast media can be injected as a large bolus dose to image the cardiac chambers and large vessels or selectively to the coronary arteries and grafts. Today, angiographic imaging and data processing use digital technologies, enabling data to be recorded and stored in digital format on compact disc, representing a significant advance from the old cine film format. Supplementary information during each procedure can be gained from haemodynamic pressure data and blood oximetry (haemoglobin oxygen saturation) from localized areas of the heart.

The most common approaches for performing the procedure are the femoral approach (using the Seldinger technique) or via a brachial cut-down. The radial approach can also be used and is becoming a preferred choice by some operators. The choice is determined by operator preference or by predisposing features of the patient's past medical history. The femoral approach is most commonly used and, additionally, would be indicated in situations involving congenital heart disease, young women who may show a propensity for coronary artery spasm, patients who have had a number of previous catheterisations via the brachial approach or situations when patients have had previous coronary bypass surgery, the latter especially when the left internal mammary artery (LIMA) has been used. This is because it is generally easier to intubate the grafts from an inferior approach and in situations involving a LIMA graft it is extremely difficult to reach using a right brachial approach (the left brachial approach may be preferable). Alternatively the brachial or radial route would be preferred where there are known tortuous iliac vessels, previous aortic–iliac surgery or in an anticoagulated patient (INR >1.5).

For the purposes of this text the cardiac catheterisation procedure can be divided into two sections, namely right heart catheterisation and left heart catheterisation. In practice, however, the majority of adult right heart cardiac catheterisation investigations are performed in conjunction with those for the left.

Right heart catheterisation. Right heart catheterisation is performed to assess and aid the diagnosis of:

- valvular abnormalities
- pulmonary hypertension
- atrial or ventricular septal defects (ASD/VSD)
- congenital heart disease.

An appropriately shaped catheter, occasionally balloon tipped to facilitate passage within the cardiac bloodstream, is introduced into the venous system with the aid of a guidewire. It is advanced via the inferior or superior vena cava (depending on approach used) into the right atrium, through the tricuspid valve and into the right ventricle. Further manoeuvring across the pulmonary valve into the pulmonary artery enables advancement into the pulmonary capillary field, the so-called pulmonary wedge (PCW) or occlusion position, enabling indirect measurement of (reflected) left atrial pressure. The left atrium is almost invariably impossible to catheterize from a left-sided approach and if specifically indicated, necessitates a trans-septal technique (from the right atrium) to be adopted from the venous approach. The advancement of the catheter is monitored under fluoroscopy and the tip location is verified from pressure waveforms. In all areas of the heart during right heart catheterisation pressure traces are recorded and blood samples may be taken for oxygen saturation levels.

In the presence of either a ventricular or atrial septal defect catheters may also enter the left heart via a right-sided approach. Catheters allow the injection of radio-opaque contrast media into the chambers and great vessels of the heart. Those most commonly recorded are aortogram and left ventricular angiogram, which will be covered in the left heart catheterisation section.

Some right heart catheterisations, particularly those for paediatric investigations and other congenital

Table 8.1 Typical normal values for systolic, diastolic and mean pressures (mmHg) together with normal blood oxygen saturation levels for different cardiac locations

Site		Pressure (mmHg)	(range)	O$_2$ sat (%)
Superior vena cava	Mean	3	(0–5)	65–75
Inferior vena cava	Mean	3	(0–5)	70–80
Right atrium	Mean	4	(0–8)	65–75
Right ventricle				
Systolic		25	(15–30)	65–75
End diastolic		4	(0–8)	
Pulmonary artery				
Systolic		25	(15–30)	65–75
Diastolic		10	(5–15)	
Mean		15	(10–20)	
Pulmonary artery wedge	Mean	10	(5–14)	
Pulmonary vein	Mean	5	(4–12)	98–100
Left atrium	Mean	7	(4–12)	95–98
Left ventricle				
Systolic		120	(90–140)	95–98
End diastolic		8	(4–15)	
Aorta				
Systolic		120	(90–140)	95–98
Diastolic		70	(60–90)	
Mean		86	(70–105)	

abnormalities, may involve the injection of contrast media to the:

- right ventricle (RV) to opacify the chamber and provide information on right ventricular function and that of the tricuspid and pulmonary valves
- pulmonary artery to provide anatomical information on the artery itself, its branches and general perfusion of the lung field.

Left heart catheterisation/coronary angiography.
Left heart catheterisation is performed to assess and aid diagnosis of:

- coronary artery disease
- bypass graft patency
- LV contractility and ejection fraction
- aortic and mitral valve disease
- aortic root, aortic arch and ascending/descending aorta anatomy (see Diagnostic Imaging: Invasive section).

Catheters of different tip design, according to need, are advanced retrogradely (i.e. against the direction of blood flow) with the assistance of a guidewire into the ascending aorta via the femoral artery and external iliac. They travel over the aortic arch and down the ascending aorta to sit just above the aortic valve. Again catheter advancement is observed under fluoroscopy with pressure wave observation. The two main aspects of left heart catheterisation are the left ventricular angiogram and coronary angiography.

Left ventricular angiogram. As previously stated, the left ventricular angiogram is performed to assess the anatomical appearance and function of the left ventricle, the extent of mitral and aortic valve competency/incompetency and, less commonly, to reveal the presence of ventricular septal defects.

The catheter is shaped so that it can be manoeuvred through the aortic valve to sit comfortably in the left ventricular cavity. On occasions this may cause some ventricular irritability and evoke ventricular ectopic beats or runs of ventricular tachycardia, which must be carefully observed. A recording is taken to measure the end-diastolic pressure, a reasonable (but not entirely reliable) indicator of the strength of left ventricular contraction.

Left ventricular function is evaluated both anatomically and physiologically. The left ventricular angiogram enables assessment of wall movement (kinesis) and myocardial contraction in respect of:

- normal function
- hypokinesia (reduced movement/contractility)
- akinesia (absent movement/contractility)
- dyskinesia (unco-ordinated movement/contractility).

This additionally provides qualitative information on the normal or ischaemic status of the regional myocardial blood supply.

On completion of the left ventriculogram the catheter is slowly pulled back from the left ventricle across the aortic valve and into the aorta whilst observing and recording the pressure wave traces to check for valvular or subvalvular obstruction. For example, in the presence of aortic stenosis the peak systolic pressure measured in the aortic root will be lower than that of the left ventricle.

Mitral and aortic regurgitation are assessed using angiography. During the left ventricular injection mitral regurgitation may be evident as contrast media refluxing into the left atrium during systole. Similarly, aortograms are used to evaluate the degree of aortic valve regurgitation as a reflux of blood back into the left ventricle during diastole. They are also useful in illustrating aortic valve flow in cases of severe aortic stenosis, where it proves impossible to traverse a heavily calcified valve or where the presence of a mechanical aortic prosthesis means it is generally unsafe to try and cross the valve. Aortograms are also useful in the diagnosis of coarctation of the aorta and aortic dissections.

Coronary angiography. The coronary anatomy varies considerably from patient to patient. For example, one main difference is exhibited by the relative dominance of the right coronary artery or left circumflex artery to the overall coronary system, whereby either may supply the posterolateral left ventricular territory. As a generalization, however, in the majority of patients, the territorial supply to the cardiac muscle by the three main coronary vessels and their respective branches will tend to be as follows (with appropriate overlap):

- left anterior descending (LAD) artery: interventricular septum (IVS), free wall and anterior surface of the LV, extending posteriorly around the apex
- left circumflex (Cx) artery; posterior and lateral LV, left atrium
- right coronary artery (RCA): right ventricle and right atrium, posterolateral and inferior LV.

During coronary angiography specially designed catheters, with tips shaped specifically to aid intubation of the left and right coronary arteries respectively, are again advanced retrogradely with the assistance of a guidewire to the ostium (the opening) of each vessel, lying just above the aortic valve. A diagrammatic representation of the coronary anatomy is shown in Figure 4.5, p. 49.

The catheters are manipulated to engage safely in the respective ostia to enable hand injection of the arteries with contrast media. Images are taken from a number of views using different X-ray image angulations to provide detailed information on the extent, site and severity of coronary artery lesions and the blood flow down each coronary artery.

Coronary artery blood flow is characterised all over the world by the same grading system known as the TIMI flow grade (Thrombolysis in Myocardial Infarction – so-called from its use in thrombolytic agent trials), as expressed in Box 8.4.

Following left heart cardiac catheterisation, if a diagnosis of CAD is made, there are different treatments available to patients depending on the severity of their disease. These therapies include percutaneous transluminal coronary angioplasty (PTCA), often in conjunction with coronary stent implantation, coronary artery bypass grafting or medical therapy. A stent is a tubular scaffold within a vessel, at a lesion site, to enlarge the lumen and support the vessel wall (Hubner 1998).

As an adjunct to coronary artery catheterisation in the context of interventional procedures, mention should be made of intravascular ultrasound (IVUS), a technique introduced over 10 years ago but only used in Britain over the last few years.

IVUS is an invasive technique for internally imaging coronary arteries (Erbel & Ge 1998), to provide detailed information about the pathology of the arterial wall. This aids the assessment of coronary artery

---

Box 8.5 Uses and disadvantages of IVUS (after Hubner 1998)
Uses ● To measure the true size of the internal vessel diameter. ● To confirm the full expansion of deployed coronary stents. ● To aid assessment of the lesion formation, which can be more severe than seen on angiography, and to aid decisions on what angioplasty equipment to use. ● To assess the result of angioplasty. *Disadvantages* ● Increased costs. ● Increased length of the procedure. ● Unable to detect thrombus within the lumen.

disease and/or the results of intervention. In the procedure an IVUS catheter is passed over a routine angioplasty guidewire and advanced into the coronary vessel. Ultrasound images of the internal wall structure and anatomy are formed and relayed to the monitor on the ultrasound machine. This enables accurate measurements of the size of the lumen and evaluation of the extent of atheromatous plaque formation to be made.

The nursing care for the patient having undergone a diagnostic cardiac catheterisation is discussed in Chapter 9.

Electrophysiological studies (EPS) and VT - stimulation studies. Cardiac electrophysiology cannot be appreciated without a basic understanding of the cardiac action potential, impulse generation/propagation, cell depolarization and repolarization, anatomy of the conduction system and pharmacological influences. The size and subject matter contained within the field of electrophysiology merits a chapter (Chapter 20) of its own so this section will limit itself to a brief description of the procedure from the nursing perspective.

The specialty has developed significantly and become increasingly more widespread over the past 10 years. Therefore, with the movement from just a few specialist centres, it is now more likely to be encountered by the cardiac nurse. Various aetiologies exist for electrophysiological abnormalities which may be congenital or acquired. The symptoms of initial patient presentation can vary anywhere from a vague sensation of palpitations to episodal presyncope or syncope and ultimately cardiac arrest.

Every effort should be made to record a full 12-lead ECG at the time of symptoms as a first step towards arrhythmia identification. This may be a

---

Box 8.4 TIMI flow grades in coronary arteries	
TIMI 0	No perfusion No antegrade flow beyond the point of occlusion
TIMI 1	Penetration with minimal perfusion Contrast fails to opacify the entire bed distal to the stenosis for the duration of the picture run
TIMI 2	Partial perfusion Contrast opacifies the entire coronary bed distal to the stenosis. However, the rate of entry and/or clearance is slower in the coronary bed distal to the obstruction than in comparable areas not perfused by the dilated vessel
TIMI 3	Complete perfusion Filling and clearance of contrast equally rapid in the coronary bed distal to stenosis as in other coronary beds

bradyarrhythmia or tachyarrhythmia. A 12-lead ECG is of particular importance when attempting to differentiate a tachyarrhythmia of supraventricular origin from one of ventricular origin. Following the appropriate associated non-invasive work-up, which may include a SAECG, echocardiogram, stress test or tilt test, a full EPS procedure should enable a full diagnosis of the culprit arrhythmia by means of testing the electrical conduction system of the heart for abnormal behaviour. Only when this classification has been accomplished can the appropriate therapy be proposed whether it be medical, pharmacological, ablative (catheter or surgical) or pacemaker/ICD implantation.

An EPS procedure involves transvenous catheterisation (although occasionally a retrograde arterial approach is indicated) with catheters advanced from a femoral or supraclavicular venous approach. The catheters are non-luminal but possess pairs of platinum electrodes, termed **bipoles**, welded to the distal end. Catheter construction may be of simple configuration with only a single electrode pair (termed **bipolar**) or variable multipolar configurations as quadpolar (4), hexapolar (6), octapolar (8) or decapolar (10). These electrode-tipped catheters are advanced to strategic points within the heart, characteristically the high right atrium (HRA), across the His bundle (near the tricuspid valve annulus), deep within the coronary sinus (CS) for left heart access and the right ventricular apex (RV). Electrograms (EGMs) are recorded from these sites as sets of bipolar signals with the multipolar catheters able to provide information over a larger intracardiac territory.

By a combination of artificial pacing manoeuvres, whilst simultaneously recording the relationships between the various EGMs, intracardiac activation sequences can be studied together with evaluation of intracardiac conduction times and tissue refractoriness. An EPS procedure is an attempt to initiate arrhythmias and identify the mechanism and location of aberrant conduction. Characterisation of arrhythmia aberrancy by this method enables determination of the most suitable and appropriate therapy for the individual patient.

Other more sophisticated mapping techniques have been devised and are very much under continued development. Whilst utilizing different technologies, the rationale behind all EP techniques is fundamentally the same, but the newest methods facilitate shorter procedure times and so reduce radiation exposure to patient and staff alike.

Sudden cardiac death (SCD) is a topic of great interest in the world of cardiac electrophysiology and, by virtue of the catastrophic nature in which patient presentation occurs, the subject of extensive research. The inextricable links with arrhythmias of ventricular origin and ICD therapy have in turn initiated development of different strategies in the management of atrial arrhythmias and serve to demonstrate the ever increasing importance of cardiac electrophysiology within cardiology.

Brief mention should be made of a more recent diagnostic modality closely linked to EPS/ablation procedures, that of intracavity echocardiography (ICE). Although at this time very much a recent concept and still in the investigative stage, ICE has the potential to improve both the diagnostic and interventional capabilities of electrophysiology. In conjunction with conventional EGM guidance and fluoroscopy, ICE techniques utilize an adapted ultrasound transducer mounted on a catheter tip to visually image intracardiac structures. By aiding the identification of anatomical regions of aberrancy and observing lesion size and formation, assistance is given to both the accuracy of catheter positioning and contact efficacy for ablation procedures, thereby reducing procedure (and fluoroscopy exposure) times.

Complications of catheterisation. Complications are always possible following any invasive procedure, although the risks associated with cardiac catheterisation are very low. Complications following or during cardiac catheterisation range from haematoma from the catheter site to an allergic reaction to the contrast used during the procedure, chest pain/unstable angina or myocardial infarction and cardiac arrest. In addition, coronary occlusion due to dissection could occur, with dislodgement of atheromatous material as emboli, thrombus formation or vessel/cavity perforation.

Patient preparation and education. High levels of anxiety may exist among patients before all procedures, especially when of an invasive nature. Part of this anxiety or apprehension can stem from the fear of the unknown. If information is given about the treatment, patients may be reassured of their recovery and some of these anxieties can be relieved. Peterson (1991) found that patients have concerns about:

- waiting time on the day of the procedure
- the actual test, lying flat on a hard table, insertion of the catheter
- possible complications, i.e. a myocardial infarction or stroke
- the outcomes of the test, medication, angioplasty, open heart surgery
- having to lie flat after the procedure

- fear of the cardiac catheterisation laboratory. It can be a frightening room with lots of modern equipment and alarm bells sounding at times.

Information is given to patients by the multidisciplinary team, quite often on the day of the procedure. However, Wilson-Barnett (1980) suggests that this may not be the best time as patients may be too distracted by other events to receive and retain information. In the 1960s, Lay & Spelman (1967) assessed some of the difficulties of the hospital as a learning environment for receiving and storing information and suggested ways to improve these.

- Patients are usually told more than they can remember. Therefore keep information succinct.
- Patients should be offered a record of what is said to them.
- Patients best remember the statements to which they attribute most importance.
- The least and most anxious patients remember less than moderately anxious patients.

As noted above, Conroy & Mulcahy (1985) mention that studies have shown that patients' knowledge is greater when written materials are added to verbal instruction. However, they also assessed the readability of the literature for cardiac care and found that four out of five of the available books and leaflets were beyond the reading ability of half the patients. This reflects the findings of other previous surveys (Doak & Doak 1980).

Therefore appropriate booklets or leaflets are an ideal way of providing patients and their relatives with information before coming into hospital but should be sent to the patient together with their admission date. Dobree (1990) found that providing patients with booklets 10 days before admission was useful and enabled the patients to take an active role in their own care. Dowling & O'Keefe (1990) noted that by providing patient booklets prior to a cardiac catherisation as little as a few days before the procedure, the majority of patients highlighted that they were more informed and more relaxed after reading the literature. However, importantly, Dowling & O'Keefe found that the booklet cannot be considered the only source of information and doctors and nurses were still vital informants to patients and their loved ones.

To take the provision of information one step further, special pre-admission clinics can be provided, with research suggesting that they can be highly successful in some hospitals. Cupple's work in 1991 indicates that the ideal time for teaching patients is between 5 and 14 days before admission. Therefore, for most pre-admis-

sion clinics, patients and their relatives are invited to attend at least a week prior to their admission.

The pre-admission clinic should ideally be nurse led and include:

- an initial clinical assessment of the patient
- a check of all patient details
- recording of baseline observations, height and weight
- recording of a 12-lead ECG
- explanation of the procedure and the care given
- discussion of risk factors, primarily regarding the procedure but with some lifestyle advice.

The purpose of the clinics is:

- to provide quality information in a relaxed atmosphere which is conducive to learning
- to fulfil the aims of providing information at least a week before admission
- to reduce patients' anxiety before admission
- to encourage family/carer involvement and to reduce their anxieties
- for nursing staff to identify those patients requiring extra support; for example, psychological, physical, social, transport and convalescence needs.

Ongoing developments in the cardiac catheterisation laboratory. There is always ongoing and improved technology being utilized in the cardiac catheter laboratory. Developments currently being investigated include the following.

- Brachytherapy. This is a procedure for 'in-stent' restenosis, whereby a radioactive source, either gamma (γ) or beta (β) radiation, delivers low-dose radiation via a wire into the affected coronary artery. This procedure has a number of safety problems and at present is only being undertaken in a limited number of British centres.
- Percutaneous transmyocardial revascularization (PTMR). This is an alternative treatment for patients with class III–IV angina and coronary artery disease who are diagnosed as unable to undergo coronary artery bypass grafting or angioplasty. The procedure is performed in the catheter lab under local anaesthetic and a laser source is used to drill micro-channels into the ischaemic myocardium to facilitate revascularization (see Chapter 26).
- Stent design and coating. There are ongoing trials to examine the effects of different coatings, e.g. anticoagulants, to both balloons and stents in attempts to reduce or prevent restenosis of the coronary arteries.

DIAGNOSTIC IMAGING

Non-invasive

The following imaging techniques are commonly described as 'non-invasive'. However, all involve either ionizing radiation, the intravenous/intra-arterial introduction of pharmaceuticals or some degree of patient discomfort. Therefore, with the possible exception of the chest X-ray, they are all more accurately described as minimally or moderately invasive.

The chest X-ray (CXR)

All X-ray imaging is possible because anatomical structures within the body have different densities. Relatively high-density structures within the chest, such as the heart and mediastinum, absorb incident X-rays more than low-density structures such as air-filled lung tissue. These differences in X-ray absorption, when recorded onto a suitable medium such as film, produce a chest X-ray.

Currently, the standard chest X-ray for cardiac applications is an erect, postero-anterior (PA) projection using high-penetration X-rays. The main advantages of this technique are:

- lower radiation dose to the patient
- increased penetration of the mediastinum, allowing more of its detail to be recorded
- minimal magnification of the heart
- reduced overall contrast, diminishing rib detail that would otherwise obscure the lungs
- shorter exposure times, reducing artefacts from respiratory and cardiac movement.

The PA chest X-ray can be supplemented with a lateral projection when three-dimensional localization of anatomical or pathological features is required. Chest X-rays are quick, straightforward and inexpensive to perform, with the basic equipment being available in most hospitals. The radiation dose to the patient is very low but must still be considered significant and no X-ray examination should be performed unless it is vital to a patient's clinical management.

The chest X-ray is used routinely in the clinical evaluation of all patients with confirmed or suspected heart disease. Its principal roles are:

- to contribute information assisting in a diagnosis of heart disease and in some cases make a specific cardiac diagnosis
- to eliminate lung pathology, such as a pneumothorax, as a cause of symptoms and to exclude any other pathology, such as a carcinoma, that could influence the patient's management
- to aid the performance of further investigations such as catheterisation and to help the cardiologist or surgeon in planning therapeutic interventions
- to monitor medical treatment following drug therapy or surgery/intervention.

The normal chest X-ray. The normal chest X-ray and the relevant anatomical landmarks are shown in Figure 5.6, p. 83. Chapter 5 offers a more indepth discussion and detailed examples of abnormalities relevant to the cardiac nurse. When examining the chest X-ray it is important to remember that left and right refer to those of the patient, not the observer. In the adult PA chest X-ray, the heart 'shadow' appears very prominently. Its right border is formed by the wall of the right atrium, its left by the wall of the left ventricle and the left atrial appendage, which is just visible below the left main bronchus. The right ventricle contributes no part to the visible outline of the heart. The ratio of the maximum width of the heart to the maximum width of the thorax – the **cardiothoracic ratio** – should not exceed 50%. Immediately above the heart, the right border of the superior mediastinum is formed by the superior vena cava and the left by the left subclavian vein, the 'knuckle-like' protrusion of the posterior aortic arch and the descending thoracic aorta. The ascending thoracic aorta and pulmonary artery are entirely concealed within the superior mediastinum.

The chest X-ray in heart disease. In patients with heart disease many anatomical changes to the heart and lungs can be detected on a chest X-ray. These can be grouped into changes in the size or contour of the heart due to haemodynamic disorders, aneurysms or tumours, secondary changes in the lungs or pulmonary vasculature, and calcification.

Heart size and contour. A cardiothoracic ratio of greater than 50% usually suggests overall cardiac dilatation and/or selective enlargement of either or both ventricles.

- Selective left ventricular enlargement causes the left heart border to appear elongated and more convex.
- Enlargement of the right ventricle can often only be recognized by the resultant displacement of the left ventricle, making it difficult to distinguish from left ventricular enlargement. However, right ventricular enlargement is frequently associated with visible enlargement of the main pulmonary artery. Right and

left ventricular enlargement can be easily distinguished on a lateral chest X-ray (obtained from the side of the patient). Anterior or posterior enlargement of the heart shadow indicates right or left ventricular enlargement in turn.

- Gross pericardial effusion can also lead to an increase in the cardiothoracic ratio but can be distinguished from ventricular enlargement by the presence of a rounded, sharply defined margin to the heart shadow, often without secondary changes to the lungs. Selective atrial enlargements generally have less effect on the cardiothoracic ratio.

- Right atrial enlargement causes visible expansion in the size and contour of the right heart border.

- Left atrial enlargement causes the left atrial appendage to appear more prominent and displaces the left main bronchus. A double shadow may also be seen through the right side of the heart.

Enlargement of the major blood vessels can also be demonstrated. Dilatation of the aorta causes widening of the superior mediastinum, sometimes with visible calcification if the dilatation is aneurysmal; dilatation of the pulmonary artery creates a prominent bulge just below the aortic 'knuckle'. Marked widening of the mediastinum, especially in association with a pleural effusion, indicates aortic dissection.

Pulmonary changes. Most heart diseases cause alterations to the pulmonary vasculature and/or secondary lung changes that can be seen on a chest X-ray. Prominent bilateral hilar shadows indicate pulmonary arterial hypertension whereas increased prominence of the vasculature in the upper lung fields suggests pulmonary venous hypertension. Severe pulmonary venous hypertension can lead to interstitial or alveolar pulmonary oedema, which can be readily distinguished by their effects on the appearance of the lungs. Interstitial oedema causes a generalized increase in their opacity (degree of opaqueness), together with loss of definition of the hili, while alveolar oedema causes widespread patchy shadowing.

Calcification. Current chest X-ray techniques may fail to demonstrate or underestimate the extent of calcifications within the heart. Consequently, calcification is not a reliable indicator of cardiac pathology. Calcification of the aorta appears as an opacity around the circumference of the aortic 'knuckle' and is seen frequently in patients over 40 years of age. Calcification in the aortic and mitral valves is also common and has the appearance of a 'C'-shaped open ring. Other sites of calcification include the

myocardium (rare, except in aneurysm), the coronary arteries and the pericardium.

Recent developments. Over the last few years there have been a number of refinements to the basic chest X-ray technique. These include the development of dedicated asymmetric film/screen combinations, which allow better visualization of the lung fields without compromising the definition of the mediastinum. A technique known as scanning equalization radiography uses a slit-collimated X-ray beam that scans across the chest optimizing the exposure for each area. However, the most significant recent developments are computed and digital radiography. Computed radiography uses a phosphor plate instead of conventional film to record incident X-rays. Following exposure, the phosphor plate is scanned with a laser and the image digitized and stored electronically. Digital radiography takes this a stage further and records incident X-rays directly with a special solid-state detector. The main advantage of these techniques is that images from a single exposure can be electronically manipulated to optimize detail in any part of the chest, without increasing the radiation dose to the patient.

Computed tomography

Computed tomography (CT) uses a finely collimated X-ray beam and an electronic detector that rotate around the patient collecting X-ray absorption data from multiple projections. A computer then reconstructs cross-sectional images from the data acquired during each 360° rotation. In this way, CT overcomes many of the limitations of conventional X-ray imaging when examining areas of the body overlaid by other structures. It is also useful when studying anatomical areas with only subtle density differences between adjacent structures, such as the mediastinum. However, adequate visualization of the blood vessels is still dependent on the intravenous introduction of contrast media and artefacts from respiratory and cardiac motion cannot be entirely eliminated. CT is relatively expensive but is widely available nonetheless, all but the smallest hospitals having access to a basic scanner. However, the radiation dose to the patient is among the highest for all imaging techniques and often exceeds several hundred times that of a chest X-ray.

Except in suspected aortic dissection, CT is rarely used as a first-line investigation for cardiac patients. It is generally used to contribute further information following abnormal chest X-ray findings. Contrast medium-enhanced CT can demonstrate not just the size and shape of the chambers of the heart but additional details within it, such as the interventricular septum, the thickness of the ventricular walls and intracavitary masses. Intracardiac calcifications can also be identified but not accurately localized. CT is particularly useful for distinguishing aneurysms of the major blood vessels from other mediastinal masses and for confirming and classifying aortic dissection. The demonstration of a double lumen in the aorta, with or without delayed filling in the false lumen, is clear evidence of an aortic dissection.

Currently, specialized techniques, such as three-dimensional CT coronary angiography, localization of intracoronary calcifications, ventricular analysis and assessment of myocardial perfusion, can only be performed using dedicated cardiac CT scanners. These scanners, which can acquire images in a fraction of a second (electron beam CT) and/or synchronize image acquisition with the cardiac cycle (ECG gating), are available in only a few of the most specialized cardiac centres.

A recent development in CT technology is helical (or spiral) CT. This allows image data to be collected from a series of continuous rotations of the X-ray tube and detector assembly. This results in the acquisition of a volume of data that can be reconstructed into images in any plane or used to create three-dimensional CT angiograms. A further development of helical CT, known as multislice helical CT, uses a split X-ray beam and detector to collect multiple image data simultaneously, significantly reducing the time required to acquire each image. This technique has the potential to rival electron beam CT and is set to become widely available.

Magnetic resonance imaging

Magnetic resonance imaging (MRI) is so fundamentally different from conventional X-ray imaging that a brief description of its basic principles is useful in order to understand its significance. The human body contains a large amount of hydrogen and consequently a large number of hydrogen nuclei or protons. In their normal state these protons, due to their intrinsic quantum mechanical properties, behave like tiny, randomly spinning dipole magnets. However, the magnetic field of a MRI scanner – typically around 30 000 times stronger than the earth's magnetic field – causes them to align and spin at a specific frequency. A radiofrequency (RF) pulse is then applied at precisely the same frequency, causing the protons to resonate and change their alignment relative to the magnetic field. When the RF is switched off the protons realign with the magnetic field, inducing a small signal in a receiver coil that surrounds the patient. A series of these signals is then reconstructed into cross-sectional images. The significance of this, in the context of cardiac imaging, is that there is no ionizing radiation dose to the patient and the inherent contrast between anatomical structures due to differences in their chemical composition can be enhanced by manipulating the RF pulse sequences. This allows the heart and blood vessels to be demonstrated without the introduction of contrast medium.

MRI is currently very expensive and not widely available. Although there are no known biological hazards and no radiation dose to the patient, MRI is **absolutely contra-indicated** for patients with implanted cardiac pacemakers and defibrillators as the strong magnetic field can interfere with their operation. Other implanted devices, such as prosthetic heart valves, sternal sutures and intravascular stents, are unlikely to be dislodged or damaged by the magnetic field but can cause considerable image artefact. Cardiac movement also causes image artefact but, just as in CT, can be overcome by synchronizing image acquisition with the cardiac cycle.

Except when investigating abnormal calcification, which cannot be demonstrated, the indications for MRI in cardiac patients are currently similar to those for CT. Its main role is in the management of patients with aortic aneurysms and dissections where the risk of surgical intervention is so great that if possible, they are treated conservatively and require frequent clinical follow-up. MR is also particularly suitable for investigating and monitoring intracardiac masses.

The development of MRI contrast media, which are inherently less toxic than X-ray contrast media and achieve adequate contrast enhancement using a much smaller injected volume, is leading to increasing interest in the use of this form of imaging in cardiac patients, particularly in MRI angiography of the aorta. Contrast-enhanced MRI can be used to perform three-dimensional MRI coronary angiography and functional studies, such as assessment of myocardial perfusion and ventricular analysis. Further applications are currently under investigation.

The role of MRI in cardiac patients is set to expand dramatically in the near future. Indeed, the potential is such that it is widely anticipated that MRI will become the primary imaging technique for most cardiac patients whose condition cannot be adequately investigated with echocardiography.

Nuclear medicine

Nuclear medicine is a functional imaging technique that records the distribution of administered radioactive pharmaceuticals within the body. The pharmaceuticals used are designed to target particular physiological processes occurring in specific organs or tissues and are known as radiopharmaceuticals. Images are obtained by detecting and recording the radioactive emissions from the radiopharmaceuticals using a γ (or scintillation) camera.

Nuclear medicine is widely available and relatively inexpensive. The overall radiation dose to the patient is approximately 10 times that of a chest X-ray but the dose to specific organs can be considerably higher.

Imaging of the heart in nuclear medicine is referred to as nuclear cardiology and its most widespread application is in the assessment of myocardial perfusion. In conventional planar nuclear cardiology, a radiopharmaceutical that is taken up by the myocardium is injected into the patient during exercise. Immediately after exercise, anterior, left anterior oblique and left lateral images of the heart are acquired. This series of images depicts the pattern of blood flow during stress. The images are then repeated after 2–4 hours, demonstrating blood flow at rest. Ischaemic areas within the myocardium are seen as 'cold spots'. A cold spot that appears on the stress images but not on the rest images indicates exercise-induced ischaemia whereas the appearance of a cold spot on both sets of images represents infarction.

Two radiopharmaceuticals are in common use for this technique: thallium-201 and technetium-99m. Thallium-201 is expensive and has a relatively long half-life (73.1 hours), which restricts the dose that can be given. Technetium-99m, on the other hand, is less expensive, has a shorter half-life (6 hours) and gives better image quality. However, it does not redistribute throughout the myocardium after rest and so a second injection is required to distinguish reversible ischaemia from infarction.

Nuclear cardiology is also frequently used to assess left ventricular function. The most common method is multigated acquisition (MUGA). A technetium-99m labelled radiopharmaceutical is injected into the patient where it attaches to haemoglobin in the red blood cells. Anterior, left anterior oblique and left lateral, ECG-gated images are then acquired. The resulting images depict the blood flow in the ventricle during systole and diastole, allowing very accurate measurement of the ejection fraction. Abnormal ventricular wall motion can also be identified.

Single photon emission computed tomography (SPECT) uses identical radiopharmaceuticals and protocols to conventional planar nuclear cardiology. The only difference is that the γ camera rotates around the patient and collects data from multiple projections. Just as in CT, a computer is used to reconstruct cross-sectional images from the information acquired during each rotation. SPECT is generally considered preferable to planar imaging as it demonstrates greater contrast between normal and abnormal areas of the myocardium and abnormalities can be more accurately localized. It is becoming more widely available despite its relatively high cost. The radiation dose to the patient is around double that of conventional nuclear cardiology.

Positron emission tomography (PET) is very different to conventional nuclear medicine. It uses a class of radiopharmaceuticals that emit positrons during their radioactive decay. These positrons collide with electrons in the body, producing two γ-rays that travel away from the collision at 180° to each other. The γ-rays are detected simultaneously by a ring of detectors encircling the patient. A computer is then used to reconstruct cross-sectional images from a series of these paired γ-rays. PET produces the highest quality images of all forms of nuclear medicine and can acquire images very much faster, allowing rapid sequential imaging. It can be used for very accurate assessment of myocardial perfusion but its high cost, both for the scanner and for the radiopharmaceuticals, currently restricts its use mainly to research protocols.

Invasive

Digital subtraction angiography

Digital subtraction angiography (DSA), like traditional angiography, relies on the introduction of contrast medium within the body vasculature to increase the density difference between the blood vessels and their surroundings. However, unlike traditional angiography, the surroundings are first electronically subtracted from each image. This allows blood vessels to be demonstrated using a lower volume of intra-arterial contrast medium and reduces the number of projections required to separate them from superimposed structures. Consequently, DSA is less invasive than conventional angiography and results in a lower radiation dose to the patient.

The main role of DSA in cardiac patients is to verify suspected aortic dissection and, where confirmed, to show the extent of the lesion. It is also commonly used to show the aortic arch as an aid to selective catheterisation of one or more of its branches.

CASE STUDIES

The following case studies are included to show how clinical evaluation combines with the use of clinical testing. As will be evident, the decisions may not necessarily be clearcut, with clinical judgement and experience accounting for much when deciding the best course for patient management.

Case study 8.1

Mr Saad Arundi is a 71-year-old Pakistani man with a 10-year history of a reported heart murmur but otherwise asymptomatic. Some 18 months ago he began to experience dyspnoea, particularly on walking uphill, and was referred by his GP to a cardiologist at his local hospital. Here an ECG revealed atrial fibrillation (AF) at rates of 50–90 bpm. Subsequent Holter monitoring suggested this to be established AF (rather than paroxysmal). An echocardiogram (echo) was reported as showing moderately good left ventricular (LV) function, mild thickening of the aortic valve cusps and mitral annulus and with mild mitral regurgitation. He was prescribed digoxin for ventricular rate control of his atrial fibrillation. On routine clinical follow-up 18 months later, the patient presented in AF with a rapid ventricular rate of 130–150 bpm and mentioned that his dyspnoea had become significantly more obvious over the recent few months. Ausculation of the heart revealed a harsh pansystolic murmur at the apex and a basal murmur radiating to the neck, suggesting aortic valve disease. Additionally, there was a suspicion of an early diastolic murmur but this was masked by the rapid AF. The lung fields were clear to auscultation and the brachial blood pressure was 170/90 mmHg. A chest X-ray suggested moderate cardiomegaly and slight pulmonary venous hypertension. There had been no history of rheumatic fever, orthopnoea, paroxysmal nocturnal dyspnoea (PND), cough, sputum, chest pain or syncope.

A further echocardiogram was requested that demonstrated mild concentric LV hypertrophy (LVH): interventricular septum (IVS) 1.5 cm, LV posterior wall 1.3 cm and a dilated LV cavity with some global impairment of systolic function (LV end diastolic dimension 6.1 cm, LV end systole 4.8 cm). The aortic valve was heavily calcified and Doppler studies showed an increased flow velocity equivalent to a calculated peak gradient of 65 mmHg. In the presence of AF a continuity equation was applied, giving a calculated valve area of 0.6 cm². The mitral valve and annulus (most notable around the insertion of the posterior leaflet) showed coincidental annular calcification with some overall reduction in cusp mobility facilitating at least moderate MR (mitral regurgitation) as indicated from colour and spectral Doppler studies. Mr Arundi responded to initial medical management and was referred for elective cardiac catheterisation. This was performed 5 months later as a day admission at the tertiary referral centre.

Coronary angiography revealed minor disease in the circumflex but otherwise essentially normal coronary arteries. Left ventricular injection showed moderately severe mitral regurgitation, obvious aortic stenosis and moderately impaired LV function. Haemodynamic pressure data showed a withdrawal pressure gradient of 60 mmHg (LV 210/30 to aorta 150/100 with an elevated pulmonary capillary wedge (LA) mean pressure of 32 mmHg and a systolic V wave of 58 mmHg.

A diagnosis of rheumatic heart disease with moderate to severe aortic stenosis and moderately severe mitral regurgitation was made. Mr Arundi was referred to the cardiothoracic surgeons for consideration of aortic and mitral valve replacement.

Case study 8.2

Mr Jim Yates is a 55-year-old Post Office worker who presented to his GP complaining of episodes of tightness across his chest on exertion. His symptoms developed whilst carrying heavy mail, causing him to stop and rest, and were particularly noticeable on cold days. The GP ordered routine blood tests, referred him to a cardiologist and prescribed sublingual GTN (glyceryl trinitrate) as an interim measure.

Mr Yates was seen in the cardiology clinic where he was assessed as overweight and found to be a moderate drinker and smoker of 30 years. Historically his grandfather had died of a 'heart attack' at age 62 years and his own father was under current treatment for angina. A resting ECG was performed showing inverted T-waves in leads II, III and aVF, indicating ischaemia of the inferior myocardial territory together with minor lateral ST changes. Subsequent blood tests revealed a significantly elevated cholesterol level and an exercise test was carried out with the patient managing 7 minutes according to the Bruce protocol. The results from this were summarized as follows.

Maximum heart rate attained 134 bpm (representing 81% of target maximum 165 bpm) with the blood pressure increasing steadily from 150/80 mmHg at rest to 205/90 mmHg at peak exercise. Towards the end of stage 2 (i.e. at $5\frac{1}{2}$ min into the exercise protocol) some tightness in the chest was reported. Within 1 min of stage 3 the chest pain had become more apparent and was accompanied by

2 mm of ST depression in the inferior ECG leads. Shortness of breath was also clearly evident and the test was terminated. When asked, Mr Yates confirmed that the pain was similar to his previous experiences and assessed this at 7 on a scale of 1–10.

A preliminary diagnosis of coronary artery disease was made and Mr Yates was placed on the waiting list for an elective coronary angiogram. In the interim period, he was commenced on aspirin (an antiplatelet agent), sotalol (a β-blocker, to reduce the heart rate and hence myocardial oxygen demand) and simvastatin (a cholesterol-lowering drug).

In due course Mr Yates reported for his day case angiogram procedure which was reported as follows.

1. Left ventricular angiogram: normal with well-preserved left ventricular function.
2. Coronary arteriograms:
   - intact left main stem (LMS)
   - left coronary artery
     - left anterior descending artery: mild irregularity only

   - left circumflex artery: no significant stenosis
- right coronary artery
  - severe localized stenosis within the proximal third of the artery with the vessel diameter assessed at 2.5–3 mm in the region of the stenosis.

Mr Yates was subsequently placed on the waiting list for an angioplasty to his right coronary artery. Two months later the procedure was performed via a right femoral arterial approach. The stenosis was predilated using a 2.5 mm diameter balloon followed by implantation of a coronary stent (3 mm diameter × 15 mm length). The result was declared successful with good anterograde blood flow down the coronary artery and no sign of residual stenosis. Mr Yates was discharged the following day on short-term clopidogrel (an antiplatelet agent) and long-term aspirin and simvastatin. He was scheduled for routine outpatient follow-up.

Mr Joel Bateman is a 60-year-old South African man who presented to the cardiac arrhythmia clinic as a new patient with a somewhat complex history following referral from his local hospital. He reported having had a myocardial infarction (MI) approximately 12 years ago at home in Cape Town and gave a lengthy history of palpitations with episodes of shortness of breath over the last 6 years. This was most noticeable over the last 18 months with some dizziness but no associated syncope. Six years ago a hospital admission due to tachycardia was needed resulting in a prescription for sotalol (β-blocker) which had been taken daily ever since.

When questioned on his exercise capabilities, Mr Bateman mentioned his ongoing attendance at the asthma/allergy clinic at his local hospital with a diagnosis of bronchiolitis obliterans requiring inhaler therapy. An incidental echocardiogram (echo) at the hospital, offered as a screening procedure by the cardiac unit some 18 months ago, revealed only moderate LV function with scarring and thinning of the interventricular septum (IVS) and anterior LV myocardial territory with possible thrombus formation at the apex. Accordingly, he was referred to the local cardiology clinic. Subsequent examination and a review of the echo led to adjustment of his medication regimen to include warfarin (an anticoagulant) and lisinopril (an ACE inhibitor) for his impaired LV function. One month later some improvement had been noted in his breathing and the sotalol dosage was reduced with a view to weaning off altogether.

However, 6 weeks later Mr Bateman suffered an acute episode of palpitations and dyspnoea accompanied by mild dizziness but without pain or syncope. This required admission via the Accident and Emergency (A&E) unit where a diagnosis of

ventricular tachycardia (VT) was made requiring DC cardioversion. Blood results were found to be normal but his original sotalol dose was recommenced and a cardiology opinion reinvited. His physical signs at that time were unremarkable, although an ECG was taken that showed sinus rhythm, left axis deviation and extensive Q-waves in leads V1–V5. A chest X-ray was essentially normal and the findings of a repeat echocardiogram were consistent with an old extensive antero-apical myocardial infarction and moderately impaired LV function with long-standing thrombus formation. A 24-hour tape revealed little more than periodic multifocal ventricular ectopics. The formal diagnosis of ischaemic heart disease complicated by VT, chronic obstructive pulmonary disease (COPD) and bronchiolitis was made.

Two weeks later Mr Bateman was again forced to attend the A&E unit with suspected VT requiring cardioversion, followed by a further similar episode 2 months later at which point amiodarone (an anti-arrhythmic) was also prescribed. Mr Bateman remained trouble free for only 3 months before presenting yet again to A&E with an episode of palpitations, moderate dyspnoea and dizziness. More detailed records were taken at this visit and the ECG showed a broad complex tachycardia at a cycle length of 400 ms, extreme left axis deviation and right bundle branch morphology. On this occasion, however, there was a spontaneous return to sinus rhythm with a resting ECG as previously reported. Some mild resting chest pain was also documented. A chest X-ray showed an enlarged heart and upper lobe blood diversion suggestive of early pulmonary oedema. To aid future management decisions and in consideration of his lack of exercise tolerance, it was decided to carry out thallium testing to evaluate the

---

Case study 8.3 *continued*

reversible status of his ischaemia. The results of this indicated reversible ischaemia in the basal and mid anterior wall with reduced muscle mass in the septum and basal inferior wall. The apex, apical inferior wall and apical anterior wall were seen to be no longer viable; 'viable' refers to effective function.

After identifying a potential for revascularization, Mr Bateman was referred to the tertiary care centre for specialist evaluation of his arrhythmia status. A SAECG demonstrated a negative result but nevertheless it was decided that as the patient was prone to confirmed VT, he must be considered a potential risk for sudden death. Ultimately his arrhythmia management would depend on the outcome of any revascularization therapy carried out, whether this be coronary angioplasty or coronary artery bypass grafting. With an encouraging thallium result, cardiac catheterisation proceeding to interventional percutaneous transluminal coronary angioplasty (PTCA)/stenting was organized on his current admission. Catheterisation revealed overall poor LV function with a large calcified antero-apical aneurysm. A large circumflex coronary artery demonstrated a tight proximal stenosis, although this was not evident in all angiographic views. The left anterior descending (LAD) artery had a long proximal stenosis with a totally occluded diagonal branch. The RCA was found to possess a complex long 50% lesion in it mid portion. On the basis of a largely

infarcted LAD territory, the circumflex lesion was identified as the target vessel and was subsequently dilated with a 3×20 mm balloon. This was followed by deployment of a 3×16 mm coronary stent, with an excellent angiographic result.

The need for subsequent anti-arrhythmic therapy and the course of action became dependent on whether a substrate for VT could still be shown to exist post revascularization. A VT stimulation study was therefore scheduled. With programmed stimulation from the right ventricular apex, ventricular tachycardia of the same morphology and rate (cycle length) to the clinical VT was found to be inducible and amenable to termination with overdrive pacing. In the context of sudden death syndrome it was decided that medical management alone would be inappropriate and 3 days later Mr Bateman was implanted with a cardioverter-defibrillator (ICD) to the left pectoral region. This was programmed for antitachycardia overdrive pacing for his VT with full defibrillation back-up. Prior to discharge from hospital an exercise test was conducted to confirm the appropriate setting of the ICD device and an echo was performed to establish new baseline function. Both support and education were offered to Mr Bateman and his wife with regard to living with the ICD. Chapter 25 offers greater detail regarding ICDs and the significance of nursing care.

CONCLUSION

This chapter has explored the variety of diagnostic investigations currently available within cardiac care. The patient who is undergoing such investigations will be offered reassurance and explanation from the team involved. However, nursing staff need to take time to provide verbal and if possible written information and to listen to the concerns of the patient and their loved ones. Health-care staff who are deciding whether to enter this area of diagnostic work will find the discussions and principles outlined in this chapter of use in offering an overview of the specialty.

REFERENCES

Conroy RM, Mulcahy R 1985 Readability of literature written for cardiac patients. Clinical Cardiology 8(2): 104–106

Cupple SA 1991 Effects of timing and reinforcement of pre-operative education on knowledge and recovery of patients having coronary artery bypass surgery. Heart and Lung 20(6): 654–660

Doak LG, Doak CC 1980 Patient comprehension profiles: recent findings and strategies. Patient Counselling and Health Education 2(3): 101–106

Dobree L 1990 Pre-operative advice for patients. Nursing Standard 4(48): 28–30

Dowling N, O'Keefe M 1990 Preparation for cardiac catheterization. Nursing Review 10(1): 15–19

Erbel R, Ge J 1998 Introduction. In: Erbel R, Roelandt J, Ge J, Gorge G (eds) Intravascular ultrasound. Martin Dunitz, London, pp. 1–9

Fogoros RN 1999 Electrophysiologic testing (practical cardiac diagnosis), 3rd edn. Blackwell Science, New York

Hubner P 1998 Guide to coronary angioplasty and stenting. Harwood Academic Publishers, Amsterdam, p. 59

Lay P, Spelman MS 1967 cited by Dowling N, O'Keefe M 1990 Preparation for cardiac catheterization. Nursing Review 10(1): 15–19

McKenzie J 1916 Principles of diagnosis and treatment in heart affections. Oxford Medical Publications, London, p. 48

Peterson M 1991 Patient anxiety before cardiac catheterization. An intervention study. Heart and Lung 20(6): 643–647

Ricciuti CG 1997 Cardiac catheterization. In: Van Riper S, Van Riper J (eds) Cardiac diagnostic tests. A guide for nurses. WB Saunders, Philidelphia, pp. 265–296

Wilson-Barnett J 1980 The prevention and alleviation of stress in patients. Nursing 10: 432–436

FURTHER READING

Chambers J 1995 Clinical echocardiography. BMJ Books, London

Cheitlin MD, Alpert JS, Armstrong WF et al 1997 ACC/AHA guidelines for the clinical application of echocardiography. A report of the American College of Cardiology/American Heart Association task force on practice guidelines (Committee on Clinical Application of Echocardiography. Developed in collaboration with the American Society of Echocardiography). Circulation 95(6): 1686–1744

Froelicher VF, Quaqlietti S 1997 Handbook of ambulatory cardiology. Lippincott-Raven, Philadelphia

Grainger RG, Allison DJ 1997 Diagnostic radiology: a textbook of medical imaging, volume 1, 3rd edn. Churchill Livingstone, Edinburgh

Giuliani ER, Fuster V, Gersh BJ, McGoon MD, McGoon DC 1991 Cardiology fundamentals and practice, volumes 1 and 2, 2nd edn. Yearbook Medical, Chicago

Julian DG (ed) 1996 Diseases of the heart, 2nd edn. WB Saunders, London

Kumar P, Clark M 1994 Clinical medicine, 3rd edn. Baillière Tindall, London

McGhie AI (ed) 2001 Handbook of non-invasive cardiac testing. Arnold, London

Wegener OH 1992 Whole body computed tomography, 2nd edn. Blackwell Science, Oxford

Cardiac conditions

This section explores the variety of cardiac conditions encountered by the nurse practitioner. Each chapter explores the epidemiology, the proposed cause and the progress of the condition. The emphasis is placed upon the increasingly empowered role of the nurse in monitoring the condition, facilitating health promotion strategies and manipulating treatments to encourage an optimum state of health.

9

Coronary heart disease: angina and acute myocardial infarction

Tom Quinn
Rosemary Webster
Richard Hatchett

Coronary heart disease (CHD) is the single most common cause of premature death in the United Kingdom (UK). The burden of CHD on patients, their families and loved ones and society as a whole is considerable. The principal clinical manifestations of CHD are angina and acute myocardial infarction. In this chapter the diagnosis, treatment and management of these conditions are discussed, together with the associated nursing care. Emerging areas of care provision such as nurse-led thrombolysis, which aims to reduce the wait to initiate this definitive treatment, are explored.

DEFINITION

Coronary heart disease (CHD) is the term used to describe the effects of a reduction or complete obstruction of the blood flow (and oxygen transport) through the coronary arteries as a result of narrowing (**atherosclerosis**) and/or blood clot (**thrombus**). Patients with CHD may be asymptomatic; however, the most common clinical manifestation is chest pain due to stable or unstable angina and acute myocardial infarction (AMI). The latter can frequently present as sudden death. In addition, CHD can result in disorders of heart rhythm (**arrhythmias**) and heart failure.

THE BURDEN OF DISEASE

Coronary heart disease remains a progressive disease and is the major cause of ill health and premature death in the developed world. As the largest single cause of death in the UK, CHD is responsible for over 135 000 deaths per year (BHF 2000), amongst the highest mortality rates in the world. Although the death rate from CHD is in fact falling, one in four men and one in five women still die from this disease (BHF 2000).

Routinely collected data from England indicate that there are over 300 000 inpatient admissions (195 679 involving men) per annum for CHD (Department of Health (DoH) 1996) out of a total 9.5 million 'all-cause' hospitalizations. CHD therefore accounts for 5% of all hospital admissions in men and 2% in women. There are both geographical and socio-economic variations in incidence and mortality from CHD. Death rates are falling faster in professional people than in unskilled manual workers, with an estimated 5000 deaths per annum resulting from this 'health gap'.

The economic consequences of CHD are considerable, as are the costs in human terms. It takes time to correlate figures but the disease cost the health service some £1.6 billion in 1996, just over half of this being accounted for by hospital care and a third by drug prescriptions. Interestingly, only 1% of costs were attributed to prevention. But health-care expenditure is only part of the cost to the taxpayer: time away from work due to CHD, lost productivity, premature death and the 'hidden costs' of non-health service care (usually provided informally by families or carers) cost the UK economy in the region of £8.5 billion in 1996. More recently, the British Heart Foundation (BHF) quoted a figure of £10 billion per year (BHF 2001). Overall, almost a fifth of production losses were due to CHD mortality, over half to CHD morbidity and a quarter to 'informal care' of CHD sufferers. More recent figures estimate that the total economic burden of CHD is now £10 000 million per annum in the UK, more than double that for any other disease for which a comparable analysis has been carried out (BHF 2000).

Given this miserable toll, it is hardly surprising that CHD features prominently in government policy. The White Paper *Saving lives: our healthier nation* (DoH 1999) set targets for a 40% reduction in deaths from CHD and cerebrovascular accident (CVA/stroke) in those under 75 years of age by the year 2010. The National Service Framework (NSF) for Coronary Heart Disease (DoH 2000a) set national standards and defined service models and monitoring arrangements for the prevention and treatment of CHD in England. The NSF, which set the scene for a 10-year programme of modernizing and improving services for CHD, represents the 'blueprint' for action required to reduce CHD mortality as set out in the White Paper. It set standards across the whole of the CHD journey, from health promotion to primary care, emergency care, specialist cardiology, cardiac surgery and rehabilitation.

PATHOPHYSIOLOGY OF CORONARY HEART DISEASE

Atherosclerosis is a complex progressive disease, associated with dynamic interactions between blood elements, alterations in blood flow and vessel wall abnormalities which several theories attempt to explain. Clinically significant abnormalities increase in number and extent during the first 15–34 years of life (Strong et al 1999).

Epidemiological evidence suggests that a variety of factors may be important in the progression of the disease. For example, studies have reported an association between atherosclerosis and certain bacterial (*Chlamydia pneumoniae* and *Helicobacter pylori*) and viral (cytomegalovirus) infections (Cheng & Rivera 1998). Insulin resistance and hyperinsulinaemia, the renin–angiotensin–aldosterone system (Malik et al 1997), elevated levels of homocysteine (Whincup et al 1999) and altered autonomic activity as a result of psychological stress (Mathews et al 1998) have also been implicated.

Atherosclerosis is characterized by the proliferation of smooth muscle cells and the accumulation of elevated protruding white lesions known as plaques in the intima of the arterial wall. Plaques consist of a lipid core and fibrous outer layer and it is the plaques with a high-fibre, low-lipid content that tend to produce the most severe stenosis (MacIsaac et al 1993). It is plaque rupture or fissuring and subsequent thrombosis that makes coronary atherosclerosis dangerous. In plaques with a high lipid concentration the fibrous cap is more likely to rupture, exposing the central core to blood flow. This exposed plaque centre is highly thrombogenic and platelets accumulate around it, ultimately resulting in the formation of a platelet thrombus and activation of the coagulation system. A thrombus superimposed on a plaque severely restricts blood flow. Clinical presentation is in part determined by the reactivity of circulating platelets and the balance between the coagulation and fibrinolytic systems (Dalager-Pedersen et al 1998).

It is not known whether acute cardiac events occur spontaneously or if they are the result of trigger factors. There is, however, a defined circadian pattern to these events with two distinct peaks, one in the early morning and one at midnight (Thompson et al 1991). This may be linked to the corresponding diurnal variation in blood viscosity and coagulability.

MYOCARDIAL ISCHAEMIA

Myocardial ischaemia results when coronary blood supply is insufficient in providing the oxygen needed to maintain myocardial tissue oxygen tension. This situation results in anaerobic respiration and is the result of an imbalance between myocardial oxygen supply and demand. Clinically, this imbalance results in an inadequate supply of oxygen to the myocardial cells, myocardial ischaemia and angina. A sudden or complete cessation of blood flow, as may result from a thrombus, results in necrosis of myocardial tissue (myocardial infarction).

Myocardial oxygen supply is generally determined by coronary artery blood flow. The fact that manifestations of ischaemia can occur at rest when there is no apparant increase in myocardial oxygen demand suggests that it is blood supply that is the significant factor. Critical restriction to blood flow occurs when the diameter of the lumen is reduced by more than half. Coronary blood flow is also determined by perfusion pressure, which is adversely affected by abnormalities in blood flow (stenosis, valvular disease), abnormalities in coronary vessel wall (atheroma, spasm) and abnormalities in the blood (anaemia, polycythaemia; the latter refers to an abnormally high level of circulating red blood cells).

Myocardial oxygen demand depends primarily on heart rate, the strength of myocardial contraction and left ventricular wall tension. The myocardium receives most of its blood supply when relaxed in diastole. As the rate increases (activity, pyrexia, arrhythmia, etc.) the duration of diastole is disproportionately decreasd compared to systole. There is therefore a reduction in coronary perfusion at a time of increased oxygen demand, with a potential for ischaemia. Sympathetic stimulation (associated with the increased heart rate) compounds the situation by increasing the force of contraction and increasing oxygen demand. Left ventricular wall tension is increased with changes in the preload and afterload. This affects the intracardiac pressures and volumes, the work of the heart and consequently myocardial oxygen demand. The preload can be defined as the end-diastolic blood volume (the volume of blood at the end of ventricular filling). The afterload is the resistance to ventricular ejection. The latter is usually a result of systemic vascular resistance, which increases as the body maintains tissue oxygen perfusion.

ANGINA

Angina is the term used to describe the discomfort that occurs during periods of myocardial ischaemia. It is a symptom, not a disease. Whilst individuals differ in their symptoms and the words used to describe them, angina classically consists of a retrosternal constricting discomfort which may radiate to either arm, the throat, the jaw, the teeth, the back or the epigastrium. It is usually a manifestation of CHD but any situation which upsets the balance between myocardial oxygen supply and demand may result in angina.

Epidemiology

Angina is the most common manifestation of CHD. It affects approximately 2 million men and women in the UK (Jackson 1997), with an estimated 22 600 new cases being diagnosed each year in the United Kingdom (Ghandi et al 1995). The British Heart Foundation has more recently quoted a figure of 2.1 million people alive in the UK with, or having had, angina, with 330 000 new cases occurring each year (BHF 2001). The prevalence increases with age in both sexes, in men from 2–5% aged 45–54 years to 11–20% aged 64–74 years, and in women 0.5–1% and 10–14% respectively. Over the age of 75 years the prevalence is the same in both sexes (Jackson 1997).

Presentation

Angina is a common symptom in both general and hospital practice. It is frequently classed as either stable or unstable.

Stable angina involves a fixed coronary artery lesion, limiting the oxygen supply at times of increased demand. Symptoms are therefore typically provoked by an activity that increases myocardial oxygen demand. Exercise/exertion (including sexual intercourse) and emotional factors are significant. The discomfort is usually relieved within 2–10 minutes by rest. Classic associated symptoms are shortness of breath, sweating, nausea, vomiting, palpitations and weakness. Symptoms tend to be worse in the morning, coinciding with a peak in blood pressure, after heavy meals and in cold weather. There is little correlation between the severity of symptoms and the disease process, although if the history is typical, the probability of CHD is high. People with stable angina are at increased risk of AMI and sudden death. It is estimated that around 10% of those presenting with anginal symptoms to their general practitioner (GP) will either have a non-fatal AMI or die from coronary causes in the following year (Ghandi et al 1995). Therefore, targeting this group with appropriate strategies is a significant part of an effective CHD management strategy.

Unstable angina is commonly associated with the rupture of an atherosclerotic plaque, accompanied by the release of vasoconstrictor substances which may induce clotting. This leads to the formation of thrombi and intermittent or prolonged obstruction of the coronary artery. Characteristically, unstable angina presents as:

- recent onset of experiencing angina symptoms (within the past 4–6 weeks)
- a change in the symptoms experienced, i.e. the discomfort has become more frequent, more easily triggered, more severe or prolonged or less responsive to nitrate therapy

- discomfort/pain and associated symptoms occurring in the absence of physical or emotional stress and lasting more than 20 minutes.

The individual may present in a variety of settings, including the GP's surgery, the accident and emergency department and the coronary care unit (CCU). This presentation may be the first manifestaion of CHD or it may occur as an abrupt change in an established pattern of chronic stable angina. Unstable angina in the first few weeks after an AMI has a particularly serious prognosis and specifically including this group of patients in the definition of unstable angina has aided management. Unstable angina is a medical emergency. Myocardial infarction or death can occur in up to a third of cases within 3 months. Predictors of high risk include:

- more than 20 minutes of chest pain at rest
- pulmonary oedema
- new or worsening mitral regurgitation
- pain at rest associated with ST changes of 1 mm or more on the 12-lead electrocardiogram (ECG)
- myocardial infarction within the previous 2 weeks (after Calvin et al 1995, Rizik et al 1995).

Diagnosis

An accurate diagnosis is an essential step in the investigation and management of angina. Diagnosis focuses on a range of factors including the nature of the symptoms, the perceived likelihood of coronary artery disease (based on the individual's cardiovascular risk profile) and the results of various diagnostic tests.

Clinical history

Obtaining a clear clinical history may be difficult, particularly if the patient is in distress or frightened. Chest pain is usually the presenting complaint, however. It has many causes and determining its aetiology can be a challenge for the practitioner. The complaint will be influenced by personality and cultural factors and a sound history plays an important role in diagnosis. Patients will have different experiences and vary in the way they describe symptoms. A pain that has become a part of everyday life will not be described in the same way as one which is of sudden onset, intense or frightening. Someone who believes they are experiencing a severe bout of indigestion will behave in a different way from one who is convinced that they are about to die as a result of a heart attack.

Research indicates that pain assessment is complex and that professionals vary in their ability to carry out and document this important apect of care (Bondestam

et al 1987, O'Connor 1995). Various tools have been used in attempts to measure cardiac pain with varying success (Standing 1997). A pain scale which asks the patient to rate the intensity of their pain on a numerical scale has been shown to be of value in quantifying pain in individual patients (Thompson et al 1994). However, it is limited in its ability to qualify the nature of the pain experienced. The use of words is important. An individual who thinks of his angina in terms of an ache or heaviness may not admit to experiencing any *pain*. Asking what they think is causing the symptom is a useful way of beginning to explore the significance of the situation for the individual concerned. Various factors influence how an individual responds to their chest pain; in particular, the time taken to seek medical advice. This is discussed later in this chapter.

It is important to establish the nature, intensity, duration, radiation of the pain and precipitating, aggravating and relieving factors. Establishing if this experience is similar to previous episodes may help clarify the situation, as will identifying associated symptoms such as shortness of breath and nausea. Some patients present atypically and may have co-existing disease which complicates diagnosis. Distinguishing between angina and oesophageal reflux can be difficult, particularly as nitrates can be effective in both instances. Signs such as hypotension and sweating, occurring as a result of non-cardiac pain, may confuse the picture. The differential diagnosis of chest pain should always be considered.

Cardiovascular risk profile

The presence of risk markers such as previous cardiac history, evidence of stenosis or previous revascularization procedures, family history of CHD, hypertension or diabetes and other established risk factors such as smoking and advancing age make it more likely that chest pain is ischaemic in origin. Blood pressure measurement, assessment of body mass index (BMI) and a record of cholesterol level should also be part of the initial assessment.

Diagnostic tests

A baseline 12-lead ECG is essential despite the insensitivity of this test. It may be normal, even in severe cases, but should be a routine investigation (Jackson 1997). If the pain appears cardiac in origin, ECGs should be repeated as often as every 30 minutes. An abnormal 12-lead ECG identifies a patient subgroup with a significantly higher risk of death or myocardial infarction. Most patients with definite unstable angina will have ST segment depression but occasionally only T-wave inversion. The ST and T-wave abnormalities classically associated with unstable angina can also occur in AMI, stress-induced stable angina, left ventricular hypertrophy and in patients taking glycosides.

If possible, an ECG should be obtained during pain. This may show ST elevation (Prinzmetal changes) or more frequently demonstrate down-sloping ST depression that resolves with resolution of the pain. Alterations in the shape of the T-wave, such as flattening, peaking and inversion, can also occur with pain. Ischaemic changes in the ECG during pain do not always correlate with angiographic findings. Some patients will subsequently have rises in levels of cardiac markers confirming myocardial infarction, usually of the non-Q wave variety. These patients should be managed in the same ways as those with unstable angina.

Levels for **biochemical cardiac markers**, which can indicate myocardial damage, should be performed on admission and again at 12 hours. Measurement of serum markers, such as myoglobin and the creatine kinase-MB (CK-MB) isoenzyme subunit, has proved beneficial in the emergency setting for detecting myocardial necrosis in patients with a non-diagnostic ECG. The cardiac troponins T and I (cTnT and cTnI) have been found to be particularly sensitive and specific measures of cardiac muscle damage. They have proven useful for the diagnosis and subsequent risk stratification of patients presenting with chest pain (Collinson 2000). Risk stratification, as discussed in Chapter 3, is the assessment of the future risk of a coronary event to an individual and has traditionally been viewed according to the clinical status; patients with elevated troponin levels have an increased risk of ischaemic complications, including sudden death (Sayre et al 1998). A bedside system is now available for measuring troponin T and I. This takes some minutes to offer a result but will obviously have an impact on providing further and more speedy evidence of myocardial damage and therefore definitive treatment. Box 9.1 provides the characteristics of cardiac enzymes and other biochemical cardiac markers.

Exercise testing with ECG monitoring, which should form part of the diagnostic screen, is only worthwhile if carried out and interpreted by trained clinicians. The Bruce protocol is most commonly used (Detrano et al 1989) and the test considered positive if there is 1 mm or more of reversible ST segment depression. False-positive tests are more common in populations with a lower incidence of CHD, including women (Melin et al 1985). A good performance on an exercise test is generally associated with a good prognosis (MacRae et al 1992).

Radionuclide studies in the form of myocardial perfusion imaging with thallium or other radionuclides have a higher diagnostic sensitivity and specificity for CHD than an exercise test (Rosanski & Berman 1987). However, they require more expensive equipment and specifically trained staff and are therefore usually reserved for cases where an exercise ECG is inconclusive or unhelpful.

Stress echocardiography improves sensitivity and specificity of a conventional exercise ECG and is comparable to myocardial perfusion imaging for diagnosis, although it is less satisfactory in estimating prognosis (O'Keefe et al 1995).

Coronary angiography, while more invasive than the tests outlined above, is regarded in many countries as a routine investigation. Angiography gives a detailed record of the coronary arteries and their anatomy, although it is not able to diagnose atheroma or myocardial ischaemia. Angiography is justified in all cases where findings would alter patient management and a ratio of 2:1 angiograms to intervention is considered reasonable. Overall mortality from coronary angiography is in the region of 1/2000 procedures and the serious complication rate is about 1% (De Bono 1993). Chapter 8 highlights in detail the specific cardiac diagnostic tests.

Referral for assessment

It has been recommended that all newly diagnosed cases of angina in patients under 70 years of age should be referred to a physician with a special interest and training in cardiology (De Bono 1999). Open access referral for exercise testing is appropriate provided there is a mechanism for expert review of test findings and consultation. Referral is also indicated where the diagnosis is in doubt or where a positive diagnosis would have major implications for the patient's livelihood. Patients should have rapid access to a cardiologist, ideally via a chest pain clinic.

Chest pain clinics

The importance of rapid-access chest pain clinics has been highlighted in the NSF for Coronary Heart Disease (DoH 2000a). This recommended that individuals who develop new symptoms of angina should be assessed by a specialist within 2 weeks of referral. It also stated that there should be at least 100 such clinics functional by 2002. Cardiology outpatient clinics and open access exercise testing are other strategies for improving GP access for advice and investigations.

Facilities for initial assessment, diagnosis and care should be easily accessible and in pleasant surroundings. As much information as possible should be available to the patient, family and carers about the illness, prognosis and the expected outcome, as well as any ongoing difficulties that might be expected. If a period of hospitalization is anticipated, a realistic date for admission is necessary. Help, information and support

---

Box 9.1 The characteristics of cardiac enzymes and other biochemical cardiac markers

Creatine kinase (CK) is found in high levels in skeletal and cardiac muscle and also in the brain. It is regarded as a highly sensitive enzyme and the gold standard for detecting AMI. CK can also be written as creatine phosphokinase (CPK). It rises and falls within 72 hours, being at its peak at 24 hours. The more specific CK-MB iso-enzyme may be measured but it will alter with events such as cardiac surgery and after strenuous exercise. CK-MB has two isoforms: MB_1 from serum and MB_2 from myocardial tissue. The normal ratio is 1.0. A ratio of MB_2/MB_1 >1.5 is diagnostic of myocardial damage. This raised ratio occurs before total CK-MB elevates with conventional testing (Swanton 1998). CK normal values: adult females 33–145 iu/l, adult males 33–186 iu/l. CK-MB: 0–12 iu/l.

Lactic dehydrogenase (LDH) elevation starts within 24–48 hours. This peaks at about 4–5 days following infarction but is useful in that it remains elevated for up to approximately 2 weeks. It is not specific to cardiac tissue and can rise in conditions such as renal disease, haemolysis/erythrocyte damage (beware of haemolysed blood samples) and liver disease. Normal values: adult male and female 266–500 iu/l. Further studies focused on the five iso-enzymes of LDH can help reduce false positives. LDH_1 is found in cardiac tissue.

Aspartate aminotransferase (AST) is also known as serum glutamic oxaloacetic transaminase (SGOT). Levels of this enzyme, which is found in approximately 70% of myocardial infarctions, rise after 8–12 hours, peaking at about 24 hours. It is less specific than CK-MB and again, it does elevate in other disorders such as liver disease and following intramuscular injections. It remains elevated for about 5 days. The normal level is approximately 10–45 iu/l.

Troponin T levels rise within 2–6 hours of myocardial damage and levels remain elevated for up to 2 weeks. It is a highly sensitive marker of myocardial damage (Murphy & Berding 1999) and can be useful in risk stratification, where there may be no apparent ECG changes. Troponin T is also a valuable prognostic indicator for patients with unstable angina (Murphy & Berding 1999). A direct correlation has been noted between raised levels and the risk of complications or death in unstable angina at the 30-day and 6-month period after elevated levels are detected (Lindahl et al 1996, Ohman et al 1996). A cut-off value of 0.1 µg/l is generally recommended in interpretation of myocardial damage.

Troponin I is rapidly released into the circulation after myocardial damage. It can be used to indicate reperfusion as levels wash into the blood and as a guide to further reinfarction. As is the case with troponin T, troponin I appears to be more specific than and as sensitive as CK-MB tests in the diagnosis of AMI in the 7–14-hour period after the onset of chest pain (Murphy & Berding 1999, Wu et al 1996). Again, it is useful in risk

stratification. Troponin I is useful and more specific in peri-operative myocardial infarction than CK-MB, because CK levels will elevate due to the muscle damage of surgery (Adams et al 1994, Murphy & Berding 1999). There are several troponin I assays available from different manufacturers which report different numerical values, primarily due to the use of different calibration materials. The quoted normal values (reference ranges), cut-off values and results seen in patients with unstable angina and myocardial infarction may therefore differ; the laboratory and/or manufacturer's literature should be consulted for guidance. Typically troponin I methods will be quoted as having a detection limit of 0.1 or 0.35 µg/l for the Bayo Immuno 1 and Dade Stratus systems respectively, the upper limit of the reference ranges being between ≤0.1 and ≤0.6 µg/l, respectively. The cut-off values quoted for these systems in patients with myocardial infarction are 0.9 and 1.5 µg/l, respectively.

Unlike other cardiac markers the troponins are undetectable in healthy subjects, therefore even small increases will indicate myocardial damage. Figure 9.3 (p. 166) demonstrates the sensitivity of troponin as a marker of myocardial damage by recommending that management can be guided by two levels, one recorded on admission and one 12 hours later. This is because cardiac troponins do take several hours to rise, so initial values may be misleading. In the case of suspected reinfarction in the acute situation, it is advisable to take a troponin level immediately to provide a baseline and then a further sample 8–12 hours later. If there is a rise from baseline, further damage has occurred consistent with reinfarction.

Myoglobin is a haem protein (Murphy & Berding 1999). It is useful as one of the earliest markers to rise due to its small molecular weight, allowing it to escape easily from damaged muscle tissue, often within a few hours of infarction. It returns to normal within approximately 36 hours. It is highly sensitive. An elevated myoglobin level has been detected in almost all patients by 6 hours of chest pain in AMI (Selker et al 1997). Two negative samples taken approximately 2 hours apart rule out the incidence of myocardial infarction in approximately 90% of cases. Selker et al (1997) go further and state that if the myoglobin has not risen in the first 3–6 hours of chest discomfort, an AMI has not occurred. However, it is also found in skeletal muscle which can be problematic in interpreting results; for example, after strenuous exercise, intramuscular (IM) injections and in renal failure (Murphy & Berding 1999). The normal levels are reported as <100 µg/l.

It is worth noting that the measurement of cardiac enzymes is gradually being replaced by the troponins due to the greater sensitivity and specificity of the latter. The transition is limited by the increased cost (and method complexity) of the newer markers despite the fact that the clinical and economic benefits are obvious.

for the patient and family/carers from an appropriate source, such as a patient support group, may help reduce uncertainty and anxiety. Figure 9.1 offers an algorithm of investigation for those with cardiac chest pain. Angiography undertaken in those considered at high risk of infarction or sudden cardiac death will indicate whether revascularisation procedures such as percutaneous transluminal coronary angioplasty (PTCA) or coronary artery bypass grafting (CABG) are required.

Patients of any age with severe, unstable or rapidly progressive symptoms, those with angina secondary to a remediable cause or with unacceptable symptoms in spite of maximal medical therapy need to be referred for specialist management.

Stable angina

The management of the patient with stable angina comprises:

Box 9.2 The National Service Framework Standard for Stable Angina (DoH 2000a)

Standard 8
People with symptoms of angina or suspected angina should receive appropriate investigation and treatment to relieve their pain and reduce their risk of coronary events.

- secondary prevention of cardiac events
- symptom control with medication
- revascularization
- rehabilitation.

Secondary prevention of cardiac events

- *Antiplatelet therapy* has been shown to significantly reduce the incidence of AMI among patients with stable angina, particularly those at increased risk of

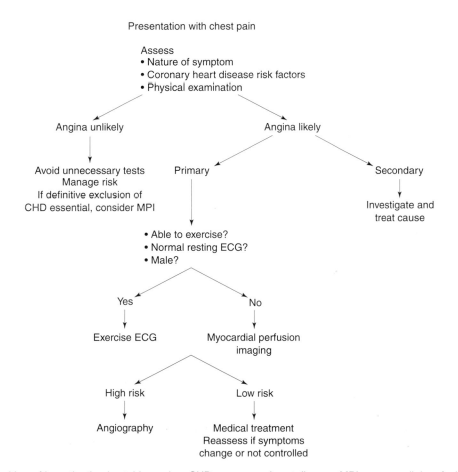

Figure 9.1 Algorithm of investigation in stable angina. CHD = coronary heart disease, MPI = myocardial perfusion imaging. (Reproduced with permission from De Bono 1999).

cardiac events (Antiplatelet Trialists' Collaboration 1994). This is usually in the form of daily aspirin therapy.

- *Lipid-lowering therapy* in the form of a statin to lower cholesterol concentration either to less than 5 mmol/l (low-density cholesterol to below 3 mmol/l) or by 30%, whichever is the greater, is recommended (DoH 2000a).

For those with familial hypercholesterolaemia, notably with high levels of low-density lipoprotein (LDL) cholesterol and who prove resistant to drug therapy, apheresis may be used. There are several systems available, but each removes blood via venous access into an extracorporeal circuit. LDH cholesterol is removed, lowering overall levels, and the blood is returned to the patient. The treatment is used for a relatively small number of patients, often with signs of premature coronary heart disease. Psychological support is needed because the treatment is often performed every few weeks to keep LDL cholesterol low.

Secondary care management usually takes place within a cardiac unit of a district general hospital, although where this institution houses a tertiary care centre, the same standards of care apply. Care for patients with stable CHD should be provided under the direction of a physician with a special interest and training in cardiology. Some patients, particularly those with diabetes, may be appropriately managed by other specialists in liaison with the local cardiologist. Facilities available for secondary care should include a full range of non-invasive diagnostic facilities, including resting and exercise ECG, ambulatory ECG and echocardiography (including both transthoracic and transoesophageal). The secondary care site should also provide a wide range of facilities for risk assessment and modification such as a lipid clinic. A designated cardiology ward, staffed by nurses trained in cardiac care and advanced life support (ALS) skills such as defibrillation, is considered essential. This helps ensure that patients with CHD obtain expert medical and nursing care and support. A CCU, again with appropriately trained nurses, is also considered essential. Close liaison between the CCU team, the resuscitation training officer and the cardiac rehabilitation service is vital.

Symptom control with medication

Many patients with mild to moderate symptoms of angina are currently managed by general physicians or GPs. Sublingual nitrates are considered standard treatment for immediate symptomatic control. A range of agents are available for background anti-anginal therapy including β-blockers, nitrates and calcium channel blockers, none of which has been proven in large trials to reduce the incidence of sudden death or non-fatal AMI. Alternative monotherapy should be considered before beginning combination therapy (DoH 2000a). There are sometimes theoretical reasons for combining two different families of anti-anginal drugs, for example β-blockers and calcium channel blockers but evidence to support the use of three or more anti-anginal agents is lacking (De Bono 1999).

In practice, the choice of agent will depend upon acceptability to individual patients. Patients need to be instructed to continue to take their anti-anginal medication unless medically advised not to do so, even if they feel their symptoms have stopped. They also need to be aware that they can take their glyceryl trinitrate (GTN) prophylactically. It is interesting to note that prescriptions issued in England for the treatment of circulatory disorders have increased markedly in recent years. Prescriptions for nitrates, vasodilators and calcium channel blockers increased from 5.1 million in 1981 to 22.6 million by 1997, while prescriptions for lipid-lowering drugs increased 15-fold in the same time period (BHF 1999). Chapter 19 provides more detailed information regarding cardiac drugs.

Non-pharmacological symptom control. Advice needs to be offered on avoiding situations that might trigger angina, such as exercising after a heavy meal, going out in the cold and intense emotional stress. Non-pharmacological approaches to symptom control in patients with frequent angina have included the use of transcutaneous electrical nerve stimulation (TENS) and spinal cord stimulation (SCS) (Anderson et al 1999, Hautvast et al 1996).

Revascularization

Coronary revascularization procedures are usually undertaken to relieve angina symptoms, although some patients may be referred for prognostic reasons. Candidates for revascularization include those with evidence of continuing extensive ischaemia or symptoms that persist despite optimal medical therapy (DoH 2000a).

Coronary artery bypass grafting (CABG). This procedure has been shown to improve symptoms and other quality-of-life indicators compared to medical treatment alone (Rogers et al 1990), although a meta-analysis of randomized trials suggests that overall benefit is confined to higher risk patients (Yusuf et al 1994).

Percutaneous transluminal coronary angioplasty (PTCA). This involves introducing a balloon catheter into the affected coronary artery and inflating the balloon within the stenosis. PTCA is superior to medical treatment in terms of symptomatic relief (RITA-2 Trial 1997), but there is no evidence of survival benefit at the present time. PTCA tends to be reserved for patients with single or two-vessel disease, in whom the short to medium-term prognosis is excellent. In this group of patients PTCA and CABG are comparable in terms of relieving symptoms and perioperative mortality is low in both groups, although patients undergoing PTCA are more likely to remain on antianginal medication and to require a repeat intervention (Pocock et al 1995). The risks associated with PTCA such as the need for emergency CABG, myocardial infarction and death are slightly higher in those with multi- as opposed to single-vessel disease and are slightly greater still in patients with unstable angina (Swanton 1998).

Centres undertaking revascularization procedures must be properly equipped and staffed, their operators competent and the cases selected appropriate (Gray et al 2000). On-site cardiac surgical cover is strongly preferred and it is recommended that PTCA procedures be confined to a tertiary cardiac centre with a minimum of 200 procedures undertaken each year and where the principal operators undertake at least 60 procedures per annum (Parker et al 1997).

The number of percutaneous revascularization interventions has increased over the past two decades, largely at the expense of medical treatment rather than surgical procedures. The indicators for the percutaneous methods have increased and no absolute contra-indications remain. The number requiring PTCA is likely to rise as more survivors from AMI subsequently require this treatment. PTCA is also increasingly being undertaken in the elderly and repeat revascularization is more common. It has been suggested, as the UK currently carries out comparatively few revascularization procedures compared to other European countries and the United States (US) (Windecker et al 1999), that the needs of the population are not being met. It had therefore been suggested that services in the UK should have aimed for 550 PTCA procedures per million population annually by the financial year 2000–1 (Gray et al 2000).

Stenting. The insertion of a temporary stent to prevent abrupt closure of the artery and longer term patency after PTCA has been shown to be superior to balloon angioplasty alone (Fischman et al 1994), reducing the need for repeat revascularization. A stent can be defined as a tiny tubular scaffold placed within a vessel, at a lesion site, to enlarge the lumen and support the vessel wall (Hubner 1998). The abandonment of post-stent systemic anticoagulation has

reduced the incidence of bleeding complications, reducing length of hospital stay and other costs associated with the monitoring of anticoagulation (Schomig et al 1996).

Glycoprotein-blocking agents. Several randomized controlled trials have demonstrated the benefits of the platelet glycoprotein IIb/IIIa inhibitors in reducing early death, non-fatal AMI and urgent revascularization when used during coronary interventions (CAPTURE 1997, EPILOG 1997, RAPPORT 1998). However, the longer term impact on requirement for repeat procedure has not been reported. Low-dose aspirin (75–325 mg/day) is recommended in patients undergoing coronary interventions, ideally administered at least one day before the procedure and continued indefinitely thereafter.

Nursing care and issues in percutaneous coronary intervention. Chapter 8 provides details of the varying cardiac diagnostic procedures. However, the nursing care for a diagnostic cardiac catheter and a PTCA do share similarities and the two are therefore discussed together here.

Diagnostic cardiac catheter. Following a diagnostic cardiac catheterisation (angiogram), the doctor will generally remove the sheaths and apply digital pressure over the femoral artery to aid closure of the puncture site. However, this may be performed by the nurse on return to the ward or unit. It is unusual to use heparin in this procedure. Pressure will be applied for at least 5 minutes, while some units state a minimum of 10 minutes (Searle & Hoff 2000), until haemostasis is achieved. Manual compression devices are occasionally used. These are usually applied as a belt around the hips and then inflated, much like a sphygmomanometer, to a value of approximately 20 mmHg above the systolic blood pressure. This enables a pad to press over the femoral area and achieve haemostasis.

There has been some debate in recent years as to how long the patient should then lie still and flat to reduce haematoma formation and aid vessel healing. Usually the patient lies flat for an hour, with one or two pillows, then moves to a sitting position, still keeping the affected leg straight. Searle & Hoff (2000), in reviewing the literature and contacting six catheter laboratories, found a variety of bedrest times ranging from 2 to 12 hours. Prolonged bedrest can be uncomfortable for the patient, resulting in back pain and the difficulties associated with using a bedpan or urinal. There is also the necessity to be able to drink, to clear the radio-opaque dye from the system. Some units therefore lay the patient at a slight angle initially, at approximately 30°. Searle & Hoff (2000) subsequently allocated patients to 3- and 2-hour bedrest periods following cardiac catheterisation. There were 696 and 680 patients in each group respectively. Both groups lay flat for 1 hour with the exception of a small number. The researchers found that early ambulation made no difference to outcomes in terms of bleeding and early haematoma formation. The patients were, however, carefully screened beforehand. Exclusion criteria included those with a platelet count $<150 \times 10^9$1 and those with uncontrolled arterial hypertension (systolic pressure above 180 mmHg).

To assist in sealing the puncture site, two types of device are available: the manual compression device as highlighted above and the vascular sealing devices (Chamberlin et al 1999). The latter, such as the Angio-Seal, are ingenious devices placed via an introducer at the end of the procedure when the sheath has been removed. A tiny biodegradable plate is pulled against the internal vessel wall by means of a Dexon suture through a collagen 'plug'. The latter is held in place on the outside of the artery wall by a tamping tube and tension spring. The patient does not have the discomfort of groin pressure, if this has been the procedure route, and does not need to keep the leg still because this is a mechanical seal. After half an hour and up to approximately 4 hours (any longer and antibiotic cover is required), the nurse removes the tension spring, cuts the suture and trims to the skin. Where an Angio-Seal has been used for a diagnostic catheter (angiogram), patients can be mobilized in an hour. They may potentially be sent home within the following hour.

Percutaneous transluminal coronary angioplasty (PTCA). Some physicians will use an oral antiplatelet drug such as clopidogrel or ticlopidine prior to the procedure if the use of stents is planned, to reduce subsequent thrombus formation and vessel closure. A glycoprotein IIb/IIIa inhibitor, such as intravenous abciximab (ReoPro), may be used during the procedure in patients considered at high risk of vessel occlusion during and after PTCA. Abciximab is in fact a monoclonal antibody, which inhibits platelet aggregation and thrombus formation. As Chapter 19 describes, it can only be given once and is used, for example, in patients where there is evidence of thrombus formation on the angiogram or in a long procedure where a large number of stents may be used. The efficacy of abciximab was initially established in the EPISTENT (1998) trial. Abciximab may be in progress on return to the coronary care area. Weight-adjusted heparin (100 u/kg) will have been used during the procedure, together with the antiplatelet drug. Sheaths should not be removed until the nurse has recorded an ACT (activated clotting time) that is within the prescribed protocol range, to prevent haemorrhage and

haematoma formation. The desired ACT will vary but may be anything from 130 to 175 seconds.

The patient will generally stay in hospital for 24 hours with a PTCA procedure but this is dependent on presenting symptoms. Some units may perform the procedure in the morning and send home in the evening or the next day in an afternoon procedure. On return from the catheter laboratory, cardiac monitoring is initiated. The nurse needs to perform a 12-lead ECG and should note any signs of chest pain and ST elevation or depression on the ECG and whether the leads correlate to the vessel of the procedure. By observing the patient's clinical signs and the monitored ECG, further 12-lead recordings can be taken and the physician or catheter lab staff notified. The colour of the leg on the side of the affected groin should be checked together with distal pulses at regular time intervals. The recording of cardiac enzymes such as CK-MB or cardiac markers such as the troponins allows the physician to note if any damage has occurred to the myocardium because of the procedure. Heart rate, blood pressure and temperature are recorded according to the unit or consultant protocol. Generally, the temperature is recorded 4 hourly, with heart rate and blood pressure recorded twice at 15-minute intervals from arrival, then half hourly on two occasions, then hourly, adjusted according to the clinical judgement of the nurse. Again, this will vary between units. At discharge an antiplatelet drug such as clopidogrel or ticlopidine orally will be prescribed to prevent vessel occlusion after PTCA. The duration will depend on physician protocol. Currently, the former drug tends to be taken for longer at between 1 and 3 months, the latter for a period of a few weeks. Aspirin is taken daily for life.

Laser angioplasty and directional or rotational atherectomy. These are two approaches which involve the physical removal of atheroma. Eximer laser coronary angioplasty (ELCA) is the most thoroughly investigated laser technology applied to coronary interventions. It uses a high-intensity, short-duration, pulsed-wave ultraviolet light applied as the catheter is advanced through the plaque. Adjunctive balloon angioplasty is required to achieve an optimal result. Rotational atherectomy reduces the plaque by drilling with a rotablator. It is particularly suitable for heavily calcified, non-dilatable vessels. The high-speed burr selectively cuts atheromatous material, leaving healthy elastic arterial wall undamaged. Rotational atherectomy has proved superior to PTCA in calcified vessels but 6-month restenosis rates were not improved and ischaemic complications were higher (Reifart et al 1997).

Enhanced external counterpulsation (EECP). This method of treating angina is non-invasive and may be offered on an outpatient basis. A series of compression cuffs around the patient's calves, plus lower and upper thighs inflate and deflate in response to particular segments of the cardiac cycle (Werner et al 1999). During the diastolic phase, the cuffs inflate upwards from the lower calves. This raises the aortic diastolic pressure with the aim of increasing the coronary perfusion pressure. During systole, rapid decompression of the cuffs produces increased left ventricular unloading, with a subsequent decrease in the cardiac workload and hence myocardial oxygen demand. It has tended to be used in those not responding to medical or surgical treatment and appears to have some beneficial long-term results (Lawson et al 2000).

Risk stratification. Risk stratification is important, both for deciding upon treatment and for the allocation of resources. Older patients are at greater risk of death or non-fatal events but may be better placed to cope with the symptoms as they undertake less physical activity and may be more stoical. Those with a family history of AMI (Barrett-Connor & Khaw 1984) or diabetes (Stamler et al 1993) are also at increased risk. Objective assessment of exercise tolerance is a more reliable predictor of risk than symptom severity (Mark et al 1994). Evidence of myocardial damage on the resting ECG or by echocardiography or perfusion imaging is associated with a worse prognosis. Angiographic evidence of the nature and distribution of coronary stenosis predicts outcome. Those patients with left main or three-vessel disease have a poorer prognosis than those with single stenosis or normal vessels on angiography (Califf et al 1988).

Waiting lists. There are significant numbers of patients on waiting lists for both investigation and intervention. These lists remain long despite political emphasis.

Scoring systems. Attempts have been made to develop 'scoring' systems to provide an equitable basis for prioritizing patients awaiting CABG (Hadorn & Holmes 1997, Naylor et al 1990), although these have been subject to some criticism (Kee et al 1998). The scoring systems tend not to distinguish between urgency and priority. However, clinicians do tend to make such distinctions when assessing individual patients and may give different weight to clinical and demographic characteristics than the published scoring systems. Patients waiting prolonged periods for surgery may require periodic reassessment of priority. Their GPs should be informed of the outcome.

Tertiary care. Increasingly, the role of the tertiary cardiac centre is seen as undertaking intervention and more complex activity (Parker et al 1997). Referral for tertiary care is indicated when revascularization by CABG or PTCA is thought to be indicated on the basis of the patient's symptoms or by objective assessment of ischaemia through non-invasive or angiographic techniques. Referral may also be indicated where there have been repeated admissions or where the diagnosis is in doubt.

Referral from secondary to tertiary cardiac care should be channelled through a cardiologist at the secondary level. Cardiac centres should be equipped with one or more catheter laboratories, cardiac theatres, a cardiac intensive care unit (or designated, staffed beds within a general intensive care unit) and associated inpatient beds. This will include a CCU with adequate bed complement to accommodate emergency admissions from the local population, as well as the additional workload arising from acute referrals from associated district hospitals. Where the cardiac centre also provides secondary care facilities for the local population, it will be necessary for there to be some duplication of facilities for non-invasive assessment. Development of further angioplasty services in non-surgical centres should only be considered in exceptional circumstances (Parker et al 1997). Facilities for further specialized cardiology and cardiac surgery, including electrophysiology, complex pacing, adult (grown up) congenital heart disease (GUCH) and paediatric cardiology, will also be required in many tertiary cardiac centres.

Resources. Manpower and financial resources, together with continuing variations in revascularization rates, remain the main obstacles to providing the high-quality service desired by the public and professions. Approximately two million people in the UK still have no access to a physician trained in cardiology (BCS 1998). More specialists are urgently needed to meet the shortfall, with published recommendations from the Royal College of Physicians of London suggesting an increase in the number of consultant cardiologists to 1/80 000 within the next few years (Royal College of Physicians 1998). It has been recommended that the ratio of cardiologists to cardiac surgeons in the tertiary centres should be 2:1 and anaesthetists: surgeons 1:1 (Parker et al 1997). Any expansion will require an increase in the number of cardiac trained nurses, technicians and support staff, although there are no clear guidelines available for these groups at the present time. Training these professionals will take a number of years, but the National Service Framework (DoH 2000a) has added impetus to these efforts.

Rehabilitation

Patients with angina are frequently not offered formal rehabilitation packages, despite national guidelines advocating that this should occur (Thompson et al 1996). Many patients find it difficult to assess the significance of their symptoms and others find the first time they need to use their GTN daunting. Time spent exploring what to do if symptoms reoccur and giving patients their own GTN when an in patient may prevent the trauma of being inappropriately admitted to hospital.

Management in primary care focuses on a programme of advice and explanation, encouragement and support in risk factor reduction and a monitoring of the patient's symptoms and progress. Practice nurses and nurse-led clinics have a key role here in optimizing health (Wiles 1997). Medical treatment includes, in most cases, low-dose aspirin, sublingual nitrates, one or more background anti-anginal agents and, where appropriate, a lipid-lowering agent. Stress management training has been shown to be effective in reducing the amount of angina symptoms experienced and in increasing exercise tolerance (Bundy et al 1994). Individualized, GP practice-based health education for patients with angina has been shown to lead to an increase in the amount of exercise and everyday activities undertaken, whilst also improving dietary habits (Cupples & McKnight 1994).

CHD is still perceived as a disease that affects men, while women may have different experiences and needs (Miklaucich 1998). Miklaucich's work suggested that in the first 2 months after a diagnosis of angina, women progressed through various stages, including distancing themselves from the need to take control over their condition, realizing and reflecting on the reality of what was happening, learning to live with their angina, including uncertainty over what to expect in the future, and eventually accepting and minimizing the effect of any limitations. Chapter 2 provides more detail regarding cardiac rehabilitation.

Sexual dysfunction in coronary heart disease

An area of growing interest and of concern in patients with CHD is that of sexual dysfunction. Interest has grown because of the links with cardiovascular disease, but also due to the potential cardiac risk of sexual activity itself (DeBusk et al 2000).

Recommendations have now been developed for clinical management of patients with this condition in cardiovascular disease (DeBusk et al 2000). It has also helped in grading patients into those who may be at risk during sexual activity. The emergence of sildenafil (Viagra) has offered hope to men with erectile dysfunction, but it cannot be used by those taking long-acting nitrates (Chew et al 2000) or with low blood pressure (<90/50 mmHg). With short-acting sublingual nitrates, sildenafil can be used but should not be taken within 24 hours of the nitrate (Chew et al 2000).

This whole area can produce anxiety for the patient and partner and impact on many other aspects of their lives. It may be an area that is difficult for the patient and even health-care staff to talk about. Specialist nurses are emerging to explore the whole issue and the options for treatment for those experiencing sexual dysfunction. It is an area that cardiac teams need to discuss in order to make provision to deal with the issue as effectively as possible.

Unstable angina

As highlighted, unstable angina is a medical emergency requiring management in the coronary care unit (CCU). Many patients experience a period of several hours of unstable angina prior to an AMI. Therefore it is important to recognize and treat the condition correctly in order to minimize this risk of progression to infarction and the consequences of the unstable angina itself, which can include heart failure and sudden death.

Assessment

The patient will typically describe their pain or discomfort as being similar to their normal angina but more severe. They may also feel sweaty and nauseous. Coronary artery spasm and thrombus formation may mean that attacks occur at rest and are not relieved by glyceryl trinitrate (GTN). The patient is likely to be anxious, particularly if normal methods of coping with angina have failed. Blood pressure and heart rate may be within normal limits, although both may rise at the onset of pain. Arrhythmias may occur as a result of myocardial ischaemia. Auscultation may reveal a third or fourth heart sound, reversed splitting of the second heart sound and transient mitral systolic murmurs. It is important to exclude AMI by obtaining serial ECGs and measuring cardiac markers and enzymes. Patients need to be continuously monitored as chest pain is not a reliable indicator of myocardial ischaemia.

The management of the patient with unstable angina comprises:

• rest and reassurance to reduce anxiety and myocardial oxygen demand

- relieving ischaemia and pain
- reducing the risk of subsequent infarction, heart failure and sudden death
- referral for investigation once symptoms have subsided, to direct further treatment.

Rest and reassurance to reduce anxiety and myocardial oxygen demand

Complete bedrest is required initially, to reduce myocardial oxygen demand. Clear and calm explanations regarding the nature of the condition, the course of treatment and investigations will reassure the patient and family/carers who may be fearful of sudden death. A quiet area near the nurses' station, together with telemetry (the use of radiowaves to transmit recordings such as the ECG from a mobile patient), will provide further reassurance. It is also important to ensure that any concerns the patient may have with regard to family or social needs are discussed and addressed, so that undue worries are alleviated.

Relieving ischaemia and pain

Oxygen therapy may benefit some patients and should be given routinely, although there is no evidence for a specific benefit other than for patients with respiratory failure or haemodynamic abnormalities.

Glyceryl trinitrate intravenously and/or β-blockers will help improve the myocardial oxygen supply–demand imbalance.

Nifedipine and other dihydropyridines (calcium channel blockers) are usually reserved for second or third-line therapy after β-blockers and nitrates, or when β-blockers are contra-indicated.

Reducing the risk of subsequent infarction, heart failure and sudden death

Heparin and aspirin have antithrombotic effects and have been shown (independently and in collaboration) to improve prognosis by preventing progression of the non-occlusive thrombus to complete occlusion (Antiplatelet Trialists' Collaboration 1994, Theroux et al 1993).

Low molecular weight heparin (enoxaparin), which is given subcutaneously, is increasingly being used for unstable coronary artery disease. This has the advantage of a more predictable anticoagulant effect than standard unfractionated heparin intravenous infusions. It is easier to administer, does not require anticoagulation monitoring and is superior in reducing mortality and serious ischaemic cardiac events (Antman et al 1999a,b, Cohen et al 1997).

Glycoprotein IIb/IIIa inhibitors, for example tirofiban (Aggrastat) and abciximab (ReoPro), are increasingly being used in unstable angina. In a recent review, Pye (2000) concluded that they are the first therapy since aspirin and heparin to improve clinical outcome. Patients with elevated troponin levels are at a higher risk and as a group may benefit from aggressive treatment with glycoprotein IIb/IIIa inhibitors and possibly revascularization (Antman et al 1996, Lindahl et al 1996, Ohman et al 1996).

More recently the National Institute for Clinical Excellence (NICE) has endorsed the use of these drugs with the release of guidelines (NICE 2000). These include their use for high risk patients with unstable angina and what is termed minor heart attack. Their use is also recommended for patients undergoing an emergency or planned percutaneous coronary intervention. This is defined as an angioplasty within the guidelines.

Restricted activities and rest in the bed or chair will help reduce myocardial oxygen demand, as will a calm approach designed to minimize anxiety and emotional stress. Thought needs to be given to the environment such as noise, light and so forth and potential visitors advised of the importance of undisturbed periods for rest. If pain persists at rest, despite optimum medical therapy, the use of an intra-aortic balloon pump (IABP) remains an option. This device increases coronary blood flow to the ischaemic area and reduces myocardial oxygen demand by decreasing resistance to blood flow in the aortic root. This ultimately reduces left ventricular end-diastolic pressure (see Chapter 18).

Referral for investigation once symptoms have subsided, to direct further treatment

Once the symptoms of unstable angina have resolved, the patient is still at risk from an unstable plaque as the endothelium remains damaged. This is a potential site for clot formation and vasoconstriction. Risk stratification is important and if the patient has angina on resuming minimal activity then they should be referred for early coronary angiography, with a view to angioplasty or bypass surgery. An exercise tolerance test and/or an assessment of myocardial perfusion and function with a thallium scan or positron emission tomography (PET) may help identify potentially reversible abnormalities. Case study 9.1 brings together the priorities of care for a patient with unstable angina.

Chest pain with normal coronary arteries

Individuals who present with atypical symptoms and insignificant history and do not respond to

Case study 9.1 Unstable angina

Mrs Jean Jones, a 62-year-old shop assistant, was admitted to the accident and emergency department suffering with shortness of breath and intermittent chest pain. This had been worsening over a 24-hour period. As is sometimes the case with unstable angina, Mrs Jones had no history of cardiac disease, although on both sides of the family it had been prevalent. On admission Mrs Jones was still experiencing chest discomfort and looked pale. Her blood pressure was 150/80 mmHg and she was tachycardic at 130 beats per minute (bpm). Reassurance was offered to Mrs Jones and her accompanying husband and oxygen of 40% was administered via a mask, with pulse oximetry revealing an arterial saturation of 95%. A 12-lead electrocardiogram (ECG) was recorded and can be seen in Figure 9.2. This revealed sinus tachycardia and a normal cardiac axis. Anterior and lateral ischaemia could be seen, from the ST depression in leads V3–V6 and leads I and aVL. No evidence of ST elevation (infarction) or pathological Q-waves (old infarction) could be noted. No other physical abnormalities were identified by medical or nursing staff.

Mrs Jones was transferred to the coronary care unit (CCU) with a diagnosis of unstable angina. The aim of treatment was to reduce and settle the symptoms medically and to prevent progression to infarction or sudden death. This was in preparation for transfer to the nearby hospital containing a catheter (angiography) laboratory, able to perform coronary angiography. Mrs Jones remained on bedrest with prescribed intravenous diamorphine 2.5–5 mg for pain relief and to reduce anxiety. Soluble aspirin 300 mg was given, with a daily maintenance dose of 150 mg commenced as an antiplatelet drug. Aspirin may reduce microthrombi formation on atherosclerotic plaque, which are known from angioscopy studies to be part of the syndrome of unstable angina (Swanton 1998).

Intravenous glyceryl trinitrate administered as an infusion and titrated against pain and the systolic blood pressure, keeping this above 100 mmHg, was commenced. The aim was then to progress to a slow-release oral form such as isosorbide mononitrate. The low molecular weight heparins such as enoxaparin and dalteparin have been shown to be of benefit in unstable angina, in reducing death, myocardial infarction and the need for revascularization (Cohen 1999). Low molecular weight heparin was therefore commenced subcutaneously. Propranolol 40 mg three times a day was prescribed, particularly in view of the tachycardia. This would assist in reducing the myocardial oxygen demand by slowing the heart rate and alleviating the symptoms.

Nursing and medical staff discussed with Mrs Jones the reasons for the chest pain and the likelihood that a coronary artery had become partly occluded by an atheromatous plaque. An anatomical model of the heart was used by both the nurse and physician to describe the procedure of coronary angiography which would guide subsequent treatment (see Chapter 8). Mrs Jones remained in the CCU for 48 hours before being transferred to the ward area for a further 3 days. By this time the symptoms had settled and Mrs Jones was discharged home with an oral nitrate, β-blocker and aspirin therapy. On return for a coronary angiography, the investigation revealed partial occlusion of the left circumflex artery. This was deemed amenable to PTCA, which was planned for 3 weeks time. Prior to this intervention an exercise tolerance test was performed to assess the degree of symptoms experienced by Mrs Jones. During the PTCA procedure, a stent was also placed to maintain vessel patency. The subsequent care and management followed that already described within this chapter.

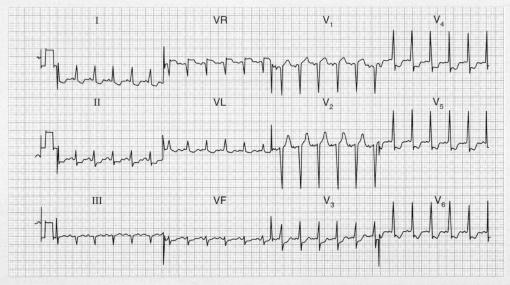

Figure 9.2 The 12-lead ECG shows both anterior and lateral ischaemia, with horizontal ST segment depression in leads V3–V4 and downward sloping depression in leads I, VL, V5–V6. (Reproduced with permission from Hampton JR 1997 100 ECG problems. Churchill Livingstone, Edinburgh.)

conventional angina management pose a problem in terms of appropriate therapy, advice and education. Inability to resolve the symptoms and doubt over the underlying cause can lead to significant psychological problems. A misdiagnosis of angina will have lifetime implications and although they are at low risk for CHD, this group warrant investigation to establish a correct diagnosis.

It is accepted that myocardial ischaemia can occur even if the evidence from angiography suggests that the main coronary arteries are normal. Small vessel ischaemia can occur in those who have diabetes, while conditions such as ventricular hypertrophy and aortic stenosis can produce subendocardial ischaemia. Moreover, there are some individuals with no evidence of either epicardial coronary atheroma or conditions known to cause small vessel disease who develop ischaemic symptoms (Holdright 1996). Syndrome X and coronary artery spasm are conditions where myocardial ischaemia may develop with 'normal' coronary arteries.

Syndrome X

Syndrome X is usually diagnosed in the presence of angina on exertion, a positive exercise test, angiographically normal coronary arteries and no evidence of coronary artery spasm. However, as there is no aetiological or pathophysiological origin implicated in the diagnosis, syndrome X is a syndrome rather than a disease. Various metabolic and endocrine factors have been implicated including hyperlipidaemia, adenosine hypersensitivity and insulin resistance. Syndrome X is more common in women and in particular peri- or postmenopausal women. Oestrogen deficiency is thought to be significant in this (Rosano et al 1995). It is possible that some patients will have a psychological origin for their problem. Abnormalities in pain perception may also be significant (Cox et al 1997).

The prognosis for those diagnosed with syndrome X is good and this needs to be emphasized. However, episodes of pain, frequent investigations, perceived loss of control and frustration may impair quality of life. Some patients may doubt their own perceptions or feel that they are not being believed. A sympathetic approach is essential with the management of noncardiac causes and the recognition and support of psychological problems, together with pain relief, are important. If the underlying cause is ischaemic, the pain may respond to angina therapy. Oestrogen therapy and administration of adenosine and imipramine have also been successful.

Coronary artery spasm

This occurs as a result of changes in the vasomotor tone of epicardial coronary arteries and was classically described by Prinzmetal et al in 1959. Underlying endothelial abnormalities are thought to be responsible for localized instability, as spasm often occurs at the sites of coronary atheroma. The spasm is usually episodic, producing transient ST elevation on the ECG. During periods of spasm, there is a significant risk of progression to infarction, although once the spasm has subsided, prognosis is good. Successful management involves calcium antagonists and nitrates. Co-existing coronary atheroma is likely and should be managed in the conventional manner as described throughout this chapter.

ACUTE MYOCARDIAL INFARCTION
Pathophysiology of acute myocardial infarction

The relationship between a reduction in coronary blood flow and subsequent damage to cardiac cells can be considered as a continuum. Unstable angina can be seen at one end and acute myocardial infarcion (AMI), affecting the full thickness of cardiac muscle, at the other. The term '**acute coronary syndrome**' is now used in practice and groups them together. To this end recommended strategies have been created to guide appropriate management (see Fig. 9.3).

Platelet aggregation, transient thrombosis and vasoconstriction may produce periodic reductions in blood flow with no permanent muscle damage. If blood flow to the myocardium is severely impaired for more than 20 minutes, then a growing area of cell necrosis develops in the affected part of the muscle. However, this may not initially affect all the muscle layers. If the period of reduction in coronary blood flow persists for more than 2 hours, the patient will invarably have a completely occlusive artery thrombus and the full muscle thickness will be involved (Willerson et al 1986). Coronary artery thrombus is found in the majority of patients dying from acute transmural myocardial infarction. In most cases of infarction, complete absence of flow in the infarct-related coronary artery as a result of thrombus is typical (De Wood et al 1980). The infarct is dependent on the degree of impairment to blood flow and may occur as a single acute episode over 6–8 hours or evolve over a period of days.

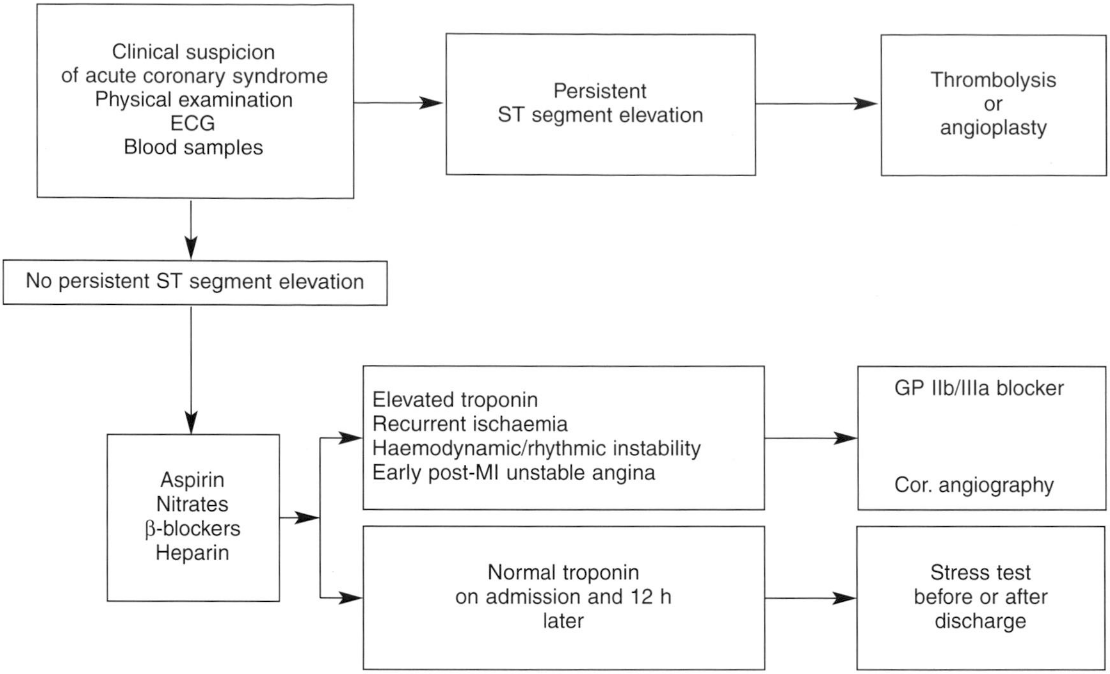

Figure 9.3 Recommended strategy in acute coronary syndrome. (Reproduced with permission from Bertrand et al 2000 European Heart Journal 21(17): 1424.)

Epidemiology

Acute myocardial infarction is a common condition accounting for the majority of CHD deaths. Of an estimated 300 000 people suffering AMI each year, about half die within 30 days of the event. Case fatality from AMI has remained largely unchanged since the 1960s and 1970s (Norris 1998), despite many advances in the knowledge of the pathophysiology of the condition and the development of effective treatments. Approximately a third of cases die before reaching hospital. Of those who do arrive at hospital 20% will not survive (Morrison et al 1997). It is estimated that there are 1.3 million people in the UK who have survived an AMI, 850 000 of whom are men (BHF 2001). This has significant psychosocial and economic implications.

Presentation

The 'classic' presentation of AMI is hard to miss: a usually middle-aged or elderly person of either sex complains of central crushing retrosternal pain, which came on at rest, lasts longer than 30 minutes and is not relieved by glyceryl trinitrate (GTN). The discomfort may radiate or localize to the neck, jaw, back and shoulders. There may be associated nausea and a

'feeling of impending doom'. Autonomic dysfunction may give rise to profuse sweating and the patient may appear cold and clammy.

The reality may differ from the patient's perceptions of what a heart attack would be like. Ruston et al (1998), in a qualitative study of patients' experiences of a cardiac event, concluded that the myth that a heart attack is a dramatic event needed to be dispelled. This study found that most patients experienced symptoms that were gradual rather than dramatic in onset and many did not use the word 'pain' to describe their experience until they were in the hospital setting.

Diagnosis

Nurses are usually the first health-care professionals the patient comes into contact with in the hospital and they have a particular responsibility to assist in the diagnosis. Diagnosis of AMI is made from the presenting history and examination, the 12-lead ECG and biochemical cardiac marker levels.

History and examination

Of those who present with chest pain, only a small percentage will be experiencing an AMI. The diagnosis of chest pain is complicated by a shared neurological pathway for thoracic and abdominal visceral organs and may be caused by a variety of gastrointestinal and musculoskeletal factors. A background of a family history of CHD and significant risk factors is the most important part of the assessment.

The initial assessment needs to be brief as the two key points to be addressed are whether the patient requires intravenous thrombolysis and if so, whether there are any contra-indications to this therapy. Patients may initially be too unwell to disclose a great deal of information. Taking a brief history and then gaining more detailed background data when the patient is feeling better may be more productive.

Physical appearance is very variable and dependent on the physical and psychological impact of the event on the particular individual. Autonomic imbalance and impaired left ventricular function may result in shortness of breath, sweating, nausea and vomiting. Auscultation may reveal arrhythmias; a muffled and diminished first heart sound and reversed splitting of the second sound. Fourth heart sounds are common, third heart sounds less so, usually reflecting left ventricular failure. The murmur of mitral incompetence is found in about 50% of patients in the early stages of AMI.

12-Lead ECG

The ECG is an essential prerequisite to determining a patient's eligibility for thrombolytic therapy and also provides an indication of the risk of adverse events. There is no single ECG change produced by myocardial ischaemia and infarction and findings will depend on the duration of ischaemia and the part of the heart affected. A typical transmural infarction will show evolving ST segment and T-wave changes with Q-wave formation. Infarction limited to the inner (subendocardial) part of the ventricular wall interferes with repolarization (and not depolarization), resulting in ST depression and deep symmetrical T-wave inversion.

Single channel recordings, such as those on defibrillator screens, are insufficient to support decision making in this regard. However, an initially normal 12-lead ECG does not of itself preclude serious heart disease (Norell et al 1992, Yusuf et al 1984). ECG findings may change over time (Adams et al 1993) and it is important to record a series of ECGs over the admission period.

Recording a 12-lead ECG should be considered a core skill for all accident and emergency (A&E) department and CCU nurses. Consistency of electrode placement is of considerable importance when performing serial ECGs. Recent advances in technology make it possible to continuously monitor the 12-lead ECG in A&E or CCU, enabling trends in patients' cardiac status to be reviewed.

Blood samples

Baseline blood tests can be taken at the same time as cannula insertion. A full blood count will detect anaemia or polycythaemia. The white cell count and erythrocyte sedimentation rate (ESR) may rise as a result of muscle necrosis. Urea and electrolyte levels are needed to assess renal function and potassium levels which are particularly significant in those taking digoxin or diuretics. Liver function tests may be abnormal in those with significant right-sided heart failure and should be measured on the initial sample along with a lipid profile and random glucose.

Cardiac enzymes and other cardiac markers

The estimation of the rise in certain intracellular cardiac enzymes, which enter the blood as the infarcting cells die, is used to confirm myocardial infarction and estimate the extent of irreversible cell damage. An enzyme rise of more than twice the normal has traditionally defined AMI. However, waiting for a cardiac enzyme result should not delay the decision for thrombolysis. The characteristics of cardiac enzymes and importantly the biochemical cardiac markers such as the troponins are summarized in Box 9.1 (p. 156).

Bedside enzyme measurement has been shown to be effective in the diagnosis of AMI (Young et al 1999). It allows diagnostic assays to be performed in locations such as the CCU where treatment can be initiated based on the results. Both troponin T and I, as well as myoglobin, can now be measured at the bedside and this is increasingly being performed in units throughout the country. There is also the potential for improved triage, risk stratification and appropriate resource utilization. Some patients who have received thrombolysis (on the grounds of history and ECG changes) may have a less than twofold enzyme rise. Here it is suggested that a diagnosis of 'threatened MI' should then be made.

Chest radiography

An initial chest X-ray film serves to exclude other causes of chest pain, such as aortic aneurysm, pneumonia and pneumothorax. If the diagnosis of myocardial infarction is unequivocal, then the chest X-ray can be delayed until after thrombolysis. A portable anteroposterior chest film is usually taken, although in otherwise fit and healthy individuals, it is reasonable to wait until the patient is well enough to have a departmental film taken.

Management

Historical context of the management of myocardial infarction

The management of patients with suspected AMI has changed profoundly since Herrick's description of the syndrome in 1912. In the early years of the 20th century patients with a myocardial infarction faced prolonged bedrest, with little therapeutic intervention bar narcotic analgesia, and the outlook was bleak. In mid-century, thrombolytic therapy to dissolve the thrombus was being used in an attempt to reduce mortality. However, the rudimentary state of understanding was to leave this life-saving treatment unavailable to the vast majority of eligible patients. Prevention of early death from ventricular fibrillation (VF) was to be of monumental significance on an absolute basis in the years following World War Two, but most patients still died before a defibrillator was available. The latter years of the century have seen significant advances in early defibrillation, infarct limitation and secondary prevention (see Boxes 9.3 and 9.4).

The main objective in the management of AMI today is prompt recanalization (re-establishing a channel) of the occluded artery, thereby enhancing myocardial perfusion and reducing infarct size. Additional therapy has the following aims (Casey et al 1998):

Box 9.3 The NSF: standards for myocardial infarction (DoH 2000a)

Standard Five
Patients with a possible heart attack should receive help from an individual equipped with and appropriately trained in the use of a defibrillator within 8 minutes of calling for help, to maximize the benefits of resuscitation should it be necessary.
Standard Six
People thought to be suffering from a heart attack should be assessed professionally and, if indicated, receive aspirin. Thrombolysis should be given within 60 minutes of calling professional help.
Standard Seven
NHS Trusts should put into place agreed protocols/systems of care so that people admitted to hospital with a proven heart attack are appropriately assessed and offered treatments of proven clinical and cost effectiveness to reduce their risk of disability and death.

Box 9.4 Interventions that patients with myocardial infarction should receive prior to hospital arrival (after the NSF for Coronary Heart Disease: DoH 2000a)

- Cardiopulmonary resuscitation and defibrillation in the event of cardiac arrest
- High concentration oxygen
- Pain relief (such as 2.5–5 mg of diamorphine intravenously; 5–10 mg of morphine intravenously with an anti-emetic)
- Aspirin (at least 300 mg orally)
- Immediate transfer to hospital

- minimizing the area of ischaemic myocardium by increasing coronary perfusion and decreasing myocardial workload
- maximizing oxygen delivery to the tissues
- controlling pain and sympathetic stimulation
- countering the detrimental effects of reperfusion
- preserving ventricular function
- reducing morbidity and mortality.

The remaining sections of this chapter describe the management of AMI by following the pathway of the individual from symptom onset to hospital discharge.

Response to symptoms

A rapid response from health professionals requires that first an individual patient, family member, carer or bystander summons help as soon as possible following symptom onset. Only then will skilled help arrive within the 'window of opportunity' for time-dependent treatments, including defibrillation and reperfusion, to exert their maximum effect. Sadly, too often the call for help is too late (Fitzpatrick et al 1992). Yet, seeking professional help in the early stages of symptoms may result in an increase in the proportion of patients developing ventricular fibrillation (VF) in the presence of emergency services personnel, improving the chances of successful resuscitation (Norris 1998, United Kingdom (UK) Heart Attack Study Collaborative Group 1998).

Factors influencing a delay in calling for help. The influence of patients' treatment-seeking behaviour on the delay to thrombolytic therapy for AMI has been demonstrated in several studies. Birkhead (1992), in an audit of 1934 patients with suspected AMI, found that the time between symptom onset and the call for help was dependent on where they were at the time and who they decided to call. The delay was longer when the patient was at home rather than a public place or at work and when they called the general practitioner

(GP) rather than the emergency services. In this study most patients called their GP and almost one quarter (23%) of patients delayed for 4 hours or longer before seeking help. Patients in rural areas were more likely to call a GP than those in urban areas.

Several other studies have reported even longer delays in seeking medical help (Dracup et al 1995, Gurwitz et al 1997, Yarzebski et al 1994) with median time from onset to presentation of between 2 and 6.5 hours. A prior history of AMI was not associated with a shorter delay in seeking help (Gurwitz et al 1997). Patient characteristics also appear significant, with older patients (Maynard et al 1989, Tresch 1998, Yarzebski et al 1994), women (Clark et al 1992, Meischke et al 1993), those from minority ethnic groups (Clark et al 1992, Crawford et al 1994) and people experiencing social and economic deprivation (Ghali et al 1993) taking longer to come under medical care.

Symptom severity may influence patient delay: patients experiencing sudden onset, severe chest pain are likely to call for help earlier (Schmidt & Borsch 1990), as are those with symptoms associated with severe left ventricular dysfunction (Rawles et al 1990, Trent et al 1995). In one series, patients who called emergency medical services in preference to their GP were more likely to have severe symptoms and develop complications (Quinn et al 1999). Calling an ambulance rather than the GP has been shown to reduce delays to CCU admission (Ahmad et al 1992). Developing symptoms in the presence of a family member (typically a spouse) has been associated with additional delay in seeking help, possibly influenced by a range of emotional factors including denial (Alonzo 1986).

Important information about the reasons why patients delay seeking medical help has been provided by a study from England (Ruston et al 1998). Patients with shorter delays described a wider range of symptoms and *limited* 'diversionary tactics' such as drinking tea or coffee or walking about in an attempt to ease symptoms. They did not generally seek the advice of other persons such as family members. Patients with longer delays tended to use a variety of measures to alleviate symptoms, including indigestion remedies and seeking reassurance from spouses and others. None of the patients in this group considered that they were having a heart attack. Patients' perception of their personal risk of heart attack prior to the onset of symptoms was inversely associated with delay. Importantly, most of the study participants suggested that their personal experience had been very different from their concept of what a 'heart attack' would be like, as portrayed by both the media and public health campaigns. This finding may have important implications for future campaigns to reduce patient delay in seeking help, since current campaigns tend to emphasize the word 'pain' yet few patients recognize the sensation as such (Treasure 1998).

Implications for high-risk patients. People with a history of AMI, angina pectoris ('pectoris' refers to the chest), heart failure, ischaemic stroke or peripheral vascular disease form a well-defined high-risk group for subsequent life-threatening coronary events. They should receive targeted education and advice on the actions to be taken if symptoms of AMI develop, as part of routine cardiac rehabilitation and secondary prevention.

To date, as highlighted, there is no evidence that patients who have suffered a prior AMI are likely to seek help earlier than those developing symptoms for the first time (Meischke et al 1993). In the United States, the National Heart Attack Alert Program (1994), a multiprofessional initiative to reduce delays to treatment for AMI, has published detailed guidelines for health professionals to support education of high-risk patients. Information given should be clearly documented in the patient's clinical records and include an 'action plan' in the event of a subsequent recurrence of symptoms and details of prescribed medication.

Educating the wider public. Given the diverse nature of any population, public health messages will need to be accessible to people from different cultures, social groups and with differing educational abilities. It would seem sensible to involve those who have been through the experience of an AMI in developing key messages. The local emergency telephone number (in the UK 999 and 112) should feature prominently, together with information on actions to be taken in the event of heart attack symptoms, including simple first aid measures and basic life support skills. Posters, leaflets and credit-card sized aides-mémoire bearing a consistent message (and translated into different languages reflecting the ethnic make-up of the target population) should be developed and widely distributed in public. National broadcast media should be encouraged to portray AMI symptoms realistically in storylines (Treasure 1998).

Prehospital care

Most deaths from AMI occur in the community (Norris 1998). The ambulance service have a well-defined role in providing a rapid response. Emergency calls are now 'triaged' to ensure that life-threatening emergencies are afforded top priority (NHS Executive 1996) with a standard having been set that by April

2001 75% of such calls would receive a response in 8 minutes (DoH 2000a). Where patients initially call their GP the most appropriate response is for a call to be placed with the ambulance control before or as the doctor travels to see the patient. The delays associated with GP involvement in the management of patients with AMI have been reported inter alia by Ahmad et al (1992) and Birkhead (1992).

Whoever attends the patient, the priorities are the same: rapid assessment of vital signs (airway, breathing, circulation) and any immediate life-saving measures.

Resuscitation. The single most important determinant of survival from non-traumatic cardiac arrest is the time elapsing from the patient collapsing to the delivery of defibrillation, if the arrhythmia requires this (Cobbe et al 1991). Since the overwhelming number of patients sustain AMI in the out-of-hospital setting (and about 75% of those in the home) (Norris 1998), the ambulance service plays a crucial role in providing a rapid response as outlined in the government's Review of Ambulance Performance Standards (NHS Executive 1996). Improving ambulance response times (including where appropriate the deployment of 'first responders' (Quinn 1999b)) will increase the proportion of cardiac arrests occurring in the presence of someone with, and trained to use, a defibrillator. In a study of three health districts (Norris 1998), the proportion of cardiac arrests 'witnessed' by ambulance crews with a defibrillator was 5%. In Seattle in the United States, famed for its effective resuscitation training programmes, 10 lives are saved per 100 000 population in out-of-hospital cardiac arrest (Cobb et al 1992), compared to three per 100 000 in Norris's (1998) study. There is clearly room for improvement.

Symptom relief. A brief assessment of the presenting condition is required to determine the nature of symptoms, including chest pain, breathlessness and nausea. Adequate analgesia is an important component of care for prognostic as well as humanitarian reasons. Pain results in sympathetic nervous stimulation, leading to an increased heart rate and a propensity for arrhythmias, peripheral constriction (increasing the afterload) and an increased myocardial contractility and oxygen demand. It is also potentially frightening for the patient and interferes with an ability to perform normal activities.

A calm, reassuring approach for both patient and family or carers is of paramount importance. Measures to alleviate pain include sublingual nitrates and intravenous diamorphine. Intramuscular injections are not indicated in AMI patients because poor peripheral circulation will make absorption of the drug unpre-

dictable. Pain relief may also be inadequate by this route and for those who subsequently receive thrombolytic therapy, there is a risk of severe haematoma. Moreover, subsequent estimation of cardiac enzyme release may be distorted by damage to the cells (see Box 9.1).

Although not proven by randomized trial, the haemodynamic effects of intravenous diamorphine are associated with a reduction in infarct size, incidence of serious arrhythmias and heart failure (Herlitz et al 1986). Diamorphine has been shown to have the quickest analgesic effect without any increase in side-effects when compared to other opiate preparations (Scott & Orr 1969). In addition, opiates possess the singular advantage (for this patient group) of reducing anxiety and fear which frequently accompany this potentially fatal condition. Ambulance paramedics in all but a few UK areas use the synthetic opioids nalbuphine and tramadol. The analgesic gas Entonox may also provide some pain relief. Medication to relieve nausea (such as metoclopramide) should be administered intravenously following opiate administration.

Oxygen should be administered to patients with suspected AMI as routine. Again, there is a paucity of evidence from randomized trials to support this course of action, but the pathophysiology of infarction suggests that supplementary oxygenation of a patient suffering from a condition associated with diminished oxygen supply to a vital organ is worthwhile. It is common practice for low-flow oxygen to be administered to most AMI patients for at least the first 24 hours. It is of course essential in patients with overt heart failure. Pulse oximetry is useful to assess adequate arterial oxygenation.

The patient should take, or be given, 300 mg of soluble aspirin to chew as soon as possible. This has been shown to enhance the effect of thrombolysis and reduce mortality and morbidity following AMI (ISIS-2 1988).

Thrombolysis. There is growing interest in the provision of thrombolytic therapy in the prehospital setting (Quinn 1999a). Indeed, this has been successfully introduced in several countries (Bouten et al 1992, GREAT Group 1992) although is not yet common practice in the UK. In the future, it is likely that thrombolytics will be initiated in some patients by ambulance paramedics prior to admission (DoH 2000b).

Transfer to hospital. This should be undertaken without delay under emergency conditions, with continuous monitoring of the patient's condition, including ECG rhythm. A defibrillator should be at the patient's side from the initial contact right up to the point of handover to hospital staff with immediate defibrillator availability.

The interface between ambulance personnel caring for a patient 'on scene' and the receiving hospital staff is an important component of the care pathway for those with suspected AMI. Direct communication between the ambulance crew and CCU staff has been reported to reduce delay in several series (Banedee & Rhodes 1998, Millar-Craig et al 1997, Prasad et al 1997) and facilitating direct admission to CCU, bypassing the A&E department, has been demonstrated as feasible (Banedee & Rhodes 1998, Millar-Craig et al 1997, Prasad et al 1997, Quinn et al 1999).

However, it is not possible for all patients with a suspected AMI to be immediately accommodated in CCU because of limited bed availability (Quinn et al 1999).

Hospital care

The majority of patients with suspected AMI are seen first in the A&E department (Birkhead et al 1999), even in those hospitals where direct CCU admission is also available. Priorities for a patient suspected of having AMI on arrival are effective analgesia and the prompt assessment and appropriate administration of thrombolytic therapy (DoH 2000a)

Most patients will arrive by ambulance, with ECG monitoring, intravenous access and oxygen therapy already in progress. A rapid initial handover should be taken from ambulance personnel, who will have gained valuable information during their own assessment and care of the patient. It is important not to underestimate the skill and contribution of ambulance staff and patients may appear in a better state than anticipated as a consequence of expert prehospital care.

A minority of patients will arrive unheralded, having made their own arrangements to get to hospital. It is essential that they are appropriately triaged and receive high priority if initial assessment suggests cardiac pain.

The patient may currently be pain free and warm as a result of analgesia and possibly correction of bradycardia by atropine. Not all patients will present with florid symptoms. Any history of recent onset or worsening chest pain, upper abdominal discomfort not readily attributable to a non-cardiac cause, makes the 'rule out AMI' approach mandatory. The history from the patient and ambulance crew should provide sufficient information on which to base prioritization.

It is essential that a formal assessment of vital signs, pain and associated symptoms be undertaken at the earliest opportunity. Rhythm disturbances causing haemodynamic compromise require urgent correction

and appropriate documentation must be instituted. Timing of events will be of importance for audit purposes (Birkhead et al 1999).

'Fast-track' strategies. Hospitals need to develop collaborative multidisciplinary systems that facilitate rapid assessment of all patients presenting with chest pain. Admission protocols, accelerated clinical pathways and admitting department triage systems mean that appropriate care is more likely. Several such strategies have been developed within the UK (Kendall & McCabe 1996, Pell et al 1992) and the nursing contribution to the immediate management of AMI is certainly becoming more significant. Nurses' decisions on the management of patients presenting with chest pain have been shown to match those of medical staff (Quinn 1995). The role of the nurse in this type of triage is one which needs to be developed further. In assessing the elements that slow down thrombolysis, it is worth analysing how many people the patient has to see, how long they take to answer pagers and attend and how many departments the patient travels through before treatment is initiated. Figure 9.4 provides an example of a triage assessment form.

The coronary care unit. Patients with AMI are best managed in a CCU. There is evidence that those cared for on a medical ward fare less well (Lawrence-Mathew et al 1994). The environment should provide continuity of care, close monitoring and a sense of security for the patient, family and carers. This will frequently be the patient's first experience of such a significant threat to their health and may be their first experience of hospitals. The environment can be alien, inhuman and even frightening (Clifford 1986). Increased patient throughput may mean that such a unit is chaotic and noisy.

Patients' perception of their CCU environment has been linked to recovery (Proctor et al 1996). Conversation as a social stressor has been implicated in increasing the heart rate of AMI patients (Baker et al 1993). Staff need to judge the timing and content of their communication with patients (Svedlund et al 1999). Strategies need to be employed to decrease sensory overload, monotony and sleep deprivation (Kinzinger 1992). Staff working in CCU need to demonstrate a calm, confident approach. Whilst needing the knowledge and experience to interpret and act on a wide variety of variables, they should also be sensitive to patient signals as seen in facial expression and body posture.

Analgesia. Ongoing pain assessment is an important part of the care of AMI and early and adequate prescribed analgesia should be given by nursing staff on

ACUTE TRIAGE ASSESSMENT

Admitted at: Time:............... Date.............   999   GP referral   TIME SYMPTOM ONSET......

CARDIAC ARREST   →   →   →   →   →   →   **YES** →   → **CCU**
↓NO

CARDIAC PAIN/SYMPTOMS			
1. Band-like pain across centre of chest	Y/N	↓	
2. Gradual onset of pain.	Y/N		
3. Pain came on at rest.	Y/N	↓	
4. Pain radiating to arms or neck or back	Y/N		
5. Episode associated with SOB	Y/N	↓	
Sweating	Y/N		
Nausea/vomiting	Y/N	*SOUNDS ACUTE*	
6. Symptoms associated with activity	Y/N	*CARDIAC* → →	**YES** → → **CCU**
7. Increasing in frequency over last few days	Y/N	↓	
8. Like previous ischaemic chest pain/		*NO*	
symptoms?	Y/N N/A		
9. Relieved by GTN?	Y/N N/A	↓	
10. Any other significant details including:			
– patient interpretation of symptoms			
– significant risk factors		↓	
– previous cardiac history suggesting			
MI/unstable angina?			
Details:	Y/N N/A	↓	

↓NO   ↓

12-LEAD ECG SHOWS ACUTE MI			
Brief details:		↓	
		ECG	
		SUGGESTIVE OF MI? →	**YES** → → **CCU**
1. Significant ST elevation?	Y/N	↓	&
2. LBBB	Y/N	*NO*	*thrombolytic*
			assessment

↓NO   ↓

ACUTE 12–LEAD ECG			
Associated with presence or <u>risk</u> of significant	Y/N	↓	
symptoms.		↓	
ECG shows (describe & tick):		↓	
* significant ischaemia			
* complete heart block		*NEEDS MONITORING/*	
* irregular heart rate		*TREATMENT ON CCU?* →	**YES** → → **CCU**
* bradycardia			
* tachycardia		↓	
Is currently experiencing (underline)			
pain, dysnoea, dizziness, palpitations,		↓	
hypotension (BP =)		*NO* ➜ ➜	
Other details:			*NO*→→ **TRANSFER**

↓NO   ↓NO

DECISION FOR <u>EARLY</u> TRANSFER TO MEDICAL WARD/EMU made at time...........by. .sig......... Grade......

ACTION taken: stay on CCU   transfer EMU   transfer ward   discharge home   TIME:

TRANSFERRED on (date)........... at (time)................ To: Home   EMU   Wd 11   Wd 2   Wd 6   Other...........

INITIAL DIAGNOSIS: MI   UNSTABLE ANGINA   STABLE ANGINA   ARRHYTHMIA   HEART FAILURE   NON-CARDIAC

FINAL DIAGNOSIS: MI   UNSTABLE ANGINA   STABLE ANGINA   ARRHYTHMIA   HEART FAILURE   NON-CARDIAC

BP = blood pressure, CCU = coronary care unit, ECG = electocardiogram, EMU = emergency medical unit, GTN = glyceryl trinitrate, LBBB = left bundle branch block, MI = myocardial infarction, SOB = shortness of breath.

Figure 9.4 An example of a triage assessment form for a patient presenting with chest pain.

their own initiative. Patients need to be aware that it is not normal or expected for them to be in pain. They should also know to whom they should report their pain. Nurses have the most contact with patients and yet various studies illustrate that pain assessment and subsequent pain management are inconsistent (Bondestam et al 1987, Meurier 1998, Meurier et al 1998, O'Connor 1995, Thompson et al 1994, Willetts 1989).

An initial intravenous dose of diamorphine 2.5 to 5 mg should be given at 1 mg per minute, followed by further 2.5 mg doses until the pain has been relieved. An anti-emetic should be administered with the opiate. Opiates act on the respiratory centre and can depress respiration, leading to a fall in respiratory rate and tidal volume. Naloxone (Narcan) should therefore be available as a potential antagonist to opiate action. Intravenous β-blockers, thrombolytics and nitrates all reduce pain, probably as a result of limiting ischaemic damage, and are likely to reduce the need for analgesic drugs. Figure 9.1 presents an algorithm of investigation for a patient presenting with chest pain (stable angina) which is suspected of being cardiac in origin.

Thrombolytic therapy

Historical context. Fletcher et al (1958) first described the feasibility of treating acute myocardial infarction patients with thrombolytic therapy to disperse thrombus and limit infarct size. Intravenous streptokinase was administered over a 30-hour period to 28 patients within 6–72 hours of symptom onset. Thrombolytic therapy did not, however, become routine treatment for myocardial infarction until the 1980s.

This delay in implementation of one of the key measures to reduce mortality and morbidity following myocardial infarction has been attributed to a number of factors. Despite Herrick's (1912) earlier observations, the belief was held among many pathologists that 'coronary thrombosis' was a secondary, rather than primary, responsible event (Roberts 1972). The primary role of thrombus was demonstrated convincingly by De Wood et al in 1980. In the two decades following Fletcher et al's (1958) observations, several studies were undertaken, but of over 30 trials comparing intravenous streptokinase with placebo or no therapy reporting between 1959 and 1988, significant benefit was seen in only six (Lau et al 1992). Lau et al's (1992) meta-analysis of these trials favoured treatment, leading to the conclusion that intravenous streptokinase could have been saving lives some years before it became a favoured treatment.

Several randomized trials of thrombolytic therapy have been reported since the 1980s. GISSI (1986) randomized 11 806 patients to streptokinase or placebo within 12 hours of symptom onset. ISIS-2 (1988) randomized 17 187 (and had a third arm assessing the effect of aspirin either alone or in combination with streptokinase). A collaborative overview of nine large, randomized trials of thrombolysis (Fibrinolytic Therapy Trialists' Collaborative Group 1994), including GISSI and ISIS-2 and involving some 58 600 patients, demonstrated highly significant mortality reduction: 30 per 1000 patients for those treated within 6 hours of symptom onset and 20 per 1000 for those treated within 7–12 hours. Benefits were largely confined to patients presenting with ST segment elevation or bundle branch block on the admission ECG.

Boersma et al (1996) presented an alternative analysis of the importance of early thrombolysis in support of the concept of a 'first golden hour' in which a substantial reduction in mortality is achievable. The relationship between treatment delay and 35-day mortality was evaluated using data from all randomized trials of at least 100 patients (the FTT group had only included trials with more than 1000 patients) comparing thrombolysis with treatment or control. Benefits of very early treatment appear striking indeed: 65 lives saved per 1000 patients treated in the first hour from symptom onset, 37 in hours 1–2 and 29 in hours 2–3. Proportional mortality reduction was significantly higher in those treated within 2 hours compared to those treated later. It has been suggested that the most appropriate place for thrombolytic treatment to be administered is not in the hospital but in the patient's home (Rawles 1997a).

The advent of thrombolysis as 'routine' treatment for such patients has prompted an increase in admissions to CCUs in the United Kingdom (Hampton & McWilliam 1992, Hampton et al 1993, Hobbs 1995, Quinn 1993). This may be a result of increased awareness among the general public and the professions that 'time is of the essence' in cases of AMI.

Thrombolysis in the A&E department. Hood et al (1998) surveyed UK A&E departments and found that thrombolytic therapy was routinely available in only 35%, raising important issues about the role of A&E staff in the management of patients with suspected AMI (Quinn 1999a). Subsequently, the National Service Framework (DoH 2000a) set a standard of 75% of A&E departments being able to provide thombolysis by 2001. Given the view that thrombolytic therapy should be afforded similar urgency to the management of cardiac arrest (Rawles 1997b), it is likely that all A&E departments will need to provide this life-saving treatment in the future. Clear local protocols for the assessment and management of patients with suspected AMI should be agreed across all relevant disciplines and departments, including the ambulance service.

Delays to thrombolysis. Four major components of delay in the hospital assessment and management of patients with suspected AMI have been identified and addressed in guidelines published in the United States by the National Heart Attack Alert Program Co-ordinating Committee (1994). These are known as the '**Four Ds**'. The principal areas of delay are:

- *D1 (Door)* representing delays in the initial assessment and triage of patients with suspected AMI presenting to hospital, whether by ambulance or otherwise
- *D2 (Data)* representing delays in recording of the initial 12-lead ECG
- *D3 (Decision)* representing delays in the decision to administer thrombolytic therapy
- *D4 (Drug)* representing delays in commencing thrombolytic therapy.

Together, the time elapsing from D1 to D4 is a component of the total 'door-to-needle' time addressed in UK national guidelines (De Bono & Hopkins 1993, Weston et al 1994, DoH 2000a). It may be worth clarifying what the various statements of time measurements indicate. The 'call-to-needle' time generally refers to the call for professional help to the initiation of thrombolytic therapy. The 'door-to-needle' time refers to the arrival at hospital to the commencement of thrombolytic therapy. The 'pain-to-needle' time, which will involve public education to recognize an infarct, refers to the commencement of chest pain to the initiation of thrombolytic treatment.

The 'Four Ds' model has been adapted for use in the UK by Quinn & Thompson (1995) but it may be more appropriate, in the light of the government standard for a 'call-to-needle' time of no more than 60 minutes (DoH 2000a), to consider the introduction of a further 'D'. This would be D0, representing initiation of the total NHS response from a patient's call for help to commencement of thrombolytic therapy. D0 and D1 have both been discussed above.

D2: Data. Evidence from a meta-analysis of large randomized trials suggests that thrombolytic therapy should be given to those patients who have 12-lead ECG evidence of ST segment elevation or bundle branch block (Fibrinolytic Therapy Trialists' Collaborative Group 1994), since these are the groups in whom thrombolytic therapy resulted in mortality reduction. No benefits were seen in patients presenting with ST depression alone or in those with a normal ECG. Indeed, in these groups, administration of thrombolytic therapy appeared to be associated with a worse outcome.

Increasingly, 12-lead ECGs are being recorded by ambulance staff prior to hospital admission. In several series (Aufderheide et al 1992, Millar-Craig et al 1997, O'Rourke et al 1992) this has resulted in reduced 'call-to-needle' time; indeed, Kereiakes et al (1992) demonstrated a halving of hospital delays to thrombolysis when the A&E staff received a cellular transmission of the ECG from the ambulance service.

D3: Decision. The decision to initiate thrombolytic therapy is, in the strictest legal sense, a medical one. However, documentation such as that from the Crown Committee (1998) does now alter the boundaries, for example through the use of agreed protocols and patient group directions, allowing appropriately assessed non-medical staff to initiate and adjust specific drug therapies. However, regardless of these issues, it is a decision that needs to be made promptly. The National Service Framework (DoH 2000a) advocated that by April 2003, 75% of eligible patients should receive thrombolysis within 20 minutes of hospital arrival. It has been proposed in recent years that appropriately trained nurses could administer thrombolytic therapy before the patient sees a doctor, thus reducing treatment delays (Caunt 1996, Quinn 1995, Somauroo et al 1999). Nurses appear to be positive about this development which can be seen as a natural progression of their role (Smallwood & Van der Woning 1999). Whoever makes the decision, the indications for thrombolytic therapy are the subject of broad professional consensus, based on good trial evidence (Fibrinolytic Therapy Triallists' Collaborative Group 1994). It is initiated on the presence of a history suggestive of cardiac pain and the presence of either ST segment elevation or bundle branch block on the 12-lead ECG (Box 9.5) provides an example of selection criteria for utilising thrombolytic therapy.

Protocols for thrombolysis do vary. However, many units now have a protocol for treating anterior myocardial infarctions with tissue plasminogen activator (alteplase), based upon the GUSTO-I (1993) trial. Anterior protocols are often age related, with the drug not administered to the elderly presenting with this type of infarction. A presentation of a low blood pressure, usually <90 mmHg, that is unresponsive to intravenous fluids is often used as an indication to use alteplase, because this drug is less likely to decrease the blood pressure further.

An 'accelerated' alteplase regimen may be used in infarctions <6 hours after the onset of chest pain. Here, the total dose is given in the usual divided format but as 15 mg in a bolus, then 50 mg over 30 minutes and 35 mg over an hour, rather than in a total of 3 hours.

Box 9.5 Selection criteria for thrombolysis with general contra-indications to therapy (adapted and updated from Quinn & Thompson 1995)

Objective: To identify patients with acute myocardial infarction (AMI) who are suitable for thrombolysis.
NB: Patients with acute chest pain should be regarded as 'at risk' of sudden deterioration and should be assessed in an area with a defibrillator readily available, irrespective of thrombolytic intentions.
History: Chest pain (or other symptoms, e.g. 'severe indigestion') of 15 minutes duration or longer, unrelieved by GTN and rest. Approximately 50% of patients with AMI have a history of prior AMI or angina.
Minutes mean myocardium! Aim for a door-to-needle time of 15–30 minutes maximum (this means thrombolysis in A&E if no CCU bed is immediately available). The door-to-needle time is the time from arrival at hospital to initiating thrombolytic therapy.

Do:
- Act rapidly
- Monitor vital signs and ECG
- Obtain intravenous access
- Obtain a 12-lead ECG
- Give intravenous analgesia/anti-emetic
- Give oxygen if pain/shock/arrhythmia
- Give aspirin 300 mg if tolerated

Do not:
- Leave unattended
- Duplicate assessments
- Send for chest X-ray
- Delay!

If ECG shows:
ST elevation >1 mm in two limb leads (I, II, III, aVL, aVF)
or
ST elevation >2 mm in two chest leads (V2–V6)
or
New left bundle branch block (fax ECG to CCU for urgent consult in cases of doubt)

...and pain onset within the last 12 hours and none of the following contra-indications (some of these will vary between units):
- known or suspected aortic aneurysm
- active bleeding
- cerebrovascular accident (CVA/stroke) or central nervous system (CNS) damage within the past year
- major surgery or traumatic injury in the past 6 months
- severe hypertension (systolic >200 mmHg, diastolic >110 mmHg) (some units will advocate immediate treatment for the presenting hypertension then reassessment for thrombolysis)
- hypotension (systolic <90 mmHg) not corrected by intravenous atropine (if bradycardia) or rhythm correction
- bleeding disorders
- traumatic/prolonged cardiopulmonary resuscitation (CPR) may appear as a contra-indication in some protocols
- guidelines may refer to *active* peptic ulcer, with a history of peptic ulcer not necessarily appearing as a contra-indication
- known oesophageal varices
- pregnancy can appear as a definite or relative contra-indication
- known hypersensitivity to streptokinase or prior administration.*
...give streptokinase at once! (1.5 mega units in 250 ml saline over 60 minutes).

*Units will have a protocol stating that streptokinase may not be given again within 12 months or this may extend to a protocol of never administering twice. This is due to antibody production to the first dose. All protocols relate to the drug being administered over 5 days ago. It takes approximately 5 days to complete antibody production to the drug.

Research trials with a single dose of a variant of TPA have taken place in patients with infarctions of <6 hours' duration (ASSENT-2 1999). This may replace divided doses in hospital protocols due to its ease of administration. In 2001 this single-dose variant was made available as tenecteplase (Dunn & Goa 2001).

D4: Drug. Although it is unquestionable that thrombolytic therapy saves lives, the choice of agent remains an issue. The thrombolytic agents in common use in the UK are: streptokinase, alteplase (rt-PA), reteplase (r-PA, Rapilysin) and anistreplase (APSAC). Of these streptokinase is the most often prescribed. Box 9.5 discusses some of the varying protocols used within units, such as the use of alteplase for anterior myocardial infarctions (GUSTO-I 1993) and those presenting with hypotension unrelieved by intravenous fluids.

Irrespective of which agent is chosen for administration (a matter of hospital policy as much as individual clinician preference), the priority is to commence administration as soon as the decision that a patient is eligible has been made. It follows that both the medication and the equipment necessary to facilitate administration are stored in a convenient place within the department where treatment is provided. Nurses working in areas where thrombolytic therapy is to be administered must possess the necessary skills in preparation and administration of intravenous drugs and the appropriate equipment, such as infusion pumps and syringe drivers, must be readily to hand.

Contra-indications for thrombolysis. As highlighted in Box 9.5, thrombolytic therapy is not without risk. The risk of haemorrhagic cerebrovascular accident

(CVA/stroke) is low (about one in 1000 patients treated) but present nonetheless and there are established contra-indications to treatment which must be excluded as part of the decision process. This requires skill in patient assessment. Patients with equivocal ECG findings, or with suspected contraindications, benefit from assessment by senior clinicians. There is need for an evaluation of the likely risks of having (or not having) the treatment, balanced against the likelihood of developing an iatrogenic complication.

Simoons et al (1993) developed a model to assist staff in estimating the risk of intracranial haemorrhage during thrombolytic therapy in a given patient. Advanced age, hypertension on admission, low body weight and treatment with alteplase were identified as being associated with increased risk. The authors stressed, however, that treatment should not be withheld from elderly and hypertensive patients, where the likely benefits from thrombolysis were judged to outweigh the risk of CVA, necessitating a judgement to be made on an individual basis. Moreover, thrombolytic therapy has been demonstrated to exert the greatest benefit in older patients, given the high case fatality in this group (ISIS-2 1988).

Diabetic patients have been shown to receive greater benefit from thrombolysis than non-diabetic patients (Fibrinolytic Therapy Trialists' Collaborative Group 1994). However, these individuals often miss out on treatment because of atypical presentation or concerns about haemorrhage from proliferate retinopathy. This is extremely rare and should not be regarded as a relative contra-indication to thrombolysis (Hammond 1998).

Hypertension should be controlled as quickly as possible, using intravenous agents such as atenolol, metoprolol or sodium nitroprusside (SNP).

Cardiopulmonary resuscitation may have been carried out in some patients prior to hospitalization. The introduction of defibrillators on emergency ambulances in the past decade has resulted in an increase in the numbers of patients surviving out-of-hospital cardiac arrest associated with AMI (Hamer et al 1993, Sedgwick et al 1993). A proportion of these will be eligible for thrombolysis. Cardiopulmonary resuscitation is not of itself a contra-indication to thrombolysis provided there is no gross trauma (e.g. flail chest). Cross et al (1991) found no clinically significant bleeding in 39 patients who underwent resuscitation before or shortly after thrombolysis.

Central venous cannulation is also a potential source of bleeding complications in patients who receive thrombolytic therapy. However, Lee et al (1995) reported a low incidence of severe bleeding complications in 56 patients who had central lines inserted before or within 24 hours of thrombolysis, concluding that thrombolysis should not be withheld solely on the basis of the presence of a central line.

The development of hospital-wide protocols together with decision support mechanisms (including arrangements for ECGs to be faxed if necessary to the CCU or to a consultant for review) are strongly recommended to ensure that patients who need thrombolytic therapy get it promptly, while safeguarding patients from inappropriate treatment.

Monitoring for complications. During administration of thrombolytics the patient will require constant observation for hypotension, the development of an allergic reaction to streptokinase (the newer agents anistreplase and reteplase are non-antigenic), onset of further pain or compromising arrhythmias. The so-called reperfusion arrhythmias, usually idioventricular in origin, are largely benign and require no treatment unless they are causing haemodynamic upset. Bradycardia, if giving rise to hypotension and syncope, is usually responsive to small doses (500 µg) of intravenous atropine. The risk of VF recedes over time but should be considered a possibility in all patients during the first few hours after symptom onset. The presence of a defibrillator and someone who can use it appropriately is, of course, mandatory. Observation of vital signs is continuous, aided in most cases by non-invasive blood pressure recordings and pulse oximetry.

Evaluation of the efficacy of thrombolysis. It is important to recognize whether thrombolysis has been successful in order that rethrombolysis or salvage (rescue) angioplasty can be considered as soon as possible. Evidence of reperfusion includes the following (Sutton & Belder 1998).

- *Resolution of chest pain* (Nicolau et al 1989), although opiate analgesia may also achieve this with the occlusion still present. An important aim of nursing care is obviously to alleviate pain.
- *Accelerated idioventricular rhythm*, although this is not a reliable indicator because the incidence of false positives is high (Doevendans et al 1995).
- *ECG criteria.* There has been much discussion over the use of ST segment resolution as an indicator of reperfusion and it is likely that eventually ECG changes will become the recognized indicator of reperfusion. ST segment resolution has been found to correlate well with outcome (30-day mortality in the INJECT trial 1995). However, there is currently debate over which leads to use, the timing after thrombolysis and the amount of ST segment resolution that is

significant. In using the lead with the most significant ST elevation on admission, failed reperfusion has been identified as less than 50% resolution of the ST segment elevation 2 hours after the initiation of thrombolytic therapy (Sutton & De Belder 1998).

- *Cardiac enzyme levels.* The peak enzyme rise of creatine kinase (CK) and its MB fraction is delayed by about 6 hours if the vessel remains occluded. However, relying on this evidence for failed thrombolysis means it can go unrecognized for up to 24 hours. Frequent venepuncture is also necessary. Troponin levels are used in some cardiac centres, although as yet there is still little evidence regarding its effectiveness as a marker for reperfusion. Myoglobin levels peak early and may therefore be more useful in the assessment of vessel patency after thrombolysis. However, myoglobin is not specific for cardiac muscle and if the patient presents late, the early peak may be missed.

The red and white clot debate. A study by Neumann et al (1998) examined 200 patients undergoing primary stenting for AMI. Doppler assessment of the infarct vessel showed a notable increase in peak velocity with the use of abciximab which is a potent glycoprotein IIb/IIIa inhibitor. As Topol (2000) indicated, this has led to a revised understanding of the reperfusion process. Currently, in using thrombolytic therapy, we may only be achieving partial clot dissolution and potentiating embolization of part of the thrombus into the microcirculation. We may be improperly focusing on the epicardial artery, when the critical supplier of perfusion to the infarct territory may be obstructed (Topol 2000). In addition, the consistency of the clot has created interest, the aforementioned red and white clot debate. The white thrombus occurs with the breach of the vessel wall, creating a platelet thrombus. The red thrombus is fibrin rich and surrounding the platelet aggregation. Traditionally, thrombolytic agents only dissolve the fibrin strands of the red clot, not addressing the white clot formation. This results in exposed thrombin, which is a potent platelet pro-aggregatory molecule (Topol 2000). Essentially, as well as not addressing the whole clot situation, we are placing the patient in a prothrombotic state.

Ongoing trials have been addressing this issue by examining combinations of intravenous glycoprotein IIb/IIIa inhibitors such as abciximab and thrombolytic agents including rt-PA and r-PA (Pye 2000). Although this may not be the complete answer, the approach is being regarded as a significant step forward in myocardial salvage. As always, time to treatment will be the issue and approaches to appropriately assess and administer such treatments will be of continued importance.

Management of failed thrombolysis.

Rethrombolysis. It is likely that the group of patients for whom thrombolysis fails are at high risk from any subsequent intervention because of the nature of the offending thrombus. Adequate analgesia and repeat thrombolysis using a different agent are often the only options available. This should be considered if the patient is still in pain and the ST segment has not resolved 60–90 minutes following thrombolysis. Some specialized centres also enhance thrombolysis with intra-aortic balloon pumping.

Salvage or rescue angioplasty. Following failed thrombolysis this has been shown to produce significant benefits in terms of reduced mortality and lower rates of severe heart failure (Ellis et al 1992). However, it is clearly not available at every hospital site. Further trials are needed to assess the relative benefits the treatment options provide.

Primary angioplasty (PTCA). Thrombolytic therapy has no effect on the residual coronary artery stenosis that remains in the majority of patients and which can contribute to re-occlusion and re-infarction. Primary angioplasty for AMI has certain benefits over thrombolysis in that it results in a higher rate of patency of the infarct-related coronary artery (consistently above 90%), lower rates of CVA and re-infarction and higher in-hospital and 30-day survival (Zijlstra et al 1999). These advantages may increase with adjunctive glycoprotein IIb/IIIa antagonist therapy (Pye 2000). The disadvantages of PTCA are that it cannot be administered outside hospital, needs an experienced team of staff to support its use (with 24-hour on-call cover) and may lose its advantages as new thrombolytic agents are developed (Chatelain & Urban 1997, Sutton & De Belder 1998). Patients should be considered if there are clear contra-indications to thrombolysis. Whilst patients at high risk, such as those with diabetes, cardiogenic shock, anterior AMI, those over 75 years and those who present within 2 hours, may fare better with angioplasty, the evidence available is insufficient to argue for the massive restructuring of cardiac services that would be required to make primary angioplasty available (Brooks 1997).

Stenting. If angioplasty is followed by abrupt re-occlusion, threatened re-occlusion and/or failure to achieve adequate blood flow, then coronary artery stenting, combined with effective postprocedural antiplatelet therapy, is an effective alternative (Neumann et al 1996, Peter et al 1999).

Adjunctive therapy. Whilst thrombolysis can reduce infarct size by restoring myocardial perfusion, with analgesics relieving pain and discomfort, additional therapy is used to optimize recovery.

β-blockers. These should be considered for all patients with AMI for at least the first year (DoH 2000a). Contra-indications include severe chronic airways disease, peripheral vascular disease, atrioventricular block, hypotension or severe left ventricular failure. β-blockers decrease myocardial oxygen demand by blocking the sympathetic stimulation of β-adrenergic receptors and may be of particular benefit to patients with hypertension and tachycardia on admission. They also have anti-arrhythmic and antiplatelet properties. Several studies (ISIS-1 1986, MIAMI 1985) have demonstrated a reduction in mortality with an intravenous β-blocker in the acute stage of infarction and they have been shown to significantly reduce the risk of further AMI. Continuing care should aim to maintain the blood pressure below 140/80 mmHg (DoH 2000a) and β-blockers may be used to achieve this.

Angiotensin-converting enzyme (ACE) inhibitors. It has been recommended that this group of drug should be prescribed to all post-AMI patients whilst in hospital and the continuing need reviewed at outpatient follow-up after 4–6 weeks. Those with symptomatic heart failure, echocardiographic evidence of left ventricular dysfunction and extensive Q-wave infarction should continue to receive this therapy (DoH 2000a). These drugs block the production of angiotensin II and therefore inhibit vasoconstriction. Given appropriately, they significantly reduce the risk of left ventricular impairment and further AMI (AIRE Study 1993, Pfeffer et al 1992). They also appear to reduce the incidence of sudden cardiac death following AMI (Domanski et al 1999). The dose should be titrated to the maximum recommended or tolerated amount. ACE inhibitors need to be used with caution in those with hypotension, renal impairment or hypersensitivity to the drug. Renal function should be assessed prior to therapy, at 7–14 days and after any increase in dose. The drug should be stopped if the creatinine rises by more than 30% (DoH 2000a).

Nitrates. Evidence for administering nitrates in the acute stage of infarction remains debatable (ISIS-4 1995). AMI is often associated with coronary artery spasm and nitrates may help in establishing vessel patency, open up collateral vessels and reverse coronary artery vasoconstriction. Administering GTN sublingually or through buccal nitrate may be of benefit, particularly if there is ST elevation on the ECG.

Heparin. This prevents coagulation by interfering with the formation of thrombin from prothrombin. It therefore prevents thrombin involvement in the conversion of fibrinogen to fibrin. It also affects platelet function. Heparin is used routinely for 24 hours after the use of clot-specific thrombolytic agents such as alteplase and reteplase.

Calcium antagonists. Verapamil has been shown to be a realistic alternative if β-blockers are contraindicated (DAVIT II 1990).

Lipid-lowering agents. The National Service Framework (DoH 2000a) recommends that patients with AMI are discharged from hospital on a statin. Statins competitively inhibit the co-enzyme involved in cholesterol synthesis, especially in the liver. They need to be used with caution in those with liver disease. A liver function test needs to be performed before and within 3 months of commencing therapy. If lipid levels are not measured on admission, it is best to wait 4 weeks, as there may be a transient lowering of cholesterol level 24 hours following AMI. The stated aim is to lower serum cholesterol concentrations either to less than 5 mmol/l (LDL to less than 3 mmol/l) or by 30%, whichever is the greater. There is evidence that taking a statin following AMI reduces mortality for up to 5 years (Sacks et al 1996, Scandinavian Simvastatin Survival Study Group 1994).

Insulin-glucose infusion. Diabetic patients account for up to 20% of the total number of individuals admitted to CCUs for suspect AMI. Mortality after AMI, both in the acute phase and during long-term follow-up, is higher for patients with diabetes mellitus than those without (Malmberg & Ryden 1988). Elevated blood glucose levels are associated with elevated free fatty acid levels and it is thought that together they have an adverse effect on myocardial function, resulting in an increase in infarct size (Hammond 1998). The DIGAMI (Diabetes and Insulin-Glucose Infusion in Acute Myocardial Infarction) study (Malmberg 1997, Malmberg et al 1995, 1999) showed that mortality was significantly reduced in those patients who received improved metabolic care by means of intensive insulin therapy. One life was saved for every nine patients treated and the benefit was sustained for at least 3 years. The therapy consisted of an insulin-glucose infusion for at least 24 hours followed by subcutaneous insulin for at least 3 months. This treatment has been shown to be cost effective (Almbrand et al 2000) and is recomended for AMI patients (including those without a previous diagnosis of diabetes) who have a blood glucose of over 11 mmol/l, unless a large volume of fluid is likely to be detrimental.

Diuretics. Acute left ventricular failure (LVF) and congestive cardiac failure are common presenting problems as well as complications of AMI. The symptoms reflect a reduced cardiac output and an increase in the venous pressure in the lungs and peripheries. Acute LVF may present quickly and be frightening for the patient and family/carers. Diuretics provide the mainstay of the management of LVF. They inhibit sodium re-absorption by the kidney and decrease intravascular volume and thereby cardiac preload. Loop diuretics, usually frusemide, are used most often. Given intravenously, they reduce venous pressure within 15 minutes. Accurate fluid balance needs to be maintained. Overdiuresis should be avoided as depleted plasma volume reactivates the renin–angiotensin–aldosterone system, leading to further fluid retention.

Complications

There are numerous complications that are possible after AMI and it is beyond the scope of this chapter to address them all. About half of AMIs will have some problem requiring additional intervention. Arrhythmias, cardiogenic shock and heart failure are covered in detail elsewhere in this book. Dressler's syndrome (postmyocardial infarction syndrome), which presents as pericarditis, is addressed in Chapter 16. Left ventricular aneurysm, acquired ventricular septal defect and mitral regurgitation are also recognized complications of AMI. The latter may manifest as mild subvalvular mitral regurgitation following inferior or posterior AMI. This is due to papillary muscle dysfunction (Swanton 1998). The risk of complications tends to be related to the size of infarct and resulting myocardial damage, along with the extent of existing coronary heart disease.

It is important to remember that anxiety and depression may also be a complication of AMI. A reassuring and positive approach involving family and carers will do much to allay fears and anxiety regarding the future.

Non-Q wave (subendocardial) infarction. A non-Q wave infarct occurs where there is incomplete thrombosis or early lysis in a coronary artery (Swanton 1998). Chest pain, ECG changes suggestive of infarct and enzyme elevation occur. The latter may be mild in comparison to a usual transmural Q-wave infarct (Swanton 1998). This type of infarct accounts for approximately 20–30% of all infarcts but importantly must be clinically followed up and investigated as there is a high 1-year mortality, a high incidence of arrhythmias and a greater incidence of postinfarct angina (Swanton 1998).

Transfer from the CCU/acute unit

Transfer from the coronary care environment needs to take place when the patient is pain free and demonstrating an acceptable and stable haemodynamic status. This is usually 18–36 hours after admission. The move needs to be planned and discussed with the patient and family or carers who may be anxious about the change in environment and routine. An up-to-date plan of care with suggested further management and expected outcomes is desirable. Patients are now often transferred to step-down wards where staff are familiar with likely problems and concerns and have the potential to provide a more seamless service. Discharge after 3 days has been suggested as possible for uncomplicated AMIs (Topol et al 1988).

Risk stratification

Prognostic assessment after AMI is important so that therapy may be optimized and treatments evaluated. Mortality is greatest in the first few weeks, the majority prior to reaching hospital. For those that survive, the annual mortality is thought to be less than 5%.

Exercise tolerance test

A predischarge exercise test may be helpful, particularly with young (in terms of the person's age) non-Q wave AMIs. Those with a strongly positive test should be considered for coronary angiography if deemed suitable for revascularization.

Box 9.6 Risk factors associated with reinfarction or sudden death following AMI (adapted from Swanton 1998)

- A history of a previous AMI
- Age > 75 years
- Poor left ventricular function as demonstrated by factors such as:
  - clinical signs such as a systolic blood pressure <100 mmHg
  - an echocardiogram showing a left ventricular ejection fraction of <40%
  - cardiomegaly on the chest X-ray (cardiothoracic ratio >50%)
- Unstable angina: rest or nocturnal angina unrelieved by GTN
- Documented VT: sustained >30 s
- Positive treadmill testing: unable to complete stage 2 of the Bruce protocol, 7 METS (METS: metabolic equivalents, a measure of oxygen consumption. The maximum oxygen consumption achieved on exercise is a good indicator of maximum cardiac performance). Add 6 min for the modified Bruce protocol, a gentler test for the postinfarct patient.
- Frequent episodes of silent ischaemia on 24-hour monitoring
- Depression of heart rate variability
- Diabetic patients

Echocardiography

This may be of help in confirming a pericardial effusion and in assessing mitral valve function if papillary muscle dysfunction or chordal rupture is suspected. It may also help determine the presence of a ventricular septal defect.

Rehabilitation

Systematic individualized rehabilitation and secondary prevention need to be offered for all AMI patients (DoH 2000a). There is now evidence that well-organized programmes designed to provide lifestyle modification that involve education, psychological

---

> **Box 9.7** The NSF: standards for suspected heart attack (DoH 2000a)
>
> NHS trusts should put in place agreed protocols and systems of care so that people admitted to hospital with proven heart attack are appropriately assessed and offered treatments of proven clinical and cost effectiveness to reduce their risk of disability and death.

---

input and exercise training may reduce mortality by as much as 25% over 3 years (Oldridge et al 1998). Chapter 2 provides an excellent overview regarding the issues of cardiac rehabilitation.

Case study 9.2 Myocardial infarction

Mr Fred Pillar is a 65-year-old man with no known history of cardiac problems. He is slightly overweight and smokes, although he has reduced this to 10 cigarettes a day. He had been feeling unwell throughout the previous evening while watching television and had gone to bed early. He was woken in the night with chest discomfort and felt the need to have his bowels open. On the toilet he felt a sudden, crushing chest pain, which he subsequently described as being like a vice restricting his chest and breathing. This radiated down his left arm, creating a tingling sensation. He managed to call out for his wife, who helped him onto the floor and called the doctor.

The general practitioner (GP) arrived to find Mr Pillar conscious, but still in a marked degree of chest pain, sweating, nauseous and ashen. The GP immediately reassured Mr Pillar and called for an emergency ambulance. He was able to administer four of the major treatment initiatives for suspected myocardial infarction prior to hospital admission: sublingual glyceryl trinitrate (GTN), 300 mg of aspirin orally, oxygen via a portable cylinder and 2.5 mg of diamorphine intravenously (with an anti-emetic). The latter relieved the pain only to a degree, so a further 2.5 mg was administered prior to the ambulance arriving. The GP could not administer thrombolytic therapy, because he did not possess a 12-lead ECG recorder for diagnosis or a defibrillator to treat potential reperfusion arrhythmias.

On the way to the hospital, the ambulance crew radioed ahead to the Accident & Emergency (A&E) department that a suspected myocardial infarction patient was being admitted. Nursing and medical staff had created a multidisciplinary protocol and integrated care pathway (ICP) to enable thrombolysis to be given quickly, appropriately and effectively. On arrival Mr Pillar was admitted immediately to the coronary care unit (CCU), where the nurse quickly performed a 12-lead electrocardiogram (ECG), while Mrs Pillar was taken to give admission details at the reception desk. She returned shortly afterwards to be with her husband. Oxygen via a face mask was administered to the patient. Reassurance and explanation were offered to both

Mr and Mrs Pillar. Figure 9.5 shows the recorded ECG.

A troponin T level was also measured by the nurse as a highly specific marker of myocardial damage. The value was slightly elevated. Another level recorded 8 hours later showed elevation indicative of severe myocardial damage. The hospital had in place an anterior protocol, meaning that patients experiencing an anterior myocardial infarction were administered alteplase based on the GUSTO-I (1993) trial. This was administered in an accelerated format due to the fact that the infarction was less than 6 hours old and was anterior in origin. This meant the total dose was administered over 1.5 hours, as opposed to 3 hours. The nurse and medical staff assessed carefully, to a set protocol, any contra-indications before administering the thrombolytic agent. Mr Pillar had no history of bleeding disorders, gastro-intestinal bleeding, cerebrovascular accident (CVA/stroke), severe hypertension or other factors such as a suspected aortic aneurysm.

Further pain relief was offered in the form of prescribed intravenous diamorphine, together with an anti-emetic. Diamorphine will also reduce the afterload and relax the patient, limiting the factors which will increase myocardial oxygen demand. The resident doctor took blood samples for urea and electrolytes, particularly potassium levels. A bolus of heparin was administered followed by a 24-hour intravenous infusion. The pulse and blood pressure were recorded frequently during thrombolysis administration and then were reduced to hourly, until the afternoon. Pain was fairly quickly relieved and ST elevation began to subside in the next one and a half hours. Reperfusion arrhythmias were noted, in the form of fairly frequent ventricular extrasystoles/ectopics. The returned potassium was noted to be 3.5 mmol/l and an oral potassium supplement was prescribed.

At an early stage, nursing staff assisted Mrs Pillar to ring her daughter and reassured her that Mr Pillar would be more comfortable now the pain relief and thrombolytic therapy had been administered. The doctor prescribed a β-blocker to commence that evening, together with an angiotensin-converting enzyme (ACE) inhibitor, the latter to be slowly titrated to a maximum dose. Aspirin, used

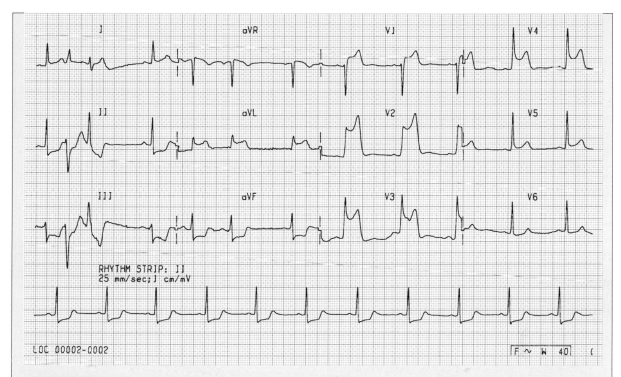

Figure 9.5 The 12-lead ECG shows clear ST elevation in the anterior leads V1–V4 with some mild elevation in V5. ST depression, sometimes known as reciprocal changes, can be noted in leads II, III and aVF. The occasional ventricular ectopic (extrasystole) beat can also be noted. ST elevation is clearly in excess of 2 mm in two chest leads, one of the usual factors in the decision to administer thrombolytic therapy. Pain onset was within the last 12 hours. This ECG was taken at 03.30 am. The GP had been called at 02.05 and arrived at the house at 02.20. (Reproduced with permission from Jenkins RD, Gerred SJ 1997 ECGs by example. Churchill Livingstone, Edinburgh.)

here as an antiplatelet drug, was also commenced at 75 mg daily. Mr Pillar's condition did not deteriorate any further. He did not experience any further chest pain, breathlessness or arrhythmias, except for the occasional ventricular extrasystole/ectopic, which lessened with the administration of the potassium supplement. He remained on bedrest for 24 hours, with all his basic nursing needs met by staff. A bedside commode was used to allow him to have his bowels open in as dignified a fashion as possible. The nursing assessment had revealed a tendency to constipation and this was addressed by the encouragement of oral fluids and a gentle laxative. It is important that patients experiencing cardiac problems are not allowed to strain at stool. This may induce the Valsalva manoeuvre and predispose to bradycardia or arrhythmias. On the second day Mr Pillar was able to sit out of bed and gently mobilize around the bed area. On the third day he was moved to the ward area, in a bay near the nurses' station. It was considered at this point unnecessary to continue cardiac monitoring.

The cardiac rehabilitation nurse was contacted and visited to discuss with Mr Pillar and his wife possible lifestyle changes and what they felt they could both realistically achieve. An appointment was made to visit the cardiac rehabilitation/health promotion unit to plan further lifestyle changes and explore Mr Pillar's condition, once he had returned home. Further medical investigation was necessary and Mr Pillar was provided with an outpatients appointment to see the consultant. There was a necessity to assess the degree of myocardial ischaemia the patient was experiencing and plan further treatment, either medical or more invasive. At this point Mr Pillar was not experiencing angina and was free of cardiac failure, therefore an exercise tolerance test was planned for early after discharge.

CONCLUSION

This chapter has reviewed the conditions of angina, unstable angina and myocardial infarction. The latter two are medical emergencies which require a co-ordinated and efficient service between all members of the multidisciplinary team, both in the hospital and community areas. There are clear advances occurring in strategy planning, allowing thrombolytic therapy to be more readily available to those who need this treatment. Hospital and community staff need to plan together to reduce the 'call-to-needle' times. This may involve breaking down old hierarchical boundaries and developing paramedic and nurse-led thrombolysis programmes based on sound education and auditing, if this is deemed the most appropriate method to implement this vital treatment. Of major significance will be the need to reduce the 'pain-to-needle' time. This is the initiation of treatment from the time the patient experiences chest pain and recognizes that a health-care professional is needed. This will involve clear education strategies aimed at the public to explain what the signs of infarction can be and will be a clear teaching challenge to the health-care profession.

The work of the catheter laboratory in areas of revascularization is currently creating great interest, with the advent of the glycoprotein IIb/IIIa inhibitor (antiplatelet) drugs. These are emerging as a viable option in reducing vessel occlusion in certain patients following coronary invasive procedures. In addition, they may offer enhancement of treatment for those receiving thrombolytic therapy. However, continuing trials will demonstrate the exact role these drugs will play in managing these conditions. Research such as the EUROASPIRE (1997) study group, which analysed the monitoring and management strategies for CHD patients, provides useful information in the impact of evidence-based medicine and care.

All the conditions and their management discussed in this chapter can and do lend themselves to innovations in the provision of nursing care. The key is communication between the varying health-care disciplines and forward-thinking managers, with the patient and improved outcomes from the condition they are experiencing as the clear endpoint. For the patient, all these advances do not change the fact that heart disease is a frightening condition and reassurance and understanding from a well-informed, efficient team underlie all approaches to care.

REFERENCES

Adams J, Trent R, Rawles J 1993 Earliest electrocardiographic evidence of myocardial infarction: implications for thrombolytic treatment. British Medical Journal 307: 409–413

Adams J, Sicard GA, Allen BT et al 1994 Diagnosis of perioperative myocardial infarction with measurement of cardiac troponin I. New England Journal of Medicine 330: 670–674

Ahmad RAS, Bond S, Burke J, Singh SP, Watson RD 1992 Patients with suspected myocardial infarction: effect of mode of referral on admission time to a coronary care unit. British Journal of General Practice 42: 145–148

AIRE study 1993 Acute Infarction Ramipril Efficacy Study Investigators. Effect of ramipril on mortality of survivors of acute myocardial infarction with clinical evidence of heart failure. Lancet 342: 821–828

Almbrand B, Johannesson M, Sjostrand B, Malmberg K, Ryden L 2000 Cost-effectiveness of intense insulin treatment after acute myocardial infarction in patients with diabetes mellitus. Results from the DIGAMI study. European Heart Journal 21: 733–739

Alonzo AA 1986 The impact of the family and lay others on care seeking during life threatening episodes of suspected coronary artery disease. Social Science and Medicine 22: 1297–1311

Anderson DJ, Jenkins C, McInally C 1999 Using spinal cord stimulation to manage angina pain. Dimensions of Critical Care Nursing 18(3): 12–13

Antiplatelet Trialists' Collaboration 1994 Collaborative overview of randomised trials of antiplatelet therapy. 1. Prevention of death, myocardial infarction, and stroke by prolonged antiplatelet therapy in various categories of patients. British Medical Journal 308: 81–106

Antman EM, Tanasijevic MJ, Thompson BW et al 1996 Cardiac specific troponin I levels to predict the risk of mortality in patients with acute coronary syndromes. New England Journal of Medicine 335: 1342–1349

Antman EM, Cohen M, Radley D et al for the TIMI IIB (Thrombolysis in Myocardial Infarction) and ESSENCE (Efficacy and Safety of Subcutaneous Enoxaparin in non-Q wave Coronary Events) Investigators 1999a Assessment of the treatment effect of enoxaparin for unstable angina/non-Q wave myocardial infarction. Circulation 100: 1602–1608

Antman EM, McCabe CH, Gurfinkel EP et al 1999b Enoxaparin prevents death and cardiac ischaemic events in unstable angina/non-Q wave myocardial infarction. Results of the Thrombolysis in Myocardial Infarction (TIMI) IIB Trial. Circulation 100: 1593–1601

ASSENT-2 1999 Single-bolus tenecteplase compared with front-loaded alteplase in acute myocardial infarction: the ASSENT-2 double-blind randomised trial. Lancet 354: 716–722

Aufderheide TP, Hendley GE, Woo J, Lawrence S, Valley V, Teichman SL 1992 A prospective evaluation of pre-hospital 12 lead ECG application in chest pain patients. Journal of Electrocardiology 24 (suppl): 8–13

Baker CF, Garvin BJ, Kennedy CW, Polivka BJ 1993 The effect of environmental sound and communication on CCU patients' heart rate and blood pressure. Research in Nursing and Health 16: 415–421

Banedee S, Rhodes WE 1998 Fast tracking of myocardial infarction by paramedics. Journal of the Royal College of Physicians of London 2: 36–38

Barrett-Connor E, Khaw KT 1984 Family history of heart attack as an independent predictor of death from cardiovascular disease. Circulation 69: 1065–1068

Birkhead JS 1992 Time delays in the provision of thrombolytic treatment in six district hospitals. British Medical Journal 305: 445–448

Birkhead J, Golacre M, Mason A, Wilkinson E, Amess M, Cleary R (eds) 1999 Health outcome indicators: myocardial infarction. Report of a working group to the Department of Health. National Centre for Health Outcomes Development, Oxford

Boersma E, Maas AC, Deckers JW, Simoons ML 1996 Early thrombolytic treatment in acute myocardial infarction: reappraisal of the golden hour. Lancet 348: 771–775

Bondestam E, Hougren K, Gaston-Johansson F, Jern S, Herlitz J, Holmberg S 1987 Pain assessment by patients and nurses in the early phase of acute myocardial infarction. Journal of Advanced Nursing 12: 677–682

Bouten MJM, Simoons ML, Hartman JAM, Van Miltenburg AM, Van der Does E, Pool J 1992 Prehospital thrombolysis with alteplase (rt-PA) in acute myocardial infarction. European Heart Journal 13: 925–931

British Cardiac Society/Royal College of Physicians of London 1998 Staffing surveys. BCS, London

British Heart Foundation 1999 Coronary heart disease statistics. British Heart Foundation, London

British Heart Foundation 2000 Coronary heart disease statistics database: annual compendium 2000. British Heart Foundation, London

British Heart Foundation 2001 Coronary heart disease statistics: morbidity supplement. British Heart Foundation, London

Brooks N 1997 Primary angioplasty in the UK: if not for all, then for whom? Heart 78 (suppl 2): 16

Bundy C, Carroll D, Wallace L, Nagle R 1994 Psychological treatment of chronic stable angina pectoris. Psychology and Health 10: 69–77

Califf RM, Mark DB, Harrell FE Jr et al 1988 Importance of clinical measures of ischaemia in the prognosis of patients with documented coronary artery disease. Journal of the American College of Cardiology 11(1): 20–26

Calvin JE, Klein LW, Van den Berg BJ et al 1995 Risk stratification in unstable angina. Prospective validation of the Braunwald classification. Journal of the American Medical Association 273: 136–141

CAPTURE Investigators 1997 Randomised placebo controlled trial of abciximab before and during coronary intervention in refractory unstable angina. The CAPTURE Study. Lancet 349: 1429–1435

Casey K, Bedker DL, Roussel-McElmeel PL 1998 Myocardial infarction: review of clinical trials and treatment strategies. Critical Care Nurse 18(2): 39–52

Caunt J 1996 The advanced nurse practitioner in CCU. Care of the Critically Ill 12(4): 136–139

Chamberlin JR, Lardi AB, McKeever LS et al 1999 Use of vascular sealing devices (VasoSeal and Perclose) versus assisted manual compression (Femostop) in transcatheter coronary interventions requiring abciximab (ReoPro). Catheterization and Cardiovascular Interventions 47(2): 143–147

Chatelain P, Urban P 1997 Is primary angioplasty feasible or will we provide a two-tier service? Heart 78 (suppl 2): 15

Cheng JW, Rivera NG 1998 Infection and atherosclerosis – focus on cytomegalovirus and chlamydia pneumoniae. Annals of Pharmacotherapy 32(12): 1310–1316

Chew KK, Stuckey BG, Thompson PL 2000 Erectile dysfunction, sildenafil and cardiovascular risk. Medical Journal of Australia 172(6): 279–283

Clark LT, Bellam SV, Shah AH, Feldman JG 1992 Analysis of pre-hospital delay among inner-city patients with symptoms of myocardial infarction: implications for therapeutic intervention. Journal of the National Medical Association 84: 931–937

Clifford C 1986 Patients, relatives and nurses in a technological environment. Intensive and Critical Care Nursing 2: 27–72

Cobb LA, Weaver WD, Fahrenbruch CE, Hallstrom AP, Copass MK 1992 Community-based interventions for sudden cardiac death. Impact limitations and changes. Circulation 85 (suppl 1): 98–102

Cobbe SM, Redmond MJ, Watson JM, Hollingworth J, Carrington DJ 1991 'Heartstart Scotland'. British Medical Journal 302: 1517–1520

Cohen M 1999 Low molecular weight heparins in the management of unstable angina/non Q wave myocardial infarction. Seminars in Thrombosis and Hemostasis 25 (suppl 3 HD): 113–121

Cohen M, Demers C, Gurtinkel EP et al 1997 A comparison of low molecular weight heparin with unfractionated heparin for unstable coronary artery disease. Efficacy and safety of subcutaneous Enoxaparin in non-Q wave coronary events study group. New England Journal of Medicine 337: 447–452

Collinson P 2000 Cardiac troponins – diagnostic, prognostic and management tools in patients admitted with suspected acute coronary syndromes. Cardiology News 3(6): 9–10

Cox ID, Salomone O, Brown SJ, Hann C, Kaski JC 1997 Serum endothelin levels in pain perception in patients with cardiac syndrome X and in healthy controls. American Journal of Cardiology 80(5): 637–640

Crawford SL, McGraw SA, Smith KW, McKinlay JB, Pierson JE 1994 Do blacks and whites differ in their use of health care for symptoms of coronary heart disease? American Journal of Public Health 84: 957–964

Cross SJ, Lee HS, Rawles JM, Jennings K 1991 Safety of thrombolysis in association with cardiopulmonary resuscitation. British Medical Journal 303: 1242

Crown Report 1998 A report on the supply and administration of medicines under group protocols. Department of Health, London

Cupples ME, McKnight A 1994 Randomised controlled trial of health promotion in general practice for patients at high cardiovascular risk. British Medical Journal 309: 993–996

Dalager-Pedersen S, Ravin HB, Falk E 1998 Atherosclerosis and acute coronary events. American Journal of Cardiology 82(10B): 37T–40T

DAVIT II (Danish Study Group on Verapamil in Myocardial Infarction) 1990 Effect of verapamil on mortality and major events after acute myocardial infarction (The Danish Verapamil Infarction Trial II). American Journal of Cardiology 66(10): 779–785

De Bono DP 1993 Complications of diagnostic cardiac catheterisation: results from 34,041 patients in the United Kingdom confidential enquiry into cardiac catheter complications. British Heart Journal 73: 297–300

De Bono D 1999 Investigation and management of stable angina: revised guidelines 1998. Heart 81: 546–555

De Bono DP, Hopkins A 1993 The investigation and management of stable angina. Report of a working party of the joint audit committee of the British Cardiac Society and the Royal College of Physicians of London. Journal of the Royal College of Physicians of London 27: 267–273

DeBusk R, Drory Y, Goldstein I et al 2000 Management of sexual dysfunction in patients with cardiovascular disease: recommendations of the Princeton Consensus Panel. American Journal of Cardiology 86(2A): 62F–68F

Department of Health 1996 Hospital episode statistics, volume 1, England, 1994–95. Department of Health, Blackpool

Department of Health 1999 Saving lives: our healthier nation. Stationery Office, London

Department of Health 2000a National Service Framework for Coronary Heart Disease. Department of Health, London

Department of Health 2000b The NHS plan: a plan for investment, a plan for reform. Department of Health, London

Detrano R, Gianrosso R, Froechlicher V 1989 The diagnostic accuracy of the exercise electrocardiogram: a meta-analysis of 22 years of research. Progress in Cardiovascular Disease 32: 173–206

De Wood MA, Spores J, Notske R, Mouser LT, Burroughs, R, Golden MS, Lang HT 1980 Prevalence of total coronary occlusion during the early hours of transmural myocardial infarction. New England Journal of Medicine 303: 897–902

Doevendans PA, Gorgels AP, Van der Zee R, Partouns J, Bar FW, Wellens HJ 1995 Electrocardiographic diagnosis of reperfusion during thrombolytic therapy in acute myocardial infarction. American Journal of Cardiology 75: 1206–1210

Domanski MJ, Exner DV, Borkowf CB et al 1999 Effect of angiotensin converting enzyme inhibition on sudden cardiac death in patients following acute myocardial infarction. A meta analysis of randomised clinical trials. Journal of the American College of Cardiology 33: 598–604

Dracup K, Moser DK, Eisenberg M, Meischke H, Alonzo AA, Braslow A 1995 Causes of delay in seeking treatment for heart attack symptoms. Social Science and Medicine 40: 379–392

Dunn CJ, Goa KL 2001 Tenecteplase: a review of its pharmacology and therapeutic efficacy in patients with myocardial infarction. American Journal of Cardiovascular Drugs 1: 51–66

Ellis SG, Van der Werf F, Ribeiro-daSilva E, Topol EJ 1992 Present status of rescue coronary angioplasty: current polarization of opinion and randomized trials. Journal of the American College of Cardiology 19: 681–686

EPILOG Investigators 1997 Platelet glycoprotein IIb/IIIa receptor blockade and low dose heparin during percutaneous coronary revascularisation. New England Journal of Medicine 336: 956–961

EPISTENT Investigators 1998 Randomised placebo-controlled and balloon angioplasty-controlled trial to assess safety of coronary stenting with use of platelet glycoprotein IIb/IIIa blockade. Lancet 352: 87–92

EUROASPIRE 1997 A European Society of Cardiology survey of secondary prevention of coronary heart disease. Principal results. European Heart Journal 18: 1569–1582

Fibrinolytic Therapy Trialists' (FTT) Collaborative Group 1994 Indications for fibrinolytic therapy in suspected acute myocardial infarction: collaborative overview of early mortality and major morbidity results from all randomised trials of more than 1000 patients. Lancet 343: 311–322

Fischman DL, Leon MB, Baim DS 1994 A randomised comparison of coronary-stent placement and balloon angioplasty in the treatment of coronary artery disease: stent restenosis study investigators. New England Journal of Medicine 331(8): 496–501

Fitzpatrick B, Watt GC, Tunstall-Pedoe H 1992 Potential impact of emergency intervention on sudden deaths from coronary heart disease in Glasgow. British Heart Journal 67: 250–254

Fletcher AP, Alkjaersig N, Smyrniotis FE, Sherry S 1958 The treatment of patients suffering from early myocardial infarction with massive and prolonged streptokinase therapy. Transcripts of the Association of American Physicians 71: 287–296

Ghali JK, Cooper RS, Kowalty I, Liao Y 1993 Delay between onset of chest pain and arrival to the coronary care unit among minority and disadvantaged patients. Journal of the National Medical Association 85: 180–184

Ghandi MM, Lampe FC, Wood DA 1995 Incidence, clinical characteristics and short term prognosis of angina pectoris. British Heart Journal 73: 193–198

GISSI-1 Gruppo Italiano per lo Studio della Streptochinasi nell'Infarto Miocardio 1986 Effectiveness of intravenous thrombolytic therapy in acute myocardial infarction. Lancet i: 397–401

Gray HH, Swanton RH, Schofield PM et al, on behalf of the Joint Working Group on Coronary Angioplasty of the British Cardiac Society and British Cardiovascular Intervention Society 2000 Coronary angioplasty: guidelines for good practice and training. Heart 83: 224–235

GREAT Group 1992 Feasibility, safety, and efficacy of domiciliary thrombolysis by general practitioners: Grampian Region Early Anistreplase Trial. British Medical Journal 305: 548–553

Gurwitz JH, McLaughlin TJ, Willison DJ et al 1997 Delayed hospital presentation in patients who have had acute myocardial infarction. Annals of Internal Medicine 126: 593–599

GUSTO-I Global utilisation of streptokinase and t-PA for occluded coronary arteries 1993 An international randomized trial comparing four thrombolytic strategies for acute myocardial infarction. New England Journal of Medicine 329: 673–682

Hadorn DC, Holmes AC 1997 The New Zealand priority criteria project. Part 2. Coronary artery bypass surgery. British Medical Journal 314: 135–138

Hamer DW, Gordon MWG, Cusack S, Robertson CE 1993 Survival from cardiac arrest in the accident and emergency department: the impact of out of hospital advisory defibrillation. Resuscitation 26: 31–36

Hammond P 1998 Management of acute myocardial infarction in the diabetic patient. Journal of Diabetic Nursing 2(2): 43–46

Hampton JR, McWilliam A 1992 Purchasing care for patients with acute myocardial infarction. Quality in Health Care 1: 68–73

Hampton P, Harrison L, Gray D 1993 Demand for hospital services following admission with suspected myocardial infarction in 1983 and 1989. Health Trends 25: 91–94

Hautvast RWM, Blanksma PK, Dejonqste MJL et al 1996 Effect of spinal cord stimulation on myocardial blood flow assessed with positron emission tomography in patients with refractory angina pectoris. American Journal of Cardiology 77: 462–467

Herlitz J, Hjalmarson A, Holmberg S et al 1986 Variability, prediction and prognostic significance of chest pain in acute myocardial infarction. Cardiology 73(1): 13–21

Herrick JB 1912 Clinical features of sudden obstruction of coronary arteries. Journal of the American Medical Association 59: 2015–2020

Hobbs R 1995 Rising emergency admissions. British Medical Journal 310: 207–208

Holdright D 1996 Chest pain with normal coronary arteries. British Journal of Hospital Medicine 56: 347–350

Hood S, Birnie D, Swan L, Hillis WS 1998 Questionnaire survey of thrombolytic treatment in accident and emergency departments in the United Kingdom. British Medical Journal 316: 274

Hubner P 1998 Guide to coronary angioplasty and stenting. Harwood Academic Publishers, Amsterdam, ch 5, p. 59

INJECT International Joint Efficacy Comparison of Thrombolytics 1995 Randomised, double blind comparison of reteplase double-bolus administration with streptokinase in acute myocardial infarction (INJECT): trial to investigate equivalence. Lancet 346: 329–336

ISIS-1 First International Study of Infarct Survival Collaborative Group 1986 Randomised trial of intravenous atenolol among 16,027 cases of suspected acute myocardial infarction. Lancet ii: 57–66

ISIS-2 Second International Study of Infarct Survival Collaborative Group 1988 Randomised trial of intravenous streptokinase, oral aspirin, both, or neither among 17 187 cases of suspected acute myocardial infarction. Lancet ii: 349–360

ISIS-4 Fourth International Study of Infarct Survival Collaborative Group 1995 A randomised factorial trial assessing early oral captopril, oral mononitrate and intravenous magnesium sulphate in 58,050 patients with suspected acute myocardial infarction. Lancet 345: 669–685

Jackson G 1997 Angina in practice. Royal Society of Medicine Press, London

Kee F, McDonald P, Kirwan JR, Patterson CC, Love AHG 1998 Urgency and priority for cardiac surgery: a clinical judgement analysis. British Medical Journal 216: 925–929

Kendall J, McCabe S 1996 The use of audit to set up a thrombolysis programme in the accident and emergency department. Journal of Accident and Emergency Medicine 13: 49–53

Kereiakes DJ, Gibler WB, Martin LH, Pieper KS, Anderson LC 1992 The Cincinnati Heart Project Study Group. Relative importance of emergency medical system transport and the pre-hospital electrocardiogram on reducing hospital time delay to therapy for acute myocardial infarction: a preliminary report from the Cincinnati Heart Project. American Heart Journal 123(4 pt 1): 835–840

Kinzinger RG 1992 Death anxiey among myocardial infarction clients in coronary care versus general medical units. Critical Care Nurse Quarterly 15: 75–79

Lau J, Antman EM, Jimenez-Silva J, Kupelnick B, Mosteller F, Chaliners TC 1992 Cumulative meta-analysis of therapeutic trials for myocardial infarction. New England Journal of Medicine 327: 248–254

Lawrence-Mathew PJ, Wilson AT, Woodmansey PA, Channer KS 1994 Unsatisfactory management of patients with myocardial infarction admitted to general medical wards. Journal of the Royal College of Physicians of London 28(1): 49–51

Lawson WE, Hui JC, Cohn PF 2000 Long-term prognosis of patients with angina treated with enhanced external counterpulsation: five-year follow-up study. Clinical Cardiology 23(4): 254–258

Lee HS, Quinn T, Boyle RM 1995 Safety of thrombolytic treatment in patients with central venous cannulation. Heart 73: 359–362

Lindahl B, Venge P, Wallentin LC for the FRISC Study Group 1996 Relation between troponin T and the risk of subsequent cardiac events in unstable coronary disease. Circulation 93(9): 1651–1657

MacIsaac AI, Thomas JD, Topol EJ 1993 Toward the quiescent coronary plaque. Journal of the American College of Cardiology 22: 1228–1241

MacRae CA, Marber MS, Keywood C, Joy M 1992 The need for invasive cardiological assessment and intervention: a ten year review. British Heart Journal 67: 200–203

Malik FS, Lavie CJ, Mehra MR, Milani RV, Re RN 1997 Renin–angiotensin system: genes to bedside. American Heart Journal 134(3): 514–526

Malmberg K 1997 Prospective randomised study of intensive insulin treatment on long term survival after acute myocardial infraction in patients with diabetes mellitus DIAGMI (Diabetes Mellitus Insulin Glucose Infusion in Acute Myocardial Infarction) study group. British Medical Journal 314: 1512–1515

Malmberg K, Ryden L 1988 Myocardial infarction in patients with diabetes mellitus. European Heart Journal 9: 259–264

Malmberg K, Ryden L, Efendic S et al 1995 A randomised trial of insulin-glucose infusion followed by subcutaneous insulin treatment in diabetic patients with acute myocardial infarction (DIGAMI study): effects on mortality at 1 year. Journal of the American College of Cardiology 26(1): 57–65

Malmberg K, Norhammer A, Wedel H, Ryden L 1999 Glycometabolic state at admission: important risk marker of mortality in conventionally treated patients with diabetes mellitus and acute myocardial infarction: long term results from the Diabetes and Insulin-Glucose Infusion in Acute Myocardial Infarction (DIGAMI) study. Circulation 99: 2626–2632

Malmberg K, Norhammer A, Wedel H, Ryden L 1999 Glycometabolic state at admission: important risk marker of mortality in conventionally treated patients with diabetes mellitus and acute myocardial infarction: long term results from the Diabetes and Insulin-Glucose Infusion in Acute Myocardial Infarction (DIGAMI) study. Circulation 99: 2626–2632

Mark DB, Nelson CL, Califf RM et al 1994 Continuing evolution of therapy for coronary artery disease. Circulation 89: 2015–2025

Mathews KA, Owens JF, Kuller LH, Sutton-Tyrrell K, Lassila HC, Wolfson SK 1998 Stress-induced pulse pressure change predicts women's carotid atherosclerosis. Stroke 29(8): 1525–1530

Maynard C, Althouse R, Olsufka M, Ritchie JL, Davis KB, Kennedy JW 1989 Early versus late hospital arrival for acute myocardial infarction in the Western Washington thrombolytic therapy trials. American Journal of Cardiology 63: 1296–1300

Meischke H, Eisenberg MS, Larsen MP 1993 Pre-hospital delay interval for patients who use emergency medical services: the effect of heart related medical conditions and demographic variables. Annals of Emergency Medicine 22(10): 1597–1601

Melin JA, Wijns W, Vanbutsele RJ et al 1985 Alternative strategies for coronary artery disease in women: demonstration of the usefulness and efficiency of probability analysis. Circulation 71(3): 535–542

Meurier CE 1998 The quality of assessment of patients with chest pain: the development of a questionnaire to audit the nursing assessment records of patients with chest pain. Journal of Advanced Nursing 27: 140–146

Meurier CE, Vincent CA, Palmer DG 1998 Perception of causes of omissions in the assessment of patients with chest pain. Journal of Advanced Nursing 28: 1012–1019

MIAMI Trial Research Group, Metoprolol in Acute Myocardial Infarction 1985 A randomised-controlled international trial. European Heart Journal 6: 199–226

Miklaucich M 1998 Limitations on life: women's lived experiences of angina. Journal of Advanced Nursing 28: 1207–1215

Millar-Craig MW, Joy AV, Adamowicz M et al 1997 Reduction in treatment delay by paramedic ECG diagnosis of myocardial infarction with direct CCU admission. Heart 78: 456–461

Morrison C, Woodward M, Leslie W, Tunstall-Pedoe H 1997 Effects of socioeconomic group on incidence of, management of, and survival after myocardial infarction and coronary death; analysis of community coronary event register. British Medical Journal 314: 541–546

Murphy MJ, Berding CB 1999 Use of measurements of myoglobin and cardiac troponins in the diagnosis of acute myocardial infarction. Critical Care Nurse 19(1): 58–66

National Heart Attack Alert Program Co-ordinating Committee 1994 Emergency department: rapid identification and treatment of patients with acute myocardial infarction. Annals of Emergency Medicine 23: 311–329

Naylor CD, Baigrie RS, Goldman BS, Basinski A 1990 Assessment of priority for coronary revascularisation procedures. Lancet 335: 1070–1073

Neumann FJ, Walter H, Richards G, Schmitt C, Schomig A 1996 Coronary Palmaz-Schatz stent implantation in acute myocardial infarction. Heart 75: 121–126

Neumann FJ, Blasini R, Schmitt C et al 1998 Effect of glycoprotein IIb/IIIa receptor blockade on recovery of coronary flow and left ventricular function after the placement of coronary-artery stents in acute myocardial infarction. Circulation 98: 2695–2701

NHS Executive 1996 Review of ambulance performance standards. Final report of steering group. NHS Executive, London

NICE 2000 NICE guidance on technologies for specialist cardiac services. The National Institute for Clinical Excellence, London

Nicolau JC, Lorga AM, Garzon SAC et al 1989 Clinical and laboratory signs of reperfusion: are they reliable? International Journal of Cardiology 25(3): 313–320

Norell M, Lythall D, Coghlan G et al 1992 Limited value of the resting electrocardiogram in assessing patients with recent onset chest pain: lessons from a chest pain clinic. British Heart Journal 7: 53–56

Norris RM 1998 Fatality outside hospital from acute coronary events in three British health districts, 1994–5. United Kingdom Heart Attack Study Collaborative Group. British Medical Journal 316: 1065–1070

O'Connor L 1995 Pain assessment by patients and nurses, and nurses notes on it, in early acute myocardial infarction: part 1. Intensive and Critical Care Nursing 11: 183–191

Ohman EM, Armstrong PW, Christensen RH et al 1996 Cardiac troponin T levels for risk stratification in acute myocardial ischaemia. New England Journal of Medicine 335: 1333–1341

O'Keefe JH, Barnhart CSS, Bateman TM 1995 Comparison of stress echocardiography and myocardial perfusion scintigraphy for diagnosing coronary artery disease and assessing its severity. American Journal of Cardiology 75: 1D–11D

Oldridge NB, Guyatt GH, Fisher ME, Rimm AA 1998 Cardiac rehabilitation after myocardial infarction: combined experience of randomised clinical trials. Journal of the American Medical Association 260: 945–950

O'Rourke MF, Cook A, Carrol G, Gallagher D, Hall J 1992 Accuracy of a portable interpretive ECG machine in diagnosis of acute evolving myocardial infarction. Australian and New Zealand Journal of Medicine 22: 9–13

Parker DJ, Balcon R, Brooks NH et al 1997 The changing interface between district hospital cardiology and the major cardiac centres. A working group of the British Cardiac Society, with the Royal College of Physicians of London, the Royal College of Physicians of Edinburgh, and the Royal College of Physicians and Surgeons of Glasgow. Heart 78: 519–523

Pell AC, Miller HC, Robertson CE, Fox KA 1992 Effect of 'fast track' admission for acute myocardial infarction on delay to thrombolysis. British Medical Journal 304: 83–87

Peter J, Yhip A, Smalling RW 1999 Primary stenting for acute myocardial infarction (review). Thrombolysis and Haemostasis 1: 160–163

Pfeffer MA, Braunwald E, Moye LA et al 1992 Effect of captopril on mortality and morbidity in patients with left ventricular dysfunction after myocardial infarction. New England Journal of Medicine 327: 669–677

Pocock SJ, Henderson RA, Rickards AF et al 1995 Meta-analysis of randomised trials combating coronary angioplasty with bypass surgery. Lancet 346: 1184–1189

Prasad N, Wright A, Hogg M, Dunn FG 1997 Direct admission to the coronary care unit by the ambulance service for patients with suspected myocardial infarction. Heart 78: 462–464

Prinzmetal M, Kennarner R, Merliss R, Wada T, Bor N 1959 Angina pectoris 1. A variant form of angina pectoris: preliminary report. American Journal of Medicine 27: 375–388

Proctor T, Yarcheski A, Oriscello RG 1996 The relationship of hospital process variables to patient outcome post myocardial infarction. International Journal of Nursing Studies 33(2): 121–130

Pye M 2000 Glycoprotein IIb/IIIa receptor blockade: the Clinical Trials in Acute Coronary Syndromes and Percutaneous Coronary Intervention. Cardiology News 3(4): 8–14

Quinn T 1993 Implications of advances in coronary care for nurses. British Journal of Nursing 2: 792

Quinn T 1995 Can nurses safely assess suitability for thrombolysis? A pilot study. Intensive and Critical Care Nursing 11: 126–129

Quinn T 1999a Thrombolysis in accident and emergency: the exception not the rule. Are we denying patients lifesaving treatment? Accident and Emergency Nursing 7: 39–41

Quinn T 1999b Improving care for patients with coronary heart disease: the crucial role of ambulance services in implementing the national service framework. Ambulance UK 14: 146–151

Quinn T, Thompson DR 1995 Administration of thrombolytic therapy to patients with acute myocardial infarction. Accident and Emergency Nursing 3: 208–214

Quinn T, Allan TF, Thompson DR, Pawelec J, Boyle RM 1999 Identification of patients suitable for direct admission to a coronary care unit by ambulance paramedics. Pre-hospital Immediate Care 3: 126–130

RAPPORT Investigators 1998 Randomised placebo controlled trial of platelet glycoprotein IIb/IIIa blockade with primary angioplasty for acute myocardial infarction. Circulation 98: 734–741

Rawles J 1997a Pre-hospital coronary care. Pre-hospital Immediate Care 1: 12–18

Rawles J 1997b Quantification of the benefit of earlier thrombolytic therapy: five year results of the Grampian Region Early Anistreplase Trial (GREAT). Journal of the American College of Cardiology 30: 1181–1186

Rawles J, Metcalfe MJ, Shirreffs C et al 1990 Association of patient delay with symptoms, cardiac enzymes, and outcome in acute myocardial infarction. European Heart Journal 11(7): 643–648

Reifart N, Vandomael M, Krajar M et al 1997 Randomized comparison of angioplasty of complex coronary lesions at a single center. Excimer laser, rotational atherectomy and balloon angioplasty comparison (ERBAC) study. Circulation 96: 91–98

RITA-2 Trial Participants 1997 Coronary angioplasty versus medical therapy: the second Randomised Intervention Treatment of Angina (RITA-2) trial. Lancet 350: 461–468

Rizik DG, Healy S, Margulis A et al 1995 A new clinical classification for hospital prognosis of unstable angina pectoris. American Journal of Cardiology 75: 993–997

Roberts WC 1972 Coronary arteries in fatal acute myocardial infarction. Circulation 45: 215–230

Rogers WJ, Coggin CJ, Gersh BJ et al 1990 Ten-year follow up of quality of life in patients randomised to receive coronary artery bypass graft surgery. Circulation 82: 1647–1658

Rosano GMC, Collins P, Kaski JC, Lindsay DC, Sarrel PM, Poole-Wilson PA 1995 Syndrome X in women is associated with oestrogen deficiency. European Heart Journal 16(5): 610–614

Rosanski A, Berman DS 1987 The efficacy of cardiovascular nuclear medicine exercise studies. Seminars in Nuclear Medicine 17: 104–120

Royal College of Physicians of London 1998 Consultant physicians working for patients Part 1: a blueprint for effective hospital practice. Journal of the Royal College of Physicians of London 32(4) (suppl 1): S1–S20

Ruston A, Clayton J, Calnan M 1998 Patients' action during their cardiac event. Qualitative study exploring differences and modifiable factors. British Medical Journal 316: 1060–1065

Sacks FM, Pieffer MA, Moye LA et al 1996 The effect of pravastatin on coronary events after myocardial infarction in patients with average cholesterol levels. New England Journal of Medicine 335: 1001–1009

Sayre MR, Kaufmann KH, Chen IW et al 1998 Measurement of cardiac troponin is an effective method for predicting complications among emergency department patients with chest pain. Annals of Emergency Medicine 31(5): 539–549

Scandinavian Simvastatin Survival Study Group 1994 Randomised trial of cholesterol lowering in 4444 patients with coronary heart disease: The Scandinavian Simvastatin Study (4S). Lancet ii: 1383–1389

Schmidt SB, Borsch MA 1990 The pre hospital phase of acute myocardial infarction in the era of thrombolysis. American Journal of Cardiology 65(22): 1411–1415

Schomig A, Neumann FJ, Kastrati A et al 1996 A randomized comparison of antiplatelet and anticoagulant therapy after the placement of coronary artery stents. New England Journal of Medicine 334: 1084–1089

Scott ME, Orr R 1969 Effects of diamorphine, methadone, morphine and pentazocine in patients with acute myocardial infarction. Lancet 1: 1065–1067

Searle M, Hoff L 2000 Bedrest after elective cardiac catheterisation. Professional Nurse 15(9): 588–591

Sedgwick MI, Dalziel K, Watson J, Carrington DJ, Cobbe SM 1993 Performance of an established system of first responder out-of-hospital defibrillation. The results of the second year of the Heartstart Scotland Project in the 'Utstein style'. Resuscitation 26(1): 75–78

Selker HP, Zanlenski RJ, Antman EM et al 1997 National heart attack alert program report. Annals of Emergency Medicine 29: 63–69

Simoons ML, Maggioni AP, Knatterud G et al 1993 Individual risk assessment for intracranial haemorrhage during thrombolytic therapy. Lancet 342: 1523–1528

Smallwood A, Van der Woning M 1999 What are the attitudes of coronary care nurses towards the introduction of nurse-initiated thrombolysis? Nursing in Critical Care 4(3): 128–132

Somauroo ID, McCarten P, Appleton B, Amadi A, Rodrigues E 1999 Effectiveness of a 'thrombolysis nurse' in shortening delay to thrombolysis in acute myocardial infarction. Journal of the Royal College of Physicians of London 33: 46–50

Stamler J, Vaccaro O, Neaton J, Wentworth D for the MRFIT Research Group 1993 Diabetes, other risk factors, and cardiovascular mortality for men screened in the multiple risk factor intervention trial. Diabetes Care 16: 434–444

Standing J 1997 Chest pain assessment tools. Journal of Clinical Nursing 6: 85–92

Strong JP, Malcom GT, McMahan CA et al 1999 Prevalence and extent of atherosclerosis in adolescents and young adults: implications for the prevention from the pathobiological determinants of atheroscleosis in youth study. Journal of the American Medical Association 281(8): 727–735

Sutton AGC, De Belder MA 1998 Acute myocardial infarction: failed thrombolysis revisited. Hospital Medicine 59: 797–802

Svedlund M, Danielson E, Norberg A 1999 Nurses' narrations about caring for inpatients with acute myocardial infarction. Intensive and Critical Care Nursing 15: 34–43

Swanton RH 1998 Cardiology, 4th edn. Blackwell Science, Oxford

Theroux P, Waters D, Qui S et al 1993 Aspirin versus heparin to prevent myocardial infarction during the acute phase of unstable angina. Circulation 88: 2045–2048

Thompson DR, Sutton TW, Jowett NI, Pohl JEF 1991 Circadian variation in the frequency of onset of chest pain in acute myocardial infarction. British Heart Journal 65: 177–178

Thompson DR, Webster RA, Sutton TW 1994 Coronary care unit patients' and nurses' ratings of intensity of ischaemic chest pain. Intensive and Critical Care Nursing 10: 83–88

Thompson DR, Bowman GS, De Bono DP, Hopkins A 1996 Cardiac rehabilitation in the United Kingdom; guidelines and audit standards. Heart 75: 89–93

Topol EJ 2000 Acute myocardial infarction: thrombolysis. Heart 83(1): 122–126

Topol EJ, Burek K, O'Neill WW 1988 A randomised controlled trial of hospital discharge three days after myocardial infarction in the era of reperfusion. New England Journal of Medicine 318: 1083–1088

Treasure T 1998 Pain is not the only feature of a heart attack. British Medical Journal 317: 602 (letter)

Trent RJ, Rose EL, Adams JN et al 1995 Delay between the onset of symptoms of acute myocardial infarction and seeking medical assistance is influenced by left ventricular function at presentation. British Heart Journal 73: 125–128

Tresch DD 1998 Management of the older patient with acute myocardial infarction: difference in clinical presentations between older and younger patients. Journal of the American Geriatric Society 46(9): 1157–1162

United Kingdom Heart Attack Study Collaborative Group 1998 Effect of time from onset of coming under care on fatality of patients with acute myocardial infarction: effect of resuscitation and thrombolytic therapy. Heart 80: 114–120

Werner D, Schneider M, Weise M, Nonnast-Daniel B, Daniel WG 1999 Pneumatic external counterpulsation: a new noninvasive method to improve organ perfusion. American Journal of Cardiology 84(8): 950–952, A7–A8

Weston CFM, Penny WJ, Julian DG on behalf of the British Heart Foundation Working Group 1994 Guidelines for the early management of patients with myocardial infarction. British Medical Journal 308: 767–771

Whincup PH, Refsum H, Perry IJ et al 1999 Serum total homocysteine and coronary heart disease: prospective study in middle-aged men. Heart 82(4): 448–454

Wiles R 1997 Empowering practice nurses in the follow-up of patients' with established heart disease: lessons from patients experiences. Journal of Advanced Nursing 26: 729–735

Willerson JT, Hillis LD, Winniford MD, Buja M 1986 Speculations regarding mechanisms responsible for acute ischaemic heart disease syndromes. Journal of the American College of Cardiology 8(1): 245–250

Willetts K 1989 Assessing cardiac pain. Nursing Times 85: 52–54

Windecker S, Maier-Rudolph W, Bonzel T et al on behalf of the European Society of Cardiology Working Group on the Coronary Circulation 1999 Interventional cardiology in Europe. European Heart Journal 20: 484–495

Wu AHB, Feng YJ, Contois JH et al 1996 Comparison of myoglobin, creatine kinase-MB, and cardiac troponin I for diagnosis of acute myocardial infarction. Annals of Clinical and Laboratory Science 26: 291–299

Yarzebski J, Goldberg RJ, Gore JM, Alpert JS 1994 Temporal trends and factors associated with extent of delay to hospital arrival in patients with acute myocardial infarction: the Worcester Heart Attack Study. American Heart Journal 128: 255–263

Young GP, Murthi P, Levitt MA, Gawad Y 1999 Serial use of bedside CKMB/myoglobin device to detect acute myocardial infarction in emergency department chest pain patients. Journal of Emergency Medicine 17(5): 769–775

Yusuf S, Pearson M, Sterry H et al 1984 The entry ECG in the early diagnosis and prognostic stratification of patients with suspected acute myocardial infarction. European Heart Journal 5(9): 690–696

Yusuf S, Zucker D, Peduzzi P et al 1994 Effect of coronary artery bypass graft surgery on survival: overview of 10-year results from randomised trials by the Coronary Artery Bypass Graft Surgery Trialists Collaboration. Lancet 344: 563–570

Zijlstra F, Hoorntje JC, De Boer MJ et al 1999 Long-term benefit of primary angioplasty as compared with thrombolytic therapy for acute myocardial infaction. New England Journal of Medicine 341: 1413–1419

FURTHER READING

BARI (Bypass Angioplasty Revascularisation Investigation) Investigators 1996 Comparison of coronary bypass surgery with angioplasty in patients with multivessel disease. New England Journal of Medicine 335: 217–225

British Cardiac Society 1994 A report of a working group of the BCS: cardiology in the district hospital. British Heart Journal 72: 303–308

Ferguson JJ, Taqi K 1999 IIb/IIIa receptor blockade in acute myocardial infarction. American Heart Journal 138(2 pt 2): S164–S170

Flischer D 1995 Fast track: early thrombolysis. British Journal of Nursing 41: 562–565

GISSI-2 1990 A factorial randomised trial of alteplase versus streptokinase and heparin versus no heparin among 12 490 patients with acute myocardial infarction. Lancet 336: 67–71

Gray D, Keating NA, Murdock J, Skene AM, Hampton JR 1993 Impact of hospital thrombolysis policy on out of hospital response to suspected myocardial infarction. Lancet 341: 654–657

GUSTO IIb Angioplasty Substudy Investigators 1997 A clinical trial comparing primary coronary angioplasty with tissue plasminogen activator for acute myocardial infarction. New England Journal of Medicine 336: 1621–1628

Mulcahy D, Knight C, Stables R, Fox K 1994 Lasers, burns, cuts, tingles and pumps. A consideration of alternative treatments for intractable angina. British Heart Journal 71(5): 406–407

Rapaport E 1991 ISIS-3: a critical analysis of the preliminary results. Journal of Myocardial Ischaemia 3: 25–32

Theobald K 1997 The experiences of spouses whose partners have suffered a myocardial infarction. Journal of Advanced Nursing 26: 595–601

Weaver WD 1995 Time to thrombolytic treatment: factors affecting delay and their influence on outcome. Journal of the American College of Cardiology 25 (7 suppl): 3S–9S

Weaver WD, Simes RJ, Betriu A et al 1997 Comparison of primary angioplasty and intravenous thrombolytic therapy for acute myocardial infarction: a quantitative review. Journal of the American Medical Association 278(23): 2093–2098

Wilmshurst P, Purchase A, Webb C, Jowett C, Quinn T 2000 Improving door to needle times with nurse initiated thrombolysis. Heart 84: 262–266

Windecker S, Meier B 2000 Intervention in coronary artery disease. Heart 83(4): 481–490

10

Chronic heart failure

Mary Gould

Chronic heart failure (CHF) is a common and debilitating condition. Mortality from coronary heart disease has declined steadily in the last 20–30 years in Western countries, yet admissions to hospital from heart failure seem to be increasing (Sharpe & Doughty 1998). In part this is due to ageing populations but it is also due to the success of treatments allowing patients with coronary heart disease to survive longer. It is now clear that mortality figures for chronic heart failure are comparable to those of malignant disease and in several cases patients fare much worse. Millane et al (2000) compared survival rates for CHF as a percentage to breast, colon and prostate cancer. At intervals of 1, 2 and 3 years the survival figures fared worse against each cancer, with the exception of those alive at 1 year following a diagnosis of colonic malignancy (Millane et al 2000). In comparing CHF with varying cancers, it should be remembered that in the latter, early detection and treatment can alter the outcome, whereas a diagnosis of chronic heart failure will result in a gradual and debilitating progression.

The incidence of CHF in the United Kingdom (UK) population is 0.3% per annum (McDonagh & Dargie 1998). The incidence is defined as the number of new cases in any given period of time and this is usually in one year. More recent figures highlight an estimated 760 000 people living with CHF and 63 000 new cases appearing each year (BHF 2001). In comparison, within the United States it is estimated that 4.6 million Americans are currently treated for heart failure and that approximately 550 000 new cases are diagnosed each year (American Heart Association 1999). Heart failure remains the only major cardiovascular disease with increasing prevalence, incidence and mortality (Gibbs et al 1998). New treatments may slow but do not arrest progression of the disease, despite the wealth of therapeutic advances. It is important also to recognize that with improved survival from therapies such as coronary artery bypass grafting, angioplasty and other revascularization and medical treatments, the community management of heart failure is likely to increase in importance. This is particularly true with the advance of nurse-led clinics and practice. On the surgical side, research continues into mechanical ventricular assist devices that can be totally contained within the body. These are likely to augment the failing cardiac function, rather than totally replace the heart (see Chapter 18).

This chapter explores the physiology of chronic heart failure, together with current investigations, management and drug therapies. The role of the nurse is explored, particularly through the emergence of heart failure clinics and more recently the recognition of the need for palliative care. Emerging treatments such as mechanical devices offer hope but may be costly, while heart transplantation suffers from a lack of donors. Nursing, therefore, is clearly emerging as an important profession in the management of this disease, defining its role in the monitoring of heart failure, health promotion strategies, the manipulation of medication and psychological support. Within this chapter the term 'heart failure' will refer to the chronic nature of the disease, as opposed to an initial, acute manifestation.

DEFINITION

Heart failure has been defined in general terms as the inability of the heart to deliver adequate oxygenated blood to the peripheral tissues to meet their metabolic demand. More specifically, it can be described as a clinical syndrome caused by an abnormality of the heart, for example a poorly contracting myocardium, and is characterized by a pattern of haemodynamic, renal, neural and hormonal responses. Common presenting features will include anxiety, tachycardia and dyspnoea. Pallor and hypotension occur in the more severe cases (Millane et al 2000).

In the late 1940s the Framingham Heart Study enrolled more than 5000 people who at the time were free of heart disease. The prevalence, incidence and prognosis of heart failure during four decades of observation have contributed greatly to the understanding of the epidemiology of this condition. The study remains ongoing. The prevalence refers to the number of existing cases of a disease at a particular point in time. It is determined both by factors that affect the occurrence of disease (incidence: I) and those that affect survival. For example, as mortality from coronary heart disease decreases and fewer people suffer premature death, the prevalence of heart failure increases. Measures of prevalence are useful in assessing the need for health care and the planning of health services.

The prevalence rate (P) is often expressed as cases per thousand or per hundred of the population and is calculated as follows:

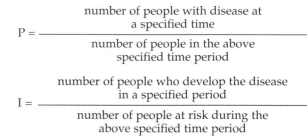

$$P = \frac{\text{number of people with disease at a specified time}}{\text{number of people in the above specified time period}}$$

$$I = \frac{\text{number of people who develop the disease in a specified period}}{\text{number of people at risk during the above specified time period}}$$

The aforementioned Framingham study in the United States revealed that the incidence of heart failure increased dramatically with advancing age and was higher in men than in women (Fig. 10.1). This was notably because of the lower incidence of coronary artery disease, the major cause of heart failure in individuals, in premenopausal women. In 1970, there were 250 000 new cases of heart failure diagnosed in the US (Abraham & Bristow 1997). In 1992, 700 000 new cases were diagnosed (O'Connell & Bristow 1994). The incidence of heart failure varies in the US from 2/1000 per year in people aged 45–54 to 30/1000 per year in people aged 85 and upwards.

Due to the varying methods of ascertainment, epidemiological data can vary widely and some cannot be compared. They do provide, however, a perspective of the size of the problem and are consistent in some respects. The prevalence of heart failure in Britain is estimated to be approximately 1.5% of the total population (Sharpe & Doughty 1998) and approximately 10% in people over 75 years (Cowie et al 1997). With patients surviving for a greater number of years following

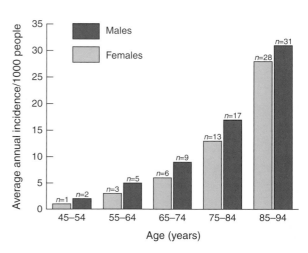

Figure 10.1 The average annual incidence of new cases of heart failure per 1000 population in the Framingham Heart Study. (Reproduced with permission from Sharpe & Doughty 1998.)

myocardial infarction and the use of thrombolysis, there are simply more patients who survive to develop heart failure at an older age. On a population level, increased survival translates to *more, not less* heart failure consultations and a greater health-care burden. Hospital admissions because of heart failure seem to have increased in the past decade (Eriksson 1995, Lenfant 1994, McMurray et al 1993). Although it is difficult to gain up-to-date figures, discharged patients with heart failure as the primary diagnosis increased by almost 60% in Scotland between 1980 and 1990 (McMurray et al 1993).

Mortality statistics do differ between countries, because different coding practices exist. In the UK in particular, where heart failure cannot be recorded on death certificates as a primary cause of death, mortality data can be of limited value. Often junior house officers are the first to be called to sign a death certificate and may not have received adequate training from senior colleagues on how to fill in these important documents precisely. Generally mortality from heart failure ranges from between 3–20 individuals per thousand, increasing to 80–160 individuals per 1000 amongst those aged 75 or over (Cowie et al 1997). These data demonstrate the pronounced impact of age on the occurrence of the disease (see Fig. 10.1).

There are some limitations in the Framingham study, especially in a study population which may not be representative of the general population as a whole. The research only tends to consist of white middle-class people, of both genders, eliminating vital data on ethnic minorities who, as this book highlights, do experience cardiovascular symptoms and severity to differing degrees.

Once heart failure is clinically diagnosed it has a high mortality rate. In the Framingham study, 37% of males and 38% of females died within 2 years of a diagnosis. These mortality rates are 4–8 times those of the general population of the same age (Kannel et al 1988, Kannel & Belanger 1991). The median survival time after the diagnosis of heart failure was 1.7 years for men and 3.2 years for women. For men the 1, 2, 5 and 10-year survival rates were 57%, 46%, 25% and 11% respectively. For women, corresponding survival rates were improved at 64%, 56%, 38% and 21%. Even following adjustment for age, survival rates were better in women. Mortality increased with advancing age in both sexes during the 40 years of follow-up of the study population and surprisingly there was no significant improvement in prognosis over that period of time. This is in sharp contrast to the considerable improvement in the prognosis of patients with coronary heart disease (Ho et al 1993a). Heart failure remains associated with a shorter life expectancy than many common types of cancer (Ho et al 1993b).

Aetiology

Heart failure is a clinical syndrome, that has a characteristic group of signs and symptoms. Any disorder that places the heart under a chronically increased volume or pressure load or which produces primary damage to the myocardium may result in heart failure. This will then comprise a constellation of signs and symptoms including fluid retention, exercise intolerance and the classic symptoms of dyspnoea and fatigue. These are all attributable to cardiac dysfunction.

Disease of the myocardium resulting in heart failure has many causes, the most common of which is atheromatous coronary artery disease and dilated cardiomyopathy. The latter, which is discussed in Chapter 11, implies an enlarged heart and reduced contractile function in the presence of normal coronary arteries. It is usually idiopathic but can be familial and linked to environmental, autoimmune or alcoholic causes (see Box 10.1).

Systolic dysfunction of the left ventricle is the most common and most important cause of heart failure in

---

Box 10.1 Some of the varied causes of heart failure

Coronary artery disease
Myocardial infarction
Ischaemia
Hypertension
Aneurysm

Cardiomyopathies
Dilated:
    Idiopathic
Environmental:
    Poisons, organophosphates
Genetic:
    Inherited
    Alcoholic
    Myocarditis

Hypertrophic
Genetic and familial

Restrictive
Amyloid
Endomyocardial fibrosis

Drugs
β-blockers
Anti-arrhythmics
Alcohol

Arrhythmias
Tachyarrhythmias
Atrial fibrillation
Bradycardias
Supraventricular (narrow complex) tachycardia (SVT)
Complete heart block

Western societies. This means a progressive decrease in myocardial contractility. It usually arises as a result of ischaemic heart disease and accounts for 70% of all cases. The incidence of heart failure as a consequence of hypertension has fallen due to improved detection and treatment, although it remains an important contributory factor to the progression of heart failure and a risk factor to the development of atherosclerosis. As Swanton (1998) highlights, by far the most common causes of heart failure in the Western world are coronary disease and hypertension.

Ischaemic heart disease appears capable of precipitating chronic heart failure by a variety of mechanisms. An infarct may impair the contractile performance of a large enough area of the left ventricle to reduce effective pump action. A generalized hypokinesis (reduced movement) of the entire left ventricle, even in areas served by relatively normal coronary arteries, can occur.

Valvular heart disease is a less frequent cause because of the successful results of valve replacement surgery in selected patients. Untreated, valve disease can lead to left and/or right ventricular hypertrophy and can eventually cause ventricular failure by an increased afterload (the resistance to ventricular ejection), such as with aortic stenosis.

Diastolic dysfunction, in which relaxation of the left ventricle is impaired, may account for up to 40% of all chronic heart failure (Mosterd et al 1999, Vasan et al 1999). This is common in the elderly where the increase in cardiac output during exercise is more dependent on the Starling mechanism than an increase in heart rate (which reduces the duration of diastole). In patients with diastolic heart failure, the stroke volume (the amount of blood ejected in each heart beat) would be greater if filling during diastole were more complete.

Heart failure can also result from systemic disease. Thyrotoxicosis, anaemia, pregnancy, beri-beri and Gram-negative septicaemia can all place excessive metabolic demands on the heart.

In summary, whatever the cause of the cardiac disease, the deterioration of ventricular function is the initial mechanism leading to heart failure.

PHYSIOLOGY

Chronic heart failure is the long-term consequence of a damaged heart, resulting in a spectrum of pathophysiological states. These can vary from those caused by a rapid impairment of pump function to the progressive and gradual impairment observed in a patient whose heart is subjected to an increased afterload or volume overload for a prolonged period. The term 'chronic' implies the persistent nature of the condition. Heart failure that carries this prefix is characterized by a punctuated course of acute exacerbations requiring hospital admission. Chronic heart failure can therefore be regarded as **compensated**, when symptoms are stable, or **decompensated**. Decompensated heart failure refers to a deterioration, which presents either as an acute episode of pulmonary oedema or as lethargy and malaise, a reduction in exercise tolerance and increasing breathlessness on exertion (Millane et al 2000). These episodes of decompensated heart failure occur as anatomical abnormalities gradually developing over time, such as myocardial remodelling.

In addition, a number of adaptive (compensatory) mechanisms will develop, allowing the patient to survive but with a continually depressed cardiac function. These include the stimulation of the renin–angiotensin–aldosterone mechanism and cardiac hypertrophy.

Cardiac performance is determined by the following factors (Fig. 10.2).

Preload (venous return)

The preload refers to the end-diastolic volume or the amount of blood left in the ventricles at the end of filling. In heart failure sodium and hence water retention, through the renin-angiotensin aldosterone mechanism, increase the preload. This will initially aid cardiac output by stretching the myocardium. This is the basis of Starling's Law of the heart. This physical law is linked to the preload and states that the more a myocardial fibre is stretched prior to its release, the greater the force of contraction. It is the 'law of elastic'. Stretching cardiac muscle fibres also increases the sensitivity of the myofilaments to calcium, which further augments force development. However, a heart will reach a point of

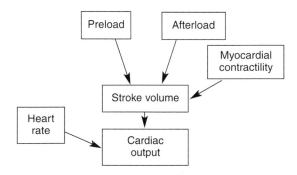

Figure 10.2 Determinants of the cardiac output.

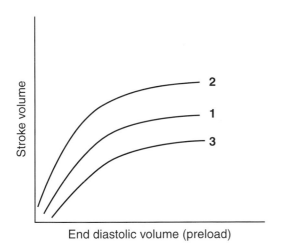

1. The relationship between stroke volume (cardiac output) and the preload in a normal ventricle. Note how there is an initial brisk response to an increasing preload, then to a lesser degree as the curve flattens.

2. The curve moves upwards and to the left with increased ventricular contraction. The stroke volume is higher for any given preload.

3. In the patient with heart failure, contractility is reduced and the stroke volume is lower for any given preload.

Figure 10.3 The ventricular function curve.

stretch where too much fluid accumulating through failure, or by intravenous infusion, will rapidly induce deterioration of function. Starling's Law is not linear. More and more fluid and myocardial stretch does not equate to a continually higher cardiac output. Those in heart failure reach this limit at an early stage.

This relationship is illustrated graphically by the Starling curve (Fig. 10.3), also known as the ventricular function curve. In heart failure, the ventricular function curve is displaced downwards and large increases in filling pressure are required to increase ventricular performance.

Afterload

This is the resistance against which the myocardium must contract. This is primarily determined by aortic impedence and systemic vascular resistance (SVR). An increase in the afterload will decrease the cardiac output. This decrease in function with further increase in end-diastolic volume and dilatation of the ventricle itself further exacerbates the problem of afterload. This

is expressed in Laplace's Law (Camm 1993) which states that the tension of the myocardium (T) is proportional to the interventricular pressure (P) multiplied by the radius (r) of the ventricular chamber; that is $T \propto$ (proportional) Pr.

The afterload generally applies to the left ventricle as only the lungs, which are valveless and offer little resistance, lie in front of the right chamber. The arterial and vasoconstriction occurring in heart failure to aid tissue perfusion add resistance to the ejecting left ventricle, augmenting the failure. This is primarily by increasing the oxygen demand of the myocardium, which is attempting to overcome the afterload.

Contractility

This refers to the quality of the myocardium and its influence on performance, independent of changes in the preload or afterload. Contractility is impaired in heart failure. Increased contractility (**positive inotropism**) can result from increased sympathetic drive. This occurs with the release of catecholamines such as adrenaline and noradrenaline, which stimulate the heart through the β-adrenergic receptors. Conversely, myocardial depressants such as hypoxia decrease myocardial contractility (**negative inotropism**).

In a normal individual, the cardiac output is matched to the body's total metabolic need. Cardiac output (CO) is equal to the product of stroke volume (SV) – the volume of blood ejected with each contraction – times the heart rate (HR).

$$CO = SV \times HR$$

The time allowed for diastolic filling must be sufficient, otherwise cardiac output will fall. The increase in heart rate is an important factor in maintaining cardiac output, but with the concomitant rise in afterload occurring in heart failure there is an increase in the myocardial oxygen requirement. This may enhance heart failure and delivery of blood to the tissues becomes insufficient and blood pressure falls. Secondly, cardiac filling pressures such as the central venous pressure (CVP) rise as the heart fails to contract and empty adequately. These basic haemodynamic changes set in motion pathophysiological (compensatory) responses to heart failure.

THE ADAPTIVE (COMPENSATORY) MECHANISMS IN CHRONIC HEART FAILURE

As the process of heart failure evolves, complex compensatory mechanisms develop. These affect not only the heart but also the peripheral circulation, the skeletal muscle and the kidneys. Neurohormonal activation in CHF results in sodium and water retention, through the renin-angiotensin–aldosterone mechanism. This increases the blood volume and pressure, as well as stretching the myocardium to increase the cardiac output (Starling's Law). These physiological changes are compensatory and aim to maintain cardiac output, blood pressure and peripheral perfusion. However, as heart failure progresses, these mechanisms are overwhelmed and represent cardiac decompensation and worsening heart failure. The renin–angiotensin–aldosterone mechanism is discussed in the section exploring renal control in Chapter 4.

In CHF one of the most important changes is that of ventricular hypertrophy. When the ventricle experiences a chronic increase in afterload, such as that imposed by arterial hypertension, aortic stenosis or pulmonary hypertension, the myocardium hypertrophies. This means it will increase in weight as a result of an enlargement of individual muscle fibres. There is also an increase in the volume of myocytes but without an increase in cell number. Collagen synthesis may also be increased. These structural changes are known as **myocardial remodelling**. Remodelling is the term used to describe molecular changes within the heart as a result of failure. It essentially involves hypertrophy of the ventricular myocyte leading to large, genetically abnormal myocardial cells that cannot contract as efficiently as normal cells. In addition, changes also occur in the interstitium, with fibrotic infiltration leading to a stiffened and less compliant myocardial wall (Albert 1999).

This results in systolic and diastolic dysfunction and impaired coronary blood flow. The degree of hypertrophy that develops can vary substantially between patients. Ventricular dilatation and remodelling start soon after the initial myocardial event. The process is progressive and does not cause symptoms for several years. The exact mechanism is unknown, but increased myocardial wall tension and activation of the renin–angiotensin–aldosterone system are potential mechanisms (McKelvie et al 1998, 1999).

Hypertrophy may be regarded as a normal compensatory mechanism which permits the heart to cope with the increased demands of heart failure. However, it does become self-defeating when it is excessive. In addition, the thickening of the fibres increases the distance by which oxygen has to diffuse from the capillaries. In response to volume overload

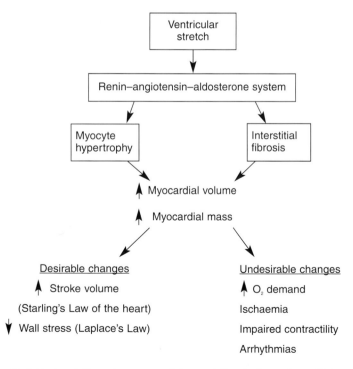

Figure 10.4 Factors influencing myocardial remodelling in the patient with heart failure.

from the hypertrophied and failed heart, dilatation occurs, increasing the ventricular blood volume. Dilatation is a normal and efficient response. However, pathological dilatation occurs when there is a myocardial disease causing decreased contractility. The ventricle must therefore be stretched to a greater extent and to a greater given volume to maintain the cardiac output.

Atrial natriuretic peptide (ANP)

ANP is released from atrial myocytes in response to stretch. Its release is proportional to the severity of heart failure, which will have increased the volume of blood in the chambers. Levels of circulating ANP are therefore elevated in heart failure and correlate with functional class prognosis and haemodynamic state. Its release has been shown to inhibit renin, aldosterone and antidiuretic hormone (ADH) secretion and results in excretion of sodium and water. ANP is counter-regulatory; its actions are largely opposite to other hormone systems activated in heart failure.

The renin–angiotensin–aldosterone system is also activated in patients with heart failure. Both the fall in cardiac output and the increase in sympathetic tone reduce an effective blood flow to the kidneys. Renin secretion subsequently occurs from the juxtaglomeru-lar cells. Renin stimulates circulating angiotensinogen to form angiotensin I. This is rapidly altered by angiotensin-converting enzyme (ACE) to form angio-tensin II, a potent vasoconstrictor. The increased levels of angiotensin II thereby assist in maintaining sys-temic blood pressure.

In addition, angiotensin II acts to increase intravas-cular volume by two mechanisms:

- stimulation of the hypothalamus, increasing thirst and therefore water intake
- an increase of aldosterone secretion from the adrenal cortex.

The latter hormone promotes sodium reabsorption from the distal convoluted tubule of the kidney into the circulation. Water follows sodium and the rise in intravascular volume increases the left ventricular preload and hence the cardiac output.

Antidiuretic hormone (ADH)

Secretion of this hormone by the posterior pituitary gland is also increased in heart failure. This is presum-ably mediated through stimulation and stretch of left atrial and arterial baroreceptors and by increased levels of angiotensin II. ADH contributes to increased intravascular volume because it promotes water reten-tion in the distal nephron. This increased intravascular volume serves to augment left ventricular preload and hence the cardiac output. Although neurohormonal activation is initially beneficial, it ultimately proves harmful. The increased circulating volume and aug-mented venous return to the heart may worsen the engorgement of the lung vasculature, exacerbating congestive pulmonary symptoms. The elevated sys-temic vascular resistance increases the afterload against which the failing left ventricle contracts and may further impair stroke volume and reduce the cardiac output.

An elevated heart rate increases metabolic demand and can therefore reduce the performance of the failing heart. Other potent vasoconstrictors such as endothelin may also contribute to the intense increase in peripheral vascular resistance.

CLASSIFICATION, SIGNS AND SYMPTOMS

Chronic heart failure (CHF) describes the long-term consequences of the damaged heart. This is evident when the patient becomes symptomatic and experi-ences exercise limitation, dyspnoea and fatigue due to a low ventricular ejection fraction and increasing diastolic volume. The signs and symptoms that characterize heart failure can be considered in the context of failure of the left or right ventricle as a pump.

The most prominent symptom of chronic left ventricular failure is dyspnoea on exertion and is largely the consequence of pulmonary congestion. If the pulmonary venous congestion exceeds 20 mmHg, there is a movement of fluid into the pulmonary inter-stitium and consequent congestion of lung tissue. The resulting reduction in pulmonary compliance contributes to an increase in the work of breathing as the patient needs to generate a greater negative intrathoracic pressure in order to move the same volume of air. The excess fluid in the interstitium compresses the walls of the bronchioles and alveoli, increasing the resistance to air flow and further adding to the effort of respiration.

In addition, an increasing lung volume (of blood) stimulates capillary receptors that mediate rapid shallow breathing. However, the patient in heart failure can suffer dyspnoea even in the absence of pulmonary congestion because reduced forward blood flow to the overworked respiratory muscles and an accumulation of lactic acid may also contribute to the breathless sensation.

Other symptoms include orthopnoea and paroxysmal nocturnal dyspnoea (PND). Orthopnoea is the sensation of laboured breathing while lying flat and is relieved by sitting upright. It results from the redistribution of intravascular blood from the gravity-dependent portions of the body (abdomen) towards the lungs after lying down. The degree of orthopnoea is generally assessed by the number of pillows on which the patient sleeps to avoid breathlessness. Sometimes it may be so marked that the patient may try to sleep upright in a chair and this they should be allowed to do if it aids comfort. PND is severe breathlessness that awakens the patient from sleep. This results from gradual reabsorption into the circulation of interstitial oedema after lying down. There is a subsequent expansion of intravascular volume and increased venous return to the heart and lungs. The failed heart and congested lungs subsequently cannot cope with this increased fluid volume. On sitting upright or standing, the sensation usually subsides.

The symptoms of heart failure comprise:

- breathlessness – initially on exertion but later at rest or manifesting as orthopnoea and PND
- fatigue
- ankle swelling – oedema.

The symptoms are often grouped by severity to produce a functional classification. The most common classification is the New York Heart Association (NYHA) category. This classification refers to exercise limitation and symptoms are seen as mild, moderate and severe, but it does not relate to prognosis.

The physical/clinical signs of heart failure include:

- tachycardia
- raised jugular venous pressure – right-sided heart failure
- pulmonary crepitations
- third heart sound
- peripheral oedema.

As with the symptoms, these signs are non-specific and further investigations are needed to establish cardiac dysfunction. The physical signs depend on severity and chronicity of the condition and can be linked and divided into right and left cardiac failure. Individuals with mild impairment may appear well, in contrast to a patient with chronic severe heart failure who may demonstrate cachexia (a frail and wasted appearance due to poor appetite and to the increased metabolic demands from the increased effort of breathing). Symptoms are often a poor guide to the true disability, as they tend to rely on the patient's own subjective assessment.

Box 10.2 New York Heart Association (NYHA) classification of heart failure

I No limitation. Ordinary physical activity does not cause undue fatigue, dyspnoea or palpitation

II Slight limitation of physical activity. Such patients are comfortable at rest. Ordinary physical activity results in fatigue, palpitation, dyspnoea or angina. However, patients can continue with everyday activities

III Marked limitation of physical activity. Although patients are comfortable at rest, less than ordinary activity will lead to symptoms, thus interfering with everyday activities such as work.

IV Inability to perform physical activity without discomfort. Symptoms such as breathlessness are present at rest. With any physical activity, increased discomfort is experienced. Unable to work.

Such interpretation can confuse the clinician or nurse, because some patients pace themselves gradually, restricting their activities to avoid symptoms. It is therefore preferable to assess tolerance and to enquire about well-defined activities, for example walking 100 feet on level ground or climbing two flights of stairs. This can be assessed easily at a clinic visit by the 6-minute walk test, which measures the distance walked over 6 minutes and uses an exertion scale for assessment immediately after the walk – the Borg Assessment (Borg 1982).

Fatigue and weakness are common but less specific features of cardiac failure and are difficult to evaluate. Possible causes of fatigue are those associated with other symptoms. Anorexia, muscle abnormalities, cardiac cachexia and depression can all influence a person's well-being and energy levels. The nutrition of patients with cardiac failure is often good in the early stages but cachexia occurs as disability increases. Loss of lean body mass is common with CHF. The weight loss may be reflected directly in the total body weight and the body mass index but may of course be distorted by fluid accumulation. If more than 10% of the lean body mass is lost this is defined as cachexia (Freeman & Roubenoff 1994). Inadequate nutrient intake but increased requirements, together with altered body metabolism, are all factors contributing to cachexia.

Oedema tends to vary in severity. It may be mild ankle to pitting oedema, affecting sacral and, in men, scrotal areas. This results in a reduction of mobility. The skin is tight and fragile, prone to injury and can result in abrasions that heal slowly due to poor tissue perfusion. Consequently, skin care must become a priority for the patient and those involved in their care. In right-sided failure, congestion of the systemic veins causes hepatomegaly and gastro-intestinal engorgement. This may again lead to anorexia, a bloated feeling and a tendency to constipation. All these factors affect a person's everyday life and interfere with personal enjoyment, consequently aggravating depression and helplessness. Ascites, an abnormal accumulation of fluid in the peritoneal cavity, may also occur in patients with severe right heart failure.

It is important to note that in the early stages of heart failure, one ventricle is usually affected more than the other. Clinical presentation will be influenced by the increase in cardiac volume and pressures behind the failed ventricle. Therefore, in left-sided failure, where the left ventricle is weakened or overloaded, pulmonary congestion will induce symptoms such as dyspnoea or orthopnoea. In right-sided failure, peripheral oedema, congestive hepatomegaly and systemic venous distension will be seen (Albert 1999).

INVESTIGATIONS FOR CHRONIC HEART FAILURE

In reality heart failure is a difficult condition to diagnose and many patients thought by general practitioners (GPs) to have heart failure may not have any demonstrable abnormality of cardiac function on objective testing (Hobbs et al 2000). A UK study showed that only 29% of 122 patients referred to a rapid access clinic with a new diagnosis of heart failure fully met the definition of heart failure by the European Society of Cardiology (Hobbs et al 2000). This may lead to community practices wanting access to echocardiography services, although issues such as the need for GPs to fully understand technical reports have to be considered (Hobbs et al 2000).

A clinical diagnosis of heart failure should always be confirmed by utilizing objective measures of left ventricular structure and function. Similarly, the underlying cause should be established in all patients. This is described as imperative by Millane et al (2000), because timely intervention may greatly improve the prognosis in selected cases, for example in those with severe aortic stenosis. The most important way to establish a diagnosis is to take a full detailed medical history and undertake a thorough medical examination, before treatment is commenced.

Chest X-ray

Depending on the cause of heart failure the chest X-ray may show cardiomegaly, defined as a cardiothoracic ratio of greater than 0.5 on the postero-anterior film. The transverse diameter of the heart is approximately 15.5 cm in a man and 14.5 cm in a woman. This ratio is used sometimes as a guide to chart improvement or deterioration of heart failure, because it measures the size of the heart relative to the thoracic cavity.

The 12-lead electrocardiogram (ECG)

This is useful in establishing ischaemia/infarction, left ventricular hypertrophy, left bundle branch block, arrhythmias such as atrial fibrillation and T-wave inversion or pathological Q-waves (see Chapters 6 and 9). If arrhythmias are suspected, the patient can then be referred for Holter monitoring or 24-hour ambulatory ECG as appropriate. An ambulatory ECG will give an indication of abnormality in everyday normal activity.

Echocardiogram

This is probably the single most useful investigation and should be used routinely for optimal diagnosis of heart failure (Cleland et al 1995, European Society of Cardiology 1997). Two-dimensional and Doppler echocardiography establishes the presence of systolic and/or diastolic impairment of the left or right ventricle. It may also reveal the aetiology, such as valve disease, cardiomyopathy, intracardiac thrombus and embolism. An ejection fraction of <45% is generally accepted as evidence of systolic dysfunction. This rapid non-invasive technique allows an accurate assessment and can be used to follow the progress of the disease. Serial measurements that show any fluctuations could depend on the operator. Therefore, if possible, the same technician should be used to eradicate operator error.

Radionuclide studies

These can be used to measure ejection fraction. Multigated acquisition (MUGA) scans are used in assessing left ventricular cavity size and wall motion abnormalities and particularly in measuring left ventricular ejection fraction. However, this information is often obtained from simple echocardiography.

Laboratory blood tests

Analysis of blood can identify underlying causes of heart failure. A full blood count to exclude anaemia and the measurement of electrolytes, particularly the serum potassium and sodium, together with measures of renal function such as urea and creatinine are useful. Electrolyte imbalance can be detected which may require correction to prevent arrhythmias such as ventricular tachycardia or fibrillation. Thyroid function abnormalities to detect thyrotoxicosis are not always easy to discern clinically. Measurement of indicators of possible ethanol ingestion such as plasma γ-glutamyl transferase activity (γ-GT) are useful in patients where the aetiology of heart failure is thought to be alcohol induced. Coronary angiography to assess coronary artery anatomy is useful when assessing the cause of heart failure.

Cardiopulmonary exercise testing

This allows a measure of the severity of the heart failure. Assessing exercise performance is one of the best ways of differentiating the grades of chronic heart failure and is a good indicator of prognosis. The single best measure is the maximal rate of oxygen uptake (VO$_2$ max) achieved during progressive exercise testing to exhaustion. This test is performed in conjunction with an ECG, haemodynamic monitoring, such as blood

pressure recording, and respiratory gas exchange measurement. The latter is via a mouthpiece, with nose clip.

Exercising testing also has the advantage of potentially differentiating between the causes of exercise-limiting symptoms. A VO$_2$ max less than 12 ml/kg/min is taken as an indicator for cardiac transplantation. Patients with a VO$_2$ max greater than 16 ml/kg/min are considered too well for transplantation. The exercise itself is performed either on a treadmill or a bicycle. The protocols vary, but it is usual that the speed and intensity will increase every 2–3 minutes. On the treadmill the patient is instructed to signal when he or she needs to stop. On the bicycle there comes a point where the patient can no longer pedal. Sometimes the patient stops exercising before reaching his or her maximal cardiopulmonary reserve, perhaps because of the development of unpleasant symptoms, such as angina, leg tiredness, breathlessness or fatigue. Submaximal endurance testing may help to assess the symptoms and quality of life of patients with mild to moderate cardiac disease.

In summary, the heart adjusts to increased demands from exercise and temporary illness by increasing its contractility and heart rate. This ability is known as the **cardiac reserve**. When this diminishes, signs and symptoms of heart failure become apparent. When cardiac reserve is exhausted, the heart compensates via:

- tachycardia
- ventricular dilatation
- ventricular hypertrophy.

When these mechanisms satisfy the metabolic demands of the body, the patient remains asymptomatic and the heart is said to be in a state of compensation. In time, the compensatory mechanisms begin to deteriorate. The cardiac muscle fibres increase in diameter and the ventricular wall thickens in an effort to provide increased contractility to move the blood against increased resistance. As the muscle thickens and becomes stronger, its demand for oxygen becomes greater. The cardiac decompensation occurs when the heart can no longer cope with the demands placed upon it. Decreased exercise tolerance is usually the first sign of decompensation.

Electrolyte imbalances in heart failure reflect complications of failure as well as the use of therapies such as diuretics. Disturbances in sodium, potassium and magnesium are particularly significant. In patients with severe heart failure an increase in total body water is reflected by a decrease in the serum sodium. Diuretics may also contribute by a real lowering of overall serum sodium if fluid intake is not restricted.

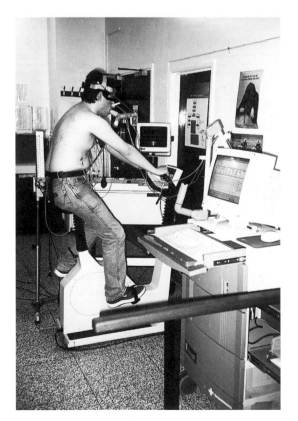

Figure 10.5 A patient undergoing a metabolic exercise test on a bicycle.

Hypokalaemia or low serum potassium and low magnesium levels may complicate heart failure as a result of the use of diuretics such as thiazides and furosemide (frusemide). These diuretics, through their mode of action, lead to excessive excretion of potassium and magnesium. Hyperkalaemia is an elevated serum potassium level and may occur secondary to depressed renal blood flow, leading to a lower glomerular filtration rate.

The prognosis of heart failure is dismal and a fatal condition with a mortality that exceeds many malignancies. In the Framingham Study, the probability of dying within 5 years of the onset of heart failure was 62% for men and 48% for women (Ho et al 1993a). One study examined for 47 months the long-term prognosis of 153 consecutive patients who presented to an Accident and Emergency (A&E) department with decompensated heart failure (Brophy et al 1994). Survival was poor, with 61% dying within the 47-month follow-up. The greatest mortality is due to refractory heart failure, but a large number of patients die suddenly, presumably due to ventricular arrhythmias. However, several studies have demonstrated that survival may be prolonged in heart failure patients with the advent of specific vasodilator drug regimens.

MEDICAL AND NURSING MANAGEMENT OF CHRONIC HEART FAILURE

Chronic heart failure requires lifelong treatment and clear co-ordination between medical, nursing and other health-care disciplines. This will mean communication, often at team meetings when the patient is hospitalized, through to clinical management meetings for community practices. Nurse-led heart failure clinics are now emerging to monitor patient progress, the response to treatment and to empower through education, thus enhancing treatment compliance. The management of heart failure itself has improved in the past two decades due to a better understanding of the pathophysiology of the condition, new diagnostic techniques, the availability of drugs such as ACE inhibitors and β-blockers and also transplantation (see Box 10.3).

Guidelines developed by the European Society of Cardiology Working Group on heart failure have helped clarify standards by which to judge the efficacy of treatments new and old (Cleland et al 1995, European Society of Cardiology 1997). Treatments must achieve one or more goals preferably without the risk of significant adverse events. The goals encompass both prevention of the development of heart failure and treatment once heart failure is present. These goals include the need to:

Box 10.3 Treatments available in heart failure

General measures which include health promotion advice and support
Smoking cessation
Reducing alcoholic intake
Dietary change, e.g. reduced salt and fat intake
Monitor fluid intake
Exercise plan
Daily weight to assess treatment effectiveness

Pharmacological options
Diuretic therapy – loop, thiazides, potassium sparing, combinations
Spironolactone
ACE inhibitors
Digoxin
Vasodilators – nitrates, hydralazine
β-blockers
Anticoagulants and/or aspirin
Anti-arrhythmics
Statins (lipid-lowering drugs)
Angiotensin II receptor inhibitors, e.g. losartan, valsartan
Positive inotropic agents (rarely used)

Surgery and invasive options
Intra-aortic balloon pump
Valve replacement/repair
Revascularization, e.g. coronary artery bypass surgery (CABG)
Implantable cardioverter defibrillator (ICD), pacemaker
Removal of ventricular aneurysm
Ventricular assist device (VAD)
Cardiomyoplasty
Cardiac transplantation
Ventricular volume reduction

General options
Counselling/education regarding symptoms, disease progress and the importance of compliance
Vaccination (such as for flu)

- improve or maintain quality of life by improvement of symptoms or prevention of them worsening
- avoid the side-effects/adverse events from treatment
- decrease the occurrence of major morbid events
- delay death.

General measures

Treatment of chronic heart failure is multifactorial and should include patient and family education, attention to dietary issues, in particular fluid and salt restriction and daily weight. Exercise training as well as optimal pharmacological management are also important issues. In episodes of decompensation, where despite treatment the patient is experiencing congestive heart failure with the associated pulmonary oedema, lethargy and malaise, skilled nursing care can work alongside the medical management to relieve symptoms. It is vitally important to reassure both patient and family or carers. It is inevitably frightening when the patient cannot catch their breath and a lack of reassurance and calmness from those around can increase fear.

Short-term bedrest is indicated to reduce metabolic demands in decompensated CHF. This will also potentiate the action of diuretics through improved renal perfusion (Millane et al 2000). Sitting the patient upright in bed and administering a high concentration of oxygen via a facemask will aid more effective breathing, providing enhanced tissue perfusion. Arterial blood gas analysis will be performed to assess the levels of oxygen and any acid base abnormalities (see Chapter 7). Humidified oxygen, notably if the patient is mouth breathing, will help reduce the drying of mucous membranes. The risks of immobility must be considered by the nursing team and low-dose subcutaneous heparin may be indicated. An infusion of an anticoagulant is not generally required. Care of the skin, particularly as peripheral oedema is likely, must be initiated and the importance of turning and relieving pressure must be explained to the patient.

Eating and drinking will be difficult and the patient may feel nauseous from oedema of the gut. Small, palatable and easily chewed meals are indicated or nutritional drinks if the former proves too much. Asking carers to bring in favourite foods is always useful practice, together with support from the dietetic team. Fluid restriction, usually to 1–1.5 litres in 24 hours, is usually implemented (Millane et al 2000). This requires careful explanation to the patient and family/carers. The patient may feel thirsty through the use of diuretics and there is a need to share out the fluid allowance to relieve thirst but to allow enough to drink throughout the 24-hour period. Graduated measuring jugs are of value in this situation. Limiting the use of salt added at table may also be of help. Salt attracts water and increases the intravascular volume.

At this stage a urinary catheter may be indicated. This will allow the accurate monitoring of the patient's fluid balance. This is primarily to assess the effectiveness of diuretic therapy, which should move the patient into a negative fluid balance. Daily weighing of the patient is vitally important, taken at the same time each day, usually before breakfast. The weight chart is a valuable method to assess the effectiveness of diuretic and other medical treatment. The fluid chart is important but it just indicates how much fluid has passed in and out. There is also the possibility that drinks become missed. The weight chart therefore provides a highly useful additional assessment.

Pharmacology

Chapter 19 provides detail regarding the drugs outlined below, but an overview of pharmacological management is presented. Management of heart failure relies on the following categories of drugs: diuretics, ACE inhibitors, β-blockers, calcium channel blockers, digoxin and anti-arrhythmics.

Diuretics

The diuretics remain the mainstay of management of oedema in heart failure. Their function is:

- to increase the activation of the sympathetic and renin–angiotensin systems
- to relieve breathlessness and oedema when overt fluid overload is present
- to promote the renal excretion of salt and water, by blocking the tubular reabsorption of sodium and chloride.

The resulting fluid loss:

- reduces the ventricular filling pressures (preload)
- produces consistent haemodynamic and symptomatic benefits in patients with heart failure
- rapidly relieves dyspnoea and peripherial oedema.

Loop diuretics. The loop diuretics such as furosemide (frusemide) induce transient venodilatation, relieving the symptoms of pulmonary oedema even before the onset of diuresis (Millane et al 2000). Furosemide (frusemide) and bumetanide act by reducing sodium and chloride reabsorption in the ascending limb of the loop of Henle. They cause a brisk and generally short-lived diuresis as the urinary concentrating power of the kidney is reduced. These agents also produce potassium loss and promote hyperuricaemia (high uric acid in the blood). Initially daily oral furosemide (frusemide) 40 mg or bumetanide 1 mg may be sufficient to control peripheral and pulmonary oedema. Some patients may require higher doses such as 80–120 mg furosemide (frusemide). More recently, attention has focused upon the varying inter- and intra-individual variability in absorption of differing loop diuretics as a possible link to cardiac decompensation (Brater 2000). This remains an area of research interest.

Thiazide diuretics. The thiazide diuretics, such as bendroflumethiaside (bendrofluazide), are mild in effect and act on the distal convoluted tubule, reducing sodium reabsorption. Potassium secretion is still enhanced, however, and the drugs are normally used to control mild heart failure in those with no renal impairment. The dose of bendroflumethiaside (bendrofluazide) is initially 5–10 mg orally in the morning and then 1–3 times a week.

Metolazone is a powerful thiazide derivative producing profound diuresis. Acting synergistically with loop diuretics, it is used in patients with persistent oedema often as a once-only dose and should be used with caution at the commencement of treatment. As little as 2.5 or 5.0 mg of metolazone, when administered in combination with a loop diuretic, can lead to several litres of additional urine output. This combination can be stronger than intravenous administration of furosemide (frusemide) and should be reserved for hospital use initially. Profound electrolyte disturbance can accompany this diuresis. A small selected number of outpatients with severe oedematous heart failure require chronic administration of metolazone, but often only 2.5 mg on alternate days or once or twice a week. Due to the aforementioned potent effects, this drug should be used with extreme caution as an outpatient treatment, at least in the initial stages of its use.

Potassium-sparing diuretics. The potassium-sparing diuretics ameliorate the loss of potassium produced by the other pharmacological agents. Spironolactone specifically inhibits an important component of the renin–angiotensin system (aldosterone). This produces a weak diuresis but with a potassium-sparing action. This drug improves prognosis in heart failure when added to the use of a diuretic and ACE inhibitor. This was noted in the recent Rales Trial (Pitt et al 1999 (see Fig. 10.7). Blockade of aldosterone receptors by spironolactone substantially reduced the risk of both morbidity and death among patients with severe heart failure.

ACE inhibitors

There is overwhelming evidence that angiotensin converting enzyme (ACE) inhibitors satisfy all the goals of effective treatment for patients with heart failure caused by left ventricular systolic dysfunction. This group of drugs has consistently shown beneficial effects on mortality, morbidity and quality of life in large-scale, prospective trials (Davies et al 2000). They are therefore indicated in all stages of symptomatic heart failure resulting from impaired left ventricular systolic function (Davies et al 2000).

Primarily, ACE inhibitors interrupt the renin–angiotensin–aldosterone cycle. In addition, they increase concentrations of the vasodilator bradykinin

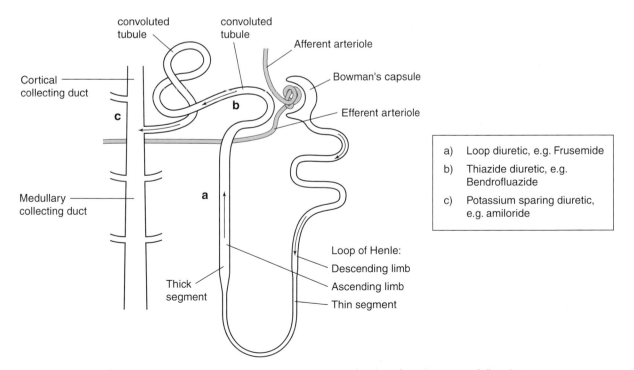

Figure 10.6 A renal nephron illustrating the areas of action of varying types of diuretics.

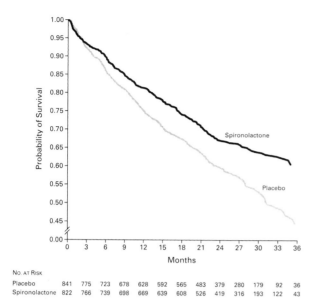

NO. AT RISK

Placebo	841	775	723	678	628	592	565	483	379	280	179	92	36
Spironolactone	822	766	739	698	669	639	608	526	419	316	193	122	43

Figure 10.7 The spironolactone/placebo survival curve in patients with severe heart failure. (Reproduced with the permission of the Massachusetts Medical Society from Pitt et al 1999. All rights reserved.)

by inhibiting its degradation (Davies et al 2000). They lower systemic vascular resistance and venous pressure, thereby reducing levels of circulating catecholamines. This improves myocardial performance. To date, only a small group of drugs such as ACE inhibitors have been shown to consistently reduce mortality and morbidity in patients with asymptomatic or symptomatic left ventricular dysfunction (McKelvie & Yusuf 1997).

The consequence of the neurohormonal effects of the ACE inhibitors is to produce venous and arterial vasodilatation. A reduction in the preload and afterload will subsequently occur, reducing the workload

of the heart to overcome these resistances. Vasodilatation also results in an increase in skeletal blood flow at rest and during exercise. The studies of ACE inhibitors have shown that they are effective in a large subset of patients with heart failure. In addition, the higher doses appear to be more effective than the lower range (ATLAS Study 1998). Many patients with heart failure who should be receiving ACE inhibitors are not and those who may be prescribed the drug often receive too low a dose (ATLAS Study 1998).

The first dose may be associated with transient hypotension and this is particularly the case in those receiving large doses of diuretics. Enalapril requires conversion to the active metabolite enalaprilat by liver enzymes. This drug therefore has a delayed onset of action and with administration of the first dose, hypotension may be forestalled for several hours. In commencing ACE inhibitor therapy, patients with mild to moderate heart failure who have normal renal function and a systolic blood pressure over 100 mmHg and who have stopped taking diuretics for at least 24 hours rarely have a problem, especially if the drug is taken before bed (Hobbs et al 2000).

Approximately 10–15% of patients taking ACE inhibitors develop a cough (Lonn & McKelvie 2000). This is due to the inhibition of bradykinin metabolism within the lung lining. Up to 4% of patients may need to have therapy withdrawn (Pitt et al 1997). In

---

Box 10.4 ACE inhibitor clinical trials

Study	Drug
CONSENSUS	Enalapril 20 mg bd versus placebo
SOLVD	Enalapril 10 mg bd versus placebo
ATLAS	Lisinopril 32.5–35 mg od versus 2.5–5.0 mg od
SAVE	Captopril 50 mg tds versus placebo
ELITE	Captopril 50 mg tds versus losartan 50 mg od
V-HeFT I	Hydralazine 300 mg versus placebo plus nitrate 160 mg
V-HeFT II	Hydralazine 300 mg versus enalapril 10 mg bd plus nitrate 160 mg
AIRE	Ramipril 5 mg bd versus placebo
TRACE	Trandolapril 4 mg od versus placebo

Box 10.5 Guidelines for commencing ACE inhibitor therapy

- Use with caution when using potassium supplements and potassium-sparing diuretics. It may be necessary to stop these. ACE inhibitors reduce aldosterone production, decreasing potassium secretion via the kidneys.
- Be cautious with or reduce the dose of diuretics before the first ACE inhibitor dose. This assists in avoiding hypotension.
- Use a small dose of the ACE inhibitor to start with. Increase after 1–2 weeks. An example starting dose may be: captopril 6.25 mg twice a day (bd), lisinopril 2.5 mg once a day (od), enalapril 2.5 mg od. Maintenance doses: captopril 25–50 mg bd, lisinopril 5–20 mg od, enalapril 10 mg bd.
- Advise the patient to reduce activity or rest for 1–2 hours after the first dose.
- Check the renal chemistry and electrolytes after 1 week and review the blood pressure.
- If stable and renal chemistry is within the normal range, increase the dose.
- Titrate to a maximum tolerated dose, with regular checks on the blood pressure. Review the renal chemistry and electrolytes.
- Consider admission to hospital to commence therapy if: severe heart failure – NYHA IV, tachycardia present, blood pressure <100 systolic.

- *Persistent cough*: due to inhibition of bradykinin
  production in the lungs *Plan*: either reduce the
  dose or change the ACE inhibitor
- *Hypotension*: the patient may experience
  dizziness/postural hypotension *Plan*: advise to take
  the tablets with food or drink
- *Hyperkalaemia*: due to a reduction in aldosterone
  Plan: reduce potassium-sparing diuretics, e.g.
  spironolactone
- *Deteriorating renal function. Plan*: regular
  monitoring of renal chemistry and/or titration of
  diuretics
- *Loss of taste or abnormal taste. Plan*: may need to
  change the ACE inhibitor if intolerable

addition, creatinine levels can rise by approximately
10–15% during therapy. This group of drugs are
contra-indicated in patients with bilateral renal artery
stenosis. This is because glomerular filtration is
reduced or abolished, leading to severe and progressive
renal failure.

The dose of ACE inhibitor is slowly increased over
the weeks until an optimal symptomatic benefit has
been reached. This may take several months (see
Box 10.6 for side-effects). Angiotensin II receptor
antagonists, such as losartan, have very similar
haemodynamic effects to ACE inhibitors but do not
affect bradykinin metabolism. They can therefore be
utilized if the patient is unable to tolerate an ACE
inhibitor.

In practice, doctors tend to prescribe lower doses of
ACE inhibitors than those used in the large mortality
trials. These trials suggest larger doses of ACE
inhibitors improve symptoms to a greater extent than
small doses, at least in patients with severe heart
failure. ACE inhibitors are therefore effective in relieving
the symptoms of chronic heart failure, increasing
exercise capacity, reducing hospitalization and reducing
mortality.

Vasodilators

Hydralazine is a direct smooth muscle relaxant, with
potent arteriolar vasodilator properties. Calcium
channel blockers also reduce afterload. The reduction
in afterload causes an increase in cardiac output and
heart rate.

Venodilators. Nitrates and hydralazine can be
combined in the long-term management of patients
with heart failure to achieve combined reduction of
preload and afterload. This combination has shown a
survival benefit in patients with symptomatic heart
failure (NYHA classes II–III) (Davies et al 2000). It has,

however, been superseded by ACE inhibition due to
the former combination being less well tolerated, with
dizziness and headaches (Davies et al 2000). Such a
combination may still be of value in patients in whom
ACE inhibitors are contra-indicated.

In Figure 10.8 line C is the patient with heart failure.
Point Ci represents severe heart failure, with a high
preload, low stroke volume and the progression into
pulmonary congestion. Cii represents the use of a
diuretic or vasodilator therapy. This reduces the high
preload but has little effect on the stroke volume. If
further diuretic or venous vasodilator therapy is used,
this can worsen the picture (Ciii). Point iv illustrates
the use of an inotrope to raise the stroke volume, while
v has utilized inotropic therapy and arteriolar/
vasodilator therapy. The latter raises the stroke
volume and lowers the high preload. Point vi represents
the careful and balanced use of an inotrope and
vasodilator therapy. It improves the situation but does
not come near to a normal heart's action.

β-blockers. Research has indicated that β-blockers
should be used more widely in the treatment of heart
failure (CIBIS-II 1999, Cleland et al 1999). Cleland et al
(1999) reviewed 25 research papers randomizing
patients with heart failure to β-blocker therapy or
control. This comprised 6511 patients. Overall β-blockers
reduced mortality by 36% (Cleland et al 1999). Until
recently β-blockers were contra-indicated in heart
failure because of their negative inotropic effects. There
is now growing acceptance that this group of drugs will
both reduce cardiac workload and may inhibit the detrimental
effects of catecholamines, as they also exhibit
anti-arrhythmic properties.

β-blockers can cause an initial exacerbation of heart
failure, therefore patients with severe failure, such
as those with NYHA class IV, should be given this

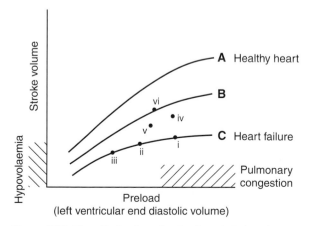

Figure 10.8 The effects of varying treatments in heart
failure on the preload and stroke volume (see text for
explanation).

treatment with caution. In the CIBIS-I trial a small sub-group of patients with severe failure did seem to obtain a mortality benefit with bisoprolol (Lechat et al 1994). More recently, two large-scale clinical trials have demonstrated conclusive evidence of the beneficial effects of β-blocker therapy on survival in chronic heart failure (CIBIS-II 1999, Merit-HF 1999). CIBIS-II enrolled 2647 patients with NYHA class III or IV symptoms and left ventricular ejection fractions of ≤35%. All-cause mortality was reduced by 32% with bisoprolol from 17.3% in the placebo group. The Merit-HF trial enrolled 3991 patients with NYHA II–IV symptoms and left ventricular ejection fractions of ≤40%. All-cause mortality was reduced by 34% with metoprolol over 1 year. This benefit was in addition to that gained with ACE inhibitor therapy.

As a result of these data, β-blocker therapy has become a part of standard therapy for patients with chronic heart failure (in addition to ACE inhibitor and diuretic therapy) (Doughty 1999). The COPERNICUS study was a large multicentre study comparing placebo and carvedilol in patients with severe heart failure, class IV. The drug was found to be beneficial. The trial was stopped early in 2000 following demonstration of a highly significant mortality benefit in patients treated with carvedilol. In addition, carvedilol has been shown to increase the ventricular ejection fraction. After 12 months of treatment this rose by 45% of the baseline (Colucci et al 1996). Secondly, after the same time period of treatment a profound decrease in ventricular mass was noted (Lowes et al 1996).

Experience is required to use β-blockers safely in heart failure and staff unused to their application in heart failure should seek the expertise of a local cardiologist (Cleland et al 1999). The first dose should preferably be administered in a clinic as an outpatient, with the patient already haemodynamically stable on standard therapy, such as a diuretic and ACE inhibitor. The aim is to start on a low dose and titrate up slowly guided by heart rate, blood pressure and renal func-tion. These should be monitered at baseline and before increasing the dose. The β-blocker should be used as part of a strategy of preventing heart failure (Cleland et al 1999). Unlike ACE inhibitors and diuretics, β-blockers are of limited use as a 'rescue' therapy in crises such as pulmonary oedema. The drugs require slow titration over weeks or months. They are most effectively and safely used in patients with milder symptoms to retard deterioration and increase the length and quality of life (Cleland et al 1999).

Calcium channel blockers. The potential benefits of these agents derive not only from their vasodilator properties but also from anti-ischaemic effects. Amlodipine has been associated with the most promising results with evidence of a mortality benefit in non-ischaemic heart failure. To date there is no compelling evidence for the use of calcium channel blockers in heart failure but their potential role in non-ischaemic cardiomyopathy requires further evaluation (see Chapter 11).

Digoxin

Digoxin is one of the oldest drugs used in heart failure and for many years it was regarded as standard therapy. Digoxin is of undoubted value in the control of atrial fibrillation, especially if this rhythm is of importance in the genesis of cardiac failure. However, its role in sinus rhythm is less certain. The Digoxin Investigation Group (DIG) trial was a major study to investigate the effect of digoxin on mortality in heart failure (DIG 1997). No effect on mortality was found in all subgroups and no particular benefit in those with severe heart failure. However, in the trial's main study group of patients assigned to digoxin or placebo, in addition to diuretics and ACE inhibitors, there were 6% fewer hospital admissions overall in the digoxin group and fewer patients were hospitalized for worsening heart failure (26.8% verses 34.7%). Digoxin's mechanism of action is discussed in Chapter

Box 10.7 The main β-blocker clinical trials			
Study	*Drug*	*NYHA grade/ejection fraction*	*Drug dose used in trial*
CIBIS-II	Bisoprolol	III–IV/≤35%	1.25–10 mg od versus placebo
MERIT-HF	Metoprolol	II–IV/≤40%	12.5 or 25 mg up to 200 mgs od versus placebo
US Carvedilol	Carvedilol	II–III/<35%	3.125 mg/6.25 mg/12.5 mg/25 mg versus placebo
COPERNICUS	Carvedilol	IV/<35% (severe heart failure)	3.125 mg/6.25 mg/12.5 mg/25 mg versus placebo

---

> **Box 10.8** The mode of action of β-blockers in heart failure
>
> - A reduction in the heart rate/blood pressure.
> - Improved diastolic relaxation.
> - Reduced oxygen consumption: slowing the heart rate can reduce myocardial oxygen demand, while prolonged diastole can increase coronary perfusion time.
> - Prevention of catecholamine toxicity: there is evidence to suggest that activation of myocardial β-receptors promotes dysfunction and death of cardiac myocytes.
> - Reduction of arrhythmias: myocardial ischaemia and a shortened duration of the action potential increase the likelihood of arrhythmias.

19. In the US and many European countries, digoxin is used widely in chronic heart failure.

Anti-arrhythmic agents

Arrhythmias are frequent in heart failure. It is tempting to think that anti-arrhythmic therapy used to suppress ventricular arrhythmias may in turn reduce the incidence of sudden death in heart failure. However, some drug treatments appear to induce more sudden deaths than they prevent (CAST 1991).

The medication regimen for heart failure is quite complex and often confusing for patients, especially when the dosages are changed and different medications prescribed. When concomitant illness arises such as chest infection requiring antibiotics, these can upset the balance and as the patient deteriorates it becomes difficult to fine tune and control symptoms without provoking side-effects. During the winter months it is appropriate, although evidence is inconclusive, for patients to consider flu vaccination in view of this tendency for and consequence of prolonged infection. Prevention of illnesses that exacerbate heart failure may also reduce direct cost and result in improved outcomes for patients with heart failure. Immunization programmes against influenza have been shown to decrease cost and improve outcome for patients with heart failure (Nichol et al 1994).

In summary, large-scale randomized controlled trials have conclusively demonstrated the efficacy of appropriate pharmacotherapy in reducing morbidity, hospitalizations and mortality in patients with heart failure (Packer et al 1996, SOLVD 1991). ACE inhibitors effectively reduce the combined endpoint of mortality and hospital admissions by 25% (Garg & Yusuf 1995), have proven cost effectiveness (McMurray & Davie

1996) and are recommended in all cases of symptomatic heart failure due to left ventricular dysfunction (AHA 1995, European Society of Cardiology 1997). Other agents which have clear indications for the reduction of morbidity, mortality or both in cardiac failure include digoxin, angiotensin II antagonists, β-blockers and more recently spironolactone (DIG 1997, Pitt et al 1999). Furthermore, evidence is accumulating on the benefits of non-pharmacological therapy, in particular exercise training (Afzal et al 1998), dietary advice and patient education, in reducing morbidity and improving functional status in chronic heart failure. This will be discussed in detail in the next section.

Surgical treatment

The more recent surgical treatments include ventricular reduction surgery – this is removal of a wedge of ventricular myocardium and as surgery remains in its infancy (Batista et al 1997). In cardiomyoplasty, the latissimus dorsi muscle is surgically wrapped around the ventricle and electrically stimulated, as an aid to left ventricular contraction (Kass 1998). The use of left ventricular assist devices (LVADs) has not been shown to affect mortality in large controlled prospective studies. However, work continues with devices such as the Jarvik 2000 Heart, in selected patients (see Chapter 18). In patients with a history of ventricular tachycardia or fibrillation, internal cardioverter defibrillators (ICDs) are effective in terminating these arrhythmias but preparation and support are needed to enable the patient and family/carers to become used to its role in their lives (see Chapter 25). Several studies have shown that resynchronization of left and right ventricular function by means of multisite pacing can result in significant haemodynamic and clinical improvement in patients with heart failure (Auricchio et al 1999). It is anticipated that multisite pacing will rapidly become a therapeutic option in subsets of patients with severe heart failure.

Cardiac transplantation has also been shown to reduce mortality. At present over 75% of patients undergoing transplantation are alive at 5 years (Millane et al 2000). This provides a better outcome than for those on optimal drug treatment for advanced heart failure. In these cases the 1-year mortality is 30–50%. Transplantation should therefore be considered for those who have an estimated 1-year survival of less than 50% (Millane et al 2000). However, there remains a shortage of donor organs and this is by no means the ultimate answer. Cardiac transplantation is discussed in detail in Chapter 23.

THE ECONOMIC IMPACT

The economic impact of chronic heart failure is excessive and is increasing over time given the extremely high cost of treatment. The high mortality, marked disability and subsequent lack of productivity of people with heart failure weigh heavily on society (O'Connell & Bristow 1994). Chronic heart failure is the most common indication for hospitalization among adults over 65 years of age and is increasing. Data from Hobbs et al (2000) examined acute admissions to a city centre hospital for patients with heart failure. The median duration of stay was 8 (range 1–96) days, with a 20% inpatient mortality. They estimate that approximately 200 000 people in the UK require admission to hospital for heart failure each year. It is always difficult to gain up-to-date figures but in 1993 in the UK, heart failure cost the NHS £360 m. The figure is probably now closer to £600 m, equivalent to 1–2% of the total NHS budget (Hobbs et al 2000).

THE JUSTIFICATION AND ROLE OF THE HEART FAILURE CLINIC

Large-scale, randomized controlled trials have conclusively demonstrated the efficacy of appropriate pharmacological therapies in reducing morbidity, hospitalization and mortality in patients with heart failure (Packer et al 1996). Numerous clinical trials have established the ACE inhibitors and β-blockers as effective for improving quality of life, by reducing the signs and symptoms of heart failure. These objectively increase exercise tolerance and prolong duration of life. Although the efficacy of ACE inhibitors has long been recognized, studies show that these agents are still underutilized in clinical practice and, furthermore, prescribing patterns depend on who looks after the patient (Philbin 1998, Smith et al 1997). In patients with mild to moderate heart failure the use of ACE inhibitors by cardiologists, general physicians and general practitioners was 80%, 71% and 60% respectively (Edep et al 1997). The underutilization of evidence-based medicines in part reflects practical difficulties with the use of such medications outside the clinical trial setting.

The typical patient with heart failure is in the community, older than 70 years and co-morbidity is common (Packer et al 1996). These patients are already taking numerous medications, rendering additional therapy difficult and unwelcome. The initiation and achievement of adequate doses of ACE inhibitors, β-blockers and other medications is often labour inten-

sive, involving dose titration, the monitoring of effects such as blood electrolytes, heart rate and blood pressure, in addition to the education of the patient regarding the nature and purpose of the treatment to ensure compliance. Extra time needs to be spent on education regarding dietary issues, weight and exercise, with attention given to the individual needs of the patient depending on social circumstances and the extent of co-morbidities. Suboptimal management, inappropriate withdrawal of therapy, excessive use of diuretics, digoxin toxicity, poor compliance, inadequate follow-up and poor social support have all been shown to be major causes of hospital re-admission in heart failure patients. A prospective study of patients in hospital with heart failure showed that 53% of early re-admissions were preventable (Vinson et al 1990).

Rich et al (1995) instigated a nurse-led, multidisciplinary intervention to reduce re-admission of patients with congestive heart failure, during the 90 days following hospital discharge. Poor compliance to treatment was seen as an area causing re-admission and the programme consisted of comprehensive education of the patient and family, a prescribed diet, social service consultation, planning for early discharge and a review of medications, together with intensive follow-up. Survival without re-admission was achieved in 91 of 142 patients, compared with 75 of 140 in the control group. The number of re-admissions for heart failure was reduced by 56.2% in the treatment group. Other-cause re-admission was also reduced by 28.5% (Rich et al 1995).

The long-term goals of heart failure management are not only to decrease mortality and morbidity but also to improve quality of life and reduce the burden on the health-care system. Expensive re-admission to hospital will increase this burden. Consequently, there is a need for specialized units to deal specifically with heart failure. Such a unit would undertake a comprehensive approach to the management of heart failure, with evidence indicating that specialty clinics may produce better clinical and economic outcomes for a variety of diseases (Zeiger et al 1991). An example can be found

---

Box 10.9 Common causes for re-admission to hospital in patients with heart failure

- Decompensated heart failure
- Poor treatment compliance
- Inadequate optimization of drug treatments
- Inadequate discharge preparation/planning/ follow-up
- Arrhythmias
- Angina/infarction
- Infections

in asthma management. Where a specialist team consisting of respiratory nurse specialists and chest physicians manage a clinic, intensive therapy, better symptomatic relief, improved exercise tolerance and decreased emergency department visits or hospitalization can be achieved, when compared with a more general care physician or nursing team (Zeiger et al 1991).

Clinics for the management of chronic heart failure are developing at a rapid rate across the UK. It is recognized that addressing all aspects of heart failure management is beyond the scope of the individual physician and therefore an effective solution demands a multidisciplinary approach that is long overdue. This comprehensive approach to the management of heart failure in a dedicated setting would include detailed assessment and history with confirmation of diagnosis, evaluation and risk stratification. It would also include management according to a defined algorithm with appropriate monitoring of electrolyte balance and kidney function. Education of the patient and their family with regard to the nature and progression of their disease would be the final holistic element. This would include the importance and necessity of medication and attention to dietary issues, in particular fluid and salt restriction, and the importance of daily weights.

This may be achieved with extended support to include the availability of telephone help and advice and a facility for unplanned outpatient assessments. To achieve these goals the heart failure clinic should consist of a multidisciplinary team. This will include a cardiologist, a cardiology specialist nurse, dietitian and pharmacist, all of whom maintain close links with the patient's general practitioner. Contact with the social services department and district nurses completes the circle (Fig. 10.9).

Several randomized and non-randomized trials have demonstrated diminution in hospitalization and reduced total medical cost, despite increased numbers of visits to clinic. Patient satisfaction was also unanimous (Cintron et al 1983). The introduction of a nurse specialist in a heart failure clinic has proved effective in reducing hospital admissions and medical costs during 1 year of follow-up compared with the year before inclusion (Cintron et al 1983) yet the important role of nurses in the management of heart failure has been relatively neglected in Britain (Hobbs et al 2000).

A study of 134 patients referred to the Vanderbilt heart failure and heart transplantation programme examined the effects on symptoms, exercise capacity and quality of life. The programme involved care by three specialist heart failure physicians, two nurse

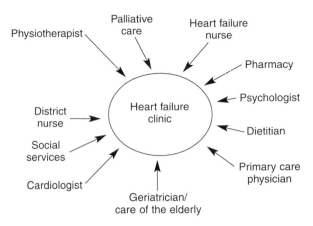

Figure 10.9 The component parts of the heart failure clinic.

co-ordinators and a home health-care team, where needed. The number of hospitalizations decreased from 210 in the year prior to referral to 104 in the year after referral. Exercise capacity was increased as measured by metabolic exercise testing. Quality of life also improved as assessed by the Minnesota Living with Heart Failure Questionnaire following 1 year in the programme (Hanumanthu et al 1997). Another study comparing the events among 51 patients in a nurse co-ordinated clinic designed to optimize chronic disease management concluded that after 6 months the frequency of follow-up clinic visits was reduced by 23% and hospitalizations by 74% when compared with the previous 6 months (West et al 1997). The intervention included education on individual disease state, sodium restriction, pharmacological therapy and warning symptoms indicating progression of heart failure. It also included behavourial techniques for improving adherence to medication and diet.

The nurse's role

This clinic should function ideally in the cardiology outpatients department. A room should be available for the cardiologist, the nurse specialist and possibly a dietitian. Ideally, the clinic should have easy access to echocardiography and ECG. On the initial referral visit the patient would be evaluated by the heart failure cardiologist. The nurse specialist will also see the patient to discuss the basics of heart failure, dietary and exercise information. A contact number will be given and appropriate situations in which the patient should contact the clinic staff would be explained. The specialist nurse plays a pivotal role in co-ordinating the care of these patients. Specific tasks of the heart failure nurse would include educating the patient regarding the importance of recognizing signs and symptoms of heart failure and discussing the nature and progress of their individual disease. The pre-scribed medications would be reviewed with the patient by the nurse.

Under specific guidelines and individual hospital policy, such as for nurse prescribing and/or patient group directions, the nurse specialist should be able to initiate and adjust the dose of specific drugs such as diuretics and ACE inhibitors. Following a protocol with appropriate training and education, the nurse would be able to perform a physical examination, order and interpret investigations such as bloods, elec-trocardiography, echocardiography and chest X-rays as appropriate. This nurse would also have the practi-cal responsibility to establish a support network for each patient: for example, dietitian, physiotherapist, general practitioner, district nurse and social services. The frequency of visits can be determined by the nurse specialist depending on the patient's clinical status. If a patient is requiring adjustment of medication, they should be seen accordingly.

The clinic may run one day a week on an appoint-ment basis and ideally a walk-in facility should exist on a daily basis at a specified time. A telephone helpline giving direct contact with the nurse specialist should be established. If patients are experiencing symptoms of worsening heart failure, they can be seen at short notice. At nights and weekends in an emer-gency situation, patients should be encouraged to either call their GP or present themselves at the nearest A&E department.

Heart failure management requires many lifestyle adjustments by patients and their families. Patients may need to make changes to their diet and daily activities that may conflict with their cultural or their long-term beliefs and desires. The onset of chronic illness such as heart failure precipitates a life transition (Moos 1982). The consequences of this condition together with fear and feelings of being a burden, may have an adverse effect on the family with ensuing guilt for the patient. The threat of losing or the loss of an income, being refused insurance and becoming a burden can create many psychosocial problems with adjustments to be made. Some degree of anxiety and depression is commonplace.

The adjustments that the patient is forced to live with, leading to new limitations and the knowledge of a shortened life expectancy, can result in a decreased quality of life. It seems that a dedicated heart failure clinic would greatly improve the medical management, together with a multidisciplinary approach providing

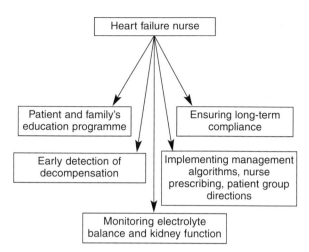

Figure 10.10 The role of the nurse in the management of patients with heart failure.

the patient with the necessary props to understand and comply with progress of the disease. The heart failure nurse plays a key role in educating and counselling the patient and the family about lifestyle modifications. Specific issues such as diet, pharmacology and exercise will be discussed in more detail.

Education on disease

In order for patients to fully co-operate with their treatment, they need to understand their disease. The heart failure nurse can provide an individually tail-ored discussion on the aetiology and basic physiology of the heart failure. Heart failure is an unfortunate term, only serving to frighten the patient. A full expla-nation of all the signs and symptoms such as breath-lessness, fatigue and those daily activities that might provoke the symptoms may help to reduce anxiety over their development. If the patient is taught to rec-ognize these symptoms as a worsening of heart failure, they can act immediately and follow a strategy.

At the initial visit to a specialist clinic, it is helpful for patients to receive a booklet or care card in order for them to record daily progress. This will help them participate in their illness. Recording of daily weight is one of the best ways for patients to monitor their condition. Patients should be encouraged to purchase scales and weigh themselves at the same time every day wearing similar garments, preferably in the morning before breakfast. They are given specific guidelines indicating that if their weight changes by more than 1–3 kg since their last recording, they should regard this as a possibility of a change in their

condition. With adequate education patients may be able to assess themselves by noting any increasing breathlessness or oedema of the ankles. They can then make a decision to inform the heart failure nurse and/or use a drop-in service.

Education on the disease process, together with issues of physiology and pharmacology, can be reinforced. If the patient is able to understand the purpose of each tablet in relation to their disease, they will become more compliant or adherent. Of course, patients cannot retain all the information in one single appointment (Mullen et al 1992). These educational sessions need to be repeated as often as necessary at the clinic on subsequent visits. More recently, Rogers et al (2000) explored patients' understanding of chronic heart failure and investigated their need for information and issues concerning communication. This study identified disease-specific barriers to effective communication, such as short-term memory loss, confusion and fatigue. They concluded that strategies to help patients ask questions, including those related to prognosis, should be developed. The outpatient department waiting area should have specific reading material available for the patient and carers to browse through and take home. This can help to clarify provided information, identify problems and concerns and promote discussion at the consultation.

The patient's family or carers play an important part and if possible should be included in the education. Chronic illness affects the whole family (Miller 1992). Evidence that it exerts a negative impact on marital couples was provided by Klein et al as early as 1967. The team discovered that levels of psychological distress and role tension reported by some spouses were equal to those of their ill partner. A process of adaptation and adjustment is necessary for the heart failure patient and his/her family or carers. The nurse specialist has an integral role in maintaining a positive attitude by lending emotional support and providing specific guidelines resulting in empowerment of the patient.

Dietary advice

Depending on the centre, a dietitian may be part of the multidisciplinary team. However, the nurse specialist should be able to provide specific information on dietary issues. Again, this should be part of the education package and written material should be available to take home. Traditionally patients with heart failure are recommended a reduced sodium diet and fluid restriction to avoid fluid overload. A reduction in salt intake to 3 g (50 mmol) is recommended for patients with mild to moderate heart failure. It has been estimated to lower systolic blood pressure by an average of 5 mmHg and 7 mmHg in those with high blood pressure (Law et al 1991).

As highlighted in Chapter 5, a large percentage of a person's sodium intake can come from processed foods. Manufacturers are facing increased pressure to reduce the sodium content of their standard products and to produce sodium alternatives but with the same tastes and technological properties of salt. The main alternative in use is potassium chloride. Evidence has shown that higher intakes of potassium are associated with lower blood pressure and hence greater protection against cerebrovascular accident (CVA/stroke)

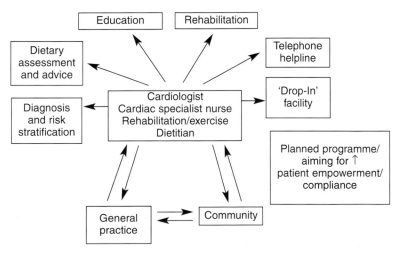

Figure 10.11 The organization of service in caring for the patient with heart failure.

(Swales 1991). However, potassium salt substitute should be taken with caution. A healthy person is able to excrete the extra potassium load whilst others may be at higher risk of developing potassium toxicity as a result of disease or drug therapy. Therefore the use of salt substitutes should not be recommended (Swales 1991).

A salt intake of 3 g per day can be achieved with no major inconvenience or loss of palatability of foods. Salt should be limited in cooking and be avoided at the table, with a careful avoidance of those products known to be high in salt, such as processed foods and snacks including crisps and peanuts. Some patients may find difficulty in understanding the difference between increased weight due to progressive heart failure and increased water retention and increased weight due to elevated food intake. It should be emphasized that increased weight coupled with increased breathlessness and/or oedema may indicate a worsening of heart failure.

Prompt advice, either via the telephone with the nurse specialist or through a visit to the clinic with subsequent alteration of the diuretics, may reduce the oedema and breathlessness and in turn reduce the weight. Recognition of dehydration must also be included in the education package. Dehydration may be caused by excessive diuresis, hot weather creating heavy perspiration and concomitant infection leading to pyrexia or diarrhoea. Increased thirst is a simple and early sign of dehydration. This may also cause the person to feel unwell, with headaches and dizziness, together with a drop in blood pressure, increasing the risk of postural hypotension. Itching and a lack of elasticity in the skin, the latter when pinching the skin on the back of the hand, are also signs of reduced fluid. An increase in fluid intake and/or a reduction in diuretics may resolve the problem.

Dietary advice should also include information on fats, cholesterol and lipid profile. This is especially pertinent if the patient has an ischaemic cause through narrowed coronary arteries. Too many dietary restrictions should be avoided as many of these patients with severe heart failure lose their appetite and suffer from anorexia and cachexia. The anorexia occurs as a result of congestion of the gastro-intestinal tract. The patient should be advised to take small frequent snacks instead of large meals. Vitamin supplementation is advisable due to inadequate nutritional intake and because of water-soluble vitamin loss associated with diuretics. This is in addition to problems of gastro-intestinal absorption of fat-soluble vitamins.

Certain ethnic groups may need individually tailored advice and counselling. Muslims, for example, have a diet very rich in salt and fats, particularly butter and ghee, a form of purified butter. Religious festivals such as Ramadan impose a complete change in diet regime when patients experience long periods of the day without any nutritional intake. There may consequently be fluctuations in body weight that require observation.

At religious gatherings the patient is open to the temptation of fatty, spicy foods. Members of the Sikh community also have a diet rich in ghee. Pickles form an essential part of their diet and these are preserved in salt. Advice here should encourage patients to opt for more grilled foods if able, taken with a salad. Sensitivity towards differences in patients' language and culture will assist in better compliance. Importance must also be placed on educating the spouse or carer, because they are likely to be involved in eating and shopping with the patient.

Alcohol

Alcohol is a well-known myocardial depressant. In cases of alcohol-induced disease such as dilated cardiomyopathy and atrial fibrillation, abstinence should be advised. In a patient who enjoys drinking socially, careful and restricted intake should be observed.

Exercise

Training increases exercise tolerance in normal subjects and in patients with ischaemic heart disease. Regular exercise is known to improve the blood lipid profiles, blood pressure and resting heart rate, decrease perceived stress and generally improve psychological status (Astrand & Rodahl 1986, Blomqvist & Saltin 1983). Patients with chronic heart failure would also benefit from this improvement in function. Such patients may be limited initially by dyspnoea or fatigue at low workloads so may be discouraged from exercise. However, with a planned and supervised programme, beneficial effects in improving exercise capacity, perceived quality of life and autonomic and skeletal muscle function have been demonstrated in chronic heart failure patients (European Heart Failure Training Group 1998, Willenheimer et al 1998).

Some of the pathophysiological processes of impaired exercise intolerance in patients with heart failure include dyspnoea on exertion and fatigue. These symptoms occur as a result of muscle fatigue, impaired cardiac output and abnormalities in skeletal muscle blood flow. This results in increased lactate pro-

duction and hence exercise intolerance (Minotti et al 1991). Exercise training seems to improve vasodilatation and muscle oxidative capacity. Current evidence suggests that patients with heart failure and no angina should be encouraged to be as active as possible. A home walking exercise programme may be an option for helping patients avoid the negative physiological and psychological consequences of inactivity. A gradual increase in distance over several months should occur while patients monitor their symptoms. Patients may feel exhausted the following day if they overexert themselves and therefore should adjust the exercise accordingly.

North et al (1990) identified exercise training as an effective treatment to improve the quality of life (QOL). Patients became more tolerant of exertion and subsequently more comfortable in performing tasks of daily living, with increasing independence, less chronic illness behaviour and less depression. Coats et al (1992) have demonstrated the potential benefits of long-term aerobic exercise for patients with stable, controlled heart failure while Koch et al (1992) noted a 63% improvement in QOL measurements amongst exercise-trained patients versus 4% improvement in controls. More recently, Kostis et al (1994) also observed a significant improvement in QOL and mood state in a similarly studied (exercise) group.

Despite the continuing emerging evidence that exercise programmes benefit patients with stable heart failure, guidelines have only recently emerged for prescribing exercise to these patients (Gianuzzi et al 2001). Based on exercise trials to date, achieving a regular exercise programme of about 3–5 days per week appears manageable for most patients with heart failure. Patients should be encouraged to keep to the same routine with their exercise habits when feeling well but to avoid exertion when experiencing symptoms of angina, arrhythmias, pulmonary congestion or recent weight gain. Additionally, it should be emphasized that exercise detraining will lead to a return of the exercise intolerance and reduced QOL previously experienced.

Most exercise trials involving patients with heart failure recommend exercise between 30 to 60 minutes per session. As with general advice to normal subjects, previously sedentary patients should start with less exercise, for example 10–15 minutes, gradually progressing to 30 minutes per session. This group may experience more fatigue initially and should be encouraged to rest briefly after a programme of exercise.

Meyer et al (1996) suggest that interval training be considered when prescribing exercise in patients with heart failure. Interval training is the ability to prolong exercise during a time period by resting at set intervals when a certain point is reached, such as a specific heart rate or point in time. It allows for a shorter exercise duration, a high physical stress on the skeletal muscles but less cardiac stress. Exercise training patients with heart failure is a specialist area because these patients require stabilization of the condition and assessment prior to commencing exercise. The choice of exercise type and level should be individualized to take into account the exercise tolerance of each patient and their programmes should be re-evaluated on a regular basis, depending on their clinical course.

Exercise training therefore represents an important and effective adjunct therapy to patients with heart failure. There are few centres in the UK offering this service as part of rehabilitation but as more heart failure clinics are established, we hope to see a multidisciplinary approach extending to exercise training.

Sexual activity

Fears regarding physical exertion may also contribute to the high prevalence of sexual difficulties in heart failure patients (Jaarsma et al 1996). In the last decade increasing recognition has occurred that sexual function is an important contributor to the QOL of cardiac patients. Health-care professionals can become pre-occupied with the diagnostic and therapeutic aspects of disease, ignoring the patient's overall well-being. Most patients find it difficult to initiate discussions on sexuality and rely on health-care professionals to do so. However, the consultation with the doctor may not include information or enquiry on sexual behaviour or function. These topics can be discussed during educational sessions either in groups or individually, giving the patient the chance to enquire directly and openly.

Anxiety or hesitancy is often expressed by the patient's partner, as they feel equally uncomfortable about stressing the patient beyond their capabilities. As early as 1970, Hellerstein & Freidman conducted a study in which subjects performed bicycle ergometry tests in the laboratory while undergoing continuous electrocardiographic monitoring. This aimed to correlate maximum oxygen uptake (VO_2 max) as assessed by the exercise test and heart rate. The heart rate information was then matched to heart rates and blood pressure measurements obtained during coitus. The maximal heart rate and blood pressure assessed during coitus (corresponding to the phase of the orgasm) ranged from 90 to 115 beats per minute. Changes in blood pressure were from 127/85 mmHg to 162/89 mmHg respectively, matching that of bicycle ergometry. This study demonstrated a mild to moderate increase in heart rate and blood pressure during the height of sexual activity.

It seems that this degree of change in haemodynamic status is one that could be tolerated by most patients with heart failure. Patients can better understand their limitations when considering and comparing normal everyday activities; for example, highlighting that the heart rate and blood pressure will increase approximately the same amount during sexual intercourse as walking up a flight or two of stairs. Fears and hesitations can be alleviated on knowing what to expect and what is usual in others.

In a study conducted by Dracup et al (1989), 71 severe heart failure patients completed the Sexual Adjustment Scale of the Psychosocial Adjustment to Illness Scale (PAIS); 76% of patients reported a marked decrease in sexual activity and 33% reported that all sexual relations had ceased. Sollano et al (1992) reported similar findings but noted that, sadly, the desire remained high. These findings suggest a need for counselling. These patients face an uncertain future and can therefore reasonably expect to be bitter and resentful, because the majority of patients believe that their sexual dissatisfaction is a part of their condition.

The poor life expectancy of heart-failed patients encourages aggressive attempts to prevent progression of ventricular dysfunction, rather than wait for treatable symptoms. The aforementioned drug regimens may have a negative impact on the QOL as a result of possible side-effects, not only on sexuality but on the physical state. Some patients may become depressed and disheartened at the large number of tablets to be taken. Emotional well-being, social and cognitive function are dependent upon the nurse's ability to establish a therapeutic dialogue with the patient. The nurse should be knowledgeable and sensitive to social class and culturally determined differences in sexual attitudes, values and practices. Sexual dysfunction may ultimately adversely affect the overall health of the individual. Sexuality is woven into the everyday life of all people and good sexual function is vital for emotional satisfaction.

PALLIATIVE CARE

An increasing interest and research into the care of the dying over the past 25 years has resulted in better symptom control, psychological support and palliative care options for people dying of cancer and their families (Higginson 1993). Yet little attention is paid to patients with heart failure, who also have a poor prognosis that severely limits their quality of life. There is evidence that palliative care teams have managed patients with heart failure successfully using the same approaches perceived as beneficial to cancer sufferers (Department of Health (DoH) 1998). However, conventional hospices and specialists in palliative care services could be overwhelmed by user demand from those in the heart failure category. Indeed, such patients do not necessarily have a clearly defined terminal phase and are inevitably more prone to sudden death than those with cancer (Gibbs et al 1998). This therefore may require both alternative or adapted planning strategies, together with further research in this area.

In the United Kingdom only one study has investigated the variety of symptoms experienced in terminal heart disease (Addington-Hall & McCarthy 1995). This was a population-based, retrospective survey of a random sample of people dying in 20 English health districts in 1990 (Gibbs et al 1998). A wide range of symptoms were experienced in those who had died from heart disease and which included heart failure. These were reported as distressing and often lasting more than 6 months (McCarthy et al 1996). In addition to dyspnoea, pain, nausea and constipation, a general low mood was common. At least one in six patients had symptoms as severe as those experienced by cancer patients who were managed in hospices or by palliative care teams. Although many were thought to have known that they were dying, open communication with health professionals was rare (McCarthy et al 1997).

Provision of palliative care remains inadequate for the cardiac population. It is seemingly available only to patients with a diagnosis of cancer and those lucky enough to live near an available service. Yet symptoms of discomfort and distress can be worse than those experienced in cancer. Although it is being increasingly recognized that palliative care is the obvious next step to be taken for patients with end-stage heart failure, the increased costs would impose a further economic burden on an overstretched health service.

A Department of Health report (DoH 1998) suggested that the advances in palliative care for cancer patients should be integrated into the care of those with clinically similar conditions to ensure an equitable service for all. Indeed, the National Service Framework (NSF) for Coronary Heart Disease has recognized that people with heart failure have a worse QOL than people with most other common medical conditions. As part of an increased awareness of the needs of this group of patients, the NSF has stated that it aims to help people with unresponsive heart failure

and other malignant presentations of CHF to receive appropriate, palliative care support (DoH 2000).

CONCLUSION

This chapter has highlighted that chronic heart failure is an increasingly prevalent condition in the United Kingdom. The long-term goals of care are not only to decrease mortality and morbidity but to improve quality of life and reduce the burden on health-care systems. Care seems to be greatly improved if delivered by specialized units that use a multidisciplinary approach. It is a chronic condition, which is a frequent cause of hospital admissions and re-admissions and therefore imposes a significant health and economic burden. Nursing is playing an increasingly dynamic

role in the management of this condition, not only in the care provided during acute episodes of the disease which require hospitalization but through a health promotion and educative role, aiming to empower patients regarding their condition and to increase medication compliance.

The emergence of the nurse-led clinic can offer much to those with this condition who are chronically ill and require lifestyle advice, with monitoring and manipulation of medication but without the need for a medical consultation each time. In addition, cardiac liaison nurses can now provide seamless care between hospital and community. Finally, palliative care teams need to be considered for a group of patients where treatments and medications may offer amelioration of symptoms, but expected lifespan is now markedly shortened.

Case study 10.1

Mrs Rita Greaves is a 70-year-old lady who had been diagnosed with chronic heart failure nearly 2 years ago. She was admitted to the Accident and Emergency (A&E) department of her local hospital at 5am, with difficulty in breathing after waking suddenly. She was also experiencing palpatations. On admission to the A&E department accompanied by her husband, the nursing staff noticed that she seemed anxious, her skin was cold and clammy and she appeared ashen. Her breathlessness made it difficult for her to speak. Nursing staff reassured both Mrs Greaves and her husband. 60% oxygen via a facemask was applied and Mrs Greaves was sat upright on the trolley to aid breathing. The doctor arrived and after an initial examination, a diagnosis of exacerbation of left ventricular failure was made. Clinical observations taken by the A&E team included a heart rate of 150 bpm and a blood pressure of 100/70 mmHg. A raised jugular venous pressure (JVP) was also noted, indicating an excess of fluid accumulating due to heart failure. Pulse oximetry revealed an arterial oxygen saturation of 90% with the oxygen mask in place and an arterial blood gas sample was also taken at this time. A chest X-ray was ordered, which subsequently showed an enlarged heart and acute pulmonary oedema (see Fig. 5.9D, p. 86).

An intravenous cannula was placed in the left hand (Mrs Greaves was right handed) and 80 mg of furosemide (frusemide) was prescribed and administered slowly. This drug will induce a diuresis to relieve pulmonary oedema and also induce transient venodilatation. The latter can lead to symptomatic improvement before the onset of diuresis (Millane et al 2000). At this time a small dose of intravenous diamorphine, 2.5 mg, was administered. This provides symptomatic relief by reducing anxiety and myocardial oxygen demand. Again, venodilatation is induced which reduces the preload (the end-diastolic volume of blood)

and thus the oxygen-demanding workload of the heart. To aid a further reduction in preload, an intravenous infusion of glyceryl trinitrate (GTN) was commenced and titrated against the presenting blood pressure. This was maintained at no lower than 100 mmHg systolic. A 12-lead ECG revealed sinus tachycardia, signs of left ventricular enlargement (tall R-waves in the left chest leads) and some inverted T-waves in the anterior leads (Fig. 10.12).

After explanation to the patient, a urinary catheter was passed to more accurately monitor the urine output. All adult patients should pass at least 0.5 ml/kg/h because this is an indication of adequate, if not optimal, tissue perfusion. It was not deemed necessary at this point to commence an inotropic agent. Following administration of the above treatment, Mrs Greaves became more settled, her breathing less laboured and pulse oximetry recordings improved. A further arterial blood gas revealed an improved PaO_2 of 10 kPa and an acid–base balance only slightly outside the normal range (base excess −3.5 mmol/l). A lowering base excess can indicate a metabolic acidosis, possibly occurring due to poor tissue perfusion and the subsequent production of lactic acid.

Mrs Greaves was transferred to the coronary care unit (CCU). Initially she remained on bedrest to reduce the heart's workload, with cardiac monitoring in place and all her basic nursing needs met by staff. A full blood count was taken to assess the level of urea and electrolytes and signs of anaemia. The serum level of potassium is particularly important. A low level, which may be induced by diuretic therapy, can result in cardiac arrhythmias and augment the effects of digoxin, which may result in undesirable side-effects such as ventricular arrhythmias. Digoxin levels were in fact taken and although the therapeutic level can overlap the level which may produce toxic effects, it was felt that these were at an acceptable measurement for Mrs Greaves (the normal range 6–8 hours post-dose is approximately 1.4–2.6 nmol/l; the range will vary between laboratories). In addition, an oral supplement of potassium was prescribed to maintain this electrolyte's level. Nursing staff ensured pressure area care was initiated and subcutaneous heparin was prescribed to reduce the risk of deep vein thrombus formation. It was important for staff to monitor Mrs Greaves' bowel habits, as she was relatively immobile at this point and had also received several doses of diamorphine, which can induce a constipating effect. A daily laxative was therefore prescribed. Daily weights were commenced before breakfast each day, as a useful way to monitor the effectiveness of therapy. The GTN infusion was discontinued after 48 hours.

Initially, Mrs Greaves had remained breathless in the CCU and a fluid restriction of 1.5 litres over 24 hours was instigated. A choice from the menu which was easily chewed and low in salt was made available to Mrs Greaves, with advice not to add further salt to the meal. This assisted in reducing excess fluid retention. The dietitian also visited to perform an assessment and offer further advice. The opportunity was also taken to perform an echocardiogram of the heart to assess the degree of further deterioration in ventricular function.

Gradually Mrs Greaves improved over the next few days. This provided the opportunity to review the current drug therapy and address the issue of patient compliance to tablets and the possibility of lifestyle advice that could augment clinical improvement. Mrs Greaves had been seen for some time by the cardiologist in clinic. She was already taking an ACE inhibitor, captopril 25 mg twice a day (bd), and had in the last month been commenced on a β-blocker, carvedilol, which was slowly being increased over the coming weeks. It was currently at a dose of 6.25 mg bd (the drug had been stopped during this period of decompensated heart failure). One tablet of spironolactone 25 mg bd was taken daily, together with daily digoxin, at a dose of 125 μg.

The hospital had recently commenced a heart failure clinic. The nurse involved in this initiative was contacted and agreed to see Mrs Greaves, initially while in hospital and subsequently when she next came to see the consultant. This clinic would be able to discuss the diagnosis with Mrs Greaves, listen to concerns, offer support and explore steps that she may take to both identify a worsening condition and prevent unnecessary deterioration. This involved discussion regarding the role of drug therapy to help augment compliance, dietary advice and issues such as planned exercise regimes to improve exercise capacity. The clinic would also be able to assess Mrs Greaves' ongoing condition and adjust medication within agreed patient group directions. The more frequent contact with the clinic enabled the consultant to be contacted at an earlier stage if marked deterioration was noted. The clinic nurse also took the opportunity to contact Mrs Greaves' own general practice. Increasingly, community practices are initiating nurse-led clinics for patients with particular ongoing conditions such as heart failure, diabetes or those in need of services such as family planning. In discussion, no such clinic was clearly under way and both hospital and community nurses agreed that the heart failure clinic would benefit Mrs Greaves and her husband.

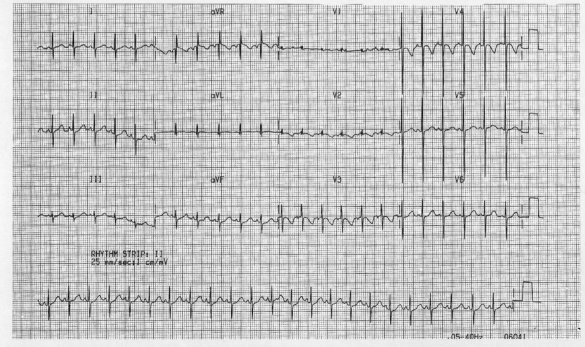

Figure 10.12 The 12-lead ECG demonstrating a sinus tachycardia (150 bpm), left ventricular hypertrophy (tall R-waves in the left chest leads) and the occasional inverted T-wave.

REFERENCES

Abraham WT, Bristow MR 1997 Specialised centres for heart failure management. Circulation 96: 2755–2757

Addington-Hall JM, McCarthy M 1995 Regional study of care for the dying: methods and sample characteristics. Palliative Medicine 9: 27–35

Afzal A, Brawner CA, Keteylan SJ 1998 Exercise training in heart failure. Progress in Cardiovascular Diseases 41: 175–190

Albert N 1999 Heart failure: the physiologic basis for current therapeutic concepts. Critical Care Nurse 13 (suppl): 1–13

American Heart Association 1995 Guidelines for the evaluation and management of heart failure. Report of the American College of Cardiology/American Heart Association Task Force on Practice Guidelines (Committee on Evaluation and Management of Heart Failure). Circulation 92(9): 2764–2784

American Heart Association 1999 Heart and stroke statistical update. American Heart Association, Dallas

Astrand P-O, Rodahl K 1986 Textbook of work physiology: physiological bases of exercise. McGraw-Hill, New York

ATLAS Study 1998 Results of the Assessment of Treatment with Lisinopril and Survival Trial (ATLAS). Presented at the 47th Annual Scientific Session of the American College of Cardiology, Atlanta, GA, April 29th

Auricchio A, Stellbrink C, Block M et al 1999 for the Pacing Therapies for Congestive Heart Failure Study Group. The Guidant Heart Failure Research Group. Effect of pacing chamber and atrioventricular delay on acute systolic function of paced patients with congestive heart failure. Circulation 99: 2993–3001

Batista RJ, Verde J, Nery P 1997 Partial left ventriculectomy to treat end-stage heart disease. Annals of Thoracic Surgery 64(3): 634–638

BHF 2001 Coronary heart disease statistics: morbidity supplement. British Heart Foundation, London

Blomqvist CG, Saltin B 1983 Cardiovascular adaptations to physical training. Annual Review of Physiology 45: 169–189

Borg GAV 1982 Psychophysical basis of perceived exertion. Medicine and Science in Sports and Exercise 14(5): 377–381

Brater DC 2000 Loop diuretics – translating pharmokinetic properties into improved clinical outcomes (abstract). Therapeutic options in CHF – focus on diuretics. Heart Failure Update, 'Venice 2000'

Brophy JM, Deslauriers G, Rouleau JL 1994 Long-term prognosis of patients presenting to the emergency room with decompensated congestive heart failure. Canadian Journal of Cardiology 10(5): 543–547

Camm AJ 1993 Cardiovascular disease In: Kumar PJ, Clark ML (eds) Clinical medicine, 2nd edn. Baillière Tindall, London, pp. 511–626

CAST Study 1991 The Cardiac Arrhythmia Suppression Trial. Mortality and morbidity in patients receiving encainide, flecainide or placebo. New England Journal of Medicine 324(12): 781–788

CIBIS-II Investigators and Committees 1999 The Cardiac Insufficiency Bisoprolol Study II (CIBIS-II): a randomised trial. Lancet 353: 9–13

Cintron G, Bigas C, Linares E, Aranda J, Hernandez E 1983 Nurse practitioner role in a chronic congestive heart failure clinic: in hospital time, costs, and patient satisfaction. Heart and Lung 12: 237–240

Cleland JGF, Erdmann E, Ferrari R et al 1995 Guidelines for the diagnosis of heart failure. European Heart Journal 16: 741–751

Cleland JGF, McGowan J, Clark A 1999 The evidence for beta blockers in heart failure (editorial). British Medical Journal 318: 824–825

Coats A, Adamopoulos S, Radaelli A et al 1992 Controlled trial of physical training in chronic heart failure. Circulation 85(6): 2119–2131

Colucci WS, Packer M, Bristow MR for the US Carvedilol Heart Failure Study Group 1996 Carvedilol inhibits clinical progression in patients with mild symptoms of heart failure. Circulation 94: 2800–2806

Cowie MR, Mosterd A, Wood DA et al 1997 The epidemiology of heart failure. European Heart Journal 18: 208–225

Davies MK, Gibbs CR, Lip GYH 2000 ABC of heart failure: management: diuretics, ACE inhibitors, and nitrates. British Medical Journal 320: 428–431

Department of Health 1998 Changing gear: guidelines for managing the last days of life in adults (HSC 1998/115). Department of Health, London

Department of Health 2000 National Service Framework for Coronary Heart Disease. Chapter 6 Heart Failure. Department of Health, London

DIG Trial 1997 The effect of digoxin on mortality and morbidity in patients with heart failure. The Digitalis Investigation Group. New England Journal of Medicine 336(8): 525–533

Doughty RN 1999 Beta-blockers for advanced heart failure – how far can you go? European Journal of Heart Failure 1(3): 259–262

Dracup KA, Walden JA, Stevenson LW 1989 Sexual activity in patients with end stage congestive heart failure. Circulation 80 (suppl II): 563

Edep ME, Shah NB, Tateo IM, Massie BM 1997 Differences between primary care physicians and cardiologists in management of congestive heart failure: relation to practice guidelines. Journal of the American College of Cardiology 30: 518–526

Eriksson H 1995 Heart failure: a growing public health problem. Journal of Internal Medicine 237(2): 135–141

European Heart Failure Training Group 1998 Experience from controlled trials of physical training in chronic heart failure. Protocol and patient factors in effectiveness in the improvement of exercise tolerance. European Heart Journal 19(3): 466–475

European Society of Cardiology 1997 The treatment of heart failure. Task Force of the Working Group on Heart Failure. European Heart Journal 18: 736–753

Freeman LM, Roubenoff R 1994 The nutritional implications of cardiac cachexia. Nutrition Reviews 52(10): 340–347

Garg R, Yusuf S 1995 Overview of randomised trials of angiotensin converting enzyme inhibitors on mortality and morbidity in patients with heart failure. Collaborative group on ACE Inhibitor Trials. Journal of the American Medical Association 273: 1450–1456

Gianuzzi P, Tavazzi L, Meyer K et al 2001 Recommendations for exercise training in chronic heart failure patients; working group report. European Heart Journal 22: 125–135

Gibbs LME, Addington-Hall J, Gibbs JSR 1998 Dying from heart failure: lessons from palliative care (editorial). British Medical Journal 317: 961–962

Hanumanthu S, Butler J, Chomsky D, Davis S, Wilson JR 1997 Effect of a heart failure programme on hospitalisation frequency and exercise tolerance. Circulation 96: 2842–2848

Hellerstein HK, Friedman EH 1970 Sexual activity and the postcoronary patient. Archives of Internal Medicine 125(6): 987–999

Higginson I 1993 Palliative care: a review of past changes and future trends. Journal of Public Health Medicine 15: 3–8

Ho KKL, Anderson KM, Kannel WB, Grossman W, Levy D 1993a Survival after onset of congestive heart failure in the Framingham Heart Study subjects. Circulation 88(1): 107–115

Ho KK, Pinsky JL, Kannel WB, Levy D 1993b The epidemiology of heart failure: the Framingham Study. Journal of the American College of Cardiology 22 (4 suppl A): 6A–13A

Hobbs FDR, Davis RC, Lip GYH 2000 ABC of heart failure: heart failure in general practice. British Medical Journal 320: 626–629

Jaarsma T, Dracup K, Walden J, Stevenson LW 1996 Sexual function in patients with advanced heart failure. Heart and Lung 25(4): 262–270

Kannel B, Belanger AJ 1991 Epidemiology of heart failure American Heart Journal 121: 951–957

Kannel WB, Plehn JF, Cupples LA 1988 Cardiac failure and sudden death in the Framingham Study. American Heart Journal 115: 869–875

Kass DA 1998 Surgical approaches to arresting or reversing chronic remodelling of the failing heart. Journal of Cardiac Failure 4(1): 57–66

Klein RF, Dean A, Bogdonoff DA 1967 The impact of illness upon the spouse. Journal of Chronic Disease 20: 241–248

Koch M, Douard H, Broustat JP 1992 The benefit of graded physical exercise in chronic heart failure. Chest 101: 231S–235S

Kostis JB, Rosen RC, Cosgrove NM et al 1994 Non pharmacological therapy improves functional and emotional status in congestive heart failure. Chest 106: 996–1001

Law MR, Frost CD, Wald NJ 1991 How much does dietary salt reduction lower blood pressure? Analysis of observational data among populations. British Medical Journal 302: 811–823

Lechat P, Jaillon P, Fontaine ML et al 1994 A randomised trial of beta blockade in heart failure. The Cardiac Insufficiency Bisoprolol study (CIBIS). Circulation 90: 1765–1773

Lenfant C 1994 Report of the Task Force on Research in Heart Failure. Circulation 90: 1118–1123

Lonn E, McKelvie R 2000 Drug treatment in heart failure. British Medical Journal 320: 1188–1192

Lowes BD, Gill EA, Rodriguez-Larrain J, Abraham WT, Bristow MR, Gilbert EM 1996 Carvedilol is associated with a reversal of remodelling in chronic heart failure. Circulation 94(8)(suppl 1): 1–407

McCarthy M, Lay M, Addington-Hall JM 1996 Dying from heart disease. Journal of the Royal College of Physicians 30: 325–328

McCarthy M, Addington-Hall JM, Lay M 1997 Communication and choice in dying from heart disease. Journal of the Royal Society of Medicine 90: 128–131

McDonagh TA, Dargie HJ 1998 Epidemiology and pathophysiology of heart failure. Medicine 26(1): 111–115

McKelvie RS, Yusuf S 1997 Large trials and meta-analysis. In: Poole-Wilson PA, Colucci WS, Massie BM, Chatterjee K, Coats A (eds) Heart failure: scientific principles and clinical practice. Churchill Livingstone, New York, pp. 597–615

McKelvie RS, Benedict CR, Yusuf S 1998 Prevention of congestive heart failure and management of asymptomatic left ventricular dysfunction. In: Yusuf S, Cairns JA, Camm AJ, Fallen EL, Gersh BJ (eds) Evidence based cardiology. BMJ Books, London, pp. 703–721

McKelvie RS, Benedict CR, Yusuf S 1999 Prevention of congestive heart failure and management of asymptomatic left ventricular dysfunction. British Medical Journal 318: 1400–1402

McMurray J, Davie E 1996 The pharmacoeconomics of ACE inhibitors in heart failure. Pharmacoeconomics 9: 186–197

McMurray J, McDonagh T, Morrison CE, Dargie HJ 1993 Trends in hospitalisation for heart failure in Scotland 1980–1990. European Heart Journal 4: 1158–1162

Merit-HF Study Group 1999 Metoprolol CR/XL in chronic heart failure. Metoprolol CR/XL randomised intervention trial in congestive heart failure (Merit-HF). Lancet 353: 2001–2007

Meyer K, Samek L, Schwaibold M et al 1996 Physical responses to different modes of interval exercise in patients with chronic heart failure – application to exercise training. European Heart Journal 17: 1040–1047

Millane T, Jackson G, Gibbs CR, Lip GYH 2000 ABC of heart failure: acute and chronic management strategies. British Medical Journal 320: 559–562

Miller JF 1992 Coping with chronic illness, overcoming powerlessness, 2nd edn. FA Davis, Philadelphia

Minotti JR, Christopher I, Oka R, Weiner MW, Lauren W, Massie BM 1991 Impaired skeletal muscle function in patients with congestive heart failure. Journal of Clinical Investigation 88: 2077–2082

Moos RH 1982 Coping with acute health crisis. In: Milton T, Green C, Meagher R (eds) Hand book of clinical health psychology. Plenum Press, New York, pp. 129–151

Mosterd A, Hoes AW, De Bruyne MC et al 1999 Prevalence of heart failure and left ventricular dysfunction in the general population: the Rotterdam Study. European Heart Journal 20(6): 447–455

Mullen PD, Mains DA, Velez R 1992 A meta-analysis of controlled trials of cardiac patient education. Patient Education and Counselling 19: 143–162

Nichol KL, Margolis KL, Wuorenma J, Von Sternberg T 1994 The efficacy and cost effectiveness of vaccination against influenza among elderly persons living in the community. New England Journal of Medicine 331: 778–784

North TC, McCullagh P, Tran ZV 1990 Effect of exercise on depression. Exercise and Sport Science Review 18: 379–415

O'Connell JB, Bristow MR 1994 Economic impact of heart failure in the United States: time for a different approach. Journal of Heart and Lung Transplantation 13: S107–S112

Packer M, Bristow MR, Cohn JN et al 1996 The effect of carvedilol on morbidity and mortality in patients with chronic heart failure. US Carvedilol Heart Failure Study Group. New England Journal of Medicine 334: 1349–1355

Philbin EF 1998 Factors determining angiotensin-converting enzyme inhibitor underutilization in heart failure in a community setting. Clinical Cardiology 21(2): 103–108

Pitt B, Segal R, Martinez FA et al 1997 Randomised trial of losartan versus captopril in patients over 65 with heart failure (Evaluation of Losartan in the Elderly Study, ELITE). Lancet 349: 747–752

Pitt B, Zannad F, Remme WJ et al for the Randomised Aldactone Evaluation Study on Mortality and Morbidity in Patients with Severe Heart Failure 1999 The effect of spironolactone on morbidity and mortality in patients with severe heart failure. New England Journal of Medicine 341(10): 709–717

Rich MW, Beckham V, Wittenberg C, Leven CL, Freedland KE, Carney RM 1995 A multi disciplinary intervention to prevent the readmission of elderly patients with congestive heart failure. New England Journal of Medicine 333(18): 1190–1195

Rogers AE, Addington-Hall JM, Abery AJ et al 2000 Knowledge and communication difficulties for patients with chronic heart failure: qualitative study. British Medical Journal 321: 605–607

Sharpe N, Doughty R 1998 Epidemiology of heart failure and ventricular dysfunction. Lancet 352 (suppl 1): S13–S17

Smith LE, Fabbri SA, Pai R, Ferry D, Heywood JT 1997 Symptomatic improvement and reduced hospitalisation for patients attending a cardiomyopathy clinic. Clinical Cardiology 20(11): 949–954

Sollano JA, Johnson J, Ahern D et al 1992 Is there sex after heart failure? Report of a prospective study of sexual desire and activity in patients with advanced symptoms

enrolled in the Promised Trial. Journal of the American College of Cardiology 164: 1868–1874

SOLVD Investigators 1991 Effect of enalapril on survival in patients with reduced left ventricular ejection fractions and congestive heart failure. New England Journal of Medicine 325: 293–302

Swales JD 1991 Salt substitutes and potassium intake. British Medical Journal 303: 1084–1085

Swanton RH 1998 Cardiology, 4th edn. Blackwell Science, Oxford

Vasan RS, Larson MG, Benjamin EF, Evans JC, Reiss CK, Levy D 1999 Congestive heart failure in subjects with normal versus reduced left ventricular ejection fraction. Journal of the American College of Cardiology 33: 1948–1955

Vinson JM, Rich MW, Sperry JC, Shah AS, McNamara T 1990 Early re-admission of elderly patients with congestive heart failure. Journal of the American Geriatric Society 38: 1290–1295

West JA, Miller NH, Parker KM et al 1997 A comprehensive management system for heart failure improves clinical outcomes and reduces medical resource utilisation. American Journal of Cardiology 79: 58–63

Willenheimer R, Erhardt L, Cline C, Rydberg E, Israelsson B 1998 Exercise training in heart failure improves quality of life and exercise capacity. European Heart Journal 19(5): 774–781

Zeiger RS, Heller S, Mellon MH, Ward J, Falkoff R, Schatz M 1991 Facilitated referral to asthma specialist reduces relapses in asthma emergency room visits. Journal of Allergy and Clinical Immunology 87: 1160–1168

FURTHER READING

Stewart S, Blue L (eds) 2001 Improving outcomes in chronic heart failure. BMJ Books, London.

11

Cardiomyopathies

Ann O'Donoghue

In the past the cardiomyopathies have been described as heart muscle disease of unknown cause and were differentiated from cardiomyopathies which developed from specific disease of the heart muscle (WHO/ISFC 1980). In 1995 the World Health Organization/International Society and Federation of Cardiology Task Force met to redefine the classifications of the cardiomyopathies (WHO/ISFC 1996). They defined them as diseases of the myocardium associated with cardiac dysfunction. These are classified as dilated cardiomyopathy (DCM), hypertrophic cardiomyopathy (HCM), arrhythmogenic right ventricular cardiomyopathy or dysplasia (ARVC/D) and restrictive cardiomyopathy (RCM). The term 'specific cardiomyopathies' is used to describe heart muscle diseases that are associated with specific systemic or cardiac disorders. There are some cardiomyopathies which do not fit into any particular group. These can present with features of more than one type of cardiomyopathy and have been termed the unclassified cardiomyopathies.

This chapter will examine the pathology, clinical presentation, management and treatment of patients with cardiomyopathy. It also aims to highlight for the cardiac nurse the psychosocial aspects that are part of the disease and the ethical issues that arise in relation to familial evaluation and genetic testing.

DILATED CARDIOMYOPATHY

Dilated cardiomyopathy (DCM) appears to be the most common of the cardiomyopathies with a prevalence of up to 40/100 000 and an annual incidence estimated at 5–8/100 000 (Codd et al 1989). However, the true prevalence of DCM is unknown as asymptomatic or mildly affected individuals are likely to escape detection. Some patients may even recover after the initial insult. DCM is characterized by:

- dilatation of the left or both ventricles (Plate 11.2)
- impaired systolic function of the left or both ventricles.

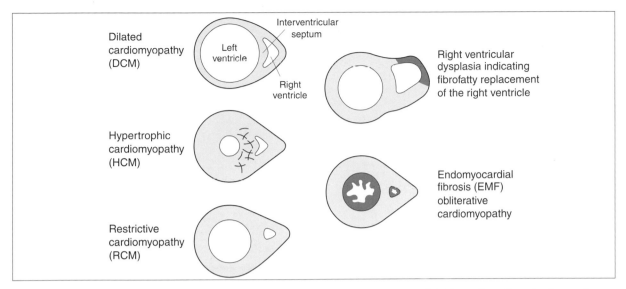

Figure 11.1 Morphological expression of different functional forms of cardiomyopathy. This illustration will assist the reader to understand the various manifestations of cardiomyopathy. It will also assist when examining the colour plates highlighting the various presentations.

Pathology

At post mortem the histological features are non-specific. In idiopathic dilated cardiomyopathy no cause is identifiable but certain features may be present. The myoctes (muscle cells) may be hypertrophied with areas of myocyte necrosis. The nuclei may be large with bizarre shapes (Plate 11.3).

Dilated cardiomyopathy is associated with the consequences of pump failure and cardiac enlargement. There is usually systolic and diastolic dysfunction of both ventricles. This may be further increased by atrial systolic abnormalities, such as atrial fibrillation or enlargement. There may be valvular regurgitation due to mitral and tricuspid annuli enlargement secondary to ventricular dilatation. Electromechanical problems can also result from left bundle branch block. Impaired systolic function can affect either left, right or both ventricles and results in poor ventricular contraction.

Historically the diagnosis has been made by demonstration of a poorly contracting ventricle with an ejection fraction of less than 40% (the normal range is usually approximately 70%) (Field et al 1973). Although there is increased myocardial mass, the ratio of left ventricular blood volume to ventricular wall thickness is much greater than that seen in patients with hypertrophic cardiomyopathy or hypertensive heart disease with diastolic dysfunction (Goodwin 1964).

Initially patients may benefit from the Frank–Starling mechanism (Starling's Law of the heart) whereby the enlarged left ventricular cavity stretches the myocardium and increases the force of contraction. The compensatory capacity of the stretched myocyte may be exceeded, however, and there may be a reduction in stroke volume. Patients may remain asymptomatic if right ventricular function and systemic vasodilator reserve are intact. Cardiac output can be maintained by an increase in heart rate and a reduction in peripheral resistance during exercise. These compensatory mechanisms eventually fail and the patient develops cardiac failure.

Most patients who present with DCM are adults but it is seen in infants and older children. Sudden death may occur at any stage. The pathogenesis of the condition is still poorly understood. Box 11.1 gives a list of various diseases and specific causes that can result in DCM.

Idiopathic dilated cardiomyopathy is a condition of unknown cause in which the heart is enlarged and contracts poorly. The familial and probable genetic basis has only recently been emphasized. Approximately 20–25% of affected individuals will have a familial autosomal dominant inheritance pattern (Michels et al 1992). In other words, if one parent has the disease, then there is a 50/50 risk that each child will inherit the single dominant gene and be affected (Fig. 11.2). Through clinical evaluation, relatives of affected family

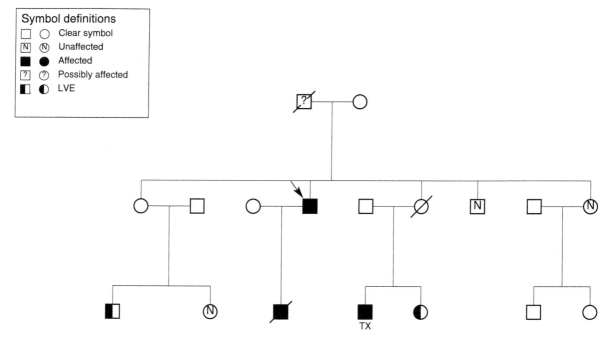

Figure 11.2 Pedigree (family tree) of dilated cardiomyopathy, left ventricular enlargement (LVE), proband (arrowed) and affected individuals. The circles represent females, squares represent males. The horizontal lines indicate a mating, vertical lines are offspring. A line through a shape indicates a death. The clear symbol indicates that the person has not been investigated or is in the process of investigation. Proband = the first person to present with the disease to clinic, whose family history or pedigree is being constructed to discover who else has and is suffering with the disease. TX = cardiac transplant.

members may be diagnosed with DCM, others may be asymptomatic, but echocardiography may reveal increased left ventricular enlargement.

Asymptomatic patients can present as young adults with cardiac enlargement before developing symptomatic heart failure, arrhythmias or thrombo-embolism (Keeling et al 1995). Baig et al (1998) demonstrated a group of asymptomatic relatives with left ventricular enlargement at family screening. These relatives were followed up over a 3-year period and 30% of them progressed to develop symptomatic dilated cardiomyopathy. Of these 30%, one patient died suddenly and one patient progressed to heart transplantation (Baig et al 1998). This suggests that familial dilated cardiomyopathy has variable and age-related penetrance. Cardiovascular evaluation of first-degree relatives should be an established practice, with the aim of identifying early disease and preventing major complications such as embolic or sudden death. Though unproven in large clinical trials, introduction of angiotensin-converting enzyme (ACE) inhibition and β-blockade drug therapy early rather than at end-stage disease may attenuate disease progression.

Preliminary data have reported several gene loci responsible for dilated cardiomyopathy but no specific gene abnormality in these loci has been identified yet. Krajinovic et al (1995) identified a large family with dilated cardiomyopathy and ventricular arrhythmias and mapped them to chromosome 9 (9q13–q22). The condition has been linked to chromosome 1q32 (Durrand et al 1995), chromosome 3 (3p22–p25) (Olson & Keating 1996) and chromosome 10 (10q21–23) (Bowels et al 1996). A rare form of dilated cardiomyopathy associated with conduction abnormalities has been linked to chromosome 1 (1p1–1q1) and was identified by Kass et al (1994). The disease affected young family members who initially developed heart block in their second and third decades of life. They then progressed to develop cardiomegaly (cardiac enlargement) and heart failure in their fifth and sixth decades. The only disease gene known so far is the dystrophin gene, which causes X-linked DCM (Stevens & Ground 1970).

Myotonic dystrophy is also found on chromosome 19 and these patients develop conduction disturbances and DCM. Viral and abnormal immune responses are

Box 11.1 WHO (1996) classification of causes of dilated cardiomyopathy

- Idiopathic
- Genetic familial:
    Autosomal dominant inheritance pattern
    Dilated cardiomyopathy and conduction disease (C1p1–1q1)
    Neuromuscular: Duchenne, Becker (Xp21), myotonic dystrophies (C19)
    Mitochondrial cardiomyopathies
    Friedreich's ataxia (rare)
- Alcoholic/toxic
- Anthracyclines
- Irradiation
- Cocaine/amphetamines
- Cobalt/heavy metals
- Viral infection:
    Coxsackie B
    Adenovirus
    Cytomegalovirus
    Varicella zoster
    Human immunodeficiency virus 1
    Hepatitis C
- Infections:
    Borrelia burgdorferi
    Chagas' disease
- Inflammatory:
    Collagen vascular disease
    Sarcoidosis
    Peripartum cardiomyopathy
- Specific cardiovascular conditions:
    Ischaemic heart disease
    Valvular disease
    Hypertensive disease
    Hypertrophic cardiomyopathy
    Incessant tachyarrhythmia
- Metabolic:
    Thyrotoxicosis
    Acromegaly
    Cushing's syndrome
    Phaeochromocytoma
    Diabetes mellitus
    Deficiencies of carnitine, thiamine, selenium and co-enzyme A
    Uraemia
    Sickle cell
    Chronic anaemias
- Pregnancy:
    Cause unknown
    Advanced maternal age
    African descent
    Multiparity and twinning are risk factors

also thought to be an underlying cause for dilated cardiomyopathy.

Myocarditis (inflammation of the myocardium) may be due to a number of causes, especially viral related, as listed in Box 11.1. Myocarditis is the most common form of inflammatory endomyocardial disease. The clinical manifestations of inflammatory heart disease span from an asymptomatic condition, where most patients with myocarditis will never be aware that they are infected and therefore will not seek medical advice, to patients who present with an acute illness often characterized by fever and cardiac failure and in some cases sudden cardiac death. The incidence of myocarditis on post mortem following sudden cardiac death in previously healthy individuals is 2.2% (Stevens & Ground 1970). When an apparently healthy young individual presents with unexplained heart failure, ventricular arrhythmia and/or ST and T-wave abnormalities on the electrocardiogram (ECG), elevated cardiac biochemical markers and in some cases elevated viral antibody titres, myocarditis should be diagnosed (Rodkey et al 1998). Endomyocardial biopsy confirms the diagnosis of myocarditis and shows acute inflammation. Treatment of myocarditis includes bedrest and an exercise restriction should be imposed. This rests the heart because in the presence of poor left ventricular function, exercise can increase the heart's workload and exacerbate the symptoms. Treatment is aimed towards alleviating any acute infection, with the management of heart failure and cardiac arrhythmias. Prognosis is usually favourable depending on the aetiology although a chronic cardiomyopathy may develop (Camm 1998).

Environmental factors may trigger a chronic immune response to cardiac antigens that results in DCM. Peripartum dilated cardiomyopathy is defined as left ventricular systolic dysfunction without apparent cause, occurring in the peripartal period. The onset can occur at any time during the third trimester of pregnancy or within the first 6 months following delivery. It is most common during the first 2 months post partum (75%) (Stevens & Ground 1970). The incidence has been reported to be anywhere between 1:1300 to 1:1500 pregnancies. Risk factors include:

- twin pregnancy
- age greater than 30 years
- multiparity
- a family history of peripartum cardiomyopathy
- African descent
- prolonged therapy with tocolytic agents (medications to decrease uterine contraction and prolong gestation).

The natural history of peripartum cardiomyopathy differs from other forms of DCM; 50% of patients will spontaneously recover, usually within the first 6 weeks to 6 months. Improvement after 6 months is unlikely while 25–50% patients die or require cardiac transplantation. Death may be due to congestive cardiac failure, arrhythmias and/or embolic events. The latter may be due to the heart's poor pumping action inducing clots. Atrial fibrillation will also increase this risk due to poor atrial emptying. It is not possible to identify those patients who are likely to improve. Other associated factors include alcohol and chemical toxicity and metabolic disorders.

Clinical presentation

Presentation is usually with heart failure, which is often progressive and can result in cardiac transplantation. DCM accounts for up to 50% of referrals for cardiac transplantation (Kaye 1993). Arrhythmias, thrombo-embolism and sudden death are common and may occur at any stage. The typical patient who presents with DCM is young or middle aged.

Left ventricular failure consists of:

- shortness of breath on exertion
- reduced exercise capacity
- fatigue
- orthopnoea (breathlessness when lying flat)
- paroxysmal nocturnal dyspnoea (sudden, night-time breathlessness, which wakes the patient).

Some patients will also display peripheral oedema and other signs of right heart failure such as abdominal distension and discomfort. Patients may present with palpitation due to atrial and/or ventricular arrhythmias. Sudden cardiac death occurs, but is an unusual initial presentation of DCM. Embolic complications may be a result of atrial arrhythmias or mural thrombi while chest pain may mimic angina due to coronary artery disease. This is due to an inability to adequately supply the myocardium with oxygen due to contractile (pump) failure. Some patients may present with no symptoms but require investigations due to an incidental finding of cardiomegaly (the most common physical sign), atrial fibrillation, left bundle branch block (LBBB) or other ECG abnormalities.

An important part of the clinical assessment is the patient's medical history as this can reveal specific causes of dilated cardiomyopathy. A family history may reveal an autosomal dominant inheritance pattern and various clinical features particular to that family. Patients who have developed DCM through a viral illness can attribute the fever to some infection, e.g. upper respiratory tract infection, gastro-intestinal infection or myalgia (muscular pain). Patients who have been exposed to toxic substances may be more difficult to identify. Those who have been exposed to irradiation and chemotherapeutic agents are evident but patients who abuse cocaine/amphetamines may be evasive about their drug history. Those who

---

Box 11.2 Clinical signs of dilated cardiomyopathy

- Left and right ventricular congestion:
  Dyspnoea at rest
  Inspiratory crepitations in the lungs
  Pleural effusions
  Occasionally cardiac asthma
  Summation gallop with 3rd and 4th heart
    sounds
  Expiratory wheezing
- Right heart failure:
  Peripheral oedema
  Ascites
  Jugular venous pressure raised
  Hepatomegaly
- Low cardiac output:
  Poor peripheral perfusion
  Systolic blood pressure reduced
- Neuroendocrine:
  Vasoconstricted peripheries
- Activation:
  Tachycardia at rest
- Cardiomegaly:
  Most common physical sign
  Left parasternal heave due to right ventricular
    enlargement
- Murmurs:
  Mitral regurgitation
  Tricuspid regurgitation
  Left bundle branch block (LBBB)
  Systolic murmurs are common with
    regurgitation but they are not loud
  Paradoxic splitting of left heart sound

---

consume excessive amounts of alcohol may also be evasive about their consumption.

The clinician can reveal other cardiac causes of DCM by taking a detailed history, thus identifying any co-existing coronary, valvular and hypertensive heart disease. The clinical examination will reveal signs that reflect cardiac enlargement and the severity of heart failure (Box 11.2).

Investigations

Electrocardiogram (ECG)

The ECG can show diffuse non-specific ST segment and T-wave changes. Sinus tachycardia may be observed in some cases which can be reversed if incessant tachyarrhythmias are slowed down. Twenty percent of patients develop atrial fibrillation. Its onset can be characterized by heart failure. Eighty percent of patients may present with left bundle branch block (LBBB) which is associated with a higher risk of death. LBBB may be due to extensive myocardial fibrosis. Asymptomatic non-sustained ventricular tachycardias may be observed on Holter monitoring recordings and are associated with a poor prognosis.

Two-dimensional and Doppler echocardiography

Echocardiography (echo) is an important non-invasive investigation for DCM. It is useful in detecting anatomical and functional abnormalities of the heart. Cardiac architecture, contractile function, haemodynamics, valve regurgitation and detection of intracardiac thrombus can be evaluated in patients with DCM.

The two-dimensional echocardiogram characteristically reveals a dilated, poorly contracting left ventricle (LV). The diagnostic echocardiographic features are increased LV end-diastolic dimensions (>5.6 cm) and severely impaired global contractile function, with LV fractional shortening of less than 25%. Blood flow within the LV is decreased because of LV dilatation and dysfunction. This may be detected by the development of spontaneous echo contrast, which increases the tendency to form thrombus in the LV, particularly at the apex (bottom of the heart).

The right ventricle (RV) is often dilated (>3.0 cm), as a result of primary failure of RV myocardial contraction or secondary to pulmonary hypertension from elevated LV diastolic pressure.

The left atrium (LA) is usually dilated (>4.0 cm) and the right atrium (RA) and inferior vena cava may be dilated, because of either the elevated RV diastolic pressure or tricuspid regurgitation. Doppler studies are useful in assessing the severity of mitral as well as tricuspid regurgitation. Mitral regurgitation secondary to dilatation of the LV is frequently noted. RV dilatation and elevation of pulmonary artery pressure result in tricuspid regurgitation. LV diastolic pressure can be estimated by the pattern of LV filling signals on Doppler study. This pattern changes as the disease progresses. It is not always easy to distinguish idiopathic DCM from DCM secondary to other causes, such as ischaemic heart disease, systemic disease and valvular disease. Echocardiographic findings including regional ventricular wall abnormalities, abnormal texture of ventricular wall and anatomical abnormalities of the valves might be helpful in searching for other causes.

In conclusion, two-dimensional and Doppler echocardiography can identify the myopathic state (myocardial function, wall thickness and so forth) and evaluate its severity and the effects of therapy. Complications associated with DCM, such as valvular regurgitation and thrombus, can also be demonstrated.

Chest X-ray

This demonstrates biventricular enlargement and cardiomegaly.

Radionuclide investigations

Multigated acquisition (MUGA) can be used to evaluate left ventricular function and ejection fraction, when echocardiography imaging is inadequate. A technetium-99m labelled radiopharmaceutical is injected into the patient and attaches to haemoglobin in the red blood cells. Anterior, left anterior oblique and left lateral, ECG-gated images are then acquired. The resulting images depict the blood flow in the ventricle during systole and diastole, allowing very accurate measurement of the ejection fraction. Abnormal ventricular wall motion can also be identified.

Thallium-201 scanning evaluates tissue perfusion and identifies areas of ischaemia and fibrosis.

VO₂ max exercise test

This test measures peak exercise oxygen consumed per minute, expressed as either an absolute value or as litres per kilogram of body weight per minute. If this is less than 10 ml/kg/min the patient will be considered for transplantation.

Blood tests

All patients should undergo routine biochemical blood screening to identify or exclude the specific causes of dilated cardiomyopathy. Table 11.1 lists the routine investigations and additional blood tests that may be ordered.

Other tests may include norepinephrine levels, creatine kinase isoforms MB2/MB1 and cardiac-specific antibodies. These remaining blood tests in a research setting may assist clinical diagnosis and characterization of the disease.

Cardiac catheterisation

Patients undergo catheterisation to exclude coronary artery disease. Right and left heart catheterisation can provide prognostic information, especially prior to cardiac transplantation. It can also monitor clinical treatment. Catheterisation in paediatric dilated cardiomyopathy can differentiate primary heart muscle disease from congenital coronary anomalies.

Endomyocardial biopsy

Endomyocardial biopsies may be taken from either ventricle. This can be used to exclude a specific cardiomyopathy and to assess viral and inflammatory involvement, usually for research purposes.

Table 11.1 Blood tests taken as part of investigations for dilated cardiomyopathy

Test	To identify	
Urea and creatinine	Uraemia	Routine
Thyroid function	Hypo/hyperthyroidism	Routine
Liver function		Routine
γ-glutamyl-transferase	Alcoholism	
Electrolytes	Hypokalaemia (a low serum potassium)	Routine
	Cushing's syndrome (overproduction of glucocorticoids by the adrenal cortex)	
Glucose	Diabetes	
	Acromegaly (excessive secretion of growth hormone in adult life)	
Full blood count	Anaemia	
Erythrocyte sedimentation rate (ESR)	Active systemic inflammation	
Mean corpuscular volume		
Specific DNA gene analysis	Familial dilated cardiomyopathy	
Serum ferritin	Haemochromatosis (chronic disease where the iron-containing pigment, haemosiderin, deposits in the liver, leading to cirrhosis)	
Sera for enteroviral neutralizing	History of viral infection	
Antibodies/IgM ELISA	Patients at high risk/low CD4 lymphocyte	
HIV1 serology	counts	
Phaeochromocytoma screen	Premature or paroxysmal hypertension	
Sickle cell screening	Afro-Caribbean patients	
Specific auto-antibody screening	Connective tissue disease	

Electrophysiology studies

This procedure may be required in the management of symptomatic arrhythmias but is not indicated as part of a routine risk stratification for sudden death.

Treatment

Patients who present with symptomatic heart failure should receive treatment which aims to relieve their symptoms, to improve their quality and duration of life. The clinical management should include the prevention and treatment of complications and in some instances the treatment of the specific causes of the condition. All patients are advised to participate in symptom-limited exercise. This is exercising but stopping if symptoms such as undue breathlessness, light-headedness, chest pain, etc. occur. It has been observed that symptom-limited exercise training leads to better peak exercise capacity and systemic oxygen uptake, through afterload reduction and improvement in diastolic function. The afterload can be defined as the resistance to the ventricular ejection of blood, usually offered by the systemic circulation constricting to maintain adequate tissue perfusion. Regular exercise is also an important factor in maintaining the patient's physiological and sociological well-being. Isometric exercise (weights, body building) is not recommended because it places an acute strain on the heart. Patients are encouraged to reduce alcohol intake and other toxins. Those with alcoholic cardiomyopathy may require thiamine replacement and correction of magnesium and phosphate deficiency.

Angiotensin-converting enzyme (ACE) inhibitors may be indicated in asymptomatic patients if their left ventricular ejection fraction is low. If there is a family history of left ventricular enlargement and poor ejection fraction, ACE inhibitors can improve the ejection fraction and halt further left ventricular enlargement (LVE) and thus improve prognosis. They may also be used in those with symptomatic heart failure to improve and prolong their quality of life.

Hydralazine and nitrates are used if the patient is intolerant of ACE inhibitors. Carvedilol or metoprolol are used if the patient presents with a tachycardia or arrhythmias. Digitalis is indicated if the patient cannot tolerate β-blockers, e.g. in asthmatics. Diuretics are given and dietary salt intake is reduced if the patient is oedematous.

Drug therapy used to control the ventricular rate will again be digoxin and/or low-dose β-blockers and calcium antagonists. All patients with atrial fibrillation should be anticoagulated in the absence of specific contra-indications. If a patient has a history of the latter together with a dilated left atrium, embolic episodes, cardiac thrombus or heart failure, anticoagulation is clearly indicated.

Patients who have documented sustained ventricular arrhythmias or who are survivors of cardiac arrest should be considered for amiodarone or an implantable cardioverter defibrillator (ICD).

Patients who fail to respond to drug therapy prescribed for ventricular arrhythmias will be considered for an ICD. This may prevent sudden death from arrhythmias by delivering a defibrillating shock from an internally placed device, which tracks the heart's electrical activity. They are unlikely to prevent progression of heart failure (see Chapter 25).

Patients who have severe dilatation and dysfunction are treated through cardiac transplantation, with some requiring mechanical circulatory support prior to this approach. Devices such as the Jarvik 2000 have also been used to augment cardiac function in those with DCM (see Chapter 18).

Patients who are refractory to medical treatment and are poor candidates for cardiac transplantation may benefit from cardiomyoplasty. Here the latissimus dorsi muscle is wrapped around the ventricle and is electrically stimulated to augment left ventricular contraction.

Patients with severe mitral regurgitation due to annular dilatation may be selected for annuloplasty. This is dilatation of the mitral valve annulus via an introduced catheter.

HYPERTROPHIC CARDIOMYOPATHY

In contrast, hypertrophic cardiomyopathy (HCM) is characterized by hypertrophy of the left and/or right ventricles without systemic or cardiac disease, although some patients may present with DCM. The most common presentation of hypertrophy is asymmetric and involves the interventricular septum (Wigle et al 1985).

HCM is predominantly a familial disease with an autosomal dominant inheritance pattern. Mutations in sarcomeric contractile protein genes have been identified as the cause of the disease (Seidman et al 1992). Clinical studies have indicated a prevalence of at least 1:500 of the general population (Maron et al 1995, Savage et al 1983). Patients can be diagnosed as result of an incidental finding such as during a medical examination for insurance cover or more routine investigations or during clinical evaluation of a family. Tragically the first presentation can be sudden death.

The incidence of sudden death in HCM is 2–4% in adults and 4–6% in children and adolescents. These figures have been collated or generated by specialist referral cardiac centres and may reflect a bias to the more severe patients. Studies from several outpatient-based populations report a lower figure of approximately 1% per annum. Data in infants with HCM are limited but sudden death is uncommon in the first decade (McKenna et al 1981, 1988). HCM accounts for up to 50% of all sudden cardiac deaths in individuals aged 25 years or less and is especially common in athletes.

HCM is characterized by:

- myocardial hypertrophy
- disorganization of myocytes and myofibrils (the thread-like structures in the cytoplasm of muscle cells)
- hyperdynamic systolic contraction/left ventricular outflow tract gradients
- diastolic dysfunction
- myocardial fibrosis/ischaemia
- arrhythmias.

Pathology

At post mortem the histological appearance of HCM shows that the cellular structure is in disarray. Myocyte disarray can be found in other cardiac diseases, e.g. aortic stenosis, congenital heart disease and hypertension, but the extent and severity of the disarray are mild in comparison to HCM, where up to 40% of the myocardium may be affected (Davis 1984). Extensive myocardial disarray and fibrosis can be found in hypertrophied myocardium dispersed amongst the relatively normal myocardium. The myocytes are usually arranged in a parallel pattern in normal muscle. In HCM the cells are disorganized, forming circles around foci of connective tissue. The myocytes can be enlarged and irregular in shape. The myofibrillar structure within the cells can also be disorganized (Plates 11.4–11.8).

Disarray is often associated with myocardial fibrosis and can cause scarring in the septum, left ventricular free wall and occasionally the papillary muscles (Maron & Roberts 1979). It is difficult, however, to assess myocardial disarray in a living person. These cellular changes are thought to be the cause of electrical instability and diastolic dysfunction (McKenna et al 1990).

Most patients with HCM have a hyperdynamic left ventricle, that ejects very forcefully with a small left ventricular cavity due to hypertrophy, which empties almost completely. The left atrium is often enlarged, reflecting the resistance to left ventricular filling due to an increased left ventricular end-diastolic pressure.

Hypertrophy of the myocardium can present in almost any pattern but commonly affects the left ventricle. The right ventricle is also involved in approximately 30% of cases. It is uncommon to have right ventricular hypertrophy alone. Asymmetric septal hypertrophy (ASH) is the most common presentation, seen in 50–60% of cases (Fig. 11.3). In ASH the interventricular septum is thicker than the posterior or left

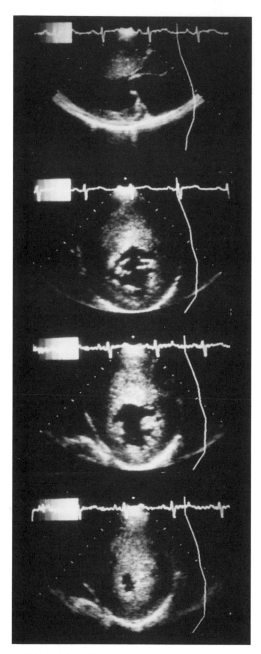

Figure 11.3 Asymmetric septal hypertrophy (ASH) with systolic anterior motion (SAM). The top picture in this two-dimensional echocardiogram demonstrates the mitral leaflet making contact with the septum, which produces regurgitation. In turn, a dilated atrium develops.

ventricular free wall. Approximately 20–25% of patients have a resting pressure gradient between the main body and outflow tract of the left ventricle. A gradient can be defined as a significant pressure difference between two chambers or a chamber and an outflow tract. The term hypertrophic obstructive cardiomyopathy (HOCM) may be used. In most cases this is accompanied by a characteristic systolic anterior motion of the anterior mitral valve leaflet during myocardial contraction. This is detected during echocardiography.

The exact mechanism of this obstruction is debatable but the most widely accepted theory is that the asymmetric septal hypertrophy and the narrowing outflow tract during systole produce a high-velocity stream of blood above the mitral valve. This causes the tip of the anterior mitral valve leaflet to be 'sucked' against the septum (SAM). This is known as the **Venturi effect** (Maron et al 1983). Abnormalities of the mitral valve and leaflet elongation may contribute to the occurrence of SAM.

Some patients may not have outflow tract obstruction at rest. They may have gradients that can be provoked by exercise or increased heart rate and manoeuvres that diminish left ventricular end-diastolic volume or augment left ventricular contractility. For the purpose of a clinical diagnosis, these patients may need to undergo manoeuvres that provoke the gradient, e.g. Valsalva (squatting) or a stress echo. The latter is where the patient is asked to exercise and then an echo is taken.

Obstructive mechanical problems result in symptoms of:

- shortness of breath
- chest pain
- presyncope (dizzy spells)
- syncope (transient loss of consciousness, due to reduced cerebral blood flow, linked here to an abnormal vascular response)
- exercise limitation
- arrhythmias.

The subsequent reduction of the mechanical outflow obstruction can result in a relief of the symptoms. Symmetric or concentric left ventricular hypertrophy with left ventricular outflow tract obstruction occurs in 20–30% of patients. In addition, some of these patients may exhibit total obliteration of the left ventricular cavity in systole (Fig. 11.4).

Apical hypertrophy (Fig. 11.5) is present in approximately 10% of patients with HCM. It seems to be more common in the Japanese than the Western population. Patients with apical hypertrophy usually do not have heart murmurs. It is also associated with giant negative (inverted) T-waves in the precordial ECG leads.

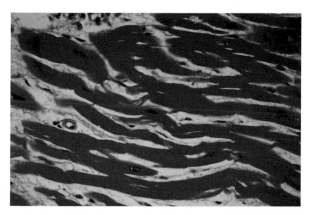

Plate 11.1 Normal heart histology from an autopsy of an elderly man who died in a road traffic accident, The mild variation in myofibre and nuclear size is usual (high power).
  This example will assist the reader in recognizing the differences which occur in the various forms of cardiomyopathy. (Reproduced with kind permission of Professor SB Lucas, Histopathology Department, St Thomas's London.)

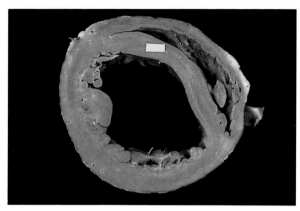

Plate 11.2 Transverse slice of the heart in dilated cardiomyopathy. Marked left ventricular cavity dilatation can be seen. (Reproduced with kind permission of Professor M J Davies. With special thanks to Dr Mary N Sheppard, The Royal Brompton Hospital, London.)

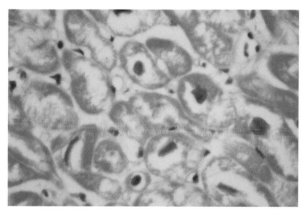

Plate 11.3 Myocyte histology in dilated cardiomyopathy. The striking feature is the loss of myofibrils, giving the myocytes an unduly vacuolated appearance (high power). (Reproduced with kind permission of Professor M J Davies. With special thanks to Dr Mary N Sheppard, The Royal Brompton Hospital, London.)

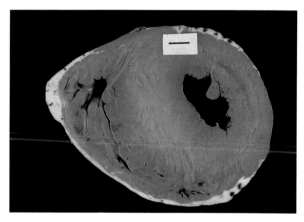

Plate 11.4 Transverse slice of HCM – asymmetric form. A very thick interventricular septum can be seen, compared with the posterior wall of the left ventricle. (Reproduced with kind permission of Professor M J Davies. With special thanks to Dr Mary N Sheppard, The Royal Brompton Hospital, London.)

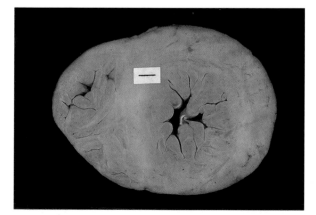

Plate 11.5 Transverse slice of HCM – symmetric form. The left ventricle has a tiny cavity and symmetric wall thickening. (Reproduced with kind permission of Professor M J Davies. With special thanks to Dr Mary N Sheppard, The Royal Brompton Hospital, London.)

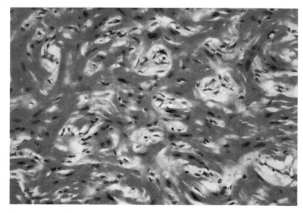

Plate 11.6 Myocyte histology in HCM. To the trained eye, the slide demonstrates the myocyte disarray typical of HCM (medium power). (Reproduced with kind permission of Professor M J Davies. With special thanks to Dr Mary N Sheppard, The Royal Brompton Hospital, London.)

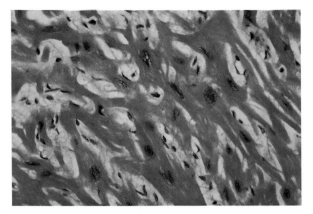

Plate 11.7 Myocyte histology in HCM. In addition to the disorganized myocyte arrangement, the concordance of wide myocytes with very large nuclei and width is a feature (high power). (Reproduced with kind permission of Professor M J Davies. With special thanks to Dr Mary N Sheppard, The Royal Brompton Hospital, London.)

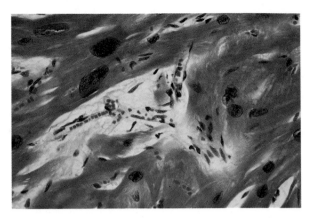

Plate 11.8 Myocyte histology in HCM. Myocytes are arranged in a circular fashion around foci of connective tissue (high power). (Reproduced with kind permission of Professor M J Davies. With special thanks to Dr Mary N Sheppard, The Royal Brompton Hospital, London.)

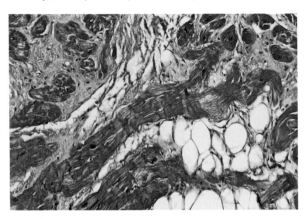

Plate 11.9 Histology of arrhythmogenic right ventricular cardiomyopathy/dysplasia. This slide shows replacement of the right ventricular myocytes with fat and fibrous tissue (high power). (Reproduced with kind permission of Professor M J Davies. With special thanks to Dr Mary N Sheppard, The Royal Brompton Hospital, London.)

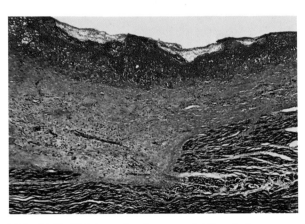

Plate 11.10 Histology of endomyocardial fibrosis (low power). (Reproduced with kind permission of Professor M J Davies. With special thanks to Dr Mary N Sheppard, The Royal Brompton Hospital, London.)

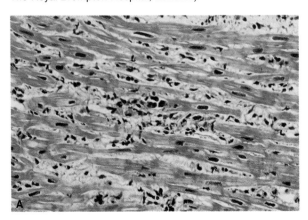
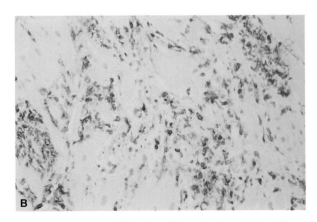

Plate 23.1 Acute rejection (working formulation category 3B). A: Myocardium showing infiltration of lymphocytes in interstitium and surrounding myocytes (H&E x200). B: Immunohistochemical staining in acute rejection showing that the infiltrate is of T-cell origin. The T-cells are identified as the brown-staining cells (streptavidin-biotin x200). (Courtesy of Dr M Burke, Consultant Histopathologist, Royal Brompton and Harefield NHS Trust.)

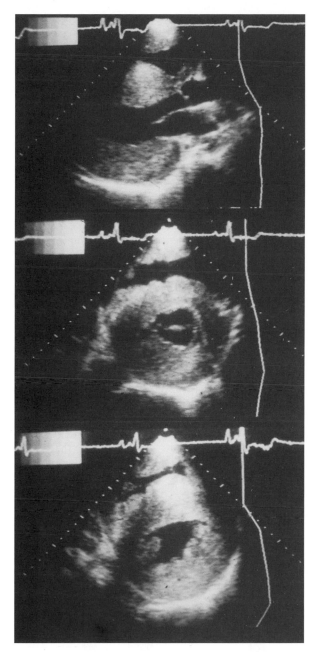

Figure 11.4 Two-dimensional echocardiogram of concentric HCM and left ventricular hypertrophy.

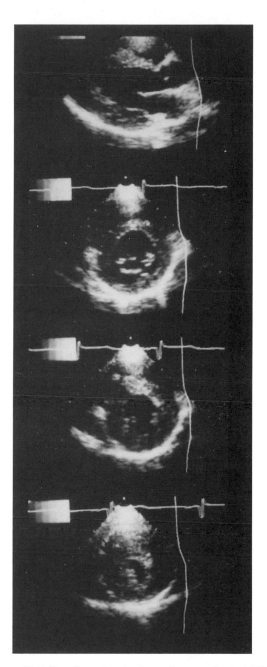

Figure 11.5 Two-dimensional echocardiogram of apical HCM.

Diastolic dysfunction occurs in up to 80% of patients. It results from a combination of impaired myocardial relaxation and reduced ventricular compliance, although the underlying mechanism is not fully understood. It is thought that chamber stiffness is increased due to an increase in muscle mass, creating a smaller ventricular cavity together with a decrease in ventricular volume. The muscle stiffness is possibly caused by myocardial fibrosis and disarray. A stiff ventricle reduces the rate of rapid filling during diastole. This subsequently results in an elevation of left ventricular end-diastolic pressures, which produces a compensatory increase in atrial systolic filling. Impaired myocardial relaxation leads to the development of progressive atrial enlargement and atrial fibrillation (Hanrath et al 1980, Wigle et al 1995).

Elevation of diastolic filling pressures may also contribute to myocardial ischaemia. This can occur in both obstructive (HOCM) and non-obstructive HCM. The exact mechanism of myocardial ischaemia is unknown. It may be due to abnormal intramural coronary arteries with decreased vasodilator capacity. There may be systolic compression of the small coronary arteries. However, an increase in myocardial mass can also result in an increase in oxygen demand. Other causes may be left ventricular outflow tract obstruction creating a greater workload to eject blood, elevated diastolic filling pressures and arrhythmias.

It is thought that myocardial ischaemia may be the cause of chest pain and dyspnoea in a majority of patients with HCM. It may also be an important trigger for arrhythmias and the development of myocardial fibrosis (Dilsizian et al 1993). Arrhythmias may be initiated by many triggers but it is thought that myocyte disarray is the main reason for the development of malignant ventricular arrhythmias which produce sudden death. The exact mechanism is unknown but the disarray may produce multiple electrical pathways which can result in ventricular fibrillation. Most sudden cardiac deaths occur following exertion, which suggests that there are other mechanisms involved such as ischaemia or excessive catecholamine release.

Genetic factors

Hypertrophic cardiomyopathy is a disorder of the sarcomeric contractile proteins. In over 80% of cases it is familial with an autosomal dominant pattern of inheritance. Familial HCM affects about 1 in 500 of the general population (Maron et al 1995, Savage et al 1983). Clinical expression can be varied even within the same family (Fig. 11.6).

Many mutations in genes encoding different cardiac sarcomeric proteins have been described in patients with HCM. These discoveries may hold an explanation for the diverse features of the disease. Box 11.3 lists some of the chromosomal loci that have been found to date. Mutations in the genes encoding the β-myosin heavy chain genes, troponin T and cardiac MyBPC probably account for approximately 50% of all reported cases. The largest number of mutations have been identified in the β-myosin heavy chain gene located on chromosome 14 (Jarcho et al 1989). Over 40 different mutations of this gene have been reported since 1989. The β-myosin heavy chain gene accounts for approximately one-third of familial HCM. α- and β-myosin heavy chain genes are expressed in high levels in the human myocardium, with β-myosin found in the ventricles and α-myosin in the atria.

Sporadic cases account for approximately 10% of HCM. Sporadic disease is usually caused by de novo cardiac heavy chain mutations (Fig. 11.7). These de novo mutations are the strongest evidence that mutations within the sarcomeric contractile protein are causative of the disease (Watkins et al 1992).

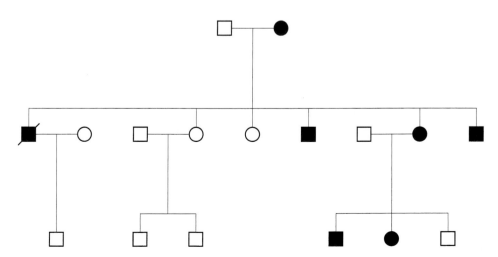

Figure 11.6 Pedigree showing autosomal dominant inheritance. The symbol definitions box and the caption for Figure 11.2 provide details of how to read a pedigree diagram.

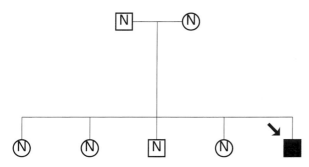

Figure 11.7 Pedigree diagram showing de novo mutation. The proband is indicated by an arrow.

Varying degrees of myocardial hypertrophy exist in patients with HCM, even among affected individuals with the same mutation, within the same family. It is thus apparent that other factors, genetic as well as environmental, must affect the degree of hypertrophy in patients with HCM. The presentation and development of cardiac hypertrophy are regulated by the renin–angiotensin system. A major component of this system is ACE (see Chapters 4 and 10) The ACE genotype DD is more common in patients from families with a high incidence of sudden death than in those without (Lechin et al 1995). It is thought that this genotype may lead to an exaggerated response to cardiac hypertrophy but this theory has yet to be proven.

HCM affects males and females equally. It does not 'skip' a generation but penetrance may be incomplete (e.g. a normal echo and abnormal ECG). The diagnosis of HCM has traditionally relied on echocardiography but in more recent years the systematic evaluation of pedigrees (family history/trees) performed in the context of molecular genetic studies has revealed that in some families with HCM, 20% of adults who carry a disease-causing gene do not fulfill conventional echocardiographic criteria (incomplete penetrance)

(McKenna et al 1997). Despite major advances in the molecular genetics of HCM, gene testing is currently reserved for studying large family pedigrees. The heterogeneity of the condition makes it impractical to offer clinical diagnostic genetic testing for all patients with HCM. In most clinical centres this remains a research-based programme.

Routine genetic testing will become generally available but it will pose a number of difficult issues. These include the ethics and practicalities of preclinical screening, insurance companies' attitude to screening and adequate pre- and post-test counselling. Therapeutic questions will include whether asymptomatic children with mutations associated with a poor prognosis should receive prophylactic therapy.

Clinical presentation

HCM can be diagnosed at any age. The majority of patients (children, adolescents and young adults) are asymptomatic or present with only mild symptoms. They may be diagnosed during family screening. In most patients with HCM there is a slow, gradual, age-related progression of symptoms and commonly adults in their fourth and fifth decades usually present with symptoms.

Chest pain

Exertional chest pain occurs in up to 30% of adults. Some may complain of atypical pain occurring at rest and after meals (Elliott et al 1996). Chest pain may be due to myocardial ischaemia.

Dyspnoea

This is a common complaint amongst adults. This is thought to be due to elevated left ventricular end-diastolic and pulmonary artery occlusion pressure

Box 11.3 Cardiac myosin heavy chain genes (CMH) in hypertrophic cardiomyopathy		
CMH1 Chromosome 14	β-myosin	Largest number of mutations with over 40 different mutations being reported since 1989.
CMH2 Chromosome 1	Troponin-T	Mild or absent left ventricular hypertrophy (LVH). Poor prognosis and high incidence of sudden cardiac death.
CMH3 Chromosome 3	α-tropomyosin	
CMH4 Chromosome 11	MyBPC	MyBPC (myosin binding protein C). Late-onset HCM in 3rd, 4th, 5th and 6th decades.
CMH5 Chromosome 7		A small group of families presented with familial HCM and WPW were linked to chromosome 7.
CMH6 Chromosome 19	Troponin I	
Chromosomes 3 and 12		The essential and regulatory myosin light chains.

(PAOP) from diastolic left ventricular dysfunction. Dyspnoea can increase with exercise due to impaired ventricular filling.

Syncope

Unexplained syncope and dizziness are present in approximately 20% of patients. Syncope may be due to arrhythmias, abnormal vascular responses during exercise or conduction system disease. The cause of syncope is rarely determined despite extensive investigation. Recurrent unexplained syncope in adolescence is associated with a higher risk of sudden death.

Palpitations/arrhythmias

These are a frequent complaint. Non-sustained, infrequent palpitations are usually due to ventricular extrasystoles/ectopics. Sustained palpitation is mostly caused by supraventricular arrhythmias.

Sudden death

Sudden death may be the first presentation of the disease. Sudden death in the first decade of life is uncommon although there are limited data in this group (Maron et al 1982). HCM is the most common cause of sudden death amongst athletes below the age of 30 years (Burke 1991, Maron et al 1980). The terminal event in most cases of sudden death is thought to be ventricular fibrillation.

Clinical signs

In the majority of patients with HCM the physical examination is unremarkable, yet it is always abnormal in patients with obstructive HCM, due to the left ventricular outflow tract obstruction.

Patients with HOCM who have a late ejection systolic murmur may be asked by the clinician to perform certain manoeuvres. This murmur reflects the late onset of the gradient as it is dependent on ventricular volume. Manoeuvres that reduce the afterload or venous return and hence ventricular volume (standing, Valsalva, nitrates) accentuate the murmur. Manoeuvres that increase the afterload and venous return (squatting, phenylephrine) reduce it. The jerky carotid pulse felt in patients with HOCM coincides with the development of the gradient.

Patients with severe left ventricular hypertrophy (LVH) display a heaving apex, which may be displaced laterally. (This may be observed by looking at the patient's chest.) A palpable double apex pulse may

also be present, caused by a chronic elevation of the left ventricular end-diastolic (LVED) pressure due to reduced myocardial compliance, which promotes more forceful atrial systole.

Investigations

The aim in HCM is to establish the diagnosis and assess those patients who may be at risk of sudden death and other complications.

Detailed family history and clinical examination

This can differentiate HCM from other conditions which can cause left ventricular hypertrophy. The clinician can establish if there is a history of multiple premature sudden deaths or recurrent syncope which can increase a patient's 'risk factor' status.

12-lead ECG

This is abnormal in the majority of patients with LVH and the abnormalities are not specific to the disease (Savage et al 1978). The ECG may be abnormal in family members who have inherited the gene but do not exhibit classic echocardiographic features. For example, children and adolescents may demonstrate ECG abnormalities several years before they display ventricular hypertrophy. The latter usually develops during periods of somatic growth, such as in the first year of life or more usually during adolescence. Children require regular investigations with ECG and two-dimensional echo during growth spurts. ECG abnormalities include right and left atrial enlargement, repolarization abnormalities and large complexes fulfilling 'voltage criteria' for LVH. Giant inverted T-waves are common in Japanese patients who present with apical hypertrophy, but they have also been described in Western patients (Yamaguchi et al 1979).

Q-waves are present in approximately 20–25% of patients. They are usually found in leads II, III and aVF and in leads V5 and V6. The exact cause of Q-waves is not fully understood but they may be due to myocardial ischaemia, abnormal septal activation and gross septal hypertrophy (Cosio et al 1980). A short P–R interval may present with a slurred upstroke resembling Wolff–Parkinson–White syndrome but accessory pathways are uncommon in patients with HCM (Frenneaux et al 1990). Left axis deviation is present in one-third of patients. Right axis deviation and right bundle branch block (RBBB) may be present when the right ventricle is hypertrophied.

Table 11.2 Comparison of differing presenting signs in obstructive and non-obstructive hypertrophic cardiomyopathy

	Obstructive HCM	Non-obstructive HCM
Carotid pulse	Initial rapid upstroke followed by a 'dip' in mid systole and a secondary rise. This coincides with the development of the gradient, producing the jerky pulse	Rapid upstroke as a result of hyperdynamic systolic function representing rapid left ventricular emptying
Ejection systolic murmur	Left ventricular outflow tract obstruction (LVOTO). This can be best heard in the left intercostal space adjacent to the left sternal edge, radiating to the aortic and mitral areas	Nil
Mitral regurgitation (MR)	Majority of patients with LVOTO present with MR. Presence suggested by length of murmur as it radiates to the axilla. Failure of closure of the mitral valve due to systolic anterior motion (SAM)	Nil

48-hour Holter monitoring

Around 20–25% of HCM patients have supraventricular arrhythmias which may be paroxysmal or sustained; 10% of patients present with atrial fibrillation at diagnosis. Most of these arrhythmias are slow in rate and the patients are asymptomatic. They occur predominantly during periods of increased vagal tone such as sleep. Some 25% of patients have episodes of non-sustained ventricular tachycardia (NSVT). The incidence of ventricular arrhythmias detected during 48-hour monitoring is age related and occurs mainly in adults. NSVT can be an increased risk marker for sudden death. Sustained ventricular tachycardia is rare.

Echocardiography

This remains the gold standard for diagnosing HCM. It evaluates anatomical and functional abnormalities underlining the presence of LVH and outflow obstruction. The most common presentation is ASH in 60% of patients, concentric (30%) and apical (10%). Other characteristic abnormalities include a small left ventricular cavity, hyperdynamic ventricle, SAM of the mitral valve and valve abnormalities. Enlarged atria and impaired diastolic function can also be seen. Doppler colour flow can determine mitral regurgitation and can measure pressure gradients. Echocardiography may not be as useful in children but they should undergo annual echocardiograms for 3–5 years during the adolescent growth spurt.

Exercise stress testing

This can be useful for obtaining functional and prognostic information. Patients with HCM have an impaired maximal oxygen ventilatory capacity (VO_2 max), which may be due to an inability to increase stroke volume during exercise. About 20–25% of patients have an abnormal blood pressure response to exercise; this is defined as a failure of the systolic blood pressure to rise by over 20 mmHg during exercise. Alternatively, it may fall from the resting baseline measurement (Frenneaux et al 1990). The mechanism for this abnormal response is unclear but it may be due to ventricular baroreceptors causing inappropriate vasodilatation. Patients under the age of 40 years who present with flat blood pressure or hypotensive responses have a higher risk of sudden death.

Chest X-ray

This may be normal or reveal cardiomegaly due to bi-atrial enlargement and left ventricular hypertrophy. Occasional mitral annular calcification can be seen while upper lobe blood diversion may be identified in patients with long-standing raised left atrial pressures.

Cardiac catheterisation

This is usually reserved for patients who require pressure measurements for severe clinical mitral regurgitation. Coronary angiography is indicated in patients with chest pain above 40 years of age to exclude underlying coronary artery disease.

Magnetic resonance imaging (MRI)

This can be useful in assessing right ventricular and apical hypertrophy in selected patients.

Treatment

Medical treatment for HCM is aimed at alleviating diastolic ventricular dysfunction, mechanical outflow obstruction if present and hyperdynamic systolic function. Symptoms and mechanisms vary from patient to patient and therefore therapy should be tailored for the individual. β-blockers are the drug of first choice if they are not contra-indicated. They work by slowing the heart rate, especially during exercise. If they are not tolerated (that is, they produce unwanted side-effects), calcium antagonists are used, notably verapamil. All these drugs can improve symptoms by:

- slowing the heart rate, especially during exercise. This reduces myocardial oxygen demand which in turn diminishes myocardial ischaemia. Time is provided for ventricular filling during diastole which improves diastolic function and relaxation
- relieving left ventricular outflow tract obstruction (LVOTO) by reducing hyperdynamic systolic function. This also increases the preload by improving diastolic filling. Improved filling will also increase the volume of blood ejected.

β-blockers appear effective in controlling arrhythmias. Calcium antagonists do not prevent fatal arrhythmias or sudden death. Disopyramide is useful in reducing outflow obstruction and symptoms in patients with severe left ventricular outflow tract gradients and SAM. This is achieved by producing a negative inotropic effect. Nifedipine should be avoided in these patients due to its potent vasodilator effects, which potentiate obstruction through a reduction in the preload, causing the ventricle to collapse in on itself more easily. Marked dehydration can do the same.

Diuretics may be used in patients with dyspnoea due to pulmonary congestion but again, care must be taken when administering these to patients with obstruction because diuresis may lead to the aforementioned dehydration and hypovolaemia, reducing the preload and aggravating the obstruction to the outflow of blood. Patients with obstructive cardiomyopathy and mitral valve abnormalities will require antibiotic prophylaxis to minimize the risk of infective endocarditis.

Surgical treatment is indicated in patients who display outflow tract gradients greater than 50 mmHg and are refractory to medical therapy. Septal myotomy and myomectomy may be considered. The perioperative mortality for this procedure ranges from 3–10% but it can provide long-term symptomatic relief for most patients. However, it does not influence prognosis.

Pacemakers have been used as an alternative to surgical treatment for the relief of outflow tract obstruc-

tion. The theory is that by pacing with a short AV delay there is an alteration in the pattern of myocardial contraction, which reduces systolic anterior motion of the mitral valve and hence LVOTO (Slade et al 1996). This procedure has varying results.

Pacemakers may also be indicated for patients who present with bradyarrhythmias or severe conduction disease. Alcohol septal ablation is a more recent cardiac procedure where absolute alcohol is injected into the first major septal artery. A small septal infarct is produced, reducing the thickness of the ventricular septum. This in turn will reduce the interventricular pressure gradient by enlarging the LV outflow tract. Preliminary results are good but the long-term effects of this procedure are awaited.

Defibrillators are indicated for patients who have symptomatic sustained ventricular arrhythmias and those who present with several risk factors for sudden death. Cardiac transplantation may be indicated for young patients who have poor left ventricular function.

Arrhythmias are a common symptom in patients with HCM. They may precipitate chest pain, dizzy spells, syncope, dyspnoea and palpitation. Amiodarone is the most effective and widely used anti-arrhythmic drug for supraventricular (narrow complex) tachycardias (SVTs), sustained symptomatic arrhythmias and ventricular tachycardias. Amiodarone does, however, have unpleasant side-effects and thyroid and liver function should be monitored regularly. Patients should also be offered advice regarding increased photosensitivity. This will include the use of sun-blocking creams and the avoidance of bright sunlight to prevent skin damage. Patients who experience recurrent or refractory SVTs may require electrophysiology studies (EPS), with a view to ablating a possible accessory pathway.

Atrial fibrillation is present in 10% of patients and is not well tolerated. Patients with severe diastolic impairment may have profound haemodynamic compromise due to loss of atrial function and contribution to the total cardiac output. If direct current (DC) cardioversion is unsuccessful, then amiodarone may restore stability. If both these methods fail, β-blockers may be used to control the ventricular rate. Patients with atrial fibrillation require anticoagulation to reduce the risk of thrombus formation due to a poorly contracting atrium.

Prognosis

The aim of clinical investigations is to determine which patients are at risk of sudden cardiac death and serious complications. Patients who fall into a high-risk category may have two or more of the following risk factors:

- a family history of premature sudden cardiac death
- hypotensive or flat blood pressure response to exercise (see above for details)
- unexplained syncope
- non-sustained or sustained ventricular arrhythmias
- severe left ventricular hypertrophy
- myocardial ischaemia
- bradyarrhythmias
- tachyarrhythmias.

Patients who are considered to be at high risk should receive prophylactic therapy such as low-dose amiodarone and/or an ICD. There is an increased incidence of exercise-related sudden death in HCM therefore aggressive physical activity and competitive sports are contra-indicated, irrespective of symptoms.

ARRHYTHMOGENIC RIGHT VENTRICULAR CARDIOMYOPATHY/DYSPLASIA

Arrhythmogenic right ventricular cardiomyopathy/dysplasia (ARVC/D) is an inherited heart muscle disease characterized by fibrofatty replacement, particularly of the right ventricle. In 30% of cases the left ventricle is also involved. Most cases are inherited in an autosomal dominant fashion with variable clinical penetrance. To date, five chromosomal loci have been reported but as yet no genetic mutations have been identified. Several families with an autosomal recessive form of the disease are described on the island of Naxos (in Greece). This 'Naxos' disease is associated with palmar–plantar keratosis (skin lesions on the palms and soles of the feet) and woolly hair (Coonar et al 1998).

Clinical presentation

ARVC/D only rarely presents in childhood, most patients developing symptoms between 15 and 40 years of age (Plate 11.9). The first presentation may be with sudden cardiac death but more typically, patients present with palpitations or synope caused by self-limiting ventricular arrhythmias arising from the right ventricle. Presentation with right ventricular failure is rare but heart failure may occur in patients with left ventricular involvement. Increasingly, patients are diagnosed incidentally or as the result of family screening following the detection of an abnormal ECG.

Investigations

Electrocardiogram (ECG)

A number of electrocardiographic features are typical of the disease. These include T-wave inversion (Fig. 11.8) and QRS prolongation (>110 ms) in leads V1–V3, and complete or incomplete RBBB. In 30% of patients a small deflection may be seen at the end of the QRS complex, the so-called **epsilon wave** (Fig. 11.9), caused by delayed after-potentials in the right ventricle.

Signal average ECG (SAECG)

This is a recording of multiple (usually more than 200) heartbeats in which the corresponding elements of the ECG signal (particularly the QRS complex) are highly amplified and superimposed on each other. The resulting tracing permits identification of very low-amplitude electrical signals believed to emanate from damaged areas of myocardium. The absence of these latter signals correlates well with a low probability of susceptibility to ventricular tachyarrhythmias (McKenna et al 1998). This is usually abnormal in patients with ARVC/D who have clinical ventricular tachycardia.

Echocardiography

If fibrofatty replacement is extensive two-dimensional echocardiography may demonstrate localized or global right ventricular dilatation, together with regional wall motion abnormalities and aneurysms of the free wall of the right ventricle. More typically, however, the echocardiogram is normal.

Right ventriculography

Radionuclide ventriculography is a form of nuclear medicine. It utilizes specifically labelled red blood cells with a radioactive substance to provide images on factors such as wall motion abnormalities and assessment of the ejection fraction. The widespread availability of echocardiography has limited its use.

Exercise testing

In some patients, symptom-limited exercise testing may be useful in the diagnosis of exercise-induced ventricular arrhythmias. It also provides an objective assessment of the functional limitation in patients with extensive fibrofatty replacement of the right and/or left ventricle.

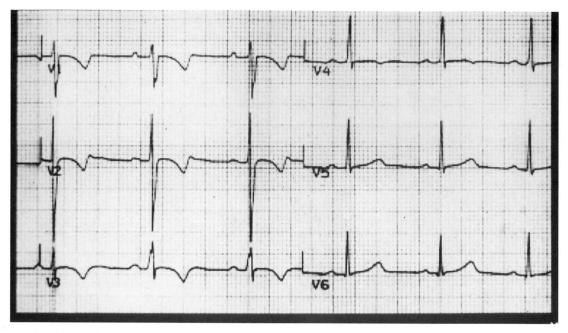

Figure 11.8 ECG in arrhythmogenic right ventricular cardiomyopathy/dysplasia (ARVC/D) in a 14-year-old male. Precordial T-wave inversion can be seen.

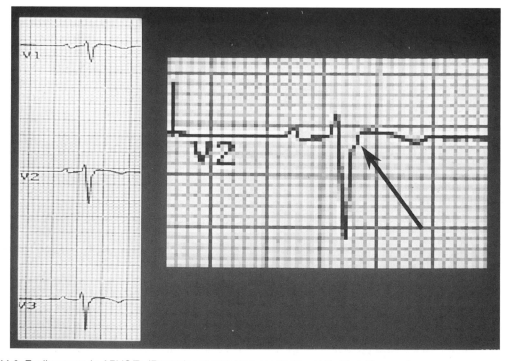

Figure 11.9 Epsilon wave in ARVC/D. (Reproduced with kind permission of Dr Mark Norman.)

48-hour Holter monitoring

The Holter is a portable instrument which the patient wears for 48 hours as it stores and records ECG tracings. This enables the clinician to observe the patient's ECG during daily life activities and detects ventricular arrhythmias.

Magnetic resonance imaging (MRI)

This can show infiltration and fatty deposits more accurately.

Treatment

There is no cure for ARVC/D but many patients have few if any symptoms and live a normal lifespan. In some patients, therapy is required to prevent disease-related complications, in particular ventricular tachy-arrhythmias and sudden death. In patients without syncope or previous cardiac arrest, symptomatic ventricular extrasystoles/ectopics or non-sustained runs of ventricular tachycardia can often be suppressed with β-blockers, in particular through using sotalol. When this is unsuccessful or when patients experience prolonged episodes of ventricular tachycardia, invasive electrophysiological testing before and after anti-arrhythmic drug therapy may be required to optimize treatment.

Radiofrequency ablation may be considered in patients with refractory but haemodynamically tolerated ventricular tachycardia. However, because of the diffuse nature of the disease, recurrence is common. ICDs may be necessary in patients with recurrent syncope, irrespective of the presence of documented ventricular arrhythmia, and are mandatory in patients who have survived cardiac arrest.

Pacemakers may be necessary in patients with conduction system disease. Conventional vasodilator and diuretic therapy should be used in patients who develop right and/or left ventricular failure. Cardiac transplantation should be considered in patients with 'end-stage' heart failure.

In summary, patients who have been evaluated and for whom treatment has been initiated for ARVC/D should be able to lead a virtually normal life. It is important that they restrict exercise activities and inform significant others in their life about their disease. Regular monitoring and review of treatment by a cardiologist is imperative.

RESTRICTIVE CARDIOMYOPATHY

Restrictive cardiomyopathy (RCM) is the rarest form of the cardiomyopathies. It is characterized by a normal or slightly enlarged heart. Restrictive filling and reduced diastolic volume of either or both ventricles results from decreased ventricular compliance (stiff ventricle) and filling. Systolic function and wall thickness are usually normal, especially early on in the course of the disease. Increased interstitial fibrosis may be present (WHO/ISFC 1980).

Restrictive cardiomyopathy may be a primary disorder due to:

- endomyocardial fibrosis
- Loeffler's cardiomyopathy
- idiopathic restrictive cardiomyopathy (aetiology unknown).

Secondary RCM can be due to:

- infiltrative disease, such as amyloidosis, sarcoidosis, post-irradiation therapy
- storage disease such as haemochromatosis, glycogen storage disease, Fabry's disease (an error of lipid metabolism which results in lipid deposition in tissues, including the heart, kidneys and blood vessels)

Pathology

Post-mortem findings include enlarged atria, mildly hypertrophied ventricles and normal ventricular cavity dimensions. Histological inspection of the myocardium may elicit the cause, such as amyloidosis and sarcoidosis. In the storage disorders, the deposits are within the cells, as with haemochromatosis and glycogen storage disease. The most common cause of RCM worldwide is endomyocardial fibrosis (Plate 11.10). The endocardium is thickened and mural thrombi may be present.

Pathophysiology

Diastolic dysfunction from impaired ventricular filling is a result of myocardial fibrosis and infiltration (amyloidosis). Impaired filling from both ventricles results in an increasing back pressure of blood on the superior and inferior vena caval and pulmonary veins. This produces clinical signs and symptoms of right and left ventricular cardiac failure respectively. Mitral and tricuspid regurgitation results from damage to the endocardium, exacerbating cardiac failure. An increased afterload and impairment of ventricular filling, together with regurgitation, produce atrial dilatation and hypertrophy.

Clinical presentation

At the time of presentation the condition is in the advanced stages. Patients present with the signs and symptoms shown in Table 11.3 depending on ventricular involvement.

The clinical signs and symptoms depend upon the degree of atrial pressure required to compensate for poor ventricular filling. This gives rise to clinical symptoms of exercise intolerance. Atrial fibrillation is common due to atrial enlargement. Ventricular arrhythmias or heart block are not uncommon in advanced cases and may be the cause of sudden death in these patients (Rodkey et al 1998).

Investigations

12-lead ECG

This usually demonstrates small voltages. There are abnormal ST segment and T-wave changes. Atrial fibrillation may be present.

Chest X-ray

This may show a normal or slightly enlarged heart.

Echocardiography

This is the main diagnostic tool in the evaluation of patients with diastolic dysfunction. It can quickly assess systolic ventricular function, atrial size and function and valvular function (Rodkey et al 1998). The atria are usually enlarged. The ventricular cavity size can be normal but in infiltrative RCM such as amyloidosis and sarcoidosis, it may be increased. Myocardial wall thickness is usually normal but again in amyloidosis, the myocardium and the interatrial septum are thickened and display a bright speckled appearance. Intramural thrombi can be identified as bright echogenic material within the ventricular cavity. There is often normal systolic function with impaired diastolic ventricular filling.

Cardiac catheterisation and haemodynamic studies

These are useful in differentiating RCM from constrictive pericarditis. Endomyocardial biopsy can be useful in diagnosing secondary RCM such as infiltrative disease (amyloidosis, sarcoidosis, post-irradiation therapy) and storage disease (haemochromatosis, glycogen storage disease, Fabry's disease). Biopsy can also be helpful in establishing primary RCM, such as endomyocardial fibrosis.

Treatment

RCM is usually in its advanced stages before it is clinically recognized. The prognosis is poor with a 2-year mortality of 35–50%. There is no specific treatment for RCM and the aim of medical therapy is to improve arrhythmias and symptoms of heart failure and to prevent mural and systemic thrombus. Pacemakers are indicated for patients with AV conduction blocks which can occur with this disease. Surgical intervention includes mitral and tricuspid

Table 11.3 Signs and symptoms of restrictive cardiomyopathy (RCM)

	Right ventricular failure	Left ventricular failure
Clinical signs	Raised central venous pressure Prominent υ waves and soft systolic murmur = tricuspid regurgitation 3rd or 4th heart sound = cardiac enlargement	3rd heart sound at apex = cardiac enlargement Murmur = mitral regurgitation
Symptoms	Peripheral oedema Ascites Abdominal pain (hepatic congestion)	Dyspnoea Orthopnoea Paroxysmal nocturnal dyspnoea

General signs of RCM
Generally patients with RCM complain of exertional dyspnoea and fatigue, as a result of reduced cardiac output due to impaired ventricular filling.
A 4th heart sound may not be present in cardiac amyloidosis as there is infiltration of the atria and this prevents effective atrial contraction. The pulse is usually regular and has a small volume.

valve repair and in severe cases cardiac transplantation should be considered.

CONCLUSION

The cardiomyopathies can have a distressing impact on a person's health-related quality of life and emotional well-being. In this chapter the pathophysiology, clinical presentation and management of the cardiomyopathies have been presented. It is important to remember that nurses will encounter patients who are living with a cardiomyopathy during different stages of its progression. Understanding this group of cardiac diseases will help the nurse evaluate the needs of individual patients and give appropriate support to the patient and their family or carers. Allowing patients access to information about their illness may dispel misconceptions and help the patient adapt to the difficulties of the disease.

Over the last 10 years, various patient support self-help groups have developed. They supply current literature and regular newsletters and patients and families benefit from local contact, advice and counselling regarding the condition. It also enables the patient and their families or carers to discuss problems and gain support and assistance in an empathic professional manner from an independent source.

Case study 11.1

History

Mrs Val Smith was a 30-year-old Caucasian female who was diagnosed with hypertrophic obstructive cardiomyopathy (HOCM). She had complained of feeling generally unwell, with pains in her arm and palpitations, especially during exercise. She was self-employed. She smoked 10–15 cigarettes per day and drank the occasional glass of wine. Her build was average and she took moderate exercise. She had two children under the age of 12 years and they had been screened for hypertrophic cardiomyopathy (HCM) and were found to have normal electrocardiograms (ECGs) and two-dimensional echocardiography (echo). The children were followed up every 3 years at the local hospital and would continue to be followed up until they had completed their growth. Mrs Smith had recently been divorced. Her mother had been diagnosed with HCM and had complained for many years of dizzy spells and palpitations. Her brother was fit and well and had a normal ECG and echo.

Physical examination

This revealed classic signs of HOCM. Her pulse was regular, in sinus rhythm and her blood pressure was 120/70 mmHg. She had a jerky pulse and a forceful apical impulse which could be felt at the fifth intercostal space, indicating dynamic left ventricular contraction. On auscultation, heart sounds 1 and 2 were normal but an ejection systolic murmur could be heard in the left intercostal space adjacent to the left sternal edge. This is consistent with a left ventricular outflow tract (LVOT) gradient. A 12-lead ECG was abnormal, showing inverted T-waves in leads I and aVL. A two-dimensional echocardiogram confirmed the diagnosis of HCM. There was a left ventricular wall thickness at the interventricular septum of 2.3 mm (normal values 0.7–1.4 mm) and at the posterior wall of 1.04 mm (normal values 0.7–1.3 mm). She had a resting gradient of 50 mmHg and had mild mitral regurgitation without systolic anterior motion of the mitral valve. Her left atrium was 4.3 mm in dimension

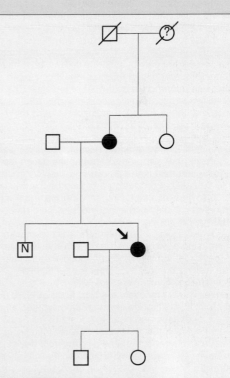

Figure 11.10 Pedigree diagram for Mrs Smith, the proband, who is indicated with an arrow.

(normal values 2.3–3.5 mm). Left ventricular systolic function was normal.

Treatment

Holter monitoring revealed that Mrs. Smith was experiencing episodes of atrial fibrillation. She was commenced on amiodarone 200 mg once a day (od) to control the frequent episodes of atrial fibrillation.

Case study 11.1 *continued*

Amiodarone controlled the symptoms for the next 14 years until Mrs Smith complained of increasing chest pain and shortness of breath after meals and walking up hills. She also complained of dizzy spells associated with palpitation. She was commenced on propranolol to relieve her symptoms.

β-blockers reduce myocardial oxygen consumption and therefore myocardial ischaemia by exerting a negatively inotropic and chronotropic effect. If the heart rate is reduced, this allows a longer time for the ventricle to fill in diastole and in turn will improve diastolic function. β-blockers reduce the hyperdynamic systolic function of the ventricle with an increase in preload from improved diastolic filling. This contributes to alleviation of left ventricular outflow tract obstruction (LVOTO). β-blockers are not effective in reducing the incidence of fatal arrhythmias or sudden death but they are effective in the treatment of symptoms in 30–60% of patients. Mrs Smith was unable to tolerate propranolol and her symptoms were persistent.

It was felt that Mrs Smith may benefit from verapamil, which is the most commonly used calcium channel antagonist in patients suffering with HCM. It has the same properties as β-blockers and it can improve exercise tolerance in over 60% of patients. She was commenced on 80 mg twice a day (bd) and could increase the dose to 240 mg slow release (SR) daily. It was felt that if after a month Mrs Smith had not noticed any significant change in her symptoms, she would be evaluated for a permanent pacemaker as a means of improving her symptoms. Verapamil reduces the rate of conduction across the atrioventricular (AV) node and has the potential of producing profound bradyarrhythmias. Mrs Smith was also taking amiodarone and it was felt that if the levels were adequate she could reduce this to 100 mg od.

Over the next 18 months Mrs Smith complained of increasing shortness of breath and chest tightness. She experienced an increase in headaches and fatigue which are well-recognized side-effects of verapamil. Amiodarone levels were well within the therapeutic range. Thyroid function and liver function tests were normal. It was time to consider the next step as all medical options had been exhausted. Mrs Smith was admitted for a trial of temporary dual chamber pacing. If this relieved her symptoms a permanent device would be implanted. A dual chamber pacemaker with short atrioventricular (AV) delay has been proposed as an alternative to surgical treatment for the relief of outflow obstruction and symptoms. The right ventricle is constantly activated from the apex. This alters the way the septum is stimulated and in turn the way the left ventricle contracts. It should reduce the LVOTO and systolic anterior motion (SAM) of the mitral valve, reducing the patient's symptoms. Pacemaker therapy is not successful for all patients with LVOTO but in Mrs Smith's case she was admitted to the ward for assessment.

After the pacemaker implantation Mrs Smith's exercise tolerance improved and she was less troubled by breathlessness and palpitations. For the next 6 months

her quality of life was good and she felt well. In the autumn she was admitted to her local hospital after experiencing an episode of fast irregular palpitation and light-headedness. The hospital staff were able to document fast atrial fibrillation with a ventricular rate of 100–150 bpm. Mrs Smith was sweaty and her blood pressure was 100/70 mmHg. She was administered 1.5 mg atenolol intravenously and the ventricular rate slowed to 80 bpm. She was still in atrial fibrillation. This reverted to sinus rhythm spontaneously 12 hours after admission and Mrs Smith was discharged home on amiodarone 100 mg od and verapamil SR 240 mg od.

Ten days later she was readmitted following further episodes of light-headedness and rapid irregular palpitations. The ECG showed atrial fibrillation with a ventricular response of 100 bpm. On this admission Mrs Smith underwent an intravenous loading dose of amiodarone and was cardioverted after 24 hours, when sinus rhythm was achieved. The patient was still having recurring episodes of paroxysmal atrial fibrillation so amiodarone was increased to 200 mg od to maintain sinus rhythm and to control the ventricular rate during breakthrough episodes. Warfarin was prescribed to reduce the incidence of thrombo-embolism. She was discharged once again and an appointment was made to attend the pacing clinic. The pacemaker was reprogrammed to a DDD mode (see Chapter 21). Her ECG showed a first-degree block with a P–R interval of 250 ms. If she developed AV block with her pacemaker in DDD mode she would receive ventricular pacing. The ventricular upper tracking rate was reprogrammed to a lower rate. Therefore if atrial fibrillation occurred this would not be tracked and paced rapidly by the pacemaker.

Over the next year Mrs Smith had a further five episodes of atrial fibrillation which reverted to sinus rhythm spontaneously. She began to experience exertional chest pain, breathlessness and lethargy. Despite medical and pacemaker therapy she had begun to experience her old symptoms. What to do next? Alcohol septal ablation was the next suggested form of treatment. This technique is a non-surgical method for reducing outflow tract obstruction in symptomatic patients who are refractory to pacemaker and medical therapy. Mrs Smith was admitted to hospital and gave consent for the procedure.

She had discontinued her warfarin 48 hours before and had commenced intravenous heparin. Alcohol septal ablation involves reduction of the left side of the ventricular septum by injecting intracoronary ethanol in the first septal coronary artery to produce a small septal infarct. Mrs Smith underwent a retrograde right and left heart catheterisation by percutaneous catheterisation of her right femoral vessel, performed under a local anaesthetic. All patients have a temporary pacing wire inserted because of the high incidence of complete heart block seen with ethanol-induced infarction. Mrs Smith already had a permanent system in place. Her gradient was measured at rest and was 60 mmHg. It increased to 150 mmHg on exercise provocation. The left main artery was intubated and visualized by giving X-ray contrast agents, which highlighted the perfused area only

Case study 11.1 *continued*

transiently. Diamorphine 2.5–5 mg was given intravenously, followed by a slow injection over 1 minute of 5 ml of ethanol into the septal vessel. The balloon was kept inflated for 5–10 minutes at the beginning of the septal artery to prevent leakage of the ethanol into the left anterior descending (LAD) artery. The balloon was deflated and the pressure gradient was measured post procedure. At rest it was 0 mmHg and during provocation 30 mmHg.

Mrs Smith was transferred to the coronary care unit (CCU) where she was haemodynamically monitored. She had cardiac enzymes taken on her return to the ward. The creatine kinase (CK) was 1190. They were repeated the following morning, with a CK recording of 1857. An echo assessed the left ventricle and the reduction of the LVOT post procedure and the following day.

Mrs Smith experienced a stable and uneventful postoperative recovery. The sheath was removed 2 hours after the procedure and she was able to get up after a further 6 hours. She could eat and drink normally. The pacemaker was checked and remained in DDD mode with a rate of 60–100 pulses per minute. Mrs Smith was discharged from hospital and provided with an outpatients appointment for 6 weeks' time.

On return to the clinic Mrs Smith was extremely well. Her symptoms had improved. She did not experience chest pain or dizzy spells. There was little improvement in her exercise capacity but the echocardiogram demonstrated no gradient. Her echocardiograph showed asymmetric septal hypertrophy (ASH) and the left

ventricle looked a little dilated. The interventricular septum measured 2.2 mm.

At her next 3-month outpatient visit Mrs Smith remained asymptomatic. She was able to cycle for 6 miles without any major problems. Her echocardiogram remained virtually the same but the left atrial dimensions were reduced from 43 mm to 36 mm since the relief of the outflow tract obstruction. She was keen to discontinue her amiodarone as this was initially commenced for atrial fibrillation. It was felt that she was less likely to have episodes of atrial fibrillation if her left atrial dimensions had returned to normal. She therefore discontinued amiodarone but remained on verapamil and warfarin. She was reviewed 3 months later and underwent an exercise test and 48-hour Holter monitoring. After this clinic visit she was followed up on a yearly basis.

Mrs Smith has enjoyed the benefits of alcohol septal ablation for 2 years. It has proved to be an effective therapy for her obstructive form of hypertrophic cardiomyopathy, where medication and pacing had failed. She remains on medication and will require yearly follow-up with:

- ECG
- two-dimensional echocardiography
- exercise testing
- 48-hour Holter monitoring.

Alcohol septal ablation appears to relieve this patient's symptoms. The preliminary results are promising, but the long-term effects still need to be assessed.

Case study 11.2

History

Tim White was a 22-year-old trainee physical instructor who had noticed that he was experiencing frequent palpitations over the last year. They lasted for less than 30 minutes and did not make him feel dizzy, sweaty or short of breath. They were not associated with chest pain and he had never lost consciousness. He did sometimes experience the palpitations after exercise. He visited his local cardiology unit to be investigated and they documented a broad complex tachycardia. He was then transferred to a specialist cardiology unit for further evaluation.

On further examination it emerged that Mr White had a strong family history of palpitations. His great grandmother frequently blacked out after a 'thumping' feeling in her chest and she died suddenly at the age of 32. She had three children (two girls and one boy). His great-great uncle collapsed and died suddenly at the age of 35 after an episode of palpitations. His grandmother had been diagnosed as having epilepsy at the age of 21. She also frequently experienced blackouts and palpitations. His aunt and mother both complained of palpitations.

Physical examination

Mr White's physical examination showed he had an athletic physique but was otherwise unremarkable. His resting electrocardiogram (ECG) showed sinus rhythm. It was unremarkable except for minor repolarization abnormalities. He had T-wave inversion across the anteroseptal leads.

His echocardiogram showed right ventricular enlargement with normal left ventricular function. There was mildly reduced septal motion giving rise to border-line shortening ejection fraction. Mr White's signal average ECG (SAECG) was positive for late potentials. As mentioned earlier SAECG is usually positive in most patients with arrhythmogenic right ventricular cardiomyopathy/dysplasia (ARVC/D) who have clinical ventricular tachycardia.

Mr White carried out his exercise test and appeared to be responding normally but during the recovery phase of the exercise test he quickly developed a non-sustained ventricular tachycardia. Prior to the exercise test he did have an episode of sustained ventricular tachycardia which had a left bundle branch block (LBBB) pattern with a right axis deviation, indicating that the ventricular ectopy came from the right ventricular free wall.

Case study 11.2 *continued*

Mr White underwent a coronary angiography which demonstrated a normal left coronary and left ventricular system. The right ventricular angiogram showed dilatation of the right chamber with areas of akinesia (no movement) in the right outflow tract and bulging in the inferior wall. Right ventricular endomyocardial biopsy specimens were taken from the septum. The right ventricular free wall is not usually biopsied because of the possibility of myocardial perforation. The results showed marked fibrosis without fatty infiltration.

Treatment

Ventricular stimulation studies were performed to determine which medication would be suitable to prevent ventricular tachycardias. Mr White was commenced on sotalol 80 mg three times a day (tds). After 72 hours of sotalol, Mr White had a repeat ventricular electrophysiology study (EPS) and ventricular tachycardias could not be induced.

Mr White was informed that he could lead a virtually normal life but he was advised not to take part in competitive sports or exercise indefinitely and to reduce his exercise programme. He was advised to reduce his alcohol intake as alcohol has a depressant effect on the heart muscle and may provoke arrhythmias. This all posed a problem for Mr White. He was in his first year at college studying to become a physical fitness instructor. In view of his family history and his clinical presentation he was grateful to have been identified as at risk of sudden death. However, Mr White and his family were extremely concerned regarding the major life changes ahead of him. It was made clear that if adequate control of his ventricular arrhythmias were achieved his outlook was favourable. He would require regular follow-up to evaluate the progression of the disease, monitoring of his exercise tolerance (via exercise test), ventricular function (echocardiograph) and arrhythmia status (ECG and 48-hour Holter monitoring).

He was discharged home on sotalol and followed up at his local hospital. Two months after being discharged from hospital, Mr White started to feel unwell on the medication. His local cardiologist reduced the oral dose from 80 mg tds to 80 mg bd. He performed a 24-hour ECG recording. This showed occasional short runs of non-sustainable ventricular tachycardia (VT). Over the next 6 months Mr White's medication was adjusted to try and reduce the episodes of non-sustained VT (NSVT) which were close to a rate of 200 bpm, the worry being that heart rates above 150 bpm are likely to lead to haemodynamic collapse. It was decided that Mr White would be reviewed during his summer vacation to try and control the rate without undue symptoms.

In the autumn Mr White was taking part in a five-a-side football match. He collapsed during the first half and the paramedic team were called. He had an indefinite period of ventricular fibrillation (estimated at approximately 5 minutes) without resuscitation measures. The ambulance crew administered defibrillation and he reverted to sinus rhythm. On admission to intensive care he had a low

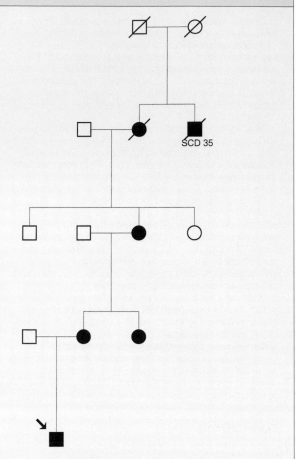

Figure 11.11 Pedigree diagram for Tim White, the proband, who is indicated with an arrow. SCD 35 = sudden cardiac death at age 35 years.

cardiac output but was in sinus rhythm. However, he did develop a sinus bradycardia with a monomorphic ventricular tachycardia. Another episode of NSVT also occurred and he was given intravenous amiodarone. He was reacting to pain, his pupils were reacting and he was able to maintain spontaneous ventilation. Neurological recovery was near complete with the exception of short-term memory loss. In view of Mr White's failed sudden cardiac death, he was transferred to the cardiac specialist centre for the insertion of an internal cardioverter defibrillator (ICD).

Mr White now has an ICD in place, following careful education and advice regarding its function (see Chapter 25). His quality of life improved dramatically and he was feeling positive and well. A year later he had made major life decisions. He wanted to marry and was considering having a family. He also wanted to travel abroad for his honeymoon and advice was given regarding malarial

> **Case study 11.2** *continued*
>
> medication as these could aggravate his ventricular arrhythmias. Mr White's symptoms had stabilized, he was enjoying his life and was fairly active. He had decided to change his career and was now employed at a desk job. As he had no further episodes of arrhythmias and his device had not discharged, he regained his driving licence. He continued to be followed up in the cardiology department, having regular checks on his ICD and evaluation of his cardiomyopathy and arrhythmia status.

REFERENCES

Baig MK, Goldman JH, Caforio AL, Coonar AS, Keeling PJ, McKenna WJ 1998 Familial dilated cardiomyopathy: cardiac abnormalities are common in asymptomatic relatives and may represent early disease. Journal of the American College of Cardiology 31(1): 195–201

Bowels KR, Gajarski R, Porter P et al 1996 Gene mapping of familial autosomal dominant dilated cardiomyopathy to chromosome 10q21–23. Journal of Clinical Investigation 98(6): 1355–1360

Burke AP, Farb A, Viramani R et al 1991 Sports-related and non-sports related sudden cardiac death in young adults. American Heart Journal 121: 568–575

Camm AJ 1998 Cardiovascular disease. In: Kumar P, Clark M (eds) Clinical medicine, 4th edn. WB Saunders, Philadelphia, pp. 625–743

Codd MB, Sugrue DD, Gersh BJ, Melton LD 1989 Epidemiology of idiopathic dilated cardiomyopathy: a population based study in Olmstead County, MN, 1975–84. Circulation 80: 564–572

Coonar AS, Protonotarios N, Tsatsopoulou A et al 1998 Gene for arrhythmogenic right ventricular cardiomyopathy with diffuse nonepidermyltic palmoplantar keratoderma and woolly hair (Naxos disease) maps to 17q21. Circulation 97: 2049–2058

Cosio FG, Moro C, Alonso M et al 1980 The Q-waves of hypertrophic cardiomyopathy. New England Journal of Medicine 302: 96–99

Davis MJ 1984 The current status of myocardial disarray in hypertrophic cardiomyopathy. British Heart Journal 51: 361–363

Dilsizian V, Bonow RO, Epstein SE, Fananapazir L 1993 Myocardial ischaemia detected by thallium scintigraphy is frequently related to cardiac arrest and syncope in young patients with hypertrophic cardiomyopathy. Journal of the American College of Cardiology 22: 796–804

Durrand JB, Bachinskill, Beiling LC et al 1995 Localization of a gene responsible for familial dilated cardiomyopathy to chromosome 1q32. Circulation 92(12): 3387–3389

Elliott PM, Kaski JC, Prasad K et al 1996 Chest pain during daily life in patients with hypertrophic cardiomyopathy: an ambulatory electrocardiographic study. European Heart Journal 17: 1056–1064

Field BJ, Baxley WA, Russell Jr RO et al 1973 Left ventricular function and hypertrophy in cardiomyopathy with depressed ejection fraction. Circulation 47: 1022–1031

Frenneaux MP, Counihan PJ, Caforio A et al 1990 Abnormal blood pressure response during exercise in hypertrophic cardiomyopathy. Circulation 82: 1995–2002

Goodwin JF 1964 Cardiac function in primary myocardial disorders. British Medical Journal 1: 1527–1533, 1595–1597

Hanrath P, Mathey DG, Siegert R, Bielgeld W 1980 Left ventricular filling patterns in different forms of left ventricular relaxation and filling patterns in different forms of left ventricular hypertrophy. An echocardiographic study. American Journal of Cardiology 45: 15–23

Jarcho JA, McKenna WJ, Pare JA et al 1989 Mapping a gene for familial hypertrophic cardiomyopathy to chromosome 14q1. New England Journal of Medicine 321: 1372–1378

Kass S, MacRae C, Graber HL et al 1994 A gene defect that causes conduction system disease and dilated cardiomyopathy maps to chromosome 1p1–1q1. Nature Genetics 7(4): 546–551

Kaye MP 1993 The Registry of International Society for Heart and Lung Transplantation: Tenth Official Report. Journal of Heart and Lung Transplantation 12(4): 541–548

Keeling PJ, Gang Y, Seo H et al 1995 Familial dilated cardiomyopathy in the United Kingdom. British Heart Journal 73(5): 417–421

Krajinovic M, Pinamonti B, Sinagra G et al 1995 Linkage of familial dilated cardiomyopathy to chromosome 9. Heart Muscle Disease Study Group. American Journal of Human Genetics 92(12): 3387–3389

Lechin M, Quinones MA, Omran A et al 1995 Angiotensin converting enzyme genotypes and left ventricular hypertrophy in patients with hypertrophic cardiomyopathy. Circulation 92: 1808–1812

Maron BJ, Roberts WC 1979 Quantitative analysis of cardiac muscle cell disorganisation in the ventricular septum of patients with hypertrophic cardiomyopathy. Circulation 59: 689–706

Maron BJ, Roberts WC, McAllister HA et al 1980 Sudden death in young athletes. Circulation 62: 218–229

Maron BJ, Tajik AJ, Ruttenberg HD et al 1982 Hypertrophic cardiomyopathy in infants: clinical features and natural history. Circulation 65: 7–17

Maron BJ, Harding AM, Spirito P et al 1983 Systolic anterior motion of the posterior mitral valve leaflet: a previous unrecognised cause of dynamic subaortic obstruction in patients with hypertrophic cardiomyopathy. Circulation 68: 282–293

Maron BJ, Gardin JM, Flack JM et al 1995 Prevalence of hypertrophic cardiomyopathy in a population of young adults: echocardiographic analysis of 4111 subjects in the CARDIA study: Coronary Artery Risk Development in (Young) Adults. Circulation 92: 785–789

McKenna WJ, Deanfield J, Faruqui A et al 1981 Prognosis in hypertrophic cardiomyopathy: role of age and clinical electrocardiograph and haemodynamic features. American Journal of Cardiology 47: 532–538

McKenna WJ, Franklin RCG, Nihoyannopoulous P et al 1988 Arrhythmia and prognosis in infants, children and adolescents with hypertrophic cardiomyopathy. Journal of the American College of Cardiology 11: 147–153

McKenna WJ, Stewart JT, Nihoyannopoulous P et al 1990 Hypertrophic cardiomyopathy without hypertrophy: two families with myocardial disarray in the absence of increased myocardial mass. British Heart Journal 63: 278–290

McKenna WJ, Spirito P, Desnos M et al 1997 Experience from clinical genetics in hypertrophic cardiomyopathy: proposal for new diagnostic criteria in adult members of affected families. Heart 77: 130–132

McKenna WJ, Perry M, Elliott PM 1998 Hypertrophic cardiomyopathy. In: Topol EJ (ed) Textbook of cardiovascular medicine. Lippincott-Raven, Philadelphia, pp. 745–764

Michels VV, Moll PP, Miller FA et al 1992 The frequency of familial dilated cardiomyopathy in a series of patients with idiopathic dilated cardiomyopathy. New England Journal of Medicine 326(2): 77–82

Olson TM, Keating MT 1996 Mapping a cardiomyopathy locus to chromosome 3p22–p25. Journal of Clinical Investigation 97(2): 528–532

Rodkey SM, Ratcliff NB, Young JB 1998 Cardiomyopathy and myocardial failure. In: Topol EJ (ed) Textbook of cardiovascular medicine. Lippincott-Raven, Philadelphia, pp. 2217–2219

Savage DD, Seides SF, Clark CE et al 1978 Electrocardiographic findings in patients with obstructive and non-obstructive hypertrophic cardiomyopathy. Circulation 58: 402–409

Savage DD, Castelli WP, Abbott RD et al 1983 Hypertrophic cardiomyopathy and its markers in the general population: the great masquerader revisited. The Framingham Study. Journal of Cardiovascular Ultrasonography 2: 41–47

Seidman CE, McKenna WJ, Watkins HC, Seidman JG 1992 Molecular genetic approaches to diagnosis and management of hypertrophic cardiomyopathy. In: Braunwald E (ed) Heart disease. A textbook of cardiovascular medicine. WB Saunders, Philadelphia, pp. 77–83

Slade AKB, Sadoul N, Shapiro L et al 1996 DDD pacing in hypertrophic cardiomyopathy: a multicentre clinical experience. Heart 75: 44–49

Stevens PJ, Ground KE 1970 Occurrence and significance of myocarditis in trauma. Aerospace Medicine 41(7): 776–780

Watkins H, Theirfelder L, Hwang D et al 1992 Sporadic hypertrophic cardiomyopathy due to de novo mutations. Journal of Clinical Investigation 90: 1666–1671

WHO/ISFC 1980 Report of the WHO/ISFC Task Force on the definition and classification of cardiomyopathies. British Heart Journal 44: 672–673

WHO/ISFC 1996 Report of the 1995 World Health Organization/International Society and Federation of Cardiology Task Force on the definition and classification of cardiomyopathies. Circulation 93: 841–842

Wigle ED, Sasson Z, Henderson MA et al 1985 Hypertrophic cardiomyopathy: the importance of the site and extent of hypertrophy: a review. Progress in Cardiovascular Disease 28(1): 1–83

Wigle ED, Rakowski H, Krimball BP, Williams WG 1995 Hypertrophic cardiomyopathy clinical spectrum and treatment. Circulation 92(7): 1680–1692

Yamaguchi H, Ishimura T, Nishiyama S et al 1979 Hypertrophic non obstructive cardiomyopathy with giant negative T-waves (apical hypertrophy): ventriculographic and echocardiographic features in 30 patients. American Journal of Cardiology 44: 401–412

CHAPTER CONTENTS

12

Congenital heart defects in adults

Adelaide Tunstill

Adults with congenital heart defects are an ever-growing population of cardiac patients. Up-to-date figures are always difficult to obtain but congenital heart disease occurs in approximately 5–8 per 1000 live births (Archer & Burch 1998). In the 1950s fewer than one in five infants with recognized congenital heart disease survived into adulthood (MacMahon et al 1953) but improvements in surgery over the past 50 years have meant that people with complex heart defects are now surviving into adulthood. However, it is only in recent years that adult congenital heart medicine has begun to be recognized as a specialty in its own right. This chapter explores the broad issues of caring for adults with congenital heart defects and highlights the more common conditions that may be encountered. The emphasis is placed upon nursing this group as a specialty aside from those with acquired heart disease, but with the need to encourage the patient to lead as normal a life as the condition allows. For many, with care, this is now achievable.

The majority of adults in a cardiology unit have what is termed 'acquired heart disease' and usually have normal cardiac anatomy but those people born with heart defects may have an altered anatomy which can result in an additional abnormal physiology. The question arises as to why this group of adults should be treated any differently from the traditional cardiac patient. For anyone who has had a chronic disease since birth, making the transition from the paediatric to the adult service is a difficult step. Congenital heart patients and their parents have complete trust in the cardiologists and cardiac surgeons who have ensured that they have reached adulthood and suddenly they need to meet and become familiar with a whole new team. This is at a time when they are also expected to become more independent, leave home, perhaps go to university or begin work.

Sparacino et al (1997) described the dilemmas of parents who have children with heart defects. The problems of normality, disclosure (whether to reveal the presence of a heart defect), uncertainty, coping strategies, social integration and the impact on the family continue to be dilemmas for these young adults. Socially they tend to fall into two categories. There are those who, because of their heart defect, may have had repeated admissions to hospital, been over-protected by their parents and grown up as 'patients'. Then there are those who have had what was thought to be corrective surgery as babies, have led fairly normal lives and who tend to deny the fact that they have a heart defect. It comes as a great shock to the latter group to discover that as adults they may once again require some sort of treatment. It is interesting to note that many of these patients are ignorant of their diagnosis and previous treatment presumably because it all occurred when they were babies (Kantoch et al 1997). There are also a number of patients who present in adulthood with previously undiagnosed defects such as an atrial septal defect or pulmonary stenosis. Infective endocarditis may be the first clue to a congenital defect or even something as catastrophic as a cerebrovascular accident (CVA) due to a thrombus passing through an atrial septal defect.

Organization of services for adult congenital heart patients needs multidisciplinary planning and input, with cardiology being the mainstay. Cardiac surgeons, anaesthetists, obstetricians, geneticists, psychologists, general practitioners (GPs), social workers and of course nurses are all part of the team. Only about 8% of these patients will need to be admitted as inpatients to a regional centre (Somerville 1996), but their state of health needs to be regularly checked as outpatients. GPs in the community cannot be expected to know everything regarding congenital heart disease but it is important that they are kept informed about individual patients in their care by the professionals in the specialist centres. This is important because for the patients, their GP is the first port of call. If admission is necessary, the district hospital requires a cardiologist with an interest in congenital heart disease and who has good contacts at regional level and can identify when to refer the patient. Therefore it can be seen that, as with all medicine, communication is of vital importance.

The great difference between those patients with acquired heart disease and those with congenital defects is the sheer complexity of the diseases in the latter. Most acquired heart problems in adults revolve around the coronary arteries and valves but the number of congenital heart defects, combinations of these defects and the various operations that have been performed in order to alleviate the symptoms is enormous.

Congenital heart patients can also develop additional problems such as polycythaemia (an abnormal increase in the number of circulating red blood cells), infective endocarditis, arrhythmias, coronary artery disease and, of course, should they become pregnant, there is the need for special care to ensure the safety of not only the mother but also the fetus.

In addition to their physical problems, such patients have social and psychological difficulties with regard to body image, peer pressure, employment difficulties and acquiring documentation such as a driving license and insurance. Females may not be able to carry a pregnancy to term. Males (and indeed females) may worry that they cannot compete on an equal footing with their peers. Will they be able to find suitable employment? If they marry, will they be able to support a family? Since the Disability and Discrimination Act (1995), employment has been less of a problem but many patients are not physically capable of undertaking a job involving manual labour. Education may have been interrupted, lessening their chances in the job market, although Gersony et al (1993) in the United States reported that those patients who had survived after surgery for aortic stenosis, pulmonary stenosis and ventricular septal defect had a quality of life similar to that of the general population. Nowadays companies providing free health insurance and running their own pension schemes may be reluctant to insure someone who may require more than the usual medical care. Inconsistencies found in insurance and job policies may be due to a lack of appropriate guidelines (Celermajer & Deanfield 1993). Help and information on these matters may be obtained from support groups, the Department of Social Security or the Citizens' Advice Bureaux.

RESTRICTIONS ON LIFESTYLE
Physical activity

Most patients with a history of congenital heart disease can lead a full and active life and do not need any restrictions. In fact, they should be encouraged to take part in activities such as swimming, cycling and low-impact aerobics. In certain conditions such as severe aortic stenosis, competitive sports are not advised. Medical investigations often include exercise testing when changes in oxygen saturations, electrocardiogram (ECG) and blood pressure are monitored, so allowing more individual advice on possible limits.

Travel

Apart from the business of trying to obtain insurance cover for travel, some patients need to take extra precautions when flying any distance. At high altitude oxygen saturations drop, so cyanosed people need to be aware of this and arrange to have supplemental oxygen available. They also require encouragement to avoid dehydration and to move around regularly because of the risk of thrombosis.

Contraception

The majority of females with congenital heart disease can use the regular methods of contraception. There are, however, some exceptions. In the cyanosed patient, polycythaemia may predispose to thrombosis so that the combined pill, which is the most effective contraceptive, may prove to be dangerous. These patients may be better with the low dose or 'mini' pill with only a small dose of progesterone. The alternative is the depot injection of progesterone which is given every 6–10 weeks. Intrauterine contraceptive coils may be effective but there is the slight risk of infection and if used, prophylactic antibiotics must be administered on insertion. The 'morning after' pill is high in oestrogen and therefore a worry for cyanosed patients because of the above risk of thrombus formation due to polycythaemia. Sterilization may be considered but the slight risks of surgery and anaesthesia mean that it should be performed in a hospital where specialist anaesthetic and cardiac care is available.

Pregnancy

Most women who are symptom free before pregnancy will be able to carry a fetus to full term safely. Pre-pregnancy counselling, ideally by both the cardiologist and the obstetrician, is important to discuss the risks and genetic implications with both parents. Because of the changes in hormone levels, extra circulating blood volume (up to an additional 50%) and the developing weight, extra strain is placed on the heart. Fortunately, with the exception of Eisenmenger syndrome, there is no increased mortality associated with pregnancy in congenital heart disease (Schmaltz et al 1999). However, in contrast, there is still considerable morbidity, due to congestive cardiac failure, thrombo-embolic complications and disturbances of rhythm (Schmaltz et al 1999). In cases of Eisenmenger syndrome, maternal morbidity is as high as 52%. This figure was noted by Gleicher et al in 1979 and today remains the same (Goodwin et al 1999). The greatest risk of death is in the peripartum period. In anyone who is cyanosed, the risk to the baby is quite high because of a lack of oxygenated blood to the placenta and it is not uncommon for these patients to suffer spontaneous abortions. The other factor which

must be taken into consideration is that if the mother does not have a good prognosis, who is going to look after the baby if she dies?

If pregnancy does occur it is important that the mother has regular clinical assessment, ideally by both a cardiologist and obstetrician to make sure that she is not developing cardiac failure, that there is no evidence of pulmonary oedema and that the baby is growing normally. She may have to be admitted to hospital to rest before the delivery. It is generally thought that cardiac patients should progress through a natural labour and a normal delivery, although they may need extra help at the end of the second stage in the way of suction or forceps. Caesarean section would be advised for the same reason as in other pregnant women. Some cardiologists recommend that antibiotics be administered once the membranes rupture but this may not be necessary if the delivery is entirely normal. A mother with a heart defect may need to stay in hospital for a few days after the birth in order to recover. As deep vein thrombosis is more common after a birth, it may be necessary to administer subcutaneous heparin until the mother is fully mobile.

In the mother with a heart defect, the risk of the fetus being similarly affected is about 2–5% (Burn et al 1998), but with fetal echocardiograms this can be checked from about 16–20 weeks. This does not necessarily mean that the pregnancy should be terminated. The mother will require great support at this time and will need the chance to talk over all possibilities, with professionals as well as family. If she decides to proceed with the pregnancy, at the very least there will be the chance for preparation. If termination is chosen, this should be performed in a hospital with anaesthetists who are experienced in caring for patients with congenital heart disease and a prophylactic course of antibiotics must be prescribed.

MEDICAL INVESTIGATIONS

Cardiac investigations have been described elsewhere (Chapter 8). For the adult with congenital heart disease the most useful diagnostic tool is probably transoesophageal echocardiography (TOE) but ECG, transthoracic echocardiography, cardiac catheterisation, angiography, electrophysiology studies (EPS), X-ray and magnetic resonance imaging (MRI) all have a part to play. MRI is particularly useful at delineating the structure of extracardiac vessels so that if coarctation or recoarctation of the aorta is suspected, MRI would be the investigation of choice. Cardiac catheterisation is needed if venous pathways are thought to be obstructed after a Senning or Mustard procedure, for instance. It must be remembered that ballooning and stenting procedures are not only used for coronary arteries. Interventional catheterisation is widely used in congenital heart medicine not only to widen and keep vessels open but also to occlude holes and vessels. Electrophysiological studies (EPS) are very often required in congenital heart patients as unfortunately many operative procedures, especially those involving the atria, undertaken in early years, have resulted in late arrhythmias. Failing ventricles are also known to cause atrial arrhythmias. Radiofrequency ablation (RFA) may offer treatment if extra pathways can be demonstrated or it may be that further surgery is required to improve the haemodynamic status. Antitachycardic pacing may also be a possible treatment. Coronary angiography must also be remembered for these patients as congenital defects do not preclude them from developing the more common adult diseases.

Nursing care following these procedures is no different than for other cardiac patients but nurses should remember that oxygen saturations, for example via oximetry, may be acceptably lower and if they have had a right or left aortopulmonary shunt it may not be possible to take the blood pressure on the affected side. It should also be noted that these patients may be more anxious because of their previous experiences.

SURGERY

Patients with congenital heart disease can present many problems. Most will have previously undergone at least one major operation. Resternotomy can be difficult especially if there is a conduit in place. A conduit is an artificial tube created to link usually a chamber to a vessel, to bypass blood around a defect. This may be adherent to the sternum and will necessitate cannulating the femoral vessels in order to establish bypass presternotomy, should there be any accidental rupture of the conduit. An antifibrinolytic agent such as aprotinin is often required for several hours postoperatively to reduce bleeding.

Myocardial preservation is difficult with hypertrophied ventricles and longer bypass times result in more postoperative complications. Many of these patients are cyanosed and as a result, organs other than the heart may be adversely affected. Renal or hepatic impairment may be a feature of the postoperative state. It should also be remembered that the cyanosed patient may need to be transfused to a higher packed cell volume (PCV). If the patient is dependent on a single ventricle, such as after a Fontan or total caval pulmonary connection procedure, then a greater filling pressure may be required. Consequently, because of high venous pressures, prolonged pleural effusion may subsequently occur. Any residual lesions may be poorly tolerated and it is usual for TOE to be carried out before chest closure to check for their presence. Postoperative arrhythmias will need immediate recognition and treatment. Once again, knowledge of the abnormal anatomy and physiology is essential when caring for this group of patients.

Finally, because of the complexity of some of these operations, success is not guaranteed and patients and families/carers need a great deal of support and patience when decisions are being made about whether or not surgery should be performed. They will require copious information, written as well as oral, and should the patient die, this support will often be needed for some time afterwards.

The following sections will identify the more common defects, possible treatment in childhood and reasons for an admission to hospital in adulthood. The nomenclature of congenital heart defects is complicated and in common with many other specialist subjects, the relevant literature is littered with the use of initials. Here it should be emphasized that CHD does not always refer to coronary heart disease, it may also mean congenital heart disease. The initials in general use will be explained.

At this point, because congenital heart defects occur while this organ is developing, it is worthwhile reviewing in diagrammatic form the fetal and adult circulations (Fig. 12.1A,B). Of note is the foramen ovale and the ductus arteriosus (Fig. 12.1A). The foramen ovale is one of two shunt systems in the fetal circulation which should close at or soon after birth. It links the right and left atria, allowing the non-functional lungs to be bypassed. The second shunt, the ductus arteriosus, transfers a large volume of blood from the pulmonary artery directly into the aorta, again bypassing the pulmonary circulation. Adequate blood is still received by the lungs to aid their development. The normal adult circulation is diagrammatically represented in Figure 12.1B.

ATRIAL SEPTAL DEFECT (ASD)

This is the most common defect found in adults. Most defects are ostium secundum defects, some are ostium primum defects and a few are sinus venosus defects (Fig. 12.2). Occasionally the foramen ovale itself remains open. Atrial fibrillation is a feature of both the pre- and postoperative condition.

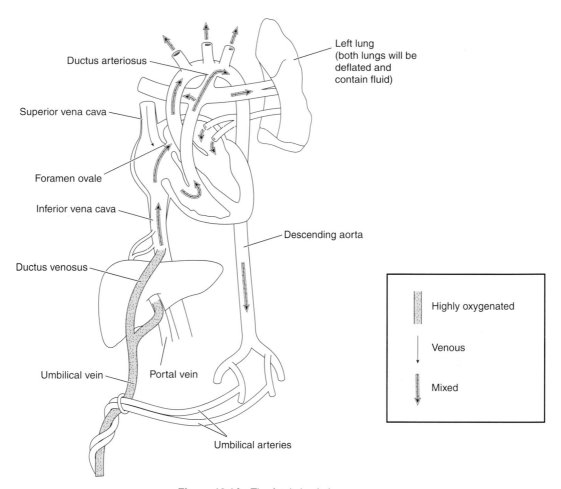

Figure 12.1A The fetal circulation.

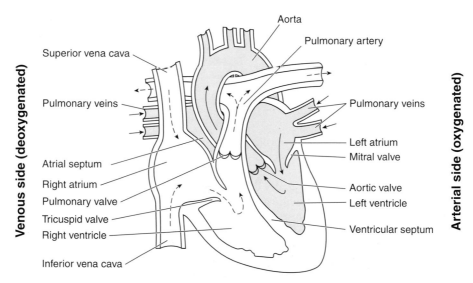

Figure 12.1B Normal adult circulation.

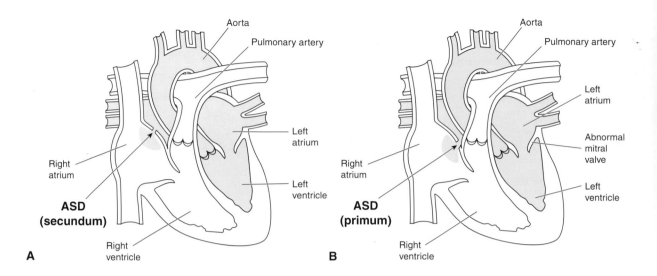

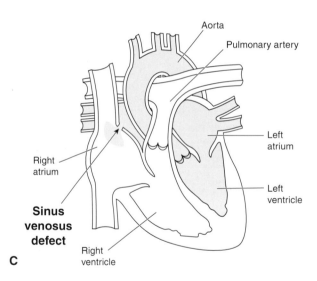

Figure 12.2 Atrial septal defect. A: Ostium secundum defect: opening in the middle of the septum – the most common ASD. B: Ostium primum defect: opening at the lower end of the atrial septum, near to the atrioventricular (AV) junction. C: Sinus venosus defect: opening is below the superior vena cava (SVC) or at the right of the inferior vena cava (IVC) junction.

Treatment in childhood

Nowadays secundum ASDs may be closed by a special device introduced via a cardiac catheter in the laboratory, such as an Amplatzer device which looks like the spokes of an open umbrella. However, the majority of adults who have had treatment as children will have had a surgical closure with either direct suture or a patch.

Reasons for admission to the adult unit

- For medical investigations.

- Initial closure either by device or surgery.
- Investigation and treatment of arrhythmias.
- Following a CVA.

ATRIOVENTRICULAR SEPTAL DEFECT (AVSD)

This defect is caused by the maldevelopment of the atrioventricular junction. There may be an atrial septal defect (an ostium primum ASD), a ventricular septal defect (VSD) or both, an abnormal common atrioventricular (AV) valve or abnormal left and right AV

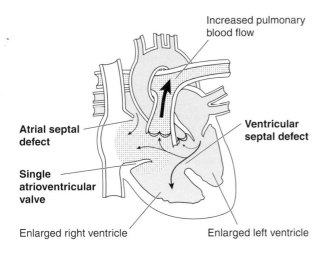

Figure 12.3 Complete atrioventricular septal defect.

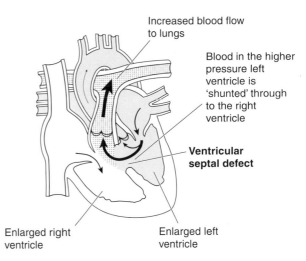

Figure 12.5 Ventricular septal defect.

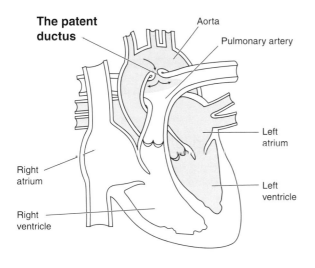

Figure 12.4 Patent ductus arteriosus.

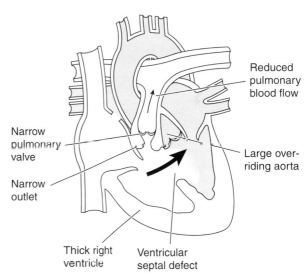

Figure 12.6 Tetralogy of Fallot.

valves (Fig. 12.3). It is termed 'complete' if there are both atrial and septal defects and 'partial' if there is only an atrial defect. The complete form is very often seen in patients with Down's syndrome.

Treatment in childhood

Complete repair with closure of the defects with patches and repair of the valves. Earlier patients may have had a 'banding' of the pulmonary artery as a first stage to reduce the amount of blood perfusing the lungs, but now early repair is recommended so as to avoid the problems of pulmonary hypertension.

Reasons for admission to the adult unit

- For medical investigations if there is a suspicion of a residual leak. These would include TOE and cardiac catheterisation and possibly EPS.
- For further surgery to close defects and to repair or replace valves. A few patients develop subaortic obstruction and this may need resection.

- Eisenmenger syndrome, if a repair has not been possible at an early age.

PATENT DUCTUS ARTERIOSUS (PDA)

The ductus arteriosus forms part of the fetal circulation linking the pulmonary artery and aorta but should close shortly after birth (Figs 12.1A and 12.4). Discovery of a moderate or large patent ductus is rare in adults as most will have been closed in infancy or childhood. A large shunt will probably be associated with Eisenmenger syndrome.

Treatment in childhood

Closure either by an umbrella-like device, coils or surgery.

Reasons for admission to the adult unit

- Investigations to rule out irreversible pulmonary hypertension.
- Device closure.
- Treatment for Eisenmenger syndrome, if symptomatic.

VENTRICULAR SEPTAL DEFECT (VSD)

This is a hole in the septum between the ventricles (Fig. 12.5). Although it is the most common heart defect found in children, about 65% of these holes close spontaneously. Others may reduce in size but never close completely. Depending on the amount of left-to-right shunting through the hole, the defect will probably have been closed early in childhood. Adults may either have an insignificant VSD and need infrequent outpatient checks along with advice about antibiotic prophylaxis or they will present with reversed shunting and pulmonary hypertension (Eisenmenger syndrome).

Treatment in childhood

If there is significant left-to-right shunting, the hole is closed either by direct suture or with a patch. Some adults will have come from the era when bypass surgery for infants was considered to be too dangerous and a palliative banding of the pulmonary artery may have been performed to cut down the flow of blood as an initial operation before closure of the defect on bypass at a later date. These patients will have a thoracotomy as well as a sternotomy scar.

Reasons for admission to the adult unit

- Medical investigation.
- Rarely, closure of a VSD either with a device or by surgery.
- Those with Eisenmenger syndrome may need regular venesection, iron therapy and, if needed, oxygen therapy. Heart/lung transplantation might be contemplated.
- Infective endocarditis is a possibility and will necessitate a course of intravenous antibiotic therapy and in rare cases surgery.

TETRALOGY OF FALLOT (TOF)

This is the most common form of cyanotic heart disease seen in adults. Fortunately, in the Western world, it is rare to see an unoperated adult with this condition but if they do reach adulthood because the circulation has been reasonably balanced, then surgery is possible.

Tetralogy of Fallot consists of four (*tetra* is Greek for four) defects. There is a subaortic ventricular septal defect, right ventricular outflow tract obstruction, over-riding of the aorta and hypertrophy of the right ventricle (Fig. 12.6).

Treatment in childhood

Palliative surgery (to increase the flow of blood to the lungs) may consist of the following procedures.

- Blalock–Taussig shunt. An anastomosis between the right or left subclavian artery and the right or left pulmonary artery via a right or left thoracotomy.
- Waterston shunt. An anastomosis between the ascending aorta and the right pulmonary artery.
- Pott's shunt. An anastomosis between the descending aorta and the left pulmonary artery.
- Brock procedure. An infundibular resection or pulmonary valvotomy.

Reparative surgery may include closure of the ventricular septal defect and relief of the right outflow tract obstruction by valvotomy, transannular patch and/or patch to pulmonary artery or by valved conduit from right ventricle to pulmonary artery.

Reasons for admission to the adult unit

- Medical investigations either as a general assessment or before further surgery.
- Further surgery after palliation.

- Further surgery after an earlier repair. The pulmonary valve may become significantly incompetent and the patient may need a homograft replacement. There might be a residual VSD and if the shunt across it is more than 1.5:1 (the pulmonary to systemic flow ratio) then intervention is advised.
- Arrhythmias requiring investigation and treatment. These may be due to haemodynamic deterioration in which case further surgery will be required.
- Balloon dilatation or stent insertion to relieve branch pulmonary artery stenosis.

COARCTATION OF AORTA (COA)

This is a narrowing of the aorta, usually just below the origin of the left subclavian artery but it may be anywhere in the aorta, even below the diaphragm (Fig. 12.7). It is usually diagnosed in infancy, when surgery is carried out. If the narrowing is not severe, then it is possible that it will not be diagnosed until adulthood. Symptoms may include headaches related to hypertension and leg cramps may develop. A bicuspid aortic valve is often present and in later life this may become calcified and stenosed and require surgery. Coarctation may be associated with Turner's syndrome in females (X0 chromosomes, a short stature, webbed neck and sterility).

Treatment in childhood

Resection of the narrowed area and an end-to-end anastomosis is the most common treatment but sometimes the left subclavian artery is used to enlarge the narrowed area and occasionally a graft replacement is necessary.

Although recoarctation may be relieved by balloon angioplasty, ballooning of native coarctation has not been so successful. It has caused intimal bleeding and aneurysm formation (Ovaert et al 1998).

Reasons for admission to the adult unit

- Medical investigations, possibly including magnetic resonance imaging (MRI).
- Surgery. Any patient presenting with coarctation or recoarctation should have some sort of intervention. Surgical repair is not so easy in adults and may incur more risk. It may be necessary for the operation to be performed on cardiopulmonary bypass or at least to have bypass standing by.

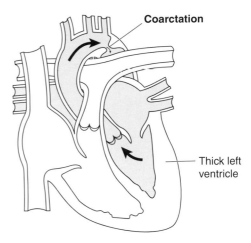

Figure 12.7 Coarctation of aorta.

- Balloon dilatation or stent insertion.
- Some patients develop aneurysms at the site of the coarctation which may in turn require surgery.
- Persistent systemic hypertension following surgery, which seems to be more common the later the repair, is treated with standard pharmacological therapy.

PULMONARY ATRESIA

Pulmonary atresia is where the pulmonary valve will not open, preventing a forward flow of blood from the right ventricle. Complete blockage of the pulmonary valve may be associated with a ventricular septal defect or an intact ventricular septum (Fig. 12.8) and a hypoplastic right ventricle. The pulmonary arteries may be of a reasonable size or be extremely narrow. Major aortopulmonary collateral arterioles (MAPCAS) may be present at birth or develop later.

Treatment in childhood

- A Blalock–Taussig shunt (an anastomosis between the subclavian artery and pulmonary artery on either side).
- A pulmonary valvotomy, either balloon or surgical.
- A valved conduit insertion between the right ventricle and pulmonary artery, closure of ventricular septal defect and ligation of collateral vessels.
- Unifocalization of collateral vessels to provide a unifocal blood supply to each lung and to encourage the growth of pulmonary arteries.

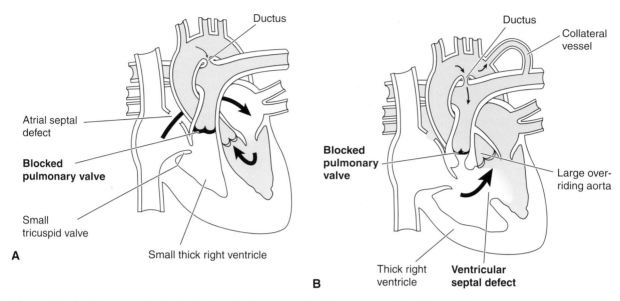

Figure 12.8 A: Pulmonary atresia – intact ventricular septum. B: Pulmonary atresia with ventricular septal defect.

- A Fontan procedure when the right atrium is anastomosed to the main pulmonary artery so that venous return is directed to the lungs, bypassing a hypoplastic right ventricle. In latter years, this operation has been modified and total caval pulmonary connection (TCPC) is more often performed.

Reasons for admission to the adult unit

- Medical investigations as a general assessment or of arrhythmias or prior to further surgery.
- For replacement of a conduit.
- For further palliative surgery such as a central shunt.
- For conversion of Fontan to TCPC circulation.

TRICUSPID ATRESIA

Absence of the tricuspid valve or extreme narrowing, possibly associated with a VSD (Fig. 12.9). An ASD allows blood to flow from the right to left atrium, then into the left ventricle and to the whole of the body. The VSD will allow some blood to flow from the left to right ventricle, and to the lungs.

Treatment in childhood

- Blalock–Taussig shunt if a VSD is not present.

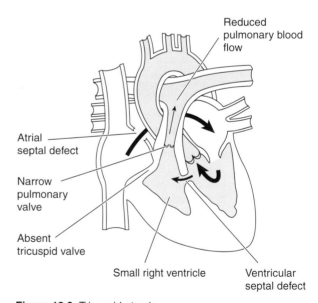

Figure 12.9 Tricuspid atresia.

- Banding of the pulmonary artery if the VSD is causing too large a shunt.
- Fontan or TCPC procedure.

Reasons for admission to the adult unit

- Medical investigation to check on the patency of systemic venous pathways or on arrhythmias.
- Further surgery.

SIMPLE TRANSPOSITION OF THE GREAT ARTERIES (TGA)

In this defect, the aorta emerges from the right ventricle and therefore pumps deoxygenated blood round the body. The pulmonary artery comes off the left ventricle and takes oxygenated blood back to the lungs (Fig. 12.10).

Treatment in childhood

In order to survive with this defect, a baby has to have a connection made between these two separate circulations and a balloon atrial septostomy is carried out soon after birth to allow some oxygenated blood into the systemic circulation. A 'switch' operation is performed within the first few weeks of life. This involves trans-section and reanastomosis of the great arteries (aorta to left ventricle and pulmonary artery to the right ventricle with coronary artery transfer).

In the 1960s and 1970s infants with TGA would have undergone either a Mustard or a Senning procedure which involved rearranging the atrial circulation so that oxygenated blood was pumped into the systemic circulation. However, the patient was still left with the right ventricle providing the systemic circulation.

In patients with complex transposition, that is TGA, a VSD and pulmonary stenosis (*left* ventricular outflow tract obstruction), the initial operation would have been a Blalock–Taussig shunt, followed by a Rastelli procedure a few years later. This operation involves closing the VSD so that the blood from the left ventricle flows into the aorta and a valved conduit is inserted between the right ventricle and the pulmonary trunk. The conduit will require replacement on at least one occasion and probably more.

Reasons for admission to the adult unit

- For medical investigations including TOE, cardiac catheterisation, EPS just to check on the right ventricular function and also to assess the venous pathways which may have become obstructed.
- Systemic or pulmonary venous pathway narrowing or obstruction requiring ballooning, stenting or even further surgery.
- Right ventricular failure requiring pharmaceutical assistance.
- Arrhythmias requiring EPS and occasionally pacemaker insertion.
- Assessment for transplantation.

For those with complex transposition, surgery to replace the homograft/conduit will be necessary.

PULMONARY STENOSIS

In this defect, there is a narrowing of the pulmonary valve or in the area above or below the valve (Fig. 12.11).

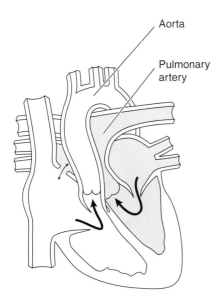

Figure 12.10 Simple transposition of the great arteries (TGA).

Aorta

Pulmonary artery

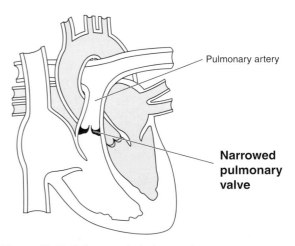

Figure 12.11 Pulmonary (valve) stenosis.

Pulmonary artery

Narrowed pulmonary valve

Treatment in childhood

Nowadays if the stenosis is significant, a balloon valvotomy is carried out to stretch the narrowed area. This procedure is carried out in the cardiac catheter laboratory. Before this treatment had been developed, any severe stenosis required surgery. Closed valvotomies (Brock procedures) were often performed in infants but open valvotomies, performed on bypass, were usually needed later.

Reasons for admission to the adult unit

- For medical investigations.
- For balloon valvotomy.
- For surgical valvotomy.
- For reintervention including balloon dilatation or valve replacement with homograft.

CONGENITALLY CORRECTED TRANSPOSITION OF THE GREAT ARTERIES (CTGA)

This should not be confused with simple transposition. In this defect, as well as the great arteries being transposed, the ventricles are also transposed so that it is usually described as atrioventricular discordance and ventriculo-arterial discordance. If there are no other defects, it should not cause problems. However, very often there is an association of other defects such as a ventricular septal defect, pulmonary stenosis, tricuspid incompetence and arrhythmias (Fig. 12.12).

Treatment in childhood

Patients with no associated defects may have managed to escape diagnosis and even those with a VSD and pulmonary stenosis may have had a balanced circulation and remained undiagnosed or at least not required surgery. Others will have become cyanosed and required a Blalock–Taussig shunt followed by a 'repair' involving closing the VSD and placing a conduit between the morphological left ventricle and the pulmonary artery. More recently, a double switch operation may have been performed. The morphological left ventricle is tunnelled through the VSD to the aorta and a valved conduit is placed between the morphological right ventricle and the pulmonary artery. An atrial 'switch' (Mustard or Senning procedure) is also necessary. Finally permanent pacing may be required for these patients who commonly develop heart block.

Reasons for admission to the adult unit

- Medical investigations.
- Initial repair.
- Replacement of conduits.
- Left atrioventricular valve repair or replacement.
- Pacemaker insertion.

AORTIC STENOSIS (AS)

This is essentially left ventricular outflow tract obstruction (LVOTO) and may occur at valvular, subvalvular and supravalvular levels. Aortic valve stenosis is usually due to a bicuspid valve and is often associated with coarctation of the aorta (Fig. 12.13).

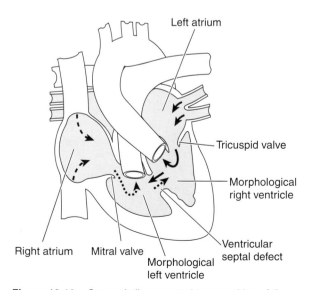

Figure 12.12 Congenitally corrected transposition of the great arteries.

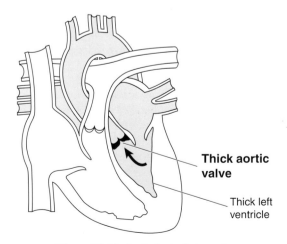

Figure 12.13 Aortic (valve) stenosis.

Supravalvular aortic stenosis is less common, is seen in Williams' syndrome (infantile hypercalcaemia, producing typical elfin features and learning difficulties) and is often associated with peripheral pulmonary artery stenoses. Subvalvular stenosis is often due to a discrete membrane or to a muscular ridge which may regrow following resection.

Treatment in childhood

In recent years, significant (i.e. a pressure gradient of >50 mmHg) valvar stenosis has been initially treated with balloon valvotomy, but most adults who have needed treatment as children will have had surgical valvotomies and, rarely, aortic valve replacements. Many of these patients will require further surgery as they grow older.

Reasons for admission to the adult unit

- For medical investigation.
- For balloon valvuloplasty.
- For surgical valvotomy or valve repair if previous surgery has resulted in incompetence. In some cases a valve replacement is necessary and others may have a Ross procedure. This involves resection of the native aortic valve and moving the patient's own pulmonary valve to the aortic position, with reimplantation of the coronary arteries. A homograft is then inserted in the right ventricular outflow tract. This latter operation has the great advantage of the patient not requiring long-term anticoagulation following the surgery whereas patients undergoing valve replacement with a mechanical valve will require warfarin for the rest of their lives.

EBSTEIN'S ANOMALY

This is an abnormality of the tricuspid valve (Fig. 12.14). It is displaced down into the right ventricle and as a result, the inflow of the right ventricle is 'atrialized', that is, the ventricular wall is thinner than usual. There may be a degree of right outflow tract obstruction, tricuspid regurgitation or stenosis, an atrial septal defect, accessory conduction pathways causing atrial tachycardias and varying degrees of cyanosis or pulmonary hypertension.

Treatment in childhood

Patients with mild Ebstein's anomaly may be asymptomatic and not require any treatment in childhood. If

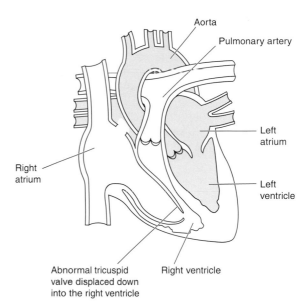

Figure 12.14 Ebstein's anomaly.

there is any right outflow tract obstruction a Blalock–Taussig shunt may have been necessary. If the tricuspid valve is incompetent every effort is made to repair the native valve but sometimes valve replacement is necessary.

If an accessory conduction pathway is present, it will be necessary to map and ablate it either at the time of surgery or in the catheter laboratory beforehand.

Reasons for admission to the adult unit

- Arrhythmias requiring EPS and possible ablation of accessory pathways.
- Surgery to repair or replace the tricuspid valve.

EISENMENGER SYNDROME

This is an extreme form of pulmonary vascular obstructive disease where there is irreversible pulmonary hypertension due to a high pulmonary vascular resistance with reversed or bidirectional shunting at great vessel, ventricular or atrial levels (Fig. 12.15). It may develop in infancy or even be present from birth.

Treatment in childhood is not usually needed. Any symptoms tend to be treated if necessary and as outlined below.

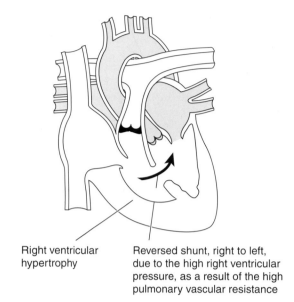

Figure 12.15 Eisenmenger syndrome.

Right ventricular hypertrophy

Reversed shunt, right to left, due to the high right ventricular pressure, as a result of the high pulmonary vascular resistance

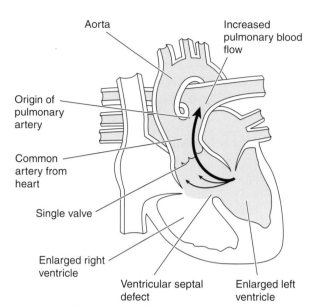

Figure 12.16 Truncus arteriosus.

Aorta

Increased pulmonary blood flow

Origin of pulmonary artery

Common artery from heart

Single valve

Enlarged right ventricle

Ventricular septal defect

Enlarged left ventricle

Reasons for admission to the adult unit

- Haemodilution. The more cyanosed the patient, the higher the haemoglobin level becomes and the greater the risk of a CVA. Under controlled conditions, venesection is carried out with the patient's blood being replaced with clear fluid. This may result in iron depletion and iron supplements may be necessary.
- Establishment of oxygen therapy.
- Assessment for heart/lung transplantation.

These patients should be advised against pregnancy as there is a 50% risk to either the mother or fetus (Connelly et al 1998).

TRUNCUS ARTERIOSUS

In this defect the aorta and pulmonary artery arise from the ventricles as one vessel and there is always a VSD (Fig. 12.16).

Treatment in childhood

Older patients may have had a palliative banding of the branch pulmonary arteries to cut down the flow of blood to the lungs but in the last 20 years babies who have been diagnosed early would have had an early 'corrective' operation with a patch to the VSD and a valved conduit inserted between the right ventricle and the small pulmonary artery.

The latter will have been dissected from the trunk. Obviously the size of a conduit used in a neonate would only be large enough for a few years and will have been replaced possibly twice before the patient reaches adulthood. These conduits, whether homografts or synthetic tubes, tend to calcify and recent research has shown that subsequent conduits do not last as long as the originals (Stark et al 1998). Some patients will have been born in an era when surgery was not contemplated and will present with Eisenmenger syndrome.

Reasons for admission to the adult unit

- For medical investigations.
- For replacement of a conduit.
- For possible ballooning or stenting of branch pulmonary arteries.
- Eisenmenger syndrome if symptomatic.

INFECTIVE ENDOCARDITIS (IE)

Despite continual advice regarding oral and skin hygiene, antibiotic prophylaxis and even with adherence to this practice, some patients will present with an unexplained illness. It is essential that if IE is suspected, blood should be taken for culture on three occasions before commencing antibiotics/antifungal agents. Echocardiography may demonstrate a vegetation: a small growth on an incompetent valve or on foreign material such as a patch or conduit. Treatment varies from centre to centre but once the organism has been identified, all will involve a period of appropriate intravenous antibiotics/antifungal agents. It may be necessary for surgery to be performed to remove or replace the infected part.

DENTAL TREATMENT

Regular dental care is essential for an adult with CHD and occasionally it may be necessary for treatment to be carried out in hospital so as to avoid any risk of infection and subsequent IE. Antibiotic prophylaxis is necessary for any procedure which may cause bleeding. The current British Heart Foundation recommendations will offer additional information in this area.

SURGERY OTHER THAN CARDIAC

It should be stressed that if patients with congenital heart disease require any form of general surgery, they may need to be admitted to a specialist centre where anaesthetists who are used to dealing with cardiac problems are readily available.

The following four case studies bring together in a more holistic fashion the broad issues of care necessary for adults with congenital heart defects. Please note that the timing and type of surgery performed in earlier years differs from that which would occur in the 21st century.

CONCLUSION

This chapter has provided an outline regarding the common congenital conditions that may be encountered by the cardiac nurse caring for adult patients. A good knowledge of the cardiac anatomy and circulation and how these alter with congenital abnormalities is vital to guide the differing nursing skills required for those used to patients with acquired heart disease.

Case study 12.1

Sarah Parker was born normally in 1966. At 3 days of age she became cyanosed and was admitted to her local regional cardiac centre for investigation. Cardiac catheterisation demonstrated transposition of the great arteries (TGA), a ventricular septal defect (VSD) and patent ductus arteriosus. She was discharged home with prescribed oral digoxin but was readmitted at 5 months with a severe chest infection. An attempt was made to perform a balloon atrial septostomy but it was not possible. At 8 months of age she was admitted to a different regional centre because her parents had moved house and again cardiac catheterisation was carried out. The foramen ovale was found to be closed, so again it was impossible to perform an atrial septostomy. She was taken to theatre and had an atrial septectomy (Blalock–Hanlon procedure), banding of the pulmonary artery and ligation of patent ductus. A tracheostomy was also performed. (In those days endotracheal tubes were still made of red rubber and if left in place for more than a few days caused tracheal stenosis. Therefore it was fairly routine to perform a tracheostomy, because plastic tracheostomy tubes had become available.)

During the postoperative phase Sarah suffered a cardiac arrest after vomiting and aspirating, but she was successfully resuscitated and eventually went home 4 weeks later. She had two more admissions with chest infections before being admitted at 3 years of age for a Mustard procedure, closure of the VSD and debanding of the pulmonary artery and again had a tracheostomy. Twelve days later after decannulation she had another cardiac arrest. This was due to granulomata in the trachea and during the course of the next 3 months she had resection of granulomata on three occasions, before eventually being successfully decannulated and discharged home.

Over the next 5 years she was readmitted on four occasions because of stridor and underwent bronchoscopy and resection of tracheal web and granulomata. At 14 years of age she was readmitted for routine investigation to check her venous pathways. Cardiac catheterisation showed mild narrowing of both the superior vena cava (SVC) and inferior vena cava (IVC) pathways and widely patent pulmonary venous pathways.

Despite these repeated admissions, she attended mainstream school and successfully completed her education. She trained as a secretary and had full-time employment. Sarah married and had two daughters with no problems. However, at the age of 33 years, she presented with arrhythmias and increasing breathlessness. She underwent a transoesphageal echocardiogram and cardiac catheterisation which demonstrated severe SVC and IVC obstruction and after discussion with her, it was decided to place a stent in the narrowed area of the IVC. She again underwent cardiac catheterisation. The SVC was dilated with a balloon and a stent was placed in her IVC following which there was no longer a gradient in either pathway. At present Sarah's arrhythmias are controlled and she is no longer breathless.

Case study 12.2

Aftar Patel was born by normal delivery, was a healthy baby and grew up very normally, attending school and further education. At the age of 26 years, he suddenly suffered a severe headache and found next morning that he could not move his right arm. He was admitted to a neurology ward where a left temporal lobe embolus was diagnosed and during examination a heart murmur was heard. The cardiologist was asked to see him and suspected an atrial septal defect (ASD). He underwent a transoesophageal echocardiogram and it confirmed that he had a moderate-sized ASD. Aftar made a full recovery from the cerebrovascular accident (CVA/stroke) but following discussion, it was decided to admit him a year later for a transcatheter device closure of his defect. The procedure was performed under antibiotic cover and heparin was administered. The following day chest X-rays were performed to check the position of the device and transthoracic echocardiography confirmed secure closure. He was discharged home on subcutaneous heparin twice daily for 5 days and thereafter just a small dose of aspirin daily. Aftar is now well and working full time.

Case study 12.3

Claire Medgrove was born with a bicuspid aortic valve discovered incidentally at a school medical examination. Apart from regular outpatient checks, she grew up quite normally and was asymptomatic. She married and before embarking on a pregnancy it was decided she should be admitted for cardiac catheterisation and angiography. This demonstrated mixed aortic valve disease and after discussion, it was decided she should undergo an aortic valve replacement. At age 27 she had a 27 mm Carpentier-Edwards valve inserted. Claire progressed well and had three children with no problems. At age 37, she started having 'dizzy spells' and found going upstairs difficult. Investigation revealed a gradient of 70 mmHg across the valve which was calcified and there was some regurgitation.

This time it was decided to perform a Ross procedure. (This involves replacing the aortic valve with the patient's own pulmonary valve and then inserting a pulmonary homograft between the right ventricle and the pulmonary artery. It has the advantage that the patient does not require long-term anticoagulation therapy.) Claire's ascending aorta was found to be rather narrow so was replaced with a synthetic tube graft. She returned from the operating theatre in heart block and so was paced. Five days postoperatively, Claire complained of pain in her right calf and chest pain. Ultrasound of the legs showed a branch popliteal vein thrombosis in her right leg. A VQ scan showed multiple bilateral microemboli in the lungs and she was therefore anticoagulated. A VQ scan is a ventilation/perfusion lung scan. This demonstrates the distribution of blood flow and ventilation in the lungs, through the scanning of gamma radiation delivered through venous injection and inhalation. She did not revert to sinus rhythm so at 10 days she had a pacemaker inserted. Because of the emboli she was discharged home on warfarin. This was discontinued 6 months later. Claire is now well and enjoying an active life with her children.

Case study 12.4

Robin Brown was born with Tetralogy of Fallot. This was diagnosed at 5 months of age when his mother reported that on occasions he screamed, became blue and seemed to lose consciousness (what may be termed a typical 'spell' associated with Tetralogy of Fallot). A right Blalock–Taussig shunt was performed and at 10 years of age he had correction. Robin was well for the next 3 years and was no longer followed up clinically for the next 23 years. He had apparently been well until a few months before presenting himself at the local hospital.

He had started to experience palpitations on exertion and these had progressed to the point where he was having great difficulty with his job as a self-employed builder. By this time he was married and had three healthy children and was worried that he was not going to be able to support the family. Medical investigation revealed a large heart and severe pulmonary regurgitation. After discussion between Robin and his family, it was decided to replace his pulmonary valve with a homograft. This was carried out and 5 months later he was able to work again.

REFERENCES

Archer N, Burch M 1998 Paediatric cardiology: an introduction. Chapman and Hall Medical, London

Burn J, Brennan P, Little J et al 1998 Recurrence risks in offspring of adults with major heart defects: results from first cohort of British collaborative study. Lancet 351: 311–316

Celermajer DS, Deanfield JE 1993 Employment and insurance for young adults with congenital heart disease. British Heart Journal 69(6): 539–543

Connelly MS, Webb GD, Somerville J et al 1998 Canadian consensus conference on congenital heart defects in the adult 1996. Journal of Cardiology 14(4): 533–597

Gersony WM, Hayes CJ, Driscoll DJ et al 1993 Second natural history study of congenital heart defects. Quality of life of patients with aortic stenosis, pulmonary stenosis or ventricular septal defect. Circulation 87 (suppl 1): 52–65

Gleicher N, Midwall J, Hochberger D, Jaffin H 1979 Eisenmenger's syndrome and pregnancy. Obstetrical and Gynecological Survey 34: 721–741

Goodwin TM, Gherman RB, Hameed A, Elkayam U 1999 Favourable response of Eisenmenger syndrome to inhaled nitric oxide during pregnancy. American Journal of Obstetrics and Gynecology 180(1 pt 1): 64–67

Kantoch MJ, Collins-Nakai RL, Medwid S, Ungstad E, Taylor DA 1997 Adult patients' knowledge about their congenital heart disease. Canadian Journal of Cardiology 13(7): 641–645

MacMahon B, McKeown T, Record RG 1953 The incidence and life expectation of children with congenital heart disease. British Heart Journal 15: 121–129

Ovaert C, Benson LN, Nykanen D, Freedom RM 1998 Transcatheter treatment of coarctation of the aorta: a review. Paediatric Cardiology 19(1): 27–44

Schmaltz AA, Neudorf U, Winkler UH 1999 Outcome of pregnancy in women with congenital heart disease. Cardiology of the Young 9(1): 88–96

Somerville J 1996 Teenagers with congenital heart disease. In: Kurtz Z, Hopkins A (eds) Services for young people with chronic disorders in their transition from childhood to adult life. Royal College of Physicians of London, pp. 59–68

Sparacino PS, Tong EM, Messias DK, Foote D, Chelsa CA, Gilliss CL 1997 The dilemmas of parents of adolescents and young adults with congenital heart disease. Heart and Lung 26(3): 187–195

Stark J, Bull C, Stajevic M, Jothi M, Elliot M, De Leval M 1998 Fate of subpulmonary homograft conduits: determinants of late homograft failure. Journal of Thoracic and Cardiovascular Surgery 115(3): 507–516

FURTHER READING

Archer N, Burch M 1998 Paediatric cardiology: an introduction. Chapman and Hall Medical, London

Deanfield JE, Gersh BJ, Warnes CA, Mair DD 1998 Congenital heart disease in adults. In: Alexander RW, Schlant RG et al (eds) Hurst's the heart, 9th edn. McGraw Hill, New York, pp. 1995–2027

Hess J, Sutherland GR 1992 Congenital heart disease in adolescents and adults. Kluwer Academic Publishers, Dordrecht

Ho SY, Baker EJ, Rigby ML, Anderson RH 1995 Colour atlas of congenital heart disease. Mosby-Wolfe, London

Jordan SC, Scott O 1989 Heart disease in paediatrics, 3rd edn. Butterworths, London

Perloff JK, Child JS (eds) 1991 Congenital heart disease in adults. WB Saunders, Philadelphia

Presbitero P, Somerville J, Stone S, Aruta E, Spiegelhalter D, Rabajoli F 1994 Pregnancy in cyanotic congenital heart disease: outcome of mother and foetus. Circulation 89(6): 2673–2676

Redington A, Shore D, Oldershaw P 1994 Congenital heart disease in adults. WB Saunders, London

Rees PG, Tunstill AM, Pope T et al 2001 Heart children, 3rd edn. HeartLine Association, Camberley

Stark J, De Leval M 1983 Surgery for congenital heart defects. Grune and Stratton, London

Webb GD, Harrison DA, Connelly MS 1996 Challenges posed by the adult patient with congenital heart disease. Advances in Internal Medicine 41: 437–495

Support groups

GUCH (Grown Up Congenital Heart Patients' Association)
c/o 12 Rectory Road
Stanford Le Hope
Essex SS17 0DL
Helpline: 0800 854759
Fax: 01375 676900

The Marfan Association UK
Rochester House
5 Aldershot Road
Fleet
Hants GU13 9NG
Tel: 01252 810472
Fax: 01252 810473

13

Valve disorders

Frances Blackburn
Beverley Bookless

Within the last 50 years there has been a noticeable change in the occurrence and incidence of valve disease. In specific terms, the decline of rheumatic fever in the Western world has led to a decrease in the numbers of patients presenting with mitral stenosis. Conversely, there has been an increase in aortic stenosis, which is a result of degenerative disease in an ageing population. Aortic regurgitation also remains relatively common and has many causes. As with other valve lesions, a decline in this condition has been observed in conjunction with the decrease in incidence of rheumatic fever (Julian et al 1996). In 1932 Campbell reported that 67% of aortic regurgitation could be attributed to rheumatic fever and 19% to syphilis yet some 50 years later, Davies (1980), in 100 cases studied, reported 26% were a result of rheumatic fever and none of syphilis. Regardless of the cause of valve disease, there are two types of stress placed on the heart: increased afterload (the resistance to ventricular ejection of blood) due to valve stenosis and insufficiency as a result of valve regurgitation.

The majority of valve disease affects the left side of the heart with the aortic and mitral valves being involved. Damage to valves in the right side of the heart is relatively rare and is often associated with left heart valve disease. An example is tricuspid stenosis which is often seen with mitral stenosis, following rheumatic fever (Guzzetta & Dossey 1992). This chapter explores the variety of presenting valve diseases, dividing the aetiogy into the left and right sides of the heart. Treatments and nursing care are discussed with each presenting condition.

HEART VALVES

The heart has four chambers; the upper two are the right and left atria and the lower two the right and left ventricles (see Chapter 4). The four heart valves aid the blood flow through the chambers in a specified direction.

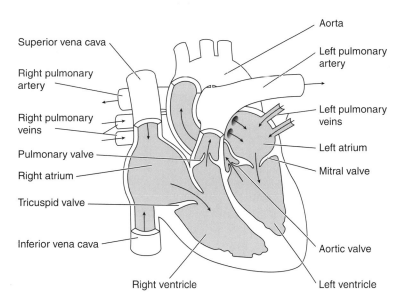

Figure 13.1 Position of the valves within the human heart.

- The **tricuspid valve** is located between the right atrium and the right ventricle. As its name suggests, the tricuspid valve has three leaflets or cusps, the anterior, posterior and septal.
- The **pulmonary valve** is between the right ventricle and the pulmonary artery. This valve has three cusps, two set anteriorly and the third in a posterior position.
- The **mitral valve** is between the left atrium and left ventricle. It has two leaflets, one anterior and one posterior. The leaflets are supported by the chordae tendineae; these are fibrous bands that pass into the two large papillary muscles of the left ventricle.
- The **aortic valve** is between the left ventricle and aorta. The aortic valve usually has three leaflets, thus it is termed tricuspid.

LEFT HEART VALVE DISEASE

THE AORTIC VALVE

Aortic stenosis

Aortic stenosis is a narrowing of the opening of the valve that obstructs the left ventricular blood flow into the aorta during systole. Over time the left ventricle becomes hypertrophied (enlarged) in order to ensure an adequate pressure of blood through the narrowed

opening into the aorta. This creates an additional problem of dilatation of the ventricle, resulting in left-sided heart failure as the ventricle finds it increasingly difficult to eject blood into the aorta. Ultimately, cardiac output and ejection fraction decrease and pulmonary hypertension develops (Rackley et al 1990).

Rheumatic fever

The incidence of rheumatic fever has declined significantly over the last 50 years in both Western Europe and the United States (US). In industrialized countries the annual incidence is around 0.5 cases per 100 000

Box 13.1 Causes of aortic valve disease

Aortic stenosis
  Rheumatic fever
  Degenerative changes
  Congenital
  Supravalvular or subvalvular aortic stenosis
Aortic regurgitation
  Rheumatic fever
  Infective endocarditis
  Syphilis
  Non-infective
  Congenital
  Non-degenerative causes, which destroy smooth muscle and elastic tissue
  Inflammatory – ankylosing spondylitis, Reiter's syndrome

children of school age. However, in developing countries rheumatic fever remains an endemic disease with an annual incidence ranging from 100 to 200 cases per 100 000 school-aged children (Olivier 2000). In these countries it remains a major cause of cardiovascular mortality.

This disease has been associated with poverty and the accompanying social factors of poor housing, overcrowding and poor diet. Rheumatic fever is caused by group A streptococcal infection of the pharynx. An improvement in social standards and economy has resulted in better housing, nutrition and less overcrowding and, along with penicillin treatment, has reduced the incidence of both rheumatic fever and consequently chronic rheumatic heart disease in the West.

Rheumatic fever causes the leaflets of the heart valves to become inflamed and oedematous. In chronic rheumatic heart disease they become fused and thickened. This may occur in an uneven manner, resulting in the valve being unable to close properly. Rheumatic aortic stenosis usually appears alongside mitral stenosis (Burckhardt et al 1996).

Degenerative disease

This usually occurs in patients over the age of 60 years and, with an ageing population, is one of the more common causes of aortic stenosis. The leaflets gradually become immobile because of the deposit of calcium. This common cause of aortic stenosis seems to be the result of normal mechanical stress over time. Although degenerative calcification extends to the leaflets from their base it does not result in fusion (Braunwald 1992). Mitral calcification and coronary artery disease often accompany it, as patients with diabetes mellitus and hypercholesterolaemia appear at higher risk (Deutscher et al 1984).

Calcification may also involve other structures of the heart, the most important being the bundle of His in the septum. This can inevitably lead to conduction problems, such as first-degree heart block and left bundle branch block (Burckhardt et al 1996). Occasionally calcium deposits can be thrown off and enter the circulation, causing infarction or ischaemia (Holley et al 1963).

Congenital

The aortic valve is normally tricuspid and the most common congenital cause of aortic stenosis is a bicuspid valve. This is the most common cause of aortic stenosis with no other associated valve disease in patients under the age of 30 years (Burckhardt et al 1996). Bicuspid valves are not commonly stenotic at birth but become so as the child grows due to the leaflets becoming fibrosed from the turbulence of blood flow over the valve. The changes occur over decades and through degenerative change stenosis results in the congenitally abnormal aortic valve (Braunwald 1992). Single or one-leaflet aortic valves are less common but are the most usual cause of severe aortic stenosis in babies. Congenital abnormalities are sometimes associated with other complications such as coarctation or patent ductus arteriosus (Campbell 1968).

Other causes

Other forms of obstructive outflow of blood through the aortic valve can occur. These include supravalvular or subvalvular aortic stenosis. Supravalvular stenosis is caused by a constricting ridge of fibrous tissue at the upper edges of the sinuses of Valsalva. Its rarer forms are associated with a condition known as hypoplastic left heart syndrome. Subvalvular aortic stenosis is characterized by a fibrous ring obstructing the outflow from the left ventricle (Burckhardt et al 1996).

Clinical symptoms

In the natural history of aortic stenosis patients do not present with problems until they are well into their fifth to seventh decades. Patients with congenital aortic stenosis often present through childhood. Those with rheumatic valve disease usually also have disease of the mitral valve, which presents before aortic stenosis (Selzer 1987). Tiredness and dizziness are the first presenting features which then become associated with a triad of characteristic symptoms: syncope (a transient loss of consciousness), angina pectoris and dyspnoea. Dyspnoea becomes a more distinct problem when left ventricular function deteriorates.

Syncope. About 25% of patients with aortic stenosis experience syncope. It usually occurs during or following exercise and is often associated with angina (Burckhardt et al 1996). Syncope is associated with reduced blood flow to the brain that occurs during exercise when peripheral vasodilatation takes place. It may result from the effects of stretching receptors in the left ventricle as the end-diastolic pressure increases. These receptors relay impulses to the vasomotor centre of the brain, which in turn prevents the normal vasoconstriction reflex associated with exercise (Brody & Abboud 1976). It can also be associated with arrhythmias, such as ventricular tachycardia (VT), ventricular fibrillation (VF) or rapid atrial fibrillation.

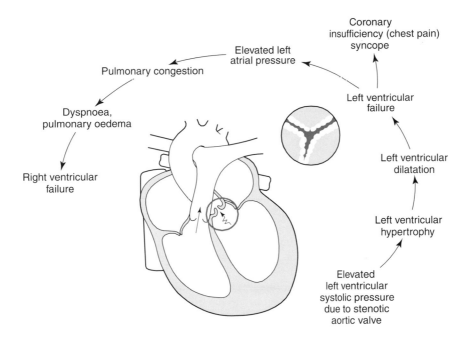

Figure 13.2 The effects of aortic stenosis. (Reproduced with permission from Guzzetta & Dossey 1992.)

Sudden death is associated with syncope and is probably a result of hypotension that accompanies the collapse. This may lead to a fatal ventricular tachycardia or fibrillation (Burckhardt et al 1996). Patients need to have an understanding of why they suddenly black out in order to be able to manage this and recognize the limitations to exercise. This is a very frightening symptom, particularly for those caring for or accompanying patients with aortic stenosis. Ventricular arrhythmias and conduction problems themselves are common in aortic stenosis, with 15–20% of sudden deaths being attributed to this in symptomatic patients (Rackley et al 1990). The arrhythmias are a result of the hypertrophied ventricle rather than the valve stenosis itself.

Angina pectoris. Angina is more common in patients with aortic stenosis than any other valve disease. It occurs in about two-thirds of patients with severe lesions and half of these have significant coronary artery disease. It is typical of the presenting features of patients with ischaemic heart disease and occurs following exertion and is relieved with rest. However, primarily it is produced by the imbalance of oxygen demand and supply rather than the usual narrowed coronary arteries. Demand for increased oxygen occurs because of the hypertrophied myocardium, while a reduction of available oxygen

occurs due to the stenotic valve reducing left ventricular output. Compression of the coronary arteries because of the abnormal pressures adds to the problem (Braunwald 1992).

Dyspnoea. This is the most common symptom experienced by patients and can be the most distressing. Breathlessness on exertion, paroxysmal dyspnoea and pulmonary oedema occur in up to 40% of patients (Kirklin & Barratt-Boyes 1993). Dyspnoea becomes much more severe in later stages of aortic stenosis and the patient is usually very distressed by this symptom which in turn exacerbates breathlessness.

Investigations

Electrocardiography (ECG). The 12-lead ECG will initially be normal, but as the disease progresses the classic signs of left ventricular hypertrophy will develop. Deep S-waves in the right precordial leads occur, together with large R-waves in the left precordial leads associated with ST segment depression and T-wave inversion. Progression of this left ventricular strain pattern is often an indication of the progression of left ventricular hypertrophy. Left axis deviation may also occur and as left ventricular function deteriorates features of left atrial overload may appear. This occurs in the form of a large negative component of the P-wave in V1 (the bifid M-shaped P-wave). Left bundle branch block (LBBB) may also develop, as may other conduction defects such as first-degree atrio-ventricular (AV) block or complete heart block. These occur as calcium invades the conduction tissues. The presence of atrial fibrillation may well indicate the presence of mitral valve disease or ischaemic heart disease, as it is unusual in pure aortic stenosis.

Echocardiography. Echocardiography (echo) re-veals thickened, non-mobile valve cusps. Evidence of calcification of the valve cusps may also be detected. The extent of left ventricular hypertrophy can also be assessed as can the presence of any left ventricular outflow tract obstruction. Obstruction at a subvalvular level is usually easily seen whilst supravalvular steno-sis may not be visualized due to difficulties in imaging the ascending aorta in adults. In aortic stenosis, as the outflow obstruction becomes more severe, left ventri-cular hypertrophy increases but the left ventricle remains small and contracts well. It is possible to correlate the degree of hypertrophy to a prediction of the aortic valve gradient. In addition, Doppler studies can in a non-invasive way assess the severity of valvu-lar obstruction and the gradient across the valve can be ascertained from the velocity of blood flow (Burckhardt et al 1996).

Chest X-ray. The chest X-ray may show a calcified valve and dilatation of the aorta distal to the obstruction. In the latter stages evidence of left ventricular enlarge-ment and pulmonary congestion may also be apparent. Radionuclide studies may be used to assess ventricular function and myocardial perfusion. By measurement of left ventricular ejection fraction at rest and during exer-cise, this technique can show deterioration of left ven-tricular function before symptoms have developed. It may also indicate impaired myocardial perfusion, sug-gesting underlying coronary artery disease.

Cardiac catheterisation. Because of advances in echocardiography, for young patients with isolated aortic stenosis cardiac catheterisation may not be necessary. However, it may be required to define the anatomy of the aortic root or aorta if abnormalities are suspected. In older patients where myocardial ischaemia or other valve lesions are suspected cardiac catheterisation is performed, especially prior to valve replacement. This can estimate the severity of the stenosis and evaluate left ventricular function. Pressure readings in the left ventricle and proximal aorta allow the gradient across the valve to be measured. However, this may not be performed if very tight aortic stenosis is suspected.

Recordings of aortic and left ventricular pressures are recorded simultaneously and the peak-to-peak

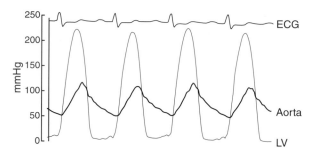

Figure 13.3 Recordings of aortic and left ventricular (LV) pressure obtained at cardiac catheterisation from a patient with severe aortic stenosis. The peak-to-peak gradient is approximately 110 mmHg. (Reproduced with permission from Julian et al 1996.)

systolic reading is used to assess the aortic gradient (Burckhardt et al 1996) (Fig. 13.3). For example, if the two readings were a systolic pressure of 180 mmHg in the left ventricle and 110 mmHg in the aorta the gradi-ent would be 70 mmHg. Coronary angiography is performed to outline the coronary circulation and identify the presence of coronary artery disease.

Medical treatment

Medical treatment is advised before symptoms develop to prevent complications and ensure valve replacement is timed appropriately. All patients should be aware of the need for antibiotic prophylaxis to prevent endocarditis for all dental and surgical pro-cedures. Patients need to be aware of symptoms that may occur. This must be balanced with reassurance about the long-term quality of life and the role they can play in maximizing this through optimizing their health behaviour. Patients without marked symptoms should have a review every 6–12 months with ECG and Doppler echocardiography to assess the progres-sion of aortic obstruction.

Patients with critical valvular obstruction should be advised to avoid vigorous athletic and physical activ-ities. This is primarily to avoid syncope and fatal arrhythmias. After symptoms develop the outlook is poor with only medical management. However, symp-toms can be treated. Cardiac failure can be controlled with diuretics and a restriction in dietary sodium. However, importantly, the use of diuretics needs to be carefully considered so as not to diminish the high preload (end diastolic volume) that the left ventricle needs to sustain the cardiac output. The use of nitrates also needs to be considered very carefully in the treat-ment of angina associated with aortic stenosis for the same reasons. Angina is said to occur in up to two-thirds of adults with severe aortic stenosis. However, only 50% will have significant coronary artery disease (Burckhardt et al 1996). Digoxin may also be used for its inotropic effect.

The use of β-blockers to slow the heart rate, therefore reducing myocardial oxygen demand and prolonging diastole, is effective. Patients with chest pain should be advised to rest initially instead of using nitrates, as this often allows the oxygen demand to reduce and coronary artery flow to increase. This therefore brings oxygen supply and demand back into balance. If pain does not ease nitrates should only be used cautiously as the aforementioned sudden reduction in preload can lead to a drop in cardiac output and syncope can occur. Patients need to be aware of the importance of reporting any presyncope or syncope and should be advised about the need to restrict activity until surgery takes place.

Aortic balloon valvuloplasty

This technique has been applied to aortic stenosis in more recent years (Cribier et al 1986). Long-term follow-up has been disappointing and therefore aortic valve replacement has remained the treatment of choice (Bernard et al 1992).

Aortic regurgitation

Aortic regurgitation is leakage of blood from the aorta back into the left ventricle during diastole. It is caused by diseases that affect the valve and its leaflets or the aortic root that affects the valve support. The most common causes are rheumatic fever (26%), infective endocarditis (21%) and degenerative changes; 23% of cases of aortic regurgitation are due to dilatation of the aortic root with dissecting aneurysm being the most common (Davies 1980).

Rheumatic aortic regurgitation

As previously described, the rheumatic process results in the valve leaflets becoming inflamed and thickened. In some cases this results in the leaflets becoming fused. If they do not, retraction occurs which has the effect of shortening them and therefore producing regurgitation. This occurs because the leaflets do not fully close the valve after diastole. There can often be combined aortic stenosis and regurgitation if the leaflets also restrict opening. It is often associated with mitral stenosis.

Infective endocarditis

This is an important cause of aortic regurgitation and is described fully in Chapter 14. Infection usually occurs upon a valve that has been previously damaged or is congenitally abnormal. Vegetation, fibrin mass, platelets, white and red blood cells, either singularly or in multiples, are found on the leaflets or the base of the valve. This causes the leaflets to tear and aneurysms can result if the surrounding tissue to the aortic valve is involved (Freeman & Hall 1996). In addition, abscesses can form which can progress to ventricular septal rupture with a left-to-right shunt of blood resulting. Coronary ischaemia can be caused by compression of the left main or right coronary artery. The conduction pathway can be involved, with AV block resulting (Burckhardt et al 1996).

Congenital

Bicuspid valves can cause regurgitation when the patient has reached adulthood, but it is not common unless associated with infective endocarditis.

Syphilis

Syphilis primarily affects the aortic root, which causes widening of the first few centimetres of the aorta. This can result in the formation of an aneurysm or in chronic cases calcification. However, as with rheumatic fever, the incidence of aortic regurgitation related to syphilis has decreased over the decades.

Inflammatory causes

Ankylosing spondylitis, rheumatoid arthritis and Reiter's syndrome are diseases that can provoke an inflammatory reaction in the aorta. Fibrosis distorts the aortic root, which can extend into the aortic leaflets. The inflammatory process can also affect the atrioventricular node, resulting in a degree of heart block (Hoffman & Leight 1965).

Non-inflammatory causes

In these cases the cause is usually unknown but degeneration of the aorta is evident which destroys the smooth muscle and elastic tissue. In some cases the aorta is concentric which leads to the valve leaflets failing to meet and therefore resulting in aortic regurgitation. Idiopathic aortic root dilatation rarely causes problems until middle age and is more commonly seen in the elderly (Burckhardt et al 1996). Most cases of aortic root dilatation are unknown; a few cases can be associated with Marfan syndrome (Sinclair et al 1960) and Erdheim disease (cystic medial necrosis) (Lewis 1965).

Dissecting aneurysm

A dissecting aneurysm involving the ascending aorta frequently produces aortic regurgitation as one of its features (Roberts & Honig 1982). The dissection usually occurs a few centimetres above the aortic valve, which tracks down to the supra-aortic ridge which compromises the aortic valve, thus resulting in regurgitation. This condition is very serious and requires surgical intervention. It can be seen on computed tomography (CT) (Fig. 13.4).

Clinical symptoms

Patients with chronic aortic regurgitation often remain symptom free for many years. However, over time the left ventricular function begins to deteriorate as a result of compensating for the incompetent valve. The patient becomes dyspnoeic, which is related to exercise. Sometimes patients with severe aortic regurgitation can be aware of a pronounced heart beat, particularly when lying down. As with aortic stenosis, the main symptoms of regurgitation are dyspnoea, tiredness and angina.

Dyspnoea. This results from an increase in left ventricular end-diastolic pressure (left-sided preload) particularly on exercise. As left heart failure progresses orthopnoea (breathlessness on lying flat) associated with paroxysmal nocturnal dyspnoea develops. In chronic cases this symptom takes many years to develop in contrast to acute aortic regurgitation, where the main presenting feature is of a sudden onset of dyspnoea (Hall & Julian 1989).

Angina pectoris. Angina does occur in pure aortic regurgitation but is more common in aortic stenosis or in a combination of both stenosis and regurgitation. It has all the features of exertional angina and is again a result of left ventricular hypertrophy (Burckhardt et al 1996). When angina does present in aortic regurgitation consideration should be given to the fact that coronary atherosclerosis may be present also. In syphilitic aortic regurgitation, angina is probably due to stenosis of the coronary ostia (Hall & Julian 1989).

Other symptoms. Abdominal pain may present, usually associated with heart failure which in the latter stages causes engorgement of the liver and hepatic system.

Investigations

Electrocardiography. The 12-lead ECG reflects the left ventricular and left atrial enlargement that occurs. This is manifest in increased QRS amplitudes, ST depression and T-wave changes. A broad P-wave in lead II and a large negative component to the P-wave in V1 (bifid) indicating left atrial enlargement is commonly seen in severe aortic regurgitation. Sinus rhythm is normally maintained with normal conduction. However, prolonged AV conduction can occur in advanced cases.

Echocardiography. An echo is useful in detecting the ventricular volume overload through measurement of increased chamber sizes. Serial studies with two-

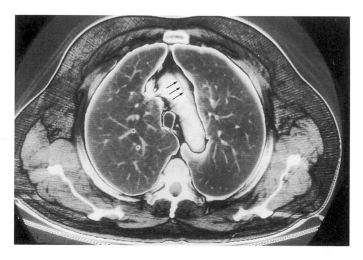

Figure 13.4 CT scan of a dissecting aneurysm. (Reproduced with permission from Julian et al 1996.)

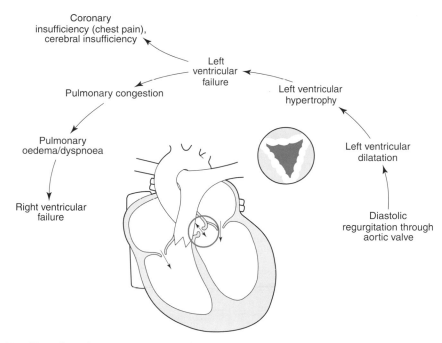

Coronary
insufficiency (chest pain),
cerebral insufficiency

Left
ventricular
failure

Left ventricular
hypertrophy

Pulmonary congestion

Pulmonary
oedema/dyspnoea

Left ventricular
dilatation

Right ventricular
failure

Diastolic
regurgitation through
aortic valve

Figure 13.5 The effect of aortic regurgitation. (Reproduced with permission from Guzzetta & Dossey 1992.)

dimensional echocardiography can identify early changes in left ventricular function. These can be useful for determining the most appropriate time for surgery. The most sensitive and accurate means of detecting even the mildest degree of aortic regurgitation is Doppler echocardiography. This can reveal aortic regurgitation that is not detectable by auscultation. Doppler studies can also determine the amount of regurgitant flow and the size of the regurgitant orifice. The appearance of the aortic root can give information about the cause of the aortic regurgitation such as aortic root dilatation due to Marfan syndrome or aortic dissection. Transoesophageal echocardiography (TOE) is superior for assessing thoracic aortic dissection and is a safe, sensitive tool and relatively atraumatic.

Chest X-ray. The chest X-ray can often show cardiac enlargement with both atrial and ventricular dilatation. The ascending aorta may be very prominent if complications such as aortic dissection have occurred. If heart failure is present then signs of pulmonary venous congestion may be evident.

Cardiac catheterisation. Cardiac catheterisation is necessary for patients who are being considered for valve replacement to assess the severity of the aortic regurgitation. It will also ascertain the degree of left ventricular dysfunction and outline the anatomy of the coronary arteries and the aortic root. Usually mild to moderate dilatation of the aortic root is seen, but this

may be severe in patients with conditions such as Marfan syndrome. The left ventriculogram will show the extent of left ventricular dilatation and impairment of wall motion. Coronary angiography can be difficult as the coronary arteries enlarge due to the high flow of blood they take to the hypertrophied left ventricle. Also dilatation of the aortic root may make it difficult to engage the coronary arteries. Cardiac catheterisation will also reveal any co-existing valve disease or cardiac abnormalities. It is also useful if there is conflicting information from non-invasive assessment methods.

Medical treatment

Aortic regurgitation is well tolerated until left ventricular function deteriorates. This means that many patients will be asymptomatic with mild or moderate aortic regurgitation. These patients often have normal or minimally elevated cardiac dimensions with the left ventricle in diastole measuring no more than 5.5 cm. These patients require no medication other than antibiotic prophylaxis for dental and surgical procedures, but should be assessed on a yearly basis, which includes echocardiography (Cavallo 1992). Some patients with severe chronic aortic regurgitation may remain asymptomatic. These patients need to be assessed every 6 months with ECG, echocardiograph and chest X-ray. Antibiotic prophylaxis is essential not only to prevent bacterial endocarditis but also to prevent infections, as fevers and subsequent arrhythmias can be very poorly tolerated. There is also a clear need to avoid heavy exertion or vigorous activity that can result in cardiac decompensation or death.

Diastolic hypertension should be controlled as it increases regurgitation. Once symptoms of dyspnoea or cardiac failure occur then diuretics may improve symptoms. Angiotensin-converting enzyme (ACE) inhibitors are also used to prevent ventricular dilatation and therefore delay the need for surgical intervention. Drugs that decrease left ventricular function are contraindicated. If angina occurs β-blockers are not appropriate as they slow the heart rate, which lengthens diastole and therefore increases regurgitation.

Symptoms may range from severe dyspnoea, needing admission to hospital for bedrest and intravenous diuretics, to mild heart failure. Nurses need to intervene and offer support as appropriate. As well as teaching patients about medication, it is important that nurses use opportunities to encourage patients to adopt and maintain healthy behaviours such as weight control and smoking cessation. Nurses can also assist patients to increase their knowledge to enable them to make informed choices as surgery approaches. The onset of symptoms is usually the indication for valve replacement as it is the only effective long-term measure. This needs to occur before irreversible left ventricular dysfunction occurs.

Surgical management of aortic valve disorders

Generally surgery is indicated when patients have developed symptoms. The outcome in symptomatic patients who do not undergo valve replacement is poor, with less than 50% alive after 2 years (O'Keefe et al 1987). Those patients who are asymptomatic with aortic stenosis but with evidence of haemodynamically severe aortic valve disease should be considered for surgery to prevent sudden death occurring. Severe aortic stenosis can be determined by a valve orifice of 0.7–0.8 cm² (Rahimtoola 1991).

The risk of sudden death is difficult to quantify. In the last 70 years the reported incidence of sudden death of patients with aortic stenosis in eight studies has ranged from 1% to 21% (Ross & Braunwald 1968). In this situation clinical judgement of the risks for the patient has to be used. The patient should be reviewed regularly with serial echocardiograms. Acute aortic regurgitation with dissection of the aorta clearly warrants urgent surgical intervention. All patients with New York Heart Association (NYHA) class III or IV heart failure should

be considered for surgery. In asymptomatic patients regular observation of deteriorating left ventricular function should be undertaken. An enlarged ventricle can be seen on chest X-ray with ECG evidence of any worsening left ventricular hypertrophy. The operative risk is slightly higher in aortic regurgitation than stenosis, 10% as compared to 6% (Scott et al 1985).

THE MITRAL VALVE

Mitral valve prolapse

Mitral valve prolapse is the most common valve disorder and in most patients is insignificant in terms of causing problems. Pocock (1987), amongst many others, has identified that mitral valve prolapse can affect up to 10% of the population. There is a strong hereditary factor, with an incidence of 25–50% in first-degree relatives (Chen et al 1983, Weiss et al 1975).

In 1963 Barlow et al demonstrated the distinctive auscultatory findings of a mid-systolic click and a late systolic murmur associated with mitral valve prolapse. This disorder is now occasionally known as Barlow's syndrome. The mitral valve can 'billow' slightly under normal conditions but extreme billowing results in what is sometimes known as a 'floppy valve'.

In severe cases mitral regurgitation occurs because the chordae becoming overly elongated (Hall & Treasure 1996). Normal heart valves have a continuous layer of collagen running down the centre, which inserts into the valve ring. This gives strength to the valve leaflet. On the atrial side of the leaflet is a spongiosa layer which is made up of myxomatous tissue (acid mucopolysaccharide). In mitral valve prolapse the leaflets become weakened by a build-up of cells in the spongiosa, which interrupts the fibrosa, hence weakening the structure. This build-up of tissue seems to be the result of abnormal collagen metabolism. This increases the quantity of acid mucopolysaccharide. The reasons for this have not been properly identified.

Box 13.2 Causes of mitral valve disease

Mitral valve prolapse
Mitral stenosis
   Rheumatic fever
   Congenital
Mitral regurgitation
   Ischaemic heart disease
   Chordal rupture
   Infective endocarditis
   Degenerative disease
   Hypertrophic cardiomyopathy

Mitral valve prolapse can also involve the whole anatomy of the mitral valve, with a weakening of the chordae tendineae through elongation and thinning and widening of the valve ring. A common result is rupture of the chordae.

Aetiology

The cause is often idiopathic but can be associated with connective tissue disorders such as Marfan syndrome, with the incidence being as high as 91% (Brown et al 1975). In addition, as already stated, there is a strong familial occurrence of mitral valve prolapse. In severe cases of ischaemic heart disease where there are abnormalities of the left ventricle or papillary muscles, the mitral valve can prolapse into the left atrium during systole.

Clinical symptoms

Most patients with mitral valve prolapse are asymptomatic but when symptoms occur they are similar to those of patients with mitral regurgitation. Tiredness and lethargy are commonly described which for unknown reasons can present over short periods of time and then disappear, only to reoccur some time later.

Anxiety and hyperventilation. These symptoms are often associated with valve prolapse. The patient may have had the murmur identified at some time during a normal physical examination and whereas this is not presenting any harm to the patient, because of the awareness a degree of neurosis can result. These patients require a great deal of reassurance from the medical and nursing team. The well-informed cardiac nurse can be invaluable in reassuring patients with this condition when it poses no threat to their health.

Chest pain. This is a common complaint and is not related to significant ECG changes or to exertion. It is described as a sharp pain under the left breast, which is not relieved by administering nitrates. The chest pain may be secondary in presentation to ischaemia of the papillary muscles caused by stress placed upon them when the valve prolapses (Buda et al 1978). The chest pain could be a result of palpitations that occasionally occur.

Palpitations, dizziness and syncope. These symptoms often present with arrhythmias and can be found in up to 40% of hospital referrals (Hall & Julian 1989).

Investigations

Electrocardiography. The ECG is usually normal, unless significant haemodynamic mitral regurgitation

is present. In 15–20% of patients, non-specific ST or T-wave changes are seen but are not diagnostic. There may also be slight prolongation of the QT interval (Cavallo 1992). A wide range of arrhythmias can also present, including atrial, supraventricular and ventricular tachyarrhythmias, atrial and ventricular ectopics, bradyarrhythmias and all types of AV block. These show no correlation to the severity, age or clinical findings. Some authors have suggested that reports of these are exaggerated and that they are no more frequent than in other individuals. (Kramer et al 1984).

Exercise stress testing and radionuclide studies. Exercise testing has a high number of false positives in patients with mitral prolapse with normal coronary arteries. Therefore other methods such as exercise thallium scanning may be more reliable.

Echocardiography. Echocardiography is the technique preferred for diagnosing mitral valve prolapse. Indeed, up to 15% of patients with no other signs will have mitral valve prolapse diagnosed by echocardiography. However, 10–25% of patients with auscultatory signs will also have no echocardiographic evidence. TOE is able to show which part of a cusp has prolapsed and whether there is chordal rupture. It can show whether surgery is required and which is most appropriate, repair or replacement. Doppler echocardiography will detect any existing mitral regurgitation.

Chest X-ray. This is usually normal unless haemodynamically significant mitral stenosis is present.

Cardiac catheterisation and coronary angiography. Cardiac catheterisation is usually normal and shows unremarkable left ventricular function unless significant mitral regurgitation is present. Left ventricular angiography can identify mitral valve prolapse although TOE is more sensitive. Coronary angiography is usually normal although the papillary muscle blood flow is sometimes hampered because of dysfunction of the valve apparatus.

Medical treatment

Most patients need no treatment, but do need reassurance that this condition is benign. If there are no symptoms with a normal 12-lead ECG with no arrhythmias, follow-up may not be required. However, some clinicians prefer to see the patient and perform echocardiography every 2–4 years. Patients with symptoms such as palpitations, dizziness or syncope should undergo 24-hour ECG and/or exercise testing as appropriate. Treatment for arrhythmias is conventional. β-blockers such as sotalol may be effective in treating ventricular arrhythmias. As pre-excitation is sometimes said to be associated with mitral valve prolapse, digoxin is used cautiously for treating supraventricular arrhythmias as its slowing action on the AV node can increase the opportunities for a re-entry circuit to occur (Hall & Treasure 1996).

Patients who complain of chest pain need to have other causes excluded, such as gastric or musculoskeletal problems. β-blockers may assist either because they treat true angina or because they can also help to relieve anxiety. Patients who have suffered a transient ischaemic attack (TIA) or a cerebrovascular accident (CVA/stroke) need to be anticoagulated in the presence of mitral regurgitation, as well as those with atrial fibrillation. Many of the symptoms patients experience can be non-specific but quite distressing. Although reassurance can help it does not relieve them. Helping patients with ongoing support and health promotion is very important, so that those patients with this usually benign condition can maintain their quality of life.

Antibiotic prophylaxis is only required if there is clinical evidence of mitral regurgitation.

Mitral stenosis

Mitral stenosis is a narrowing of the mitral valve orifice that reduces blood flow into the left ventricle during diastole. Abnormalities in both diastolic and systolic left ventricular function occur because the main problem associated with mitral stenosis is obstruction of blood flow from the left atrium (Hall & Treasure 1996).

Increased pressure in the left atrium eventually results in pressure within the pulmonary vessels, causing pulmonary hypertension and damage to the pulmonary system (Rackley et al 1991). The right ventricle hypertrophies as a result of the increased pulmonary pressure in order to maintain adequate cardiac output. Mitral stenosis is nearly always a result of rheumatic heart disease. The incidence in Western Europe and the US has declined dramatically and mitral stenosis tends to be seen in the middle aged and elderly. In rare cases it can be congenital in nature. Other less common causes are associated with systemic lupus erythematosus, malignant carcinoid and rheumatic arthritis (Bortolotti et al 1984).

The long-term effects of rheumatic valve disease leave the leaflets thickened and shortened. Inflammatory changes which cause fibrosis also result in thickening and fusion of the chordae tendineae. Inflammation along the leaflets can also result in fusion and therefore reduce the valve opening. In severe cases regurgitation also presents as the leaflets and chordae tendineae become shortened. Fibrosis can also occur in the left ventricle and scarring results in a poorly contracting ventricle.

Clinical signs and symptoms

Many patients remain asymptomatic for years and it is only with major insult upon the circulatory system, such as pregnancy or the development of atrial

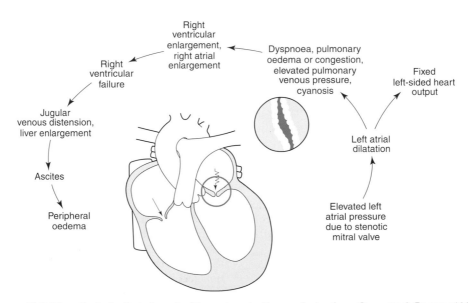

Figure 13.6 The effect of mitral stenosis. (Reproduced with permission from Guzzetta & Dossey 1992.)

fibrillation, that more severe symptoms develop. Through listening to patients and understanding their particular concerns, the nurse can help them to come to terms with their disease and manage the symptoms accordingly.

Dyspnoea. This is the most common symptom in mitral stenosis. It is usually a result of exercise but in severe cases can be present at rest. This is a very distressing symptom for patients who need to be able to understand the causes and therefore be in a position to manage it. The breathlessness results from pulmonary congestion, oedema and chronic changes to the lungs. The lungs become 'stiff' and this affects gaseous exchange and the vital capacity. In addition, the onset of atrial fibrillation can precipitate dyspnoea and present with an acute episode of pulmonary oedema.

Orthopnoea sometimes accompanied by paroxysmal nocturnal dyspnoea are later symptoms, which suggests that there is chronic lung damage. The blood flow through the atria becomes sluggish due to the poorly functioning mitral valve and increases the risk of emboli formation. Pulmonary emboli can also be a cause of dyspnoea (Hall & Treasure 1996).

Cough. This is a commonly described symptom of mitral valve disease and is associated with pulmonary congestion and can be worse at night. In addition, the cough may present because the enlarged left atrium presses on the left bronchial tree, causing some constriction, although this is quite rare. Sometimes a pink, frothy expectorant can result and once again this suggests pulmonary congestion. Patients with mitral stenosis who also smoke can more readily develop chronic bronchitis (Hall & Julian 1989). Excessive coughing at night can exacerbate tiredness and general fatigue as a result of a poor sleeping pattern. Advice to patients regarding sleeping position is important in order for them to maximize their periods of rest. Patients should be advised to sleep and rest in an upright position supported with pillows.

Haemoptysis. Haemoptysis (the expectoration of blood from the respiratory system) occurs in about 10% of patients with mitral stenosis. This symptom can occur late in the disease and can also be severe although this is quite rare. It is a result of increased pressure within the pulmonary capillaries due to the hindering of forward-flowing blood by the failing mitral valve. It tends to be associated with pulmonary oedema. In chronic mitral stenosis bronchial vein varicosities can be produced which then rupture. In very severe cases when atrial fibrillation is present pulmonary emboli may form which can also result in haemoptysis (Hall & Julian 1989).

Palpitations. This symptom is common and can present early. It is often a result of atrial premature beats (ectopics) and, in later disease, the presence of atrial fibrillation. This can be an unpleasant symptom for the patient.

Tiredness. This is another common symptom and can be more of a problem to some patients than breathlessness. It is often a result of reduced cardiac output. Patients frequently do not recognize fatigue as a major contributing factor to their disease until after treatment, when this symptom improves dramatically.

Angina pectoris. Some patients experience chest pain that is not associated with angina but may be caused by right ventricular hypertension (Ross 1961). However, angina pectoris reported with mitral valve disease is increasing as the years go by; this could be because investigation for coronary heart disease is becoming more common prior to surgical treatment. In 1955 Stuckley reported an incidence of 8.5% whereas in 1984 Ramsdale et al noted angina in 28% of patients. Also those presenting with mitral stenosis are older and therefore the incidence of accompanying coronary heart disease is likely to be more common. In Ramsdale et al's studies 62% of patients had accompanying coronary heart disease. Angina pain may also be the result of coronary embolization (Oakley et al 1961).

Dysphagia and hoarseness. Dysphagia can be present because of pressure upon the oesophagus from the dilated left atrium. This is a very rare occurrence and therefore other causes of dysphagia should not be overlooked. Another rare symptom is hoarseness, due to compression of the laryngeal nerve between the dilated main left pulmonary artery and the aorta (Dorward & Kerr 1982).

Characteristic physical signs. Mitral stenosis does create distinctive physical signs in patients that nurses can readily recognize. Typically patients develop mitral facies which is a bluey-purple coloration of the cheeks, characteristically in the shape of butterfly wings. This is usually present in patients with chronic valve disease and can be seen where there is a reduced cardiac output. However, it is most often associated with mitral valve disease.

Investigations

Electrocardiography. Changes on the ECG reflect the pathophysiological response to mitral stenosis. The most striking change observed on the ECG is P-mitrale; this is due to left atrial enlargement, which produces a wide notched (bifid) P-wave, predominantly in lead II; 90% of patients who are still in sinus rhythm when surgery is being considered have ECG

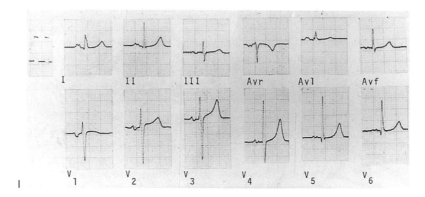

I

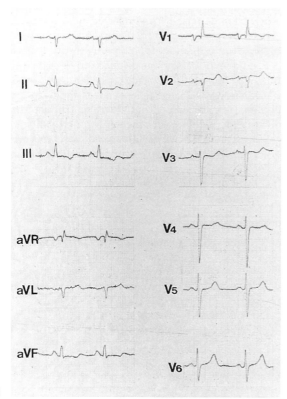

II

Figure 13.7 ECG of a patient with mitral stenosis. Evidence of left atrial hypertrophy is demonstrated on the ECG by a broad notched P-wave seen in leads I and II (P-mitrale) and a large negative component to the P-wave in V1.
(Reproduced with permission from Julian et al 1996.)

cardiac catheterisation is not needed from a diagnostic point of view. Imaging can provide very accurate information about the abnormal movement and thickening of the mitral valve leaflets. This can enable decisions about the suitability of percutaneous balloon valvuloplasty, surgical valvotomy, repair or replacement to be taken. Echocardiography also demonstrates the degree of left atrial enlargement and the stages of right ventricular enlargement. Quantification of the mitral valve area is used to assess the severity of mitral stenosis. In diastole the whole of the orifice can often be visualized; alternatively Doppler ultrasound is used to measure the rate of flow across the stenotic orifice. Higher rates of flow indicate more severe degrees of stenosis. Exercise testing or stress echocardiography is sometimes used to evaluate the symptomatic response and assess functional capacity.

Chest X-ray. The chest X-ray may be normal in the presence of mild mitral stenosis. As this progresses the chest X-ray can reveal changes due to the effects of left atrial hypertension; these include a double shadow due to left atrial enlargement, altered pulmonary venous pattern, prominent pulmonary arteries and an enlarged right ventricle.

Cardiac catheterisation. Cardiac catheterisation is performed to assess the severity of the stenosis and the effects of this upon the heart. These include cardiac output, the diastolic pressure gradient between the left atrium and left ventricle and the area of the mitral valve orifice. The pressure gradient is assessed by measuring simultaneously left atrial pressure (either using a pulmonary artery (PA) catheter wedge pressure (see Chapter 5) or directly with a trans-septal approach) and left ventricular pressure. If the cardiac

evidence of left atrial enlargement (Hall & Treasure 1996). Right axis deviation may also be observed as pulmonary hypertension develops and becomes severe. Tall R-waves in the right precordial leads develop as right ventricular hypertrophy worsens. The QRS complex is usually normal. Atrial fibrillation develops in more than a third of patients with mitral stenosis as a consequence of atrial enlargement (Goldberger 1989).

Echocardiography. Echocardiography in mitral valve disease can provide enough information so that output is normal and the pressure gradient is significant (>15 mmHg in diastole or >5–10 mmHg end diastolic) then pressure readings alone can be used. This may be unreliable if the cardiac output is significantly increased or decreased and other calculations may be needed.

In some patients results do not seem to reflect the expected severity. However, asking the patient to perform gentle exercise on the table (arm bends or leg raises), thereby increasing cardiac output, will demonstrate a rapid rise in left atrial pressure and cross-valve gradient. This falls at the end of exercise. Right heart catheterisation is often performed to measure mean pulmonary artery pressure and therefore determine pulmonary vascular resistance. Right ventricular pressures are also measured (Grossman & Baim 1986).

Medical treatment

The medical treatment of mitral stenosis is aimed at prevention of complications rather than cure. With time, surgical intervention or balloon valvuloplasty is required to alter the obstruction of flow across the stenotic valve. Prophylactic antibiotics are usually given to patients prior to dental or surgical procedures to prevent endocarditis or recurrence of rheumatic fever.

Patients need to be aware of likely symptoms they may begin to experience as the valve disease progresses and left-sided heart failure and eventually right-sided heart failure or atrial fibrillation occur. If patients are asymptomatic they still need support and education to optimize their health choices. Patients with mitral stenosis can be reassured about their ability to lead a normal life whilst asymptomatic, but may need to avoid excessive exertion and be informed that following the development of symptoms, surgery can offer real improvements and preserve their quality of life. Nurses can also help encourage and educate patients about the benefits of maintaining healthy behaviours and the value to be gained by remaining physically active, not smoking or being overweight.

Medical treatment can often help relieve or palliate symptoms once they occur. Initially breathlessness will occur during strenuous exertion but once this is more limiting, diuretics and ACE inhibitors are usually prescribed to reduce preload and relieve venous congestion. Advice regarding a low sodium dietary intake should also be offered and discussed. Pulmonary hypertension, although not treatable itself, can be reduced by the treatment of heart failure.

If or when atrial fibrillation occurs, digoxin is usually indicated to control the heart rate. Attempts to restore sinus rhythm with direct current (DC) cardioversion may initially be successful but as the atria enlarge and become more arrhythmogenic this is less likely. Once atrial fibrillation has become sustained, anticoagulation with a drug such as warfarin is needed to prevent the development of atrial thrombus due to pooling and stasis of blood within the atria. Incorrectly managed, this can lead to embolic events. Patients will need education about the need to monitor their anticoagulation regularly and information related to the specific anticoagulant used (Box 13.3).

It is essential that the international normalised ratio (INR), used to assess the degree of anticoagulation, is monitored; this needs to be daily or on alternate days initially, then at longer intervals. Patients and carers should be given an oral anticoagulation treatment book which, as well as including details of the prescribed dose and treatment, should contain written information as shown in Box 13.4.

Women of childbearing age with mitral stenosis need to be aware of the need for close supervision during pregnancy and often require additional emotional support and information about their condition

---

Box 13.3 Oral anticoagulation

Patients with valve disease often require oral anticoagulation because of the risk of systemic embolization due to atrial fibrillation or to prevent emboli developing on mechanical prosthetic valves.

Warfarin is the drug of choice, with other oral anticoagulation such as acenocoumarol (nicoumalone) or phenindione rarely being used. Oral anticoagulation antagonizes the effects of vitamin K and takes at least 48–72 hours to achieve a full effect. If patients need to be anticoagulated immediately or need to be able to have their clotting altered rapidly, for example to have cardiac catheterisation performed, they may need an intravenous agent such as heparin.

The usual adult commencement dose of warfarin is 10 mg daily for 2 days. The subsequent dose depends on the patient's INR (prothrombin time expressed as the **international normalised ratio**). The maintenance dose should be taken at the same time each day and is usually between 3 and 9 mg.

Target INR

- INR 2.5 for atrial fibrillation, cardioversion and rheumatic mitral valve disease.
- INR 3.5 for mechanical prosthetic valves.

Target values are now recommended rather than ranges. An INR within 0.5 of the target is said to be acceptable, while larger variations need dose adjustment (BNF 2001). NB: Oral anticoagulants are damaging to the fetus (teratogenic).

Box 13.4 Advice for patients regarding oral anticoagulation treatment

Do:
- carry the booklet at all times
- keep all hospital/clinic appointments
- inform the doctor of bruising or bleeding problems, e.g. bleeding gums, red or dark brown stools
- remind your doctor or dentist of any anticoagulation treatment
- take your tablets at the same time each day.

Don't:
- miss a dose of anticoagulation
- take an extra dose of anticoagulation
- run out of tablets
- take aspirin
- go on crash diets or start binge eating
- take more than moderate amounts of alcohol.

---

and treatment options if they become pregnant (Hall & Treasure 1996). Patients with mild mitral stenosis or mitral or aortic regurgitation usually remain fit and cope well during pregnancy, although they may notice increasing breathlessness because of the increased circulatory burden. Patients with more severe mitral stenosis may need hospitalization for bedrest and possibly surgical intervention, which can be very distressing for the patient and their family or loved ones. For patients with known severe mitral stenosis mitral valvotomy may be considered prior to conception but frequently it is only diagnosed because of the onset of symptoms during pregnancy (Hall & Treasure 1996).

Percutaneous mitral balloon valvuloplasty/commisurotomy

Percutaneous mitral balloon valvuloplasty has become an alternative to surgical mitral valvotomy. It is most successful when applied to non-calcified non-regurgitant stenosed valves and is performed using a standard cardiac catheter approach. Patients would normally be admitted on the day prior to the procedure and need a pre-procedure echocardiograph both to visualize the valve and to screen for atrial thrombus. This could be displaced during the procedure and produce an embolic event. Patients may have already had a previous cardiac catheter and so be aware of the sights and sounds they will experience in the radiodiagnostic rooms. However, they will still need explanations of the procedure and the risks.

Of primary importance are discussions regarding the risk of producing mitral regurgitation that will need surgical intervention, sometimes urgently. Peripheral venous access is also required prior to the procedure. Sedatives are normally administered orally as premedication. Further opiates or sedatives can then be administered intravenously as needed during the procedure. The procedure is carried out transvenously; the intra-atrial septum is punctured and the site enlarged with a small dilatation catheter to allow the passage of the larger valvuloplasty balloon through the septum. It is then positioned across the stenotic mitral valve. When the balloon is inflated the fused commissures are separated, thus enlarging the mitral valve orifice. Occasionally, as highlighted above, this can lead to the development of mitral regurgitation.

Most patients can be discharged from hospital the next day following echocardiography, which assesses mitral valve function. Up to one-third will also have a small left-to-right atrial shunt as a result of the puncture of the septum. This is not usually a significant haemodynamic problem. Follow-up clinical assessment at 6 months generally shows preservation of the enlarged mitral valve orifice, with resulting physiological improvements in filling pressure and pulmonary vascular resistance. Long-term restenosis rates are comparable to surgical valvotomy (Braunwald 1994).

As well as preserving the patient's quality of life and improving symptoms, this approach is obviously much less invasive for patients and also delays the need for cardiac surgery. However, for those patients whose valve is not suitable for percutaneous balloon valvuloplasty, surgical intervention is the primary treatment.

Mitral regurgitation

This is the leakage of blood during systole, from the left ventricular stroke volume back into the left atrium. Although in the past most mitral regurgitation was a result of rheumatic disease, non-rheumatic causes are now more prevalent. The two most common causes of mitral regurgitation in the elderly population are ischaemic heart disease and chordal rupture (Hall & Treasure 1996).

Ischaemic heart disease

Mitral regurgitation has been described in up to 30% of patients undergoing surgery for coronary artery disease (Gahl et al 1977). A dramatic form of mitral regurgitation is a result of papillary muscle rupture during acute myocardial infarction resulting in acute left-sided heart failure. However, this occurs in less than 1% of patients suffering a myocardial infarction (Hall & Treasure 1996).

Papillary muscle dysfunction, rather than rupture, occurs in about 10% of patients who have had an acute

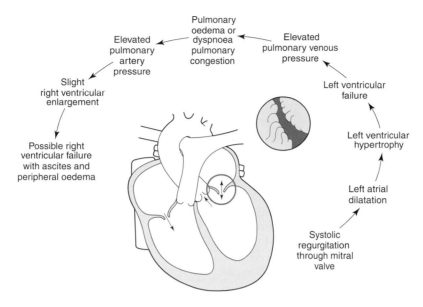

Pulmonary
oedema or
dyspnoea
pulmonary
congestion

Elevated
pulmonary
artery
pressure

Elevated
pulmonary venous
pressure

Slight
right ventricular
enlargement

Left ventricular
failure

Possible right
ventricular failure
with ascites and
peripheral oedema

Left ventricular
hypertrophy

Left atrial
dilatation

Systolic
regurgitation
through mitral
valve

Figure 13.8 The effect of mitral regurgitation. (Reproduced with permission from Guzzetta & Dossey 1992.)

myocardial infarction (Lehmann et al 1992). This type of regurgitation is often transitory and resolves after a few weeks. The acute phase, however, can produce very severe regurgitation that may warrant urgent valve replacement. These patients also experience impaired left ventricular function, which can improve following coronary artery grafting. A small number of patients do progress to have continuing problems with mitral regurgitation several months afterwards and also require valve replacement (Hall & Treasure 1996).

Chordal rupture

This is an important cause of mitral regurgitation and is associated with old age. In some cases the cause of the rupture is unclear but is often connected with mitral valve prolapse and 'floppy' mitral valves. It is up to five times more common in men than women (Grenadier et al 1985). The rupture may be due to fibrosis of the papillary muscle, which leads to increased tension in the chordae.

Infective endocarditis

This should always be suspected when there is a worsening situation of mitral regurgitation. Infective endocarditis usually produces regurgitation by perforation of the valve leaflets. The infective process can also cause chordal rupture due to erosion of the chordae tendineae (Hall & Treasure 1996).

Degenerative disease

The mitral valve often calcifies in the elderly and this is more common in women than men (Korn et al 1962, Pomerance 1970). It often co exists with aortic stenosis and can have an increased prevalence in patients with chronic renal failure with secondary hyperparathyroidism, hypertension and diabetes (De Pace et al 1981).

Hypertrophic cardiomyopathy

Some patients experiencing this condition also have some mitral regurgitation, which occasionally requires valve replacement (Hall & Treasure 1996).

Clinical symptoms

These are similar to those already described in mitral stenosis. In acute mitral regurgitation there is a sudden increase in pulmonary venous pressure. The normal lungs are not prepared for such an event and therefore the patient becomes acutely aware of being breathless on mild exercise and at rest. This is accompanied by other symptoms of pulmonary congestion such as a cough and orthopnoea. This type of patient is usually under medical observation because of having suffered an acute myocardial infarction. Sometimes the patient may complain of right hyperchondrial pain due to congestion of the liver, with nausea and anorexia.

Chest pain is not usually a feature but severe fatigue is experienced. In chronic mitral regurgitation the symptoms take weeks, months or years to develop. Symptoms of left atrial pressure, such as a cough at night, present. If congestive heart failure follows, the ankles become swollen (Hall & Julian 1989). Atrial fibrillation may present in up to 30% of patients. This can be linked to the size of the left atrium (Henry et al 1976).

Investigations

Electrocardiography. The ECG in chronic mitral regurgitation may be normal. As the condition progresses signs of left ventricular hypertrophy as well as left atrial dilatation appear. Left atrial enlargement produced by chronic severe mitral regurgitation is usually associated with atrial fibrillation. Exercise testing may be used to evaluate functional reserve and assess symptoms of chronic mitral regurgitation. A decline in exercise tolerance is seen as the left ventricle performance deteriorates.

Echocardiography. Echocardiography has become so refined that cardiac catheterisation is rarely undertaken to establish a diagnosis. Echocardiography will always identify a rheumatic valve causing regurgitation and it will often identify other reasons such as infective endocarditis or mitral valve prolapse, development of a flail valve due to ruptured chordae or papillary muscle and calcification of the mitral annulus. It also assists in assessing the haemodynamic consequences rather than determining severity of regurgitation.

Doppler and colour flow Doppler echocardiography can be used to determine severity of regurgitant flow. This and TOE often show whether mitral valve replacement or repair is appropriate. Assessment of left ventricular function non-invasively by echocardiography is vital, as it is important that any deterioration is detected early and surgery can be planned before left ventricular function is permanently damaged. Increased left atrial size and reduced left ventricular function suggest that chronic mitral regurgitation is severe. In this group the mortality following surgery is higher (Hall & Treasure 1996). In acute mitral regurgitation the left atrial size is often normal, as it has not had time to enlarge.

Chest X-ray. The chest X-ray reveals an increase in cardiac shadow that indicates left ventricular and left atrial enlargement, when mitral regurgitation is significant. The left atrium can sometimes enlarge and extend into the right side of chest, compressing the right bronchus and causing atelectasis.

Cardiac catheterisation. Assessment by high-quality echocardiography is as accurate as that performed invasively by cardiac catheterisation. However, some patients are difficult to assess non-invasively, so cardiac catheterisation is performed to determine the degree of mitral regurgitation and to assess left ventricular function. Injecting radio-opaque contrast medium into the left ventricle assists greatly in the confirmation and quantification of mitral regurgitation. Left ventriculography is of particular value in assessing the severity of mitral regurgitation, which complicates mitral stenosis, and shows the reflux of dye into the left atria from the left ventricle. The presence of left ventricular failure may be confirmed by finding a high left ventricular end-diastolic pressure. In all cases, coronary angiography is important prior to surgery, as coronary disease may be the underlying cause of the regurgitation.

Medical treatment

Medical treatment is utilized to treat symptoms dependent on severity. Following initial diagnosis, if patients are asymptomatic they need advice about antibiotic prophylaxis and early recognition of symptoms. Patients also need reassurance about long-term prognosis and should be encouraged to maintain as healthy a lifestyle as possible. Once symptoms appear, physical activities that produce extreme fatigue and/or dyspnoea will need to be restricted.

Congestive cardiac failure can be initially controlled with diuretics and vasodilators. ACE inhibitors can be used to decrease afterload and help relieve symptoms of left-sided failure. Symptoms vary in severity. Some patients will need to be hospitalized for treatment with intravenous diuretics and bedrest.

Nurses may need to give full support, but must be sensitive in allowing patients to maintain some independence within their own limitations. Some patients may be very hesitant about surgery and appropriate support and listening from nursing staff is essential for as fully informed decisions as possible to be made. Patients may be admitted electively a few days prior to surgery for bedrest and medication to optimize their condition.

It is important that hypertension is controlled, as high systemic vascular resistance can increase regurgitation. If atrial fibrillation has occurred, then ventricular rate control is usually achieved with digoxin. It may also be used for its positive inotropic effects, strengthening cardiac output, even when patients are in sinus rhythm. Anticoagulation may also be needed if atrial fibrillation is present, patients have evidence of intracardiac thrombus or have experienced an embolic event.

Surgical management of mitral valve disorders

Indications for surgery

In most cases pure mitral stenosis can be managed by balloon valvotomy. Surgery is used in cases where balloon valvotomy has failed or where the valve is not suitable for this type of procedure.

In chronic mitral regurgitation the decision for surgical replacement is a difficult one. One school of thought is that patients can have this problem for many years without major deterioration. If the patient does not complain of a poor quality of life this could be seen as being asymptomatic. However, mitral regurgitation has a detrimental effect upon left ventricular function and in the early stages the left ventricle itself compensates by thickening. Eventually the ventricle becomes dilated due to the increased blood volume and function deteriorates, leaving the patient disabled in terms of symptoms and quality of life. Surgical intervention at this latter stage often produces little or no improvement in symptoms (Hall & Treasure 1996).

In severe mitral regurgitation the chest X-ray will show an enlarged heart. Figure 13.9 displays the enlarged left ventricle before surgery and then the recovery made following mitral valve replacement. The ECG will demonstrate left ventricular hypertrophy and left atrial abnormality (Carabello 1998).

Moderate to severe mitral regurgitation (NYHA classes II and IV) merits surgical intervention. If left to deteriorate, symptoms worsen and surgical outcome is poor. In the decision-making process to refer for surgery, symptom severity is important. Often patients tolerate and learn to live with symptoms, adapting their lifestyle accordingly. A worsening exercise tolerance often indicates deteriorating left ventricular function (Hochreiter et al 1986).

The onset of persistent atrial fibrillation also indicates a deterioration of ventricular function and a decrease in cardiac output and is a good indicator that surgery is required. Surgical replacement should be undertaken before there is irreversible left ventricular damage. Close follow-up of these patients with serial echocardiograms should highlight left ventricular

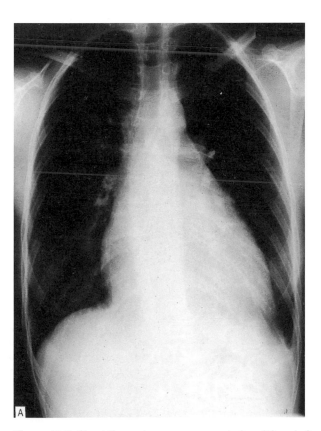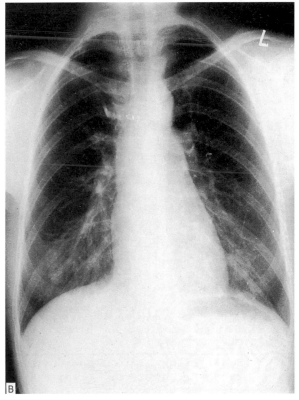

Figure 13.9 Chest X-ray of a young woman before (A) and after (B) surgery for mitral regurgitation. (Reproduced with permission from Julian et al 1996.)

damage before it becomes irretrievable. When the end-systolic dimension is >45 mm, surgical intervention should be performed to prevent further irreversible left ventricular dysfunction (Carabello 1998).

Acute mitral regurgitation is always symptomatic. Mild cases can be successfully treated medically but most cases of acute mitral regurgitation are very acute and require urgent surgical intervention.

In determining the correct timing for surgical replacement, the degree of symptoms experienced needs to be assessed. When the NYHA class II symptoms develop mortality increases and surgery should be performed before class III symptoms occur. Also, the development of pulmonary hypertension increases the surgical risk and therefore valve replacement should be considered before the pulmonary artery systolic pressure is > 50 mmHg (Crawford et al 1990).

Mitral valve repair

The advancement in surgical techniques has reduced the risk for patients with mitral regurgitation. Early operation for this type of valve disorder should be considered. Valve replacement with a prosthesis was often postponed until the patient's condition had become severe. This often left the patient with left ventricular dysfunction and all the risks associated with having a prosthesis: risks of infection, thromboembolic attacks, mechanical device failure and the need to be anticoagulated. However, this type of surgery is now becoming more prevalent. Patients considered for repair are not usually as well advanced in their disease as those that will require valve replacement. Table 13.1 illustrates patient survival at 5 and 10 years following the two alternative surgical approaches for mitral valve disorders.

Types of valve prosthesis

In the last 40–50 years many different valves have been developed and used. They are basically divided into two groups: bioprosthetic and mechanical. Bioprosthetic valves are made from human or animal tissue and are similar to the natural heart valves. Mechanical valves are made from materials such as carbon or metallic alloys and in no way resemble the human equivalent. It can usually be said that any valve replacement does not function as well as the natural heart valves.

Bioprosthetic valves. There are several glutaraldehyde-treated porcine and pericardial valves. The porcine valve or pericardium is sterilized and strengthened by the glutaraldehyde. One of the more commonly used is the Carpentier-Edwards bioprosthesis (Fig. 13.10).

The porcine aortic valve is mounted onto a frame with a suitable suturing material to enable the surgeon to secure the new valve in place. The risk of thromboembolic attacks is small and therefore the use of anticoagulation therapy is not required. The only exception to this would be if the patient had persistent atrial fibrillation, which readily encourages clot formation in the atria.

Glutaraldehyde-treated pericardial valves have been modified over recent years and clinical performance can be compared to that of porcine valves (Frater et al 1992, Wheatley et al 1995). Homografts, valves taken from cadaver donors, are also used but are difficult to acquire. Tissue valve banks have been established in some cities and permission sought to remove valves from hearts not suitable for transplantation. In some cases this may be from hearts being replaced but which have otherwise normal valves.

Table 13.1 Patients free from re-operation following mitral valve repair, in comparison to mitral valve replacement (after Enriquez-Sarano et al 1994)

	Valve repair (n = 195)	Valve replacement (n = 214)
5 years post-op	90%	93%
10 years post-op	75%	80%

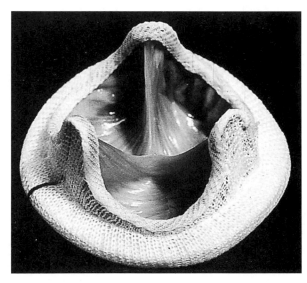

Figure 13.10 Carpentier-Edwards porcine bioprosthetic valve. (Reproduced with permission from Julian et al 1996.)

Mechanical valves. The design and development of these valves have changed considerably over the last 40 years. There are three main designs, all having different mechanisms for opening and closing to allow blood flow (Figs 13.11–13.13). The main disadvantage of the mechanical valve is that patients need to be anticoagulated to prevent thromboembolic episodes (see Box 13.3).

Choice of valves

Life expectancy needs to be considered when selecting the type of valve used in replacement. Bioprosthetic valves do become calcified and the need for re-operation to replace these valves is high after 10 years. This may be the reason for the tendency to use mechanical valves. Patients in whom anticoagulation therapy is

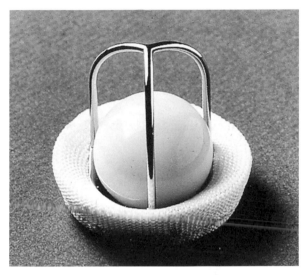

Figure 13.11 Starr-Edwards caged ball valve. (Reproduced with permission from Julian et al 1996.)

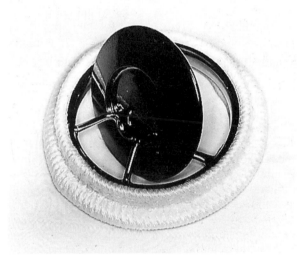

Figure 13.12 Björk-Shiley disc valve. (Reproduced with permission from Julian et al 1996.)

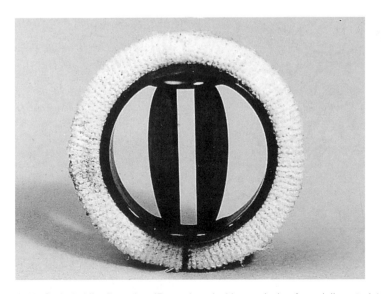

Figure 13.13 St Jude bileaflet valve. (Reproduced with permission from Julian et al 1996.)

contra-indicated and young women who may wish to start a family clearly have no choice but to have a bioprosthetic valve inserted. As these patients are generally young, they face the prospect of revision surgery.

Current practice generally demonstrates that patients under the age of 70 years have a mechanical valve inserted and those over have a bioprosthesis (Wheatley 1996). Despite the above issues, the choice of type of valve used is often dictated by the surgeon's preference. There are differing opinions in this area and there is no easy way to decide, unless there are fairly clear indications for one particular choice over another (Wheatley 1996).

Nursing patients following valve surgery

The patient undergoes a median sternotomy and valve replacement or repair with the utilization of cardiopulmonary bypass. The peri- and postoperative care is similar to that for any cardiac surgical patient and is discussed in detail in Chapter 22. The patient who has undergone a mechanical valve replacement has to become accustomed to hearing the 'click' of the mechanical device. Some patients initially find this quite intrusive and it is more prominent at night. Initially patients can at times become alarmed that there is something wrong and therefore may require reassurance from the nurse that they will learn to live with the sound of the new valve. Further education will be necessary for the patient who requires anticoagulation therapy. This is to ensure compliance but also for the patient to be able to identify any problems that may arise and to understand the need for regular surveillance.

Quality of life following valve replacement

Cardiac surgical nursing can be one of the most rewarding in terms of the physical improvement and relief of symptoms these patients experience. A study conducted by Walter et al (1992) concluded that heart valve replacement has benefits in all aspects of quality of life. There is a reduction in the symptoms of fatigue, dyspnoea and chest pain and an improvement in depression because the lack of physical ability is greatly alleviated following replacement. Life following bioprosthesis replacement, even for those faced with the possibility of further surgery within 10–15 years, is preferable for a small group of patients who do not have to live with the 'click' of the mechanical valve and the lifelong prospect of anticoagulation therapy.

With improvements in health care and the increasing numbers of elderly patients, there has been an increase in those presenting with problems that are treated without question in the younger population. Tseng et al (1997) concluded that aortic valve replacement can be performed in patients over the age of 70 years with acceptably low mortality, good long-term results and an excellent quality of life.

RIGHT HEART VALVE DISEASE

Disease of the tricuspid and pulmonary valves in the right side of the heart is much less common than that of the mitral and aortic valves but is worth highlighting.

TRICUSPID VALVE DISORDERS

Tricuspid stenosis

Tricuspid stenosis is nearly always associated with rheumatic heart disease but in isolation is quite rare and is often accompanied with mitral and aortic valve involvement. As with other valves, stenosis occurs because of fusion of the leaflets. This then tends to calcify or fibrose but usually to a lesser degree than mitral or aortic stenosis. When there is significant tricuspid stenosis the right atrium becomes hypertrophied. When associated with mitral valve disease, the blood flow into the right ventricle and lungs is also restricted.

Clinical symptoms

Symptoms of right sided heart failure include ankle oedema and abdominal pain and swelling. There is also excessive tiredness and reduced exercise tolerance. All these features are a result of venous congestion because of restriction in the forward flow of blood. Other clinical symptoms associated with mitral valve disease are present, such as dyspnoea and orthopnoea. The patient is usually in sinus rhythm but the pulse is of poor volume.

Investigations

Electrocardiography. The only finding on the ECG related to tricuspid stenosis is due to the development of right atrial hypertrophy. This is manifest by a tall peaked P-wave, which is 3 mm or more in height. It is usually most prominent in leads II, III, aVF and V1 (P-pulmonale). There is no evidence of right ventricu-

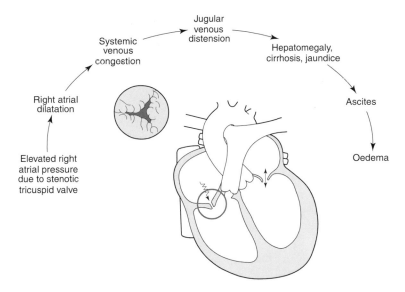

Figure 13.14 The effect of tricuspid stenosis. (Reproduced with permission from Guzzetta & Dossey 1992.)

lar hypertrophy and the QRS complex may be small and in some cases will be smaller than the P-wave.

Echocardiography. The tricuspid valve is often difficult to visualize and a cross-sectional technique is needed. This often only reveals the anterior and septal cusps but will allow any thickening of the cusps and limitation of movement to be detected. These findings are not specific to rheumatic tricuspid valve disease. Discovery of a tricuspid valve with a restricted and doming movement towards the right ventricle in diastole makes diagnosis more certain. The severity of tricuspid stenosis is best assessed using Doppler echocardiography, which appears to have a good correlation between the pressure gradient obtained by this technique and cardiac catheterisation (Hall & Treasure 1996).

Chest X-ray. The chest X-ray notably shows marked enlargement of the right atrium and changes associated with mitral valve disease are common.

Cardiac catheterisation. The cross-valve gradient is often small and difficult to measure accurately. When the gradient exceeds 2 mmHg some degree of tricuspid stenosis is present. Severe stenosis, where the valve opening area is less than 1 cm^2, usually leads to a mean gradient greater than 5 mmHg. Injection of contrast medium into the right atrium shows enormous enlargement of the chamber, thickening of the tricuspid valve and a thin high-velocity jet of contrast into the right ventricle, in comparison to the broad low-velocity jet seen in the normal valve.

Medical treatment

Diuretics can relieve retained fluid in the form of peripheral oedema or ascites. Arrhythmias are treated as for mitral valve disease. Balloon valvuloplasty has been attempted in some cases but may lead to tricuspid regurgitation, which still leads to long-term symptoms. A conservative medical management is often utilized unless other valve surgery is being planned. Antibiotic prophylaxis is often considered for surgical or dental procedures.

Tricuspid regurgitation

This is extremely rare and most causes of tricuspid regurgitation occur as a result of the widening of the tricuspid outlet secondary to right ventricular dilatation, which increases the tricuspid ring. Very rarely, malignancy or trauma may cause tricuspid regurgitation. In addition, any condition that increases pulmonary vascular resistance can have an effect upon the tricuspid valve (Hall & Nitter-Hauge 1996).

Clinical symptoms

These are similar to those already described but patients often complain of facial bloating when they bend down. This is because of venous congestion. In addition, nausea and vomiting are prominent due to further abdominal congestion. In advanced stages this may lead to jaundice and extreme oedema formation.

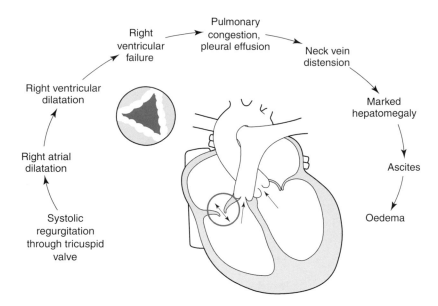

Figure 13.15 The effect of tricuspid regurgitation. (Reproduced with permission from Guzzetta & Dossey 1992.)

Investigations

Electrocardiography. This shows no typical changes. Any that do occur relate to the condition and process that has caused the functional tricuspid regurgitation to occur.

Echocardiography. The echocardiogram reveals right ventricular dilatation. Septal motion is usually reversed. This is non-specific and is due to the volume overload of the right ventricle. Doppler echocardiography is very accurate and sensitive at diagnosing tricuspid regurgitation; indeed, it may detect it in normal subjects. In functional tricuspid regurgitation valve cusps usually appear normal. When the aetiology is organic, the echocardiogram may show the cause, such as vegetation in infective endocarditis or a congenital abnormality such as Ebstein's anomaly.

Chest X-ray. The chest X-ray often shows enlargement of the right atrium and ventricle due to the volume overload.

Cardiac catheterisation. If tricuspid regurgitation is haemodynamically significant, right atrial pressure is increased substantially. Right ventricular end-diastolic pressure is raised in most cases. The right atrial pressure rises on inspiration or exercise and then fails to fall as quickly as it would in normal subjects. When tricuspid regurgitation is severe the pressure tracing in the right atrium can resemble the right ventricle.

Medical treatment

Tricuspid regurgitation is often well tolerated even when severe. If organic tricuspid regurgitation has led to fluid accumulation such as peripheral oedema or ascites, diuretics usually relieve the symptoms. Functional tricuspid regurgitation frequently resolves if the primary causes are treated. If the cause is left ventricular dysfunction, the regurgitation may disappear if the left ventricular failure can be adequately treated. Once the tricuspid valve becomes competent again, left ventricular function further improves as cardiac output increases, renal perfusion improves and peripheral oedema disappears more readily. Patients with peripheral oedema and ascites need help and support because of the decreased mobility and fatigue they will be experiencing. Advice about resting and limb elevation is important and bedrest is a useful adjunct to medical treatment if oedema or ascites is severe. Restriction of fluid intake may be necessary during treatment to control acute oedema. The issue of salt restriction should also be discussed with patients to further reduce fluid accumulation. If atrial fibrillation occurs it is treated with digoxin.

PULMONARY VALVE DISORDERS

Problems with the pulmonary valve are usually congenital (see Chapter 12) and acquired disease is extremely rare. The most common cause of acquired pulmonary valve disease is carcinoid heart disease, where there is obstruction from the right ventricle extending up to the pulmonary valve due to fibrous tissue.

Investigations

Electrocardiography. Unexpected findings on the ECG indicating right ventricular hypertrophy may suggest pulmonary stenosis and a possible underlying cause of pulmonary hypertension.

Echocardiography. This may be helpful as it can show the cause of right ventricular outflow obstruction, such as a mass in the outflow tract or vegetation on the pulmonary valve. Cross-sectional echocardiography will show right ventricular hypertrophy. Doppler techniques are helpful, as they will show the increased velocity of flow across the obstruction. This will allow an assessment of the severity of pulmonary stenosis. The echo will show an increase in pulmonary artery dimensions when pulmonary regurgitation is secondary to either pulmonary hypertension or idiopathic dilatation of the pulmonary artery. If the degree of regurgitation is severe, right ventricular volume overload will also be seen. Doppler techniques are very sensitive and will detect pulmonary regurgitation. Doppler also allows a semiquantitative estimate of the severity to be obtained from the size of the regurgitant jet seen on colour flow imaging (Hall & Treasure 1996).

Chest X-ray. In cases of pulmonary stenosis there are no usual features on the chest X-ray, but it may show a cause such as a mediastinal tumour or aortic aneurysm. In pulmonary regurgitation there may be evidence of dilatation of the main pulmonary artery and when the lesion is severe there may also be enlargement of the right ventricle.

Cardiac catheterisation. This may be needed to confirm the pressure gradient across the right ventricular outflow tract. If a tumour is suspected great care needs to be taken not to dislodge any tissue.

Management

This is dependent upon the underlying cause. Pulmonary regurgitation seldom requires treatment in its own right.

CONCLUSION

This chapter has illustrated the causes, clinical signs and medical and surgical management of valve disorders. The causes have altered over the last 50 years from rheumatic fever to degeneration in the ageing population. However, in the developing world rheumatic fever continues to be a major cause.

Problems with the heart valves can be very debilitating for patients. The symptoms can be distressing and deterioration can be rapid. Surgical repair or replacement is the treatment of choice. The quality of life for these patients improves dramatically.

Nursing the patient following valve replacement can be one of the most rewarding aspects of cardiac nursing. The patient is admitted with a very limited exercise tolerance, they are breathless and often very weary because they have interrupted sleep due to pulmonary congestion. Once the valve is replaced this all changes and the patient can often resume a normal life.

Case study 13.1

Mrs Ada Moore is a 68-year-old widow. She was referred by her general practitioner (GP) to the cardiologist at her local district general hospital (DGH) when 65 years of age. This was with a history of 16 months of breathlessness that had responded well to oral bendroflumethiazide (bendrofluazide). She did not complain of any chest pain and slept flat. However, Mrs Moore did complain of a wheeze that was not associated with an upper respiratory tract infection. Her exercise tolerance was between 50–100 yards on the flat. There was nothing significant in her past medical history, in particular no history of rheumatic fever. Her heart rate was normal and she was in sinus rhythm.

An echocardiogram at this time showed a heavily calcified mitral valve with mitral regurgitation and mild stenosis. There was no evidence of mitral valve prolapse. The mitral valve area was 1.68 cm^2 with reduction in leaflet movement. The aortic valve was also calcified with mild aortic regurgitation but no stenosis. There was overall reasonable function of the left ventricle.

It was decided that Mrs Moore would be reviewed by the cardiologist in 1 year's time and would continue to be monitored by her GP. Her medication was to continue with bendroflumethiazide (bendrofluazide) 5 mg daily.

As often happens in patients with valve disorders, Mrs Moore deteriorated and only 2 months after her first consultation was referred back to the cardiologist. She had become much more short of breath and had been experiencing angina. She was no longer able to go upstairs without anginal-type pain and having to stop to rest. She had some ankle swelling, paroxysmal nocturnal dyspnoea and wheeze. Her medication had been altered to bendroflumethiazide (bendrofluazide) 10 mg, propranolol 60 mg daily and nifedipine 30 mg was also added. There was no improvement with furosemide (frusemide).

A repeat echocardiogram showed calcified aortic and mitral valves, with moderate mitral regurgitation and stenosis, moderate aortic regurgitation with severe aortic stenosis, the transaortic gradient being 112 mmHg and the mitral valve area now 1.4 cm². This result was considerably worse than the previous echo performed only 2 months earlier which did not show any aortic stenosis at that time. This gives a clear illustration of how patients suddenly deteriorate and need regular follow-up. It must also be said that Mrs Moore was a very stoical lady and needed a great deal of encouragement from her daughter to admit that she was not well. There was no reported history of syncope in this case.

It was decided following this consultation to assess Mrs Moore more fully and plans were made to admit her as soon as possible for a right and left heart catheterisation and coronary angiography. Only 2 weeks later Mrs Moore experienced an upper respiratory tract infection, which made her symptoms much worse. She had a temperature of 38.1°C with bilateral basal crepitations on sounding of her chest. She was very short of breath at rest. She was admitted to the DGH and 2 days later transferred to the tertiary centre for further investigation and management.

Mrs Moore underwent cardiac catheterisation, which showed unobstructed coronary arteries. An aortogram showed a heavily calcified aortic valve with reduced cusp movement and mild to moderate aortic regurgitation.

There was also a heavily calcified mitral valve but good left ventricular function. A repeat echo also confirmed previous findings.

Mrs Moore was referred to the surgical team for valve replacement on this admission. She stayed on the cardiology ward on medication until surgery was performed, remaining in sinus rhythm, while all her other symptoms persisted. The evening before Mrs Moore's surgery she was visited by the anaesthetist and her recovery phase was fully explained to her. She was given a premedication of temazepam 20 mg and commenced prophylactic antibiotics (flucloxacillin).

Six days after her transfer to the tertiary centre Mrs Moore had an aortic and mitral valve replacement. The surgeon chose mechanical valves. The operation was straightforward and she recovered overnight on the intensive care unit. She required a low dose of isoprenaline and glyceryl trinitrate (GTN) to maintain the haemodynamic pressures within the desired parameters, but this recovery period was uncomplicated. She was extubated 8 hours postoperatively and was given oxygen at 5 l/min via a face mask. Mrs Moore was orientated but drowsy and responding to commands. The isoprenaline was reduced with no effect on the pressures. She was transferred to the postoperative ward the morning following her bilateral valve replacement.

The postoperative phase commenced with Mrs Moore making steady progress. She still had a mediastinal drain in place on return to the ward and had intravenous fluid therapy in progress, but was tolerating small amounts of oral liquids. The intravenous therapy was discontinued the same evening. Mrs Moore also had atrial and ventricular pacing wires in place, set on a demand rate at 90 beats per minute (bpm) with an underlying rhythm present. She was also administered IV morphine for pain relief. Observations were recorded 2 hourly overnight and they remained very stable and within the desired parameters.

The following day, postoperative day 2, Mrs Moore's chest drain was removed. However, the chest X-ray revealed a pneumothorax and the chest drain was re-inserted. The sternal wound was dry so the dressing was removed. Mrs Moore was tolerating fluids well but had little appetite. She also developed atrial fibrillation and was commenced upon digoxin. This is a common postoperative complication. She was also commenced on warfarin that she would need to take for the rest of her life to prevent clots forming on the mechanical valves.

On the third postoperative day the intercostal drain was removed. Mrs Moore was mobilizing well and managing her personal hygiene independently. Her heart beat remained irregular but apex and radial pulses were synchronized. She was only requiring paracetemol for pain relief. She continued to make steady progress and was discharged home on her eighth postoperative day. During this time the digoxin was discontinued as she had reverted back into sinus rhythm.

Mrs Moore was discharged home on warfarin, the INR to be maintained at around 3. This was monitored regularly at the anticoagulation clinic.

It is over 2 years since Mrs Moore had her aortic and mitral valve replacements. She has kept very well and leads a normal life. She has recommenced the voluntary work she did before her symptoms deteriorated. In fact, she 'pulled' her right knee a year ago at a keep fit class. She was reviewed at 6 weeks by the surgeons and discharged back to the care of the DGH cardiologist who reviews Mrs Moore on an annual basis.

This case study clearly demonstrates how quickly patients with valve disorders can deteriorate yet how, following surgical replacement, there can be a dramatic improvement in their quality of life.

REFERENCES

Barlow JB, Pocock WA, Marchand P, Denny M 1963 The significance of late systolic murmurs. American Heart Journal 66(4): 443–452

Bernard Y, Etievent J, Mourand JL et al 1992 Long-term results of percutaneous aortic valvuloplasty compared with aortic valve replacement in patients more than 75 years old. Journal of the American College of Cardiologists 20(4): 796–801

BNF 2001 British National Formulary, 41st edn. British Medical Association and the Royal Pharmaceutical Society of Great Britain, London

Bortolotti U, Valente M, Agozzino L, Mazzucco A, Thiene G 1984 Rheumatoid mitral stenosis requiring valve replacement. American Heart Journal 107(5 part 1): 1049–1051

Braunwald E 1992 Heart diseases, 4th edn. WB Saunders, Philadelphia

Braunwald E 1994 Valvular heart disease. In: Isselacher KJ et al (eds) Harrison's principles of internal medicine, 13th edn. McGraw Hill, New York, pp. 1052–1065

Brody MJ, Abboud FM 1976 Tissue perfusion. In: Frohlich ED (ed) Pathophysiology, 2nd edn. JB Lippincott, Philadelphia

Brown OR, De Mots H, Kloster FE, Roberts A, Menashe VD, Beals RK 1975 Aortic root dilatation and mitral valve prolapse in Marfan's syndrome: an echocardiographic study. Circulation 52(4): 651–657

Buda AJ, Levene DL, Myers MG, Chisholm AW, Shane SJ 1978 Coronary artery spasm and mitral valve prolapse. American Heart Journal 95(4): 457–462

Burckhardt D, Hoffman A, Bryan AJ 1996 Aortic valve disease. In: Julian DG, Camm AJ, Fox KM, Hall RJC, Poole-Wilson PA (eds) Diseases of the heart, 2nd edn. WB Saunders, London, pp. 763–765, 778

Campbell M 1932 Aortic valvular disease. British Medical Journal 1(32): 8

Campbell M 1968 Calcific aortic stenosis and congenital bicuspid aortic valves. British Heart Journal 30(5): 606–616

Carabello BA 1998 Mitral valve disease. In: Yusuf S, Cairns JA, Camm AJ, Fallen EL, Gersh BJ (eds) Evidence based cardiology. BMJ Books, London, pp. 798–810

Cavallo GAO 1992 The person with valvular heart disease. In: Guzzetta CE, Dossey BM (eds) Cardiovascular nursing. Mosby Year-book, St Louis, pp. 358–393

Chen WW, Chan FL, Wong PH, Chow JS 1983 Familial occurrence of mitral valve prolapse: is it related to the straight back syndrome? British Heart Journal 50(1): 97–110

Crawford MH, Souchek J, Oprian CA et al 1990 Determinants of survival and left ventricular performance after mitral valve replacement. Department of Veterans Affairs Cooperative Study on Valvular Heart Disease. Circulation 81(4): 1173–1181

Cribier A, Savin T, Saoudi N, Rocha P, Berland J, Letac B 1986 Percutaneous transluminal valvuloplasty of acquired aortic stenosis in elderly patients: an alternative view to valve replacements? Lancet 1: 63–67

Davies MJ 1980 Pathology of cardiac valves. Butterworth, London

De Pace NL, Rohrer AH, Kotler MN, Brezin JH, Parry WR 1981 Rapidly progressing, massive mitral annular calcification. Occurrence in a patient with chronic renal failure. Archives of Internal Medicine 141(12): 1663–1665

Deutscher S, Rockette HE, Krishnaswami V 1984 Diabetes and hypercholesterolemia among patients with calcific aortic stenosis. Journal of Chronic Diseases 379(5): 407–415

Dorward AJ, Kerr JW 1982 Left vocal cord paralysis and chronic obstructive airways disease. British Journal of Diseases of the Chest 76(3): 306–308

Enriquez-Sarano M, Tajik AJ, Schaff HV, Orszulak TA, Bailey KR, Frye RL 1994 Echocardiographic prediction of survival after surgical correction of organic mitral regurgitation. Circulation 90(2): 830–837

Frater RW, Salomon NW, Rainer WG, Cosgrove DM 3rd, Wickham E 1992 The Carpentier-Edwards pericardial aortic valve: intermediate results. Annals of Thoracic Surgery 53(5): 764–771

Freeman R, Hall RJC 1996 Infective endocarditis. In: Julian DG, Camm AJ, Fox KM, Hall RJC, Poole-Wilson PA (eds) Diseases of the heart, 2nd edn. WB Saunders, London, p. 894

Gahl K, Sutton R, Pearson M, Caspari P, Lairet A, McDonald L 1977 Mitral regurgitation in coronary heart disease. British Heart Journal 39(1): 13–18

Goldberger E 1989 Textbook of clinical cardiology. Mosby, St Louis

Grenadier E, Keidar S, Sahn DJ et al 1985 Ruptured mitral chordae tendineae may be a frequent and insignificant complication in the mitral valve prolapse syndrome. European Heart Journal 6(12): 1006–1015

Grossman W, Baim DS 1986 Profiles in valvular heart disease. In: Grossman W (ed) Cardiac catheterisation and angiography. Lea and Febiger, Philadelphia, pp. 557–581

Guzzetta CE, Dossey BM 1992 Cardiovascular nursing: holistic practice. Mosby, St Louis

Hall RJC, Julian DG 1989 Diseases of cardiac valves. Churchill Livingstone, Edinburgh

Hall RJC, Nitter-Hauge S 1996 Other valve disorders. In: Julian DG, Camm AJ, Fox KM, Hall RJC, Poole-Wilson PA (eds) Diseases of the heart, 2nd edn. WB Saunders, London, pp. 853–871

Hall RJC, Treasure T 1996 Mitral valve disease. In: Julian DG, Camm AJ, Fox KM, Hall RJC, Poole-Wilson PA (eds) Diseases of the heart, 2nd edn. WB Saunders, London, pp. 801–803, 813–815, 825

Henry WL, Morganroth J, Pearlman AS et al 1976 Relation between echocardiographically determined left atrial size and atrial fibrillation. Circulation 53(2): 273–279

Hochreiter C, Niles N, Devereux RB, Kligfield P, Borer JS 1986 Mitral regurgitation; the relationship of non invasive descriptors of right and left ventricular performance of clinical and hemodynamic findings to prognosis in medically and surgically treated patients. Circulation 73(5): 900–912

Hoffman FG, Leight L 1965 Complete atrioventricular block associated with rheumatoid disease. American Journal of Cardiology 16(4): 585–592

Holley KE, Bahn RC, McGoon DC, Mankin HT 1963 Spontaneous calcific embolisation associated with calcific aortic stenosis. Circulation 27: 197–202

Julian DG, Camm AJ, Fox KM, Hall RJC, Poole-Wilson PA (eds) 1996 Diseases of the heart, 2nd edn. WB Saunders, London

Kirklin JW, Barratt-Boyes BG 1993 Cardiac surgery, 2nd edn. Churchill Livingstone, New York, chapter 12 (vol 1), pp. 491–571

Korn D, De Santis RW, Sell S 1962 Massive calcification of the mitral annulus. New England Journal of Medicine 267: 900

Kramer HM, Kligfield P, Devereux RB, Savage DD, Kramer-Fox R 1984 Arrhythmias in mitral valve prolapse: effect of selection bias. Annals of Internal Medicine 144(12): 2360–2364

Lehmann KG, Francis CK, Dodge HT 1992 Mitral regurgitation in early myocardial infarction. Incidence, clinical detection, and prognostic implications. TIMI Study Group. Annals of Internal Medicine 117(1): 10–17

Lewis MG 1965 Idiopathic medionecrosis causing aortic incompetence. British Medical Journal 1: 1478

Oakley C, Yusuf R, Hoffman A 1961 Coronary embolism and angina in mitral stenosis. British Heart Journal 23: 357

O'Keefe JH Jr, Vlietstra RE, Bailey KR, Holmes DR Jr 1987 Natural history of candidates for balloon aortic valvuloplasty. Mayo Clinic Proceedings 62(11): 986–991

Olivier C 2000 Rheumatic fever: is it still a problem? Journal of Antimicrobial Chemotherapy 45: 13–21

Pocock WA 1987 Mitral leaflet billowing and prolapse. In: Barlow JB (ed) Perspectives on the mitral valve. FA Davies, Philadelphia, pp. 45–112

Pomerance A 1970 Pathological and clinical study of calcification of the mitral valve ring. Journal of Clinical Pathology 23(4): 354–361

Rackley CE, Edwards JE, Wallace RB, Katz NM 1990 Aortic valve disease. In: Hurst JW, Schlant RC, Rackley CE et al (eds) The heart, 7th edn. McGraw-Hill, New York, pp. 795–819

Rackley CE, Edwards JE, Karp RB 1991 Mitral stenosis. In: Hurst JW, Schlant RC, Rackley CE et al (eds) The heart, 7th edn. McGraw-Hill, New York, pp. 820–851

Rahimtoola SH 1991 Perspective on valvular heart disease. Update II. In: Koebe S, Dacks S (eds) Era in cardiovascular medicine. Elsevier, New York, pp. 45–70

Ramsdale DR, Bennett DH, Bray CL, Ward C, Beton DC, Faragher EB 1984 Angina, coronary risk factors and coronary artery disease in patients with valvular heart disease. A prospective study. European Heart Journal 5(9): 714–726

Roberts WC, Honig HS 1982 The spectrum of cardiovascular disease in the Marfan syndrome. A clinico-morphologic study of 18 necropsy patients and comparison to 151 previously reported necropsy patients. American Heart Journal 104(1): 115–135

Ross J, Braunwald E 1968 Aortic stenosis. Circulation 38(1 suppl): 61–67

Ross RS 1961 Right ventricular hypertension as a cause of precordial pain. American Heart Journal 61: 134

Scott WC, Miller DC, Haverich A et al 1985 Determinants of operative mortality for patients undergoing aortic valve replacement. Discriminant analysis of 1,479 operations. Journal of Thoracic and Cardiovascular Surgery 89(3): 400–413

Selzer A 1987 Changing aspects of the natural history of valvular aortic stenosis. New England Journal of Medicine 317(2): 91–98

Sinclair RJG, Kitchin AH, Turner RWD 1960 The Marfan syndrome. Quarterly Journal of Medicine 29: 19

Stuckley D 1955 Cardiac pain in association with mitral stenosis. British Heart Journal 17: 397–408

Tseng EE, Lee CA, Cameron DE 1997 Aortic valve replacement in the elderly. Risk factors and long-term results. Annals of Surgery 225(6): 793–802, discussion 802–804

Walter PJ, Mohan R, Amsel BJ 1992 Quality of life after heart valve replacement. Journal of Heart Valve Disease 1(1): 34–41

Weiss AN, Mimbs JW, Ludbrook PA, Sobel BE 1975 Echocardiographic detection of mitral valve prolapse. Exclusion of false positive diagnosis and determination of inheritance. Circulation 52(6): 1091–1096

Wheatley DJ 1996 Surgery for valvular heart disease: techniques and materials. In: Julian DG, Camm AJ, Fox KM, Hall RJC, Poole-Wilson PA (eds) Diseases of the heart, 2nd edn. WB Saunders, London, p. 878

Wheatley DJ, Tolland MM, Pathi V et al 1995 Randomised, prospective evaluation of a new pericardial heart valve: outcome after seven years. European Journal of Cardiothoracic Surgery 9(5): 259–267, discussion 267–268

14

Infective endocarditis

Sue Mason

Infective endocarditis (IE) occurs when micro-organisms colonize the endocardial surface of the heart and valves, causing tissue destruction (Nunley & Perlman 1993). The endocardium is a thin, delicate membrane of endocardial cells, lining the surface of the atria, ventricles, valves and chordae tendineae. The disease occurs when the endocardium is compromised by endothelial damage and as a consequence blood-borne micro-organisms adhere to the damaged endocardium and proliferate. The hallmark of IE is a platelet–fibrin–bacteria mass known as a **vegetation** (Marrie 1987). This chapter explores the causes and presentation of infective endocarditis and focuses particularly on the nursing care to prevent an occurrence of the disease in those vulnerable to its development. The emergence of home-based antibiotic therapy is examined as an option for certain groups of patients presenting with IE.

EPIDEMIOLOGY AND HISTORY

Infective endocarditis is not a notifiable disease in the UK so its true incidence is not known. However, the Office of Population Censuses and Surveys records approximately 200 deaths per year from IE (Prasad & Fraser 1995). In contrast, the incidence of IE in the USA is known and estimated at one in 1000 hospital admissions (Steckelberg et al 1990). It has been identified that there are 10 000–20 000 new cases each year (Bayer et al 1991). Despite these statistics it is acknowledged that it is a relatively rare disease with Bayer & Scheld (2000) citing 1.7 per 100 000 person-years in a prospective survey in the USA. This they describe as analogous with the UK. Swanton (1998) has highlighted that 1500 cases of IE occur in the UK each year. The first account of IE was provided by Osler in 1885 (Bansal 1995) and before the advent of antibiotics the disease was considered fatal. Although this is not the case today, IE is still considered a serious occurrence with an associated mortality of 10–20% and a 5-year survival of only 50–60% (Nunley & Perlman 1993).

CLASSIFICATION

The classification of IE is based upon the clinical presentation of the disease, its course, progression and the causative organisms and their associated virulence. Previously, IE was categorized as acute or subacute depending on the duration of the illness and the presence or absence of systemic toxicity. Due to the overlap of these two categories, the distinction is now difficult to make and so the generic term infective endocarditis is used. There still remains the view, however, that this term is imprecise as it covers all cardiac pathogens responsible for endocarditis, but does not provide a useful clinical correlation relating to clinical presentation or virulence of the infecting micro-organism (Cunha et al 1996). Therefore the original classifications will be described.

A patient with acute bacterial endocarditis (ABE) presents classically in acute illness with a high temperature, rigors and manifestations of septic emboli but no initial heart murmur. The responsible organisms are consequently virulent. Conversely, subacute bacterial endocarditis (SBE) presents with a low-grade pyrexia and is caused by organisms which are far less virulent.

Acute bacterial endocarditis (ABE)

This usually occurs on normal heart valves and is caused by particularly virulent micro-organisms (for example, *Staphylococcus aureus*). The valve is rapidly destroyed following the onset of symptoms. A regurgitant heart murmur of striking intensity develops in the vast majority of these patients.

Nosocomial acute bacterial endocarditis

Acute endocarditis acquired whilst in hospital is termed nosocomial acute bacterial endocarditis. Intravascular and intracardiac catheters and devices can be implicated in this type of acute endocarditis.

Subacute bacterial endocarditis (SBE)

This usually occurs on previously damaged valves with the causative organisms originating from the body's normal flora, for example the oral cavity. It progresses more slowly than acute bacterial endocarditis.

Other classifications

Culture-negative infective endocarditis

The most common reason for persistently negative blood cultures is the administration of antibiotics, which can result in negative results for 1 month after administration (Oakley 1995). However, other causes can include fastidious organisms such as Brucella and Legionella, which can take up to 3 weeks to culture, cell-dependent organisms such as Chlamydia and Coxiella, fungi or a major immune reaction (Oakley 1995). If a clinical diagnosis is made but cultures remain negative, treatment should be instigated.

Prosthetic valve endocarditis (PVE)

The incidence of PVE is about 4% (Almirante Gragera et al 1998). PVE is any infection on parts of a mechanical or biological valve substitute or on a reconstructed native heart valve. Infection develops at the interface between the sewing ring of the prosthesis and the valve annulus and extends into the annular tissue, leading to the development of an abscess and consequent tissue necrosis. This allows the sutures anchoring the prosthesis to pull free, which then causes the valve to leak.

Patients with PVE are classified into early-onset and late-onset groupings.

- Early onset – endocarditis develops when the infection occurs in the perioperative valve replacement period. The mortality is high ranging from 40% to 60% (Chastre & Trouillet 1995).
- Late onset – endocarditis develops 60 days after surgery due to another initiating event (Horstkotte et al 1995).

PATHOLOGY

Native or prosthetic heart valves are most commonly affected but infection may also occur on the mural endocardium or in septal defects.

Lesions of IE form by alterations in blood flow creating areas of trauma on the endothelial surface. Circulating platelets and fibrin become deposited on damaged subendothelial collagen, leading to a non-bacterial thrombotic vegetation.

Vegetations grow by repetitive layering of platelets and fibrin, most commonly occurring in the mitral and aortic valve regions, downstream from areas of high pressure. These vegetations occur on regurgitant rather than stenotic valves and on the low pressure side, thus occurring on the atrial side of the mitral valve and the ventricular side of the aortic valve. The vegetations tend to be large, several centimetres in size, single or multiple, friable and often project from the valve cusps. Their colour varies from pink, red, yellow or green in the early stages to grey after

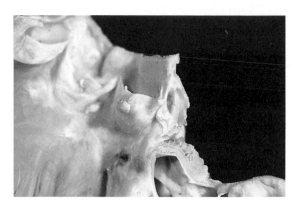

Figure 14.1 Vegetations of infective endocarditis on an aortic valve. (Reproduced with kind permission of Dr Mary N Sheppard, Royal Brompton Hospital, London.)

healing. Clumps of these vegetations are sometimes referred to as verrucae (Burden & Rodgers 1988). The vegetation interferes with the normal alignment of the valve cusps resulting in incomplete closure and regurgitation.

If micro-organisms invade the bloodstream through, for example, infection or an invasive procedure, they become enmeshed in the growing vegetation and colonize. The infection causes the valve to become insufficient by either destroying the valve leaflets or rupturing the valve-supporting structures.

CLINICAL PRESENTATION

IE is a complex multifaceted disease that may affect any organ. Although a wide variety of clinical manifestations can be present, resulting in a varied clinical presentation for each patient, symptoms tend to include fever, sweats, chills, anorexia, fatigue, weight loss, arthralgia, arthritis, myalgia and back pain. Hence patients with IE often describe flu-like symptoms. As highlighted, the temperature is usually low grade unless an organism such as *Staphylococcus aureus* is responsible and then a high fever and rigors may occur. Damage to the heart is usually seen as a later consequence rather than an initial presentation. On examination a heart murmur, splenomegaly, mucosal, cutaneous and retinal changes can be seen. About 80–95% of patients who develop IE have heart murmurs. Furthermore, over 90% of patients with IE will present with a murmur (Matthews 1994).

Approximately one-third of patients present with neurological symptoms caused by a cerebrovascular accident (CVA/stroke), transient ischaemic attack or brain abscess (Nunley & Perlman 1993). This presentation will form part of the diagnosis along with the iso-

lation of causative organisims in the blood cultures. These signs and symptoms are related to bacteraemia, acute valvulitis, peripheral emboli and immunological vascular phenomena.

Signs of heart failure such as dyspnoea, orthopnoea (breathlessness on lying flat), coughing, paroxysmal nocturnal dyspnoea, pulmonary oedema and a third heart sound may occur. As more patients are presenting acutely with virulent valvular pathogens such as Staphylococcus, there is a reduced frequency of certain dependent peripheral stigmata of IE such as splinter haemorrhages. Acute dyspnoea, pleuritic chest pain, cough and haemoptysis indicate pulmonary embolus which can occur with tricuspid endocarditis. It has been suggested that IE should be considered when there is an insidious onset of congestive cardiac failure, acute neurological changes and an acute onset of arthralgia or myalgia (pain in one or more muscles).

Infection can progress through the following mechanisms.

- *Bacteraemia.* Micro-organisms discharged into the bloodstream cause fever, sweats, fatigue and anorexia. These circulating micro-organisms continue to re-seed the original vegetation, therefore perpetuating the infection.
- *Local infiltration*, when the micro-organisms within the vegetation cause necrosis of the valve cusp tissue leading to aneurysm and rupture of the chordae tendineae. This can cause cardiac conduction abnormalities (for example, prolonged P–R interval) and pericarditis.
- *Embolism.* Infected vegetation fragments break off and enter the bloodstream. These can then lodge in any organ causing infarction, for example in the retina, brain, coronary arteries, kidneys, spleen, intestine and lungs. In the case of embolic retinal artery occlusion, this can cause sudden blindness or in the case of embolization of the mesenteric artery, it can lead to ischaemic bowel and abdominal pain. Oral and cutaneous petechiae and subungular splinter haemorrhages are also manifestations of emboli appearing as dark, red streaky lines found in the distal third of the nail beds.
- *Immune complexes* occur when circulating micro-organisms produce an antibody response. These complexes can cause glomerulonephritis, synovitis and vasculitis. Osler's nodes, which are erythematous purple tender nodules (2–15 mm) on pads of toes and fingers, and Janeway lesions, which are non-tender erythematous lesions on palms and soles, are both skin manifestations of this immune complex response.

PREDISPOSING FACTORS

Historically, IE was believed to be a potential health problem primarily affecting patients with rheumatic heart disease, congenital heart disease or syphilis. This pattern has now changed and includes patients with a variety of other health disorders including prosthetic valve replacement and degenerative heart disorders, including mitral valve prolapse (Trausch 1988).

There is also a shift towards patients acquiring IE who previously had normal valves, as well as reduced incidence of acute rheumatic fever and consequently rheumatic heart disease. In 20–40% of cases no predisposing factors are found (Trausch 1988). Similarly, the mode of entry of the organisms has not been apparent in many patients with IE.

Similarly, there is an increasing incidence in the elderly population and in intravenous (IV) drug abusers. As lifespan continues to lengthen, the former is likely to continue. In this elderly population degenerative heart disease such as mitral or aortic valve calcification and congenital heart disease, specifically bicuspid aortic valve, are now important predisposing lesions. Also patients with congenital heart disease are now living longer and more elderly patients are having surgical interventions such as prosthetic valve replacement and permanent pacemaker implantation. The average age of patients with IE is now 58 years and it is more common in men than women (Griffin et al 1985).

The mitral valve is more commonly affected than the aortic valve but prognosis is poorer in aortic valve involvement. Mitral valve prolapse is one of the most common predisposing cardiac disorders.

In recent years there has been an overall increase in medical and surgical interventions that predispose to bacteraemic episodes, for example, the increased use of equipment such as the pulmonary artery (PA) catheter, arteriovenous shunts and other treatment modalities. Certain disease states where the body's defences are less likely to cope with invasion of microorganisms, such as serious burns, neoplasms, renal failure, haematological disorders and cirrhosis in the setting of bacteraemia, can lead to IE.

Cardiac diseases that are known to predispose to IE usually exhibit specific haemodynamic factors. These include a narrow orifice, with a pressure gradient resulting in a high-velocity abnormal jet stream flowing from an area of high pressure to low pressure causing damage to the endocardial surface. Platelet–fibrin deposition occurs and this is then a focus for infection. To apply this principle in the case of ventricular septal defect (VSD), it is the small haemodynamically restrictive defect which has a high systolic pressure gradient between the left and right ventricles which has the highest risk; that is, lesions occurring around the orifice on the right ventricular side or at the site where the jet impacts on the wall of the right ventricle. Conversely atrial septal defects (ASD) rarely become affected as there is an absence of a pressure gradient and velocity jet between the atria.

Patients with a prior history of IE have a higher chance of recurrent endocarditis in the future. This has been referred to as endocarditis diathesis (Durack 1977), which implies that such patients have a weakness for the disease.

Intravenous drug abusers

This specific subgroup of patients usually present acutely with right-sided valvular infection caused by *Staphylococcus aureus*. The classic peripheral stigmata of IE are absent because these signs usually require left-sided valvular involvement. Instead, these patients present with fever and pulmonary emboli. Cure rates of 85–95% have been reported for right-sided endocarditis in the setting of intravenous drug abuse (Bayer et al 1991).

COMPLICATIONS

IE remains an important and life-threatening infection despite improvements in diagnosis and management. The mortality rate ranges between 20% and 30% (and is as high as 40–70% in the elderly). If left untreated it will almost always result in death (Delahaye et al 1995). The reasons for this high mortality include failure to prevent the disease, late recognition once the disease is present and ineffective antibiotic therapy. Congestive cardiac failure is the most common cause of death in IE (Matthews 1994). In right-sided endocarditis the mortality rate is not so grim, with rates under 7% being reported (Bayer et al 1991).

During the initial phase of IE the mortality is high, but after 1 year the risk of dying is low although not quite at the rate of the general population (Delahaye et al 1995).

Intracranial mycotic aneurysm (also known as infective or bacterial aneurysm)

Intracranial mycotic aneurysm (IMA) is a rare complication, occurring in 2–10% of cases (Kong & Chan 1995). It arises when a blood-borne infective embolus lodges in a cerebral artery. Infectious and inflammatory processes lead to a weakening of the arterial wall, causing a cerebral mycotic aneurysm. These can occur singularly or in multiples. The risk of the aneurysm rupturing is about 1–2% and when this occurs it is usually catastrophic, causing subarachnoid haemorrhage, intraventricular haemorrhage or intracerebral destruction of the brain (Kong & Chan 1995). A patient with IMA will usually be asymptomatic until it ruptures. Some patients may complain of headache, lethargy, neck discomfort and other neurological deficits attributed to the location of the aneurysm. A diagnosis can be made by cerebral angiography.

Mortality from surgical intervention will depend on a number of factors, including the haemodynamic status of the patient, the severity of the lesion, type of endocarditis (native or prosthetic), causative organism and the type of surgery required. The mortality rate varies from 5% to 30% (Acar et al 1995).

The term 'new' IE refers to a recurrence of the disease after the previous episode has healed. This is usually due to a different micro-organism and occurs more than 6 months later (Delahaye et al 1995).

MICROBIOLOGY

The bacteria Streptococcus and Staphylococcus still account for the most attributable causative organisms (Nunley & Perlman 1993). However, there is a change in organisms causing IE from *Streptococcus viridans* to staphylococci and enterococci. In addition, there is an increase in penicillin-resistant streptococci, enterococci resistant to β-lactams, aminoglycosides and methicillin-resistant staphylococci.

Streptococci

- *Streptococcus viridans*. These organisms are part of the normal flora of the oral cavity. When the oral mucosa is breached (for example in dental work) these organisms are able to enter the bloodstream. Congenital or acquired valvular disease is the main predisposing factor for *Streptococcus viridans* endocarditis. In these cases clinical symptoms occur approximately 2 weeks after the bacteria have infected the valve.
- *Streptococcus bovis*. Patients who have this type of endocarditis are likely to have an underlying bowel disorder, including cancer. Therefore these patients should always be screened to exclude carcinoma of the colon. However, this organism is relatively rare (Matthews 1994).
- *Streptococcus pneumoniae*. This rare cause is often associated with the underlying diseases of alcoholism and diabetes, without prior valve disease. It can quickly cause destruction of the aortic valve and abscess formation.

Enterococci

Enterococci cause 5–10% of IE (Kunkel 1995). The incidence of *Enterococcus faecalis* is on the increase (Matthews 1994); this organism normally inhabits the gastro-intestinal and genito-urinary tracts. The types of patient this is likely to affect are elderly men following genito-urinary manipulation or young women after childbirth, gynaecological procedures or abortion.

Staphylococci

Staphylococcus aureus accounts for at least 20% of native valve endocarditis (Bansal 1995). It is the most common cause in IV drug abusers.

This organism has the ability to infect a previously normal valve and cause an acute illness. Consequently, it leads to suppurative complications such as myocardial abscess, valve ring abscess and purulent pericarditis.

Staphylococcus epidermidis is the most common cause of prosthetic valve endocarditis.

Other organisms

Aerobic Gram-negative bacilli such as Enterobacter, Klebsiella and Proteus species have all been reported as causing IE. Similarly other culprits include the HACEK group which are part of the oropharyngeal flora (Haemophilus species, *Actinobacillus actinomycetemcomitans*, *Cardiobacterium hominis*, *Eikenella corrodens*, Kingella species). Gram-positive bacilli such as diphtheroid are an important cause of prosthetic valve endocarditis, particularly in IV drug abusers (Rubinstein & Lang 1995).

Fungi

The main organisms implicated in this group are *Candida albicans* and *Aspergillus*, occurring mainly in patients with a prosthetic valve or an intravenous device in place. Large friable vegetations and emboli occurring in large vessels are common in this group. Prognosis is poor, with survival being around 50% (Rubinstein & Lang 1995).

INVESTIGATIONS

The diverse presentation of the disease means that diagnosis can be difficult. There are three aspects of investigation which need to be considered prior to diagnosis. These have been referred to as Duke's diagnostic criteria (Bansal 1995).

- Clinical presentation
- Microbiology
- Echocardiography

A preliminary diagnosis can be made after a detailed history is taken and physical examination is performed. In assessing the heart by auscultation, murmurs should be identified in terms of timing, location, configuration, intensity, pitch, quality and radiation. Review of dental, urological, gynaecological and surgical interventions is particularly important in identifying the potential source of the infection in suspected cases of IE.

The single most important laboratory test is the blood culture. Three sets of blood cultures need to be obtained with at least hourly intervals, within a 24-hour period, prior to the initiation of antibiotics. It is important to consider careful skin preparation when taking the cultures as common skin flora such as *Staphylococcus epidermidis* and diphtheroid can cause endocarditis and also contaminate the samples. Another important consideration is that culture-negative endocarditis is possible, with the most common cause being previous antimicrobial therapy. Also, some bacteria are slow growing (from the HACEK group) and may require 3–4 weeks of culturing.

If a patient presents with fever, anaemia, heart murmur and embolic phenomena (FAME) IE must be considered as a distinct possibility. Normocytic anaemia is quite frequent in subacute IE in response to a fairly chronic illness. The standard blood tests should be taken. The erythrocyte sedimentation rate (ESR) will be elevated if the endocarditis is acute. Urinalysis is performed to assess for microscopic haematuria, pyuria, red blood cell casts and proteinuria.

A computed tomography (CT) scan of the head should be performed if the patient has any neurological signs and symptoms. A transthoracic echo is performed to assess the function of the valves and location of any vegetations. The development and refinement of two-dimensional transthoracic echocardiography has led to an improved overall sensitivity of approximately 70% in establishing the presence of vegetations, depending on the size of the valve and the type (Bayer et al 1991).

The major advance in terms of investigations has to be the development of transoesophageal echocardiography (TOE). This investigation identifies valvular changes earlier and more precisely as it has a greater sensitivity in detecting vegetations compared with the transthoracic technique (Daniel et al 1991). Also the TOE is able to assess for valvular perforation, regurgitation, aneurysm and abscess formation.

A chest X-ray is performed to assess for signs of congestive cardiac failure.

An electrocardiogram (ECG) is performed to assess for cardiac arrhythmias, evidence of left or right ventricular hypertrophy or conduction abnormalities. Conduction abnormalities may suggest the development of a septal abscess.

THE ROLE OF THE NURSE

The seriousness of this disease undoubtedly highlights the importance of the nursing role in caring for patients with IE. Due to its numerous complications and life-threatening nature it is important that nurses understand the disease process in order to assess and plan appropriate nursing care. If a nurse lacks knowledge of certain aspects of this disease and its implications for the patient, complacency may occur, particularly when a patient has recovered from the acute phase of the illness.

The main aspects of nursing care focus upon the antibiotic administration regimen but must include meeting the psychological and emotional needs of both the patient and those close to them, due to a prolonged hospital stay. A social assessment should be undertaken and a care plan formulated in order to reflect the individual needs of the patient and the above issues, notably the psychological effects of a prolonged hospital stay away from family life and work.

In caring for the patient the nurse needs to monitor the effects of the antibiotics, how the patient is responding to treatment and the occurrence of side-effects. Observation of the patient's physical health is important in order to monitor for worsening of the condition. In some instances it may be necessary to prepare the patient for emergency surgery, so from the point of diagnosis of IE, the nurse needs to begin the educational process so that the patient and family/carers know what to expect if this approach is required urgently.

Patient teaching regarding IE needs to include individual patient predisposing factors and the relationship to future susceptibility, prophylaxis and dental care. Therefore, the goal of the nurse in preparing the patient for discharge is to decrease the potential for recurrence of infection by increasing the patient's and family/carers' knowledge of endocarditis. Appreciating the importance of prophylactic antibiotic therapy before undergoing any invasive procedures such as dental work or surgery is imperative for the patient. Empowerment is an important issue, with patients needing to understand that they have responsibility for their own health and therefore should inform doctors and dentists of the need for antibiotic prophylaxis.

TREATMENT

The treatment of IE consists of high doses of antibiotics active against the infecting organism; these are usually given intravenously to ensure bioavailability, high serum concentrations and good penetration into the vegetations. As a result, oral antibiotics are not recommended for initial treatment of IE. The main aim of medical treatment is to sterilize the vegetation (Besnier & Choutet 1995). Surgery to replace the valve is necessary when moderate to severe heart failure develops as a result of valve dysfunction (Francioli et al 1992). For many patients with IE, surgery is an essential therapeutic option, with 60% of patients requiring surgery at some point, 20–30% initially and 30–40% during the following 5–8 years (Delahaye et al 1995).

The goals of surgery are to correct valvular dysfunction, remove infected tissue, purge and seal abscess cavities, close any fistulas and remove mobile vegetations which can cause systemic emboli (Acar et al 1995). For many patients surgery offers a way of stabilizing cardiac haemodynamics, eradicating infection and reducing mortality (Chastre & Trouillet 1995). The most appropriate time for surgery depends on the haemodynamic status of the patient. An emergency approach is needed when refractory heart failure occurs due to valvular lesions, intracardiac fistulas or high-grade cardiac conduction abnormalities secondary to septal abscesses.

Studies have demonstrated the use of once-daily preparations such as ceftriaxone (Francioli et al 1992). Changes are occurring in the approach to treatment for IE, with the development of shorter courses, oral and once-a-day regimens and outpatient programmes. Antimicrobial susceptibility of the infecting organism is determined once blood cultures are found to be positive. Once three or four sets of blood cultures have been sent and the clinical diagnosis has been made, antibiotic treatment should be instigated.

Penicillin is the most commonly used antibiotic but erythromycin, vancomycin, gentamicin, ceftriaxone or teicoplanin may also be utilized depending on the organism. The treatment choice for Staphylococcus is penicillin and an aminoglycoside. In general, penicillin and gentamicin are used for subacute endocarditis and flucloxacillin and gentamicin if the onset is acute. Vancomycin, rifampicin and gentamicin are indicated if a prosthetic valve is implicated, because these patients are likely to have methicillin-resistant staphylococci. It is important that the patient is monitored carefully whilst on treatment, particularly by auscultation of the heart as a changing murmur may indicate valvular destruction.

In treating IV drug abusers with an uncomplicated disease process, 2 weeks' therapy may be enough and surgery may not be needed. As Staphylococcus is the dominant causative organism in IV drug abusers, penicillin and an aminoglycoside is the treatment of choice. The main problem with this group of patients is the issue of compliance with a lengthy therapy. If the condition is left sided, 4–6 weeks of treatment is required to prevent relapse or failure and surgery may be indicated if there are significant systemic emboli or heart failure (Besnier & Choutet 1995).

It is worth considering the effects of prolonged antimicrobial therapy. These may include interstitial nephritis, phlebitis, superinfections, skin rash, diarrhoea, drug fever, haemolytic anaemia, leucopenia and ototoxicity and nephrotoxicity if aminoglycosides are used. Therefore serum concentrations must be measured regularly to prevent some of these potential effects. Similarly, it is important to ensure efficient and effective concentrations are maintained.

PREVENTIVE MEASURES

Clearly, prevention is better than diagnosis and treatment. However, the employment of antibiotic prophylaxis is controversial. It is worth considering the following, as preventive measures are based upon these principles.

Oral cavity

The oral cavity is a point of entry into the bloodstream for micro-organisms. The presence of gum disease is highly likely to introduce bacteria by this route even before dental extraction. Interestingly, this is supported by the fact that edentulous people do not seem to be exempt from acquiring IE. However, chewing, brushing and irrigation during dental procedures have all been shown to produce positive blood cultures (Wahl 1994). In addition, there is a recognized association between dental extraction and bacteraemia and endocarditis. However, this correlation is not as strong as once thought and it has been shown that dental procedures only contribute to a small proportion of all cases of IE (Bayliss et al 1983).

Risk reduction is therefore concerned with ensuring that those at risk receive teaching on the importance of regular dental examination and appointments with the dental hygienist. The importance of the prevention of dental and gum disease cannot be overemphasized, with the encouragement of avoiding sugary foods, which contribute to dental caries. Careful brushing with a soft bristle toothbrush at least twice a day should be advocated.

Skin and nail care

Special consideration needs to be given to teenagers who are particularly prone to acne, focusing on controlling the skin condition and reducing infection. Similarly, at risk patients should be aware of how nail biting can lead to paronychia, which is a source of bacteraemia. Psoriasis may also be a possible source of infection.

Invasive procedures and operations

Orotracheal intubation, rigid bronchoscopy, endoscopy with biopsy, barium enema and urological procedures all pose a significant risk if a patient has a predisposing factor for IE. Cardiac catheterization surprisingly offers only a low risk due to the aseptic approach employed. TOE, which is a particularly pertinent investigation for patients with valve disease, also has a low risk. Therefore, risk reduction involves weighing up the risks against the benefits when considering referring a susceptible patient for an invasive procedure or operation.

Contraception

It is advisable to avoid using intrauterine devices in patients with congenital heart defects or other heart diseases predisposing to IE.

Cardiac surgery

A number of factors associated with cardiac surgery can present as a significant risk for IE. The underlying heart disease and prosthetic valve are the obvious risk factors but also a urinary catheter, an endotracheal tube and invasive haemodynamic monitoring can pose a threat. Similarly, pneumonia or a urinary tract infection can place the patient at risk. Micro-organisms such as *Staphylococcus epidermidis* and *Staphylococcus aureus* have the opportunity to enter the body through the wounds so antibiotic prophylaxis is utilized by most cardiac surgeons.

Intravenous drug abusers

The risk of recurrence is high in this group of patients. This can be reduced partly by teaching skin cleansing before injecting. However, the most effective preventive approach is for abusers to give up their addiction.

Box 14.1 Risk categories for the development of infective endocarditis

High risk
- Prosthetic valves, conduit, cardiac surgical patches
- Surgically created systemic to pulmonary shunts
- Previous endocarditis

Intermediate risk
- Acquired or congenital valvular dysfunction
- Hypertrophic obstructive cardiomyopathy (HOCM)
- Congenital shunts (other than atrial septal defects)
- Arteriovenous shunt (haemodialysis)
- Mitral valve prolapse (if regurgitation is present)

Low risk
- Uncomplicated atrial septal defect
- Mild valvular pulmonic stenosis
- Indwelling cardiac pacemakers

It is generally thought that the risk of developing IE can be stratified into three main areas (Box 14.1).

HOME INTRAVENOUS ANTIBIOTIC THERAPY

Traditionally the lengthy hospital stay for intravenous antibiotic treatment has been referred to as an antibiotic sentence (Williams 1995). Reflecting on my own clinical experience, it does appear that removal from work and family roles for an extended period contributes to patients' feelings of depression, loss of self-esteem, emotional stress, financial concerns, disruption to the family unit, lack of sleep and the psychological effects of seeing other patients admitted and discharged.

Bernstein (1992) identified how the growth and acceptance of home care in the USA has provided an alternative to institutionalization for large numbers of patients. However, the situation is very different in Britain with only slow progress being made in this area. Despite this, there are early signs of shifting boundaries between primary and secondary care with examples of hospital-at-home schemes developing to avoid hospital admission or to facilitate early discharge.

In relation to IE, home intravenous antibiotic therapy (HIVAT) appears to be limited to patients with penicillin-sensitive streptococcal infection. Kunkel (1995) suggests that patients with this type of endocarditis who have low risks of complications are ideal candidates for a HIVAT programme. The reason why Staphylococcus tends to be inappropriate to such programmes is the increased frequency of complications such as heart failure, valvular decompensation and embolic episodes (Williams 1995).

Coker & Lampert (1990) postulate that one of the focuses of HIVAT is the promotion of independence and self-care. Similarly, Cohen (1997) suggests that people with serious illnesses often feel more in control if they can manage part of their own care. There appear to be three ways to develop HIVAT for a patient group: by teaching patients or a family member/carer to self administer the IV antibiotics; by the patient attending the outpatient department for their treatment; or by a nurse administering the antibiotics in the patient's home (Williams 1995).

It is worth reflecting on the benefits of HIVAT programmes as outlined in Box 14.2.

It has been proposed that with proper training, many patients well enough to be at home are capable of administering their own medications (Masoorli 1996). I would suggest that fundamental to the successful implementation of a HIVAT programme is the development of a comprehensive teaching programme for patients. Coker & Lampert (1990) endorse this view when stating that to allow patients to learn the complex skills and information required to self administer home infusion therapy and to subsequently lessen patients' anxiety, teaching must be comprehensive and augmented by formal written instructions.

Education is particularly important for patients with IE, primarily in relation to minimizing the risk of re-infection. Nunley & Perlman (1993) identified that 15–25% of cases of IE are associated with invasive dental, gastro-intestinal and genito-urinary procedures in patients with underlying valvular disease. Therefore the importance of a patient understanding the need for prophylactic antibiotics is essential. Trausch (1988) highlights, perhaps logically, that patient education may in fact be life saving.

In order for learning to occur within such a teaching programme, a trusting relationship between the nurse as teacher and the patient needs to exist (Niederpruem 1989). This implies a change in the nurse's role from a provider of care to a somewhat passive recipient,

to one of educator and facilitator with the aim of empowerment. In developing a self-administration teaching programme the patient will learn at three levels. There is a need to understand the necessity for intravenous antibiotics in the home setting (cognitive), a change in attitude from being a receiver of care to being an active provider of care (affective) and the mastering of skills to self administer the medications (psychomotor) (Niederpruem 1989).

It has been highlighted that there may be difficulties in teaching patients. Wood (1991), for example, has concerns over teaching sick people, mentioning specifically the effects of anxiety, drugs and biochemical imbalance on mental concentration. Therefore a patient must be medically stable and well enough to embark on such a programme. This has to be considered in determining the initial criteria for admission to the programme and similarly, the teaching style and approach must also recognize these concerns. A further consideration is the importance of reinforcing information which enables the patient to identify and prioritize the important details (Miner 1994).

Ward (1990) claims that patients who appear confident in the hospital setting may not feel the same in the home environment away from the security and support of the nursing staff. Careful individualized discharge planning, with the nurse gradually reducing the support while in hospital, should be explained and advocated. To enhance what is taught several writers endorse the aforementioned written instructions or a checklist as a guide (Masoorli 1996, Ward 1990). Consideration of the educational and reading level of the patient may therefore preclude some individuals from safely being able to participate in a HIVAT programme. Alternative approaches with the assistance of videos have been suggested as a way of making the learning process easier for the patient (Masoorli 1996).

However, despite all these strategies, the anxiety associated with the transition from hospital to home will not be totally eradicated by the teaching and learning process and other support mechanisms need to be in place. Box 14.3 suggests the learning outcomes that may be incorporated in the implementation of a HIVAT programme.

The length of the supervision and teaching will be tailored to each individual patient but it is anticipated that patients will require at least 5 days' initial training and assessment of competence (Conway 1996). I propose that the aim of the teaching programme is to lead the patient along a continuum from dependence on the nurse to independence, where the patient (with the assistance of significant carers as required) will be self caring in administering his or her intravenous

---

Box 14.2 Primary aims of the HIVAT programme

- To improve the quality of life for patients with IE
- To potentially limit what would be long periods in hospital
- To potentially reduce the risk of hospital-acquired infection
- To provide the convenience of treatment in the comfort of their own home
- To enable greater involvement of the patient/carers and increased flexibility in the administration of treatment

---

Box 14.3 Suggested patient learning outcomes in a HIVAT endocarditis programme

The patient will:
1. Demonstrate understanding of:
   - the function of the heart and valves
   - what infective endocarditis is
   - why he is at risk.
2. be able to identify the symptoms associated with infection and the importance of reporting to his doctor.
3. be able to monitor his own temperature.
4. be able to test his own urine and record and recognize results of concern.
5. be able to monitor his weight.
6. demonstrate an understanding of the importance of seeking advice regarding birth control (applicable to women).
7. demonstrate an understanding of the importance of preventive health (e.g. good dental hygiene, prophylactic antibiotics).
8. demonstrate competence and safety in caring for an intravenous catheter including:
   - recognizing problems or complications, e.g. phlebitis, catheter blockage
   - knowing the action to take if a problem arises
   - care of the dressing
   - demonstration of effective hand hygiene.
9. demonstrate a broad knowledge of how antibiotics work.
10. demonstrate competence and safety in preparing and administering the intravenous medication including:
    - preparation of the equipment
    - how to obtain further supplies of equipment
    - principles of an aseptic technique and infection control principles
    - the reconstitution of the antibiotics
    - the method and speed of administration
    - minimizing the risks of air embolism.

---

antibiotics. Therefore, the patient must be totally independent in these skills prior to hospital discharge.

Fay & Evans (1997) believe that adequate care, support and supervision are vital if the concept of home intravenous therapy is to be widely accepted. Patient confidence appears to be central to experiencing physical and emotional comfort whilst receiving HIVAT. I suggest that the linchpin to this confidence is a clear understanding of the treatment through education.

Wood (1991) argues that patients may feel frightened but having access to someone who understands their problems and treatment may relieve many of these anxieties. Whether the supporting hospital has staff who are designated to answer concerns regarding the HIVAT programme or whether the practice or district nurse team offer competent advice is a further and important consideration which emphasizes the need for effective liaison between hospital and community services. It would seem logical to utilize community colleagues as advisors when forming the team who will initiate the programme. A further consideration is that the problems which in hospital seemed trivial may be overwhelming when at home. Thus careful discharge planning is the key to the management of HIVAT (Kayley 1996).

Patients with IE may feel particular concerns over their disease. Scrima (1987) demonstrates this in highlighting how patients with IE may experience real fear associated with their critical illness. Miner (1994) goes further in suggesting that increasing patients' knowledge of their disease, with a consequent raising of the awareness of morbidity and mortality, may lead to an exacerbation of helplessness and fear. This raises uncomfortable issues concerning how much information a patient should be given. There is the danger that health-care professionals can be paternalistic and make personal judgements about the amount and type of information given to patients and their families or carers. In my view, patients' rights to knowledge of their health and disease process are to be respected and health-care professionals should be guided by what the patient wants to know. This should be reflected in the teaching programme for patients with IE.

The literature seems to indicate that patients require follow-up every 3 days to evaluate catheter patency, monitor the infection and identify problems with self-administration, as well as evidence of phlebitis (Poretz et al 1982, Sarisley 1987). The aforementioned importance of knowing whom to contact should the patient experience a difficulty is highlighted within the literature (Wood 1991). Alongside professional guidance and help, patients will also need support from their family and/or carers. Kunkel (1995) recommends that patients with IE participating in a HIVAT programme should not live alone but have a reliable person available for support and observation.

CONCLUSION

IE is a complex and potentially life-threatening condition. This chapter has highlighted the variety of patients at risk and the many factors which can predispose to the development of IE. One of the primary roles of the cardiac nurse, in both the hospital and the community, is the empowerment of the patient and carers to allow an understanding of the disease and to facilitate personal care and monitoring, with the ultimate aim of avoiding IE.

Home intravenous antibiotic therapy may offer an opportunity to avoid the potential of infection in hospital and facilitate empowerment. However, it is only suitable for a small group of IE patients, who present with few if any complications. An effective planned teaching programme focusing on facilitating knowledge, rather than a pure didactic approach, and one linked to specific learning outcomes appears to be the key. It will be interesting to see if emerging research demonstrates a reduction in the subsequent occurrence of IE and improved patient satisfaction, through a process of empowerment with HIVAT programmes.

REFERENCES

Acar J, Michel PL, Varenne O, Michaud P, Rafik T 1995 Surgical treatment of infective endocarditis. European Heart Journal 16 (suppl B): 94–98

Almirante Gragera B, Tornos Mas MP, Soler-Soler J 1998 Prosthetic valve endocarditis. Revista Espanola de Cardiologia 51 (suppl 2): 58–63

Bansal RC 1995 Infective endocarditis. Medical Clinics of North America 79(5): 1205–1240

Bayer AS, Scheld WM 2000 Endocarditis and intravascular infections. In: Mandeu GL, Bennett JE, Dolin R (eds) Mandell, Douglas and Bennett's principles and practice of infectious diseases, 5th edn. Churchill Livingstone, Philadelphia, pp. 857–902

Bayer AS, Hutter AM, Wilson WR 1991 Current management of infective endocarditis. Patient Care 25(2): 15–18, 21–23, 28

Bayliss R, Clarke C, Oakley C, Somerville W, Whitfield AG 1983 The teeth and infective endocarditis. British Heart Journal 50(6): 506–512

Bernstein LH 1992 Marketing home IV antibiotics therapy to physicians. Caring 11(5): 50–52, 54, 56

Besnier JM, Choutet P 1995 Medical treatment of infective endocarditis: general principles. European Heart Journal 16 (suppl B): 72–74

Burden LL, Rodgers JC 1988 Endocarditis: when bacteria invade the heart. Registered Nurse 51(12): 38–46

Chastre J, Trouillet JL 1995 Early infective endocarditis on prosthetic valves. European Heart Journal 16 (suppl B): 32–38

Cohen P 1997 Intravenous therapy at home. Nursing Times 93(15): 42–44

Coker M, Lampert A 1990 Teaching checklist for home infusion therapy. Oncology Nursing Forum 17(6): 923–926

Conway A 1996 Home intravenous therapy for bronchiectasis patients. Nursing Times 92(45): 34–35

Cunha BA, Gill MV, Lazar JM 1996 Acute infective endocarditis. Infectious Disease Clinics of North America 10(4): 811–834

Daniel WG, Mugge A, Martin RP et al 1991 Improvement in the diagnosis of abscesses associated with endocarditis by TOE. New England Journal of Medicine 324: 795

Delahaye E, Erochard R, De Geuigney C et al 1995 The long term prognosis of infective endocarditis. European Heart Journal 16 (suppl B): 48–53

Durack DT 1977 Experience with prevention of experimental endocarditis. In: Kaplan EL, Taranta AV (eds) Infective endocarditis: an American Heart Association Symposium. American Heart Association Monograph No. 52. American Heart Association, Dallas, pp. 28–32

Fay L, Evans M 1997 Direct line to home. Nursing Times 93(37): 29–30

Francioli P, Etienne J, Hoigne R, Thys JP, Gerber A 1992 Treatment of streptococcal endocarditis with a single daily dose of ceftriaxone for 4 weeks: efficacy and outpatient treatment feasibility. Journal of the American Medical Association 267: 264–267

Griffin MR, Wilson WR, Edwards WD et al 1985 Infective endocarditis: Olmstead County Minnesota 1950 through 1980. Journal of the American Medical Association 254: 1199–1202

Horstkotte D, Piper C, Niehues R, Wierner M, Schulthesis P 1995 Late prosthetic valve endocarditis. European Heart Journal 16 (suppl B): 39–47

Kayley J 1996 Use of IV antibiotics at home. Community Nurse 2(7): 15–16

Kong K, Chan K 1995 Ruptured intracranial mycotic aneurysm: a rare cause of intracranial haemorrhage. Archives of Physical Medicine and Rehabilitation 76(3): 287–289

Kunkel MJ 1995 Out-patient treatment of endocarditis. Presented at the Infectious Disease Society Annual Meeting, September, San Francisco, CA

Marrie TJ 1987 Infective endocarditis: nursing considerations. Critical Care Nurse 7(2): 31–36, 38–43, 46

Masuorli S 1996 Home IV therapy comes of age. Registered Nurse 59(10): 22–26

Matthews D 1994 The prevention and diagnosis of infective endocarditis. Nurse Practitioner 19(8): 53–60

Miner PA 1994 Infective endocarditis: implications for care of the adult with congenital heart disease. Nursing Clinics of North America 29(2): 269–283

Niederpruem MS 1989 Factors affecting compliance in the home IV antibiotic therapy client. Journal of Intravenous Nursing 12(3): 136–142

Nunley DL, Perlman PE 1993 Endocarditis: changing trends in epidemiology, clinical and microbiological spectrum. Postgraduate Medicine 93(5): 235–238, 241–244, 247

Oakley CM 1995 The medical treatment of culture-negative infective endocarditis. European Heart Journal 16 (suppl B): 90–93

Poretz DM, Eron LJ, Goldenberg RI et al 1982 Intravenous antibiotic therapy in an outpatient setting. Journal of the American Medical Association 248(3): 336–339

Prasad A, Fraser AG 1995 Prevention of infective endocarditis: enthusiasm tempered by realism. British Journal of Hospital Medicine 54(7): 341–346

Rubinstein E, Lang R 1995 Fungal endocarditis. European Heart Journal 16 (suppl B): 84–89

Sarisley C 1987 Designing a teaching program for outpatient antibiotic therapy. Journal of Nursing Staff Development 3(3): 128–135

Scrima DA 1987 Infective endocarditis: nursing considerations. Critical Care Nurse 7(2): 47–50, 52, 54–56

Steckelberg JM, Melton LJ 3rd, Ilstrup DM et al 1990 Influence of referral bias on the apparent clinical spectrum of infective endocarditis. American Journal of Medicine 88(6): 582–588

Swanton RH 1998 Cardiology, 4th edn. Blackwell Science, Oxford

Trausch PA 1988 Infective endocarditis: nursing care and prevention. Progress in Cardiovascular Nursing 3(2): 45–53

Wahl MJ 1994 Myths of dental induced endocarditis. Archives of Internal Medicine 154(2): 137–144

Ward L 1990 Patient teaching for home IV therapy. Registered Nurse 53(4): 86, 88

Williams DN 1995 Home IV antibiotic therapy (HIVAT): indications, patients and antimicrobial agents. International Journal of Antimicrobial Agents 5: 3–8

Wood S 1991 Extending the principle of self care intravenous therapy in the community. Professional Nurse 6(9): 543–544, 546, 548–549

15

Aortic aneurysm

Jane Young
Lianne Daniels

The diagnosis of aortic aneurysm falls into two categories: aortic aneurysm and dissecting aortic aneurysm. This chapter will deal with each independently but will link together the nursing management of both conditions. The medical management is twofold. First, it will involve careful nursing monitoring and evaluation of the effectiveness of drug therapy. The second approach is surgical, involving all the skills required for nursing patients following major cardiac surgery. The care for both calls for the nurses' skills in rehabilitation and health education, particularly as hypertension may be a concomitant condition, to achieve the maximum outcome for the patient and family/carers.

AORTIC ANEURYSM

The definition of aortic aneurysm has perhaps best been described as a permanent localized dilatation of the aorta, having a diameter at least 1.5 times that of the expected normal diameter of that given aortic segment (Johnston et al 1991). The condition is more common in men and can be localized or diffuse along the length of the aorta; 74% of aortic aneurysms are abdominal with only 23% being thoracic (Burress 1993). However, as this is primarily a cardiac text, this chapter will focus upon thoracic aortic aneurysms with no reference to the abdominal variety.

An aneurysm can be unnoticed until it has reached an extensive size or can spontaneously rupture with an associated mortality of 76%, with or without treatment, in the first 24 hours. Burress (1993) suggests that aneurysms are strongly associated with atherosclerosis in approximately 96% of cases. As such, they can be regarded as part of the general process of systemic atherosclerosis. Within the subgroup of risk factors for aortic aneurysm, hypertension is the most common. As Lindsay et al (1998) state, hypertension exposes weaknesses that might otherwise not be manifest and in addition, probably accelerates degeneration of the

> **Box 15.1** Aetiology of aortic aneurysm
>
> - Atherosclerosis
> - Connective tissue disease, e.g. muscular dystrophy, scleroderma (progressive systemic sclerosis), the Marfan syndrome (Chapter 17 provides further details regarding this latter group of patients)
> - Degenerative diseases, e.g. medial necrosis
> - Trauma
> - Inflammatory diseases, e.g. aortitis
> - Malignancy
> - Bacterial – mycotic aneurysm (an aneurysm caused by an infected embolus, which weakens the blood vessel walls)

aortic wall. Any mechanism that can weaken the wall of the aorta can cause aortic dilatation and aneurysm formation.

Aortic aneurysms are divided, for descriptive purposes, into three main groups.

1. *Fusiform aneurysm* – a dilatation of the whole circumference of the aortic wall, uniform in shape. This is often due to a weakness in the vessel wall
2. *Saccular aneurysm* – a bulge at a segment of the aortic wall, more localized. This can be accompanied by thrombus formation. Saccular aneurysms frequently follow aortic dissection when operative repair is not carried out (Lindsay et al 1998).
3. *False aneurysm* – not a true aneurysm but a collection of blood and connective tissue external to the aortic wall. The cause can be a contained rupture of the aortic wall. Another term for false aneurym is pseudo-aneurysm.

Whether the aneurysm is fusiform or saccular, and many are not pure examples of either, its lumen virtually always contains laminated thrombus. Such clots may be extensive enough to fill a saccular aneurysm or to cover the circumference of a fusiform aneurysm (Lindsay et al 1998). Thoracic aneurysms are classified by the portion of aorta involved, such as the ascending, arch or descending thoracic aorta (Isselbacher et al 1997).

Clinical presentation

The clinical presentation of thoracic aortic aneurysm is diverse and dependent on location and the expansion rate of the aneurysm. Pressler & McNamara (1985), in reviewing 260 cases of thoracic aortic aneurysm, described 40% of patients as being asymptomatic at the time of diagnosis and this still appears true today. The presentation may be incidental to another routine physical examination or chest X-ray. This is particularly true of descending thoracic or abdominal aortic aneurysms.

Aneurysms of the ascending aorta tend to be fusiform and may cause aortic valve regurgitation due to dilatation of the aortic root, with the associated symptoms of congestive cardiac failure. A local mass effect from an ascending or aortic arch aneurysm may cause obstruction of the superior vena cava, leading to engorged neck and superficial veins, cyanosis and oedema of the face, neck and arms. Aneurysms of the aortic arch may also cause compression of the trachea, bronchi and laryngeal nerve, producing symptoms of dyspnoea, hoarseness, dysphagia and pain. Large airway obstruction may produce a dry cough and haemoptysis.

Aneurysms of the descending aorta are often asymptomatic until they reach a large size, pain being

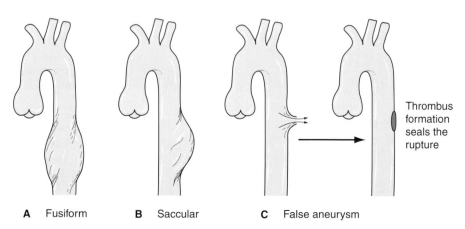

| **A** Fusiform | **B** Saccular | **C** False aneurysm |

Thrombus formation seals the rupture

Figure 15.1 Aortic aneurysms. A: Fusiform. B: Saccular. C: False.

the most common symptom. This is described as steady and continuous, due to the direct compression of other intrathoracic structures or erosion of localized bones, for example the ribs. Rupture of the aneurysm will produce severe pain, life-threatening haemoptysis or haematemesis with haemodynamic collapse. It was noted in a study of 1510 patients treated for aortic aneurysms at all levels that nearly 13% were found to have multiple aneurysms. More than half of those with thoracic aneurysms had other lesions, with 12% of those with abdominal aneurysms having thoracic aneurysms. Therefore examination of the entire aorta is always prudent practice (Crawford & Cohen 1982, Isselbacher et al 1997).

Diagnosis

The diagnosis is made on a precise clinical examination and history. Further investigation is necessary to identify the cause of the symptoms and distinguish type, site and extent of the aneurysm to decide the future management. There are six main investigations available to assist with diagnosis, although the patient may only require two or three.

Chest X-ray

This is the initial investigation, which is routine for the vast majority of patients admitted to hospital with chest symptoms. The X-ray may reveal widening of the mediastinum, enlargement of the aortic knob or displacement of the trachea (Fig. 15.2). Saccular aneurysms or smaller aneurysms may go undetected and cannot be excluded by chest X-ray alone. The chest X-ray is an easily performed, mobile and adaptable non-invasive investigation, allowing the patient to be in a variety of positions or indeed places such as the Accident and Emergency Department, X-ray or the cardiac care unit.

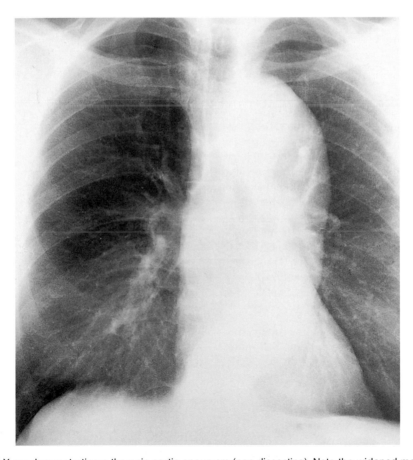

Figure 15.2 Chest X-ray demonstrating a thoracic aortic aneurysm (non-dissecting). Note the widened mediastinum. (Reproduced with permission from Corne et al 1997.)

Computed axial tomography

Computed axial tomography (CAT scan) can be performed using contrast dye to enhance the results. A known allergy to the contrast would be a major contra-indication but except for this, the only other limitation is the availability of the equipment in the hospital. This investigation does provide very accurate information on location and size of the aneurysm.

Magnetic resonance imaging

Magnetic resonance imaging (MRI scan) is a more recent advancement and produces accurate information. The use is limited in patients who suffer claustrophobia because the scanning involves lying in a narrow tunnel for some time, possibly as long as 45 minutes. Sedation may overcome this problem but patients may still find it intolerable. Haemodynamically unstable patients would not be suitable for MRI scanning because monitoring and safety, for example maintenance of a compromised airway or haemodynamics, could not easily be maintained. Some metal implants, for example pacemakers and certain metal valves, prohibit the investigation because the process uses powerful magnets. The radiology/radiography department always has relevant information available.

Transoesophageal echocardiography

Transoesophageal echocardiography (TOE) is useful for accurate diagnosis and particularly good for diagnosing dissecting aortic aneurysms for which it has emerged as the investigation of choice. The investigation can be performed at the bedside under sedation. Caution must be taken in patients with impaired respiratory function. There have been some studies suggesting that TOE does have restricted view in the area of the ascending aorta and vessels of the head and neck, when imaging a suspected acute aortic dissection (Francis et al 1994, Nienaber et al 1992, Reid & Gillespie 1994).

Transthoracic echocardiography

This is not very accurate for identifying aneurysms, particularly in the descending aorta, but is a quick, non-invasive and mobile investigation for early, speedy assessment. It is not a definitive diagnosis.

Aortography

Aortography may be performed to identify the aneurysm and associated vessels. This involves injecting radio-opaque dye into the aorta to identify the aneurysm, usually via the femoral artery and is per-formed under local anaesthetic. It is an invasive procedure with associated risks and not all patients are suitable. Contra-indications include renal impairment (due to the introduction of the dye into the bloodstream), peripheral vascular disease and left ventricular dysfunction. Aortography is rarely performed today because more accurate and less invasive investigations are available.

Medical management

Thoracic aortic aneurysms are often asymptomatic and only identified through routine investigation. Consequently the management of the condition is usually medical when the situation is not acute. The management primarily involves the control of pre-existing hypertension. Disruption of the arterial wall structure by the aneurysm can lead to the formation of thrombus, with an associated increase in the risk of emboli. Therefore anticoagulation is used if thrombus formation is suspected. Aspirin may be used to prevent increases in thrombus size and emboli. Long-term management involves 6-monthly monitoring to assess the aneurysm size.

The optimal timing for surgical repair of an aortic aneurysm remains uncertain. Several issues have to be considered. Isselbacher et al (1997) highlight the fact that there are limited data on the normal history of thoracic aneurysms, notably the outcome of surgical intervention. In addition, the high incidence of co-existing cardiovascular disease in this group means that many patients die of other cardiovascular causes before their aneurysm ruptures. The risks of surgery also have to be considered. The aforementioned authors recommend surgery when the thoracic aortic aneurysm reaches 6 cm or larger, or 7 cm or larger in those considered a high surgical risk (Isselbacher et al 1997). The full medical management will be described below, when discussing dissecting aortic aneurysms.

In the acute situation of rupture, surgery is the only immediate option because delay increases the already high mortality rate. Emergency and elective surgery incorporates excision of the aneurysm and replacement of the aortic wall with an artificial graft. The goals of nursing care, both in the acute phase and long term, are similar for aortic aneurysm and dissecting aortic aneurysm. Again, these will be discussed in depth below.

DISSECTING AORTIC ANEURYSM

Thoracic aortic dissection is one of the acute life-threatening emergencies. Lindsay et al (1998) define aortic dissection as longitudinal cleavage of the aortic media by a dissecting column of blood. If untreated, 20% of all the patients will die in the initial 24 hours and 90% in the first week (Isselbacher et al 1997). In initiating treatment, either conventional or surgical, the survival rate increases to 25% in the first 14 days. The occurrence of this condition has been estimated as 10–20 cases per million population (Burress 1993).

The predisposing factors associated with thoracic aortic dissection are varied but the most common factor is aortic medial degeneration. With advancing age the aortic media undergoes characteristic histologic changes (Lindsay et al 1998): fragmentation of elastic fibres and loss of smooth muscle cell nuclei, so-called medial necrosis. Collagenous tissue and basophilic ground substance replace these lost medial components (Schlatmann & Becker 1977). An elevated blood pressure or evidence of its existence can be found in 80% of patients (Lindsay et al 1998, Spittell et al 1993). Twenty percent of patients with dissection involving the ascending aorta present with hypotension (Lindsay et al 1998). The peak incidence of aortic dissection is in the 60–70 age group, with men outnumbering women by a ratio of 3:1 (Isselbacher et al 1997). Trauma is an increasing factor and this form of aneurysm accounts for 15–20% of all fatalities associated with high-speed accidents. Box 15.2 highlights the predisposing factors for this type of aortic aneurysm.

Altered anatomy and physiology

A dissecting aortic thoracic aneurysm is caused by a tear in the intimal layer of the aortic wall, allowing blood to be pushed into the medial layer. This produces a haematoma and a false channel. With each ventricular contraction blood is pushed down the aorta and into the false lumen. The pressure will cause the tear to lengthen and potentially rupture the aortic wall.

A fusiform or false aneurysm may be present prior to dissection but it is not a prerequisite for dissection to occur. The position of the entry tear classifies the different types of dissection. There are two classification groups, De Bakey and Stanford, which are used internationally to describe the location of the dissection and consequently further management (Box 15.3).

The tear in the aorta can actually form a flap which moves with blood flow within the lumen of the aorta. It is often the identifying feature on any of the described investigations. The flap is also a method of identifying the entry tear and therefore site of the dissection, enabling typing to occur which is vital for deciding between medical or surgical management.

Clinical presentation

The symptoms displayed by patients with a dissecting aortic aneurysm can be diverse, involving different systems of the body depending on the course of the dissection. The most common symptom is pain which is characteristically described as of sudden onset with literally a tearing sensation in the chest. It is usually retrosternal, radiating through to the back, neck and left chest (Swanton 1998). The pain does not build in intensity, unlike other cardiac conditions; it is at its most intense from the start (Lindsay et al 1998). The pain may often be unrelieved by opiates. Associated symptoms include nausea, vomiting and sweating and occasionally syncope occurs. Anterior chest wall pain is more common in proximal dissections and posterior chest wall pain is associated with distal dissections. The pain can also move along the tract of the dissection. This dissection may extend to the renal arteries producing lumbar pain, haematuria and possibly renal failure itself.

If the peripheral arteries are involved, the affected limb may demonstrate pain, paraesthesia (numbness and tingling) and vascular insufficiency with coldness and reduced or absent pulses. If arms are affected, unequal blood pressures may result in each arm, the systolic difference being greater than 20 mmHg. Occlusion of the anterior spinal artery by the dissection may result in paraplegia.

Hypertension is seen in more than 90% of those with distal aortic dissection but is less common in proximal dissection (Isselbacher et al 1997). However, hypotension may occur as a presenting symptom with associated tachycardia, sweating and cold, clammy skin due to hypovolaemia. Hypotension occurs much more commonly among those with proximal rather than

---

Box 15.2 Predisposing factors for dissecting thoracic aortic aneurysm

- Hypertension
- Atherosclerosis
- Medial degeneration
- Age
- Marfan syndrome
- Aortitis
- Coarctation
- Trauma
- Turner's syndrome
- Iatrogenic factors
  - Left-heart cardiac catheter procedures
  - Intra-aortic balloon pump
  - Aortic cannulation on bypass

Box 15.3 Classification for dissecting thoracic aortic aneurysm

De Bakey (classification well known but less used today)
Type I   Ascending and descending aorta involved, can extend to
             the whole aorta
Type II   Tear in ascending aorta only
Type III   Tear below origin of the left subclavian artery, descending
             aorta only and extending down

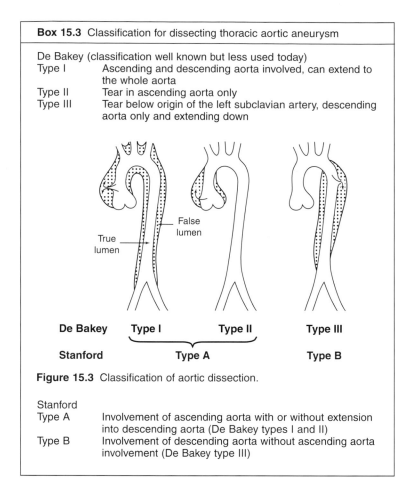

Figure 15.3 Classification of aortic dissection.

Stanford
Type A   Involvement of ascending aorta with or without extension
             into descending aorta (De Bakey types I and II)
Type B   Involvement of descending aorta without ascending aorta
             involvement (De Bakey type III)

---

distal aortic dissection. This is usually the result of cardiac tamponade, intrapleural rupture or intraperitoneal rupture (Isselbacher et al 1997). If cardiac tamponade is present (compression of the heart chambers), associated symptoms of dyspnoea, tachycardia and hypotension will be demonstrated. Neurological symptoms of aortic regurgitation may develop when the dissection involves the aortic valve, which occurs in two-thirds of proximal dissections. Symptoms may develop when the dissection includes the carotid arteries producing syncope, cerebrovascular accident (CVA/stroke) and coma.

Aortic dissection can demonstrate the electrocardiogram (ECG) changes of left ventricular hypertrophy if the patient has been hypertensive but in cases where the dissection results from medial necrosis of the aorta, without preceding hypertension, the ECG will be normal. If the dissection occludes a coronary artery the ECG changes of an infarction may develop (Hampton 1989). The clinical history and detailed recording of

signs and symptoms are vital to identify which diagnosis applies. This is particularly important when the current management of acute myocardial infarction

---

Box 15.4 Clinical presentation in dissecting thoracic aortic aneurysm

- Chest and back pain (tearing, ripping, crushing)
- Syncope, CVA, coma
- Nausea, vomiting
- Lumbar pain
- Haematuria
- Paraesthesia
- Paraplegia
- Limb coldness
- Reduced/absent peripheral pulses
- Unequal blood pressure
- Hypertension/hypotension
- Dyspnoea – left ventricular failure, cardiac tamponade
- Tachycardia

involves administering a thrombolytic agent with the associated risk of bleeding and would also be contra-indicated for surgical intervention.

Diagnosis

The investigations required to confirm diagnosis are the same as for aortic aneurysm but are performed in the acute setting with a potentially haemodynamically unstable patient. This factor has a large influence on which investigation is performed. The most accurate investigation is TOE to clearly identify the tear/flap and enable classification of the type of dissection. Clinical examination usually reveals the extent of involvement of the dissection but sometimes MRI scanning may be performed to show the extent of the descending aortic dissection. If TOE is unavailable then MRI scanning is the next most appropriate investigation, although monitoring of the haemodynamic status can be difficult.

Immediate investigations, performed on admission, will be a chest X-ray and a 12-lead ECG. The chest X-ray may show a widened mediastinum suggestive of dissection and cardiomegaly (enlarged heart). The aortic shadow on X-ray is abnormal in 80–90% of cases (Lindsay et al 1998). In proximal dissection, for example, protrusion can be seen on the right side of the mediastinum. If the aortic valve is compromised, evidence of left ventricular failure and pulmonary oedema may exist. As highlighted, the ECG can demonstrate several changes which will all provide information. It may show the acute changes of ST elevation or non-specific T-wave changes if a coronary artery is occluded. Left ventricular hypertrophy may be found if pre-existing hypertension exists. Generalized small amplitude complexes may support a diagnosis of cardiac tamponade.

Medical management

The immediate therapy is always medical and this is primarily to control the blood pressure. If hypotension exists, intravenous fluid and drug therapy will be instituted until the blood pressure is improved. Hypertension, the more common presenting situation, requires immediate drug therapy to reduce the haemodynamic stress on the aortic wall and thus slow or stop the dissection extending or a haematoma forming. Lowering the systemic arterial pressure reduces the velocity, therefore reducing myocardial contractility and thus aortic wall stress. First-line drug therapy is to use an intravenous β-blocker which reduces both blood velocity and pres-

---

> **Box 15.5** Management guidelines for dissecting thoracic aortic aneurysm
>
> - Surgical intervention for Stanford type A, De Bakey types I and II
> - Medical management for Stanford type B, De Bakey type III

---

sure. If the patient is unable to tolerate a β-blocker, for example due to left ventricular failure, chronic obstructive pulmonary disease or asthma, a potent vasodilator must be used. This may be intravenous sodium nitroprusside (SNP). Control of the blood pressure is extremely important to improve the outcome and reduce mortality. The incidence of late rupture of dissecting aortic aneurysms is dramatically increased if blood pressure control is not achieved.

In the long term, both forms of treatment will require monitoring and management of the underlying cause, predominantly the close control of the blood pressure.

Nursing management

The main goals of nursing management of a patient presenting with acute thoracic aortic dissection are:

- immediate assessment to identify clinical features to aid diagnosis
- assessment of pain and adequate prescribed analgesia
- to stabilize and monitor the clinical condition, to prevent progression
- to provide psychological support to the patient and family/carers
- to prepare the patient and family/carers for long-term management.

The patient is admitted directly to a critical care environment. The immediate assessment on admission includes the usual temperature, pulse, heart rhythm and, vitally important in this situation, the blood pressure. The blood pressure will be recorded in the right and left arm to identify any deficit. If a deficit is identified, suggesting dissection before the origin of the left subclavian artery, the recording of the higher blood pressure is used for any future management decisions. An assessment of the volume and presence of all peripheral pulses is performed and clearly documented, so any change can be immediately noted. Neurological assessment should be performed and continued if a deficit is identified.

The location, nature, duration and description of any existing pain are established and the intensity as judged by the patient is recorded. This is frequently helped by the use of the local pain analogue. This enables the nurse to monitor the effect of pain relief with the patient and institute further treatment if the desired response is not achieved. Capturing a clear history of the pain, in conjunction with the medical staff, can prompt the diagnosis of aortic dissection. The location and movement of the pain can help to identify the site of the tear and the potential extension of the dissection.

The use of analgesia should be immediate because the pain is often extremely severe. Intravenous opiates would be the drug of choice, with repeated doses until pain control is achieved, providing respiratory observations are satisfactory. An anti-emetic would also be prescribed with the opiate. At this point, oral pain relief is inappropriate due to the slow onset of action. In addition, the patient will have nothing by mouth to prepare for investigation and potential surgery. Alleviation of pain is vital, to ensure the patient is comfortable, to assist with blood pressure control and to encourage the patient to have confidence in the health-care team which in turn can help to reduce anxiety and consequently blood pressure. In addition, the use of opiates is encouraged because of the associated sedative effect and the slight vasodilatation achieved, both of which encourage a reduction in blood pressure.

Close monitoring of the oxygen saturation levels via pulse oximetry must be instituted and continued. This helps identify any respiratory difficulty, in conjunction with observing the respiratory rate, which may indicate pulmonary oedema. Oxygen therapy via a mask would also be advocated. Any expectoration from the patient must be observed for haemoptysis. Hypotension must be treated immediately, as highlighted, with the use of intravenous fluid replacement. Hypotension may indicate cardiac tamponade or rupture and if confirmed, immediate transfer for surgery would then be indicated. More commonly, as discussed, hypertension is the main problem. Control of blood pressure reduces potential extension of the dissection and the risk of aortic valve rupture. Consequently it assists in pain control. The nursing team **must** maintain the systolic blood pressure within the agreed parameters, which are usually below 100–120 mmHg, with a mean arterial pressure (MAP) of 60–75 mmHg. However, this must be high enough to maintain organ perfusion, particularly of renal and cerebral areas.

The intravenous drug therapy is titrated according to the blood pressure response, which indicates that very frequent observations are required. The use of an arterial line is advocated for several reasons. It ensures accurate recording of the blood pressure, allowing rapid identification of instability and lability. It also reduces disturbance to the patient, minimizing the sleep deprivation that may otherwise result where such frequent manual recordings are taken, possibly over several days. Arterial blood gases can also be easily obtained, without the need to repeatedly draw blood from an artery with a needle and heparinized syringe (arterial stab).

After 48–72 hours the slow, cautious and closely monitored transfer from intravenous to oral therapy will occur, providing the patient has not received surgical intervention. Preparation for investigation and potential surgery predominantly involves full and clear explanation to the patient and family/carers about the investigations, diagnosis and future management, whether surgical or medical. Clear, continuous explanation of all procedures is essential to reduce anxiety. It is important to include carers wherever possible and allow open visiting to help ease their anxieties and concerns.

Close observation of the fluid balance is vital to ensure that the renal function is being maintained. Hypertensive patients can be very susceptible to a drop in blood pressure, easily compromising renal perfusion. A strict record of urine output is important and may require the insertion of an indwelling urinary catheter to achieve this.

The lowering of blood pressure may compromise cerebral perfusion. In both instances, a compromise of renal or cerebral function may result in medical staff altering the blood pressure parameters to improve perfusion. During this acute stage, the patient will predominantly be on bedrest and consequently will require all basic nursing needs to be met, in addition to a great deal of psychological support.

When the blood pressure is controlled on oral medication (the systolic arterial pressure maintained below 140 mmHg), no further episodes of pain have occurred and renal function is stabilized, the patient is ready for transfer to the ward environment. This is a difficult time for the patient and their loved ones with the security of the critical care unit being removed. It is important to explain that the condition is stable, healing has begun and the monitoring will continue on the ward but not through invasive techniques. Preparation for the transfer can be vital in reducing anxiety. Time and sensitivity need to be applied for a smooth transfer.

Once in the ward environment, a gradual approach towards self-care is instituted. Progressively, discharge and any arrangements required are identified with the patient and family/carers.

One of the most important aspects of self-care is the understanding and correct administration of all the specific drugs required to maintain good blood pressure control. An efficient and proactive method of ensuring compliance and understanding is a ward-based drug self-administration programme. This allows the patient to take the responsibility for medication with adequate support and explanation so that by the discharge date the patient is well educated regarding the required medication. If the patient is unable to self-medicate, it is important that family/carers are involved and fully understand the drug therapy.

While the patient is on the ward nursing staff should assess the previous lifestyle and identify risk factors.

Case study 15.1

Mr Bill Critchley, a 72-year-old man, was admitted to the coronary care unit (CCU) with a presenting history of back pain and collapse. An in-depth history revealed that the back pain, located between the shoulder blades, had developed suddenly while he was mowing the lawn. He described the pain as tearing and excruciating. It was associated with profuse sweating and giddiness. It had lessened in intensity, but still remained severe.

Assessment
On admission, Mr Critchley was pale and sweating, with cool peripheries and a pain analogue of 7/10. He was dyspnoeic at rest, with a respiratory rate of 24 breaths per minute (bpm). Oxygen saturations measured by pulse oximetry were 89%. All peripheral pulses were palpable and his blood pressure in the right and left arms was equal at 190/105 mmHg. The ECG revealed sinus tachycardia and a heart rate of 118 bpm. The chest X-ray indicated some evidence of pulmonary oedema, together with dilatation of the ascending aorta. A raised jugular venous pressure (JVP) was noted, indicating congestive cardiac failure, together with a systolic murmur heard on auscultation. The latter suggested the presence of aortic regurgitation.

Past medical history
- Hypertension for 15 years treated with β-blockers. A CVA 10 years ago with a full recovery.
- Drug therapy: atenolol orally 100 mg once daily.

Risk factors
Mr Critchley smoked 30 cigarettes a day, with a positive family history of heart disease. Cholesterol unknown.

Immediate management
Pain relief was instituted immediately: diamorphine 5 mg intravenously followed by two further doses of 2.5 mg until the pain was controlled. An anti-emetic was also prescribed. Intravenous furosemide (frusemide) 80 mg was given to alleviate the pulmonary oedema and to reduce the blood pressure. This also allowed a central line to be placed in the internal jugular vein in the neck. A urinary catheter was inserted for close monitoring of the urine output, which was satisfactory at >0.5 ml/kg/h. Following the furosemide (frusemide), there was an immediate diuresis of 200 ml followed by 100–150 ml/h.

An intravenous β-blocker is usually the first-line treatment to reduce presenting hypertension. However, in this case the management of hypertension was commenced using a sodium nitroprusside (SNP) infusion via the central line. β-blockers were contraindicated due to the presence of pulmonary oedema. In such situations, their use may exacerbate heart failure. The dose of SNP was titrated according to the blood pressure, aiming to maintain the systolic pressure at 100–110 mmHg. Oxygen therapy via a humidified system of 35% was commenced to maintain oxygen saturations of 95–100%. Full explanations of all procedures were provided and priority given to the patient's comfort and anxiety. His relatives were kept fully informed of the situation.

Investigations
Transthoracic echocardiography was performed, which revealed severe aortic regurgitation and a dilated aortic root. TOE again revealed severe aortic regurgitation, a dilated aortic root and a dissection flap in the arch of the aorta above the subclavian artery branch. An entrance tear was identified in the aortic arch and limited to this area. A diagnosis was made of acute aortic dissection De Bakey type II (Stanford type A) and the cardiac surgeons were contacted. Finally, a MRI scan was performed to detect the exit site and notably the extent of the dissection, which was confined to the aortic arch.

Management
The situation was carefully explained to Mr Critchley and his family and the suggested management of immediate cardiac surgery was discussed. The family were with Mr Critchley as much as possible prior to surgery. The need for speed restricted a full discussion of the postoperative management.

Mr Critchley was transferred to theatre and underwent an aortic valve and root replacement. A long and complicated postoperative course was endured but eventually he was discharged home after 4 weeks with a follow-up appointment for 2 weeks in the first instance and arrangement for cardiac rehabilitation in the near future. The importance of smoking cessation and blood pressure management was discussed at length with Mr Critchley and his family. An ongoing plan of action and support was offered, as Mr Critchley expressed a desire to stop smoking. The general practitioner was fully informed of the patient's diagnosis and management. After 3 months of home care from his family and community nurses, Mr Critchley was making good progress, tending to his garden and enjoying family life. He continues to be seen at the cardiac outpatients department every 6 months for clinical monitoring of his health and well-being.

Health education and promotion can begin, emphasizing the importance of lifestyle changes, for example smoking cessation and weight reduction, two major predisposing factors to hypertension. Involvement of the family or carers is very important to support and encourage the patient to maintain the lifestyle changes.

Follow-up after discharge will eventually be 6 monthly to monitor the blood pressure, the dissection, aneurysm formation and resolution of haematoma, ensuring that healing is progressing. This will also occur through the local general practitioner as deemed appropriate. Referral to cardiac rehabilitation, if available, can enhance positive lifestyle changes and maximize the quality of life following a major psychological and physical insult to the system.

CONCLUSION

This chapter has highlighted the seriousness of aortic aneurysm and aortic dissection. The condition challenges all the skills available to the nurse, ranging from intensive critical nursing to education and rehabilitation. The nurse is integral to the management of these conditions by maximizing the potential for a positive outcome. This is achieved through monitoring of haemodynamic parameters and a knowledge of the full range of symptoms that may identify deterioration, such as renal, neurological and peripheral vascular changes. Education and rehabilitation are vital to ensure that the maximum quality of life is achieved for the patient and carers to reduce further incidence.

REFERENCES

Burress N 1993 Aortic dissection: diagnosis and acute care management. Cardiovascular Nursing 29(6): 41–51

Corne J et al 1997 The chest X-ray made easy. Churchill Livingstone, Edinburgh

Crawford ES, Cohen ES 1982 Aortic aneurysm: a multifocal disease. Archives of Surgery 117(11): 1393–1400

Francis CM, Sutherland GR, Turnbill CM 1994 Imaging methods used in aortic dissection. British Medical Journal 308: 136–137

Hampton JR 1989 The ECG in practice. Churchill Livingstone, Edinburgh

Isselbacher EM, Eagle KA, Desanctis RW 1997 Diseases of the aorta. In: Braunwald E (ed) Heart disease, 5th edn. WB Saunders, Philadelphia, pp. 1546–1581

Johnston KW, Rutherford RB, Tilson MD et al 1991 Suggested standards for reporting on arterial aortic aneurysms. Journal of Vascular Surgery 13(3): 452–458

Lindsay J Jr, Beall AC Jr, De Bakey ME 1998 Diagnosis and treatment of diseases of the aorta. In: Alexander RW, Schlant RC, Fuster V, O'Rourke RA, Roberts R,

Sonnenblick EH (eds) Hurst's the heart. McGraw-Hill, New York, pp. 2461–2582

Nienaber CA, Spielmann RP, Von Kodolitsch Y et al 1992 Diagnosis of thoracic dissection: magnetic resonance imaging verses transoesophageal echocardiography. Circulation 85: 434–447

Pressler V, McNamara JJ 1985 Aneurysm of the thoracic aorta: review of 260 cases. Journal of Thoracic and Cardiovascular Surgery 89(1): 50–54

Reid JH, Gillespie IN 1994 Imaging methods used in acute aortic dissection (letter). British Medical Journal 308: 535–536

Schlatmann TJM, Becker AE 1977 Histologic changes in the normal aging aorta: implications for dissecting aortic aneurysm. American Journal of Cardiology 39(1): 13–20

Spittell PC, Spittell JA Jr, Joyce JW et al 1993 Clinical features and differential diagnosis of aortic dissection: experiences with 236 cases (1980–1990). Mayo Clinic Proceedings 68(7): 642–651

Swanton RH 1998 Cardiology, 4th edn. Blackwell Science, Oxford

FURTHER READING

Sansevero AC, Ruddy Y 1996 Managing aortic dissections. A critical care challenge. Critical Care Nurse 16(5): 44–50

16

Pericarditis and myocarditis

Jane Young
Lianne Daniels

This chapter will explore the variety of conditions which make up pericardial disease. The aetiology, presentation, diagnosis and management will be discussed, together with the specific nursing care required to meet patients' and carers' needs. In addition, myocarditis, an inflammatory condition of the myocardium, will be explained, with an exploration of the associated care.

PERICARDIAL DISEASE

Pericardial disease is an umbrella term for clinical conditions which affect the pericardium and the pericardial space. Three conditions are discussed here: acute pericarditis, constrictive pericarditis and pericardial effusion. The aetiology is identical for each clinical condition. The diagnosis, management and nursing care for each will be dealt with separately.

Infections causing pericardial disease have greatly reduced in incidence over the last 30 years, due to the overall improvement in social conditions and antibiotics which have more successfully treated the predisposing infections. However, in the current environment of increasing numbers of immunosuppressed patients, such as with transplantation, chemotherapy treatment and acquired immune deficiency syndrome (AIDS), pericardial disease as a result of infection could potentially increase. In addition, immunosuppression can cause the symptoms of pericardial disease to be masked and consequently the infection can become overwhelming before it is identified.

Aetiology of pericardial disease

The varied aetiology of pericardial disease is listed in Box 16.1.

ACUTE PERICARDITIS

Acute pericarditis is defined as an inflammatory reaction involving the visceral and parietal layers of the

---

Box 16.1   The aetiology of pericardial disease

- Acute idiopathic pericardial disease
- Infectious – bacterial, viral, fungal and parasitic
- Connective tissue diseases
- Collagen diseases, e.g. systemic lupus erythematosus (SLE), polyarteritis nodosa (PAN), scleroderma (progressive systemic sclerosis)
- Acute rheumatic fever
- Rheumatoid arthritis and ankylosing spondylitis
- Post open heart surgery, e.g. valve replacement, coronary artery bypass surgery
- Bleeding into pericardium (haemopericardium), e.g. trauma, dissecting aortic aneurysm, hereditary haemorrhagic diathesis, anticoagulation
- Post myocardial infarction
- Miscellaneous, e.g. uraemia, radiation, sarcoidosis, myxoedema, amyloidosis and malignancy (usually metastases)

---

pericardium, the membrane enveloping the heart. The inflammatory process irritates the epicardium, the visceral layer of the pericardium, which is responsible for the main clinical symptom of pain. Pericarditis is always a symptom of another disease process which must be diagnosed and treated appropriately.

The range of aetiology is shown in Box 16.1. The most common causes of acute pericarditis include idiopathic or viral pericarditis, uraemia, bacterial infection, acute myocardial infarction and pericardiotomy associated with cardiac surgery (Lorell 1997). Three specific causes, idiopathic pericarditis, post cardiac surgery and post myocardial infarction, are discussed in more detail. Acute idiopathic pericarditis is generally benign, starts abruptly and is usually self-limiting. It is thought to be caused by viral infection, with young men more commonly affected following upper respiratory tract infections, e.g. Pseudomonas, aspergillosis, rickettsia.

Pericarditis following cardiac surgery occurs in approximately 10–40% of patients postoperatively (Prince & Cunha 1997). It often develops 2–3 weeks after surgery and again is usually self-limiting. However, it can occur within 2–3 days of cardiac surgery, with non-specific chest pain, pyrexia, pain on inspiration and transient but generalized ST segment elevation on the 12-lead ECG. The condition can vary in intensity and duration, over a course of usually 2–4 weeks.

Myocardial infarction (MI) causes acute pericarditis in approximately 20% of patients (Camm 1998). It frequently occurs in the first few days after an acute MI, especially following anterior wall infarction. Anterior MIs have larger areas of necrotic damage and greater ischaemic zones. Anti-inflammatory medication is usually a successful treatment. Post myocardial infarc-

tion syndrome (Dressler's syndrome) is a recognized late complication. It occurs in approximately 1–5% of infarcts (Swanton 1998), presenting as pericarditis that develops from 2 weeks to a few months post MI. It is thought to be caused by an auto-immune response to damaged cardiac tissue and is regarded as a chronic condition (Swanton 1998). It is more common after a second or subsequent MI. Anti-inflammatory medication, including systemic corticosteroids, may be necessary (Camm 1998). Anticoagulation should generally be discontinued in the presence of Dressler's syndrome (Alexander et al 1998).

Pericarditis can be dry or effusive, together with a high erythrocyte sedimentation rate (ESR), anaemia and fever. Effusive pericarditis produces an effusion and potential cardiac tamponade. The latter, defined as a compression on the heart from fluid accumulating in the pericardium, provokes different signs and symptoms and a distinctive line of treatment and care. This is discussed in depth later in the chapter.

Clinical presentation

The most prominent and common symptom of pericarditis is pain in the chest. Careful assessment of the chest pain, type, location, radiation, nature and intensity can lead the clinician to make an early and relatively accurate diagnosis. The chest pain is classically described as of sudden onset. It is retrosternal in most cases, but differs from the pain of an MI in its sharp quality, which is aggravated by deep inspiration, coughing and changes in posture (particularly lying flat) (Timmis et al 1997). It may be relieved by sitting forward and shallow breathing. It is not associated with nausea and vomiting, but may induce sweating due to the intensity. The location of the pain is often diffuse, across the precordium with radiation to the intrascapular region and the neck. Tachypnoea is often associated with pericarditis due to the restriction on respiration from the pain.

A pericardial friction rub is heard on auscultation, usually at the lower left sternal border (Marinella 1998). *The friction rub can still be heard when the breath is held, which is unlike a pleural rub which is only present on breathing.* It has been described as creaky, sounding like a pair of old shoes. Associated symptoms that assist in building the clinical picture are pyrexia, due to the inflammatory process, restlessness and malaise.

Investigations

The 12-lead ECG may demonstrate concave ST elevation in all leads and occasionally a depressed PR

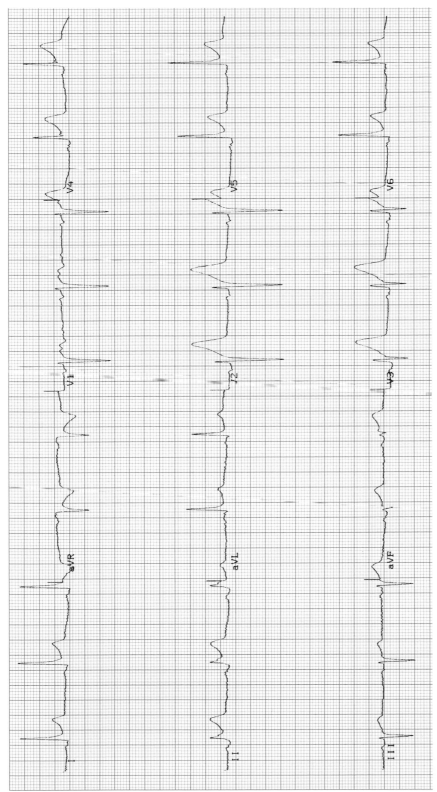

Figure 16.1 12-lead ECG from a patient with acute pericarditis. Note the concave upwards, saddle-shaped ST elevation in multiple leads. This occurred one week after a MI. (Reproduced with permission from Jenkins & Gerred 1997.)

segment may be present, but there is no reciprocal depression. Low-voltage complexes, reduced in height, may indicate an effusion. T-wave changes can also be seen but are generally non-specific (Dugan 1998, Marinella 1998). Swanton (1998) highlights that ECG changes are generally non-specific and may show T-wave inversion only. The presence of pathological Q-waves indicates a myocardial infarction which can be the underlying cause of the pericarditis. ECG changes of acute MI can appear similar, but an accurate history and physical examination will usually exclude this (Marinella 1998). In pericarditis the ST segment is *concave* upwards and described as 'saddle shaped' while it is usually *convex* upwards in infarction (Swanton 1998). Echocardiography will not demonstrate any particular feature unless fluid is present in the pericardial space.

The ESR and the white blood count are raised but these are also elevated in most of the causes of pericarditis.

A Mantoux test should be performed if tuberculosis is suspected.

Clinical management

Most cases of pericarditis are self-limiting. After diagnosis is established, reassurance can be given to the individual about the cause of the pain, which in itself can help the situation. Anxiety and apprehension caused by the symptoms, particularly pain, can worsen the situation and make the pain more severe or less well tolerated. Adequate analgesia must be provided and the most effective are non-steroidal anti-inflammatory drugs. This is providing the individual can tolerate this group of drugs and has no preceding gastric problems and a stable renal function. Opiates are not helpful because they do not successfully relieve the pain but merely sedate. If the pericarditis is prolonged in duration, a course of steroids may be required to resolve the situation. This is particularly true in Dressler's syndrome which can be resistant to resolution with the above management.

Rest is an important part of the clinical and nursing management, to reduce the inflammatory process and lessen the pain. Adequate fluid and nutritional input is important during the active inflammatory process of the condition.

Reducing the fever will assist in increasing patient comfort and this can be achieved through adequate loose clothing, oral fluids and antipyretic drugs such as paracetamol.

The management also incorporates clinical observations to detect the complications of pericardial effusion

and/or cardiac tamponade developing. Discontinuing anticoagulation, a treatment that may be used in myocardial infarction, will reduce the potential of haemorrhage into the pericardial space, which could lead to effusion and/or cardiac tamponade.

Cardiac tamponade is the gradual compression of the heart by fluid, usually in the pericardial sac. The patient will become increasingly restless, with a tachycardia, lowering blood pressure, but initially elevated central venous pressure (CVP) due to cardiac constriction. Circulatory collapse can eventually occur, the speed depending on the degree of constriction.

General clinical observation of the overall condition of the patient and strict recording of fluid balance are included in the monitoring process (Bennett 1990). This will include monitoring the ECG for signs of tachycardia and low-amplitude complexes. How often the temperature, pulse and respirations (TPR) should be recorded is difficult to decide. If the patient is clearly recovering, with few symptoms and is regarded as convalescing, recordings may be every 4 hours while in hospital. During the more acute phase, hourly recorded observations may be needed to detect any signs of cardiac compromise. Clinical observations should always be initiated based on the assessment skills of the nursing and medical team and not just on routine practice.

One of the most important steps in the clinical management of pericarditis is to establish the underlying cause of the condition and ensure that appropriate treatment is instituted. Pericarditis alone is a relatively simple condition to treat but the underlying cause may be far more complex. If the pericarditis is associated with or develops to effusion, the treatment becomes more invasive.

CONSTRICTIVE PERICARDITIS

Constrictive pericarditis is characterized by a thickening and fibrosed pericardium which impairs ventricular filling, by impeding diastolic relaxation, and results in elevated heart pressures. The incidence of constrictive pericarditis is difficult to establish, but what is known is the change in aetiology in the Western world over the last 50 years. Tuberculosis used to be a major cause, but advances in public health knowledge have reduced this considerably.

Altered anatomy and physiology

Constrictive pericarditis usually begins as an acute pericarditis with pericardial effusion. The effusion slowly progresses to the subacute phase of reabsorption, followed by chronic inflammation, fibrous scarring and thickening of the pericardium. This closes the pericardial space, leading to fusion of the visceral and parietal layers of the pericardium, causing rigidity and inelasticity. The restriction of the inelastic pericardium reduces filling of the heart chambers and consequently impairs cardiac output. This leads to the associated symptoms of right and left heart failure.

Clinical presentation

The clinical course of the condition can vary greatly, from a symptomatic problem to a life-threatening constriction. The extent of the constriction and how long it has been present dictate the symptoms. The patient may complain of chest pain, central or pleuritic, and dyspnoea, with anorexia and fatigue. In long-standing situations abdominal swelling and discomfort may be present due to hepatomegaly and ascites. The patient will appear unwell with all the symptoms of heart failure. A knowledge of any pre-existing diagnosis may assist with the current diagnosis; for example, malignancy, connective tissue disorders or previous radiotherapy.

Investigations

Physical examination will reveal potential signs of right and left heart failure.

- The chest X-ray may be normal. Indeed, the combination of a normal heart size and signs of severe right-sided failure is suggestive of constriction (Timmis et al 1997).
- A 12-lead ECG may be unremarkable or demonstrate widespread low-voltage QRS complex and non-specific T-wave changes. Atrial fibrillation is present in approximately one-third of patients.
- An echocardiogram will demonstrate the thickened pericardium.
- Magnetic resonance imaging (MRI) will differentiate between constrictive pericarditis and restrictive cardiomyopathy (see Chapter 11), also demonstrating dilated vena cavae and hepatic veins.

Clinical management

Although diuretic therapy may be of temporary benefit (Swanton 1998), the treatment for constrictive pericarditis is usually surgical pericardiectomy. This involves stripping the pericardium from the apex to the base of both ventricles. This is major surgery and the postoperative management is similar to any cardiac surgical procedure. Early mortality has been cited as approximately 11% (Arsan et al 1994) while in the most extreme cases of severe long-standing constrictive pericarditis, with profound cachexia and liver dysfunction, it may be that treatment with a diuretic and digitalis is preferable. Ling et al (1999) reviewed 135 patients who had undergone pericardiectomy and compared them to a historical cohort. There was a noted increase in the frequency of constrictive pericarditis due to cardiac surgery, mediastinal radiation and presentation in older patients. The perioperative mortality had decreased to 6% from a previous 14% (Ling et al 1999).

Medical management would involve maximizing cardiac function pre-operatively, reducing the extent of heart failure and improving the overall physical condition of the patient, addressing any anorexia and malnutrition.

Nursing management

The nursing management of the patient with constrictive pericarditis involves controlling the symptoms and preventing deterioration in preparation for the surgical procedure. Close monitoring of the response to heart failure treatment is important to assess beneficial improvement. Clinical observation of any deterioration in cardiac function through the blood pressure, pulse, rhythm, respiratory function and fluid balance is vital. Oxygen therapy may be required and appropriate positioning of the patient will maximize respiratory function. Adequate pain relief is important to improve respiratory capability and, most importantly, for patient comfort. A full explanation of the condition and treatment plan to the patient and family/carers is vital to both ensure informed co-operation and reduce anxiety. The explanation concerning surgery is also important to assist in improving the postoperative course.

PERICARDIAL EFFUSION

A pericardial effusion is the gradual or sudden accumulation of fluid in the intrapericardial space between the visceral and parietal layers of the pericardium. This normally accommodates 15–20 ml of fluid. A rapid accumulation of fluid leads to critical elevation of pressure, impeding diastolic relaxation of both ventricles equally (Timmis et al 1997). This will lead to cardiac compression and the symptoms of cardiac tamponade. However, if the fluid accumulation is gradual, as much as 2 l of fluid can accumulate before symptoms occur. This is because gradual accumulation of fluid allows progressive stretching of the pericardial sac (Timmis et al 1997).

Rapid diagnosis of the effusion will lead to early treatment and potentially improved long-term results. Large pericardial effusions are frequently associated with serious underlying illnesses such as malignancy and uraemia. Chronic pericardial effusions are associated with abdominal ascites, pleural effusions and heart failure.

Clinical presentation

The signs and symptoms of pericardial effusion become evident only as a small effusion progresses in size and are those of a decreased cardiac output, due to cardiac tamponade (see Box 16.2).

Additional symptoms the patient may experience are dull continuous chest pain or pressure and nausea and vomiting due to abdominal pressure increase, particularly in the presence of abdominal ascites.

Clinical management

The immediate treatment to relieve the symptoms of pericardial effusion, with or without cardiac tamponade, is a pericardial tap (pericardiocentesis). It is important to remember that the condition of the patient may be critical with near cardiopulmonary collapse.

The procedure involves the physician inserting a cannula into the pericardial space and aspirating the fluid, followed by the insertion of a J-tipped pericardial drain for further drainage. Full explanation prior to the procedure, explaining the benefits to the patient, will help to alleviate anxiety. It must be emphasized that a local anaesthetic will be used so that the pain felt will be minimal.

The procedure is performed utilizing an aseptic technique and usually involves X-ray control or echocardiographic guidance to ensure accurate loca-

---

Box 16.3 Investigations for pericardial effusion

- Chest X-ray – normal or enlarged heart if effusion greater than 250 ml
- ECG – low-voltage QRS complexes and non-specific T-wave changes
- Echocardiography – the definitive diagnostic test:
    Enlarged pericardial space >1 cm
    Right atrial collapse during diastole
    Right ventricular collapse during diastole
    Left ventricular collapse post cardiac surgery
    (Posterior effusions, anterior wall adhered to sternum)

---

tion of the needle. It is possible to attach the ECG to the needle to monitor the position. When the needle reaches the epicardium, ST elevation will result, so the needle is withdrawn slightly for aspiration. However, this method of locating the needle position is rarely used. During the procedure careful haemodynamic monitoring is required to detect deterioration and complication; this includes continuous observation of cardiac rhythm, respiratory rate and oxygen saturation levels via pulse oximetry.

Collection of samples of pericardial aspirate is important to assist with the final diagnosis, particularly if malignancy is suspected. The colour and consistency of the fluid can give initial clues to diagnosis. The fluid is normally straw coloured and clear but may be bloodstained, cloudy or contain pus when there is an active disease and infection process.

Insertion of the drain permits free drainage, which overcomes the problem of rapid reaccumulation of fluid. It is important that the drain patency is regularly checked and maintained. Frequent movement of the patient is necessary to ensure any pockets of fluid are moved for maximum drainage. Much of the nursing care of the patient with pericardial effusion is aimed at managing the underlying condition and helping the patient and family/carers accept and understand the diagnosis and future management.

Pericardial effusions that are prone to recurrence require repeated aspiration. This is particularly true of effusions associated with malignancy. A further management approach is therefore the creation of a hole or

---

Box 16.2 The signs and symptoms of cardiac tamponade

- Increasing dyspnoea and restlessness
- Hypotension
- Tachycardia – atrial tachycardias are common
- An initially raised or rising central venous pressure (CVP)
- Cyanosis
- Oliguria/anuria
- Raised jugular venous pressure
- Pulsus paradoxus (an inspiratory decline in systolic blood pressure exceeding 10 mmHg)
- Tachycardia and reduced amplitude of ECG complexes

Box 16.4 The complications of pericardial aspiration

- Cardiac perforation
- Dysrhythmias
- Infection
- Haemorrhage

window in the pericardium to allow continuous drainage of fluid into the right or left pleural space and eventual reabsorption. The two layers of pericardium eventually adhere to each other because the lubricating fluid is absent.

Surgical pericardiectomy can be performed, which involves removal of the majority of the parietal pericardium to allow drainage into the right or left pleural cavities. The mortality rate at 30 days can be as high as 60% as this is a palliative procedure, with the patients tending to be very ill and debilitated at this stage, with severe underlying disease.

Balloon pericardiotomy is a relatively new alternative, non-surgical technique. It utilizes a catheter and the percutaneous, subxiphoid approach. A balloon is threaded over a guidewire into the pericardium, inflated, then deflated and withdrawn, creating a pericardial window (Galli et al 1995, Jackson 1994, Law et al 1997). The procedure is performed using fluoroscopic (X-ray) and echocardiographic guidance. It is of particular benefit for patients who are suffering malignant recurrent pericardial effusion, who have a reduced life expectancy and are having to undergo repeated pericardiocentesis to drain the fluid. In these cases it can be a useful, palliative and successful procedure, producing excellent symptom relief.

MYOCARDITIS

Myocarditis is an inflammatory process affecting the myocardium and causing a wide range of symptoms from a flu-like syndrome to heart failure and death. It is said to be present when the heart is involved in an inflammatory process, often caused by an infectious agent (Wynne & Braunwald 1997). The aetiology is diverse and can broadly be divided into infectious and non-infectious causes. Box 16.5 is not an exhaustive list.

The true incidence is unknown, as a substantial proportion of patients with probable myocarditis have subclinical, self-limiting symptoms with a rapid and complete recovery and therefore never seek medical attention. Of those that do present, 80% of causes are viral in origin, principally from the coxsackie B group of viruses (Burke & Mattson Porth 1994). The disease

---

Box 16.5   Causes of myocarditis

Infectious

Viral

Rickettsia
Coxsackie A and B
Hepatitis B
Mumps
Rabies
Lassa fever
Rheumatic fever
Influenza A and B
Rubella
Polio virus
Adenovirus
Human immunodeficiency virus (HIV)
Epstein–Barr virus

Bacterial

Legionella
Clostridia
Diphtheria
Pneumococcus
Neisseria meningitidis
Streptococcus species
Salmonella
Pseudomonas

Fungal

Candidiasis
Aspergillosis
Blastomycosis

Others

Toxoplasma gondii (intracellular protozoon)
Trypanosoma species (protozoa infection)
Chagas' disease (*Trypanosoma cruzi*)

Non-infectious

Systemic disease

Systemic lupus erythematosus
Sarcoidosis
Ulcerative colitis
Crohn's disease
Cardiac rejection (e.g. following
    transplantation)
Giant cell myocarditis
Peripartum myocarditis
Thyrotoxicosis
Phaeochromocytoma (tumours of
the sympathetic nervous system)

Drug-induced

Cocaine
Alcohol
Arsenic
Catecholamines
Cyclophosphamides
Interleukin 2

process may be either localized to an isolated region of the myocardium or diffuse, affecting the whole myocardium (both ventricles), and may lead to chronic dilated cardiomyopathy. The subsequent heart failure that ensues from myocarditis-induced cardiomyopathy is a highly complex multisystem disorder generating much current interest, discussion and research (see Chapter 11).

Myocarditis is a potentially life-threatening condition which predominantly affects previously fit young adult males. Ideally, early diagnosis and treatment is essential as this influences the outcome (Richardson et al 1995), although the diagnosis is made difficult due to a lack of specific clinical signs.

Altered anatomy and physiology

The histological changes in myocarditis are non-specific with lymphocyte infiltration resulting in a generalized inflammatory picture. The subsequent change may cause myocytic necrosis, vascular and interstitial autonomic nerve injury and dysfunction. The widespread pattern of damage can give rise to numerous clinical manifestations such as dysrhythmias and impaired myocardial function. Myocarditis has been said to occur in four phases: fulminant, acute, chronic active or chronic persistent.

Clinical presentation

The clinical presentations of myocarditis are variable (Mancini & Beniaminovitz 2001). Most patients seek medical attention when they start to experience chest pain and/or dyspnoea. Some cases present with acute or chronic cardiac failure, cardiogenic shock or an apparent myocardial infarction. During the acute or inflammatory phase, common symptoms include those which are non-specific and flu-like, chest pain, palpitations, dyspnoea, syncope, fatigue and fever. Other presentations may include a history of previous upper respiratory tract or gastro-intestinal infection. Systemic or pulmonary thrombo-embolic disease is associated with myocarditis (Mancini & Beniaminovitz 2001).

Physical examination may reveal soft heart sounds on auscultation, a prominent third heart sound, gallop rhythm, pericardial friction rub, transient murmurs, elevated jugular venous pressure, pulmonary crepitations and peripheral oedema.

Diagnosis

An accurate clinical history is an important aid to diagnosis in myocarditis, because clinical examination usually reveals non-specific signs.

12-lead ECG

This may reveal numerous abnormalities ranging from minor ST and T-wave segment changes to evidence of left ventricular hypertrophy, left atrial enlargement, left bundle branch block and atrial fibrillation (AF) in patients with a more protracted duration of illness. Atrioventricular block or ventricular arrhythmia can occur. Myocarditis is a known cause of sudden death (Mancini & Beniaminovitz 2001).

Chest X-ray

This may show non-specific indications of cardiac failure such as cardiomegaly, pulmonary venous congestion, Kerley B lines, pleural effusion and pericardial effusion, depending on the progress and virulence of the underlying disease process.

Echocardiography

This can assist in the detection and qualification of myocardial dysfunction. Dilated right and left ventricles are commonly seen and the ejection fraction can be estimated which can be a guide to disease progression or diagnosis. Echocardiography may also show mitral regurgitation, mural thrombosis and pericardial effusion.

Blood tests

Elevated creatinine phosphokinase, CK-MB and troponin T are markers of myocardial cell damage in clinically suspected myocarditis.

Viral titres are performed routinely to identify any causative organism.

Magnetic resonance imaging (MRI)

This demonstrates the localization, activity and extent of inflammation.

Radionuclide ventriculography

This may be used to help quantify ejection fraction and wall motion abnormalities, which can be a guide to the stage and prognosis of the disease.

Endomyocardial biopsies

These can diagnose myocarditis and the extent of the lesion (Wodniecki et al 1990). A negative biopsy result does not necessarily eliminate myocarditis, due to different diagnostic criteria, interpretation of results and the stage of the disease process when the biopsy was taken. Sequential biopsies may confirm 'active' and 'healed' myocarditis. Active inflammatory disease may be identified through the presence of myofibril degeneration and increased interstitial lymphocytes.

Virus in the stool, throat, blood, myocardium or pericardial fluid may identify viral myocarditis.

Treatment

Ideally the goal of treating myocarditis is to identify the specific cause and treat accordingly; for example, appropriate antibiotic therapy for bacterial causes. If the patient presents with left ventricular dysfunction, the management is similar to that for other forms of congestive heart failure (O'Connell & Renlund 1998). Most management, however, is generally aimed at relieving symptoms and trying to prevent further deterioration of the clinical condition. The role of many drugs in treating myocarditis is a subject receiving continuous research. Drugs that may exacerbate myocarditis or depress myocardial function, such as those with negative inotropic properties, for example calcium channel blockers, should be avoided. Immunosuppressants are only recommended for those with biopsy-proven myocarditis that has not responded to conventional therapy and who are awaiting cardiac transplantation.

Management of heart failure will include conventional treatment with diuretics, angiotensin-converting enzyme (ACE) inhibitors, β-blockers and digoxin. Other forms of treatment in severe haemodynamic compromise can include the use of the intra-aortic balloon pump, left ventricular assist devices (LVADs), cardiomyoplasty and heart transplantation.

Nursing care is focused upon symptomatic relief, bedrest, management of the fluid balance and restriction of activity. This aims to decrease the myocardial workload until the fever and cardiac symptoms subside (Savoia & Oxman 1990). Increased exercise during the acute phase is associated with further inflammatory and necrotic lesions. Assessment and recordings of the heart rate, blood pressure, respiration and temperature are all maintained. Close monitoring of these parameters is important to identify deterioration at an early stage and initiate treatment promptly. A convalescent period of 6 months is recommended from the onset of clinical manifestations and, potentially, further rehabilitation before returning to a full active life.

Explanation is important to the patient and family/carers. However, it may be very difficult to be specific about treatment and prognosis due to the disease process being unpredictable, with a 'wait and see' approach. The patient and family/carers will need information at a regular and clear pace, relevant to the clinical state being experienced. Serious illness could be apparent and discussion regarding transplantation at this point may be necessary. However, the disease process may only be producing mild symptoms with eventual resolution so discussion about the potential problems may be inappropriate.

CONCLUSION

This chapter has explored the variety of conditions encompassing pericardial disease, in addition to myocarditis. The conditions can be both frightening and debilitating for the patient and reassurance and explanation are needed for both patient and family/carers. This requires the nurse to be fully aware of the treatment options and the stage of disease that the patient is experiencing. Nursing skills will also include monitoring for early signs of cardiac compromise due to the disease process, notably the occurrence of cardiac tamponade. In addition, it can be seen that, particularly with pericardial effusion, this area of cardiac nursing crosses into the domain of oncology. The cardiac team may be called upon to provide palliative care to those with advanced malignancy and this necessitates the kindness and understanding that should be a part of all nursing care.

Case study 16.1

John Cheng was an 18-year-old boy, admitted to the coronary care unit (CCU) from a referring hospital. He was studying at university and one week previously had suddenly developed ankle oedema and dyspnoea. John had no previous significant cardiac history; the only episode of note was a viral illness 3 weeks prior to admission with a temperature, sore throat and general malaise, which had lasted for 4 days. During his admission to the referring hospital, he had suffered an episode of ventricular fibrillation (VF) requiring immediate defibrillation. Following this event John was transferred to the tertiary centre.

On arrival, John's circulation demonstrated peripheral shutdown, his skin was cold and clammy and he was dyspnoeic at rest. Arterial oxygen saturation via pulse oximetry was 82% on room air. John had a very low urine output of only 500 ml in the previous 24 hours. A urinary catheter was already in place with a urometer and for the preceding 2 hours he had become anuric. His blood pressure was 72/40 mmHg, he was in a sinus tachycardia, with a temperature of 38.4°C and a heart rate of 130 bpm. Intravenous inotropic support was in progress and was slowly being increased. It was also decided to electively mechanically ventilate John to increase tissue oxygenation and reduce the oxygen demand.

Investigations

The electrocardiogram (ECG) showed sinus tachycardia with diffuse ST segment elevation and T-wave inversion. The chest X-ray showed widespread pulmonary oedema and a slightly enlarged heart. A transthoracic echocardiogram revealed global hypokinesis (reduced muscle movement) with an estimated ejection fraction of only 15%.

Blood tests revealed normal serum sodium and potassium levels, with urea at 20 mmol/l and creatinine 250 mmol/l. A full blood count (FBC) revealed a white blood count (WBC) of 22×10^{-9}/l (normal range $4-11 \times$ 10^{-9}/l), indicating the presence of infection. Blood was sent for culture and viral titres analysis, together with a throat swab to identify the possible cause.

A pulmonary artery (PA) catheter was passed and revealed a central venous pressure of 16 mmHg, a high systemic vascular resistance of 2100 dynes/sec/cm^{-5}, a pulmonary capillary occlusion ('wedge') pressure of 22 mmHg and a cardiac output of 3.2 l/min. NB: Chapters 5 and 18 provide further detail of this monitoring device.

Diagnosis

Acute myocarditis with cardiogenic shock.

Management

The priority in clinical management was to stabilize John's condition, preventing further deterioration and to augment the cardiac output, which at this stage was 3.1 l/min. Cardiac transplantation was considered the only viable option and this was explained and discussed with John's parents, to aid their understanding of the severity of the situation and the plan of treatment. Although he was ventilated, the prospect of transplantation was also discussed with John. A transplant centre was contacted and accepted him as their patient. All necessary details were faxed.

In the interim, inotropic support was maximized and an intra-aortic balloon pump was inserted. This improved the myocardial and renal perfusion and increased the cardiac and urinary output. Intravenous furosemide (frusemide) was continued and a morphine infusion was commenced to provide symptomatic relief.

John was transferred to the transplant centre. Fifteen minutes after arrival he suffered a further cardiac arrest, but was successfully resuscitated. He underwent preparation for transplantation as described in Chapter 23 and although his haemodynamic status remained unchanged, requiring the intra-aortic balloon pump, any further left ventricular assist device (LVAD) was not required. A cardiac transplant was performed 3 weeks later and John made a steady but full recovery.

REFERENCES

Alexander RW, Pratt CM, Roberts R 1998 Diagnosis and management of patients with acute myocardial infarction. In: Alexander RW, Schlant RC, Fuster V, O'Rourke RA, Roberts R, Sonnenblick EH (eds) Hurst's the heart. McGraw-Hill, New York, pp. 1345–1433

Arsan S, Mercan S, Sarigul A et al 1994 Long-term experience with pericardiectomy: analysis of 105 consecutive patients. Thoracic and Cardiovascular Surgeon 42(6): 340–344

Bennett SJ 1990 Pericarditis: nursing care makes the difference. Advances in Clinical Care 5(6): 32–34

Burke L, Mattson Porth C 1994 Alterations in cardiac function. In: Mattson Porth C (ed) Pathophysiology concepts of altered health status, 4th edn. JB Lippincott, Philadelphia, p. 445

Camm AJ 1998 Cardiovascular disease. In: Kumar PJ, Clark ML (ed) Clinical medicine: a textbook for medical students and doctors. WB Saunders, London, pp. 625–744

Dugan KJ 1998 Caring for patients with pericarditis. Nursing 28(3): 50–51

Galli M, Politi A, Pedretti F, Castiglioni B, Zerboni S 1995 Percutaneous balloon pericardiotomy for malignant pericardial tamponade. Chest 108(6): 1499–1501

Jackson G 1994 Cardiology update: balloon pericardiotomy. Nursing Standard 8(35): 52–53

Jenkins RD, Gerred SJ 1997 ECGs by example. Churchill Livingstone, Edinburgh

Law DA, Haque R, Jain A 1997 Percutaneous balloon pericardiotomy: non-surgical treatment for patients with cardiac tamponade. West Virginia Medical Journal 93(6): 310–312

Ling LH, Oh JK, Schaff HV 1999 Constrictive pericarditis in the modern era: evolving clinical spectrum and impact on outcome after pericardiectomy. Circulation 100(3): 1380–1386

Lorell BH 1997 Pericardial disease In: Braunwald E (ed) Heart disease: a textbook of cardiovascular medicine, 5th edn. WB Saunders, Philadelphia, vol 2, pp. 1478–1534

Mancini DM, Beniaminovitz A 2001 Myocarditis and specific cardiomyopathies: endocrine disease and alcohol. In: Fuster V, Alexander RW, O'Rourke RA et al (eds) Hurst's the heart, 10th edn. McGraw-Hill, New York, pp. 2001–2032

Marinella MA 1998 Electrocardiographic manifestations and differential diagnosis of acute pericarditis. American Family Physician 57(4): 699–704

O'Connell JB, Renlund DG 1998 Myocarditis and specific cardiomyopathies. In: Alexander RW, Schlant RC, Fuster V, O'Rourke RA, Roberts R, Sonnenblick EH (eds) Hurst's the heart, 9th edn. McGraw-Hill, New York, pp. 1591–1607

Prince SE, Cunha BA 1997 Post pericardiotomy syndrome. Heart and Lung 26(2): 165–168

Richardson PJ, Why HJF, Maisch B 1995 Myocarditis, myopericarditis and dilated cardiomyopathy. In: Julian DG, Camm AJ, Fox KM, Hall RJC, Poole-Wilson PA (eds) Disease of the heart, 2nd edn. WB Saunders, London, pp. 489–505

Savioa MC, Oxman MC 1990 Myocarditis, pericarditis and mediastinitis. In: Mandell GL, Douglas RG, Bennett JE (eds) Principles and practice of infectious disease, 3rd edn. Churchill Livingstone, Edinburgh, pp. 727–728

Swanton RH 1998 Cardiology, 4th edn. Blackwell Science, Oxford

Timmis AD, Nathan AW, Sullivan I 1997 Essentials of cardiology, 3rd edn. Blackwell Science, London, pp. 161–171

Wodniecki J, Polonski L, Szygula E, Szczurek Z, Szczurek K, Tendera M 1990 Value of endomyocardial biopsy in the assessment of the degree of the changes in myocarditis. Kardiologia Polska 33(1): 12–18

Wynne J, Braunwald E 1997 The cardiomyopathies and myocarditides. In: Braunwald E (ed) Heart disease: a textbook of cardiovascular medicine, 5th edn. WB Saunders, Philadelphia, vol 2, pp. 1404–1463

FURTHER READING

Mangan CM 1992 Malignant pericardial effusions: pathophysiology and clinical correlates. Oncology Nursing Forum 19(8): 1215–1221

Mattson Porth C (ed) 1990 Pathophysiology concepts of altered health status, 5th edn. JB Lippincott, Philadelphia

Mayberry-Toth B, Landron S 1989 Complications associated with acute myocardial infarction. Critical Care Nursing Quarterly 12(2): 49–63

Monaghan MJ 1993 Practical echocardiography and Doppler. John Wiley, New York, pp. 67–71

Narula J, Khaw BA, Dec GW Jr et al 1993 Brief report: recognition of acute myocarditis masquerading as acute myocardial infarction. New England Journal of Medicine 328(2): 100–104

Pisani BA, Carlquist JF, Taylor DO, Anderson JL 1998 Acute myocarditis and dilated cardiomyopathy. In: Yusuf S, Cairns JA, Camm AJ, Fallen EL, Gersh BJ (eds) Evidence based cardiology. BMJ Books, London, pp. 671–697

Prince SE, Cunha BA 1997 Post pericardiotomy syndrome. Heart and Lung 26(2): 165–168

Spodick DH 1985 Acute pericardial disease. Heart and Lung 14(6): 599–604

Spodick DH 2001 Pericardial disease. In: Braunwald E, Zipes DP, Libby P (eds) Heart disease: a textbook of cardiovascular medicine, vol 2. WB Saunders, Philadelphia, pp. 1823–1876

Turk M 1989 Acute pericarditis in post myocardial infarction patients. Critical Care Nursing Quarterly 12(3): 34–38

17

The Marfan syndrome

Glen Brice

Marfan syndrome is one of the most common heritable disorders of connective tissue. It affects many body systems, but predominantly the heart (aortic dissection, mitral valve prolapse), the eyes (dislocated lenses) and skeleton (scoliosis) (Kainulainen & Peltonen 1993). Before the advent of modern medical and surgical therapy many patients had a significantly shortened lifespan with the vast majority of patients dying from a cardiovascular cause (Murdoch et al 1972). This chapter reviews the incidence, presentation and, importantly, the various treatment options available to the patient presenting with this condition. The latter section focuses upon the nursing care and support required for both patient and carers.

Marfan syndrome occurs in approximately 1 in 5000 births (Dietz & Pyeritz 1995), affects all racial groups and has wide clinical variability, both between and within families (Pyeritz 1993). In approximately 75% of cases Marfan syndrome is inherited from an affected parent (dominant inheritance), whilst in the remaining 25% there is no previous family history, the condition arising as the result of a new mutation (Pyeritz 1993). It is now established that the Marfan syndrome is caused by mutations in the gene FBN1, responsible for the production of fibrillin-1, a large protein which is a major component of microfibrils in connective tissues (Kainulainen et al 1990).

In general the cardiac conditions encountered by the nurse caring for the Marfan patient will be similar to those seen in other patients with aortic aneurysm or dissection, valvular disease and heart failure. However, the earlier age of onset, heritability and associated conditions (scoliosis, ectopia lentis) can have implications particularly in terms of long-term follow-up, psychological care of the patient and the future health of close relatives.

HISTORY

The first description of manifestations of the syndrome was made more than 100 years ago by Professor AB

Marfan, a renowned professor of paediatrics in Paris (Marfan 1896, cited by Pyeritz 1993). In his publication he described the case of a 5-year-old girl, Gabrielle P, who had disproportionately long, thin limbs and digits together with underdeveloped musculature. She also suffered from contractures of the fingers and knees.

Over the years various other investigators published on the subject, adding to and at times confusing the phenotype. The hereditary nature of Marfan syndrome was first described in 1931 (Acierno 1994), but it was not until the 1940s that the true prevalence and type of cardiovascular manifestations were accurately described.

In 1990 the exact molecular cause of Marfan syndrome was discovered following an international collaborative effort which resulted in the finding of the causative gene for fibrillin-1 on chromosome 15 (Kainulainen et al 1990).

CLINICAL FEATURES

Marfan syndrome is a multisystem disorder which involves mainly the cardiovascular, ophthalmic and musculoskeletal systems. There is broad clinical spectrum of disease from the near normal to the severely affected neonatal or infantile Marfan patient. Clinical features may appear from birth to old age and tend to be progressive, particularly during the rapid growth phases such as puberty.

Cardiovascular system

The reduced life expectancy seen in many Marfan patients is a direct result of the cardiovascular manifestations of the disease, with over 90% of premature deaths recorded in one study due to aortic dissection, aortic regurgitation and congestive cardiac failure (Murdoch et al 1972).

The first reported cardiovascular manifestations of Marfan syndrome involved the mitral valve (Piper & Irvine-Jones 1926) but with the widespread introduction of echocardiography in the 1970s the extent and natural history of the cardiac anomalies seen in Marfan syndrome were documented.

In the normal population, mitral valve prolapse affects approximately 3% of individuals and is generally benign (Devereux et al 1989) but amongst Marfan patients it is found in around 75% of individuals on echocardiographic (echo) examination. More than 25% of those affected will show progression of the prolapse leading to mitral regurgitation (Pyeritz & Wappel 1983) which, if severe enough, will require mitral valve repair or replacement (see Chapters 13 and 22).

Histologically the mitral valve often shows redundancy of the leaflets, stretching of the chordae tendineae and dilatation of the annulus (fibrous ring in which the valve rests). Calcification of the valve annulus has also been reported to occur at a greater rate than in the general population (Roberts & Honig 1982).

The aorta in the Marfan patient may develop a variety of abnormalities, all of which share the feature of dilatation, with the ascending portion the most commonly affected. This may be because it is the part which normally has the highest proportion of fibrillin-containing elastic fibres, which are deficient or abnormal in Marfan patients. The ascending aorta is also the site most exposed to the haemodynamic forces generated by the left ventricle. The weakened connective tissue in the aortic wall leads to progressive dilatation under the influence of both the level of blood pressure and the rate of rise of the blood pressure during systole (De Belder et al 1989). Enlargement of the sinuses of Valsalva, which leads to aortic regurgitation and possible left heart failure, may occur early in life or occasionally before birth (Morse et al 1990). It has been estimated that 10–15% of Marfan patients will develop significant aortic regurgitation or dissection before the age of 21 years (Pyeritz et al 1982).

Histological examination of Marfan aortas often shows massive medial degeneration (sometimes described as 'cystic medial necrosis') and loss of elastic tissue leading directly to dilatation (see Fig. 17.1).

A study of Marfan patients using ambulatory electrocardiograms (ECGs) has shown premature ventricular and atrial contractions, QT segment lengthening and ST depression to be more prevalent than in the normal control population (Savolainen et al 1997).

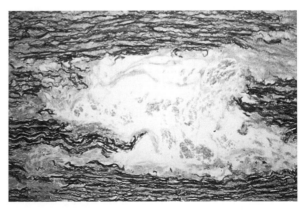

Figure 17.1 Specimen of aorta from a Marfan patient showing loss of elastic tissues from the media (middle layer).

Axis deviation may also occur due to rotation of the heart, secondary to severe pectus excavatum (sunken chest) or thoracic lordosis (excessive anteroposterior curvature of the spine) (Pyeritz 1996).

Musculoskeletal system

Mean height in Marfan syndrome patients tends to be greater than that of the general population and of any unaffected family members. The arms and legs are also disproportionately long, a sign which Marfan called dolichostenomelia. Arachnodactyly (long thin fingers) occurs often but is largely a subjective measure. Attempts to use metacarpal index (length to width ratio of hand bones) as a diagnostic tool have demonstrated a lack of sensitivity and specificity (Thomas et al 1996).

The wrist sign (overlapping of the thumb and fifth finger when placed around the wrist) and thumb sign (extension of the thumb well past the ulnar border when apposed across the palm) have also been used in diagnosis but are relatively non-specific.

Scoliosis is found in at least 50% of Marfan patients and may be severe and progressive. As in other varieties of scoliosis, the curvature tends to increase with growth and may eventually threaten the health and mobility of the patient through restrictive pulmonary disease and back pain. A scoliosis of less than 10° by the end of the pubertal growth spurt is unlikely to progress (Pyeritz 1993). Pectus excavatum (sunken chest) and pectus carinatum (pigeon chest) or a combination of both occur commonly. Protrusio acetabulae, in which the femoral head protrudes through the acetabulum into the pelvis, probably occurs in up to 50% of Marfan patients in which the skeletal manifestations are severe (Steel 1996). This can cause severe hip pain.

Marfan patients, often thought to have universally lax joints, can in fact have normal mobility or even flexion contractures (Pyeritz 1993).

Ocular system

Dislocation of the ocular lens (ectopia lentis), myopia (short-sightedness) and retinal detachment are the most common ocular manifestations seen in Marfan syndrome. Lens dislocation is found in approximately 60–70% of patients and in at least 50% of these cases is detected before the age of 5 years (Calver & Jones 1995). The ocular lens is normally held in place by fibrillin-rich fibres fixed to the ciliary muscle. As these are weakened by a lack of fibrillin, in many patients the lens is not held securely and dislocates (Fig. 17.2).

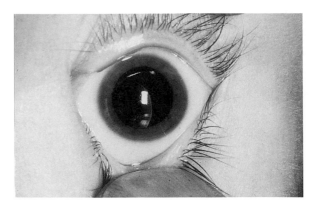

Figure 17.2 Lens dislocation as seen in many Marfan patients.

In most cases the dislocated lens is not removed unless visual acuity is reduced due to either cataract or awkward displacement of the lens.

Varying degrees of axial myopia, in which there is an increased front-to-back diameter of the eyeball, occurs in a large proportion of patients, with around 10% having severe myopia.

Retinal detachment is known to be associated with connective tissue disorders, myopia and lens dislocation, all of which are associated with Marfan syndrome. Up to 10% of Marfan patients may be affected by retinal detachment and of these the vast majority will also have suffered previous lens dislocation (Calver & Jones 1995).

Other systems

The skin may be affected in Marfan patients, with severe stretch marks (striae atrophica) often appearing during the pubertal growth spurt and pregnancy. Inguinal and incisional hernias are relatively common and recurrence after surgical repair is often reported by patients (Pyeritz 1993).

Spontaneous pneumothorax is the most commonly occurring pulmonary manifestation. In one study 11% of patients had suffered a spontaneous pneumothorax and in all but one case the problem had recurred (Wood et al 1984). With the increasing use of magnetic resonance imaging (MRI) scanning, reports of a high incidence of dural ectasia (widening of the spinal canal) have appeared (Raftopoulos et al 1993).

DIAGNOSTIC CRITERIA

In the years following Professor Marfan's initial description, additional manifestations were recog-

Box 17.1 Diagnostic criteria

For the first case in a family
- If the family/genetic history is not contributory, major criteria in two different organ systems and the involvement of a third system.
- If a mutation known to cause Marfan syndrome in others is detected, one major criterion in an organ system and involvement of a second.

For a relative of the first case
- Presence of a major criterion in the family history and involvement of a second organ system.

Skeletal system

Major criteria
Presence of at least four of the following manifestations.
- Pectus carinatum (pigeon chest)
- Pectus excavatum (sunken chest) requiring surgery
- Reduced upper segment to lower segment ratio or armspan to height ratio greater than 1.05
- Wrist and thumb signs
- Scoliosis of >20° or spondylolisthesis (forward displacement of a vertebra over a lower segment, usually in the lumbar region)
- Reduced extension of the elbows
- Flat feet
- Protrusio acetabulae (deepened hip sockets) of any degree

Minor criteria
- Pectus excavatum of moderate severity
- Joint hypermobility
- Highly arched palate
- Characteristic facial appearance (long thin face, receding lower jaw, anti-mongoloid eye slant)

Ocular system

Major criteria
- Ectopia lentis (dislocation of the ocular lens)

Minor criteria
- Abnormally flat cornea
- Increased axial length of globe
- Hypoplastic iris or hypoplastic ciliary muscle

Cardiovascular system

Major criteria
- Dilatation of the ascending aorta with or without aortic regurgitation and involving at least the sinuses of Valsalva
- Dissection of the ascending aorta

Minor criteria
- Mitral valve prolapse with or without mitral regurgitation
- Dilatation of the main pulmonary artery below the age of 40 years
- Calcification of the mitral annulus below the age of 40 years
- Dilatation or dissection of the descending thoracic or abdominal aorta below the age of 50 years

Pulmonary system

Major criteria
- None

Minor criteria
- Spontaneous pneumothorax
- Apical blebs ('blisters' on the apex of the lung which may rupture, leading to pneumothorax)

Skin and integument

Major criteria
- None

Minor criteria
- Striae atrophica (stretch marks) not associated with marked weight changes or pregnancy
- Recurrent or incisional hernia

Dura

Major criteria
- Lumbosacral dural ectasia (widening of the spinal canal due to weakness of the connective tissues in the dura mater) by computed tomography (CT) or MRI scan

Minor criteria
- None

Family/genetic history

Major criteria
- Having a parent, child or sibling who meets the diagnostic criteria independently
- Presence of a mutation in FBN1 known to cause the Marfan syndrome
- Inheritance of genetic markers known to be associated with Marfan syndrome (linkage to chromosome 15q)

Minor criteria
- None

nized as frequent components of Marfan syndrome. However, before 1988 there were no clearly established diagnostic criteria for diagnosing a patient as suffering from the syndrome. In 1986 a committee of international consultants identified such diagnostic criteria for the most common heritable disorders of connective tissue, including Marfan syndrome (Beighton et al 1988). These criteria were a marked improvement but with the increasing use of scanning and molecular techniques, revision was necessary (De Paepe et al 1996).

Clearly it is not easy to memorize such a detailed set of diagnostic criteria so if there is a high index of suspicion the patient should be referred to the nearest specialist centre for definitive diagnosis. A good rule of thumb to remember is that if the patient is classically affected in two out of three major organ systems (ocular, cardiovascular, skeletal) then specialist advice should be sought. Indicators of increased risk include new mutation (i.e. first affected in family), family history of early dissection, male sex and extreme physical characteristics (Child 1997a).

GENETICS

Marfan syndrome is inherited in an autosomal dominant fashion. In other words, if one parent has the Marfan syndrome then there is a 50/50 risk that each child will inherit the single dominant gene and be affected (Fig. 17.3).

In most instances the child will be affected to the same degree as those in the preceding generations though intrafamilial variation is large (Pyeritz & McKusick 1979). On average 1 in 10 children will be severely affected, requiring surgery for eye, heart or skeletal problems early in life (Child 1997a).

Marfan syndrome does not skip generations and therefore those 'at-risk' members of a family must be examined by an experienced practitioner for physical signs to determine whether they are carrying the gene or not. Those children who do not inherit the gene cannot pass it on.

In 1986 the protein fibrillin-1 was discovered (Sakai et al 1986). Fibrillin-1 is a large protein found primarily in structures which must resist load and strain, hence its presence in the aorta, skin and the suspensory ligament of the eye. Following the discovery of the connection between fibrillin-1 and Marfan syndrome (Kainulainen et al 1990), it was hoped that a simple genetic test could be developed for screening patients. This has not proved possible to date due to the large number of different mutations found (Hayward & Brock 1997), the large size of the gene and often low probability of detecting a change (approximately 17–78%) in the DNA even in those severely affected (Hayward et al 1997). However, within a family, if a mutation is located this can be used to test other members of the family and obviate the necessity for regular clinical follow-up of individuals not carrying the mutation. To date, more than 100 mutations have been reported in patients suffering from Marfan syndrome. With very few exceptions, each mutation has proved to be unique and only found in other affected members of the same family (Collod-Beroud et al 1997). Due to the well-described variation in expression between and within families it is not normally possible to give prognostic information based on the type or site of mutation. The inability to find a mutation in FBN1 or a molecular abnormality in fibrillin-1 does not exclude the diagnosis of Marfan syndrome in someone who meets the clinical criteria.

Following the discovery of the link between Marfan syndrome and the fibrillin protein, it was speculated that individuals with the isolated features of the syndrome may also have mutations in the fibrillin gene (Milewicz 1994). This becomes important when screening patients referred with a possible diagnosis of Marfan syndrome. Approximately 70% of those referred to the Marfan syndrome and related disorders clinic at St George's Hospital, London for screening do not fulfil the criteria for Marfan syndrome but do require a diagnosis. There are a number of conditions which share some of the features of Marfan syndrome

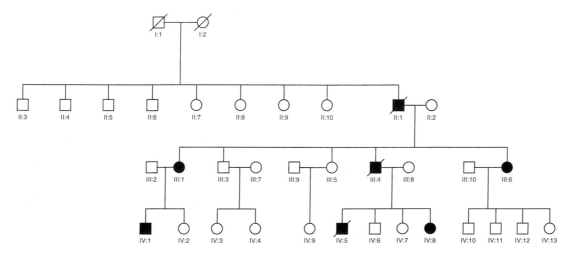

Figure 17.3 Pedigree diagram of Marfan family demonstrating dominant inheritance. Note risk to children of either sex of an affected parent, male-to-male transmission and probable new mutation in individual II-1. Males are denoted by squares and females by circles. Deceased individuals are denoted by a diagonal line through the symbol.

but can normally be excluded by looking at inheritance patterns and type and severity of signs present in the patient.

It has now been reported that mutations in the fibrillin gene are implicated in isolated ectopia lentis (dislocated lenses) (Lonqvist et al 1994), ascending aortic aneurysm (Francke et al 1995) and thoracic aortic aneurysm (Milewicz et al 1996). Many of these patients are tall and thin (marfanoid).

NEONATAL OR INFANTILE MARFAN SYNDROME

Infrequently Marfan syndrome is diagnosed in infancy, in which case the child is severely affected and is normally the first affected in the family (new mutation). Cardiac pathology in these cases tends to be present at birth with progressively worsening mitral

> **Case study 17.1**
>
> John Sims, a male child, was referred to the Marfan clinic for confirmation of the diagnosis of Marfan syndrome. Neither parent was affected on close clinical examination. John weighed 3.6 kg at birth with dysmorphic features including redundant skin on the forehead, wide nasal bridge, low-set ears, down-turned mouth, long body and limbs with long fingers and the thumb flexed across the palm. Contractures of the knees and elbows were present. Slight pectus excavatum was noted along with lower thoracic kyphosis (spinal curvature). An echocardiogram revealed a dilated aortic root, mild anterior mitral valve prolapse, mitral regurgitation and tricuspid regurgitation.
>
> By the age of 1 year John was able to put some weight on his feet and swimming was suggested as a means of both strengthening his musculature and improving his contractures. His kyphosis had become slightly more prominent and the use of a soft brace was recommended to allow the lower lobes of the lung to expand. Loud rhonchi were audible without the aid of a stethoscope and were reported by the parents to be present even in the absence of a cold. His aortic root size had not markedly enlarged by the age of 1 year.
>
> A blood sample was taken from John and a mutation found within exon 25 of the fibrillin gene, one of those included in the so-called neonatal region. This has allowed confirmation that neither parent carries the mutation and would allow screening of any future pregnancies to rule out a rare recurrence. The risk of recurrence in families such as this with both parents clinically normal is near the population risk (1 in 5000). However, gonadal mosaicism (mutation in the reproductive cells not causing Marfan syndrome in the parent), which may lead to more than one affected child being born to unaffected parents, should be considered (Rantamaki et al 1999).

regurgitation and aortic root dilatation (Morse et al 1990). Patients often do not survive beyond the age of 5 years with the cause of death being cardiac failure. A number of mutations have been described in these patients and thus far all have occurred in exons 24–32 (exon = gene segments which code for amino acids) of the fibrillin gene (Kainulainen et al 1994, Nijbroek et al 1995, Putnam et al 1996).

MEDICAL MANAGEMENT

The treatment of the Marfan patient has progressed rapidly over the past two decades with all manifestations now treatable, increasing both length and quality of life even for those severely affected. Screening for Marfan syndrome is best offered in a centre in which all manifestations of the disease can be assessed, preferably on the same visit, by a specialist with experience of the syndrome. Follow-up visits, where feasible, should also occur at the same centre to allow a rapport to be built up with the patient and family. Meticulous records of height, weight, presence and degree of scoliosis and aortic root size should be kept for comparison on subsequent visits. Screening by echocardiography should be carried out on the first clinic visit and then yearly in an uncomplicated case. More frequent reviews are required if there is evidence of a dilating aortic root or severe mitral regurgitation. Measurements may be taken at several points along the aorta, most commonly in the sinuses of Valsalva, sinotubular junction and aortic arch (Fig. 17.4). Wherever possible, the same operator should perform the echocardiogram in order to reduce intra-observer error in reporting on the cardiac manifestations.

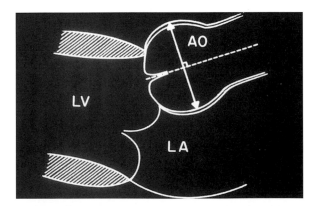

Figure 17.4 Diagram showing point at which aortic root diameter is commonly measured in the sinus of Valsalva, at the tip of the open aortic valve cusps.

Routine screening of the Marfan patient is normally performed with transthoracic echocardiography although transoesophageal echocardiograms and MRI scans are becoming more widely available and offer better sensitivity in diagnosing changes in dimensions and detection of dissections.

If mitral valve prolapse is present and a murmur is evident then antibiotics should be prescribed prior to surgical or dental procedures.

Referral to a cardiac surgeon familiar with Marfan syndrome patients is recommended when the aortic root size is greater than 4.5 cm, with a view to prophylactic aortic root replacement surgery if the aorta continues to dilate to 5 cm. There is controversy regarding at what aortic root diameter surgery should be performed. It is a major operation for a potentially catastrophic complication and, as the British Heart Foundation clinical guide highlights, replacement will be recommended at a diameter greater than 5 cm, 5.5 cm or 6 cm depending on the author (Child & Briggs 2001). However, early referral allows time for the patient to undergo any further investigations the surgeon may require. Adequate warning of the impending operation also allows the patient to come to terms with the diagnosis, arrange time off work or school and ask any questions which may be relevant. The early use of β-blocking therapy has shown clear benefits to many but not all Marfan patients, with a reduction in the rate of progression of aortic root dilatation (Haouzi et al 1997, Salim et al 1994, Shore et al 1994). β-blocker therapy should commence at the first sign of aortic root dilatation, with the dose titrated to the largest which can be tolerated by the patient. The aim is not only to reduce the blood pressure but also to reduce the rate at which the systolic pressure is reached. If β-blockers are contraindicated, alternative antihypertensive therapy may be used but clinical trials specifically involving Marfan patients have not been undertaken.

A full skeletal assessment should also be performed to provide a baseline measurement of height and weight and the presence or absence of scoliosis or pectus deformities. Any abnormalities of the spine or chest may worsen or appear during the accelerated growth period around puberty and the involvement of other professionals such as physiotherapists and orthopaedic and thoracic surgeons may be necessary. The question of whether to retard growth may arise in some cases. This problem has not been addressed directly in Marfan patients, primarily due to the small number of patients involved. Referral to an endocrinologist with expertise in this field is essential if this treatment is considered.

Box 17.2 Overview of management

- Regular examination by one co-ordinating physician
- Periodic multidisciplinary evaluation as follows:
  - ophthalmic: between birth and 6 months; annually thereafter
  - orthopaedic: monitoring for scoliosis, pectus deformity, flat feet to age 20
  - cardiovascular: newborn, every 2 years to age 11 then annually
  - psychosocial: after diagnosis and again during adolescence
  - genetic counselling: at first diagnosis and again with partner
- Periodic ECG and echocardiogram focusing on dysrhythmias, mitral valve prolapse and aortic root diameter
- Chest X-ray focusing on apical blebs
- Echo, CT or MRI scan of entire aorta–baseline assessment in all adults and again periodically if dilatation or dissection present
- Antibiotics prior to surgery or dental care for endocarditis prophylaxis
- β-blockers at first sign of dilatation
- Restriction of strenuous activities
- Surgical repair of aortic aneurysm when widest diameter exceeds 5 cm

---

SURGICAL TREATMENT

The prognosis in Marfan syndrome for both adult and paediatric patients is primarily related to the cardiovascular complications. Aneurysmal dilatation of the ascending aorta is the most serious consequence of Marfan syndrome and in many cases requires surgical treatment to prevent catastrophic rupture. Aneurysms may occur at any point on the aorta but classically occur at the aortic root, just distal to the aortic valve. Regular monitoring with echocardiography and MRI scanning is used to determine the correct time to offer elective replacement of the aorta (Barron & Pepper 1997). Elective aortic root replacement should be recommended if the aortic root has reached 5 cm but intervening earlier may be warranted in cases where there is a family history of dissection at smaller aortic root dimensions. Patients undergoing elective replacement of the aorta have a significantly reduced surgical mortality (1.8%) and morbidity compared with those having emergency operations (9.8%). This underlines the need for close follow-up of patients, with particular regard to the aortic root measurement. The overall survival in a study of patients having undergone surgical repair was 65% at 20 years (Gott et al 1996).

In addition to the technique of complete replacement of the aorta first described by Bentall (Bentall &

De Bono 1968), a valve-sparing operation, first described in 1979 (Yacoub et al 1998), is available at a limited number of centres throughout the world. This procedure allows the patient to retain their native aortic valve, obviating the necessity for lifelong anticoagulation. It also virtually eliminates the risk of thrombo-embolism and reduces the risk of endocarditis (Gott et al 1996). Further details on surgical procedures can be found in Chapters 15 and 22.

Operating on patients with Marfan syndrome after aortic dissection has already developed is often too late. Not only are the operative morbidity and mortality rates high but in many cases only the area involving the intimal tear and surrounding dissection can be replaced. The pathological process, which often extends distal to the aortic arch into the descending aorta, is not addressed, raising the probability of complications at a later date. If there are no contra-indications, β-blockers are normally commenced or continued following surgery, reducing the risk of further cardiovascular complications. Acute dissection with its origin distal to the left subclavian artery should be managed medically with reduction of blood pressure until the patient stabilizes. If, however, there is progressive dilatation, limb ischaemia or signs of new dissection then repair may be indicated (Pyeritz 1993). It is now possible to replace the complete aorta in staged operations in those patients in whom the dilatation is not confined to the ascending part of the aorta (Crawford et al 1984).

Case study 17.2

A 63-year-old man had been clinically monitored for many years following his initial presentation with bilateral dislocated lenses and detached retinas. On examination he was 6'5" (193 cm) tall with a high-arched palate, pectus carinatum, kyphoscoliosis, large ears and loose joints (Fig. 17.5).

His family history included the death of seven family members (Fig. 17.6) from aortic complications at ages ranging from 17 to 50 years.

His aortic root size was measured regularly and showed progressive dilatation to a size of 4.8 cm. Surgery was recommended when the aortic size reached 5.5 cm. For 4 years the aortic root size did not increase beyond 4.8 cm. However, sadly the patient developed an acute dissection of the ascending aorta and died. It is possible that in this case, although there was no increase in size of the aorta, the fibres in the aorta were ageing and deteriorating, leading to the dissection. Despite the terrible family history of dissection there were no echocardiographic measurements from other family members to use as a guide to clinical decision making for this man.

The surgical treatment of mitral regurgitation associated with Marfan syndrome remains controversial because of the underlying degenerative process which may be present in the valve. Replacement of the valve will remove all abnormal tissue whilst a repair operation may fail in the long term due to degeneration of the abnormal tissues. The cause of regurgitation in the majority of cases is leaflet prolapse, with annulus dilatation accounting for the remainder. Bearing in mind the concerns of repairing a fundamentally defective valve, in the majority of cases mitral valve repair is still the preferred surgical option with low surgical morbidity and good long-term results (Fuzellier et al 1998). This approach also obviates the necessity for long-term anticoagulation unless atrial fibrillation is present.

PREGNANCY IN MARFAN SYNDROME

Improved surgical and medical management of patients with Marfan syndrome have permitted many more affected female patients to reach child-bearing age. The risk of transmitting the condition to the child, the possibilities of prenatal diagnosis and the obstetric risk to the mother should be discussed with the prospective parents. If pregnancy is contra-indicated, the alternatives of adoption, fostering, egg or sperm donation or surrogate pregnancy may be considered (Child 1997b).

Before embarking on pregnancy, women with Marfan syndrome should be fully assessed for cardiological problems and general health. Those women with minimal cardiac involvement (aortic root diameter less than 4.0 cm and with no significant aortic or mitral regurgitation) should be counselled that there is a low risk of serious complications (Lipscomb et al 1997, Pyeritz 1981, Rossiter et al 1995). The major complications to be borne in mind include endocarditis, aortic dissection and congestive cardiac failure. Patients with substantial cardiac complications, including those who have undergone aortic root or valve replacement or who have an aortic root measurement of more than 4 cm, are advised that pregnancy would carry a high risk of further complications.

Bearing in mind the risks involved in many Marfan pregnancies, the process should be carefully monitored by both a cardiologist and an obstetrician knowledgeable about the possible complications. If aortic dilatation is detected, bedrest and β-blockers should be prescribed, with consideration given to early delivery if the pregnancy has progressed far enough, to reduce cardiac stress. Labour and delivery should be managed in a manner designed to keep cardiac stress

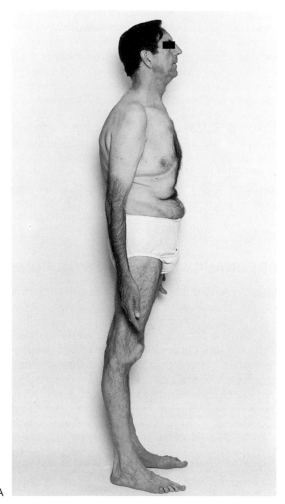

A

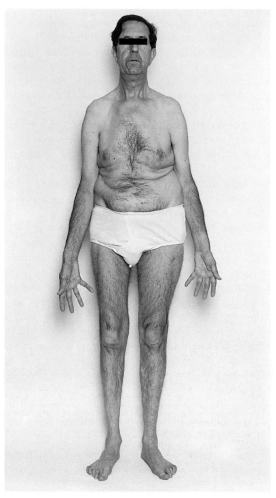

B

Figure 17.5 **A,B:** This man, the subject of case study 17.2, demonstrates tall, thin habitus with long arms, kyphosis, antimongoloid slant to eyes, large ears and feet. Hyperextension of the knees is also evident.

to a minimum (Gordon & Johnson 1993). This is normally an uninduced labour with vaginal delivery. Caesarean section should not be routinely performed but if the aortic root size is larger than 4.5 cm or there is significant aortic regurgitation, delivery at 39 weeks by induction or caesarean section should be considered (Child 1997b).

β-blocking drugs are effective antihypertensive agents in pregnancy with no known teratogenic (causing fetal abnormalities) effects. Some side-effects, such as bradycardia and apnoea, have been reported in babies whose mothers have been prescribed β-blockers but these need to be measured against the reduction in risk to the mother (Oakley & De Swiet

1997). Certainly if the aortic root begins to dilate at any time during the pregnancy, β-blockers should be commenced.

It should also be borne in mind that aortic dissection can occur in the mother without further dilatation from the size at conception (Brice et al 1996). Consequently, any signs of severe chest or abdominal pain should be treated as possible aortic dissection with immediate ultrasound assessment of the entire aorta (Child 1997b).

No pregnant Marfan patient can be reassured that pregnancy is uniformly safe or can be taken lightly, but the risks can be markedly reduced if current recommendations are followed.

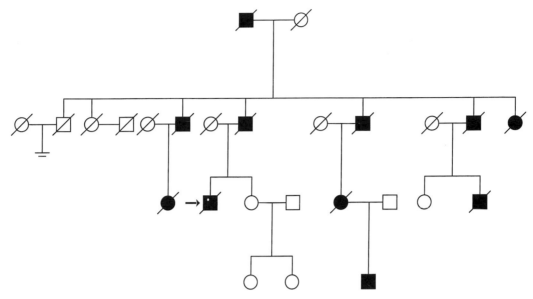

Figure 17.6 Pedigree diagram of the subject of case study 17.2 (arrowed) with those affected by Marfan syndrome marked in black.

Case study 17.3

Jill, a 27-year-old patient became pregnant and presented to the clinic for assessment. She was carefully monitored with echocardiography at all subsequent outpatient appointments. Blood pressure measurements remained within normal limits. Aortic root measurements during the course of the pregnancy ranged from 4.0 to 4.6 cm. At 37 weeks' gestation, Jill reported severe chest pains and was admitted to a specialist centre for assessment. A transoesophageal echo showed a dissection of the ascending aorta and emergency surgery combined with caesarean section was planned. Unfortunately, whilst awaiting transfer to cardiac theatre, Jill suffered a cardiopulmonary arrest and although it was possible to perform an emergency caesarean section and save the child, the mother could not be resuscitated. No warning signs could be elicited from reviewing the medical notes of the patient. The aorta, although enlarged, had not dilated further through pregnancy. Jill's father had died at the age of 37 years from aortic dissection but as this was a post-mortem diagnosis there were no records on which to base a prognosis for his daughter. The baby was not affected by Marfan syndrome.

NURSING CARE

The cardiac manifestations of Marfan syndrome are also common in isolation in the general population and therefore treatments will not be unfamiliar to the cardiac nurse. It is, however, necessary to bear in mind that these patients suffer a collection of abnormalities, many of which will require repeated treatment throughout their lives and possible prolonged hospital stays. It is often reassuring for these regular attenders to be seen by a nurse familiar both with their care and also with the special problems of the Marfan patient.

Practical day-to-day help in terms of longer beds (and operating tables) to accommodate a generally taller stature and pressure-relieving equipment to reduce the risk of pressure sores in these generally thin patients will be appreciated. Easy fatiguability is sometimes a feature of Marfan syndrome and this needs to be taken into account, particularly following surgery and during the rehabilitation process after leaving hospital. The possibility of reduced visual acuity in those with ocular manifestations should also be borne in mind.

The diagnosis of Marfan syndrome in any member of a family may have implications for other relatives who will require screening as described earlier. Occasionally this is overlooked, sometimes with disastrous results. The diagnosis of Marfan syndrome affects the entire family with each individual requiring time to adjust to the diagnosis, making allowances for the condition whilst maintaining individual self-fulfillment. When the diagnosis of Marfan syndrome is made in a newborn, couples may experience a temporary strain in their relationship. During this period of adaptation they need to communicate their hopes and fears to each other. Questions commonly asked during this period of adjustment include 'Why did this happen to us?', 'Do I have Marfan syndrome?', 'What is the risk of a second child having the syndrome?' and 'Is there a cure?'. The answers to these questions vary from case to case and stock answers cannot be given. Family history, age at diagnosis and degree of expression need to be taken into account before correct counselling can be given.

Parents of an affected child should be reassured that treatment is available for all aspects of Marfan syndrome and, as far as possible, the child should lead as normal a life as they are able, being a child first and Marfan syndrome sufferer second. Unaffected brothers and sisters also need support. They may feel guilty that they have 'escaped' Marfan syndrome or may be fearful that they too will become affected or have children of their own who will inherit the condition. Many of these concerns can easily be allayed with careful examination and explanations.

Siblings may in some cases resent the extra attention given to the affected child and the fact that they have to compensate by doing jobs the affected child cannot do. During the pubertal growth spurt from 10 to 20 years, features of Marfan syndrome may appear for the first time or worsen. The child realizes that they are different from their peers and may have severe difficulties with body image, for example due to a severe pectus deformity. A prolonged period of dependency may occur because of the problems of independent existence. Conversely some young adults may react by trying to prove they are normal, for example by playing highly competitive or dangerous sports. Reactions to a diagnosis in a partner range from total acceptance to temporary rejection. Experienced counselling may be required. The reaction of the partner often depends on whether the diagnosis is made before or after marriage and/or before or after children have been born.

When a diagnosis of Marfan syndrome has been made this often involves accepting loss: loss of health, self-image, career prospects and perhaps loss of a job postoperatively. Again, expert counselling may be required to help the individual to come to terms with the diagnosis and possible treatment. The psychological stresses are similar to those suffered by any patient with a long-term disabling condition. There is a chance that some patients may become cardiac hypochondriacs due to the need for regular follow-up in a cardiac unit. They should be reassured that sudden catastrophic cardiac events rarely occur in patients who are being closely monitored. Jobs, life insurance, mortgages and pensions may be difficult to obtain but this will vary with the degree to which the patient is affected.

A study (Van Tongerloo & De Paepe 1998) evaluated the psychological effects of Marfan syndrome, examining specific items such as schooling, occupation choices, self-image and social behaviour. The results showed that the disease had a significant effect on the daily physical activities, schooling and job opportunities of those affected. Most were teased by their peer group due to their abnormal habitus, leading to an introvert personality in many cases. The risks associated with child bearing also represented a major concern. Nevertheless, most patients had come to terms with their disease and considered themselves happy most of the time.

Genetic counselling is available for each family member and other supportive and educational counselling is also possible for those who wish it. Peer group counselling, especially for those at crisis points during their lives, such as immediately before and after cardiac surgery, is now available. In addition, the Marfan Association UK, through its nationwide support groups, offers information, resources and referrals for those who are in need (Box 17.3). Research is being actively pursued in many centres throughout the world to find better treatments and earlier diagnosis, offering hope for an increased quality of life and a normal lifespan.

Box 17.3 Support group

The Marfan Association UK
Rochester House
5 Aldershort Rd
Fleet
Hants GU13 9NG
Tel: 01252 810472
Fax: 01252 810473

REFERENCES

Acierno LJ 1994 The history of cardiology. Parthenon Publishing, New York, pp. 413–414

Barron D, Pepper J 1997 Aortic dissection – management and prevention. British Journal of Cardiology 4(1): 25–28

Beighton P, De Paepe A, Danks D et al 1988 International nosology of heritable disorders of connective tissue, Berlin 1986. American Journal of Medical Genetics 29: 581–594

Bentall H, De Bono A 1968 A technique for complete replacement of the ascending aorta. Thorax 23: 338–339

Brice G, Treasure T, Pumphrey C, Leech G, Child A 1996 Serial echocardiography is of limited value in predicting aortic dissection in pregnant Marfan patients. European Journal of Pediatrics 155: 745

Calver DM, Jones B 1995 Ocular manifestations and their management. In: Child A, Birdwood G (eds) The Marfan syndrome – a clinical guide. British Heart Foundation, London, pp. 9–10

Child AH 1997a Marfan syndrome – current medical and genetic knowledge: how to treat and when. Journal of Cardiovascular Surgery 12: 131–136

Child AH 1997b Management of pregnancy in Marfan syndrome, Ehlers–Danlos syndrome, and other connective tissue disorders. In: Oakley C (ed) Heart disease in pregnancy. BMJ Books, London, pp. 153–162

Child AH, Briggs MJ 2001 The Marfan syndrome: a clinical guide. British Heart Foundation, London

Collod-Beroud G, Beroud C, Ades L et al 1997 Marfan database (second edition): software and database for the analysis of mutations in the FBN1 gene. Nucleic Acids Research 25(1): 147–150

Crawford ES, Crawford JL, Stowe CL, Safi HJ 1984 Total aortic replacement for chronic aortic dissection occurring in patients with and without Marfan's syndrome. Annals of Surgery 199(3): 358–362

De Belder MA, Child AH, Pumphrey CW 1989 The timing of aortic root replacement in Marfan's syndrome. Cardiovascular Medicine 8(3): 67–70

De Paepe A, Devereux RB, Dietz HC, Hennekam RCM, Pyeritz RE 1996 Revised diagnostic criteria for the Marfan syndrome. American Journal of Human Genetics 62: 417–426

Devereux RB, Kawkins I, Kligfield P 1989 Mitral valve prolapse: causes, clinical manifestations and management. Annals of Internal Medicine 111: 305–314

Dietz HC, Pyeritz R 1995 Mutations in the human gene for fibrillin-1 (FBN-1) in the Marfan syndrome and related disorders. Human Molecular Genetics 4: 1799–1809

Francke U, Bery M, Tynan K et al 1995 A Gly1127Ser mutation in an EGF-like domain of the fibrillin gene is a risk factor for ascending aortic aneurysm and dissection. American Journal of Human Genetics 56: 1287–1296

Fuzellier JF, Chauvaud SM, Fornes P et al 1998 Surgical management of mitral regurgitation associated with Marfan's syndrome. Annals of Thoracic Surgery 66(1): 68–72

Gordon CF, Johnson MD 1993 Anaesthetic management of the pregnant patient with Marfan syndrome. Journal of Clinical Anaesthesia 5: 248–251

Gott V, Laschinger J, Cameron D et al 1996 The Marfan syndrome and the cardiovascular surgeon. European Journal of Cardiothoracic Surgery 10: 149–158

Haouzi A, Berglund H, Pelikan P, Maurer G, Siegel R 1997 Heterogeneous aortic response to acute β adrenergic blockade in Marfan syndrome. American Heart Journal 133: 60–63

Hayward C, Brock D 1997 Fibrillin-1 mutations in Marfan syndrome and other type-1 fibrillinopathies. Human Mutation 10(6): 415–423

Hayward C, Porteus ME, Brock D 1997 Mutation screening of all 65 exons of the fibrillin-1 gene in 60 patients with Marfan syndrome: report of 12 novel mutations. Human Mutation 10(4): 280–289

Kainulainen K, Peltonen L 1993 Marfan syndrome: molecular pathogenesis. In: Verma RS (series ed) Advances in Genome Biology 2: 113–133. Jai Press, London

Kainulainen K, Pulkkinen L, Savolainen A, Kaitila I, Peltonen L 1990 Location on chromosome 15 of the gene causing Marfan syndrome. New England Journal of Medicine 323: 935–939

Kainulainen K, Karttunen L, Puhakka L, Sakai L, Peltonen L 1994 Mutations in the fibrillin gene responsible for dominant ectopia lentis and neonatal Marfan syndrome. Nature Genetics 6: 64–69

Lipscomb KJ, Smith JC, Clarke B, Donnai P, Harris R 1997 Outcome of pregnancy in women with Marfan's syndrome. British Journal of Obstetrics and Gynaecology 104(2): 201–206

Lonqvist L, Child A, Kainulainen K, Davison R, Puhakka L, Peltonen L 1994 A novel mutation of the fibrillin gene causing ectopia lentis. Genomics 19(3): 573–576

Milewicz D 1994 Identification of defects in the fibrillin gene and protein. Texas Heart Institute Journal 21: 22–29

Milewicz DM, Michael K, Fisher N, Coselli JS, Markello T, Biddinger A 1996 Fibrillin-1 (FBN1) mutations in patients with thoracic aortic aneurysms. Circulation 94(11): 2708–2711

Morse R, Rockenmacher S, Pyeritz R et al 1990 Diagnosis and management of infantile Marfan syndrome. Pediatrics 86: 888–895

Murdoch JL, Walker BA, Halpern BL, Kuzma JW, McKusick VA 1972 Life expectancy and causes of death in the Marfan syndrome. New England Journal of Medicine 286: 804–808

Nijbroek G, Sood S, McIntosh I et al 1995 Fifteen novel FBN1 mutations causing Marfan syndrome detected by heteroduplex analysis of genomic amplicons. American Journal of Human Genetics 57(1): 8–21

Oakley C, De Swiet M 1997 Antihypertensive drugs. In: Oakley C (ed) Heart disease in pregnancy. BMJ Books, London, pp. 330–335

Piper RK, Irvine-Jones E 1926 Arachnodactylia and its association with congenital heart disease: report of a case and review of the literature. American Journal of Diseases in Childhood 31: 832–839

Putnam E, Cho M, Zinn AB, Towbin JA, Byers PH, Milewicz DM 1996 Delineation of the Marfan phenotype associated with mutations in exons 23–32 of the FBN1 gene. American Journal of Human Genetics 62(3): 233–242

Pyeritz R 1981 Maternal and fetal complications of pregnancy in the Marfan syndrome. American Journal of Medicine 7: 784–790

Pyeritz R 1993 The Marfan syndrome. In: Royce P, Steinmann B (eds) Connective tissue and its heritable disorders. Wiley-Liss, New York, pp. 437–468

Pyeritz R 1996 Marfan syndrome and other disorders of fibrillins and microfibrilogenesis. In: Rimoin DL, Connor JM, Pyeritz R (eds) Principles and practice of medical genetics, 3rd edn. Churchill Livingstone, New York, pp. 1027–1066

Pyeritz R, McKusick VA 1979 The Marfan syndrome: diagnosis and management. New England Journal of Medicine 300: 772–777

Pyeritz R, Wappel MA 1983 Mitral valve dysfunction in the Marfan syndrome: clinical and echocardiographic study of prevalence and natural history. American Journal of Medicine 74: 797–807

Pyeritz R, Gott VL, McDonald GR et al 1982 Surgical repair of the Marfan aorta: technique, indications and complications. Johns Hopkins Medical Journal 151(2): 71–82

Raftopoulos C, Delecluse F, Braude P, Rodesh C, Brotchi J 1993 Anterior sacral meningocele and Marfan syndrome: a review. Acta Chirurgica Belgica 93(1): 1–7

Rantamaki T, Kaitila I, Syvanen A, Lukka M, Peltonen L 1999 Recurrence of Marfan syndrome as a result of parental germ-line mosaicism for an FBN1 mutation. American Journal of Human Genetics 64(4): 993–1001

Roberts WC, Honig HS 1982 The spectrum of cardiovascular disease in the Marfan syndrome: a clinico-morphologic study of 18 necropsy patients and comparison to 151 previously reported necropsy patients. American Heart Journal 104(1): 115–135

Rossiter J, Repke J, Morales A, Murphy E, Pyeritz R 1995 A prospective longitudinal evaluation of pregnancy in the Marfan syndrome. American Journal of Obstetrics and Gynecology 173: 1599–1606

Sakai L, Keene D, Engvall E 1986 Fibrillin, a new 350-KD glycoprotein, is a component of extracellular microfibrils. Journal of Cell Biology 103: 2499–2510

Salim M, Alpert B, Ward J, Pyeritz R 1994 Effect of beta-adrenergic blockade on aortic root rate of dilation in the Marfan syndrome. American Journal of Cardiology 74: 629–633

Savolainen A, Kupari M, Toivonen L, Kaitila I, Viitasalo M 1997 Abnormal ambulatory electrocardiographic findings in patients with Marfan syndrome. Journal of Internal Medicine 241(3): 221–226

Shore J, Berger KR, Murphy EA, Pyeritz R 1994 Progression of aortic dilatation and the benefit of long term β-adrenergic blockade in Marfan's syndrome. New England Journal of Medicine 330: 1335–1341

Steel HH 1996 Protrusio acetabuli: its occurrence in the completely expressed Marfan syndrome and its musculoskeletal component and a procedure to arrest the course of protrusion in the growing pelvis. Journal of Pediatric Orthopedics 16(6): 704–718

Thomas S, Younger K, Child A, Wilson A 1996 Is the metacarpal index useful in the diagnosis of Marfan syndrome? Clinical Radiology 51(8): 570–574

Van Tongerloo A, De Paepe A 1998 Psychosocial adaption in adolescents and young adults with Marfan syndrome: an exploratory study. Journal of Medical Genetics 35(5): 405–409

Wood J, Bellamy D, Child A, Citron KM 1984 Pulmonary disease in patients with Marfan syndrome. Thorax 39: 780–784

Yacoub MH, Gehle P, Chandrasekaran V, Birks EJ, Child A, Radley-Smith R 1998 Late results of a valve-preserving operation in patients with aneurysms of the ascending aorta and root. Journal of Thoracic and Cardiovascular Surgery 115(5): 1080–1090

Management of care

This section allows the opportunity for the nurse to understand and explore the variety of management issues related to the care of the cardiac patient/client and their loved ones. The skill of manipulating haemodynamics to optimise tissue perfusion, proceeds to detailed discussion regarding complex areas such as electrophysiology studies, cardiopulmonary resuscitation, the support of those with internal cardioverter defibrillators and the role of complementary therapies.

18

Augmenting the cardiac output in adults

Richard Hatchett
Claire Bennett

A major role of the cardiac care nurse is the augmentation or increase of the patient's cardiac output, with the aim of optimizing tissue oxygenation. This may, for example, be for a patient whose cardiac function has decreased following cardiac surgery or for the cardiology patient experiencing left ventricular failure. Primarily, optimization involves the choice of three approaches: intravenous colloids and occasionally crystalloids, creating a passive stretching of the myocardium to increase cardiac output, the use of inotropic agents to directly stimulate the heart and finally and less commonly, the implementation of cardiac assist devices, notably the intra-aortic balloon pump (IABP).

The choice of method will be dictated by the presenting clinical data and the perceived benefits to the patient of each approach. The role of the cardiac nurse as part of the health-care team is to practise safe, informed care, through an understanding of both the advantages and disadvantages of each approach based on the clinical scenario encountered.

This chapter explores the three principles and utilizes a case study approach throughout the text, allowing the reader to consider a variety of presenting clinical data and appropriate haemodynamic manipulation. Although the IABP is the most usual mechanical aid to a low cardiac output, the range of ventricular assist devices (VADs) in clinical use will be explored. In addition, the attempt to develop a VAD that is totally implantable, to support those with chronic heart failure, is highlighted. Chapter 5 explores the variety of monitoring devices currently in use and should be read in conjunction with this section, if these devices are unfamiliar to you.

Manipulating haemodynamics is a clear example of the potential for the ever-present practice–theory gap. The skill cannot be learnt purely in a classroom, as it is a problem-solving exercise which involves the holistic consideration of a whole variety of presenting clinical data. Yet without the theory, the parameters are merely monitored figures and the potential to safely optimize tissue perfusion is lost.

In considering the broad principles of haemodynamic manipulation, an understanding of three initial terms is required: preload, Starling's Law of the heart and afterload. The preload is the end-diastolic volume or the amount of blood remaining in the ventricles at the end of filling, just before systole (ejection). If the preload is high, it may indicate poor myocardial contractility and the inability of the heart to eject blood forward. Conversely, within monitored parameters, the preload may be manipulated and increased by intravenous fluids to stretch the myocardium and augment the cardiac output.

Starling's Law of the heart is a physical law, closely linked to the preload. It states that, within physiological limits, the greater a myocardial fibre is stretched before its release, the greater the force of contractility. The contraction is proportional to the initial fibre length (Hinds & Watson 1996). Hence, if the preload is raised through intravenous fluids, Starling's Law is utilized to increase that cardiac output. Obviously you cannot keep filling a patient with intravenous fluids and increasing the cardiac output as the heart will eventually become too full of fluid and the cardiac output will diminish. The decline of the stroke volume as this limit is reached is shown in Figure 10.3 (p. 193). It is therefore important to closely monitor the response of the filling pressures, such as the central venous pressure (CVP), to filling as much as the amount of fluid being administered.

The afterload is simply the resistance to ventricular ejection of blood. The term generally refers to the left ventricle because in front of this chamber lies the entire arterial and venous system. This will inevitably offer some resistance to create an adequate blood pressure and deliver optimum oxygen and nutrients to the tissues. However, in any situation where a disruption in cardiac function is encountered, contriction of peripheral vessels due to neurogenic and more long-term catecholamine stimulation (adrenaline (epinephrine), noradrenaline (norepinephrine) and dopamine) may result in an undesirably high afterload. In contrast the right ventricle pumps to the lungs which contain no valves and therefore the afterload is negligible. The exception may be in conditions presenting with pulmonary hypertension (elevated pressure in the pulmonary artery) or in diffuse and chronic lung disease.

In manipulating haemodynamics, one other factor is important and is linked to the above issues. Myocardial oxygen demand will markedly increase in the presence of two factors: a tachycardia and an increased afterload. This is significant because whichever principle is utilized to augment the cardiac output, to some degree these two factors will have a bearing. Increasing the myocardial oxygen demand in the critically ill cardiac or intensive care patient may have detrimental effects with regards to the heart's pumping action and can prove arrythmogenic.

MANIPULATING HAEMODYNAMICS

The myriad of issues regarding the augmentation of the cardiac output cannot all be discussed within this chapter. However, the following case studies provide some of the issues and discussion points in relation to the three principle approach. References are provided throughout to guide the reader to more detailed reading.

The issue of whether crystalloids or colloids should be administered to expand plasma volume is controversial and is known as the colloid/crystalloid debate. A crystalloid is a water-based solution, such as 0.9% sodium chloride, 5% dextrose or Hartmann's solution. Colloids are solutions with particles in suspension.

Crystalloids are valuable as hydration for the patient and will expand the intravascular volume. However, they move rapidly from the intravascular space into the interstitial area. A volume of 3–4 times that of a colloid may be required to expand the intravascular volume (Hinds & Watson 1996). The concern is that such a move may precipitate complications such as pulmonary oedema. Colloids, either synthetic such as the gelatins (Gelofusine, Haemaccel) or more natural solutions such as human albumin 4.5%, remain in the intravascular space for a greater amount of time, the latter far longer than the former two although it is more expensive. Yet this may also present the problem of preventing fluid moving into dehydrated interstitial and intracellular areas.

If the colloid is able to pass into the interstitial area it may draw more fluid with it by osmosis and further and unpredictably augment the fluid volume. The use of a crystalloid will encourage a diuresis while Haemaccel and Gelofusine through an osmotic effect within the kidneys are also recognized as mild diuretics.

In all the discussion regarding colloids and crystalloids, what is clear is that in severe haemorrhage, volume replacement is more important than red blood cell replacement. Human beings may survive up to an 80% loss of red blood cells, provided normovolaemia is maintained, but only a total volume loss of approximately 30% (Isbister 1997).

Case study 18.1

John Jackson, an 80 kg, 55-year-old man, is admitted with an inferior myocardial infarction to the coronary care unit. Nursing staff assess the patient correctly for the contra-indications to thrombolytic therapy. Streptokinase is administered but after 20 minutes John becomes cold and clammy to touch, expresses feelings of nausea and suffers two large episodes of haematemesis. After half an hour in the unit the following clinical signs were recorded.

- Skin pale, clammy and cool to touch
- Heart rate 130 bpm
- Blood pressure 75/40 mmHg
- Mean arterial pressure (MAP) 57 mmHg
- Urinary output 20 ml/h

It is unlikely that a pulmonary artery (PA) catheter would be passed in this situation, as the underlying problem is not an issue of poor contractility but severe hypovolaemia due to the unexpected and massive bleeding. Thrombolytic therapy also precludes such invasive line insertion. The tachycardia, low blood pressure and MAP reflect this volume depletion. The low urinary output highlights that blood is actively being shunted away from the kidneys to the vital organs, resulting in severe oliguria. At the present time it is impossible to ascertain whether the vital organs are adequately perfused. A urinary output of at least 0.5 ml/kg/h would suggest vital organ perfusion, as the kidneys receive a blood supply to produce urine, after vital organ perfusion. If a PA catheter were passed it would indicate a high systemic vascular resistance (SVR) as the peripheral vessels are constricted in an attempt to maintain the blood pressure. This is indicated by the

cool, clammy skin. The cardiac output and index would also be low.

Mr Jackson requires intravenous fluids to replace the volume depleted, which would be administered quickly but with care due to the underlying myocardial infarction. A recording of the central venous pressure (CVP) of the heart would be useful to guide intravenous fluid filling, which will utilize Starling's Law. Fluids can be rapidly administered and the CVP used as a guide to the nearing of an acceptable infused volume. However, as highlighted, the use of thrombolytic agents prevents passing this line. Administering intravenous fluids, and this is likely to be blood due to the large volume loss, will be accompanied by an improvement in skin colour and temperature, an increased urine output as blood returns to the kidneys, a rise in blood pressure and a reduced tachycardia.

Due to the time needed to prepare blood products, the nursing staff are likely in the initial stages to administer a colloid with a short half-life, such as Gelofusine or Hae-maccel. This will expand the depleted intravascular space and offer room for blood to be administered when pre-pared, due to the aforementioned product's short half-life.

What would be wholly inappropriate here would be to commence an inotropic agent, even though in this severe state the cardiac output is low. Such a drug would certainly raise the cardiac output but apart from not addressing the underlying problem, it would markedly increase the myocardial oxygen demand. The heart, already starved of oxygen due to acute blood loss, would be forced to work harder with a limited circulating volume to utilize. Ideally this man requires blood and a crystalloid as a hydration fluid.

THE USE OF INOTROPIC AGENTS

A positive inotrope is a chemical agent, usually given by continuous intravenous administration, which increases myocardial contractility, primarily through effects on the β1-adrenergic receptors. Many are also chronotropes, which means they increase the heart rate. The latter is desirable as the cardiac output is created from the stroke volume (the amount of blood ejected in one heart beat) × the heart rate. However, as previously mentioned, increasing the heart rate will increase the myocardial oxygen demand.

All inotropes, except digoxin, are chronotropic to a degree. Digoxin is not used in cardiogenic shock for a variety of reasons. It has a slow onset of action and is therefore difficult to titrate to the presenting clinical data and in addition, its toxic effects overlap its thera-peutic range. In addition to their chronotropic effects, inotropes will generally increase oxygen demand through direct stimulation of β1-adrenergic receptors in the heart. If they raise the afterload in an attempt to increase the blood pressure, as with inotropic dopamine, this may further add to the problem.

The subsequent choice of an inotrope is based on the properties of the drug and the clinical presentation. Personal preference will also have some bearing. Dopamine in its inotropic dose, above approximately 3–5 µg/kg/min, may be inappropriate for Mr Jackson. In line with all inotropes, it will increase cardiac contractility and output through stimulation of β1-adrenergic receptors in the heart, but it does create an unwanted peripheral vasoconstriction through the release of noradrenaline.

Mr Jackson's systemic vascular resistance (SVR) is already high as a compensatory mechanism and to raise this further with inotropic dopamine may be foolhardy. Dobutamine is probably a better choice. It increases cardiac output and again is chronotropic, although this may be more dose related. However, to a degree it dilates the peripheral vessels which will decrease the afterload and would be more welcome. Alternative inotropes may be milrinone (Primacor), a phosphodiesterase inhibitor with a similar effect to dobutamine, in that it augments cardiac output while reducing total peripheral resistance (Shipley &

Case study 18.2

Fred Jones, a 75 kg man, is admitted to the cardiac intensive care unit following coronary artery bypass grafting. Initially on return he appeared to be improving adequately, slowly warming with gentle intravenous fluid replacement. Gradually his monitored clinical observations began to alter, with a diminishing urinary output and deteriorating arterial blood gases, despite 50% oxygen being administered via the ventilator. A PA catheter was passed and after 4 hours in intensive care the following haemodynamic results were recorded.

- Skin pale, clammy and cool to touch
- Heart rate 130 bpm
- Blood pressure 105/55 mmHg
- MAP 72 mmHg
- CVP 15 mmHg
- Urinary output 15 ml/h
- PA pressure 32/21 mmHg
- Pulmonary artery occlusion pressure (PAOP) 22 mmHg
- Cardiac output 3.4 l/min
- Cardiac index 2.2 l/min/m²
- Systemic vascular resistance (SVR) 2160 dynes/sec/cm⁻⁵
- Mixed venous saturation (SVO₂) 60%

In the first instance, note the similarities between this case and John Jackson. Both have cool clammy skin, a tachycardia and low urinary and cardiac outputs. Yet the causes are very different and require different management. In nursing Mr Jones you would be aware of the history of cardiac surgery and that he was not in a state of severe hypovolaemia. Following open heart surgery, it is often difficult to ascertain how much blood has been lost in theatres but it would be replaced intraoperatively.

The key difference here lies in the fluid pressures of CVP, PA and PAOP. These demonstrate that the poorly perfused tissues, as demonstrated by the cool, clammy skin, low urinary output and probable poor blood gases, are due to failing myocardial contractility. Mr Jackson cannot effectively pump forward the fluid already present in his body and this has resulted in severely elevated CVP and PAOP pressures. To utilize the first principle of augmenting the cardiac output, that is intravenous fluid therapy, would be wholly inappropriate and indeed dangerous in that it would markedly worsen the situation. If the CVP and PAOP pressures had been within the low to normal range, careful intravenous fluid therapy may have been considered. As the pressure limits have been reached and in fact exceeded, it would now seem appropriate to consider inotropic support and possibly an IABP.

Note that although the cardiac output is low, the compensatory mechanisms of neurogenic and catecholamine release have maintained the blood pressure relatively well through peripheral vessel constriction, but this doesn't mean that tissue oxygen delivery is necessarily adequate. At this point some cardiologists and intensivists may consider a small dose of an intravenous nitrate. Its administration would be carefully guided by the urinary output and blood pressure, as the latter parameter may be lowered to an unacceptable level by subsequent vasodilatation. A nitrate's benefit would be increased coronary perfusion through vessel dilatation and an 'offloading' of the heart. This means that vasodilatation would reduce the blood returning to the heart, thus reducing the preload, with the consequent reduction in workload diminishing myocardial oxygen demand. This may ultimately improve contractility and cardiac function.

Hastillo 1996). Adrenaline (epinephrine) may be used in lower doses (0.04–0.1 µg/kg/min) as it has a dilatory action, but in higher doses will again actively constrict peripheral vessels.

At this point it is worth mentioning that dopamine essentially behaves rather like two different drugs at its lower and higher dose ranges. At approximately 2.5 µg/kg/min it dilates the renal vasculature ('renal dopamine'), increasing blood flow and urinary output (Cuthbertson & Noble 1997). It may also decrease renal metabolism, through inhibition of the sodium–potassium pump, thereby decreasing the occurrence of acute tubular necrosis which is associated with poor glomerular oxygenation (Evans 1998). Dopamine may be of value in preventing acute renal failure (ARF) while attempts are made to augment and maintain the cardiac output. Recently, the role of renal dopamine has become questionable as studies are still required to determine whether ARF really is avoided by the use of this drug (Cuthbertson & Noble 1997, Evans 1998, Park 1997). There is also concern that deficits in

intravenous fluid filling may be masked by a forced diuresis. In addition, dopamine itself may have certain unwanted side-effects such as an impairment of the immune response (Cuthbertson & Noble 1997).

As discussed above, in higher doses an inotropic range is encountered with a somewhat problematic arterial and vasoconstriction. Certainly as an inotrope, dopamine is perhaps best reserved for low cardiac output–hypotensive states. Chapter 19 explores inotropes in more detail but Table 18.1 offers an overview of the main properties. Papers which explore the subject of inotropic support include Graver (1992), Singer (1993), Peppers (1995) and Evans (1998).

THE INTRA-AORTIC BALLOON PUMP

Figure 18.1 illustrates the placement of the intra-aortic balloon pump, the third principle. This is a left ventricular assist device, but more accurately it is a counterpulsation device assisting during the diastolic phase of the cardiac cycle. It consists of a helium-filled

Table 18.1 Main properties of the primary intravenous inotropes

Inotropic agent	β1 action	α1 action	Dopaminergic dilatory action
Adrenaline (epinephrine)	Potent increase in myocardial contractility	Strong arterial constriction in higher doses. Peripheral vasodilatation in lower doses	Can actively shunt blood away from renal vasculature
Noradrenaline (norepinephrine)	Increase in myocardial contractility, strong chronotropic effect, potent potential for arrhythmias	Potent arterial constriction. No peripheral vasodilatation	No effect
Dopamine	Increase in myocardial contractility in higher doses (see text), mild chronotropic effect, potential for arrhythmias	Mild to potent effects on arterial constriction depending on dose (see text). Some peripheral vasodilatation	Renal vasculature dilated in lower doses (see text)
Dobutamine	Increase in myocardial contractility, mild chronotropic response, mild arrhythmia potential (dose related)	Limited α effects. Mild vasodilatation	No effect

Milrinone (Primacor) is a phosphodiesterase inhibitor. It increases myocardial contraction, has little chronotropic effect, while supraventricular (narrow complex) tachycardia and ventricular arrhythmias have been reported during use. Vasodilatation is generally greater than with dobutamine.

balloon placed, in theatre or under sterile conditions, into the descending femoral artery. The balloon sits just below the aortic arch. The device has its own ECG leads which are securely attached to the patient. It is usually the R-wave of the ECG complex which triggers the balloon to rapidly inflate and deflate within each cardiac cycle (Quaal 1984).

Following left ventricular ejection and during diastole, the balloon rapidly inflates just after the aortic valve has snapped shut (counterpulsation). This is signified by the dicrotic notch on the arterial trace (Fig. 18.2). Blood ejected into the aorta from the previous ventricular ejection is therefore rapidly dispersed, as the balloon inflates. This serves two purposes. First, oxygen-rich blood is dispersed upwards, around the coronary and cerebral arteries, increasing perfusion. Second, as the balloon rapidly deflates before the next ventricular ejection, the afterload is markedly decreased. The ventricle can then eject blood with much greater ease. These actions increase myocardial oxygen supply and, through afterload manipulation, also decrease the demand. This all aids effective cardiac output (Wojner 1994).

When fluid therapy is utilized, it is usual to reach the parameter limits before commencing inotropes. However, the IABP tends to be used in conjunction with inotropic therapy, rather than taking this form of pharmaceutical approach to the therapeutic limit. The two approaches are complementary. The device is not suitable for all patients and is contra-indicated where

marked aortic regurgitation or damage to the aorta, for example through aneurysm, is present (Hinds & Watson 1996). An IABP would seem an appropriate device for Fred Jones (Case study 18.2) until an improvement in the presenting clinical data.

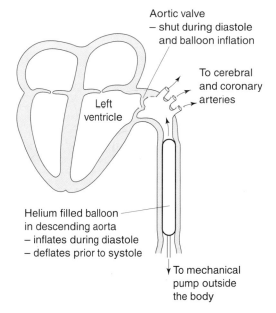

Figure 18.1 Placement of the intra-aortic balloon pump. (Reproduced with permission from Hatchett 1998.)

**Unassisted and assisted IABP
arterial waveform**

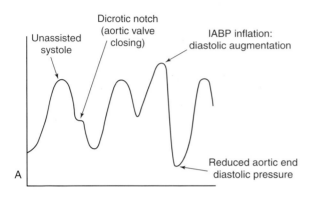

A

IABP Inflation

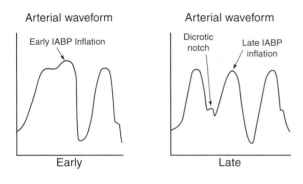

IABP Deflation

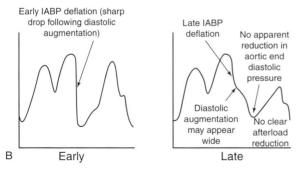

B

The timing on the ballon pump console can
be altered to rectify the above problems

Figure 18.2 Arterial waveform demonstrating (A) unassisted
and assisted waveform from the intra-aortic balloon pump and
(B) late and early inflation and deflation. There is a need to
adjust the timing of the balloon on the machine's console by
observing the arterial trace so that inflation occurs just after
the aortic valve has shut (the dicrotic notch), while deflation
occurs before the next ventricular ejection of blood (systole).

THE VENTRICULAR ASSIST DEVICES

If the patient deteriorates to a condition which is unresponsive to drug therapy and the use of short-term
mechanical support, such as the IABP, further mechanical assistance may be required. The broad aim of all the
ventricular assist devices (VADs) is to sustain
systemic circulation, eliminate left ventricular wall
tension (thereby reducing oxygen demand), increase
coronary perfusion and enhance right ventricular function. This is indicated for those in severe cardiac failure
resulting from a reduction in myocardial contractility,
secondary to ischaemic or myopathic heart disease.

The devices currently available for offering such
support can be classified in three ways.

- Extracorporeal or inplantable devices
- Univentricular or biventricular support
- Via the type of device mechanism and its function

In general the extracorporeal systems are used for
shorter periods of support than the implantable
systems, which may be used for medium and long-
term use (Barron & Pepper 1998).

Extracorporeal devices

Extracorporeal or external devices consist of a blood
pump that is placed outside the body, with the inflow
cannula draining blood from the patient to the pump,
while the outflow cannula drains blood back from the
pump to the patient. Both the inflow and the outflow
cannulae have to exit through the patient's skin.
Extracorporeal devices can create pulsatile or non-
pulsatile flow.

First-generation centrifugal vortex pumps such as the
Bio-Medicus (Bio-Medicus Inc, Eden Prairie, MN) are
still being used today. These VADs were designed for
use after cardiotomy and are utilized for their simplicity,
accessibility and relative ease of applicability. Centrifugal pumps provide a non-pulsatile flow generated
from the centrifugal force created by the electrically
powered magnetic impeller. Complications associated
with centrifugal pumps are bleeding, sepsis and
thrombo-embolism. Centrifugal pumps can be used for
7–10 days and can support the right and left ventricle.

Pulsatile flow is created by blood pumps that are
pneumatic, pulsatile devices. They generally comprise
an inflow cannula from either the left atrial appendage
or left ventricular apex to the blood pump and an
outflow cannula from the blood pump to the aorta,
and a drive console to provide the pneumatic power. If
the patient also requires right heart support to create a
biventricular system (BIVAD), cannulation of the right

atrium and pulmonary artery is also required (Reedy 1993). As these pumps are extracorporeal, either placed on the skin surface of the abdominal wall (such as the Thoratec device: see Fig. 18.3) or mounted at the side of the patient's bed (such as the ABIOMED BVS® 5000), mobility is quite severely restricted. The Berlin Heart, designed by Hetzer and colleagues in Europe, can be used as a biventricular or ventricular assist device. It allows for mobility and has also been scaled down for paediatric use (Stiller et al 1998).

Implantable/internal devices

With implantable or internal devices the blood pump and the inflow and outflow cannulae to the pump are placed within the body. A driveline that carries the power and/or the pneumatic line exits through the

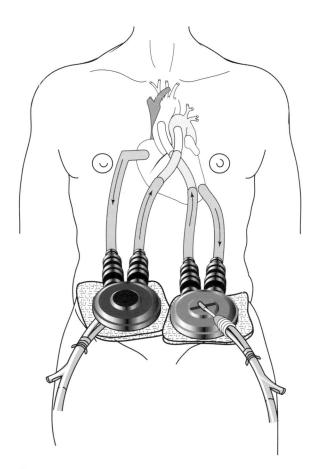

Figure 18.3 The Thoratec pneumatic biventricular assist device. (Reproduced with permission of Mosby Inc from Ready JE 1993 Heart & Lung 22(1): 72.)

skin. Internal devices can create pulsatile or non-pulsatile flow.

The Hemopump® is a temporary device able to provide ventricular support without major surgical intervention. It is usually inserted via the femoral artery, retrogradely through the aortic valve, into the left ventricle. It may also be inserted via a sternotomy incision. It is based on the principle of the Archimedes screw, in the form of a miniaturized axial flow pump. This sits in the left ventricle where the rotating head is able to provide up to 4.7 l/min of non-pulsatile flow. This is without the need for synchronization, or any contribution, from the left ventricle (Wampler et al 1991).

Among the currently available implantable systems for long-term support of the left ventricle are the Novacor pump (Baxter Healthcare Corporation, Oakland, CA) and the HeartMate (Thermo Cardiosystems Inc, Woburn, MA). Both are pusher plate devices and have been successfully used as a bridge to transplantation and more recently as a bridge to recovery (Mann & Willerson 1998). The pump is usually placed within the abdominal cavity with external connection to a power source and a vent to allow air displacement as the pump diaphragm moves.

The Novacor system (Fig. 18.4) is an electrically powered blood pump with a dual pusher plate system (Pennington et al 1995). The two plates are brought together by magnets which propel blood out of a smooth polyurethane blood sac, whilst bovine pericardial valves encourage unidirectional flow. The pump has a maximum stroke volume of 70 ml and can pump in excess of 10 l/min. The electric driveline connects from the pump to a portable controller and battery system and is able to operate in 'fill-to-empty', 'ECG synchronous' and 'fixed rate' modes. The patient is anticoagulated with warfarin and aspirin to minimize thrombo-embolic problems from the inflow conduit and the smooth polyurethane sac (Westaby & Katsumata 1997).

The HeartMate also consists of an implantable pusher plate blood pump. However, the blood sac interior surface has a textured blood-contacting surface of sintered titanium as it is believed that this promotes a pseudo-neointimal lining, negating the need for anticoagulation. Porcine valves are present on the inflow and outflow tract to provide unidirectional flow. It has a maximum stroke volume of 83 ml with a pump output of up to 11 l/min. As with the Novacor pump, the HeartMate operates in two different modes, 'fixed rate' and 'auto' mode which relies on venous drainage, enabling it to follow normal physiology. The pump ejects when it reaches 90% filling and the rate is altered automatically with activity. The HeartMate can

Implantable centrifugal pumps are under development with the AB-180 (Cardiac Assist Technologies Inc, Pittsburgh, PA) serving as an example. This device is small in size and weight with a very small blood contact surface area that requires no systemic anti-coagulation with heparin.

More recently, the Jarvik 2000 Heart has been developed. This is an intraventricular axial impeller pump which weighs only 85 g and is thumb size. It is implanted into the left ventricular apex of the failing heart, is totally silent and can provide a cardiac output of up to 10 l/min at a mean aortic pressure of >80 mmHg (Fig. 18.5). Blood entering the left ventricle is withdrawn via a Dacron graft to the descending aorta whilst normal physiological blood flow in and out of the heart is allowed to continue. The pump offloads the heart (essentially reducing the preload and high filling pressures) and adjustable flow allows the heart to provide a proportion of the cardiac output

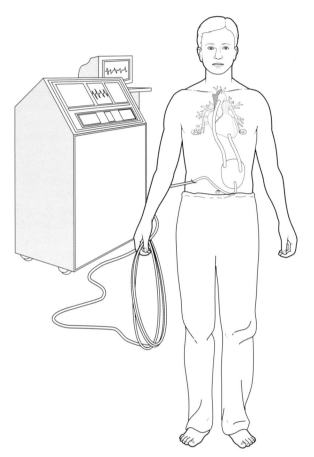

Figure 18.4 The Novacor electrical left ventricular assist device. (Reproduced with permission of Mosby Inc from Ready JE 1993 Heart & Lung 22(1): 72.)

be driven by either air or electricity. The vented electrical system uses a low-speed motor to drive the pusher plate. In the newer model, the electric driveline and vent, which allows air to transfer in and out of the motor chamber, are combined with the power source generated from a portable battery pack or bedside console (Poirier 1997).

Currently, researchers have not yet developed a clinically acceptable, implantable compliance chamber that can be wholly encompassed in the human body. Consequently, the current pulsatile pumps must still be vented externally. These devices also still require a transcutaneous power line. The successful development of a cardiac assist device which could be completely intracorporeal with the use of transcutaneous power would enhance their usage greatly as complications from infection should be reduced.

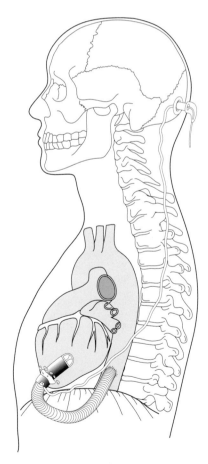

Figure 18.5 The Jarvik 2000 impeller pump. (Reproduced with permission from Mosby Year Book Inc.)

and pulsatility (Westaby & Katsumata 1997). There are several other implantable axial flow impeller pumps available, such as the Baylor (NASA) and the Nimbus (Pittsburgh).

The pump rotates at between 8000 and 12 000 rpm maintaining flows with a range of 1–10 l/min. This high flow stream of blood reduces the potential for thrombus formation and haemolysis (Westaby et al 1997).

As with previous devices, a fully implantable system with a transcutaneous power source will not be realized for some time. However, in Oxford an innovative system has been developed using a skull-mounted percutaneous titanium pedestal to transmit the power line. This aims to avoid driveline infections along with other surface infections, as similarly placed cochlear implants have been shown to resist infection for more than 15 years (Westaby et al 1997).

For those patients who are unsuitable for transplantation and left ventricular assist, a total artificial heart (TAH) may be the final answer. With this system the heart is completely excised and replaced orthotopically with a biventricular mechanical pump, which is anastomosed to the great vessels. As yet, the development of such a device has proved difficult for researchers in this field.

Probably the best known TAH is the CardioWest Heart (Jarvik 7 TAH) which, when implanted for permanent use in the 1980s, produced encouraging haemodynamic results, but thrombo-embolism and infection were serious problems. With technological improvements, the previously encountered neurological and bleeding complications were significantly reduced and the pump was subsequently used as a bridge to transplantation in biventricular failure

(Copeland et al 1986). There are several other TAHs that have been used such as the Akutsu, the Liotta, the Utah and Phoenix. More recently, three other devices have undergone evaluation: The AbioCor™ Implantable Replacement Heart (ABIOMED) at the Texas Heart Institute; the Nimbus Heart at the Cleveland Clinic; and the Sarns/3M Health Care Heart at Pennsylvania State University.

Indications for use

The decision to institute mechanical circulatory assist is based on evidence of deteriorating end-organ function, despite maximal pharmacological therapy and/or IABP support. The broad group of patients who require VADs are generally those who cannot be weaned from cardiopulmonary bypass and those with established heart failure either as a result of chronic cardiomyopathy or massive acute myocardial infarction. The general indications and haemodynamic criteria for the application of circulatory assist devices are summarized in Box 18.1. Patient selection is the most important determinant of success with the use of VADs, therefore there are many contra-indications to be considered before implant. These are shown in Box 18.2 and are very similar to those routinely followed for cardiac transplantation.

Specific nursing care for patients with ventricular assist devices

The nursing care of a patient with a VAD has fundamental similarities to the needs of any other critically ill patients. However, there are also many specific needs

---

Box 18.1 General indications for the use of VADs in acute, chronic or biventricular failure

Indications

- Acute myocardial ischaemia or infarction in patients with coronary artery disease, e.g. post-ischaemic stunned myocardium, myocardial infarction, viral myocarditis or protozoal infections

- Left ventricular or biventricular failure with failure to wean from cardiopulmonary bypass after technically successful cardiac surgery

- Primary myocardial disorders leading to chronic congestive heart failure, e.g. chronic ischaemic cardiomyopathy, idiopathic dilated cardiomyopathy and myocarditis

Haemodynamic indications

- Cardiac index <2.0 l/min/m^2

- Systolic blood pressure <90 mmHg

- Systemic vascular resistance >2100 dyne/s/cm^{-5}

- Pulmonary capillary (occlusion) wedge pressure LVAD, right atrial pressure (RVAD) or both (BIVAD) >20–25 mmHg

- Urine output <20 ml/h

Indications for use will usually be dictated by a combination of the above, along with individual assessment

---

Box 18.2 General contra-indications for VADs

- Septicaemia or other systemic infection
- Chronic renal failure
- Severe liver dysfunction with coagulopathy, cirrhosis or portal hypertension
- Evidence of malignant disease
- History of thrombo-embolic events
- Fixed pulmonary hypertension
- Chronic obstructive pulmonary disease (COPD) or severe emphysema
- Active peptic ulcer disease
- Contra-indications to anticoagulation therapy
- Severe peripheral vascular disease or cerebral vascular disease
- Implanted mechanical heart valve – thrombus formation on the valve or mechanical failure of the valve can occur with the VAD. Thrombus formation is more likely to occur with the aortic valve, because it will not open adequately if the left ventricle is fully offloaded by the device
- Ventricular/atrial septal defect
- Morbid obesity
- Drug or alcohol addiction
- Inadequate psychosocial support
- Presence of other conditions that might limit long-term survival
- High probability of patient non-compliance, e.g. taking anticoagulation, caring for the battery life, etc.
- Blood dyscrasia

---

to focus upon. The critical care nurse, in collaboration with the surgeons, physicians, perfusionists and other members of the multidisciplinary team, has a challenging role in the care of these patients. The number who receive assist devices at any designated hospital tends to be quite small. Consequently it is important that the team is composed of members used to managing this type of patient. The main priorities of care are continuous haemodynamic monitoring and observing for and preventing potential complications.

The nurse continually assesses the patient's response to the VAD flow by monitoring arterial pressure, CVP and cardiac output studies, which are performed using a pulmonary artery (PA) flotation catheter for the LVAD patient. Continuous cardiac output monitoring can be used but it is inaccurate for the right ventricular assist device (RVAD) patient, as blood flow is being diverted from the right ventricle. Here the Fick principle may be used to determine the cardiac output. This calculates the cardiac output via a formula utilizing direct measurement of arterial oxygen content, mixed venous oxygen content and the consumption of oxygen by the body (VO_2). Alternatively, the majority of the pumps have a constant, digitally displayed cardiac output figure.

Most pumps are able to deliver 5–6 l/min, although the aim is usually 2–4 l/min. To maximize flow and prevent atrial collapse around the cannula, it is essential that the patient's circulating volume is optimized. Therefore, an essential nursing intervention is to redress any volume imbalance adequately without creating fluid overload. As highlighted, the CVP and other indicators of filling pressure are vitally important in this monitoring process. The VAD patient is likely to be receiving inotrope and vasodilatory support and will require close monitoring and titration of these drugs, particularly once the device is functioning. This is because the drugs can usually be reduced when the pump is operational.

Bleeding is a common complication with VAD patients. This is thought to be related to a combination of the prolonged cardiopulmonary bypass, the need for anticoagulation and the multiple cannulation sites (Coombs 1993). The intensive care nurse is able to observe for potential bleeding by close monitoring of the chest and abdominal (pump site) tube drainage and the presence of blood loss from cannulation sites and incisions.

Regular assessment of the serum coagulation studies is performed to observe for prolonged coagulation rates and reduced haemoglobin/ haematocrit and platelet levels. However, protocol and device requirements will vary. A continuous and adequate stock of blood, clotting factors and platelets is needed and the nurse responsible must be aware of the availability of blood and blood products (Coombs 1993).

Cardiac tamponade may also occur as a result of excessive bleeding. It is important for the nurse to recognize the signs at an early stage and instigate appropriate treatment. The signs, which are well described throughout this book, include a tachycardia, rising atrial and pulmonary pressures with a reduction in the MAP and cardiac/pump output (the VAD filling is impeded). This will be followed by a marked haemodynamic improvement once the chest is reopened and the collected blood is evacuated. Inevitably, there is a fine line to be maintained between excessive bleeding and thrombus formation. Because of the risk of micro-emboli travelling to major organs and causing infarction, anticoagulation therapy is important. The nurse should maintain a close assessment of the patient's peripheral perfusion and neurological and respiratory status, changes in which may indicate that a thrombo-embolic event has occurred. Anticoagulation therapy usually commences with an intravenous infusion of heparin or low molecular weight dextran. This is followed by either aspirin and dipyridamole or warfarin.

However, some of the VADs utilize textured linings which allow a pseudo-neointimal lining to form, which has been found to decrease the risk of thrombus formation (Poirier 1997). This reduces the need for anticoagulation therapy.

Infection continues to be the most common complication related to long-term VAD therapy. Effective treatment is difficult and without early transplantation, mortality may be high. Therefore, if the infection persists despite maximal antibiotic therapy, it may be necessary to remove the device or an infected bioprosthetic valve to eradicate it (Massad & McCarthy 1997). Infection may occur at the sternal site, the pump pocket and the driveline site. The latter connects the patient with the external power supply. A strict aseptic technique is of paramount importance in wound care. Daily wound dressings are required in line with individual

unit protocols. This allows regular observation of sites for signs of infection. Prophylactic antibiotic therapy is utilized. The nurse needs to monitor chest and pump pocket drainage and send samples for culture and sensitivity as required. Any signs and symptoms of infection should be reported, such as a raised white cell count, elevating temperature and redness, swelling and exudate at any site (English 1989).

Dysrhythmias may be a potential problem. Patients supported by the VAD actually tolerate ventricular tachycardia/fibrillation very well. However, it is necessary to treat prolonged episodes, because there may be a risk of clot formation in the native ventricular chambers and pump. Patients on BIVAD therapy can maintain near normal parameters during dysrhythmic or asystolic episodes. Should cardiac arrest occur, cardiac compressions are not recommended as there is

---

Case study 18.3

Peter Jones, a 27-year-old, 70 kg male was admitted to the coronary care unit (CCU) with progressive left ventricular failure. A central line was inserted and an echocardiogram performed. Reassurance and explanation regarding all that was occurring were offered to Mr Jones and his parents, who had arrived with him at the hospital. The echo revealed a grossly dilated and hypokinetic left ventricle. An initial assessment and clinical observations revealed:

- skin pale and clammy to touch
- respiratory rate 32/min
- heart rate 125 bpm
- blood pressure 85/45 mmHg
- CVP 16 mmHg
- urine output 20 ml/h.

An initial diagnosis of acute left ventricular failure was made. The above observations appeared to reflect poor tissue perfusion due to reduced myocardial contractility. Therefore, a PA catheter was inserted shortly afterwards, enabling a closer observation of Mr Jones' left ventricular function. The results were as follows.

- Pulmonary artery pressure (PAP) 44/28 mmHg
- Pulmonary capillary wedge pressure (PCWP) 27 mmHg
- Cardiac output (CO) 3.2 l/min.
- Cardiac index (CI) 2.1 l/min/m^2
- SVR 1900 dynes/sec/cm^{-5}

These results provided further indication that Mr Jones was unable to support his own circulating volume due to the ineffectiveness of his myocardial function. Clearly, assistance to improve the cardiac output was required.

Following transfer to the intensive care unit, inotropic support was introduced, a urinary catheter was passed to more accurately monitor the urinary output and an IABP was inserted. Intravenous fluid therapy was positively avoided.

The cardiac output improved slightly to 3.35 l/min but he began to have sustained runs of ventricular

tachycardia (VT) coupled with a renewed deterioration in his cardiac output. Amiodarone was added, improving the dysrhythmias but not improving the cardiac output. Despite intravenous dobutamine, dopamine utilized at a low renal dilatory dose, fluid restriction and diuretics, Mr Jones' arterial blood gases were deteriorating due to increasing pulmonary oedema. A repeat echo confirmed that there was no improvement in ventricular function and the latest PA catheter measurements revealed:

- PAP 55/30 mmHg
- PCWP 29 mmHg
- CO 3.1 l/min
- CI 2.0 l/min/m^2
- SVR 2100 dynes/sec/cm^{-5}

Mr Jones was referred to the cardiac transplant team for emergency transplantation. After discussion, they decided to opt for an LVAD implant as early organ availability could not be relied upon and the patient was deteriorating to the point where he may not survive to transplantation. Surgery to implant the device went smoothly and he was admitted to cardiac surgical intensive care for postoperative management. He was extubated on the first postoperative day, requiring only 40% inspired oxygen via the face mask with excellent arterial blood gas results. Chest and abdominal drainage was minimal, allowing the chest drains to be removed after 48 hours. All inotropic support was discontinued by day 3, leaving only intravenous dopamine at a renal dilatory dose in progress. Haemodynamically, Mr Jones was now able to maintain a systolic blood pressure of 110 mmHg, generating much improved renal and tissue perfusion. On day 3 he began taking diet and fluids and to mobilize around the bed area. By day 5 Mr Jones was transferred to the ward where he stayed for a further 48 hours, when a suitable organ became available. He finally returned to theatre for a successful cardiac transplant and continued to make a steady, but uneventful postoperative recovery.

the potential to dislodge the cannula. If external defibrillation is required standard techniques may be used (Coombs 1993).

As previously mentioned, other nursing issues are very similar to those which relate to critically ill patients. However, there may be additional psychological issues because the VAD patient and family/carers are likely to have many emotive concerns that need to be addressed. The insertion of an 'artificial heart' and being so near to death can precipitate many crises for the patient and those significant to them. The nurse and the rest of the health-care team can provide education regarding the various procedures occurring and the equipment in use, with constant updates about the patient's condition. This will serve to promote early emotional and psychological adaptation (Lewandowski 1995). It is important also to remember the education and orientation of staff who are new to nursing patients with these devices. The concept of a conscious patient who is pulseless with a non-recordable blood pressure, due to the non-pulsatile nature of some devices, requires adjustment for both patient and health-care team members new to the procedure. Technically, the nurse has to re-examine how adequate tissue perfusion is assessed and recognize that an undulating arterial trace, if this is monitored, may be acceptable with the non-pulsatile device and not indicative of inaccurate monitoring or a dampened trace. When the assistance the device is offering is reduced, if this is the clinical plan, then a more familiar arterial pattern and blood pressure will return.

The weaning process

Long-term VAD therapy as a bridge to transplantation has led to the crucial discovery that in some patients it allows for myocardial recovery. Levin et al (1995) reported that after prolonged support it was apparent that some of the native hearts with end-stage dilated cardiomyopathy had reverted to normal size and weight. This has meant that rather than the pump being explanted at the time of transplantation, there has arisen the potential for the pump to be weaned to removal, without a subsequent transplant.

The nurse will become involved in this weaning process, which would normally take place gradually when there is suspected ventricular improvement, inotropic support is minimal and there is haemodynamic stability. The process itself varies according to which pump is being used, although the principle remains the same. The pump assistance is withdrawn gradually, allowing the native heart to take over, increasing the levels of the cardiac workload. Throughout the weaning process various studies are performed to monitor the state of myocardial function. These will include cardiac output studies and transthoracic/oesophageal echocardiography, some of which are performed with the pump switched off for short periods.

CONCLUSION

This chapter has taken a pragmatic approach to the manipulation of haemodynamics to augment the cardiac output. A three-stage approach is suggested. The early section focused upon the use of intravenous fluids to passively stretch the myocardium, when monitored filling pressures allow this, utilizing the principle of Starling's Law of the heart to augment the preload. Inotropes, chemical agents that stimulate myocardial contractility, can be introduced when maximal fluid therapy does not improve tissue perfusion or fluids are contraindicated, as in case studies 18.2 and 18.3. The intra-aortic balloon pump augments tissue perfusion by providing counterpulsation, displacing aortic blood during diastole.

The final section examined the variety of ventricular assist devices being developed and the hope for an artificial heart housed totally within the body. The finding that a heart which has developed cardiomyopathy, when totally rested by utilization of the ventricular assist device, may in fact not require transplantation is of enormous value for the use of these devices. As noted in Chapter 5, it is important to emphasize the value of understanding how monitored pressures and clinical assessment can guide the indication for and use of each of the three processes to augment tissue perfusion.

REFERENCES

Barron D, Pepper J 1998 Mechanical circulatory support. British Journal of Cardiology 5(3): 140–148

Coombs M 1993 Ventricular assist devices for the failing heart: a nursing focus. Intensive and Critical Care Nursing 9: 17–23

Copeland JG, Levinson MM, Smith R et al 1986 The total artificial heart as bridge to transplantation: a report of two cases. Journal of the American Medical Association 256(21): 2991–2995

Cuthbertson BH, Noble DW 1997 Dopamine in oliguria. British Medical Journal 314: 690–691

English MA 1989 Preventing complications of ventricular assist devices. Dimensions of Critical Care Nursing 8: 330–336

Evans D 1998 Inotropic therapy – current controversies and future directions. Nursing in Critical Care 3(1): 8–11

Graver J 1992 Inotropes – an overview. Intensive and Critical Care Nursing 8: 169–179

Hatchett R 1998 The principles of augmenting the cardiac output in adults. Intensive and Critical Care Nursing 14(5): 244–251

Hinds CJ, Watson D 1996 Intensive care: a concise textbook, 2nd edn. WB Saunders, London

Isbister JP 1997 Blood transfusion. In: Oh TE (ed) Intensive care manual, 4th edn. Butterworth Heinemann, London, pp. 741–753

Levin HR, Oz MC, Chen JM, Packer M, Rose EA, Burkhoff D 1995 Reversal of chronic ventricular dilatation in patients with end stage cardiomyopathy by prolonged mechanical offloading. Circulation 91: 2717–2720

Lewandowski AV 1995 The bridge to cardiac transplantation: ventricular assist devices. Advanced Technology 14(1): 17–25

Mann DL, Willerson MD 1998 Left ventricular assist devices and the failing heart. A bridge to recovery, a permanent assist device or a bridge too far? Circulation 98: 2367–2369

Massad MG, McCarthy PM 1997 Will permanent LVADs be better than heart transplantation? European Journal of Cardio-thoracic Surgery 11 (suppl): S11–17

McCarthy T, Wheeldon D 1991 Towards an artificial heart: medium-to long term cardiopulmonary support devices. Hospimedica 10: 44–50

Park G 1997 Controlled trials in the critically ill. Care of the Critically Ill 13(1): 6

Pennington DG, Portner PM, Swartz MT 1995 Clinical experience with the Novacor left ventricular assist system. In: Lewis T, Graham TR (eds) Mechanical circulatory support. Edward Arnold, London, pp. 225–226

Peppers M 1995 Inotropes for heart failure. Emergency 27(7): 18–25

Poirier VL 1997 The HeartMate left ventricular assist system: worldwide clinical results. European Journal of Cardio-thoracic Surgery 11 (suppl): S39–44

Quaal SJ 1984 Comprehensive intra-aortic balloon pumping. CV Mosby, St Louis

Reedy JE 1993 Transfer of a patient with a ventricular assist device to a non-critical care area. Heart and Lung 22: 71–76

Shipley JB, Hastillo A 1996 Review: Milrinone: basic and clinical pharmacology and acute and chronic management. American Journal of the Medical Sciences 311(6): 286–291

Singer M 1993 The management of acute heart failure – an iconoclastic view. Care of the Critically Ill 9(1): 11–16

Stiller B, Dähnert I, Weng YG, Hennig E, Hetzer R, Lange PE 1998 Children may survive severe myocarditis with prolonged use of biventricular assist devices. Heart 82: 237–240

Wampler RK, Frazier OH, Lansing AM et al 1991 Treatment of cardiogenic shock with the Hemopump left ventricular assist device. Annals of Thoracic Surgery 52(3): 506–513

Westaby S, Katsumata T 1997 Long-term implantable circulatory support. British Journal of Hospital Medicine 57(7): 333–338

Westaby S, Katsumata T, Evans R, Pigott D, Taggart D, Jarvik RK 1997 The Jarvik 2000 Oxford system: increasing the scope of mechanical circulatory support. Journal of Thoracic and Cardiovascular Surgery 114: 1–8

Wojner AW 1994 Assessing the five points of the intra-aortic balloon pump waveform. Critical Care Nurse 14(3): 48–52

The pharmacological management of the cardiac patient

Prashant Sanghani
Lynda Filer

In recent years deaths rates from coronary heart disease (CHD) have been declining but it persists as the most common cause of premature death in the United Kingdom (UK). Twenty-six percent of premature deaths in men and 16% in women are caused by CHD (BHF 2000) and it remains an incurable and progressive disease. The use of drugs therefore offers an opportunity to ameliorate symptoms, assist in secondary prevention and in some cases reduce the risk of death. For example, there is good evidence that the use of β-blockers is associated with a reduction in morbidity and mortality following myocardial infarction (Freemantle et al 1999, Owen 1998).

Some pharmacological agents do add years to life but the vast majority improve the quality of the remaining years. In conjunction with surgical techniques, pharmacology still offers our greatest weapon in fighting the disease in those where it has already developed. The aim of this overview chapter is to demonstrate how one drug can be chosen on a rational basis in the treatment of cardiac-associated conditions. An example of this would be making the most appropriate choice from the many β-blockers currently licensed for use within the UK.

This question of choice is easy to answer when there are large randomized controlled trials demonstrating positive clinical outcomes for an individual drug or combination of drugs. However, as more evidence is collated, there seems to be little difference in the actions of drugs within the same group. The only difference appears to be in the commencing and maintenance doses of these agents. This is the case for β-blockers, angiotensin-converting enzyme (ACE) inhibitors and most recently the statins.

When a beneficial class effect is recognized, how should a choice be made of one individual agent over another? This chapter will specifically highlight clinically significant pharmacological (receptor level), biopharmaceutical (absorption, distribution, metabolism and elimination) and pharmaceutical (dose form and formulation) differences between agents in the same class.

Although this chapter will not discuss general pharmacology in depth, each section begins with a brief description of the uses of the agent(s) and is followed by the differential pharmacology, biopharmaceutical and pharmaceutical properties.

The bases of the sections are derived from the British National Formulary (BNF) which is released on a 6-monthly publication cycle by the British Medical Association and the Royal Pharmaceutical Society of Great Britain. Only the agents considered less suitable for prescribing are omitted here; that is, those agents which are not considered a first choice, although their use may be justified in certain circumstances.

The drug classes discussed are:

- positive inotropic agents
- sympathomimetics
- vasodilator antihypertensive agents
- centrally acting antihypertensive agents
- diuretics
- anti-arrhythmic agents
- β-blockers
- drugs affecting the renin–angiotensin system
- nitrates
- calcium channel blockers
- anticoagulants: heparin, including low molecular weight heparins
- antiplatelet agents
- thrombolytic agents
- lipid-regulating agents.

POSITIVE INOTROPIC AGENTS

- Cardiac glycosides
- Phosphodiesterase inhibitors

Cardiac glycosides

Currently licensed in the UK: digoxin and digitoxin.

Uses

Cardiac glycosides provide inotropic support, thereby increasing the force of myocardial contraction. They also possess negative chronotropic activity (reducing the heart rate) via a reduction of conductivity within the atrioventricular (AV) node. As a result, digoxin and digitoxin are typically used as adjunct therapy to diuretics and ACE inhibitors in heart failure and for ventricular rate control in chronic atrial fibrillation.

Differential pharmacology

Digitoxin, which is rarely used clinically in the UK, undergoes hepatic transformation to digoxin. Thus, the two agents have the same pharmacological action.

At the molecular level they both inhibit myocardial sodium/potassium adenosine triphosphate (ATP)ase. Often written as $Na^+/K^+ATPase$, this is an enzyme that is involved in maintaining the resting membrane potential by providing the energy to pump sodium (Na^+) ions out and potassium (K^+) ions into the cell. A pump is required as these ions are moving against their concentration gradient. The result of inhibiting this enzyme is an increase in intracellular sodium ions. This then leads to the inhibition of the sodium/calcium (Na^+/Ca^{2+}) exchanger.

The Na^+/Ca^{2+} exchanger is also a membrane-bound pumping system but it aids the movement of Na^+ ions into the cell in exchange for pumping calcium (Ca^{2+}) ions out. Therefore no calcium is pumped out, leading to an increase in this intracellular ion. This increase in calcium allows for increased actin–myosin interaction within cardiac myocytes, leading to an increased force of contraction (positive inotropic effect). The negative chronotropic effect of this group of drugs occurs through an increase in the vagal tone to the heart; vagus nerve stimulation slows the heart rate.

Of clinical significance for both agents is the need to avoid hypokalaemia (low serum potassium levels), hypomagnesaemia and hypercalcaemia during use as these predispose the myocardium to increased cardiac glycoside effect, resulting in toxicity. Conversely, hyperkalaemia can render the myocardium relatively resistant to the pharmacological effects. The clinically significant differences between these agents lie in their biopharmaceutical properties.

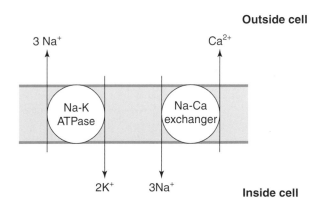

Figure 19.1 Cellular mechanism for cardiac glycosides.

Differential biopharmaceutical properties

Digoxin has poor oral bio-availability and is also metabolized to inactive metabolites by *Eubacterium lentum*, an enteric bacterium present in approximately 10% of the general population. Digoxin has a narrow therapeutic window and is primarily cleared renally, making dosage adjustment in renal impairment critical.

Digitoxin, however, is completely absorbed and its dosing is unaffected by renal function. Therefore, there is no need to reduce the dose in renal failure. However, the drug is rarely used in this situation.

Both agents have long half-lives, making them suitable for once-a-day dosing but also necessitating the use of loading doses if therapeutic effects are required urgently. The half-life is the time taken for the concentration of a drug to decrease by half. This is primarily influenced by elimination through the renal system.

Differential pharmaceutical properties

Digoxin is available as tablets, elixir and injection. Digitoxin is available as tablets only.

Phosphodiesterase inhibitors

Currently licensed in the UK: enoximone and milrinone (Primacor).

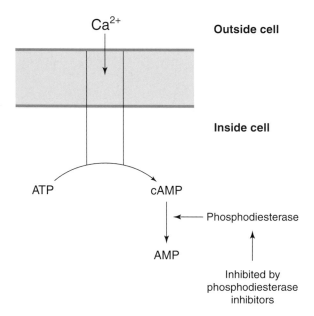

Figure 19.2 Phosphodiesterase inhibition.

Uses

When used in acute cardiac failure, enoximone and milrinone increase the cardiac output. They also reduce the pulmonary capillary occlusion (wedge) pressure (measured via a pulmonary artery (PA) catheter) and the peripheral vascular resistance. However, there is little evidence of mortality reduction.

Differential pharmacology

Both of these agents are relatively specific inhibitors for phosphodiesterase isoenzyme III (compared with the non-specific xanthines, theophylline and caffeine) and there is little to differentiate them.

Phosphodiesterase inhibitors increase cardiac output by increasing cardiac muscle contraction. This is achieved by increasing intracellular calcium levels through the opening of calcium channels that allows the ion outside to enter the cell. The opening of these channels is stimulated by a product of ATP, called cAMP (cyclic adenosine monophosphate). cAMP is then converted to AMP by phosphodiesterase enzymes. If these enzymes are blocked by phosphodiesterase inhibitors, then cAMP is not broken down, the calcium channels are stimulated and more calcium enters the cell (Fig. 19.2).

Differential biopharmaceutical properties

None.

Differential pharmaceutical properties

Enoximone must be administered using plastic apparatus as the use of glass encourages crystal formation.

SYMPATHOMIMETICS

- Inotropic sympathomimetics
- Vasoconstrictor sympathomimetics

Inotropic sympathomimetics

Currently licensed in the UK: dopamine, dobutamine, dopexamine and isoprenaline.

Uses

Dobutamine and dopamine act on the cardiac muscle and increase contractility with little effect on the heart rate. Dopexamine also provides a positive inotropic effect but also increases renal perfusion by causing vasodilatation. Isoprenaline increases both

Table 19.1 Main properties of the primary intravenous inotropes

Inotropic agent	β1 action	α1 action	Dopaminergic dilatory action
Adrenaline (epinephrine)	Potent increase in myocardial contractility	Strong arterial constriction in higher doses. Peripheral vasodilatation in lower doses	Can actively shunt blood away from renal vasculature
Noradrenaline (norepinephrine)	Increase in myocardial contractility, strong chronotropic effect, potent potential for arrhythmias	Potent arterial constriction. No peripheral vasodilatation	No effect
Dopamine	Increase in myocardial contractility in higher doses (see text), mild chronotropic effect, potential for arrhythmias	Mild to potent effects on arterial constriction depending on dose (see text). Some peripheral vasodilatation	Renal vasculature dilated in lower doses (see text)
Dobutamine	Increase in myocardial contractility, mild chronotropic response, mild arrhythmia potential (dose related)	Limited α effects. Mild vasodilatation	No effect

Milrinone (Primacor) is a phosphodiesterase inhibitor. It increases myocardial contraction, has little chronotropic effect, while supraventricular (narrow complex) tachycardia and ventricular arrhythmias have been reported during use. Vasodilatation is generally greater than with dobutamine.

heart rate and contractility and is now only used as an emergency treatment of heart block or severe bradycardia.

Depending on the haemodynamic status, the profound hypotension of cardiogenic shock and the subsequent poor cardiac output may be improved by the use of adrenaline (epinephrine), dobutamine or dopamine (see Table 19.1). In septic shock and the systemic inflammatory response syndrome (SIRS), the latter mimicking the former but where initially no septic focus can be isolated, fluid replacement and inotropic support may fail to maintain the blood pressure and consequently noradrenaline (norepinephrine) may be used.

Differential pharmacology

At low infusion rates (<5 μg/kg/min) the main action of dopamine is exerted via D1 dopaminergic receptors, resulting in an increased renal perfusion by dilating the renal vasculature, subsequently increasing the glomerular filtration and sodium (Na^+) excretion. Consequently, it is used in the management of cardiogenic and hypovolaemic shock to encourage a diuresis and protect the kidneys starved of an adequate blood flow. More recently, there has been some controversy regarding the use of this lower 'renal dose' of dopamine (Cuthbertson & Noble 1997, Evans 1998). This indicates a need for

research to confirm that acute renal failure can be avoided by the use of this drug. Some centres now advocate correcting the patient's blood pressure to pre-shock levels as a method of ensuring sufficient renal perfusion.

Infusion rates of 5–10 μg/kg/min act almost like another drug, stimulating β1-receptors in two ways: directly stimulating the receptors and also inducing noradrenaline (norepinephrine) release from nerve terminals, which then acts on β1-receptors. This increases the force of myocardial contraction and thus the cardiac output, without having a significant effect on the peripheral vascular resistance.

At rates higher than 10 μg/kg/min, the α-adrenergic receptors are the primary sites of stimulation (Graver 1992). There is therefore an increase in peripheral vasoconstriction and this can lead to an exacerbation of cardiac failure. Due to the increase in peripheral vasoconstriction, inotropic dopamine, that is the higher dose range, is best reserved for patients exhibiting a low cardiac output and hypotensive state. There have been incidents where patients have experienced severe ischaemia in fingers and toes due to the vasoconstrictory effects.

Dobutamine used clinically consists of a racemic mixture that affects both α- and β-adrenergic receptors. A racemic mixture is a mixture of molecules (enantiomers) that can be built as mirror images but then possess different pharmacological properties.

The (−) enantiomer is an α1-agonist whilst the (+) enantiomer is an α1-antagonist. Both enantiomers are β1- and β2-agonists (with the (+) enantiomer about 10 times more potent). In clinical practice the effects of β stimulation are most clearly visible and displayed by positive inotropic effect and little chronotropic change. The lack of an increased afterload (resistance to ventricular ejection, usually caused by vessel constriction) when using dobutamine, which is a result of the agonist–antagonist α1 activity, makes it a better choice over dopamine in patients with acute cardiac failure who have not responded to oral vasodilators and diuretics. It does, however, mean that little change in the blood pressure may be noted but increased cardiac output will result in better tissue and organ perfusion. If there is need to elevate the blood pressure, dobutamine may not be the ideal choice. It is important to realize that a blood pressure within the normal range, perhaps augmented by vessel constriction, does not necessarily equate to an adequate cardiac output.

Dopexamine mainly stimulates β2-receptors and peripheral dopamine receptors. This increases renal perfusion, decreases afterload and improves cardiac output. There is a mild positive inotropic action with little vasoconstriction and dopexamine may be used post cardiac surgery.

Isoprenaline is a potent, non-selective β-agonist with very little effect on α-receptors. As highlighted, as a result of its positive inotropic and particularly its chronotropic effects, isoprenaline is used in emergencies to stimulate heart rate in patients with bradycardia or heart block.

Differential biopharmaceutical properties

All of these agents are effective only when given intravenously. Notably, dopamine is a substrate for monoamine oxidase (MAO) and catechol-O-methyl transferase and so not only is it ineffective when taken orally but its actions can also be augmented when used in a patient who has been treated with MAO inhibitor antidepressants.

Differential pharmaceutical properties

All only available as injection.

Chapter 18 directly applies the use of inotropic agents to clinical situations and is a useful adjunct to this section. Table 19.1, which is reproduced from that chapter, provides a useful guide in comparing inotropic agents.

Vasoconstrictor sympathomimetics

Currently licensed in the UK: ephedrine, metaraminol, methoxamine, adrenaline (epinephrine), noradrenaline (norepinephrine), phenylephrine.

Uses

Vasoconstrictor sympathomimetics raise the blood pressure for a short period of time by acting on α-adrenergic receptors to constrict peripheral vessels. Although they can be used as an emergency method of raising blood pressure, they carry the risk of decreasing blood flow through vital organs such as the kidneys. Ephedrine or methoxamine is used in addition to intravenous fluids, oxygen and elevation of the legs to correct hypotension following spinal and epidural anaesthesia. Ephedrine, in addition to causing vasoconstriction, also increases the heart rate and so is useful in the management of associated bradycardia. Methoxamine is most appropriate to use when hypotension exists in association with a tachycardia. The potent action of adrenaline (see Table 19.1) is used notably in cardiopulmonary resuscitation to increase myocardial and cerebral perfusion pressure (Resuscitation Council (UK) 2000).

Differential pharmacology

All act directly on α-receptors, although metaraminol also acts indirectly by displacing endogenous noradrenaline (norepinephrine) and thus has a longer duration of action. By increasing peripheral resistance they bring about a rise in blood pressure. However, this does not usually bring about a tachycardia as there is a reflex increase in vagal tone except when using ephedrine, which via its β-agonist actions can maintain or increase the heart rate. For this reason, it is used in spinal anaesthesia. Noradrenaline (norepinephrine) primarily stimulates the α-adrenergic receptors in the peripheries, constricting the blood vessels and raising the blood pressure. The beneficial effects of vasoconstriction brought about by these agents needs to be considered alongside the decreased perfusion of the organs, such as the kidney. Also, as in many cases of shock, the patient's peripheral circulation is already often naturally constricted and the use of these agents in shock is not warranted.

Differential biopharmaceutical properties

None.

Differential pharmaceutical properties

None.

VASODILATOR ANTIHYPERTENSIVE AGENTS

Currently licensed in the UK: hydralazine, minoxidil, sodium nitroprusside.

Uses

These vasodilators are powerful, especially when used with β-blockers and a thiazide diuretic. They cause a sudden hypotension when first used and so must be carefully administered.

Hydralazine, if used alone, causes an increase in heart rate and fluid retention. Sodium nitroprusside is useful to control hypertensive crises, for example immediately after cardiac surgery. Minoxidil, due to its adverse effect of increasing hair growth, is not recommended for women. It is used topically as a hair growth agent, effective in certain patient groups. Also it must be used in conjunction with a β-blocker and potent diuretic, usually furosemide (frusemide), to offset the increased cardiac output, tachycardia and fluid retention.

Differential pharmacology

Hydralazine dilates the arteries but not veins, via an unclear mechanism. There is a resultant reflex tachycardia that renders this agent of little use as monotherapy. Minoxidil appears to open potassium channels in smooth muscle membranes and thus brings about vasodilatation. As with hydralazine, this is limited to arteries. Sodium nitroprusside, in addition to the arterial dilating properties of the other two agents, also dilates venous vessels, probably via activation of nitric oxide (NO). The reduction in preload and afterload makes this agent a very powerful treatment for hypertensive emergencies and severe cardiac failure.

Differential biopharmaceutical properties

Hydralazine undergoes extensive metabolism by enzymes in the liver and as a result the bioavailability and duration of action are dependent on the status of the patient with respect to liver enzyme function. Minoxidil has a half-life of just 4 hours but the production of an active metabolite, minoxidil sulphate, results in hypotensive effects lasting 24 hours. Sodium nitroprusside's effects last no more than 10 minutes, making it necessary to administer it as a continuous infusion.

Differential pharmaceutical properties

Hydralazine is available as tablets and injection, minoxidil as tablets only and sodium nitroprusside as injection only. As the physical stability is low, sodium nitroprusside infusion must be freshly made and protected from light to prevent photodegradation to cyanide (Galbraith et al 1999).

CENTRALLY ACTING ANTIHYPERTENSIVE AGENTS

Currently licensed in the UK: methyldopa, moxonidine.

Uses

Methyldopa is safe for use in asthmatics, in heart failure and in pregnancy. Side-effects are minimal if daily doses are below 1 g. For mild to moderate essential hypertension, moxonidine can be used, particularly when other established agents have failed to lower the blood pressure.

Differential pharmacology

Methyldopa is a prodrug (a drug that needs to be converted from an inactive form to an active form). It is converted to methylnoradrenaline, which replaces noradrenaline, thus depleting its stores. As methylnoradrenaline is as potent a vasoconstrictor as noradrenaline, its antihypertensive effects are not those of a peripheral action. Instead, methylnoradrenaline acts centrally to inhibit adrenergic neural outflow, probably via α2 stimulation. This stops adrenergic signals to the peripheral system. Alpha 2-receptors occur on neurons in the central nervous system (CNS) and presynaptic nerve terminals in both the central and peripheral nervous systems. The results of this receptor action are a reduction in peripheral resistance without much change in cardiac output and heart rate.

Unfortunately, methyldopa's central effects also produce centrally derived side-effects, including transient sedation, depression, galactorrhoea (inappropriate secretion of milk) and parkinsonian signs. Other side-effects include hepatotoxicity with or without fever. Moxonidine is centrally acting as well but via imadazoline receptors and α2-receptors. Its main role is in add-on or substitution therapy in hypertensive patients who are uncontrolled on or who are intolerant of β-blockers, ACE inhibitors and calcium channel blockers.

Differential biopharmaceutical properties

As methyldopa has quite an involved mode of action, its effects last far longer than its plasma levels would suggest. It is suitable for once-a-day or twice-a-day dosing. Moxonidine has a short half-life (1–3 hours) but produces two active but relatively weak metabolites. Moxonidine and its metabolites are renally excreted and the agent often needs to be given twice a day.

Differential pharmaceutical properties

Methyldopa is available as oral formulations and injection, while moxonidine is available as tablets only.

DIURETICS

- Thiazide and related diuretics
- Loop diuretics
- Potassium-sparing diuretics

Thiazide and related diuretics

Currently licensed in the UK: bendroflumethiazide (bendrofluazide), chlortalidone, cyclopenthiazide, hydrochlorothiazide, hydroflumethiazide, indapamide, mefruside, metolazone, polythiazide, xipamide.

Uses

These agents are reasonably powerful diuretics usually administered in the morning or early afternoon, so the patient does not have to wake up at night to pass urine. When used in hypertension, low doses provide equal antihypertensive effects as higher doses. Higher doses additionally increase adverse effects and so should be avoided. Occasionally, thiazides have been used to reduce oedema due to chronic heart failure.

Differential pharmacology

Chlortalidone, indapamide, metolazone and xipamide are sulphonamides but have qualitatively similar actions to the thiazides (benzothiadiazines). They are therefore known as the thiazide-like diuretics. All the agents inhibit sodium chloride reabsorption in the distal convoluted tubule but the thiazide-like agents, being acids, are secreted into the proximal tubule by the organic acid secretory system of the kidney. They may therefore compete with urea excretion, causing an increase in uraemia. Metolazone is a relatively weak

diuretic when used alone but produces a considerable synergy when used with loop diuretics.

Differential biopharmaceutical properties

The thiazide-like agents generally have a slower onset of action and longer half-life. Indeed, chlortalidone, with a half-life of 44 hours, can be given every other day in clinical practice. Although the relative potencies of all the agents vary by 250-fold and the bio-availabilities alter from 10% (the lipophobic chlortalidone) to nearly 100%, these factors are normalized by the use of different dose amounts.

Differential pharmaceutical properties

None.

Loop diuretics

Currently licensed in the UK: furosemide (frusemide), bumetanide, torasemide.

Uses

These very powerful diuretics relieve pulmonary oedema caused by left ventricular failure. Preload reduction and improvements in breathlessness occur quickly following intravenous administration. Loop diuretics can also be used for the management of chronic heart failure and are effective in patients with very poor renal function. When combined with thiazides, they are even effective in the treatment of diuretic-resistant oedema.

Differential pharmacology

There is none regarding efficacy but allergic reactions (skin rash and, rarely, interstitial nephritis) have been reported with furosemide (frusemide) therapy and myalgia (muscle pain) with bumetanide.

Differential biopharmaceutical properties

Oral absorption of torasemide is rapid and its onset of action comparable to the intravenous use of furosemide (frusemide) or bumetanide with a peak effect within 30 minutes (BNF 2001). When used intravenously, the latter two must be given slowly (less than 4 mg/min for furosemide (frusemide) and not more than 2 mg every 20 minutes for bumetanide) to avoid ototoxicity (damage to the eighth cranial nerve in the ear, causing hearing impairment).

Differential pharmaceutical properties

Furosemide (frusemide) and bumetanide are available in both tablet and intravenous forms. Torasemide is available only as a tablet.

Potassium-sparing diuretics

Currently licensed in the UK: amiloride, triamterene, spironolactone.

Uses

These weak diuretics are useful in maintaining serum potassium concentration when used in combination with the more potent thiazide and loop diuretics. Spironolactone potentiates these more potent diuretics by inhibiting aldosterone. This latter property makes it particularly useful in the treatment of oedema due to cirrhosis of the liver. It can also be used for chronic heart failure, especially if associated with hepatic engorgement. Naturally, spironolactone has a role in the management of primary hyperaldosteronism (Conn's syndrome).

Differential pharmacology

All three agents antagonize the effects of aldosterone at the cortical collecting tubule and late distal tubule of the kidney. However, amiloride and triamterene do so by inhibition of sodium (Na^+) transport in the luminal membrane whereas spironolactone directly antagonizes the mineralocorticoid receptors.

Differential biopharmaceutical properties

Spironolactone undergoes substantial metabolism in the liver and its full effects take many days to materialize. Triamterene undergoes substantial metabolism and so needs to be administered more frequently than amiloride.

Differential pharmaceutical properties

Spironolactone is not available as as injection.

ANTI-ARRHYTHMIC AGENTS

- Drugs for supraventricular (narrow complex) arrhythmias
- Drugs for supraventricular and ventricular arrhythmias
- Drugs for ventricular arrhythmias

Drugs for supraventricular (narrow complex) arrhythmias

Currently licensed in the UK: adenosine, cardiac glycosides (see p. 349), verapamil.

Uses

Adenosine is widely used for terminating paroxysmal supraventricular tachycardia (PSVT) and as a diagnostic agent in narrow QRS complex or wide-complex tachycardia of uncertain cause.

Cardiac glycosides are useful in atrial fibrillation, although occasionally used, with little success, in atrial flutter and for chemical cardioversion.

Verapamil is used for the treatment of re-entrant supraventricular tachycardia and can be used to control the ventricular rate in atrial fibrillation and flutter. Verapamil must **not** be used in Wolff–Parkinson–White syndrome, in which there is an accessory conduction pathway that bypasses the atrioventricular (AV) node. The AV node normally acts as a gate in atrial fibrillation (AF), preventing the rapid atrial rate passing to the ventricles. If the AV node is inhibited by verapamil and AF develops, then the rapid impulses from the atria can easily pass through the accessory pathway at a very fast rate to the ventricles, resulting in a fast ventricular rate and possibly ventricular fibrillation (VF).

Differential pharmacology

These three agents are all in different drug classes and their pharmacological actions are thus well differentiated. Adenosine reduces sinus rate temporarily and increases the refractory period in the AV node. It is therefore sometimes termed an AV blocker. These effects come about through the reduction of calcium (Ca^{2+}) currents via inhibition of intracellular cyclic AMP. See p. 349 for the pharmacology of cardiac glycosides.

Verapamil blocks activated and inactivated calcium channels and thus has a more marked effect on the sino-atrial (SA) and AV nodes. The reason for this is that these tissues fire impulses more frequently, are less completely polarized at rest and are activated exclusively by calcium current in comparison with other myocardial tissue. Verapamil thus prolongs the effective refractory period during AV conduction and similarly for SA conduction. However, this can be over-run by the reflex tachycardia induced by the small vasodilatation effect of verapamil on arterial vessels.

Differential biopharmaceutical properties

Adenosine, given as 3 mg then increased to 6 mg and further still to 12 mg as appropriate, has a short duration of action, with a half-life of just 6–8 seconds. However, its effects are prolonged in patients taking dipyridamole which is an adenosine uptake inhibitor. Conversely, doses may need to be increased in patients who have recently taken theophylline or caffeine, because these antagonize the adenosine receptor.

Verapamil possesses clinically important hepatic enzyme inhibitory properties. Its use can double the normal therapeutic digoxin concentrations and therefore a lower dose of digoxin is needed. Verapamil also potentiates the action of warfarin and as a consequence, the dose of the latter drug needs to be reduced. Unlike adenosine, verapamil can cause bradycardia when given after β-blockers.

Differential pharmaceutical properties

None. All are available intravenously for the treatment of supraventricular arrhythmias.

Drugs for supraventricular and ventricular arrhythmias

Currently licensed in the UK: amiodarone, disopyramide, flecainide, procainamide, propafenone, quinidine.

There have been various clinical trials investigating the use of anti-arrhythmic therapy. The results from CAST-1 (1989), a study of pharmacological agents for ventricular arrhythmias, demonstrated that more patients died in the group that were treated with flecanide than placebo. CAST-2 (1992), also studying ventricular arrhythmia treatment, was terminated at an early stage because the anti-arrhythmic moracizine was associated with an increase in mortality. However, the problem with any drug trial involving life-threatening arrhythmias is that mortality will occur anyway due to the underlying illness and this makes the effects of drug therapies harder to evaluate. Further technical advances that have proved efficacious, such as internal cardioverter defibrillators (ICDs), make the use of new unproven anti-arrhythmics difficult to trial effectively.

Uses

Amiodarone is used in the treatment of Wolff–Parkinson–White syndrome and should only be used for other arrhythmias if other drugs are ineffective or contra-indicated. Disopyramide, given intravenously, can be used to control post myocardial infarct arrhythmias but it can inhibit cardiac contractility.

Flecianide may be of use in seriously symptomatic ventricular arrhythmias, paroxysmal AF and junctional re-entry tachycardias.

Procainamide can be used acutely to control ventricular arrhythmias but problems are associated with its long-term use (see Differential Pharmacology below).

Propafenone is used for both prophylaxis and treatment of supraventricular and ventricular arrhythmias but its β-blocker activity can reduce its usefulness (see Differential Pharmacology below).

Quinidine is effective in the prophylaxis of supraventricular and ventricular arrhythmias but, like all of the above, can be pro-arrhythmogenic and therefore must be used by specialists or with specialist involvement.

Differential pharmacology

Classification of anti-arrhythmics has previously been related to their effects on active myocardial cells. The Vaughan Williams classification (Box 19.1) has been considered to be of limited clinical use as several agents, including adrenaline (epinephrine), isoprenaline, digoxin, amiodarone and adenosine, do not easily fit into the classifications. The Task Force of the Working group on Arrhythmias of the European Society of Cardiology (1991) has suggested a more flexible system recognizing effects as arising from

---

Box 19.1 The Vaughan Williams (1970) classification of anti-arrhythmics (example agents have been added in brackets)

Class 1 agents inhibit the fast sodium channels. Also known as the membrane-stabilizing agents or fast sodium channel blockers. This grouping is further broken into three categories.
1. Class 1a agents block the sodium channel and delay repolarization (quinidine).
2. Class 1b agents block the fast sodium channel, accelerate repolarization and decrease action potential duration (lidocaine (lignocaine)).
3. Class 1c agents produce a pronounced sodium channel blockade with little effect upon repolarization (flecainide).

Class 2 agents block sympathetic stimulation (propranolol).

Class 3 agents prolong the action potential (amiodarone, bretylium and sotalol).

Class 4 agents act as calcium channel blockers (verapamil).

actions on channels, pumps, receptors and other sites. This system classifies arrhythmias by their mechanism but is not well known and has not been adopted in preference to the Vaughan Williams classification. Consequently, it is this latter system to which reference is made in this section.

Amiodarone, originally an anti-anginal agent, is a structural analogue of thyroid hormone. By blocking sodium (Na^+) and potassium (K^+) channels, amiodarone prolongs refractoriness of all myocardial tissues and thus prolongs the action potential. It is also a weak calcium channel blocker and a non-competitive inhibitor of β-adrenergic receptors. Amiodarone is concentrated in tissue and skin and can be found in virtually every organ. The eyes are usually first to be affected and the presence of light brown crystals can be detected in the cornea after just a few weeks of therapy. These deposits normally affect the patient's night vision and can cause halos to be seen in the peripheral visual fields.

Skin deposits result in hypersensitization to strong light, developing a slate-grey coloration to the skin. It is this side-effect that is most likely to result in withdrawing the drug (Swanton 1997). Common neurological effects include paraesthesia, tremor, ataxia and headaches. Both hypothyroidism and hyperthyroidism can occur, with the iodine content of the local water determining which one. Hepatocellular necrosis, constipation and pulmonary fibrosis also occur in 5% of cases (Swanton 1997). The latter can be fatal and also may be easily missed as dyspnoea occurs with worsening heart failure. The lung changes can be reversed if the condition is noted early and the drug treatment stopped (Swanton 1997).

Nonetheless, when amiodarone is used intravenously it is well tolerated, producing very few side-effects. It interacts significantly with warfarin, theophylline and digoxin. With the latter agent, there is a pharmacokinetic interaction; that is, the clearance of digoxin is reduced along with the volume of distribution, resulting in raised digoxin levels. Additionally there is a pharmacodynamic interaction with both agents working on the AV node.

Quinidine binds to and blocks sodium channels. However, because recovery is slower and less complete in depolarized tissue, quinidine increases the refractory period and depresses the excitability of depolarized tissue more than normal tissue. Therefore the pacemaker rate, especially ectopic pacemaker, and conduction of stimulated tissue are depressed.

Electrocardiogram (ECG) changes include a lengthening of the Q–T interval and, as is well known, this effect is linked with torsade de pointes (a form of ventricular tachycardia seen on the ECG), which is estimated to occur in 2–8% of patients taking this agent. This adverse effect even occurs at normal or low plasma levels of quinidine. Quinidine also possess α-adrenoreceptor blocking properties and so causes vasodilatation and reflex tachycardia, particularly when given intravenously. This effect is not helped by quinidine's antimuscarinic properties which, by inhibiting vagal stimulus, can create an increased sinus rate and AV conduction. Unfortunately, in atrial flutter the ratio of atrial:ventricular conduction can drop to 1:1, causing a dramatic increase in ventricular response. This effect can be prevented by using verapamil or digoxin.

Disopyramide resembles quinidine pharmacologically but possesses even greater antimuscarinic effects and so is not recommended for use in patients with cardiac failure, glaucoma or prostatic hypertrophy.

Flecainide is a potent blocker of sodium (Na^+) and potassium (K^+) channels and, unlike quinidine, it has no antimuscarinic activity. However, even at usual therapeutic doses it can cause exacerbation of arrhythmias in patients with pre-existing ventricular tachyarrhythmias and in those with previous myocardial infarction and ventricular ectopy.

Procainamide pharmacology is similar to quinidine, although it may be less effective in suppressing pacemaker activity and more effective in reducing conduction in depolarized tissue. Unlike quinidine, there is less vagal inhibition via antimuscarinic activity and so depression of the SA and AV nodes is greater. Procainamide also causes less vasodilatation and any hypotension observed is usually due to an excessively high infusion rate. Long-term use of procainamide can lead to a systemic lupus erythematosus-like syndrome. Although renal lupus is rarely seen, arthralgia, pleuritis, pericarditis and parenchymal pulmonary disease have been noted occasionally in patients receiving long-term therapy.

Propafenone is structurally similar to propranolol but possesses weak β-adrenoreceptor blocking activity. Its anti-arrhythmic activity resembles quinidine and its sodium channel-blocking properties are similar to flecainide.

Differential biopharmaceutical properties

Amiodarone has a remarkable half-life of up to 100 days. A plasma level of 1–2 mg/l can be used as a guide to therapeutic concentration but myocardial levels are actually some 30 times this concentration and using clinical effect is recommended for assessing effectiveness of therapy. However, as amiodarone side-effects are related to duration and dose, the serum level can be used when considering a reduction of the maintenance dose in order to reduce overall exposure. Once-daily dosing is adequate and in fact, if a dose were missed for several days there would be little clinical significance. An unfortunate corollary to the long half-life is that side-effects persist for many months after stopping therapy.

The half-life, as previously defined, is the time taken for the concentration of a drug to decrease by half. This is primarily influenced by elimination through the renal system. If a drug's concentration is 500 µg/l at a timed point and this reduces to 250 µg/l in 3 hours, then the half-life of the drug is 3 hours. This assists in deciding when repeat doses should be administered. Figure 19.3 demonstrates the development of a steady-state concentration of a drug. The steady state is the minimally effective therapeutic concentration. Figure 19.3 illustrates why a drug takes 4–5 half-lives to reach a steady state. In addition, it demonstrates why a drug with a longer half-life will take longer to reach its steady state. Therefore, with a drug such as amiodarone which has an extremely long half-life, a large loading dose needs to be administered followed by smaller maintenance doses to achieve the desired therapeutic effect.

Quinidine is rapidly absorbed when taken orally and then mostly metabolized by the liver, with 20% being excreted unchanged. The resultant half-life is 6 hours. A therapeutic plasma concentration range of 3–5 µg/l can assist dosing when assessing a patient for non-compliance or suspected toxicity.

Disopyramide has a bio-availability of just 50% but it is extensively protein bound and so, as the dosage is increased, available binding sites decrease and a non-linear rise in free, active drug is seen. Therefore plasma levels of total drug do not reflect the pharmacological activity. Dosage must be reduced in patients with renal dysfunction because it is principally renally excreted. Its half-life is usually 6–8 hours.

Flecainide is well absorbed and is cleared by both hepatic and renal routes. Its half-life is 20 hours which allows once-daily dosing at higher doses.

Procainamide has a major active metabolite, N-acetylprocainamide, that possesses class 3 activity (see Box 19.1). Accumulation of this metabolite has been suggested to cause torsade de pointes and is particularly likely in patients with renal dysfunction in whom the usual half-life of 3–4 hours is increased. As the metabolite is more slowly eliminated than the parent compound, it accumulates more slowly and so after treating for some weeks it can help to measure serum levels of both in order to optimize the safe use of procainamide.

Propafenone usually has a half-life of 5 hours but this can be increased to 17 hours in individuals who are poor metabolizers.

Differential pharmaceutical properties

Amiodarone is available as injection and tablets, quinidine as slow-release tablets only, disopyramide as an injection, tablets and slow-release tablets, flecainide as injection and tablets, procainamide as injection and tablets, propafenone as tablets only.

Drugs for ventricular arrhythmias

Currently licensed in the UK: bretylium, lidocaine (lignocaine), mexiletine, moracizine, tocainide.

Uses

Bretylium is only used as an anti-arrhythmic drug in resuscitation and this is quite rare.

Lidocaine (lignocaine) is relatively safe and should be considered first for emergency use such as in haemodynamically unstable ventricular tachycardia, within the advanced life support algorithm (see Chapter 24), post myocardial infarction and for the treatment of ventricular arrhythmias caused by digoxin, phenothiazines or tricyclics.

Mexiletine may be given as a slow intravenous injection if lidocaine (lignocaine) is ineffective. Tocainide is restricted for use in circumstances where

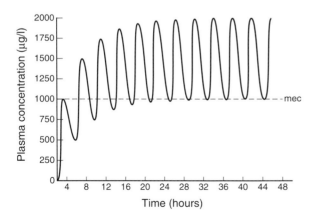

mec = the minimum effective concentration of a drug which is therapeutically beneficial

Figure 19.3 Development of steady-state concentration for a drug with a short half-life.

other treatment has failed or is inappropriate, because it possesses the potential to cause serious side-effects (see below).

Moracizine is only available as tablets on a named-patient basis for those already stabilized on the drug.

Phenytoin was used in ventricular arrhythmias caused by cardiac glycosides but this use is now obsolete.

Differential pharmacology

Bretylium is a sympathetic ganglion-blocking agent and effectively produces a chemical sympathectomy by depressing noradrenaline (norepinephrine) release. The resulting hypotensive effect can be problematic (see below). Bretylium increases the ventricular fibrillation threshold, by prolonging the duration of the action potential and the effective refractory period (ERP) in ventricular muscle and Purkinje fibres.

Lidocaine (lignocaine) depresses spontaneous phase 4 depolarization in the action potential. It has little effect in action potential duration and, as with other class 1 agents, its action is reduced in patients with hypokalaemia. Thus it is important to correct this electrolyte concentration. As one would expect, high doses of lidocaine (lignocaine) can produce bradycardia and hypotension.

Mexiletine is a class 1b agent and has effects similar to those of lidocaine (lignocaine). It produces very little decrease in left ventricular contractility and, in comparison with the other agents, is relatively safe to use in patients with congestive cardiac failure. However, this drug is fat soluble (lipophilic) which allows it ready access to the central nervous system (CNS).

Tocainide has a structure based on lidocaine (lignocaine) and possesses similar pharmacological actions. Heart failure is rarely precipitated but patients and their carers must be told how to recognize the signs of blood or pulmonary disorders, such as aplastic anaemia, interstitial pneumonitis and fibrosing alveolitis, and to seek medical attention as this agent has life-threatening side-effects. Nurses administering this drug should make it their responsibility to prepare teaching packs for both staff and patients that address these issues.

Differential biopharmaceutical properties

Bretylium is effective when used both intramuscularly and intravenously but the intravenous route should only be used if there is doubt as to the adequacy of perfusion of the skeletal muscles, which may impair the absorption. The onset of action after intravenous (IV) use is approximately 2–3 minutes and after intramuscular (IM) use 15–60 minutes. Therefore during a cardiopulmonary resuscitation attempt it may be necessary to continue for some time before the drug's anti-arrhythmic effects are realized.

Lidocaine (lignocaine) when given as a bolus dose produces effects for 5–10 minutes. Therefore the infusion should be started when the bolus is administered. Used this way, there is little drop in the plasma concentration whilst the initial dose is excreted. The therapeutic range of 1.4–6 mg/l can be used but CNS side-effects, including convulsions, can occur at levels above 5 mg/l. The clearance of lidocaine (lignocaine) is reduced in hepatic failure, reduced hepatic perfusion and congestive cardiac failure and here the dose may need to be halved.

Mexiletine is reasonably well absorbed orally and produces peak levels 2–4 hours after being taken. The relatively short half-life of 9 hours can be lengthened to over 24 hours in patients with renal failure. Aiming for plasma levels between 0.75 and 2 mg/l can help dosing but this agent is lipophilic and thus easily crosses the blood–brain barrier, producing an array of neurological side-effects. These include confusion, tremor, diplopia (double vision), paraesthesia, ataxia and nystagmus (tremor of the eyes). Plasma levels are reduced in patients who are taking phenytoin or rifampicin concomitantly.

Tocainide absorption from the stomach is almost 100%. Peak plasma levels are produced in 1–1.5 hours and the usual half-life is around 12 hours. This can be increased to 30 hours in patients with renal failure.

Differential pharmaceutical properties

Bretylium and lidocaine (lignocaine) are only available by injection. Mexiletine is available as ordinary tablets which are given four times a day, slow-release tablets given twice a day and also as an injection. Tocainide is only available as tablets.

β-BLOCKERS

Currently licensed in the UK: propranolol, acebutolol, atenolol, betaxolol, bisoprolol, carvedilol, celiprolol, esmolol, labetalol, metoprolol, nadolol, oxprenolol, pindolol, sotalol, timalol.

Uses

β-Blockers block the β-adrenoreceptors in the heart, peripheral vasculature, bronchi, pancreas and liver.

There are two β-receptor subtypes: β1 and β2. By blocking β1 receptors in the heart, the heart rate is slowed and thus oxygen demand is decreased.

β-Blockers are effective in controlling hypertension and anginal pain and are considered essential in post acute myocardial infarction as secondary prophylaxis. They also have a minor role as anti-arrhythmics, more commonly in controlling the ventricular response in atrial fibrillation, and most recently have been seen in the management of heart failure.

Differential pharmacology

The most well-known differentials are that of receptor selectivity (whether β1 and β2 or primarily just β1) as well as the presence of partial agonist activity, also known as intrinsic sympathomimetic activity. The clinical significance of the former includes less bronchoconstriction in susceptible patients (e.g. asthmatics) and reduced and fewer metabolic complications, including reduction of glycogenesis, weight gain and altered blood lipid profile, manifested as an increased serum triglyceride and reduced high-density lipoprotein:low-density lipoprotein (HDL:LDL) ratio.

However, it must be noted that even the β1 (and hence cardiac) selective antagonists also inhibit β2-receptors. β2-Receptors are found in several organs, including the lungs, and inhibition of β2-receptors causes bronchoconstriction. This inhibition is clinically insignificant at lower doses but at higher blood levels, the selective agents lose this property. These agents are therefore not known as cardiospecific and are still to be avoided in patients with asthma unless the risk:benefit ratio is favourable.

Intrinsic sympathomimetic activity is a property of acebutolol, oxprenolol, pindolol and celiprolol, with the first two having agonist activity on β1-receptors and the last two on β2-receptors. The purported advantages of intrinsic sympathomimetic activity include reduced bradycardia and reduced peripheral vasoconstriction but such effects have proved of little clinical benefit in practice. Sotalol has specific anti-arrhythmic properties and is no longer licensed for use in angina, hypertension or post myocardial infarction. Sotalol's effects on prolonging the action potential and Q–T interval on the ECG have given it a place in the prophylaxis of paroxysmal supraventricular arrhythmias. It is also effective in suppressing ventricular ectopics and non-sustained ventricular tachycardia.

Carvedilol, labetalol, pindolol and celiprolol, in addition to their β-antagonist actions, all possess arteriolar vasodilating actions, carvedilol and labetalol by α-blockade and pindolol and celiprolol via their partial β2-agonist activity. These β-blockers may be of use in patients suffering from cold extremities but are also likely to produce postural hypotension. Carvedilol additionally possesses anti-oxidant properties and is licensed for use in heart failure in patients under hospital supervision. However, positive clinical outcomes from the use of β-blockers in (carefully selected) patients with heart failure may be a class effect. Outcomes of trials using β-blockers without such differentiating properties will help to provide further answers.

Differential biopharmaceutical properties

All β-blockers are either predominantly lipid soluble or water soluble. Lipid-soluble agents readily cross the blood–brain barrier (thus exerting CNS-related side-effects) and are hepatically metabolized (hence exhibiting short to medium half-lives). Conversely, the lipophobic agents are less (but still to some degree) associated with central side-effects and, being renally excreted, display medium to long half-lives. They accumulate in renal impairment unless appropriately reduced doses are employed.

Esmolol is used intravenously and has a short duration of action, being rapidly metabolized by enzymes in erythrocytes. It is useful in the short-term management of atrial flutter, atrial fibrillation, sinus tachycardia or hypertension, especially in the peri-operative period.

Differential pharmaceutical properties

Propranolol, atenolol, labetalol, metoprolol and sotalol are all available in oral forms and injection. Esmolol is only available as an injection and the others only in oral forms. Propranolol, metoprolol and oxprenolol also come in slow-release formulations.

DRUGS AFFECTING THE RENIN–ANGIOTENSIN SYSTEM

- Angiotensin-converting enzyme (ACE) inhibitors
- Angiotensin II antagonists

ACE inhibitors

Currently licensed in the UK: captopril, cilazapril, enalapril, fosinopril, lisinopril, moexipril, perindopril, quinapril, ramipril, trandolapril.

Uses

ACE inhibitors are well established for use in cardiac failure, particularly in prevention of left ventricular hypertrophy following myocardial infarction and in the management of hypertension, particularly in patients with diabetes with early signs of renal damage.

Differential pharmacology

Although the different drugs vary considerably in potency, this is taken into account in the different doses that are recommended, i.e. higher potency drugs are available in smaller doses than the weaker agents. All agents inhibit the conversion of angiotensin I to angiotensin II and there is little to differentiate them on pharmacological grounds.

Angiotensin II is a potent vasoconstrictor, which increases the afterload to a failing heart and stimulates aldosterone secretion. This results in an increase in renal sodium re-absorption and thus an increased fluid load within the patient, exacerbating a failing heart.

Differential biopharmaceutical properties

All ACE inhibitors except captopril and lisinopril are metabolized to more potent metabolites as they pass through the liver. Thus the effects of these ACE inhibitors needs to be monitored more closely when used in patients with hepatic impairment. All ACE inhibitors are principally eliminated through the kidney and so need dosage adjustments in renal failure. Although the liver and the kidneys eliminate moexipril and fosinopril, they too may require dosage adjustment as determined by clinical effects. An ACE inhibitor such as captopril with a short half-life (3 hours) should be used to test for ACE inhibitor response so that any adverse effects during assessment are short lived. The test usually consists of giving a patient an oral dose of 6.25 mg of captopril and then monitoring the blood pressure every 15–30 minutes for 4 hours.

Differential pharmaceutical properties

None.

Angiotensin II antagonists

Currently licensed in the UK: candesartan, irbesartan, losartan, valsartan.

Uses

All these agents appear effective in the management of hypertension. Trials are ongoing with some of these agents for use in heart failure.

Differential pharmacology

All these agents inhibit the action of angiotensin II on its receptor site and so have little to differentiate them on pharmacological grounds.

Differential biopharmaceutical properties

Although these agents have different durations of action and different trough and peak ratios, i.e. blood pressure control between doses is variable, they are all licensed as once-a-day preparations for the treatment of hypertension.

Differential pharmaceutical properties

None.

NITRATES

Currently licensed in the UK: glyceryl trinitrate (GTN), isosorbide dinitrate, isosorbide mononitrate, pentaerithrityl tetranitrate.

Uses

These agents have a well-established role in the treatment and prophylaxis of stable angina pain and are valuable in unstable angina, particularly when given intravenously. Nitrates can also be used in the treatment of left ventricular failure.

Differential pharmacology

All these agents release nitric oxide (NO) in vascular smooth muscle target tissues and this brings about predominantly venodilatation and some arterial dilatation. The effect of venodilatation is to reduce venous return, thus reducing the preload and therefore the oxygen demand of the myocardium. This reduces the angina pain experienced. All can contribute to a non-specific nitrate tolerance. Side-effects from nitrates include headache, flushing, dizziness and, with higher doses, hypotension, all due to the vasodilatory effects. All of these are diminished after the first few days of therapy. As a result of the similarity in pharmacology, the agents are chosen depending on their duration of action and formulation available.

Differential biopharmaceutical properties

Glyceryl trinitrate undergoes extensive 'first-pass' metabolism. The first-pass effect refers to the initial metabolism of oral drugs by the gastro-intestinal (GI) tract and the liver. From the GI tract, drugs pass via the portal vein through the liver, before reaching the general circulation. Therefore, a drug such as GTN, which is extensively metabolized by the liver, is regarded as having a high first-pass effect, as the amount that would reach the circulation for therapeutic effect is negligible. This renders the oral route ineffective. Sublingual administration is a direct route to the bloodstream via the oral mucosa. GTN's duration of action is no more than 20–30 minutes. This duration of action can be increased to 24 hours when using transdermal patches. As with all the other forms of nitrate, it is recommended that an 8-hour nitrate-free period be employed within every 24 hours, to minimize tolerance.

Isosorbide dinitrate can be used sublingually and has been formulated to be taken orally, in which case it is metabolized to isosorbide mononitrate. Conventional isosorbide dinitrate tablets require dosing three times a day, but the slow-release brands are effective over 12 hours. Isosorbide mononitrate intrinsically has a duration of 12 hours and its slow-release formulations need only be taken once a day, as they can provide nitrate cover for 16 hours. Pentaerithrityl tetranitrate is used orally and undergoes biotransformation to tri-, di- and mononitrate. It has no advantages over isosorbide mononitrate. When used intravenously, the effect of tolerance appears to be overcome by achieving substantially higher serum levels.

Differential pharmaceutical properties

GTN is available as sublingual tablets and spray, buccal tablets (dissolved in the mouth between the upper lip and gum), intravenous preparations, transdermal patches and as an ointment which is applied but not rubbed in. Isosorbide dinitrate is available as a sublingual spray and tablet, a modified-release preparation, intravenously and as a transdermal spray. Isosorbide mononitrate is available orally and as a modified-release preparation. Pentaerithrityl tetranitrate can be found as an oral preparation but this drug has recently been discontinued.

CALCIUM CHANNEL BLOCKERS

Currently licensed in the UK: amlodipine, diltiazem, felodipine, isradipine, lacidipine, lercanidipine, nicardipine, nifedipine, nislodipine, verapamil.

Uses

These agents are used for the management of hypertension and stable angina, while verapamil has a role in the treatment of some arrhythmias.

Differential pharmacology

All calcium channel blockers reduce the calcium flow through slow calcium channels of active cell membranes and thus affect myocardial cells, specialized conduction tissues and cells of vascular smooth muscle. As can be seen from the above uses, these agents do not form a homogeneous group.

Nifedipine and the other calcium channel blockers in the same class (the dihydropyridines) are more selective as vasodilators and produce very little cardiac depression. Diltiazem has intermediate actions. The dihydropyridines produce a reflex tachycardia that can contribute to ischaemic pain, as a result of the increased cardiac workload and hence oxygen demand. This dihydropyridine-induced reflex tachycardia is more problematic in the elderly in whom the body's response to the resultant hypotension is diminished. In this group the drop in blood pressure is not easily overcome. The concurrent use of β-blockers would counter this tachycardia and so this combination is quite suitable.

The negative inotropic properties (reduced myocardial contraction) of diltiazem and verapamil prevent any reflex tachycardia when these agents are used. Of course, it is evident that verapamil has the greatest effect on the heart from its use as an anti-arrhythmic agent. For this reason, β-blockers should be avoided in patients being administered verapamil (and used with caution in patients on diltiazem), as there is a risk of inducing bradycardia and heart block.

In terms of adverse drug reactions, the dihydropyridines have the highest incidence of vascular side-effects, with headache, dizziness and flushing being common. This is particularly so with the immediate release formulations which have a short half-life. The dihydropyridines, and in particular nifedipine, also produce a diuretic-resistant oedema. With regard to contraction, the lower oesophageal sphincter is inhibited by calcium channel blockers and all the agents are known to cause gastric reflux, whilst verapamil additionally causes constipation.

The effect of using β-blockers with these agents highlights the differential properties of this drug and unsurprisingly, verapamil also commonly causes problems when used with digoxin. However, in this case, it is not only due to the common action at the AV node but also because verapamil can increase digoxin levels. Although the cardiac-depressive actions of verapamil are dose dependent and therefore potentially easily avoided, hypotension and arrhythmias are commonly induced when it is used intravenously and particularly in patients following a myocardial infarction.

Differential biopharmaceutical properties

Verapamil undergoes extensive first-pass metabolism and only 20% of an oral dose is available systemically. When used intravenously, the liver is bypassed and so the dose necessary is much lower. If used in patients with hepatic dysfunction, the dose used would need to be further reduced. Verapamil has a half-life of 7 hours, whilst the other agents have half-lives that vary between 1.5 and 64 hours. Those with short half-lives may need to be taken up to three times a day but many, including amlodipine, felodipine, isradipine, lacidipine and lercanidipine, can be taken daily. Following metabolism, most agents produce active metabolites but these are always less potent than the parent compound.

A common use of nifedipine capsules has been to break them open and use them sublingually when attempting to reduce a severely raised blood pressure in a patient. Although this is effective and a reduction in blood pressure is observed within 10 minutes, the onset of action is actually no faster than if the capsule is taken orally (Schumann 1991). Nonetheless, the former method has a place when the patient is unable to swallow.

On a practical note, many of the calcium channel blockers which have intrinsically short half-lives have been formulated into twice-a-day, slow-release or controlled-release (CR) tablets or capsules and also into once-a-day (extra long or longer acting) tablets or capsules. As these various formulations have not been shown to have the same clinical effect, it is necessary to know the brand of calcium channel blocker being prescribed and all attempts should be made to keep a patient on the same brand.

Differential pharmaceutical properties

All are available as oral preparations. Diltiazem is available as a longer-acting formulation while nicardipine, nifedipine and verapamil are available as modified-release preparations. Verapamil is also available as an intravenous preparation.

ANTICOAGULANTS

- Low molecular weight heparins
- Oral anticoagulants

Low molecular weight heparins

Currently licensed in the UK: certoparin, dalteparin (Fragmin), enoxaparin, tinzaparin.

Uses

These agents are used for the prophylaxis and treatment of deep vein thrombosis (DVT), pulmonary embolism (PE) and unstable angina. Although not all these agents are licensed for every indication, this will change as manufacturers seek wider uses for their products.

Differential pharmacology

Although each agent has an individual structure and molecular size, they all act via inhibition of factor Xa and are clinical indistinguishable.

Differential biopharmaceutical properties

Again these agents are very similar and all have advantages over the more traditional infusion of unfractionated heparin. These advantages include dosing by subcutaneous injection and the reduced need to monitor activated partial thromboplastin time (APTT). In fact, there is no routine haematological monitoring required for efficacy when used at the recommended doses.

Differential pharmaceutical properties

All agents are available in preloaded syringes of varying amounts. Dalteparin and tinzaparin are further available in ampoules of varying sizes and tinzaparin alone is available in a multidose vial.

Oral anticoagulants

Currently licensed in the UK: warfarin, nicoumalone, phenindione.

Uses

These agents are used for the prophylaxis of DVT and PE, particularly in patients with atrial fibrillation or in patients with a mechanical heart valve. They are also used before elective direct current (DC) cardioversion.

It is vital that all patients on anticoagulation therapy are advised to report any excessive bleeding or bruising to their general practitioner (GP), hospital doctor or nurse and are warned that any cuts or grazes will take longer to stop bleeding. Extra care is needed in activities such as playing sports or gardening, dealing with family pets that may scratch and tasks such as wet shaving. The latter requires additional caution and the advice to alter to an electric shaver if possible. A variety of leaflets are available from the anticoagulation clinics.

Differential pharmacology

None. They all inhibit the hepatic manufacture of vitamin K-dependent clotting factors, namely II, VII, IX and X. However, serious hypersensitivity reactions can occur with any agent, in which case another may be tried. Warfarin is by far the most widely used oral anticoagulant, with both nicoumalone and phenindione rarely being utilized.

Differential biopharmaceutical properties

None. All are well absorbed and affected significantly by vitamin K in the diet and by drugs which affect the liver enzymes responsible for metabolism. INR monitoring is essential to assess the effect on blood clotting. This is carried out for patients prescribed the drug over a longer period, at an anticoagulation clinic, where blood samples are taken and the prescribed dose altered in a booklet kept by the patient. There is debate about the target value for the INR and this should be based on the reason for anticoagulation. The various uses of the INR are highlighted within specific chapters in this book.

Differential pharmaceutical properties

None, all available as tablets.

ANTIPLATELET AGENTS

Currently licensed in the UK: aspirin, clopidogrel, dipyridamole, abciximab, ticlopidine.

Uses

Since platelet aggregation is essential in the early stages of thrombus formation, these antiplatelet aggregating agents have their primary role in the prevention of myocardial infarction and ischaemic cerebrovascular accident (CVA/stroke). Some of these, such as ticlopidine, are also effective in reducing the re-occlusion of arteries following stent insertion.

In addition, within the next few years we can expect agents such as abciximab (ReoPro) to be used in conjunction with thrombolytic agents to reduce the mortality of myocardial infarction. Numerous investigators have shown that the glycoprotein (GP) IIb/IIIa integrin mediates the 'final common pathway' in platelet aggregation (Pye 2000). This paper provides a useful overview of the use of GP IIb/IIIa antagonists such as abciximab during coronary interventions such as angioplasty to reduce vessel occlusion and the emerging trials in conjunction with thrombolytic agents for acute ST elevation myocardial infarction.

Differential pharmacology

Aspirin acts inside platelets, blocking synthesis of thromboxane A2 from arachidonic acid. In doing this, it reduces the aggregating properties of the platelet and because the inhibition is irreversible, the effect lasts for the 7–10-day lifespan of the platelet. However, platelet aggregation can be stimulated by other means and newer drugs have been developed to produce a more complete inhibition, principally by working on or at the key glycoprotein receptor IIb/IIIa site, which is found on the surface of platelets and is the site to which fibrin binds.

Clopidogrel and ticlopidine are structurally related and act by inhibiting the expression of the GP IIb/IIIa receptor. Ticlopidine has a slow onset of action despite producing an active metabolite and produces a maximal effect in 3–7 days. This agent also produces undesirable adverse effects including rash, diarrhoea and, more seriously, neutropenia and agranulocytosis. Clopidogrel also produces rash and diarrhoea but despite being more potent, rarely causes haematological abnormalities. Whilst these two agents inhibit the activation of the GP IIb/IIIa receptor, abciximab is a monoclonal antibody Fab fragment which specifically binds to this receptor and so prevents its availability to initiate clotting. However, this agent is immunogenic and so can only be used once in the same patient.

All the agents discussed have proven antiplatelet aggregating properties, whereas dipyridamole appears to work well when used in combination with another antiplatelet aggregating agent, such as aspirin. Dipyridamole works via many ill-defined mechanisms but is a weak inhibitor itself.

Differential biopharmaceutical properties

Aspirin is well absorbed orally and generally well tolerated. Patients who report gastric irritation can be effectively treated with a suitable proton pump inhibitor, such as omeprazole or landsoprazole. Ticlopidine is excreted renally and a dose adjustment is needed in patients with poor renal function.

Differential pharmaceutical properties

Aspirin, clopidogrel and ticlopidine are available as tablets, dipyridamole as tablets and injection while abciximab is only available as a once-only injection.

THROMBOLYTIC AGENTS

Currently licensed in the UK: alteplase (rt-PA), anistreplase, reteplase, streptokinase, tenecteplase.

Uses

These agents are used for the treatment of myocardial infarction and pulmonary embolism. The majority of cardiac nurses now know the importance of initiating prescribed thrombolytic agents as soon as possible after diagnosis and assessment for contra-indications. After a coronary artery becomes occluded, the amount of myocardium salvaged by clot lysis (breakdown) and subsequent reperfusion is linked critically to the speed of initiating thrombolytic therapy. The mega trials for thrombolysis, which have included many thousands of patients, extend back to the mid-1980s and the GISSI trial in 1986. This demonstrated a 39% reduction in 12-month mortality for patients treated with streptokinase within 1 hour of suspected myocardial infarction (see Chapter 9).

Since the initial trials, subsequent research has demonstrated the benefits of administering aspirin with a thrombolytic agent in infarction (ISIS-2 1988) and the use of β-blockers (Freemantle et al 1999, ISIS-1 1986, Nuttall et al 2000), although the latter still appears underused (Owen 1998). Further trials began comparing varying thrombolytic regimens and GUSTO-1 (1993) demonstrated that accelerated alteplase (that is, the total dose administered over 1.5 hours) was significantly superior in terms of mortality benefit to both streptokinase regimens and to alteplase plus streptokinase. Some questions were unanswered, such as whether the mortality benefits lasted over time. The choice of agent is not always clearcut and will be dictated by factors such as whether streptokinase has been administered previously, inhibiting its use again due to antibody production, the location of the infarct, the presence of hypotension and the risk of adverse effects, such as intracranial bleeding, in more aggressive regimens and, of course, cost. Chapter 9 explores in more detail these ongoing trials, the choice of agent and contra-indications to therapy. Innovations designed to rapidly assess the patient and initiate appropriate thrombolytic therapy are also explored. These include the concept of nurse-led thrombolysis programmes.

Differential pharmacology

All these agents bring about the lysis (breakdown) of a thrombus by converting plasminogen to plasmin. Streptokinase possesses no intrinsic enzymatic activity but by exposing an active site on fibrinogen, it brings about the breakdown of the chain to fibrin. Anistreplase is a streptomycin–lysplasminogen complex that should allow it to 'target' a thrombus more accurately but in practice, systemic fibrinolysis still occurs. Both of these agents are immunogenic and so can only be used once in any one patient.

Alteplase and reteplase possess enzymatic activities of their own and effectively bring about thrombolysis.

Streptokinase and anistreplase are not thrombus specific, unlike alteplase and reteplase. Nonetheless, there is little clinical difference between these agents with respect to systemic bleeding. Other adverse effects include hypotension and low-grade fever with streptokinase and anistreplase. In 2001 a single-dose variant of alteplase (tenecteplase) became available.

Differential biopharmaceutical properties

All agents are given intravenously and the agents' short half-lives result in their administration time being 60–90 minutes. The exceptions are reteplase, which can be given as two single bolus doses, and anistreplase, which is given as a single 5-minute bolus. Tenecteplase is administered as a single weight-related bolus dose over 5–10 seconds.

Differential pharmaceutical properties

None. All are available as injection only.

LIPID-REGULATING DRUGS

- Anion exchange resins
- Clofibrate group
- Statins
- Nicotinic acid group

Anion exchange resins

Currently licensed in the UK: colestyramine, colestipol.

Uses

Used for the management of hypercholesterolaemia, in particular type IIa hyperlipidaemia.

Differential pharmacology

None. Both bind bile salts in the intestine and prevent re-absorption of the bile in the terminal ileum. Thus the body synthesizes more bile salts from cholesterol, thereby reducing the hepatic stores. There is an unfortunate increase in triglycerides.

Differential biopharmaceutical properties

None. These agents do not work systemically and so although there are no systemic side-effects, there are common complaints of gastro-intestinal upset, constipation and abdominal fullness. Also, as the exchange resin can cause a decrease in the absorption of many drugs, for example digoxin, fat-soluble vitamins and warfarin, these must be taken 1 hour before or 6 hours after the resin.

Differential pharmaceutical properties

None. Both are available as powders/granules in a sachet.

Clofibrate group

Currently licensed in the UK: clofibrate, bezafibrate, ciprofibrate, fenofibrate and gemfibrozil.

Uses

These agents decrease LDL cholesterol, whose levels are linked to the development of coronary heart disease, increase HDL cholesterol, which is a protective factor, but mainly they decrease triglycerides.

Differential pharmacology

There is little difference between these agents. They all stimulate lipoprotein lipase and so increase the hydrolysis of triglycerides. The exact mechanism of action is unclear. Unusually, one agent in this group, clofibrate, causes an adverse effect that is unique in the group – it increases the chances of developing gallstones by increasing cholesterol secretion through the bile duct. As a result this agent should only be used in patients who have had a cholecystectomy.

Differential biopharmaceutical properties

None.

Differential pharmaceutical properties

None. All are available as tablets or capsules.

Statins

Currently licensed in the UK: atorvastatin, cerivastatin, fluvastatin, pravastatin, simvastatin.

Uses

All agents in this group are effective in reducing total cholesterol levels, while atorvastatin can also lower triglycerides. Only some have shown that these biochemical modifications result in clinically important reduction in morbidity and mortality. However, there is an increased move towards thinking that these clinical effects are a group effect. This suggests that they could occur with any of the agents.

Differential pharmacology

None. All act by inhibiting 3-hydroxy 3-methylglutaryl co-enzyme A (HMG CoA) reductase, although atorvastatin is the most potent, reduces cholesterol levels faster and affects triglycerides, as mentioned.

Differential biopharmaceutical properties

The enzyme HMG CoA is most active during the night and should be taken at this time for maximal effect. However, this does not appear to be necessary for atorvastatin, which has a particularly long half-life.

Differential pharmaceutical properties

None.

Nicotinic acid group

Currently licensed in the UK: acipimox, nicotinic acid.

Uses

These agents lower cholesterol and triglycerides and increase HDL cholesterol, a protective factor for coronary heart disease.

Differential pharmacology

Both work in adipose tissue to decrease the supply of triglycerides to the liver. Prostaglandin-mediated vasodilatation causes flushing, dizziness, headaches, palpitations and pruritus (itching) but these effects, which are more marked with nicotinic acid, can be obviated by reducing the starting dose or by taking aspirin 75 mg 30 minutes before the nicotinic acid. Although acipimox has a better side-effect profile, it is also less effective.

Differential biopharmaceutical properties

None.

Differential pharmaceutical properties

None.

Combining classes of lipid-lowering agents: a warning from the Committee for the Safety of Medicines (CSM)

The CSM has advised that rhabdomyolysis (a condition of acute renal failure via a variety of factors such as poisoning, excessive myoglobin release from skeletal muscle as in crush injuries and hyperthermia) can be associated with lipid-regulating drugs, such as the fibrates and statins. This appears to be extremely rare but may be increased in those with renal impairment and possibly in those with hypothyroidism. Concomitant treatment with a fibrate and a statin may also be associated with an increased risk of serious muscle toxicity.

CONCLUSION

This chapter has attempted to illustrate how it is possible to differentiate between agents that appear similar, from within a group of their class. In some cases, the differences are marked, for example with the calcium channel blockers. This makes it questionable as to why such different agents are classified similarly. Conversely, there is little to separate the low molecular weight heparins in terms of their pharmacological, biopharmaceutical or pharmaceutical properties. Yet even here not all of the agents are licensed for every indication and so a simple choice can be made – use a licensed product.

However, there must be methods of choosing between agents that are just too similar, such as the clofibrate group. It may be possible to differentiate between agents by using information from reputable randomized controlled trials. If the evidence exists and

is pertinent to the patient group, it is difficult to argue against the trial data. Indeed, if we consider our responsibilities under clinical governance, it may be considered negligent to do so.

Nonetheless, there is always another great practicality to bear in mind and that is, naturally, cost. Simply put, we all need to make the most of the resources available and so we are, in effect, helped to make a choice when the three properties described throughout this chapter and the issue of licensing fail to differentiate the drugs. If all the agents are the same, with no clinically significant differences, choose the cheapest.

This neatly places the choice of an agent into a framework that is easy to use, but the reality is that the evidence is never clearcut. All agents will produce side-effects as well as beneficial effects. How can you quantify, in monetary terms, the cost of a side-effect, beneficial effect and quality and quantity of life? This is an area of economic analysis termed pharmacoeconomics which, although highly relevant to cardiac care, is outside the remit of this chapter.

As to the future, individual chapters within this text highlight the pharmacological directions that we can expect which will affect nursing and medical practice. These include the use of β-blocker therapy in heart failure and the emergence of the glycoprotein IIb/IIIa antagonists for patients at high risk of coronary occlusion during coronary invasive procedures. The latter group of drugs may also be used in the management of infarction, with concomitant use of the traditional thrombolytics. Thrombolytics themselves may undergo changes in the way they are administered, in terms of speed and number of doses. In the future, drugs used in a familiar and 'traditional' role may well emerge as a new and alternative cardiac therapy. The role of nursing is to meet these changes with innovative, often multidisciplinary strategies to implement and monitor treatments for patients who are living with cardiac conditions.

REFERENCES

British Heart Foundation 2000 Coronary heart disease statistics database: annual compendium 2000. British Heart Foundation, London

British National Formulary 2001 41st edn. British Medical Association and the Royal Pharmaceutical Society of Great Britain, London

CAST-1 (Cardiac Arrhythmia Suppression Trial) 1989 New England Journal of Medicine 321: 406–412

CAST-2 (Cardiac Arrhythmia Suppression Trial) 1992 New England Journal of Medicine 327: 227–233

Cuthbertson BH, Noble DW 1997 Dopamine in oliguria. British Medical Journal 314: 690–691

Evans D 1998 Inotropic therapy – current controversies and future directions. Nursing in Critical Care 3(1): 8–11

Freemantle N, Cleland J, Young P, Mason J, Harrison J 1999 Beta blockade after myocardial infarction: systemic review and meta regression analysis. British Medical Journal 318: 1730–1737

Galbraith A, Bullock S, Manias E, Hunt B, Richards A 1999 Fundamentals of pharmacology: a text for nurses and health professionals. Addison Wesley Longman, Harlow

GISSI (Gruppo Italiano per lo Studio della Streptochinasi nell Infarcto Miocardico) 1986 Lancet i: 397–401

Graver J 1992 Inotropes – an overview. Intensive and Critical Care Nursing 8: 169–179

GUSTO-1 1993 Global utilisation of streptokinase and t-PA for occluded coronary arteries. New England Journal of Medicine 329: 673–682, 1615–1622

ISIS-1 (International Study of Infarct Survival Collaborative Group) 1986 Randomised trial of intravenous atenolol among 16,027 cases of suspected acute myocardial infarction. Lancet ii: 57–66

ISIS-2 (International Study of Infarct Survival) 1988 Lancet ii: 349–360

Nuttall SL, Toescu V, Kendall MJ 2000 Beta blockers have a key role in reducing morbidity and mortality after infarction. British Medical Journal 320: 581

Owen A 1998 Intravenous beta blockade in acute myocardial infarction. British Medical Journal 317: 226–227

Pye M 2000 Glycoprotein IIb/IIIa receptor blockade: the clinical trials in acute coronary syndromes and percutaneous coronary intervention. Cardiology 3(4): 8–14

Resuscitation Council (UK) 2000 Resuscitation Council guidelines. Resuscitation Council, London

Schumann D 1991 Sublingual nifedipine controversy in drug delivery. Dimensions in Critical Care Nursing 10: 314–320

Swanton H 1997 Amiodarone. British Journal of Hospital Medicine 58(7): 329–332

Task Force of the Working Group on Arrhythmias of the European Society of Cardiology 1991 The 'Sicilian Gambit'. A new approach to the classification of anti-arrhythmic drugs based on their actions on arrhythmogenic mechanisms. European Heart Journal 12: 1112–1131

Vaughan Williams EM 1970 Classification of anti-arrhythmic drugs. In: Sandhoe E, Flensted-Jensen E, Loesen KH (eds) Symposium on cardiac arrhythmias. AB Astra, Sodertalje, Sweden, p. 449

FURTHER READING

ABPI 1998–99 Compendium of data sheets and summaries of product characteristics. Datapharm Publications, London

Hardman JG, Limbird LE 1996 Goodman & Gilman's the pharmacological basis of therapeutics, 9th edn. McGraw-Hill, New York

Laurence DR, Bennett PN, Brown MJ 1997 Clinical pharmacology, 8th edn. Churchill Livingstone, Edinburgh

Page CP, Curtis MJ, Sutter MC, Walker MJA, Hoffman BB 1997 Integrated pharmacology. Mosby, London

Rang HP, Dale MM, Ritter JM 1999 Pharmacology, 4th edn. Churchill Livingstone, Edinburgh

20

Electrophysiology studies

Angela Bygrave

Until recently electrophysiology remained the domain of large teaching hospitals and academic institutions. Furthermore, electrophysiologists were viewed with some curiosity and specialized electrophysiology (EP) nurses were unheard of. Cardiology is a rapidly changing medical specialty and electrophysiology is no exception. With the increase in nurse specialists and indeed consultant nurses, it may not be long before the field of electrophysiology benefits from such practitioners.

Cardiac electrophysiology simply refers to the electrical conduction system of the heart. An electrophysiological study (EPS) is an invasive procedure performed in order to diagnose and potentially treat disorders of the heart's electrical system. Therefore an EP study may be categorized as either a diagnostic procedure or a therapeutic one, although frequently both are performed as one in a single session. The disorders of electrical function usually manifest as arrhythmias, which may be a form of bradycardia or tachycardia and may produce a variety of symptoms in each individual. It would be useful to be familiar with Chapter 4 with regard to the anatomy and physiology of the heart which will help to provide a deeper understanding of electrophysiology.

Figure 20.1 shows the important electrophysiological structures of the heart.

THE PROCESS OF REFERRAL

It is important to understand the process by which a patient ultimately has an EP study performed. This process may take place in a number of ways. A common symptom may be episodes of palpitation, causing the patient to visit their general practitioner (GP). Often patients do not seek help until their symptoms become more frequent or severe. Other symptoms may be breathlessness, fatigue, chest pain, presyncope or syncope (a transient loss of consciousness, due to interrupted cerebral blood flow). The

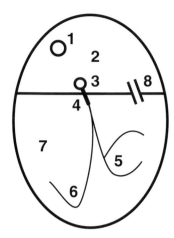

1. Sino-atrial node (SAN)
2. Atrial myocardium
3. Atrioventricular node (AVN)
4. His bundle penetrating the AV ring
5. Left bundle branch, dividing into anterior and posterior hemibundles (LBB, LAH and LPH)
6. Right bundle branch (RBB)
7. Purkinje fibres and ventricular myocardium
8. (where present – accessory pathway)

Figure 20.1 Electrophysiology structures of the heart.

patient may then be referred to the local hospital for an outpatient clinic visit. Apart from the routine medical history, the physician will take a detailed history of the nature of all the symptoms, including the frequency of symptoms, whether they start and finish suddenly or gradually, when they occur, for example in the daytime or during the night, whether they occur at rest, during exercise or after exercise or whether there is a temporary pattern to the symptoms.

It will also be useful to know if the symptom of palpitation itself is regular or irregular in nature. The patient may be asked to tap out the rhythm in order to determine this point. Women may be asked if the symptoms occur during certain times of their menstrual cycle (known as catamenial symptoms). Certain foods or drinks may exacerbate symptoms (alcohol is a prime example here). Furthermore, the doctor will want to know the severity of the symptoms and a scale of 1–10 may be used as a rough guide.

Physicians should ask what coping strategies the patient may use to either alleviate or terminate symptoms. Certain patients may find vagal manoeuvres, such as the Valsalva manoeuvre, successful in terminating an episode. Others may try a variety of methods, such as drinking ice cold water, lying down, deep breathing or even vigorous exercise. It will be

useful to enquire when the symptoms first appeared, how long they last and the interval between episodes. During a typical outpatient visit a 12-lead electrocardiogram (ECG) will be performed, in order to rule out an obvious abnormality.

At this point documentation of the symptoms is the next step, unless they are associated with syncope in which case EPS should be recommended. Recording a 24- or 48-hour Holter or using an event recorder (see Chapter 8) typically achieves documentation, if symptoms are infrequent. It is always useful to obtain a 12-lead ECG during symptoms and patients are often encouraged to attempt this by visiting their local Accident and Emergency (A&E) department or GP surgery during episodes of the symptoms.

Once ECG documentation of symptoms has been achieved, and providing it is appropriate to do so, anti-arrhythmic medication may be commenced in an attempt to reduce the frequency or severity of the symptoms (see Chapter 19). Usually, if symptoms persist or become more severe or frequent or side-effects from the medication occur, the patient will be referred for further investigation. The patient may also request referral if the prospect of taking long-term medication does not appeal. This referral may be to a tertiary centre with specialized arrhythmia services.

At this point the individual may undergo treadmill exercise testing (see Chapter 8), echocardiography, signal-averaged ECG, further Holter recordings and, if appropriate, left and right heart catheterisation with coronary angiography. Naturally the extent of these investigations will depend very much on the nature of the symptoms, the age of the patient and concurrent illnesses. A number of patients will never follow such a pathway of referral to an electrophysiologist; examples of such patients include those who suffer out-of-hospital cardiac arrest and those suffering from arrhythmias following other cardiac conditions, for example myocardial infarction. These patients may be admitted to their local hospital and then referred directly to an EP centre. There will always be patients who have never suffered illness until an acute cardiac event brings them into contact with a cardiologist (such as failed sudden cardiac death).

INDICATIONS FOR THE EP STUDY
Supraventricular tachycardias

Patients with a history of supraventricular tachycardia (SVT) are the most common group referred to cardiac electrophysiologists. The tendency is for the tachycardia

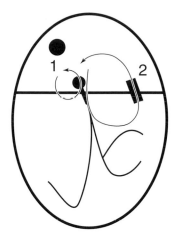

1. AV nodal re-entry
   tachycardia (AVNRT)

2. AV re-entry
   tachycardia (AVRT)
   orthodromic, down
   the AV node and up
   the accessory pathway

Figure 20.2 Atrioventricular re-entry tachycardia (AVRT)
and atrioventricular nodal re-entry tachycardia (AVNRT)
mechanisms.

to be paroxysmal (i.e. episodic) and it is therefore
frequently referred to as paroxysmal supraventricular
tachycardia (PSVT). Typically, individuals present with
narrow complex tachycardia, where the QRS duration
is less than 0.12 s. A narrow complex tachycardia is
most often due to a form of re-entry conduction (see Fig.
20.2) and PSVT is typically seen in young healthy
patients who do not have heart disease (Fogoros 1995).

An EP study may be required in order to establish
the diagnosis and guide therapy. The urgency of referral to an electrophysiologist will largely depend on the
symptoms of each individual. This type of arrhythmia
may be subdivided according to the mechanism.

Atrioventricular nodal re-entry tachycardia

Atrioventricular nodal re-entry tachycardia (AVNRT)
occurs in patients with two rather than one pathway
within the atrioventricular (AV) node region. This
allows the occurrence of re-entry. Conduction travels
antegradely (down) one pathway and retrogradely
(back up) the other pathway. Typical AVNRT is usually
induced from an atrial premature beat (ectopic) that
travels down the slow pathway and up the fast

pathway (see Glossary). An individual with AVNRT
may be referred for electrophysiological assessment
when symptoms become troublesome. Diagnosis via
an EP study may help the choice of drug therapy and
determine the benefits and risks of ablation therapy. A
small number of patients may present with collapse
due to AVNRT, in which case an EP study will almost
certainly be warranted.

Atrioventricular re-entry tachycardia

Atrioventricular re-entry tachycardia (AVRT) is the
typical arrhythmia of patients with Wolff–Parkinson–
White syndrome (WPW). The ECG demonstration of
the presence of an extra connection conducting
between an atrium and a ventricle, but outside the AV
node region, was first described in 1930 (Wolff et al
1930) as a short P–R interval and an abnormal QRS
morphology with a slurred upstroke, thus giving rise
to the appearance of a delta (δ) wave on the ECG.
AVRT most commonly is **orthodromic**; this term refers
to a tachycardia which moves in a forward direction
down the AV node and up through the accessory
pathway. Again, conduction occurs antegradely and
normally through the AV node and then retrogradely
via the accessory pathway back to the atria (Ward &
Camm 1987). This usually gives rise to a narrow
complex re-entry tachycardia, although occasionally
bundle branch block aberration occurs resulting in a
broad complex tachycardia. Orthodromic AVRT is
therefore seen in individuals who do not have overt
pre-excitation but have an accessory pathway which
only conducts retrogradely. The accessory pathway is
known as 'concealed' and the ECG in sinus rhythm is
normal.

Less frequently, tachycardia may be **antidromic**,
when AV antegrade conduction travels down via the
accessory pathway and retrograde conduction occurs
up via the AV node. This gives rise to a broad complex
tachycardia with a slurred upstroke to the QRS
complex.

Another arrhythmia seen in patients with WPW is
atrial fibrillation, which is a particular problem as conduction via the accessory pathway may be particularly
rapid, thus causing haemodynamic instability or even
ventricular fibrillation (VF). This arrhythmia is known
as pre-excited atrial fibrillation and often requires
prompt cardioversion.

Atrial fibrillation and atrial flutter

Details of these arrhythmias can be found in Chapter
6. Ordinarily a patient with atrial fibrillation (AF) may

not be referred for an EP study. However, if conventional management strategies fail and symptoms are particularly troublesome, an EP study may be useful in considering new forms of therapy. Other indications for referral are arrhythmias that are co-existent, for example atrial tachycardia and pre-excitation. An example of new therapy for AF is the atrial defibrillator. This is an implantable device with defibrillator leads in the right atrium and in the coronary sinus, between which an R-wave synchronized shock may be delivered to cardiovert AF. A third lead is situated in the right ventricle, which can provide back-up pacing if required (Ayers et al 1994).

Other reasons for performing an EP study in patients with AF include cases where there is a suspicion of an atrial ectopic focus triggering the arrhythmia, especially paroxysmal AF. It may be possible to identify and locate this focus during an EP study, which may be suitable for ablation therapy. Furthermore, the electrophysiologist may analyse the potential of new forms and/or sites of pacing to prevent the onset of AF. Electrophysiological assessment may be required in atrial flutter if termination by pacing is to be considered or if radiofrequency ablation of the flutter circuit is a therapeutic option.

Atrial tachycardia

This may be due to re-entry or to an abnormal ectopic focus or foci within the atria, known as **enhanced automaticity**. In the automatic form, the tachycardia will 'warm up', where the rate increases after initial induction. The re-entrant form often occurs in patients with atrial scars, such as following cardiac surgery. Although discrete P-waves are seen, they generally differ in appearance from the sinus beat P-waves. An EP study may be warranted to further define the tachycardia mechanism and site of origin or when an ECG diagnosis is not available.

Ventricular tachycardias

There are many different presentations of ventricular tachycardia (VT), with symptoms varying from sudden cardiac death to paroxysmal palpitation. The ECG during tachycardia will give clues to the diagnosis of VT rather than SVT with aberrant conduction and these include a QRS of greater than 0.14 seconds (Schamroth 1990) and AV dissociation. VT is most commonly the result of ischaemic myocardial damage but is also seen in the presence of dilated or hypertrophic cardiomyopathy, arrhythmogenic right ventricular cardiomyopathy (ARVC) (see Chapter 11),

long QT syndrome and metabolic disturbance and in the absence of apparent cardiac disease, where it is known as normal heart VT (NHVT). VT may be identified at EPS as the cause of an out-of-hospital cardiac arrest. Assessment of the need for and efficacy of treatments, such as drugs, ablation and implantable cardioverter defibrillators (ICDs), in patients with actual or suspected VT or VF is an important reason for EP referral.

Syncope

Syncope is defined as the sudden and complete loss of consciousness, with a full recovery within a few minutes (Darling 1994). The causes of syncope are many but following inconclusive non-invasive investigations, i.e. tilt table testing, Holter monitoring, exercise testing and neurological assessment, an EP study may be recommended. This is a challenging situation for the electrophysiologist, who has to assess whether the cause of syncope is arrhythmogenic, due to either tachycardia or bradycardia.

Bradycardias

Bradycardia has a variety of causes including drugs, metabolic disorders and disorders in any part of the conduction system. Sinus node disease and AV block are the most common examples of conduction system disease resulting in bradycardia. Detailed EP evaluation is rarely indicated to determine the nature of such conduction disease.

PREPARATION OF THE PATIENT
Psychological

The psychological preparation of the patient undergoing an electrophysiological study is paramount. Co-operation from the patient is crucial for this type of invasive investigation. It is also important to consider that whilst some patients may tolerate their symptoms, others may find them extremely uncomfortable and distressing and the thought of having symptoms reproduced in the EP laboratory will upset them.

The majority of EP procedures are carried out under light sedation as anaesthetic agents may interfere with the mechanism and induction of the arrhythmia under investigation. Patients have many fears and anxieties concerning not only the investigation but also their cardiac condition, the implications of the diagnosis and broader issues surrounding family and work.

One example could be the case of an aircraft pilot, who may be otherwise fit and well, but found to have an abnormal ECG at routine health screening. Let us consider that the ECG reveals pre-excitation, as in the Wolff–Parkinson–White syndrome, but he has never suffered any symptoms of palpitation, presyncope or syncope. In order to retain his pilot's licence, and therefore his livelihood, an EP study may be recommended. This individual may find the prospect of such an investigation extremely stressful, particularly in the absence of previous symptoms. Another individual may be anxious about the possibility of being given the diagnosis of ventricular tachycardia, with the consequence that the risk of sudden death is higher than in other conditions.

In 1992 Connelly examined the stressors which patients undergoing EP studies faced. She found that family concerns were a major worry. In addition, issues relating to their illness and time spent in hospital caused anxiety. Furthermore, requiring cardioversion during the EPS was a concern, although not ranked as the most stressful element of the whole experience. Connelly concluded that because such patients are faced with so many new experiences, they often do not appreciate the full implications of their illness at the time of hospitalization.

Psychological preparation of the patient undergoing EP studies should commence as early as possible. This may mean at the first outpatient clinic visit when the investigation is first considered. The doctor should give an explanation of the procedure, including complications, risks and implications for future management. However, nurses can play a major part in the explanation of the procedure. This information may come from the outpatient nurse, cardiac nurse or arrhythmia nurse specialist, depending on the availability of such resources. It is often helpful to utilize teaching aids such as simple anatomical pictures or models, information booklets and videos.

On occasions it may be possible to arrange for a patient who has undergone EPS to meet with an individual about to experience the procedure. Obviously, in this situation, careful selection and supervision by the nurse will be necessary in order to allay fears, rather than increase them. It is useful to include the family or those close to the patient in regard to the provision of information. Effective communication between the nurse and patient is essential, particularly as several health-care professionals may be involved in their care. Patients who are given information in the outpatient clinic will benefit from an information booklet to take home, with relevant contact numbers enabling them to make future enquiries. A follow-up telephone call by the appropriate nurse may be a useful method for identifying concerns and allaying fears.

Informed consent

Patients must be given a full explanation of the procedure with the opportunity to ask questions. They should be asked to sign a consent form, which must accompany them to the EP laboratory. They may visit the laboratory prior to the study and meet the EP team (electrophysiologist, nurse, radiographer and technician) and familiarize themselves with the surroundings. It should be explained that the EP team will be wearing theatre clothing and lead aprons, which may be intimidating for some patients. The EP laboratory may contain equipment which looks complicated and of a highly technical nature.

The patient should also be told about the level of pain to expect; for example, the local anaesthetic will cause a stinging sensation and the area becomes numb. They will be aware of a pushing sensation when venous access is achieved. The positioning of the wires may be completely painless, although some patients report a momentary discomfort at this point. Furthermore, wire positioning may be sufficient to induce tachycardia, a frightening expectation for many patients, particularly those who have collapsed or required cardioversion in the past. It is absolutely essential that patients are informed before the EP study that tachycardia induction is frequently a necessary part of the procedure. Although this may cause anxiety, it should be explained that tachycardia will be induced under controlled conditions and that termination of the arrhythmia will be achieved swiftly, if necessary by pacing. On occasions cardioversion by transthoracic shock may be required if an unstable cardiac rhythm is induced. However, this will occur promptly, may be preceded by sedation and patients should be reassured accordingly.

If a patient is particularly anxious, sedation may be given intravenously, such as a benzodiazepine, e.g. midazolam or diazepam. However, large quantities of sedation should be avoided as tachycardia induction may be made more difficult. Oxygen saturation and blood pressure monitoring are necessary, particularly if sedation has been used. There is continuous ECG monitoring. The patient will be required to confirm that the symptoms of induced tachycardia match the clinical symptoms. Occasionally, an opiate may be used, frequently diamorphine, with the addition of an anti-emetic, such as metoclopramide. A general anaesthetic will generally only be used in children undergoing EPS.

Physical preparation

The following are usually required.

- Medical notes including details of full physical examination, medical history and family history, history of alcohol and drug use, history of allergies.
- A 12-lead ECG in sinus rhythm and during symptoms (usually tachycardia). Not always possible, but very useful.
- Holter monitor recordings.
- Echocardiography.
- Full blood count, clotting screen and urea and electrolytes.
- Preparation of the site, shave of the right and left groin. Occasionally the subclavian or internal jugular veins are used, in which case shave if necessary.
- Removal of dentures if loose; they are kept in if they are a good fit (Colquhoun et al 1999).
- A pregnancy test for women of child-bearing potential, due to the risks to the fetus associated with the use of X-rays during the procedure.
- A 'drug-free state'. Anti-arrhythmic medication should generally be discontinued for at least five half-lives prior to the EP study, as these drugs may alter cardiac electrophysiology and suppress tachycardia. Medication will not be discontinued if testing the efficacy of a drug, in the case of VT.
- Nil by mouth for 4–6 hours before the procedure, in case intubation is required. However, starving a patient for longer than 6 hours may cause dehydration and make venous access difficult.
- An intravenous cannula will be positioned in one of the veins in the arm.
- Skin preparation prior to ECG monitoring. This may involve shaving, cleaning the skin with an alcohol wipe and gentle exfoliation in order to record a clear ECG signal.
- A baseline recording of blood pressure and heart rate. Usually blood pressure is recorded conventionally but a high-risk patient, such as those likely to experience VT or VF, may require arterial blood pressure monitoring.
- Skin preparation with an antiseptic solution (chlorhexidine or iodine based).
- Sterile drapes surrounding the site. The drapes will reach from the patient's neck to the feet.

COMPLICATIONS

Despite the complex and invasive nature of EP studies, the complication rate is considered to be low. The majority of complications are associated with the introduction of catheters into the veins. These include bleeding or bruising, thrombo-embolism and infection. The induction of tachycardias associated with haemodynamic collapse, e.g. polymorphic VT or VF, may occur but is dealt with by transthoracic shock. Chen et al (1996) reported that 12 out of 1643 patients experienced VF whilst undergoing electrophysiological procedures. Other serious complications include pericardial effusion and tamponade but these are extremely rare in diagnostic EP studies and, if at all, more likely to be seen in elderly patients (Chen et al 1996).

THE DIAGNOSTIC ELECTROPHYSIOLOGICAL PROCEDURE IN DETAIL

These studies are generally performed in a specified procedure room such as a cardiac catheterisation laboratory or electrophysiological laboratory. The electrode catheters or 'wires' are inserted under aseptic conditions using fluoroscopic (direct viewing via X-ray) control. The purpose of the study is to identify abnormalities of cardiac electrical conduction by recording and pacing from intracardiac signals at various sites within the heart. The safety issues during the EP study are a crucial part of the diagnostic process. All emergency equipment, including the defibrillator, oxygen, suction and airway tray, must be checked and documented prior to each laboratory session. The personnel involved in performing the study should be trained and qualified in the skills of advanced life support. Furthermore, the relevant personnel (manufacturer or medical physics department) should check and maintain all electrical equipment in good working order on a regular basis. The radiation exposure must comply with radiation protection guidelines and the exposure to patients and staff must be limited, where possible. As the study will be performed under aseptic conditions, sterility of relevant areas is paramount.

Once the patient is prepared, physically and psychologically, the study will commence. The Seldinger technique is usually applied in order to introduce the catheter electrodes. This involves injecting local anaesthetic (lidocaine (lignocaine) 1% or 2%) around the relevant femoral vessel (usually the right femoral vein). The vein is punctured with a needle, a guidewire is inserted through the needle into the vessel and an introducer sheath advanced over the guidewire. Several introducer sheaths may be inserted into the vessel. It is not a standard procedure to cannulate an artery for an EP study, although this may be done if arterial blood pressure monitoring is required or if signals are necessary from the left side of the heart. At this point the catheter electrodes are inserted, using fluoroscopic guidance, into the right side of the heart.

Catheter electrode positioning

A variety of catheter electrodes are available with different curve shapes, tip spacing and poles (number of electrodes) (Fig. 20.3).

Generally quadrapolar (4) catheter electrodes are used, to allow sensing from the proximal and pacing from the distal bipoles (2). The standard wire positions include the high right atrium (HRA), which refers to the right atrial appendage. A second wire is usually positioned in the right ventricular apex (RVA), although this may subsequently be repositioned into the right ventricular outflow tract (RVOT) in studies

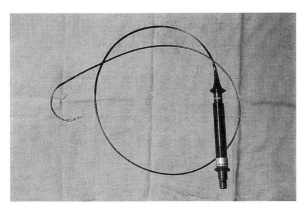

Figure 20.3 Catheter electrode. (Reproduced with permission of St George's Hospital Medical School.)

involving induction of ventricular tachycardia. Adequate positioning of this wire is paramount, as it is required for back-up pacing in the event of bradycardia or complete heart block. The His bundle electrogram (HBE) is located by passing the electrode across the tricuspid valve in its anterior and septal portion. A small potential or 'spike' will be seen between the atrial and ventricular signals as the electrode is advanced and then withdrawn slowly to achieve clearer recordings. This intracardiac signal enables studies of AV nodal function and because conduction is seen from the atria, His and ventricle, it is often the most important catheter position in the EP study (Fig. 20.4).

The fourth electrode is positioned in the coronary sinus, which enables recording and pacing from the left atrium. In this position, signals will be seen from the left atrium and ventricle. The coronary sinus ostium (or opening) is located in the medial posterior septum of the right atrium (Singer 1997), in the AV groove. It is often said to be most easily positioned from a superior approach (superior vena cava), although it is possible to place it from the femoral vein, using a steerable catheter and in the hands of an experienced operator (Fig. 20.5).

The intracardiac signals are displayed simultaneously with selected ECG signals, on a multichannel recorder (Figs 20.6, 20.7). These signals are stored for later retrieval and analysis, as review of the study may be necessary in order to obtain a correct diagnosis.

Issues of recording and pacing

'Normal' measurements may vary according to age (Ward & Camm 1987).

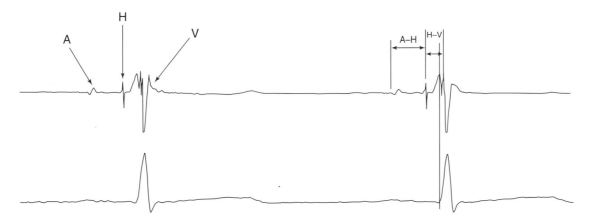

Figure 20.4 His bundle electrogram.

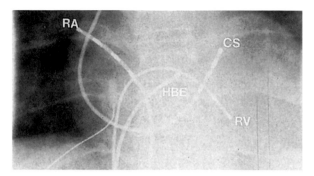

Figure 20.5 X-ray showing fourth electrode position. (Reproduced with permission from Grace et al 1993.)

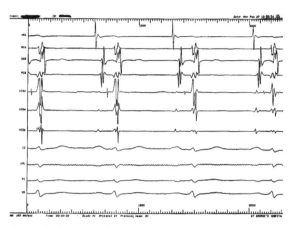

Figure 20.6 Intracardiac signals of basic EP intervals. (Reproduced with permission of St George's Hospital Medical School.)

Baseline conduction intervals

The PR, RR, intervals, QRS duration and QT interval are measured from the surface ECG. The PA interval is a measure of intra-atrial conduction, from the onset of the P-wave on the surface ECG to the onset of atrial conduction in the His bundle electrogram recorded with the His bundle catheter (Josephson 1993). The PA interval is normally 25–55 ms (Ward & Camm 1987).

The AH interval is an indication of AV nodal conduction and is measured from the atrial electrogram recorded on the His bundle catheter to the onset of the His electrogram (see Fig. 20.7). Values of 60–125 ms are considered normal (Josephson 1993).

The HV interval is a measure of conduction time from the His bundle to the ventricle, indicated by the onset of the His signal to the onset of the ventricular signal recorded by the His bundle catheter. Normal values are 35–55 ms.

Pacing

Pacing protocols vary according to the laboratory but generally include evaluations of ventricular, atrial, SA and AV nodal conduction and attempts to induce tachycardia. The endpoint of the study is to acquire a complete understanding of the patient's conduction system and to define any abnormal rhythms. The clinical relevance of an induced tachycardia depends in part on whether the symptoms are similar to clinical (i.e. spontaneous) episodes. This means that the tachycardia induced in the laboratory should correlate with the patient's symptoms. For this reason the patient should be co-operative and be given the correct quantity of sedation in order to maintain comfort but coupled with the ability to communicate with the physician or nurse.

Incremental pacing means pacing at a gradually increasing rate, to observe the response in the conduction intervals. Pacing from the ventricle in this way will determine the presence of ventriculo-atrial (VA), that is, retrograde conduction, which is present in 40–90% of the population. Furthermore, changes in atrial activation will be seen and the presence of a concealed accessory pathway may be revealed. Refractory periods (when depolarization cannot occur) will be measured in both the ventricle and atrium. Refractoriness indicates the response of the myocardial tissue to premature paced impulses. Typically, the effective refractory period (ERP) is determined as part of the electrophysiology protocol, although measurements of the functional refractory period and relative refractory period are possible. The ERP is defined as the longest coupling interval (the time between successive paced beats) for which an impulse fails to propagate (stimulate to depolarize) through that tissue (Fogoros 1995, Josephson 1993).

The ventricular effective refractory period (VERP) is determined by pacing the ventricle at a certain cycle length (e.g. 600 ms or 100 bpm), for a certain number of impulses (e.g. eight) and then delivering an earlier or premature stimulus. The point at which the stimulus no longer captures the ventricular myocardium in order to deplorize it is the ERP. This process may be repeated at other cycle lengths, depending on the patient's intrinsic heart rate. A normal VERP is in the range of 170–290 ms (Josephson 1993).

Atrial pacing will determine 'antegrade' conduction, which is conduction from the atria to the ventricles. This may be normal, delayed or absent. There may be sudden increases in the A–H (atri–His) interval

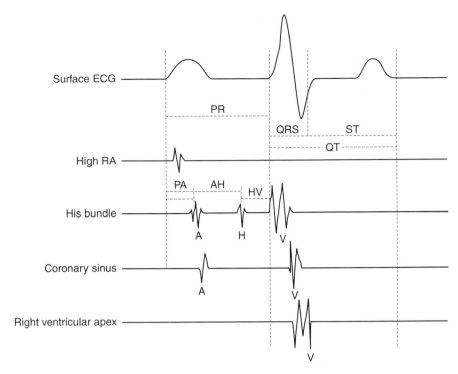

Figure 20.7 EP intervals.

noted through small changes in the paced beats delivered, indicating AV nodal duality (two pathways in the AV node). The refractory period of the atria is determined in a similar manner to that of the ventricle. The AV nodal refractory period is also quantified by examining each premature beat to observe when one fails to conduct through the AV node. Sinus node function is evaluated by the measurement of the sinus node recovery time (SNRT). The SNRT is measured by suppressing the sinus node using overdrive atrial pacing. The pacing rate is set just above the sinus rate and continued for at least 30 seconds. Pacing is stopped abruptly and the time taken from the last paced beat to the first spontaneous sinus beat is the SNRT. As normal sinus rates vary, this measurement may be repeated at various cycle lengths and corrected for the underlying sinus rate, by subtraction of the sinus cycle length from the SNRT preceding the pacing. Pacing gives rise to the SNRT by suppressing the sinus node and observing the time from the last paced beat to the first sinus beat (as explained above). A normal CSNRT (C=corrected) is less than 550 ms (Darling 1994).

The refractory periods within the atrium are measured by pacing the right atrium in the same way that

ventricular refractory periods are achieved. The atrium is paced at a fixed rate for a determined number of beats and an earlier impulse delivered until it no longer captures. This method will give rise to the atrial ERP (AERP), which is normally in the range of 150–360 ms (Josephson 1993). Again various cycle lengths may be used as part of the EP protocol.

AV nodal conduction is determined by assessing the AV nodal ERP (AVNERP), by pacing the high right atrium for a number of impulses and delivering an earlier impulse until block through the AV node occurs. A normal AVNERP will range between 230–425 ms (Josephson 1993). This method may also be applied in terms of retrograde conduction, by pacing the ventricle and assessing the retrograde refractory period of the AV node. This is achieved by observing for conduction occurring backwards from the ventricles, through the AV node, to the atria.

In addition, AV nodal conduction is determined by evaluating the point at which the AV node blocks conduction. This is known as the Wenkebach cycle length. It is performed both antegradely by pacing the atrium and retrogradely by pacing the ventricle. In each case incremental pacing commences with a stepwise increase in the pacing rate (ramp pacing). The pacing rate increases until the point at which block occurs. In regard to the antegrade Wenkebach, the A–H interval will increase with the pacing rate until Wenkebach block is seen. There are various influences on AV conduction, for example the autonomic nervous system and the presence of accessory nodal pathways, which mean that the AV Wenkebach point may occur normally in the range of 500–350 ms (Josephson 1993). These figure are the correct way round because 500 ms is a slower rate than 350 ms. The retrograde Wenkebach is seen as a cessation of VA conduction.

Tachycardia induction

An important component of the EP study is the induction of tachycardia, where appropriate. It is desirable to have documented evidence of the 'clinical' or spontaneous tachycardia in the form of a 12-lead ECG. Therefore, should tachycardia occur during the study, the ECG recording may be compared to the 'clinical'

example. This is especially important in patients with VT, who may suffer from more than one form or circuit of VT (Fig. 20.8). The aim of inducing tachycardia during the EP study is to observe the onset, cycle length, activation sequence, termination and effects of tachycardia.

A variety of pacing protocols to induce tachycardia may be utilized. Typically, pacing the atria will initiate a SVT and ventricular pacing will induce a VT. Various stimulation protocols are used but typically they will consist of a stepwise approach, becoming more aggressive as the protocol progresses. Table 20.1 is an example of a typical VT stimulation protocol. This protocol works by pacing the ventricle in an increasingly aggressive manner, in order to induce VT. For example, stage 1 indicates that while in sinus rhythm, one ventricular premature beat is introduced, until it does not capture or becomes refractory. This is the equivalent of a patient experiencing a ventricular ectopic in an everyday situation.

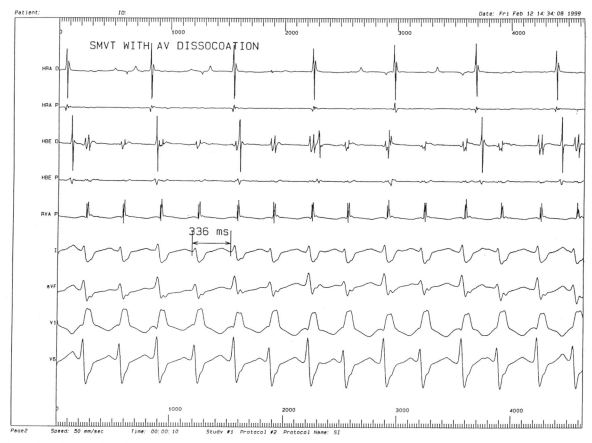

Figure 20.8 Intracardiac signals of single morphology VT. (Reproduced with permission of St George's Hospital Medical School.)

At the other end of the protocol, stage 12 involves pacing at 400 ms (or 150 bpm) for eight beats, followed by three ventricular premature beats. The stage at which VT is induced is an endpoint. In other words, if VT is induced at stage 1, it means that the arrhythmia is easily inducible, so there is no value in going on to the next stage. If VT is not induced at all, the patient's VT is known as non-inducible. Generally speaking this is an encouraging sign and may mean that the patient is less likely to experience VT in a clinical situation than someone who has VT induced at an early stage.

If pacing should fail to induce tachycardia, isoprenaline may be given as an infusion in a concentration of 10 μg/ml or as a bolus of up to 5–10 μg. Doses of around 3 μg per minute may be titrated in order to increase the sinus rate to >100 bpm. The patient is warned that they will feel their heart racing and 'thumping', as if they were exercising. Some patients feel hot and agitated at this point. However, the isoprenaline is usually administered for only a few minutes and the short half-life means that the effects disappear within approximately 10 minutes. Care should be taken in patients with ischaemic heart disease, as this form of 'stress' on the heart may aggravate pre-existing ischaemia.

The role of the EP nurse is crucial during tachycardia induction in terms of patient safety. Observation of the patient's level of consciousness, blood pressure and degree of comfort, including evidence of chest pain, are all important factors which will be communicated to the electrophysiologist. If, for example, the blood pressure is low and the patient feels dizzy, the electrophysiologist may need to terminate the tachycardia promptly. Termination of tachycardia usually consists of pacing, either single, double or triple pre-

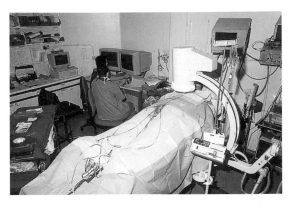

Figure 20.9 An EP study in progress. (Reproduced with permission of St George's Hospital Medical School.)

mature beats, or overdrive, or burst pacing with or without a combination of premature impulses. These kinds of anti-tachycardia pacing are not only important in terms of restoring the patient to sinus rhythm in the laboratory but also in terms of future management, particularly if an ICD is a consideration for treatment of VT (see Chapter 25). Occasionally, drugs may need to be administered if pacing fails to terminate the tachycardia. Adenosine intravenously in a bolus may be given for AVRT or AVNRT, as it blocks AV nodal conduction. The advantage of using this medication is the short half-life, which will not alter cardiac electrophysiology for the remainder of the EP study. Should AF persist, cardioversion by shock or drugs may be required to restore sinus rhythm. If pulseless VT or VF is induced, immediate defibrillation is required, after which the patient will need reassurance and explanation.

POST-PROCEDURE CARE

Following the recording, pacing, tachycardia induction and termination (if appropriate), a diagnosis is obtained. The wires are withdrawn and, providing heparin has not been administered, the sheaths are removed. Digital pressure is applied to prevent haematoma formation. The patient is transferred to the ward and remains on bedrest for at least 2 hours for femoral venous cannulation and 4 hours for arterial punctures. These puncture sites are covered with a small dressing and observed for signs of bleeding, swelling and inflammation. Those patients with a subclavian puncture site will require a chest X-ray to detect the presence of a pneumothorax.

The blood pressure, heart and respiratory rate should be recorded and assessed on return to the

Table 20.1 Wellens' protocol (after Wellens et al 1985)

Stage	Drive cycle	Premature beats
1	Sinus rhythm	1
2	Sinus rhythm	2
3	600 ms	1
4	600 ms	2
5	500 ms	1
6	500 ms	2
7	400 ms	1
8	400 ms	2
9	Sinus rhythm	3
10	600 ms	3
11	500 ms	3
12	400 ms	3

600 milliseconds (ms) = 100 beats per minute (bpm)
500 ms = 125 bpm
400 ms = 150 bpm

ward. It may be necessary to monitor the heart rhythm, depending on the diagnosis. Particular attention is given to those patients who have received sedation with regard to their level of consciousness, respiratory pattern and haemodynamic status. These individuals may have some difficulty in recalling the EP study and information regarding the diagnosis, due to the amnesic effects of certain medication. It is therefore important that the facts relating to the diagnosis and future management are discussed at an appropriate time.

Hereafter therapy may involve medication, device therapy (pacemaker, ICD), surgery, catheter ablation or a combination of these. The treatment options will be discussed with the individual in terms of benefits, side-effects, expected outcomes and waiting-list times for certain procedures. Patients may require education regarding medication, in terms of dose, administration and side-effects.

Depending on the management plan, the patient may be discharged on the day of the EP study or indeed undergo an appropriate procedure, such as catheter ablation, serial drug testing or surgery. If discharged, the patient may return to normal activities the following day but avoid strenuous activity for a week in order for the puncture site to heal sufficiently.

CATHETER ABLATION

History

The first human cardiac ablation occurred by accident in 1979. A patient undergoing an EP study sustained complete AV block during direct current defibrillation, where the defibrillator paddles came into contact with the terminal pins of an ordinary electrode catheter (Vedel et al 1979).

High-energy direct current (DC), that which comes from a defibrillator, was one of the early methods used. Catheter electrode construction was not yet sophisticated enough to withstand high-energy delivery, so this later changed to low-energy DC. The disadvantages of these methods are:

● DC energy is painful, so a general anaesthetic is required
● the lesion formed is large and difficult to direct or aim so viable tissue may be destroyed.

Borggrefe et al first used radiofrequency (RF) energy in the treatment of cardiac arrhythmias in 1987. Radiofrequency is high-energy alternating current, which works by causing cell damage via resistive

heating up to 55°C in the area of the catheter tip. This has certain advantages over DC energy, which is painful and less easily tolerated by the patient. It is currently the energy source used by the majority of electrophysiologists.

The delivery of RF energy produces discrete, concentrated areas of damage, which means that careful mapping is required in order to destroy the target site. Furthermore, long-term success also depends on the delivery of RF energy for up to 60 seconds, which means that the catheter has to be maintained in a stable position for that time.

Generally most electrophysiologists will use a temperature-controlled catheter with a sensor in the tip during the ablation procedure. Tissue temperatures of up to 55°C are required in order to cause myocardial cell necrosis at the catheter tip. Once a successful ablation procedure has been performed, a waiting period of up to 30 minutes is necessary to verify that success has been maintained. This may be confirmed by attempting to induce the clinical tachycardia by pacing or pre- and post-isoprenaline administration. (Isoprenaline increases the heart rate and may induce tachycardia.) Other methods of demonstrating successful ablation may be employed. In WPW the δ wave will disappear from the ECG. In the case of concealed accessory pathways, adenosine may be given during ventricular pacing to cause temporary retrograde block in the AV node. The continued presence of a retrograde pathway is thus demonstrated on the ECG by retrograde conduction via the pathway whereas successful ablation is indicated by VA block on the ECG.

Indications

Wolff–Parkinson–White syndrome and concealed accessory pathways

The reasons for performing ablation in these cases are shown in Box 20.1 (see also Case study 20.1)

Atrioventricular nodal re-entry tachycardia

The presence of AVNRT refractory to drug therapy is an indication to ablate one of the atrial inputs to the AV node. These are the 'fast' and 'slow' pathways. In the early years of ablation techniques, the 'fast' pathway was ablated but the risk of complete AV block was high due to the proximity of the compact AV node. Currently it is usual to ablate the 'slow' pathway.

> **Box 20.1** Clinical indications for an ablation procedure
>
> • An atrial arrhythmia, such as AF, conducted via the pathway resulting in a high ventricular rate.
> • AV re-entrant tachycardia which proves refractory to drug therapy.
> • Individuals who are unable to or do not wish to take drug therapy (e.g. women wishing to conceive in the future).
> • Individuals who have a δ wave on the ECG without tachycardia, whose profession excludes such ECG abnormalities (e.g. airline pilots). Such people may have a δ wave on the surface ECG but never have experienced palpitation. Strictly speaking, they would be classed as having a pre-excited ECG but not the WPW syndrome. (These patients only come to attention during routine medical screenings, for example in their job.) Location of the accessory pathway may be anywhere around the AV rings and the most common site is on the left (i.e. mitral) free wall. Success rates of accessory pathway ablation are high and vary between 95–100% depending on their location and the experience of the electrophysiologist.

Atrial fibrillation (AF)

There are patients who suffer severe symptoms associated with AF in whom medication and/or DC shock fails to either cardiovert or control the ventricular rate. In these extreme cases it may be necessary to completely ablate the AV node and implant a permanent pacemaker system. In permanent AF this should be a ventricular device but a dual-chamber device may be used in paroxysmal AF. Although not a curative procedure, this approach has been shown to improve the quality of life in certain individuals (Brignole et al 1994).

Atrial flutter

Common or typical atrial flutter may be ablated by creating a 'line of conduction block', consisting of several adjacent lesions across the isthmus in the right atrium between the tricuspid annulus and the inferior vena cava. The line of RF lesions is continued until both clockwise and counter-clockwise block can be demonstrated. Success rates vary but are generally considered to be around 90% in typical flutter.

Automatic atrial tachycardia

It is possible to ablate the site of origin in these tachycardias, although it may be generally more difficult to locate the precise area. However, this may be a life-

saving procedure in those patients who present with incessant atrial tachycardia and a tachycardia-induced dilated cardiomyopathy. This is because the cardiomyopathy may resolve after restoration and maintenance of sinus rhythm. In patients with paroxysms of atrial tachycardia, where drug therapy has failed or is inappropriate, catheter ablation may be indicated. With recent advances in technology leading to more sophisticated cardiac mapping techniques, locating the tachycardia focus and successful ablation is becoming more frequent.

Ventricular tachycardia

Ventricular tachycardia (VT) is a notoriously difficult arrhythmia to manage, particularly when it occurs in the context of ischaemic heart disease. The success of ablating this tachycardia depends on various factors. The VT ideally has to be inducible and tolerated haemodynamically to allow continual mapping. If VT is not readily inducible from the outset, a technique called pace mapping is used. This involves positioning the catheter electrode in the ventricle and pacing the heart at the same cycle length as the tachycardia. A 12-lead ECG of the paced rhythm is recorded and compared to a 12-lead recording during clinical tachycardia. The catheter is then manoeuvred in order to achieve the same QRS morphology of paced rhythm as the tachycardia.

Successful pace mapping indicates that the catheter is positioned in the relevant area for ablation. This may be a treatment option in those patients suffering from normal heart VT; in other words, VT in the absence of cardiac disease. These patients tend to have relatively haemodynamically stable VT with a single morphology (arising from one site in the ventricle). This means that it is possible to locate discrete areas suitable for ablation. Those patients with VT due to coronary artery disease may be considered for catheter ablation if other treatment options, i.e. drugs or surgery, are not feasible. One difficulty in these cases is that there may be multiple circuits of re-entrant VT due to ischaemic heart disease, which makes ablation difficult.

Nursing considerations of the ablation procedure

Before the procedure

The preparation necessary for the EP study will apply equally to the catheter ablation procedure. There are, however, additional points to consider. Patients will vary in their needs depending on the length of time since the onset of symptoms, diagnosis and time on the waiting list for the procedure. Most important is the issue of informed consent. The electrophysiologist will discuss the procedure in detail, providing success rates for the particular type of ablation and potential benefits and risks. The patient will undoubtedly feel some anxiety regarding the ablation and it is therefore crucial that the nurse involved with the individual patient spends time allaying fears and answering any queries. The use of anatomical models, simplified diagrams and educational videos may be helpful at this stage.

Perhaps the most common issue is the potential risk of catheter-induced complete AV block requiring subsequent permanent pacemaker implantation. This applies to patients with AVNRT and with accessory pathways close to the AV node. The risk in AVNRT should be 2%. As in the case of the EP study, the patient is made aware of the necessity to lie in one position for possibly 2 hours or more. Whatever the individual's situation, the patient must have the relevant details explained, thus enabling him or her to make an informed decision before signing the consent form. Additionally, consent for a general anaesthetic may be sought, in the event that either cardioversion or DC energy as an ablation source is required. A general anaesthetic is used for ablations using DC energy, because, as highlighted, it causes pain and discomfort to the patient. Additional skin preparation may be necessary to facilitate the use of the adhesive grounding pad, which is placed on the upper part of the patient's back and forms part of the RF current circuit.

If arterial access is required or venous access is needed in lengthy procedures, anticoagulation will be given in the form of heparin. Therefore, relevant coagulation results, such as the international normalised ratio (INR) or prothrombin time, may be sought. Any anti-arrhythmic medication will be discontinued for at least five half-lives, because it may alter cardiac conduction.

After the procedure

The ablation catheters and sheaths will be removed at the end of the procedure, unless heparin has been administered. Usually arterial sheaths are not removed until 4 hours after the last dose of heparin. Bedrest is maintained for approximately 4 hours post arterial sheath removal. The puncture sites are observed for signs of bleeding and haematoma formation, which should be reported immediately. The pedal pulses (in the feet) should be checked frequently (initially quarter-hourly) to assess for an adequate peripheral circulation in the lower limbs, in addition to the blood pressure and heart rate. Signs of cardiac tamponade, such as increasing heart rate, raised jugular venous pressure, decreasing blood pressure and restlessness, should be reported immediately and an urgent echocardiogram sought.

If sedation has been administered during the procedure, oxygen saturations are monitored via oximetry until the patient is fully conscious. It may be necessary to monitor the heart rate for some hours after the procedure to display any rhythm disturbances. A 12-lead ECG should be recorded on return to the ward and prior to discharge. Special consideration should be given to new ST and T-wave changes developing after the procedure which, at this point, may be an indication of myocardial damage caused by the ablation.

Obvious changes such as first, second or third degree AV block, inappropriate bradycardia or tachycardia or the return of a δ wave (short P–R interval, slurred upstroke of the R-wave and QRS >0.12 s), indicating the return of accessory pathway conduction, should be brought to the attention of the doctor. Most centres discharge patients on the day of or the day following the ablation procedure. Patients are advised to return to normal activities, including employment, after a few days.

It is important to explain that following such a procedure, some patients are more aware of their heart beat and some have the feeling of presentient palpitation; in other words, the feeling that their palpitations are about to begin again. This is possibly the sensation of ectopic beats, previously the initiating factor in tachycardia. Some individuals are aware of 'missed beats' or an irregularity of the heart. Similarly these feelings are most likely to be ectopic activity and generally become less frequent over a few weeks. However, patients should be told to report any sustained tachycardia and, if possible, to visit their GP or local hospital to obtain a 12-lead ECG during symptoms.

Aspirin 150 mg per day is given for up to 3 months following the procedure, to prevent clot formation at the ablation site. Centres vary on anticoagulation protocols. Patients are generally seen in the outpatient clinic 1–2 months after the procedure.

Complications

It is important to know that the complication rate of catheter ablation, as with electrophysiological studies, is low. Complications of the ablation procedure are primarily related to the catheterisation process, as with the diagnostic electrophysiological study. However, there are additional complications associated with the therapeutic application of RF energy. The most serious of these are those associated with myocardial perforation caused by excessive RF delivery or irreversible destruction of viable conduction tissue. Damage to the pericardium, cardiac tamponade, pericardial effusion and pericarditis occur in less than 1% of patients, but for this reason an echocardiogram may be requested after the ablation procedure and prior to discharge from hospital.

The patient may develop ischaemic changes ranging from angina to infarction. Damage to other cardiac structures, such as the coronary arteries and valves, is a rare but potential hazard. The induction of non-clinical tachycardias, such as polymorphic VT or VF, may occur but these are dealt with promptly. The Multicenter European Radiofrequency Ablation Survey reported an overall complication rate (i.e. not just related to the heart itself) of 5.1% (MERFS 1993). A large single-centre study in China revealed a complication rate of 3.1%, although this rate increased to 6.1% in those patients aged over 75 years (Chen et al 1996).

THE FUTURE

Electrophysiology is an exciting and evolving area of cardiology. In the mid 1980s it was hard to imagine that ablation would become a relatively straightforward and routine treatment for relevant patients. Future advances are not always easy to predict. However, advances in catheter design are likely. These catheters may include features which facilitate positioning and increased stability of the catheter during energy delivery, therefore decreasing the procedure time and potentially reducing associated complications. The use of alternative power sources, such as cryo-ablation, and safe methods of cooling are also possible. More sophisticated mapping techniques and non-contact mapping are probable, thus enabling the treatment of more complex arrhythmias.

Current challenges appear to be the curative treatment of atrial fibrillation and ventricular tachycardia. Abolishing the electrical substrate of atrial fibrilla-

tion, using a catheter maze approach, may provide symptomatic relief and increased quality of life for many sufferers. However, the success of such therapy may depend on the utilization of new methods other than fluoroscopy-guided mapping to identify and select sites for treatment. One of these is intracardiac ultrasound, which offers much more accurate localization of key anatomical landmarks such as the crista terminalis (a muscular ridge in the wall of the right atrium), coronary sinus ostium (the opening of the coronary sinus, a major vein receiving most of the venous blood from the heart) and the pulmonary vein orifices.

Successful ablation of VT due to coronary artery disease would be a welcome advance for this often difficult to treat and life-threatening arrhythmia. However, the effect of such developments has to be considered. The workload of electrophysiology centres would dramatically increase, which may necessitate increased funding for expansion of existing services or the development of new EP centres.

CONCLUSION

Electrophysiological studies and catheter ablation are performed in patients with a variety of arrhythmias. The pattern of referral of such patients to an electrophysiologist may depend largely on local practice. Furthermore, patients likely to be referred are those with seriously symptomatic arrhythmias, rhythm disturbances refractory to drug therapy or those individuals who can no longer tolerate medication due to side-effects. The role of the cardiac nurse in caring for patients undergoing such procedures is vital. Broadly speaking, this role includes the education and provision of information and the awareness of potential complications in order to maintain patient safety.

Catheter ablation can be a complex procedure, which requires the close collaboration of nurses, physicians, technicians and radiographers in order to achieve a successful outcome. It has high success rates, low morbidity and extremely low mortality rates. It is widely becoming the treatment of choice for patients with certain tachyarrhythmias, particularly those of supraventricular origin. The procedure is relatively short in duration, usually lasting a few hours. Ultimately it offers a cure for the patient, compared to a lifetime of anti-arrhythmic drugs or device implantation.

Case study 20.1 Catheter ablation of an accessory pathway due to Wolff–Parkinson–White syndrome (WPW)

Peter Cross, a 25-year-old plumber, was admitted to the Accident and Emergency (A&E) department of his local hospital, with dizziness and palpitation. These symptoms had occurred once previously, 5 years ago, at which time he sought no medical advice. On this occasion the symptoms were of sudden onset and did not terminate spontaneously. He is otherwise fit and well and lives with his wife and young child. On admission to the A&E department, a medical history was taken and a 12-lead ECG was recorded. Figure 20.10 illustrates the rhythm strip recording from Mr Cross.

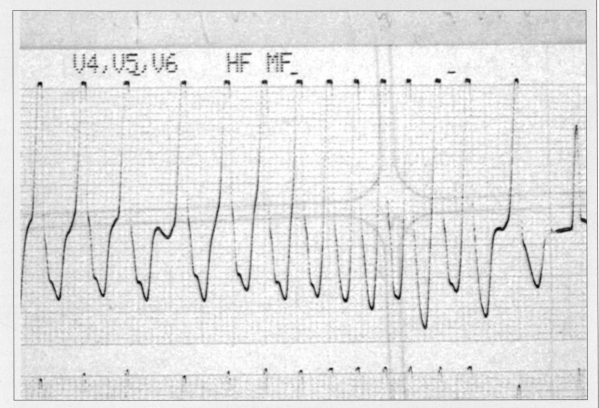

Figure 20.10 Rhythm strip recording of pre-excited AF. (Reproduced with permission from Grace et al 1993.)

The ECG was described at the time as a wide complex tachycardia, possibly ventricular in origin. The initial aim was to restore the tachycardia to sinus rhythm. Therefore, adenosine was given intravenously (IV), in incremental doses, from 6 to 18 mg, with no change in the rhythm. Lidocaine (lignocaine) IV 200 mg was further given with no success. A cardiological opinion was sought and cardioversion recommended and duly carried out, after administration of a general anaesthetic.

Mr Cross was admitted to the coronary care unit (CCU) and was seen by the cardiologists, who felt that the tachycardia recorded on admission was not ventricular tachycardia but atrial fibrillation (AF) in association with ventricular pre-excitation. This means that if atrial fibrillation occurs, it will be conducted through the accessory pathway at a rapid rate, as pathways do not have the slowing properties of the AV node. This rapid ventricular rate may cause haemodynamic collapse or, as in this case,

Case study 20.1 *continued*

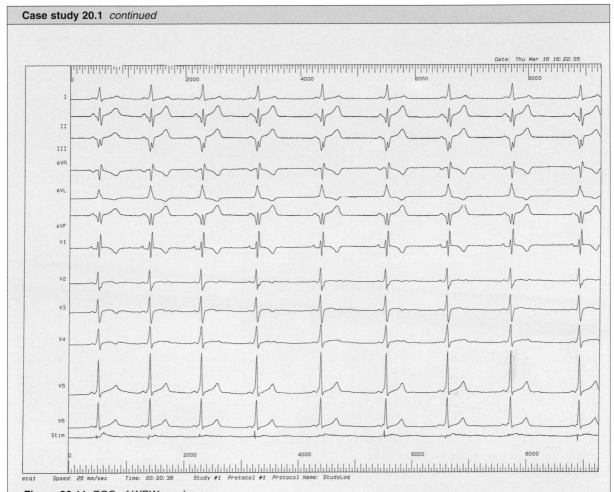

Figure 20.11 ECG of WPW syndrome.

symptoms of palpitation and dizziness. Once cardioverted, the ECG in sinus rhythm was reviewed and a diagnosis of Wolff–Parkinson–White (WPW) syndrome was made. The ECG in Figure 20.11 indicates the short P–R interval of WPW syndrome and the δ wave (slurred upstroke on the QRS complex) clearly visible in leads V2–V4.

An urgent electrophysiological study was recommended to confirm the diagnosis with subsequent ablation using radiofrequency (RF) energy a likely outcome. Two days later the electrophysiological study was performed. The right femoral vein was punctured. The intracardiac electrograms during pacing and sinus rhythm indicated an accessory pathway. During mapping, the pathway was found to be in a right posteroseptal position. RF energy was delivered at this location, during which time pre-excitation disappeared after 3 seconds. The intracardiac electrograms in Figure 20.12 indicate this point.

The disappearance of pre-excitation indicates that the accessory pathway has been abolished. In order to verify this, ventricular pacing is performed, which should indicate blocked conduction from ventricle to atria (known as VA block). However, if there is no VA block, this does not necessarily mean that the pathway is present; it may just mean that conduction from ventricle to atria is still possible via the normal conduction system. In this situation, a bolus of adenosine IV may be given, during sinus rhythm.

Case study 20.1 *continued*

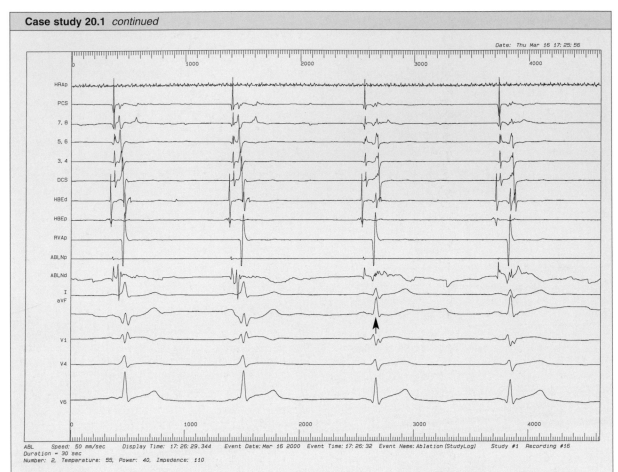

Figure 20.12 Intracardiac electrograms indicating the moment of ablation. The arrow indicates this point most clearly on the ECG, with a change in the shape of the complex.

Adenosine will block AV nodal conduction and, if present, preferential conduction will occur down the accessory pathway, indicated by a broad complex QRS on the surface ECG. This pattern will only be seen for a few seconds as the half-life of adenosine is so short. In this case, the absence of retrograde conduction indicates that the pathway has been abolished and the procedure is considered a success.

Mr Cross returned to the ward and was given the usual postablation care. The following day he was discharged home on aspirin 150 mg per day for 3 months. He was seen in the outpatient clinic 6 weeks later. An ECG recorded at the time is shown in Figure 20.13.

Case study 20.1 *continued*

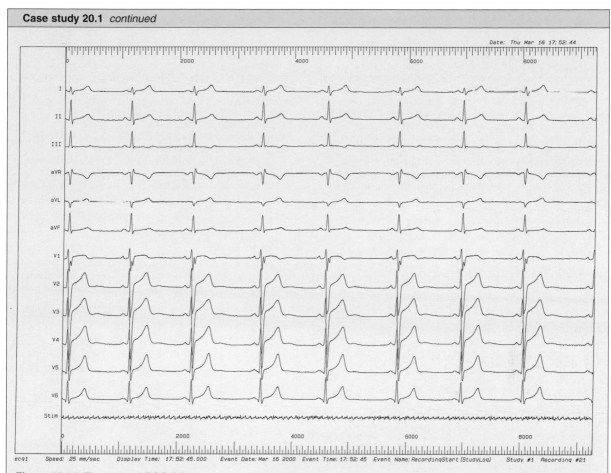

Date: Thu Mar 16 17:52:44

I

II

III

aVR

aVL

aVF

V1

V2

V3

V4

V5

V6

Stim

ecg1   Speed: 25 mm/sec   Display Time: 17:52:45.000   Event Date: Mar 16 2000 Event Time: 17:52:45 Event Name: RecordingStart (StudyLog)   Study #1   Recording #21

Figure 20.13 The 12-lead ECG following successful ablation.

The absence of symptoms after the ablation procedure and the normal ECG mean that the accessory pathway has disappeared. Mr Cross is now considered cured and has been discharged from the clinic.

Case study 20.2 Ventricular tachycardia

Anne Cant, a 26-year-old teacher, was referred to an EP centre with a 7-year history of palpitation. These episodes occurred 2–3 times per month and were described as feeling 'very fast'. Other symptoms included dizziness and, on one occasion, syncope. Various anti-arrhythmics had been tried, all producing either side-effects or lack of efficacy. As the symptoms had become more frequent, the consultant electrophysiologist suggested electrophysiological studies followed by catheter ablation as a treatment option. Initially a diagnostic EP study was performed in order to identify the origin of the palpitation. During wire insertion, sustained broad complex tachycardia was initiated. This tachycardia had a right bundle branch block pattern, right axis deviation and a cycle length of 340 ms, meaning a rate of 177 bpm. The atrial electrograms confirmed the presence of AV dissociation, meaning that the ventricles are working independently of the atrial impulses. These factors are consistent with sustained monomorphic VT, possibly arising from one of the fascicles in the ventricle. The VT terminated spontaneously, thus enabling the EP study to continue. Baseline conduction intervals were normal and the examination of the rest of the conduction system proved to be unremarkable. VT was re-induced and terminated by two ventricular extra stimuli (Fig. 20.14).

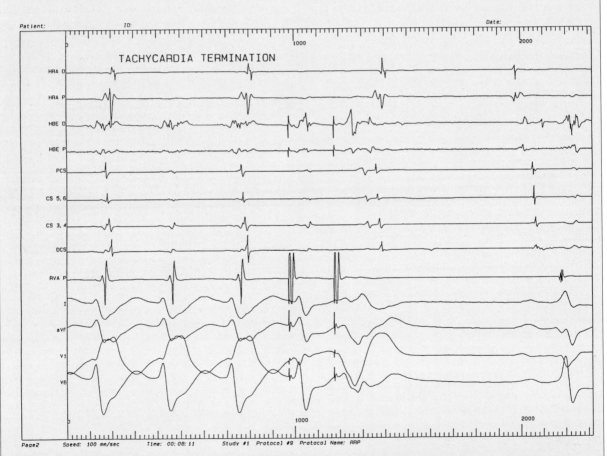

Figure 20.14 Intracardiac signals of termination of VT. (Reproduced with permission of St George's Hospital Medical School.)

Case study 20.2 *continued*

The results of the diagnostic part of the study were discussed with the patient and it was decided that ablation of the VT was to proceed. Following placement of a sheath in the right femoral artery, an ablation catheter was positioned into the left ventricle via the aorta. Anticoagulation in the form of heparin 5000 iu was given to prevent clot formation in the left ventricle. The VT was found to originate from the anterior base of the left ventricular septum. Three applications of RF energy were delivered to this site and the tachycardia, which had previously been easily inducible, was now non-inducible. Therefore a successful ablation was complete.

Anne returned to the ward after a procedure lasting 3 hours. She was offered something to drink and a light meal. Her cardiovascular observations were all normal. The femoral sheaths were removed 4 hours after the administration of heparin, in order to avoid haematoma formation. She remained on bedrest for an additional 4 hours. The following day, Anne was given a 6-week outpatient appointment and discharged home on aspirin 150 mg per day for 3 months.

REFERENCES

Ayers GM, Griffin JC, Flina MB 1994 An implantable atrial defibrillator: initial experience with a novel device. Pacing and Clinical Electrophysiology 17: 769

Borggrefe M, Budde T, Podczeck A, Breithardt G 1987 High frequency alternating current ablation of an accessory pathway in humans. Journal of the American College of Cardiology 10(3): 576–582

Brignole M, Gianfranchi L, Menozzi C et al 1994 Influence of atrioventricular junction radiofrequency ablation in patients with chronic atrial fibrillation and flutter on quality of life and cardiac performance. American Journal of Cardiology 74(3): 242–246

Chen SA, Chiang CE, Tai CT, Cheng CC 1996 Complications of diagnostic electrophysiological studies and radiofrequency catheter ablation in patients with tachyarrhythmias: an eight year survey of 3966 consecutive procedures in a tertiary referral center. American Journal of Cardiology 88(1): 41–46

Colquhoun M, Handley AJ, Evans TR 1999 ABC of resuscitation. BMJ Books, London

Connelly AG 1992 An examination of stressors in the patient undergoing cardiac electrophysiologic studies. Heart and Lung 21(4): 335–341

Darling EJ (ed) 1994 Overview of electrophysiologic testing. Critical Care Clinics of North America 6(1): 1–13

Fogoros RN 1995 Electrophysiologic testing, 2nd edn. Blackwell Science, Boston

Grace AA, Hall JA, Schofield PM 1993 Cardiology. Churchill Livingstone, Edinburgh.

Josephson ME 1993 Clinical cardiac electrophysiology: techniques and interpretations, 2nd edn. Lea and Febiger, Philadelphia

Multicentre European Radiofrequency Survey (MERFS) 1993 Complications of radiofrequency catheter ablation of arrhythmias. The MERFS Investigators of the Working Group on Arrhythmias of the European Society of Cardiology. European Heart Journal 14(12): 1644–1653

Schamroth L 1990 An introduction to electrophysiology, 7th edn. Blackwell Science, Oxford

Singer I (ed) 1997 Interventional electrophysiology. Lippincott, Williams and Wilkins, Baltimore

Vedel J, Frank R, Fontaine G, Fournial JF, Grosgogeat Y 1979 Permanent intra-hisian atrioventricular block induced during right intraventricular exploration. Archives des Maladies du Coeur et des Vaisseaux 72(1): 107–112

Ward DE, Camm AJ 1987 Clinical electrophysiology of the heart. Edward Arnold, London

Wellens HJ, Bruganda P, Stevenson WG 1985 Programmed electrical stimulation of the heart in patients with life-threatening ventricular arrhythmias: what is the significance of induced arrhythmias and what is the correct stimulation protocol? Circulation 72(1): 1–7

Wolff L, Parkinson J, White PD 1930 Bundle branch block with short PR interval in healthy young people prone to paroxysmal tachycardia. American Heart Journal 5: 685

FURTHER READING

Hummel, JD, Kalbfleish SJ, Dillon JM 1999 Pocket guide to electrophysiology. WB Saunders, London

Zara AL, Rose MR (eds) 2000 An introduction to cardiac physiology. Gordon and Breach, Amsterdam

GLOSSARY OF TERMS

Antegrade refers to the forward direction of conduction from atria to the ventricles.

Automatic tachycardia. This mechanism is less common than re-entry. It refers to an abnormal focus firing rapidly and initiating a tachycardia.

Decremental. Where conduction delay occurs, as in the atrio-ventricular (AV) node, it is considered to be decremental.

Effective refractory period. The most commonly used refractory period. It refers to the point at which a premature impulse no longer captures the myocardial tissue to initiate conduction.

It is defined as the longest coupling interval which fails to produce a response.

Morphology. This refers to the ECG pattern of presentation of an arrhythmia, in particular ventricular tachycardia. The awareness of the morphology of a clinical tachycardia may assist the correct diagnosis of those induced in the electrophysiology laboratory.

Non-clinical tachycardia. A tachyarrhythmia initiated in the electrophysiology laboratory, which does not match the patient's symptoms, or a previously documented tachycardia may be described as non-clinical. It may be of little clinical significance and makes diagnosis difficult. This emphasizes the need to record a 12-lead ECG of the tachycardia if at all possible during the familiar symptoms.

Re-entry. The majority of tachycardias are caused by this mechanism. It requires a circuit capable of sustaining a tachycardia within the heart and a premature impulse arriving at a critical moment. Typically, this means the presence of two pathways, with distinct conduction velocities, coupled with the initiation of an appropriately timed premature impulse.

Retrograde refers to the reverse direction of conduction from ventricle to atria.

21

Care of patients requiring cardiac pacing

Maree Barnett

This chapter reviews the indications for cardiac pacing and the various systems available, both temporary and permanent. The conduction system within the heart is revisited to ensure the reader can relate the principles of cardiac pacing to the altered physiology. The chapter assumes a broader pre-existing knowledge of the action potential of a cardiac myocyte and the normal electrocardiogram (ECG) complexes and intervals. Knowledge of the ECG's manifestation of abnormalities is essential for rapid intervention and treatment of the cardiac patient. These areas can be explored in detail in other chapters within this text, notably Chapters 4 and 6.

THE ANATOMY AND PHYSIOLOGY OF THE CARDIAC CONDUCTION SYSTEM

Embryological development

The heart is a derivative of the mesoderm, one of three primitive layers of cells, which begins to develop before the third week of gestation. From the mesodermal cells a pair of endothelial tubes develop (sometimes called the **cardial tube**). These then form a common tube termed the **primitive heart tube**. Five distinct regions begin to develop: the ventricle, bulbus cordis, atrium, sinus venosus and truncus arteriosus. The initial shape is that of a U and then a more sophisticated S shape is taken on. Contraction of the primitive heart begins by day 22 when blood is forced through the tubular heart. At the seventh week partitioning of the heart occurs, the atrium dividing into right and left with an opening between called the foramen ovale. The intraventricular septum also develops, forming the right and left ventricles, and the bulbus cordis and truncus arteriosus divide into two vessels. The aorta arises from the left ventricle, the pulmonary trunk from the right ventricle and the superior and inferior vena cavae develop from the venous end of the primitive heart tube.

Nodal tissue develops in the wall of the sinus venosus. Part of this structure is included in the formation of the right atrium where nodal tissue condenses to form the sino-atrial (SA) node. This is situated close to the entry of the superior vena cava. Another concentration of nodal tissue occurs at the right atrioventricular orifice forming the atrioventricular (AV) node. The bundle of His develops separately as the interventricular septum is created by infolding of myocardial cells along the interventricular groove. The open edge of the septum contains myocardial cells which will become conducting tissue at a later date (Guyton & Hall 1996). The histochemical distinctiveness of the conducting tissue has allowed it to be distinguished at an early stage of gestation. The earliest identification of the sinus node has been at 32 days from ovulation. The atrioventricular bundle has been identified at 33 days and the AV node at 37 days.

At a late stage of gestation and before closure of the interventricular foramen, the conduction tissue lying beneath the foramen enlarges to become the bundle of His. At the anterior margin of the foramen the bundle divides into the right and left bundle branches. These then extend down the right and left sides of the interventricular septum. The atria are separated from the ventricles by a fibrous ring to which the valves are attached. This structure is electrically inert and acts as an insulator, preventing electrical impulses from crossing.

Once this process is complete the AV bundle is the only tissue capable of the conduction of action potentials from the atria to the ventricles. In abnormal physiology such as the Wolff–Parkinson–White (WPW) syndrome, one or more accessory pathway(s) develop allowing the initiation of the conduction pathways, without the heart rate protection afforded by the AV node. These accessory pathways can form laterally (left lateral being the most common) or run close to the AV node (see Chapter 20).

Cardiac cells are self-excitable, autorhythmic cells, able to repeatedly and rhythmically generate action potentials. The **action potential** refers to the generation of electrical impulses due to changes in the inward and outward flow of ions, through a cell membrane. **Depolarization** is the point when a cell's interior is maximally charged with positive ions. Cardiac cells can achieve the creation of an electrical impulse without an external stimulus and are said to have the property of **automaticity**. All cardiac cells have the potential to depolarize eventually without a stimulus. But it is the cells within areas such as the SA node, AV node/junction and Purkinje system, dispersing electrical impulses through the ventricles, which will achieve

this more quickly. This is due to a greater cell membrane permeability to potassium and calcium (Paul & Hebra 1998).

These cells have two functions:

● to act as a pacemaker, essentially setting the heart rate. The SA node is the dominant pacemaker in health
● to form the conduction system. This is the route that action potentials take to reach all heart muscle cells and thereby co-ordinate the pump action of the heart.

For a more detailed overview of the physiology of the action potential, please refer to Chapter 4.

The conduction system

In normal circumstances the conduction system stimulates the heart to fill and empty its chambers of blood in a controlled manner. When the conduction system works correctly, the atria of the heart contract about one-sixth of a second ahead of ventricular contraction. The ventricular chambers contract simultaneously, so that sufficient pressure generation can expel blood into the systemic circulation (Guyton & Hall 1996) (see Fig. 21.1).

The sino-atrial (SA) node

The sino-atrial (SA) node is a dense network of collagen that contains pacemaker (P) cells which initiate electrical impulses. Transitional cells are found between the P cells and ordinary atrial myocardial cells. Specialized tracts are also found fanning out from the node across the atria. Anatomically, the human SA node is spindle shaped and measures about $20 \times 3 \times 1$ mm (Opie 1998). It is situated on the superior lateral wall of the right atrium, inferior and lateral to the superior vena cava. In the general population 55% of people have the blood supply to the SA node emerging from the proximal few centimetres of the right coronary artery (RCA). The remaining 45% have the proximal few millimetres of the left circumflex artery (LCX) supplying the blood. The left sinus node artery arises from the LCX ramus and this comes in from the adjacent atrial epicardium, encircling and penetrating the centre of the sinus node.

The SA node has the highest rate of spontaneous depolarization. It is therefore known as the primary pacemaker of the heart, because it can generate an electrical impulse faster than other pacemaker cells (Paul & Hebra 1998). In health, it will initiate conduction, while its proximity to the SA nodal artery allows

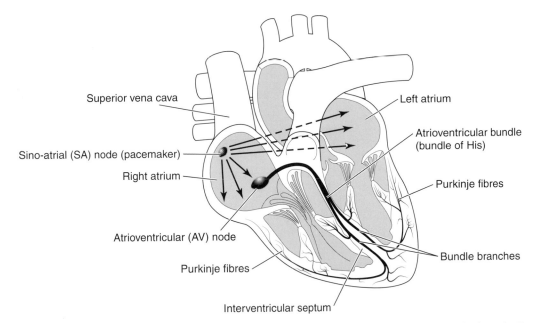

Figure 21.1 The conduction system of the heart. A fibrous ring supporting the valves prevents electrical conduction passing from the atria to the ventricles, except via the AV node and the bundle of His. In health, the depolarization wave is initiated by the SA node. It passes through the atrial myocardium to the AV node. Here, after a short pause, it passes to the bundle of His and into the right and left bundle branches. The Purkinje fibres facilitate rapid ventricular depolarization.

for continuous metabolic monitoring and instantaneous adjustments of the heart rate as required, due to hormonal and neural influence.

The mechanism for sinus node rhythmicity stems primarily from differences in the action potential compared to those in ventricular muscle fibre. Sinus node fibres have a lesser negativity of the resting potential which is only 60 millivolts compared to 90 millivolts in ventricular muscle. When the membrane potential remains less negative than 60 millivolts the fast sodium channels are inactivated. Sodium ions leak toward the interior of the sinus node fibres through multiple membrane channels and this change causes an increase in membrane potential. If it reaches about 40 millivolts calcium channels become activated and calcium and sodium ions rush in, causing depolarization. Cells in the SA node have the fastest phase 4 activity; basically at rest, they are very close to the depolarization threshold (Paul & Hebra 1998). Therefore they are the normal pacemaker of the heart. It is the inherent leakiness of the sinus node fibres to sodium ions that causes their self-excitation (Guyton & Hall 1996) (Fig. 21.2).

The cells, however, do not remain depolarized due to the calcium and sodium channels closing within 100–150 ms. Therefore the influx of calcium and sodium ions ceases and a large number of potassium

channels open. This allows out large quantities of positive potassium ions which produce an increased negativity in the fibre. This is termed **hyperpolarization** and causes the resting membrane potential to reduce to 60 millivolts. The resting potential rises slowly again once the potassium channels open.

The action potential from the sinus node travels across both atria via gap junctions in the intercalated discs of atrial fibres. In addition, there are three internodal pathways named anterior, middle and posterior internodal pathways which contain specialized conduction fibre mixed with atrial muscle. The action potential travels at a speed of 0.05 s/50 ms to the AV node.

The sinus node generates 90–100 action potentials per minute without the influence of the autonomic nervous system. The release of acetylcholine by the parasympathetic system (primarily but not exclusively the vagus nerve) increases the permeability of the fibre membranes to potassium, which causes increased negativity (hyperpolarization) and less excitability. Therefore the vagus nerve has an inhibitory action on the heart rate.

The atrioventricular node

The AV node is a subendocardial structure, containing a collagenous network of pacemaker cells, atrial tran-

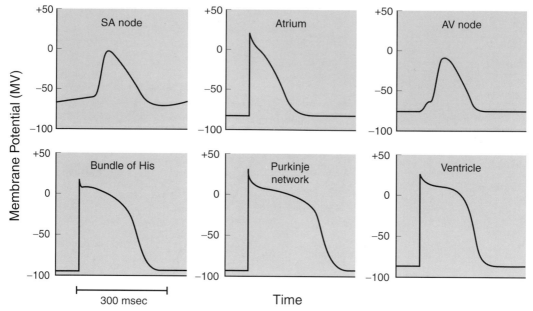

Figure 21.2 Automaticity of the action potential in pacing sites within the heart. (Reproduced with permission from Paul & Hebra 1998.)

sitional cells, ordinary myocardial cells and Purkinjie fibres. It arises from the apex of the penetrating U turn made by either the right or left coronary artery crossing the crux of the heart. This is an accepted angiographic landmark since James's work in the late 1960s (James 1968). The U turn lies just below the ostium of the coronary sinus and its apex is only a few millimetres from the AV node. The AV node lies on the posterior septal wall of the right atrium behind the tricuspid valve, adjacent to the opening of the coronary sinus. The specialized conduction tracts from the SA node all converge on this point.

In 90% of people the right coronary artery supplies the AV node and the first few millimetres of the AV bundle of His, the other 10% being supplied by the LCX. Collateral circulation is supplied by Kugel's artery. Once the impulse reaches the AV node there is a 0.09 second delay before it reaches the AV bundle of His. This is due to the fibres in the AV node having a smaller diameter which therefore produces a similar effect to a highway where three lanes converge to two. In addition, Guyton & Hall (1996) discuss three other factors: the low voltage to drive the ions, greater resistance to the movement of ions caused by few gap junctions connecting the successive fibres, and autonomic enervation (literally, to deprive of nervous strength). This delay allows emptying of the atria and ventricular filling and allows time for the AV node to act as

a filter, preventing the ventricular rate becoming too rapid in response to atrial tachycardia.

The Purkinje system

These fibres come from the distal AV node, converge to form the AV bundle of His (following the membranous septum to the start of the muscular septum) and then they divide into the right and left bundle branches which spread out across the ventricles. The left and right bundle branches lie beneath the endocardium of each side of the septum. The left bundle branch is a large sheet of fibres with two main parts feeding the anterior and posterior papillary muscles. This facilitates their contraction which occurs before the contraction of the ventricular free wall and therefore prevents mitral regurgitation. Purkinjie fibres are divided into separate threads by a collagenous structure. Few pacemaker cells are found here.

Box 21.1 Guyton & Hall's (1996) figures for velocity

- Sinus node to AV node – 1 m/s
- AV node – 0.05 m/s; 0.09 s delay
- AV node to Purkinje system – 0.02 m/s, 1/12 that of normal cardiac muscle
- Purkinje fibres – 1.5–4 m/s, 6 times normal cardiac muscle

This longitudinal dissociation of electrical impulses allows the diagnosis of specific conduction defects. They are different from the rest of the system in that they are very large fibres and can pass on action potentials at a rate of up to 4.0 m/s. This is the mechanism by which the cardiac impulse is spread throughout the entire ventricular system. Autonomic enervation is sparse, with the blood supply usually coming from the AV nodal artery or septal branches of the left anterior descending (LAD) artery.

The ability to transmit electrical impulses quickly is thought to be due to increased permeability of the gap junctions at the intercalated discs, between the successive cardiac cells that make up the Purkinje fibres. As previously highlighted, the AV bundle of His is the only electrical connection between the atria and ventricles because the fibrous rings and sheets of connective tissue act as an electrical insulation between the atria and ventricles. An impulse cannot travel across this fibrous structure.

Autonomic control of heart rate

Sympathetic system

The cardiovascular centre in the brain's medulla oblongata receives input data from the limbic system and cerebral cortex. Sympathetic fibres from the medulla oblongata travel via the spinal cord to the thoracic region of the cord, where cardiac accelerator nerves branch off to the sinus node, AV node and most parts of the myocardium. Impulses in the cardiac accelerator nerves release noradrenaline (norepinephrine) which binds to β1-receptors on cardiac muscle fibres. This then speeds up the sinus and AV node fibres' rate of spontaneous depolarization. Contractile fibres throughout the atria and ventricles are acted upon by norepinephrine (noradrenaline) which enhances calcium ion (Ca^{++}) entry through the voltage-gated slow Ca^{++} channels and thus increases contractility. This in turn increases the ejection of blood in systole. The rate of maximum stimulation is 250 beats per minute (bpm) which has been demonstrated by electrophysiological study using norepinephrine. An increase in sympathetic tone enhances automaticity in the pacemaker cells, resulting in their ability to fire more quickly with increasing velocity. This leads to a decrease in action potential duration and a decrease in refractory time.

Parasympathetic system

Cranial nerve X (vagus) innervates the sinus node, AV node and the atrial myocardium. As previously mentioned, the release of acetylcholine decreases the heart rate by causing depolarization and a slowing of the rate of spontaneous depolarization in autorhythmic fibres. There are very few vagal fibres in ventricular muscle.

Ions

Any metabolic imbalance caused by a disease process can cause electrolyte imbalance. Sodium and potassium are important to the production of the action potential. High levels of potassium and sodium decrease heart rate and contractility. Excess sodium will block calcium inflow during cardiac action potentials and decreases the force of contraction. Excess levels of potassium block the generation of action potentials. Acidosis or alkalosis all affect the body's ability to excrete and retain essential ions.

THE HISTORY OF PACEMAKER TECHNOLOGY

The survival rates of patients with bradyarrhythmias was radically altered by the arrival of pacemaker technology. In 1958 the first pacemakers were implanted in humans. They were single-chamber, fixed-rate devices which could not sense the intrinsic electrical activity of the heart. The early pacemakers used zinc mercuric oxide cells in the pulse generators and the lead was made up of multistrand stainless steel epicardial wires in a Teflon cover. Pacemaker implantation was a major operation, requiring left anterior thoracotomy to expose the myocardium.

Jeffrey & Parsonnet (1998) summarized the major problems associated with pacing in the 1960s as fractures of lead wires, leakage of body fluids into the pulse generator causing it to short circuit (early batteries released hydrogen gas and therefore could not be sealed), the threshold (the point at which the pacemaker's electrical stimulus depolarizes the myocardial cells) rising beyond the output capability of the pulse generator, thoracotomy required for implant, competition between the intrinsic electrical activity of the heart and that of the stimulus provided by the pulse generator, early battery exhaustion (attempts had been made to develop a nuclear generator using plutonium 238) and the time commitment required for the clinical follow-up of the patient, from the medical and technical point of view.

The past 40 years have seen dramatic strides in the treatment of patients with pacemaker implantations. Demand devices, batteries which allow the pulse generator to be sealed and a decrease in the size of the

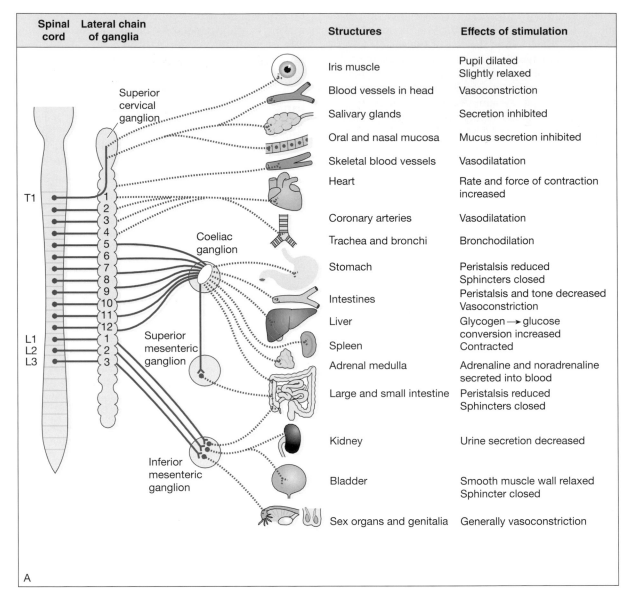

Spinal cord	Lateral chain of ganglia		Structures	Effects of stimulation
	Superior cervical ganglion		Iris muscle	Pupil dilated Slightly relaxed
			Blood vessels in head	Vasoconstriction
			Salivary glands	Secretion inhibited
			Oral and nasal mucosa	Mucus secretion inhibited
			Skeletal blood vessels	Vasodilatation
T1	1 2 3 4 5 6 7 8 9 10 11 12		Heart	Rate and force of contraction increased
			Coronary arteries	Vasodilatation
		Coeliac ganglion	Trachea and bronchi	Bronchodilation
			Stomach	Peristalsis reduced Sphincters closed
			Intestines	Peristalsis and tone decreased Vasoconstriction
			Liver	Glycogen → glucose conversion increased
L1 L2 L3	1 2 3	Superior mesenteric ganglion	Spleen	Contracted
			Adrenal medulla	Adrenaline and noradrenaline secreted into blood
			Large and small intestine	Peristalsis reduced Sphincters closed
			Kidney	Urine secretion decreased
		Inferior mesenteric ganglion	Bladder	Smooth muscle wall relaxed Sphincter closed
			Sex organs and genitalia	Generally vasoconstriction

A

Figure 21.3 The connections of the sympathetic (A) and parasympathetic (B) nervous systems. (Reproduced with permission from Wilson K 1996 Ross and Wilson's anatomy and physiology in health and illness, 8th edn. Churchill Livingstone, Edinburgh.)

batteries have all changed the patient outcomes for the better. It was the decrease in the size of the pulse generator which led to pectoral implants becoming possible. This enabled implantation to be undertaken using local anaesthetic and with this came the added bonus of early discharge. In addition, the method by which patients are clinically followed up is constantly improving. For example, the use of transtelephonic device checks is becoming more common for checking

factors such as battery life. However, this approach tends to be more common in countries with large geographic regions such as the United States.

HOW DOES CARDIAC PACING WORK?

An artificial pacemaker delivers an electrical stimulus which excites the myocardial cells. The inherent properties of cardiac muscle cells (automaticity and

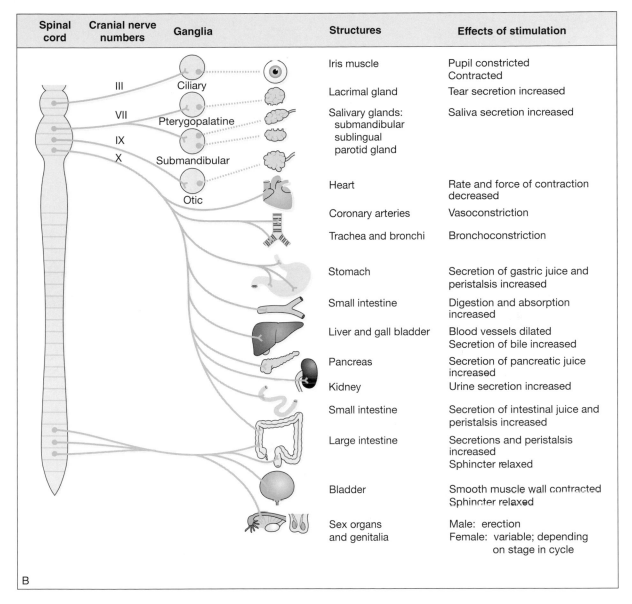

Spinal cord	Cranial nerve numbers	Ganglia		Structures	Effects of stimulation
	III	Ciliary		Iris muscle	Pupil constricted Contracted
	VII	Pterygopalatine		Lacrimal gland	Tear secretion increased
	IX	Submandibular		Salivary glands: submandibular sublingual parotid gland	Saliva secretion increased
	X	Otic		Heart	Rate and force of contraction decreased
				Coronary arteries	Vasoconstriction
				Trachea and bronchi	Bronchoconstriction
				Stomach	Secretion of gastric juice and peristalsis increased
				Small intestine	Digestion and absorption increased
				Liver and gall bladder	Blood vessels dilated Secretion of bile increased
				Pancreas	Secretion of pancreatic juice increased
				Kidney	Urine secretion increased
				Small intestine	Secretion of intestinal juice and peristalsis increased
				Large intestine	Secretions and peristalsis increased Sphincter relaxed
				Bladder	Smooth muscle wall contracted Sphincter relaxed
				Sex organs and genitalia	Male: erection Female: variable; depending on stage in cycle

B

Figure 21.3 *continued*

rhythmicity) make this possible. The pacing stimulus must be of sufficient amplitude and duration to initiate a self-perpetuating wave of action potentials that move away from the site of stimulation. Providing the myocardium is of adequate health, this will cause a contraction. The pacing system needs both a negative (cathode) and positive (anode) pole to complete the electric circuit. The stimulating electrical impulse is conducted to the heart by a pacing lead. There are two types of pacing: bipolar and unipolar.

Unipolar pacing has one electrode, containing one insulated electrical wire which is negative (the cathode) at the tip. The positive pole (the anode) is the can of the pulse generator, with the electrolyte system and tissues of the body completing the circuit (Fig. 21.4). This produces on the surface ECG a very large pacing spike.

Bipolar pacing has an electrode with two insulated wires in a plastic coating at the end of which are two ring electrodes, the distal of which is negative (the

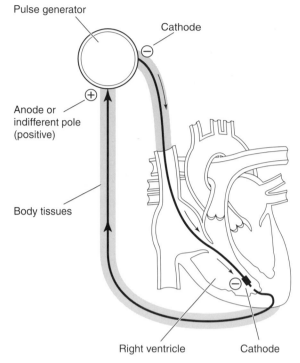

Figure 21.4 A unipolar pacing system (ventricular pacing).

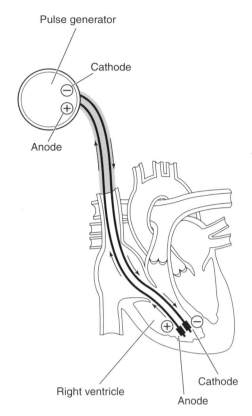

Figure 21.5 A bipolar pacing system (ventricular pacing).

cathode) and the proximal, about 1 cm from the tip, is the positive electrode (the anode) (Fig. 21.5). On the surface ECG only a small pacing spike is seen.

For successful pacing to take place several key elements must be present.

The pulse generator

The pulse generator has five main elements. The box/casing in which it is housed (depending on whether the pacing system is intended to be permanent or temporary), the power source, output, timer and sensing circuits. In recent permanent systems, telemetry circuits are now available.

The power source

Cardiac pacing requires a power source in the form of a chemical battery. Today lithium–iodine cell batteries are the most common. A chemical battery provides energy by moving electrons from the anodal element (this provides the supply of electrons) to the cathodal element (this receives the electrons). In today's lithium–iodine cell, lithium provides the electrons and iodine acts as the cathode and receives them. At the battery terminals the anode gives up electrons and is

positively charged and the cathode accepts electrons and is negatively charged. Electrons are carried from the anodal terminal of the battery to cathodal terminal when the circuit is complete.

The battery has a material separating the anodal and cathodal element called the **electrolyte** which acts as a conductor of ionic movement and as a barrier to the transfer of electrons. In lithium–iodine batteries the electrolyte is a semisolid layer of lithium iodine which increases in thickness over the life of the cell (Kay 1996). This development allowed manufacturers to hermetically seal the pacemaker, thus preventing body fluids from seeping into the batteries and causing pacemaker failure.

An important aspect of the batteries now used in pacemakers is their ability to predict end of battery life. Early pacemakers were prone to fail suddenly and without warning but with the lithium batteries of today it is possible to predict when the pacemaker will fail. This allows time to admit a patient for pacemaker replacement in a planned manner.

The battery voltage of the lithium–iodine cell is 2.8 V at implant and at the end of life (90% depleted), the battery has decreased to around 1.8 V (Kay 1996). Technicians determine this by applying calculations to magnet-related pacing rates. Amplitude and duration of output plus frequency of use all affect battery duration.

Output circuits

Output circuits control the delivery of the electric current generated by the battery to the myocardium. The stimulus comes from the discharge of a capacitor to the anode and cathode of the pacing leads. The impulse from the capacitor is described as having leading and trailing edges which is a description of the voltage waveform.

Timing circuits

These circuits control rate and recovery times. They are responsible for pacing cycle length, pulse duration, AV interval and sensing refractory and alert periods. This is achieved by a crystal oscillator that generates signals with frequency in the kHz range. There is also a fail-safe element in a rate-limiting circuit that prevents the pacing rate from exceeding an upper rate limit in the very rare event of device failure; it is usually set at 220 bpm.

Sensing circuits

These circuits allow the pacing system to recognize and analyse inherent cardiac signals. The intracardiac electrogram is conducted from the electrodes to the sensing circuit of the pulse generator. Two processes are applied, amplification and filtering. Once this is finished the signals are compared with the reference voltage to see if the signal exceeds a threshold detection level. Signals with amplitude greater than sensitivity threshold are sensed as intracardiac events, those below the level considered as noise. The signals determined as intracardiac events are marked by an output that is sent to the timing circuit.

The sensing circuits are also responsible for protecting the pulse generator from things such as electromagnetic interference, defibrillation or electrocautery which produce high levels of electrical energy. The protection is achieved by a device called a Zener diode which sends excess energy back through pacing leads to the myocardium. The sensing circuits also make sure that T-waves or retrograde atrial activity are not sensed as ventricular activity, thus inhibiting the pacemaker function.

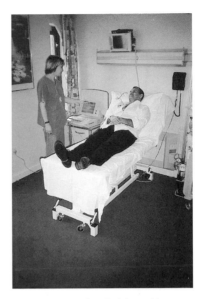

Figure 21.6 A patient and technician with a pacemaker programmer.

Telemetry circuit

These are found in programmable pulse generators. They can respond to radiofrequency signals emitted from an external programmer and two-way communication is possible. Information that can be transmitted includes pulse amplitude and duration, lead impedance, battery impedance and amount of current being delivered.

Electrodes

None of the functions held within a pulse generator is of any use unless there is an electrode able to make direct contact with the heart. This is the conduit through which information about spontaneous intracardiac signals gets back to the sensing circuits and in addition it delivers the pacing stimulus to the heart. The coiled wire is enclosed in an insulated casing. The permanent (more rigid) and temporary (soft, highly flexible) electrodes look and feel quite different.

Connecting cable leads (temporary systems only)

In permanent pacing systems the lead connects directly to the pulse generator. Some temporary electrodes are also able to be connected directly to the pulse generator and male patients in particular find these easier to deal with, as they slip easily into the pocket of pyjamas. This allows greater mobility for the patient while decreasing the risks associated with bedrest. In the United Kingdom (UK), however, most cardiac units use two main types of temporary system; the alternative to the above system is a large box which can hang on the head of the bed but still requires a connecting cable from pulse generator to electrode. This may increase troubleshooting time when searching for connection faults. However, mobile patients also tend to swing the cable around or leave it trailing behind which poses a significant clinical risk.

INDICATIONS FOR CARDIAC PACING

Conditions causing conduction abnormalities include myocardial infarction (MI). Here, ischaemia to the SA or AV node is often combined with an increase in vagal tone in other parts of the system, leading to permanent or transient abnormalities. Cardiac surgery where trauma leads to oedema, particularly during valve surgery, may also interfere with the conduction system. Drug toxicity or inappropriate prescribing may contribute to delays in conduction. Fibrosis or sclerosis of the conduction system from sarcoid or Lenegre's heart disease (degenerative fibrosis and calcification of the distal conduction system) and calcification of the aortic or mitral valves may rarely interfere with conduction. Congenital heart block, electrolyte imbalance such as hypokalaemia or myocarditis may all require pacing on a temporary or permanent basis.

Abnormalities in the conduction system of the heart fall into two broad categories:

- bradyarrhythmias – the heart rate is too slow
- tachyarrhythmias – the heart rate is too fast.

Fogoros (1995) divided bradyarrhythmias into two subdivisions: the failure of pacemaker cells to generate appropriate impulses (disorders of automaticity) and failure to propagate electrical impulses (heart block).

Sinus bradycardia

The SA node is producing an insufficient number of electrical impulses. This may be due to idiopathic conduction tissue disease or ischaemia but it should be remembered that it may be a benign process at work. A slow rate may not be due to a disease process in the conducting system; athletes in endurance sports have been noted to have resting heart rates of 30–40 bpm. It is also important to establish whether it is sinus rhythm. Drugs such as calcium antagonists will suppress sinus node function. The effect of the parasympathetic nervous system dampens the sinus rate by anything up to 50% in some circumstances in young patients with high vagal tone. Treatment depends on the cause (Fig. 21.7).

Sick sinus syndrome

This can be defined as abnormal SA node function. It may be familial or congenital and can occur in

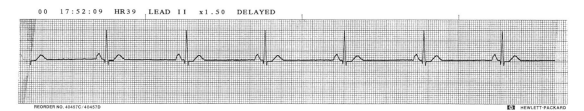

Figure 21.7 Rhythm strip for sinus bradycardia.

SICK SINUS SYNDROME

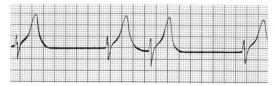 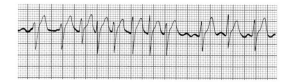

Figure 21.8 Rhythm strip for sick sinus syndrome. The left trace shows a 'silent atrium' with junctional escape beats. The right trace shows episodes of junctional tachycardia which can occur, causing unpleasant palpitations. (Reproduced with permission from Hampton J 1986 The ECG in practice. Churchill Livingstone, Edinburgh.)

ischaemic, rheumatic, hypertensive or infiltrative cardiac disease. However, it is frequently idiopathic (no recognizable cause) (Hampton 1998). It is common to see AV junctional escape beats or AV junctional rhythms taking over.

Heart block

Inhibition or failure of the electrical impulse generated in the SA node to be conducted through the conduction system to the ventricles. This can occur because of an abnormality of conduction velocity or complete refractoriness in the conduction system.

First-degree heart block

All impulses reach the ventricles. Delay occurs in the intra-atrial conduction to the AV node. The P–R interval represents this and therefore is greater than 0.20 seconds in duration (Fig. 21.9).

Sino-atrial block. The sinus node initiates an impulse but it fails to conduct the atrial myocardium. The following discharge from the sinus node triggers atrial depolarization at the normal time so the ECG trace will show a missed beat double that of the normal cycle length (Fig. 21.10). If this occurs often, it can be misdiagnosed as 2:1 heart block.

Second-degree heart block

Conduction to the ventricles is intermittent.

Mobitz type I (Wenckebach). A level of block is found in the AV node and the surface ECG shows a gradual lengthening of the P–R interval in the run-up to a non-conducted impulse (no QRS seen on surface ECG). The cycle usually repeats itself (Fig. 21.11). This is most commonly seen following an inferior myocardial infarction and, unless the patient is symptomatic, is usually observed in the coronary care unit (CCU) for several days before any decision on pace-

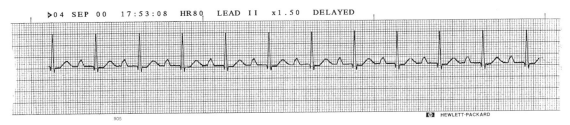

Figure 21.9 Rhythm strip for first-degree heart block. Note the prolonged P–R interval.

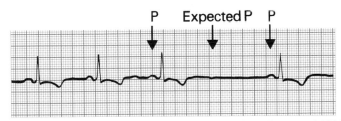

Figure 21.10 Rhythm strip for sino-atrial block. (Reproduced with permission from Hampton J 1986 The ECG in practice. Churchill Livingstone, Edinburgh.)

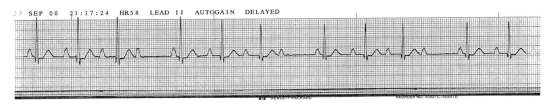

Figure 21.11 Rhythm strip for second-degree heart block, Mobitz type I (Wenckebach phenomenon). Note that in a cycle the P–R interval becomes progressively longer, before a P-wave becomes non-conducted (no following QRS complex). The cycle then starts again.

maker implantation is made. In most cases it resolves by itself.

Mobitz type II. This is suggestive of disease in the His–Purkinje system and is due to intermittent failure of an atrial impulse to conduct. There is no change in the P–R interval. Some P-waves are followed by a QRS complex, others are not. Patient symptoms depend on the ventricular rate generated. This rhythm is associated with progression to complete heart block and is an indication for pacemaker implantation (Fig. 21.12).

2:1 Second-degree AV block. Every second P-wave is conducted to the ventricles. It is considered a more stable rhythm and there is much debate over the need for permanent pacing (Fig. 21.13).

Third-degree heart block

This is described as atrial and ventricular activity independent of each other. Atrial impulses conducted do not reach the ventricles. The ventricles release their own

> *As a general rule, the lower in the conduction system the escape pacemaker is, the slower the ventricular rate.*

slow escape impulses. Consequently, no relationship in conduction between atria and ventricles can be found (Fig. 21.14). The level of block affects prognosis. A narrow QRS complex indicates that the pacemaker cell is at the level of the AV node whereas a broad complex (>120 ms) suggests the escape pacemaker is in the Purkinje system or is a ventricular muscle pacemaker cell.

Congenital complete heart block does occur but complete heart block is seen more often in the elderly where degenerative disease of the conduction system is present or following an ischaemic event such as an anterior myocardial infarction. In these circumstances it is a poor prognostic indicator. The other main group of patients are those with ongoing inflammatory disease processes.

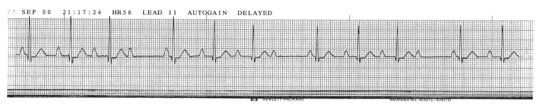

Figure 21.12 Rhythm strip for second-degree heart block, Mobitz type II. (Reproduced with permission from Hampton J 1997 The ECG made easy, 5th edn. Churchill Livingstone, Edinburgh.)

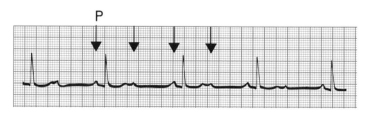

Figure 21.13 Rhythm strip for 2:1 second-degree AV block. Note the conducted beats have a normal P–R interval, but alternate P waves are not followed by a QRS. (Reproduced with permission from Hampton J 1986 The ECG in practice. Churchill Livingstone, Edinburgh.)

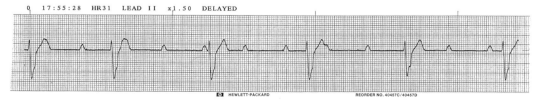

Figure 21.14 Rhythm strip for third-degree (complete) heart block. Note the slow ventricular escape beats and the total lack of association between the P-waves (atrial activity) and the wide bizarre QRS complexes (ventricular activity).

There is often confusion over the terms AV dissociation and third-degree heart block. AV dissociation is present when the atria and ventricles are being controlled by two separate independent rhythms. In complete heart block the atrial rate is faster than the ventricular rate. However, it is possible to have an accelerated junctional pacemaker over-ride normal sinus rhythm and it would not be true to say that complete heart block was present.

Trifascicular block

By definition, trifascicular block is a blockage in the right bundle branch and the two fascicles of the left branch. This will present with complete heart block, requiring pacing. However, it can be a more gradual process, perhaps with right bundle branch block (RBBB) and commonly an initial blockage of the left anterior fascicle. The aim is to understand the risk of progression to trifascicular block and the requirement for pacing.

Asystole with persistent P-waves

This presentation, commonly referred to as ventricular standstill, can be seen in a patient who is pacemaker dependent and receiving ventricular pacing which is abruptly switched off or if the pulse generator fails completely. A Stoke Adams attack, where the patient collapses with loss of consciousness, will ensue. A ventricular escape rhythm may arise but in the example in Figure 21.15, full resuscitation was required.

Other indications for cardiac pacing

Pacing for long QT syndrome

Patients with this syndrome usually present to a CCU with a history of collapse. When an event is witnessed in the hospital a polymorphic tachycardia with the QRS complexes undulating about the baseline is seen. This is termed torsades de pointes. The problem is prolonged myocardial repolarization which is shown on the surface ECG by a prolonged Q–T interval. The aim of pacing is to increase the ventricular rate, which in the normal individual would shorten the Q–T interval and eliminate late potentials, which are thought to be one of the initiating factors in torsades de pointes. β-Blockers have been of benefit in this syndrome but if given alone, they could worsen the condition as they significantly slow the heart rate.

Pacing for neurally mediated syncope

These patients usually present for permanent pacing, having been through many investigations. The patient has abnormal autonomic control of their circulation with exaggerated response from the sympathetic nervous system. This diagnosis is made by a tilt-table test. Patients are tilted for various lengths of time. In the normal patient α- and β-adrenergic tone is increased as the baroreceptors are stimulated, therefore compensating for venous return and preventing syncope (a transient loss of consciousness, due to reduced cerebral blood flow). In an abnormal response tilting triggers hypervagaltonia and activates a Bezold Jarisch reflex. This decreases contractility of the left ventricle and decreases cardiac blood supply which leads to excessive stimulation of the receptors responsible for vagal reflex (Kapoor et al 1994).

Pacing in patients with hypertrophic obstructive cardiomyopathy (HOCM)

These patients may be admitted for a trial of pacing using a temporary pacing system or may go straight to the catheter laboratory where the trial and permanent insertion can be carried out in one visit. The aim of pacing these patients is to induce paradoxical septal motion with the ventricular septum moving away from rather than toward the anterior leaflet of the mitral valve and left ventricular outflow tract during systole (Fananapazi et al 1992). This is best achieved by using a dual-chamber pacemaker (which can pace both atria and the ventricle in a way close to normal human physiology) and programming a short P–R interval <125 ms to induce early right ventricular and

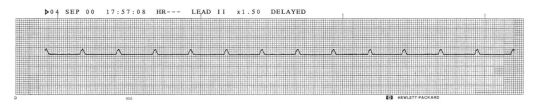

▷04 SEP 00   17:57:08   HR---   LEAD II   x1.50   DELAYED

Figure 21.15 Asystole with persistent P-waves (commonly referred to as ventricular standstill).

septal activation and therefore a maximum amount of wall motion dysynchrony (Ellenbogen 1996). This should haemodynamically reduce left ventricular cavity obstruction which occurs in this condition and thus decrease the left ventricular outflow tract gradient. This is not always successful and in some patients their condition is made worse. Therefore, a trial of pacing is important and should be carried out in a specialist centre where expertise has been gained (see Chapter 11).

CARDIAC PACING SYSTEMS

Temporary cardiac pacing

Transcutaneous (external) cardiac pacing

This method of pacing for emergency situations has become readily available over the last 5 years with many defibrillators having the facility to do this. Its use in paediatrics is increasing and good results have been reported.

Transcutaneous cardiac pacing is non-invasive and delivers electricity from the external power source (usually part of the external defibrillator). This causes the depolarization of excitable myocardial tissue by pulsed electrical current conducted through the chest wall, between electrodes adherent to the skin. These electrodes are self-adhesive, about 4 or 5 inches in diameter and are pre-impregnated with conducting gel. For effective capture the anterior chest electrode has to be of negative polarity. If the negative electrode is placed posteriorly capture may not be obtained and the patient will find it acutely painful if they are conscious.

The anterior (negative) electrode is centred over the cardiac apex at the V3 position along the left sternal border. The posterior (positive) electrode is positioned level with the inferior aspect of the scapula, between the spine and right or left scapula. Positioning over bone will increase the threshold. If capture is not achieved the positive electrode can be moved to the V6 position in an attempt to achieve capture.

Position of electrodes. The external pacing generator within the defibrillator generates up to 200 mA of current per pulse and a long pulse duration of 20–40 ms tries to balance the need for capture without overstimulating skeletal muscles and local nerves which cause the patient distress (Wood & Ellenbogen 1996). If failure to capture occurs, the most likely causes are electrode position, skin/electrode contacts, electricity failure (make sure the device is plugged in; in the initial emergency situation plugging in the device can be forgotten) or battery failure (if the patient is pacing frequently battery depletion will be rapid). In the event of failure, increasing the pulse width (the specific period of time over which the programmed output is delivered) should also be tried. Some devices are now using an oscillating band technique which has shown a higher level of capture.

Pain is a common complaint from the conscious patient and this is made worse by shaving the chest or back in an effort to increase contact. The salt from sweat also causes increased pain with each stimulus. All that can be done is to wash and dry the skin frequently and avoid shaving the skin if at all possible. Because of the above issues, this pacing device should only be used as a temporary measure.

Transvenous pacing

This is a common procedure in coronary care units across the country. It is usually performed only when the patient is haemodynamically compromised by bradycardia or for arrhythmia suppression or termination by antitachycardiac pacing.

At least three members of the multidisciplinary team are required for the procedure: doctor, nurse and radiographer. The area in which insertion can take place depends on what sort of pacing catheter it is. If it is a flotation catheter then it can be carried out on the CCU or acute unit but if X-ray is required then an appropriate leaded area is required. Some units have this just off the CCU but in others the patient has to be transferred to the catheter laboratory, theatre or X-ray department. If transfer is required a portable defibrillator to monitor the patient, plus all emergency equipment, is necessary. Wherever the procedure is carried out it is important to have oxygen, suction and defibrillator present and ready for use.

The procedure is carried out under local anaesthetic, but it is considered preferable that the patient has had

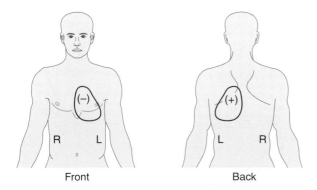

Front   Back

Figure 21.16 The position of external electrode pads for transcutaneous cardiac pacing.

nothing to eat for the previous 2–4 hours (practice varies in different cardiac units). The need for a transvenous wire suggests that the patient is unstable and ventricular irritation can occur during the procedure. In extreme cases ventricular tachycardia or ventricular fibrillation can occur or a loss of effective cardiac output from extreme bradycardia. It is common, of course, for the patient to be admitted to casualty having eaten and in this event careful attention must be paid to maintaining a safe airway. Some physicians prefer a nasogastric tube to be passed to eliminate the risk of vomiting and inhalation during the procedure. It is therefore important to ascertain when the patient last ate, if at all possible.

An intravenous catheter electrode is positioned endocardially, via the subclavian or external jugular venous route, and this is then connected to an external generator by a lead connector. Two types are seen: bipolar electrodes, where both anode and cathode are intracardiac, and unipolar (rare) where one pole is extracardiac. This is ideally the anode and is attached to the skin surface.

Atrial (paces and senses in the atria only), ventricular (paces and senses in the ventricle only) and dual-chamber (paces and senses in both chambers) pacing can all be achieved with temporary pacing electrodes. Bipolar temporary pacing is the most common type seen in the UK. Platinum-coated electrodes are used with the distal electrode comprising the tip of the catheter. The catheter is made of a rigid woven polyester so that it can be manipulated into position by fluoroscopic (X-ray) guidance. The other method of inserting a bipolar electrode is by using a flow-directed balloon catheter. This is made of flexible plastic and is floated in much the same way as a pulmonary artery (PA) catheter (see Chapter 5), but stopping when it reaches the right ventricle. Lang et al (1981) argued that in general hospitals these catheters provide shorter insertion times and may be safer to use. Some PA lines have pacing electrodes incorporated into them in the atrial and ventricular positions. They are difficult to fix in position as they move when the balloon is inflated for pulmonary capillary wedge pressure readings and loss of capture can occur. This is therefore not an ideal method of pacing.

Most temporary pacemaker generators use disposable batteries (9 volt battery often found in telemetry receivers or the AA batteries found in personal stereos) to produce a constant current. Current output from 0.1 to 20 mA is possible and the pulse width can be changed within short parameters of 1–2 ms. Sensitivity settings vary from 0.1 mV to asynchronous pacing. If the sensitivity level is too low then electronic

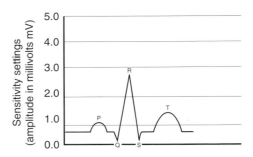

Figure 21.17 Cardiac pacing sensitivity setting in relation to the QRS complex.

circuits may pick up T-waves as inherent ventricular activity and inhibit the pacemaker. If it is set too high it will not pick up the R-waves and may cause the pacemaker to pace inappropriately. The sensitivity setting on temporary pacing boxes often causes confusion.

To increase the sensitivity, a lower sensitivity threshold is used. To decrease it, a higher sensitivity threshold is used. Put simply, we are drawing a line *above* which the pacemaker will count and interpret. Double counting of heart rate often appears on ordinary cardiac monitors in the CCU when a similar circuit counts the T-waves as well as the R-waves of the QRS (Fig. 21.17).

Insertion sites. The most common approach used is via the right external jugular or left subclavian veins (Fig. 21.18). This approach allows the most stable positioning of wires, whereas in the femoral vein or brachial routes electrode stability is a major problem as the patient moves. These routes are often favoured by inexperienced doctors as the likelihood of pneumothorax or inadvertent carotid or subclavian artery puncture is avoided.

The electrode is positioned in the right ventricular apex (VVI pacing), right atrial appendage (AAI pacing) or both in the case of dual-chamber pacing (DDD pacing).

Connection to the pulse generator. In bipolar systems, the distal pole serves as the cathode (negative). The pacing box sometimes has active or distal on it. Whatever terminology is used, DAN is a good acronym to remember: Distal Active Negative. For example, if the electrode has negative (–) on it, it must be connected to the distal or active connection on the pacing box. The proximal pole serves as the anode (positive).

In unipolar systems, the negative cathode (–) is intracardiac and the positive anode (+) is secured to a subcutaneous wire electrode or via patch electrode to the skin.

Right external jugular vein

Right subclavian vein

Left subclavian vein

Cephalic vein

Heart

Brachial vein

Femoral vein

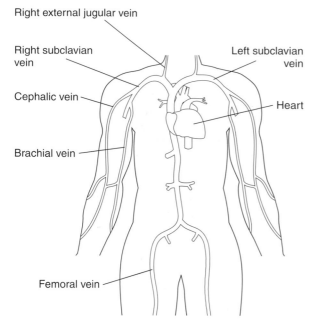

Figure 21.18 Commonly used vessels for temporary cardiac pacing.

Complications of insertion of temporary pacing wires include:

- haemo/pneumothorax
- rupture of major blood vessels
- perforation of right ventricle
- VT/VF induced with manipulation of the catheter
- infection.

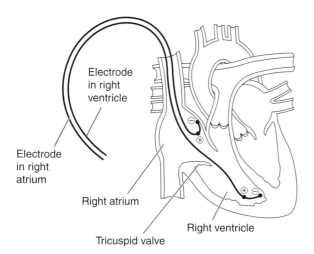

Electrode in right ventricle

Electrode in right atrium

Right atrium

Tricuspid valve

Right ventricle

Figure 21.19 The position of bipolar atrial and ventricular pacing electrodes.

Threshold testing. This is usually carried out by the nurse at the time of insertion and on a daily basis thereafter. Threshold testing is only possible because of the fundamental characteristic of myocardial contractility. When the heart is stimulated by an electrical impulse it responds either completely or not at all. The lowest electrical energy that will cause myocardial contraction is called the threshold.

The threshold can be affected by the duration of the stimulating pulse (pulse width), the output voltage, how long the wire has been in position and by the inflammatory response at the electrode/tissue interface (see Permanent pacemakers, p. 411).

Procedure for testing the threshold in a temporary pacing system. Equipment required:

- cardiac monitor
- spare pulse generator (pacing box) and connectors
- defibrillator and advanced life support equipment nearby, including oxygen and suction facilities.

Explain what you are about to do to the patient. Some patients are very sensitive to changes in pacing rate, especially if pacing dependent.

Make sure the patient is lying on a bed. It is poor practice to carry out this procedure sitting on a chair next to the monitor as some patients become dizzy very quickly and may fall and injure themselves. If the patient is not pacing all the time you need to turn the pacing sensing rate up to 5–10 beats above the intrinsic rate. Before you do this it is important to consider the patient's underlying aetiology. If the patient has had a recent myocardial infarction it may be inappropriate to turn up the rate. If the rate requires exceeding 80 bpm, medical staff should be consulted before this is attempted. The risk would involve increasing the heart rate and therefore the myocardial oxygen demand and in the ischaemic patient this could be detrimental to the cardiac functioning. Once continuous pacing is observed the output dial is slowly turned down until loss of capture is seen, then raised slowly until capture returns (Fig. 21.21).

The point at which capture returns is the threshold and is measured in volts in the UK. Current practice is to place the output dial on 2.5–3 times the threshold level. For example, a threshold of 2 volts means the output dial should be set on 6 volts to give a safe margin. Documentation should include the threshold, underlying rhythm seen, if any, and the output that the pulse generator is finally set to. The threshold should be checked on a daily basis and also at any time the pacemaker appears to be malfunctioning.

Procedure for testing sensitivity threshold in a temporary pacing system. This is performed more rarely in the UK

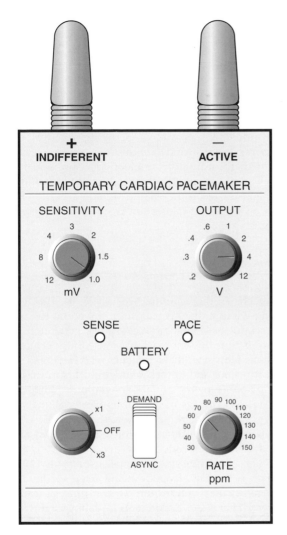

Figure 21.20 Temporary pacing box.

The equipment required for sensitivity testing and explanation to the patient are as for threshold testing.

In this situation it is necessary to be able to see the patient's own intrinsic rate and therefore the usual practice is to turn the pacing rate down to 5–10 beats below the inherent rate. Again, common sense must prevail. If the patient's underlying rhythm is only a ventricular escape at 20 bpm, turning the rate down will cause the patient to be severely symptomatic and at risk. If pacing is operating in the normal manner it is debatable whether this procedure is necessary at all (cardiac units vary).

The sensitivity dial is turned until the sensing indicator light (usually green) flashes with each intrinsic R-wave. It is then turned in the opposite direction until the pacing indicator light (usually red) begins to flash. Move the dial back in the other direction until the first sensed beat occurs and this is the sensitivity threshold. This is measured in mV in the UK. Documentation should be of the sensitivity threshold and what the sensitivity setting was finally set to.

Good practice guidelines.

- Any patient with a temporary pacing wire in place should remain on 4-hourly temperature observation, regardless of the length of time they have been apyrexial. Infection in these patients tends to present quickly and is potentially fatal.
- Check before commencing temporary pacing that you have two pulse generators (pacing boxes), which have been maintained and the date of the last battery change is marked. Once a patient has had a temporary system connected it is important that there is another pacing box and connector cable on the ward/unit in case of device failure. When patients are transferred to other wards often this is forgotten.
- Any pacing box which has been dropped or had water spilt on it must be sent back to a medical electronics department to be checked.
- Vases of flowers are usually not permitted in the CCU/ITU area, but are sometimes permitted in the

and is only likely to occur in a situation where the patient has a temporary dual-chamber pacing system in place.

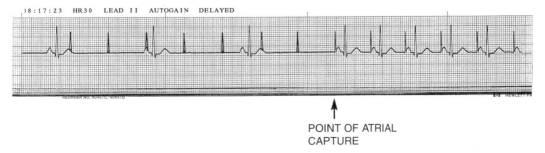

POINT OF ATRIAL CAPTURE

Figure 21.21 Rhythm strip illustrating point of atrial capture in temporary cardiac pacing.

ward. Patients with temporary systems should have the risk of the vase falling over and water getting into the pacing box explained.

- Ensure that the terminal connections are covered in insulating material such as the finger of a rubber glove to prevent microshocks passing down the electrode into the heart. Make sure the tape is easy to remove; that is, not wound round repeatedly as this can lead to the loss of valuable time trying to reconnect in an emergency. ECG electrodes should never be used to cover the ends as they contain conducting gel and have a metal connection which could produce the same effect. Night-clothes are often made of brushed nylon or similar substances and these create significant amounts of static. Bed linen also develops a static charge. It is not uncommon to see the connections between the pacing wire and connector cable incorrectly set, leaving the terminal exposed. If there is a need for defibrillation, the box should be switched off and the device checked by a technician as soon as possible after the event.

It is essential that all electrical equipment the patient uses is properly earthed. Appliances used in the home such as hairdryers may only have two pins and are not earthed. Most hospitals have a policy of sending all electrical equipment the patient uses for checking by an electrician. The patient should be cardiac monitored at all times and, if mobile, should not leave the unit or step-down area. This point should be discussed at the earliest opportunity with patients as they often feel well once the rhythm disturbance is controlled. This applies even if the patient has the pacing wires capped off. A temporary wire in the right ventricle which can move about quite freely, causing ventricular irritation and ventricular tachycardia or fibrillation, is a possibility.

Removal of temporary wires. In those patients in whom a central venous access route has been used, it is important to remember that the risk of air embolism is the same as for any central venous catheter. The patient should be supine or in a slight Trendelenburg position (head down) (Mennim et al 1992). During the removal of the catheter, it is advisable to monitor the patient via the ECG, as it is possible to irritate the myocardium and cause ventricular arrhythmias on exit of the wire. In the case of ventricular pacing the catheter is positioned in the right ventricle and must pass through the tricuspid valve. The catheter can become stuck here but in this event, pressure should not be applied as this can damage the valve. Medical assistance should be called and the catheter removed with fluoroscopic guidance.

The entry site should be covered by an air-occlusive dressing. Gauze is not air occlusive. The dressing should then remain in place for at least 24 hours to allow healing over the entry site. All temporary wires are now disposable and it is usual practice to send the tip for microscopy, to detect organisms likely to cause infection. If a positive result is returned, the patient can be closely observed and treated with antibiotics as appropriate. Observations following removal of a temporary wire include continuous cardiac monitoring, with recording of the blood pressure and heart rate. The site should be observed for leakage and the temperature recording should remain 4 hourly for 2 days, to ensure any infection is detected at an early stage.

Epicardial pacing

In the early days of pacing this was a common approach. A thoracotomy was used to attach the pacing wires to the myocardium, threading the leads down into the abdomen to the pulse generator. It is rare today for this approach to be used for permanent systems. However, those patients who have had successful pacing and no problems with this in the past may come in for replacement of the pulse generator. The decrease in size of new units brings about problems with movement and stress on the leads so it is common for the pulse generator to be removed and a new system put in endocardially.

Today's epicardial pacing most usually involves a temporary pacing electrode being fixed to the atrial and ventricular epicardium at the time of cardiac surgery. This is not uncommon in valve surgery. The electrodes are usually stainless steel wires coated with Teflon. Practice varies amongst surgeons depending upon the operation performed and whilst in years past all cardiac surgical patients had epicardial pacing wires in place, nowadays most patients don't have any at all. The wires are paired to each chamber and passed through the skin in the subxiphoid region. Ideally they should be labelled but in reality they rarely are. This is poor practice and should be addressed as a clinical risk issue. Documentation should be found in the operation notes completed by the surgeon at the time of the procedure.

Atrial pacing wires generally come out in the right subcostal region and ventricular wires in the left subcostal regions. If only one epicardial wire is inserted and pacing is required, the pacing loop is achieved by using a needle through the subcutaneous tissue with a crocodile clip attachment leading to the pulse generator. When pacing is required a careful check on the threshold each day is needed, because this climbs rapidly over the first week and may exceed the output of the pulse generator.

The connections at the ends of the electrodes are fragile and if the insulation is peeled away two tiny mircofilaments can be seen. In an emergency, where the patient is pacing dependent and the end of the pacing wire breaks, these microfilaments will achieve pacing if connected to an old-style junction box. This should not be carried on for longer than it takes to place a transvenous system as the filament progressively breaks and the danger of microshock is present. It is important to cover electrodes not in use with a non-conductive rubber glove finger to prevent microshock.

Transthoracic pacing

Direct percutaneous introduction of wire electrodes into the ventricular chamber is used only in cardiac arrest situations, where asystole is present with P-waves and transcutaneous pacing has been ineffective and transvenous pacing cannot be achieved quickly.

A myocardial pacing wire is threaded through a percutaneous cardiac needle. An electrode capable of going through this small diameter is used. The needle punctures the right ventricle and verification of its position is by aspiration. Once this is confirmed the electrode is advanced into the ventricle. Most of the prepacked kits on the market have a system where on deployment the electrode flares out and hooks itself in place. The needle/introducer is then withdrawn, leaving the pacing wire behind. Ideally, during insertion, the end of the pacing catheter should be connected by alligator clamps on to a V lead on an ECG machine/monitor. Myocardial contact is indicated by ST elevation at the time of contact. The electrode is then connected by crocodile clips to the pulse generator. Some of the kits allow the electrode to connect directly to the pulse generator. The usual approach is subxiphoid.

Ideally the distal intraventricular electrode acts as the cathode and the proximal electrode is the anode. The distal electrode does not have to be in contact with the endocardium for capture, but this is the ideal. Unipolar transthoracic intraventricular pacing uses a subcutaneous needle as the anode.

Transoesophageal pacing

The close proximity of the oesophagus to the posterior wall of the left atrium makes atrial capture possible in the general population. This is useful in terminating some arrhythmias, particularly where drugs or X-rays are not suitable, such as with pregnant women. Ventricular pacing can be achieved in some people but most patients have difficulty with pain.

Table 21.1 Common capture problems in temporary pacing systems

Problem	Action to be taken
Threshold exceeding output	Recheck the threshold and increase the output. If the threshold is greater than the output refer to medical staff and prepare for replacement of the temporary wire.
Lead displacement	This is usually confirmed by chest X-ray, if it is not clear the wire has been pulled out some distance. Depending on the cause, prepare for repositioning or replacement. Some temporary systems now have sterile sleeves covering the insertion site which allows for repositioning. It is useful to put a mark or piece of tape to demonstrate the length of wire protruding from the neck.
Myocardial infarction	Necrotic tissue is unable to propagate an impulse. The position of the electrode will have to be moved.
Excessive fibrosis at the electrode site	This is unlikely to occur unless the electrode has been in position for several weeks and the cause of failure to capture is an increase in the threshold above the output of the temporary pacing box. Some temporary boxes allow a delivery of up to 15–20 V. It is worth checking to see if one of these can be obtained. The question to be asked is why this pacing wire has been in so long; the known risk of systemic infection must be considered.
Electrolyte imbalance	Potassium levels should be checked on a regular basis when temporary wires are in place, so that appropriate action can be taken at an early stage, not when an emergency situation has already developed.
Myocardial perforation	This is often present with a loss of capture, but the patient may be hiccuping or coughing from diaphragmatic stimulation. Repositioning of the wire should be carried out immediately and the patient observed for signs of cardiac tamponade (see Chapter 22).

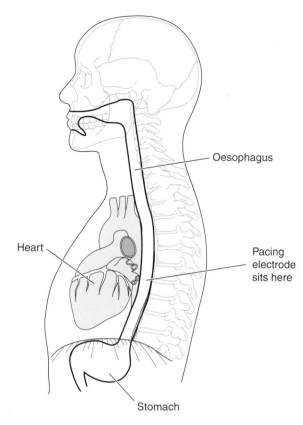

Figure 21.22 Lateral view of the electrode position for transoesophageal cardiac pacing.

Trouble shooting

Failure to capture. Failure to depolarize the myocardium due to the delivery of an ineffective pacing stimulus. On the ECG, pacemaker spikes are not followed by P-waves or a QRS complex, depending on the pacing mode. Signs and symptoms demonstrated by the patient are bradycardia, hypotension, dyspnoea, chest pain, dizziness, fatigue and collapse.

Safe practice dictates that whenever a patient with a temporary wire is in hospital all equipment necessary for immediate replacement of any part of the pacing system should be present. This includes, where possible, facilities for transcutaneous pacing which can be commenced by nursing staff in most cardiac units following completion of the advanced life support (ALS) training programme. It is important to notify the appropriate member of the medical team as soon as a problem is detected (Fig. 21.23).

Failure to sense. Sensing is the ability of the circuitry in the pulse generator to recognize the intrinsic electrical activity (intracardiac signals) of the heart and inhibit a pacing impulse release. In failure to sense, the pacemaker does not inhibit when spontaneous beats occur, resulting in competition between the artificial and natural pacemaker. The danger to the patient is that a pacing spike may fall on the T-wave of a sinus beat (the effect is an artificial R-on-T ectopic) which, if occurring in the vulnerable period of the T-wave, may induce ventricular tachycardia or fibrillation. The main symptom patients complain of is palpitations as paced and inherent rhythms compete. On the ECG tracing, pacing spikes can be seen coming in at inappropriate times. Failure to sense (Fig. 21.24) may be caused by damage to the pacing wire, the sensing threshold being set too high, critical positioning of the wire tip or other equipment failure (Jenkins & Gerred 1997) (Table 21.2).

Use of temporary pacing wires for control of arrhythmias

Transvenous pacing wires are used in cardiac units for the control of ventricular tachycardia (VT), making the assumption that VT is a re-entrant tachyarrhythmia.

Table 21.2 Common reasons for mal-sensing in temporary pacing systems

Occurrences	Action to be taken
Battery depletion	Check battery and maintenance sticker. If in doubt change pulse generator.
Sensitivity setting incorrect	This is often the cause, as it is the most confusing concept related to temporary pacing. Check sensitivity threshold and reset as necessary.
Change in sensitivity threshold due to increasing oedema or fibrosis at the electrode site	Recheck sensitivity threshold.
Myocardial infarction	Electrode may now be in contact with necrotic tissue which does not conduct impulses. Repositioning is necessary.
Poor contact between the electrode, lead connectors and pacing box	Check and change as necessary. Ensure that all connection sites are properly insulated.

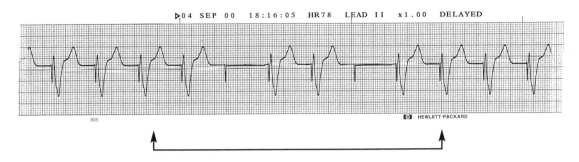

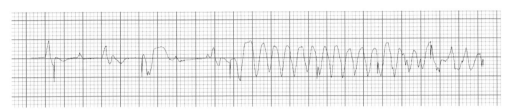

Figure 21.23 Rhythm strip for failure to capture in cardiac pacing. Note that a pacing spike is not followed by either a P-wave (atrial pacing) or a QRS complex (ventricular pacing).

Figure 21.24 Rhythm strip for failure to sense in cardiac pacing. In this example the pacemaker continues to fire despite the presence of spontaneous myocardial depolarization. This is hazardous because, as shown here, the pacemaker has discharged while the ventricle was repolarizing (R-on-T phenomenon), causing ventricular tachycardia. (Reproduced with permission from Jenkins RD, Gerred SJ 1997 ECGs by example. Churchill Livingstone, Edinburgh.)

For a re-entry circuit to exist, three key criteria have to be met (Fogoros 1995). Two conducting pathways must run parallel to one another and be connected proximally and distally by conduction tissue to form a potential circuit. One of the pathways (A) must have a refractory period substantially longer than that of the other pathway (B). Pathway B with the shorter refractory period, must conduct electrical impulses more slowly. If these three preconditions are all met a premature stimulus at a critical time (when pathway B is ready to accept an impulse, pathway A is still refractory and the slow conduction through B gives A time to recover) will initiate a re-entry circuit.

Antitachycardia pacing operates on the principle that an appropriately timed impulse can enter the circuit during re-entry tachycardia and collide with the re-entrant impulse, stopping the arrhythmia. The pacing rate is determined by the tachycardia rate and should be around 15% higher (Josephson et al 1987). Only burst pacing (this has a constant cycle length – the time between each impulse generated is the same) is possible with a temporary pacing system, but during electrophysiology studies (EPS) or when using an internal cardioverter defibrillator (ICD), there is a facility to shorten the coupling interval with each successive beat. This enables the ICD to be programmed

to each patient's own individual tachycardia. It has been estimated that 90% of spontaneous episodes of VT can be pace terminated (Gillis et al 1993).

Permanent pacemakers

Today these devices are inserted almost exclusively under local anaesthetic. The pacing electrode is introduced through the cephalic vein (using a cutdown procedure) or by a direct subclavian puncture (using a stylet, introducer and internal vessel dilator to introduce the lead). The pulse generator weight varies depending on the manufacturing company but usually weighs between 25 and 35 g and is 0.5 cm thick. The battery lasts 8–12 years depending on use. It can be programmed using radiofrequency devices that look very similar to the wands used in airports or, more recently, like the mouse of a computer.

The electrodes are made of platinum or carbon with the distal cathodal electrode specially treated to reduce electrical resistance. Pacing leads are grouped into two main types. First, active fixation leads where the electrodes have a screw or branch-like device at the tip to prevent catheter movement. This development has significantly decreased the length of stay of patients in hospital, while allowing more freedom of movement of the arm on the affected side. The second group are the passive fixation leads where no penetration of the myocardium occurs. The lead usually has tines (finger-like projections, from the end of the electrode) to wedge the lead within the trabeculae of the right ventricle. In atrial pacing catheters the distinctive J shape helps positioning in the right atrial appendage.

Once the electrode has been successfully implanted, the following occurs in a cascade manner (Kay 1996).

- Tissue reaction to lead – acute injury to cell membranes.
- Myocardial oedema – coating of electrode by platelets and fibrin.
- Cellular inflammatory reaction – infiltration by leucocytes and mononuclear cells.
- Macrophages attack interface between pacing electrode and myocardium.
- Extracellular release of proteolytic enzymes and free O_2 radicals resulting in acceleration of tissue injury under electrode.
- More macrophages and then fibroblasts move into the myocardium.
- Fibroblasts in the myocardium begin producing collagen.
- Development of fibrotic capsule around electrode.

The end result of this process is that the electrode is now not in direct contact with the excitable myocardial tissue. Some passive fixation electrodes have a silicone core impregnated with dexamethasone which works by decreasing the inflammatory response of the cardiac tissue.

The change in the threshold in permanent leads reflects the above process. During the first 24 hours there is an acute rise, continuing over the next 5 days and peaking a week after implant. The threshold then comes down to less than the peak at a week. How much will depend upon what electrodes are used as they vary in size and shape and chemical composition.

The surface structure, stability of the electrode/myocardial interface, the flexibility of the lead, autonomic tone, circulating catecholamines, potassium levels, acid–base balance and what drugs the patient is taking will also affect the threshold. Whether the electrode has tines or a 'screw-in' fixation device will affect what happens at the myocardial interface.

The concomitant treatment of the patient will also affect the threshold. For example, in those patients with tachy-brady syndrome, drug therapy to slow down the heart rate will not commence until the pacemaker is in place. β-Blockers are frequently used and can increase the threshold. Close clinical follow-up of the permanent system over the months and years is important, because pacing stimulus, amplitude and duration have a profound effect on the battery life of the device. The safety margin is important, but should not be set unnecessarily high.

One way in which battery life can be prolonged is by using a programmable feature called **hysteresis**. Hysteresis is the period between the last intrinsic beat and the next paced beat. For example, if the pacing rate is set at 60 bpm the pacemaker would normally be programmed to initiate pacing when the heart rate drops below 60 bpm even if this was 58 bpm. If a hys-

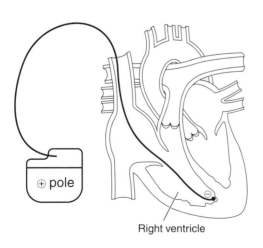 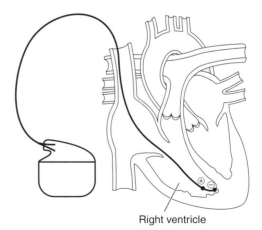

Right ventricle   Right ventricle

A Unipolar pacing   **B** Bipolar pacing

Both are VVI systems

Figure 21.25 Unipolar (A) and bipolar (B) permanent cardiac pacing systems.

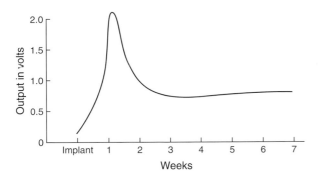

Figure 21.26 The change in the pacing threshold in a patient with a permanent pacemaker implant.

Box 21.2 Code letters to classify cardiac pacing modes

For positions I–IV	*Position V*
A = atrium	P = pacing
V = ventricle	S = shock
D = dual	D = pacing and shock
(atrium and ventricle)	O = none
O = none	
T = trigger pacing	
I = inhibit pacing	
P = programmability of	
rate or output	
M = multiprogrammable	
C = communicating	
R = rate responsive	

teresis of 20 is programmed, then the heart rate would need to drop to 40 bpm before pacing at 60 bpm was initiated. The art in setting this rate revolves around the need to balance patient symptoms and the battery life of the pacemaker, so the patient does not have to undergo repeated early replacement of the pulse generator. A lower heart rate at night when the patient is sleeping or if the patient has atrial fibrillation, where the rhythm is irregularly irregular, are two common examples of where the hysteresis setting can be useful.

In 1974 an international generic code was developed to standardize the way in which pacemakers could be described. Initially there were three positions but in 1985 this was expanded to five with the development of programmable devices and ICD devices.

The five categories are:

- chamber paced
- chamber sensed
- response to sensing
- programmable features
- antitachyarrhythmia functions.

Recently a sixth position was proposed to describe follow-up properties, i.e. transtelephonic. The code positions are arranged in sequence I, II, III, IV and V across the top. Underneath, code letters describe a function or characteristic. Only one letter is possible for each position (Box 21.2).

VVI pacing

V (ventricular chamber paced), V (ventricular chamber sensed), I (inhibit pacing/the response to sensing).

In the UK this is still the most common form of permanent pacing. The pacing electrode is positioned in the right ventricle. On sensing a spontaneous ventricu-

lar beat, the pacemaker is inhibited. Pacing is at a set rate. It is appropriate to mention pacemaker syndrome at this point. Some patients return with symptoms not unlike those they suffered before insertion of a VVI system and in some cases they describe feeling much worse. Symptoms include dizziness, presyncope and syncope, weakness, fatigue and shortness of breath. The most likely cause is AV synchrony which can cause systemic hypotension and AV valve regurgitation. This leads to a decrease in cardiac output and to pulmonary congestion. In some patients pulsation is seen at the neck. These are called cannon A-waves and are due to atrial contraction against closed AV valves (Fig. 21.27).

VVIR

V (ventricular chamber paced), V (ventricular chamber sensed), I (inhibit pacing/the response to sensing), R (rate responsive).

This mode paces and senses in the ventricule. A sensed beat inhibits the pacing stimulus, but there is also a sensor implanted which allows the ventricular response to increase due to additional demand, such as in exercise. Sensors available include motion sensors, which use low-frequency vibration (4 Hz). Here, a piezo-electric ceramic crystal is situated on the pulse generator case. The sensed vibration is converted to an electrical signal. An inappropriate response to vibration can occur such as sitting in a helicopter or vigorous swimming. The pacemaker response is to produce a rapid increase in rate.

Respiration sensors use minute volume and changes in transthoracic impedance (between pacing lead, auxiliary subcutaneous lead implanted over the anterior chest wall and the pulse generator) as triggers. Temperature sensors work via a right ventricle

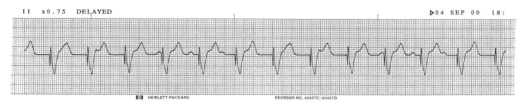

Figure 21.27 Rhythm strip for VVI cardiac pacing. Note the pacing spike occurring before each bizarre QRS complex.

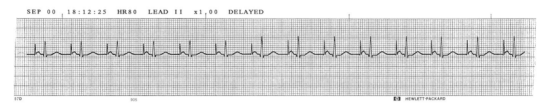

Figure 21.28 Rhythm strip for AAI cardiac pacing. Note the pacing spike before the P-wave and a normally conducted QRS complex.

thermistor similar to that found in pulmonary artery thermodilution catheters.

Recent studies on physiologic sensors include those looking at Q–T interval, stroke volume, O_2 saturation and blood pH.

AAI

A (atrial chamber paced), A (atrial chamber sensed), I (inhibit pacing/the response to sensing).

The pacing electrode is placed in the right atrial appendage. If a P-wave is sensed then the pacemaker will inhibit. The pacing rate is set. This form of pacing is only useful in patients without AV block. It provides AV synchrony and thus maximum cardiac output (Fig. 21.28).

DDD

D (dual chamber pacing), D (dual chamber sensed), D (dual chamber inhibit pacing/the response to sensing).

This mode uses two bipolar pacing electrodes, one in the right atrial appendage and the other in the right ventricular apex. The pacemaker senses and paces both chambers. A sensed beat in the atrium inhibits the atrial pacing stimulus and if no inherent activity is sensed after the programmed AV interval, a ventricular paced stimulus will follow. DDD pacing is able to provide a rate response by sensing intrinsic atrial activity and tracking the heart rate by pacing the ventricles at the same rate. It is a common mistake to assume a DDD

pacemaker is not working when this complex activity varies from beat to beat. For example, the first beat has a normal P-wave but no ventricular activity is sensed therefore you see a paced ventricular complex. The second complex may have no P-wave sensed therefore an atrial pacing spike is seen but this does conduct normally and a normal QRS complex follows and in the third beat no inherent activity is sensed therefore both atrial and ventricular pacing spikes are seen (Fig. 21.29).

DDD pacing offers the nearest approximation to normal function and with today's rate-responsive pacemakers, most patients feel almost as though they have normal conduction. It is important, however, not to say they will feel exactly as though they did not have a pacemaker. This sets up unrealistic expectations. One possible drawback is that a small number of patients may have intact ventriculo-atrial conduction and a pacemaker-mediated tachycardia (PMT) may occur. Ventricular pacing causes a retrograde (travelling backwards) impulse to be transmitted to the atrium where it is sensed by the atrial lead and interpreted by the pacemaker as an intrinsic atrial beat. When no inherent activity is found the pacemaker then triggers another ventricular paced beat creating a tachycardia. In the acute situation the application of a magnet stops atrial sensing and interrupts the tachycardia. The use of the DDI mode of pacing can prevent this from occurring. Both the atria and ventricle are sensed and paced but when the atrial rate goes over the upper rate limit, a ventricular response does not follow; that is, the ventricular rate is fixed. The downside is that the normal response in ventricular rate

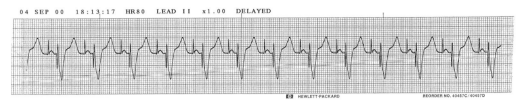

04 SEP 00   18:13:17   HR80   LEAD II   x1.00   DELAYED

HEWLETT-PACKARD   REORDER NO. 40457C/40457D

Figure 21.29 Rhythm strip for DDD cardiac pacing. Note the pacing spike before both the P-wave and the wide QRS complex.

does not occur during exercise. The atrial rate increases but the ventricular rate cannot follow.

A pacing mode of DDDR is possible in the more sophisticated pacemakers. The pacemaker senses and stimulates both atria and ventricle. The stimulation rate is controlled by setting an upper rate limit and the rate can respond to a sensor up to the upper rate limit. A minimum rate is also set.

DVI paces both the atria and the ventricle but senses only in the ventricle. The pacemaker is inhibited and timing reset by inherent ventricular activity, but ignores the inherent atrial rate.

One programmable feature that can help the pacemaker mimic normal physiological function is that of rate smoothing. This stops an abrupt change in heart rate; for example, if a patient has an atrial tachycardia the response will be immediate but not up to the exact atrial rate. A percentage rate increase is used, e.g. 12% increase in rate rather than 30% immediately. This will only apply up to the set upper rate limit, beyond which there will be no further response from the pacemaker. It is important to know if this facility has been programmed, as it often leads to an interpretation that the pacemaker is functioning inadequately.

A sensing problem that happens rarely in DDD units is called crosstalk. Crosstalk means incorrect sensing by the ventricular sensing circuitry of the atrial pacing stimulus which then inhibits ventricular pacing, resulting in long pauses. This can also happen in AAI or VVI systems when sensing of the intracardiac signal from the other chambers can result in inappropriate inhibition.

NURSING MANAGEMENT

Temporary dual-chamber pacing system (AV sequential pacing)

There are occasions when the patient will return to the acute coronary or intensive care unit with a dual-chamber temporary pacing system. It appears that the majority of nursing staff do not routinely adjust or manipulate these pacing systems. However, with

appropriate education and assessment this may inevitably become the case. Certainly, as with all equipment, a working knowledge is required to ensure optimal treatment. Figure 21.30 illustrates a typical dual-chamber system, which is capable of a variety of pacing modes. Four wires will complete two circuits, one in the right atrium and one in the right ventricle. The following is a brief overview of the pacing box itself.

The pacemaker box is switched ON from a recessed switch on the left hand side of the unit. Switching the unit on automatically selects the DDD mode at standard values. Moving the switch forward to the LOCK position locks out the keypad, so that further changes to the programme cannot be made without first moving the switch back to the ON position. A visible and audible warning is given if the keypad is pressed whilst in the LOCK position.

In Figure 21.30 the pacing output in both the atrial and ventricular chambers is set to 5.0 volts (V). This is a standard setting for the device. In assessing the appropriate output to programme, the threshold should be assessed (see p. 406) and the output adjusted to provide an ample safety margin: the greater of 5.0 V or three times the threshold value. Battery conservation is not a valid concern in temporary pacing.

When the rate button is pressed, a cursor should flash by the rate which in Figure 21.30 is set at 60 pulses per minute (ppm). The positive and negative keys can then be used to elevate or lower the rate. Again, if excessively low or high rates are set, a message may appear in the screen offering a warning before these 'out of normal range' rates can be applied.

The mode button allows the type of pacing to be altered. In Figure 21.30 it is set on DDD (the dual-chamber pacing mode). Most machines allow you to browse the options via the arrow up and down keys, then to press the mode again to change and confirm it.

The atrial sensitivity level is set at 1.0 mV and 2.0 mV in the ventricle. This again is a standard setting

A

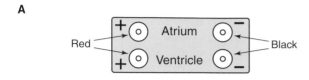

B

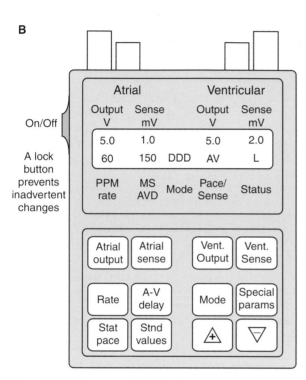

Figure 21.30 Temporary dual-chamber pacing system.

and indicates that the machine will only sense electrical elements of the complex above this mV level. If the sensitivity value is set too low (i.e. the system is more sensitive), interference, such as electrical 'noise' from surrounding appliances, may be sensed and interpreted as normal cardiac conduction. This is termed 'oversensing' and would inappropriately inhibit pacing. If the sensitivity value is set too high (i.e. the system is less sensitive) there is a risk that no part of the QRS complex will be sensed. This is termed 'undersensing' and can result in inappropriate pacing in the presence of an intrinsic rhythm.

The sensitivity level is altered by pressing the atrial sense or ventricular sense keys, which produces a flashing cursor over the respective sensitivity value. The arrow up or down keys at the bottom right of the machine can be used to alter these levels. An adequate

safety margin should also be added to the sensitivity level, to ensure reliable sensing. If excessively low or high sensitivity values are selected, the machine will display a visual and audible warning before proceeding to the 'out of range' values.

The AV delay (AVD) is defined as the time interval between an atrial output pulse and a ventricular output pulse. The standard value for the AVD is 150 ms. If the system detects intrinsic atrial activity it initiates a PV delay, whereby the machine automatically shortens the programmed AVD by 25 ms. The AVD can be increased or decreased to suit haemodynamic or electrophysiological requirements and changing this parameter can significantly influence a patient's stroke volume and therefore cardiac output. The machine may automatically adjust the AVD in dual-chamber modes when the rate is changed.

The pace/sense window in Figure 21.30 indicates AV. This is a flashing sign which indicates what the pacemaker's status is at that time. It is important to always be guided by the ECG tracing on the monitor to know the exact pacing action but this figure will also assist. A flashing A and then V indicates that the atria and then the ventricle are being paced, after the aforementioned AV delay (AV sequential pacing). A flashing PR indicates an intrinsic P-wave from the patient and an intrinsic R-wave. This would mean no pacing was occurring and could be sinus rhythm.

A flashing AR would indicate a paced atrium, followed by an intrinsic R-wave. This would indicate atrial pacing with intrinsic conduction to the ventricle. A flashing PV indicates an intrinsic P-wave followed by a paced ventricle (i.e. the pacemaker is 'tracking' the intrinsic atrial rate).

The flashing occurs with the sensing or pacing, therefore the faster the flashing, the faster the rate. Different pacing modes allow different combinations of pacing and sensing in each or both chambers. It is important to have a good knowledge of a pacing mode's benefits and limitations before adjusting.

Other indicators displayed in the status window include:

- L – indicates a low battery
- N – indicates interference ('noise') has been detected
- B – indicates the pacemaker is performing 2:1 block in the presence of a high atrial rate
- W – indicates the device is performing what may be termed the 'electronic Wenckebach phenomenon' in the presence of high atrial rate. The ECG pattern for the Wenckebach phenomenon can be found elsewhere in this text (p. 401)

- S – shows the device is performing ventricular safety pacing.

The stat pace button is used when the doctor or nurse becomes confused regarding what pacing the machine is achieving. It will automatically switch the device to the DDI mode with standard settings but with a higher output and pulse width. This should ensure that the pacemaker captures immediately, without further adjustment, provided the pacing threshold is not grossly elevated. It should be used if an adjustment of pacing suddenly results in a haemodynamically unstable patient.

The standard values button is similar to the stat pace button. It can be used in a haemodynamically stable patient to return to the preset standard values for the device. The standard value button will not change the pacing mode, only the parameters within that mode.

The special parameters button is rarely used and offers pacing options outside the normal values or choices. To cycle through these options, press the special parameters key and press again to advance to the next option. Adjusting is performed in the usual manner with the plus/minus keys. Some more common uses are as follows.

By pressing 'special parameters', it will ask you to press the atrial and ventricular output keys together. In doing this all pacing function is inhibited but only while the buttons are pressed. This allows the underlying rhythm to be seen without switching off the box. Releasing the buttons restores pacing at the programmed modality.

The memorize recall choice allow the box to memorize the settings when the arrow up (+) key is pressed. When the box is next switched on, the special parameters button can be pressed, followed by the arrow down (–) button and the memorized programme will be applied.

The Atr PW and Vnt PW allow the atrial and ventricular pulse widths to be altered. The pulse width, as previously discussed, is the period of time over which the programmed output is delivered. There is little indication to alter this. However, the pulse width can be increased to facilitate capture in a patient with a high capture threshold. Also, if using a unipolar pacing system, a high capture threshold can cause muscle 'twitching' in the area of the indifferent electrode. By increasing the pulse width, the output can be reduced (hopefully reducing/eliminating any twitching) whilst maintaining an appropriate safety margin. Note that it is recommended to perform a capture threshold test after adjusting the pulse width or

output values to ensure an appropriate safety margin is programmed.

The rapid pacing option allows a high rate to be delivered on the atrial channel. This can be used, for example, to 'overdrive' and terminate an atrial tachycardia. Once the desired rate is selected, pressing the rate key will deliver that rate in AOO mode for as long as the rate key is pressed. Releasing the rate key restores the pacer function to its previous programme. Care should be exercised when using this option and it should only be attempted under medical guidance/supervison.

The PVARP (post ventricular atrial refractory period) forms part of the pacemaker's refractory period. It is a period of time after a ventricular sensed or paced event whereby the atrial channel is made refractory (i.e. cannot respond to any sensed events). It can be used to prevent the tracking of premature atrial ectopics and is very useful in the prevention and termination of PMTs. This, as previously highlighted, is caused by a retrograde impulse from a ventricular ectopic or paced ventricular event travelling retrogradely to the atria via the AV node and being sensed by the device as a sensed atrial event. The pacemaker's response to a sensed atrial event (in DDD mode) is to deliver a ventricular pace after the programmed AVD. Therefore the pacemaker 'tracks' this retrograde event and a cycle of paced ventricle following retrograde P-wave results in a 'loop' tachycardia, usually at the upper tracking rate of the pacemaker.

By programming the PVARP to a value longer than the V–A time of the retrogradely conducted beat, the PMT can be terminated. However, lengthening the PVARP will also limit the maximum tracking rate of the pacemaker, so care should be exercised in adjusting this parameter. The pacemaker may have other algorithms for the prevention of PMTs, but the PVARP is the most accessible to the prescriber and can be the easiest way of preventing inappropriate tachycardia. The standard PVARP value is 250 ms.

The ventricular refractory period is rarely altered. If shortened, the upper rate of the device can be increased. If lengthened significantly, the upper rate of the device can be limited. If refractory settings compromise the selection of higher rates, a prompt to reduce the refractory period is displayed.

The MTR is the maximum tracking rate. In DDD mode it defines the maximum rate to which intrinsic atrial activity will be tracked by ventricular pacing. It is preset at 120 ppm and can be adjusted to facilitate higher rate tracking. It is a frequently adjusted parameter on paediatric patients, where higher rates are required. If intrinsic atrial activity occurs at rates faster than the programmed MTR, then the pacemaker will not track all of these events 1:1, but exhibit upper rate behaviour which is manifested as the 'electronic Wenckebach phenomenon' and then 2:1 block of the sensed atrial events. By observing the status window, the upper rate behaviour can be observed.

Care of the temporary dual-chamber pacing system

The pacemaker unit usually runs on two 9 V batteries. The battery life will vary according to mode, output level and pacing demand. Typically the pacemaker will operate continuously at standard DDD settings on two new batteries (for example, Duracell model MN1604) for about 1.5 weeks. Low battery condition is displayed in the status window followed by an audible tone and warning message every 4 minutes. At this time the batteries **must** be changed. To facilitate battery change whilst the pacemaker is in use, the pacemaker will continue to work at its programmed settings with one battery (provided the batteries are changed as soon as the low battery warning is given). If the programmed settings have not been saved, removing both batteries simultaneously will result in a reset of the pacemaker parameters to the standard settings. It is therefore recommended to change the batteries one at a time whilst the pacemaker is connected to the patient. If low battery warnings are ignored, abrupt loss of pacing may occur. Additionally, the batteries should be changed routinely every time the pacemaker is removed from a patient and prepared for the next.

The pacemaker unit is durable and water resistant (it is not water proof). For cleaning, a damp cloth or sponge (dampened in warm water with a non-abrasive detergent) is recommended. Immersion is contraindicated. Additionally, it must not be sterilized using steam autoclaving or γ radiation methods.

Great care should be exercised when using diathermy/cautery equipment with patients with pacing systems. Adequate monitoring must be used and an asynchronous pacing mode should be selected where appropriate. Additionally care should be exercised in the placing of defibrillatory electrodes. The pacemaker is protected against defibrillatory discharges, but the paddles must be positioned well away from the pacing leads.

The pacemaker should be inspected prior to connection to the patient. If it appears damaged or the casing is compromised, the unit should not be used.

It is recommended that prior to handling the pacing leads or pacemaker, the operator should first touch some part of the patient's skin at a site remote to the pacemaker lead. This is to equalize the electrostatic potential between the operator and the patient. Following on, the pacemaker and leads should not be placed in close proximity to high-powered mains-operated or high-powered field-generating equipment. This minimizes any risk of artefact detection or any signal conduction/induction through the pacing system (which can induce serious arrhythmias).

Permanent pacemaker insertion

Patient preparation

It is crucial to assess the patient's individual needs before pacemaker insertion and highlight any particular issues, for example working with industrial magnets, which will impact on their lifestyle. It is important to know the medical indications for insertion of a permanent pacemaker as this will guide your preparation of the patient. Within our own organization we have developed an integrated care pathway (ICP) and guidelines for a minimum information which is set for all patients. The first documentation required after biographical details is the indication for pacing and documentation of same. From this we prepare the patient for informed consent by using the following checklist, which must be signed and dated by the nurse once the information has been given.

- Cardiac anatomy and physiology of the heart and conduction system.
- Type of conducting problem the person is experiencing.
- The purpose of the pacemaker and how it will work in the patient's own circumstances.
- Catheter laboratory layout, X-ray machinery, local anaesthetic, possibility of palpitations.
- Guide to length of time in the laboratory.
- Immediate postprocedure care, length of bedrest, movement limitations, treatment of pain and discomfort.
- Wound size and site, cardiac monitoring, chest X-ray and drugs (antibiotic prohylaxis).
- Discharge arrangements and social circumstances.

Physical preparation. If the patient has been in hospital for some time, such as following a myocardial infarction, and has required temporary pacing, it is essential that the electrodes used for monitoring are not placed over a prospective pulse generator site. The conducting gel and/or the adhesive used to keep them in place is irritant to most skins and often causes abrasion to the skin, thus setting up an increased possibility of infection. This is often forgotten and a clean site is impossible to find.

Minimal shaving should be carried out on the day of the procedure and only if the patient's chest is particularly hairy. The patient should also have a shower or bath at this time. It is usual to place intravenous access on the opposite side to the pulse generator so that in the event of an emergency the physician and other team members are not competing for the same side of the patient.

The last food or drink should be taken 2–4 hours prior to the procedure depending on the cardiac unit policy. Adequate hydration is extremely important. A dehydrated patient will not only feel unwell but is also more likely to become confused, especially if elderly, and venous access at the time of procedure is likely to be more difficult. This may then increase the risk of complications, such as a pneumothorax.

Informed consent is obtained. It is important that the patient is not promised an unrealistic outcome and this is especially true when the indication for pacing is not definitive. Syncope in the elderly, for example, can have a myriad of causes and whilst a conduction abnormality is found on the ECG, there is no guarantee that this is the cause of their syncope. The expression 'feeling as good as new' in a population where VVI pacing is still the most common form is unrealistic, for reasons described previously.

The hand which is dominant for the patient is important information and usual practice places the pulse generator on the opposite side. This may not always be possible, for example in those women who have had radical mastectomy, but does aid comfort if it can be achieved. Premedication varies between institutions. It is common to find a narcotic such as Omnopon and an anti-emetic such as metoclopramide written up with intravenous (IV) or intramuscular (IM) antibiotics. Pacemaker insertion is considered to be a fairly routine procedure but the risk of a severe infection such as endocarditis remains, with a mortality rate similar to those patients with other causes of endocarditis (Klug et al 1997). Many patients already have a temporary wire in place and it is important to make sure that this has not become infected, leading to a risk that this will extend to the permanent system. A meta-analysis recently published (Da Costa et al 1998a) analysed the available findings of 2023 patients in randomized trials. The results suggested that systemic antibiotic prophylaxis significantly reduced the incidence of potentially serious infective complications after permanent pacemaker implantation.

The patient is then taken to the laboratory, which should be prepared under strict aseptic conditions when any implant is being carried out. The nurse in charge of the catheter laboratory should ensure that no extraneous personnel are wandering in and out unnecessarily. DaCosta et al's (1998b) prospective study concluded that pacemaker infection was due mainly to local contamination during the implant procedure, so procedures in the catheter laboratory need to adhere to strict infection control practices. It is important to introduce the patient to the nurse/technician/radiographer and physician performing the implant. The patient is awake throughout the procedure and may be anxious.

After the procedure

On return to the ward/unit, the nursing handover should include which route was used (subclavian vein access requires a chest X-ray following the procedure to rule out a pneumothorax), the name of the device, the mode of pacing and rate limits. The mode of pacing described previously is key information for the cardiac nurse because without this information it is impossible to make a judgement on whether the device is working properly.

The patient should be attached to a cardiac monitor and a rhythm established. The cardiac monitors have several filters which minimize outside 'noise' from muscle movement. Unipolar spikes are large and hard to miss but bipolar spikes, as previously mentioned, are small and may completely disappear. Today's modern monitoring systems counteract this effect by having a special circuit which looks for pacing spikes. It is important to activate them. On the new touch screens it usually states 'pacing on/off'. This should be turned to ON and left like that regardless of whether the patient is using the pacemaker device.

The wound site should be checked for bleeding or haematoma. Marking the dressing with biro is to be discouraged as this breaks the integrity of the dressing and can lead to infection. A diagram in the nursing notes is just as informative.

Recorded clinical observations vary between units and will depend on the status of the patient when they return to the ward/unit. Those patients who have been heavily sedated or are bleeding from their wound need more frequent observations. Cardiac monitoring is continuous but blood pressure should not be less than $\frac{1}{2}$ hourly for the first 2 hours and hourly for another two. Recording of the temperature should remain 4 hourly until the patient's discharge, as this is usually the first sign of infection.

Current practice for bedrest varies depending upon consultant choice. Movement of the arm on the affected side is restricted to avoid excessive upward vigorous activity that could conceivably displace the electrode. This is less likely to occur where a screw-in electrode is used. It is also vital to ensure that the patient does not stop moving his arm altogether, thus risking development of a frozen shoulder which can take many months of physiotherapy to improve. The elderly are at particular risk.

Observations of the wound site in the first few hours after implantation aim to note signs of haemorrhage or haematoma. It is important to inspect the whole chest when the patient returns to the ward. The amount of swelling around the site is an important observation to make and document. Haematoma formation can occur over several hours and is often at an advanced stage before action is taken. Pneumothorax and haemothorax are the other major complications. The patient usually complains of breathlessness and sometimes pain on inspiration. If this occurs the patient needs rapid assessment and intervention (usually the insertion of a chest drain). The patient should have their ECG rhythm monitored for at least the first few hours after implant to ensure normal function of the pacemaker.

Nursing use of magnets for assessment of permanent pacemaker function varies between cardiac units. Each unit should have a clear protocol in place. Each

Table 21.3 Troubleshooting in the immediate postoperative period following permanent pacemaker insertion

Problem	Likely cause	Action
Pacing spikes present with failure to capture	Lead dislodgement or poor position, output incorrectly set, damage to insulation of lead at time of implant	If patient loses output perform ALS procedures. Inform medical staff: application of magnet to check response, chest X-ray to check position. Alert technical staff regarding the need for a programming check
Pacing spikes present but failure to sense	Sensitivity setting incorrect, connection between lead and pulse generator not secure; rarely, fault in pulse generator, inadvertent setting of pulse generator on fixed rate	Urgent action required due to danger of R-on-T phenomenon. Inform technical and medical staff immediately. Have magnet available
Pacing spikes absent	Appropriate inhibition due to patient's own inherent rate above pacing rate. Failure of pulse generator or leads not screwed in properly at time of procedure, crosstalk, monitor not set up for pacing	Assess patient, perform ECG, check cardiac monitor set up to display pacing spikes, change monitoring lead. Inform medical staff if a problem with pacemaker function
Oversensing	Inappropriate sensitivity setting	Call cardiac technician and inform medical staff
Electromagnetic interference	Rare in current practice, as large motors are the main cause	Check local area, particularly if building work going on in adjacent wards. All equipment in contact with the patient should be earthed
Failure of impulse generation	Device failure or lead not connected to pulse generator	This can only be ascertained by a technical check. From a nursing point of view treat as for loss of capture
Variation in rate when pacing all the time	Battery failure of pulse generator or pacing set on rate response mode and responding to given sensor	Check pacemaker and mode set. If not in rate response mode, inform technical and medical staff
Stimulation of diaphragm (hiccups)	Perforation of right ventricle	Inform medical staff, chest X-ray to confirm position, watch for signs of pericardial tamponade

pacemaker has an individual response to magnet application. Magnets over or close to pulse generator circuitry convert pacing to fixed (asynchronous) mode by temporarily disconnecting the sensing circuitry in most modes. This is useful for the diagnosis of problems relating to sensing and can ensure pacing in situations where electromagnetic interference can inhibit output, for example when a patient requires emergency surgery that needs electrocautery and they are pacing dependent. A magnet also allows the pacemaker to be tested at routine clinical follow-up, when the patient is in their own rhythm and it is inhibited.

Many patients have surprisingly little pain following the procedure. This is in part due to the local anaesthetic infiltrated into the area but this will diminish and it is important to ask the patient if they are experiencing discomfort. Length of stay in hospital in the UK will vary between a day case and a one- or two-night stay.

Ensure that the patient has had a chest X-ray (PA and lateral) which is deliberately overpenetrated to look at lead position. A pacing check is sometimes performed in the catheter laboratory, but documentation of this will be found in the medical notes. It is essential that this is confirmed before the patient goes home. Medication for discharge is commonly the completion of a course of antibiotics.

Prior to discharge patients and their carers, as necessary, should receive advice on the care of the wound and suture removal (usually 5–7 days unless glue has been used for sealing the wound), exercising the affected shoulder and resuming work. This is dependent upon the job they do, a heavy labour-intensive job such as building, for example, taking much longer than a desk-based job. Advice does at present seem to vary between hospital, consultant and general practitioner.

Current DVLA regulations state that the patient must refrain from driving for one week after a pacemaker insertion or box change, unless the indication for pacing occurred following myocardial infarction (MI) when the restrictions for MI apply. There are many myths surrounding pacemaker implantation, the most common being around the use of microwaves and airport security equipment. The concern with these devices stems from the electromagnetic interference caused. Microwaves are safe providing they are not leaking and today's microwaves will not function with the door open so safety issues have been addressed. Recent studies have shown that in the electromagnetic field of an airport metal detector or a theft control device, a small proportion of patients' pacemakers will change the mode they are working in. In airport metal detectors, the metal casing of the device will set off the alarm. It is important that patients travelling carry their pacemaker card with them at all times.

It is often not possible for patients to avoid these devices in shops as in many instances there is no other way in. Patients should be instructed to walk briskly through and away from them. Mobile phones are safe as long as the phone is not placed over the pulse generator. One habit to be discouraged is the no-hands approach, holding the phone between the shoulder and ear on the affected side by shrugging the shoulder toward the neck. This places the phone almost directly over the pulse generator if on the implant side.

Other common sources of electromagnetic interference include radar stations, large motors and dental ultrasonic cleaners used for a 'scale and polish'. This procedure can be carried out using manual instruments only.

Management of clinical problems of the pacemaker patient

Electrocautery, as used in theatre, can cause the pacemaker to inhibit inappropriately and in extreme cases VT or ventricular fibrillation (VF) can be induced. The patient should be monitored at all times. Cardioversion/defibrillation can damage a permanent pacemaker. The paddles should be placed as far away from the pulse generator as possible and close attention paid to good contact with the gel pads. If possible, the anteroposterior paddle position should be used. The pacemaker should be checked as soon as practicable after the procedure.

Magnetic resonance imaging (MRI) scanners should be avoided totally (see Chapter 8).

Radiation therapy may damage the pacemaker circuitry. If possible, shielding should be used but it may be necessary to move the pulse generator out of harm's way in cases of lung and breast cancer.

Special considerations

The population for pacemaker insertion is elderly and therefore the mobility of the patient may be restricted. Oversedation during device implantation should be avoided as this often causes confusion in the elderly patient who is in unfamiliar circumstances. Poor discharge planning, particularly around transport home, often leads to longer lengths of stay than necessary on medical grounds.

Patients taking anticoagulation therapy require careful preparation and clinical follow-up, particularly if they have artificial heart valves in place. The risk of clot formation versus bleeding into the pacemaker pocket is always a difficult clinical issue. These patients are usually admitted several days before implant and converted onto heparin which is then stopped 6–12 hours before the procedure. Following the procedure, at least 24 hours without any prescribed anticoagulation is usual but after this, consultant preference varies. The international normalised ratio (INR), which assesses the speed of blood clotting, needs to be greater than 2.5 before discharge, if the patient has an artificial valve in place.

Case study 21.1

Mr Jim Stone, a 60-year-old man, was admitted to the CCU with an anterior MI. He had been suffering chest pain intermittently since just before breakfast. Despite thrombolytic treatment, Mr Stone's heart rate dropped to approximately 30 bpm during the night; the rhythm was regular but the QRS complex had become wider. He was haemodynamically compromised, with a blood pressure reading of 80/65 mmHg and cool, clammy skin. The 12-lead ECG can be seen in Figure 21.31.

Any change where the patient has become haemodynamically compromised requires the medical staff to be notified straight away. Observations of vital signs should be increased in frequency whilst waiting for the medical team to arrive. During the nursing assessment, if a 12-lead ECG takes time to arrange, a long rhythm strip should be obtained from the monitoring equipment, as this can provide valuable information regarding the pattern and occurrence of any arrhythmia. All too often by the time medical staff or the 12-lead ECG machine arrives the arrhythmia has resolved, only to reappear once the team leave. Complete heart block in a patient suffering from an anterior MI is a poor prognostic sign, as it indicates that a large section of the left ventricle has been destroyed.

Despite attempting transvenous pacing, Mr Stone deteriorated over the next few days and died shortly afterwards.

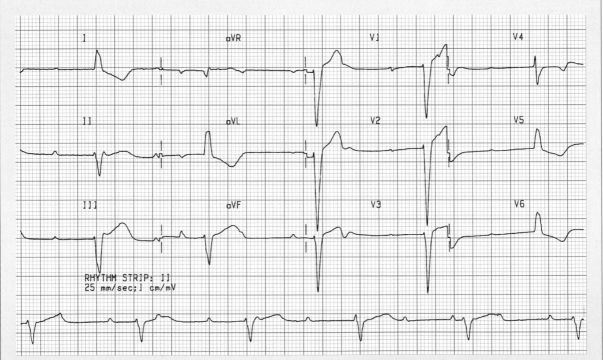

Figure 21.31 12-lead ECG indicating third-degree (complete) heart block. Note the dissociation between the P-waves and the QRS complexes, indicating a block between the atria and ventricles, and the slow, wide QRS complexes initiated from within the ventricles and maintaining a low cardiac output. (Reproduced with permission from Jenkins RD, Gerred SJ 1998 ECGs by example. Churchill Livingstone, Edinburgh.)

Case study 21.2

Mrs Jean Smythe, a 55-year-old housewife, had been referred to her local hospital with increasing shortness of breath, palpitations and on two occasions she had fainted (syncope), once when out with friends and once when running for a bus. While in hospital awaiting a 24-hour ECG tape, she again experienced palpitations. The CCU nurse caring for Mrs Smythe took the 12-lead ECG shown in Figure 21.32.

An initial diagnosis of sick sinus syndrome was made. This was later confirmed by a 24-hour Holter ECG recording. The term sick sinus syndrome covers a number of abnormalities. These can include spontaneous sinus bradycardia, sinus arrest or SA exit block, paroxysms of regular or irregular atrial tachycardia and inadequate heart rate response to exercise (Jenkins & Gerred 1997). Mrs Smythe initially had a temporary atrial pacing wire placed, before being referred for a permanent (AAI) system. She has now retuned home, following education regarding areas such as signs of possible pacemaker malfunction and situations that may affect device function. The heart rate is now appropriate and well controlled and Mrs Smythe is clinically reviewed periodically as an outpatient to assess the pacemaker function.

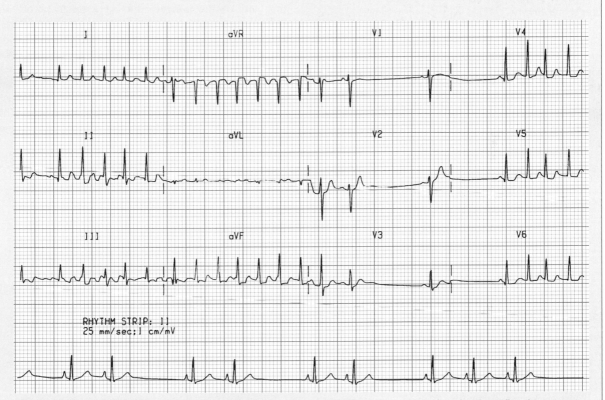

Figure 21.32 12-lead ECG demonstrating sick sinus syndrome. Note the spontaneous sinus bradycardia, sinus arrest and paroxysms of regular or irregular atrial tachyarrhythmias. (Reproduced with permission from Jenkins RD, Gerred SJ 1998 ECGs by example, Churchill Livingstone, Edinburgh.)

Late complications of permanent pacemaker insertion

Infection. This may occur in the immediate postoperative period or many months after implantation. It is important that patients understand that no matter how long ago they had their pacemaker implanted, they should contact the pacemaker clinic as soon as the signs and symptoms of infection occur. This could be pain, swelling or discharge from the site. All too often an essentially superficial infection has been treated with several sets of antibiotics and becomes much more deepseated before contact with the pacemaker centre is made.

Erosion. This is often a problem that occurs some months after surgery and is more common in thin patients. The only course of action is to reposition the pulse generator more deeply. Care should be taken to check that the pocket is not infected and swabs should be taken and sent for microscopy.

Thrombosis. This may occur in the first few days following implant and usually after the patient has returned home. This should be suspected if patients contact the hospital complaining of a swollen arm or neck or if their hand and arm are looking blue or dusky (Li-Jen Lin et al 1998). Engorgement of the superficial veins of the upper limb, usually on the side of the pulse generator, may be seen. Treatment depends on which vessel is involved. Anticoagulation practices tend to vary.

Patient manipulation of the pacemaker ('twiddler's syndrome'). This can occur when the pacemaker pocket allows undue movement of the pacemaker casing. As today's devices become smaller the pocket from the previous pacemaker has extra room in it. The patient is able to turn it over and over again. This leads to twisting of the lead and fracture in some instances. Treatment involves fashioning a new pocket.

Allergic reaction. This is very uncommon.

CONCLUSION

This chapter has explored the altered physiology and indications for both temporary and permanent pacemaker devices. There is a clear requirement for any nurse involved in caring for patients with pacemakers to understand not only the type of device and settings but also how this should manifest on the ECG tracing. There is a need to understand the causes and consequences of pacemaker failure while the patient is within the unit and quickly and promptly address these should they occur. At worst, this may mean initiating advanced life support skills. The pacemaker will become an integral part of the patient's life so assessment of the patient's and carer's knowledge and subsequent education is of major importance. This will aim to primarily ensure that any complications or pacemaker malfunction are quickly and effectively managed. A planned and agreed teaching strategy, incorporated into an integrated care pathway (ICP) if these are used, will assist in standardizing both the information and the quality of care provided to each patient. Evaluation of the above measures is of importance.

REFERENCES

DaCosta A, Kirkorian G, Chucherat M et al 1998a Antibiotic prophylaxis for permanent pacemaker implantation: a meta analysis. Circulation 97(18): 1796–1801

DaCosta A, Lelievre H, Kirkorian G et al 1998b Role of the preaxilliary flora in pacemaker infection – a prospective study. Circulation 97(18): 1791–1795

Ellenbogen KA 1996 Cardiac pacing, 2nd edn. Blackwell Science, Cambridge, MA

Fananapazi L, Canno RO, Tripodi D, Panza JA 1992 Impact of dual chamber pacing in patients with OHCM with symptoms refractory to verapamil and beta-adrenergic blocker therapy. Circulation 85: 2149–2161

Fogoros RN 1995 Electrophysiologic testing, 2nd edn. Blackwell Science, Cambridge, MA

Gillis AM, Leitch JW, Sheldon RS et al 1993 A prospective randomized comparison of autodecremental pacing to burst pacing in device therapy for chronic ventricular tachycardia secondary to coronary artery disease. American Journal of Cardiology 72(15): 1146–1151

Guyton A, Hall J 1996 Textbook of medical physiology. WB Saunders, Philadelphia

Hampton JR 1998 The ECG in practice, 3rd edn. Churchill Livingstone, Edinburgh

James T 1968 A useful landmark for interpreting angiocardiograms. Radiology 75: 804

Jeffrey K, Parsonnet V 1998 Cardiac pacing 1960–1985. A quarter of a century of medical and industrial innovation. Circulation 97(19): 1978–1991

Jenkins RD, Gerred SJ 1997 ECGs by example. Churchill Livingstone, Edinburgh

Josephson ME, Almendral JM, Buxton AE 1987 Mechanisms of ventricular tachycardia. Circulation 75 (4 pt 2): 41–47

Kapoor WN, Smith MA, Miller NL 1994 Upright tilt testing in evaluating syncope: a comprehensive literature review. American Journal of Medicine 97(1): 78–88

Kay G 1996 Basic concepts of pacing. In: Ellenbogen K (ed) Cardiac pacing, 2nd edn. Blackwell Science, Cambridge, MA, pp. 37–123

Klug D, Lacroix D, Savoye C 1997 Systemic infection related to endocarditis on pacemaker leads: clinical presentation and management. Circulation 95(8): 2098–2107

Lang R, David B, Klien HO 1981 The use of the balloon tipped floating catheter in temporary transvenous cardiac pacing. PACE 4: 491–496

Lin L-J, Lin J-L, Wei-Chuan Tsai et al 1998 Venous access thrombosis detected by transcutaneous vascular ultrasound in patients with single polyurethane lead permanent pacemaker. PACE 21: 396–400

Mennim P, Coyle CF, Taylor JD 1992 Venous air embolism associated with removal of central venous catheter. British Journal of Medicine 301: 171–172

Opie LH 1998 The heart: physiology from cell to circulation. Lippincott-Raven, Philadelphia

Paul S, Hebra JD 1998 The nurse's guide to cardiac rhythm interpretation: implications for patient care. WB Saunders, Philadelphia

Wood M, Ellenbogen K 1996 Temporary cardiac pacing. In: Ellenbogen K (ed) Cardiac pacing, 2nd edn. Blackwell Science, Cambridge, MA

FURTHER READING

Berne M, Levy M 1981 Cardiovascular physiology. CV Mosby, St Louis

Berstein AD, Parsonnet V 1996 Pacing practices in the United States: the 1993 survey. PACE 19: 576

Haskell RJ, French WJ 1986 Optimum AV interval in dual chamber pacemakers. PACE 9: 670–675

Hickey J, Quimette R 1996 Advanced practice nursing: changing roles and clinical application. Lippincott, Philadelphia

Hildick-Smith DJ, Lowe MD, Newell SA et al 1998 Ventricular pacemaker upgrade: experience, complications and recommendations. Heart 79(4): 383–387

Kacet S, Lekieffre J 1997 Systemic infection related to endocarditis on pacemaker leads: clinical presentation and management. Circulation 95: 2098–2107

Schuppel R, Buchele G, Batz L, Koenig W 1998 Sex differences in selection of pacemakers: retrospective observational study. British Medical Journal 316(7143): 1492–1495

Tortora G, Brabowski S 1996 Principles of anatomy and physiology. HarperCollins, New York

22

Nursing management of the cardiac surgical patient

Sarah Fisher
Gill Walsh
Nigel Cross

Cardiac surgery is no longer the phenomenon it was some 30 years ago, when the first coronary artery bypass graft (CABG) surgery was performed. It has since become commonplace and cardiothoracic centres often work with an almost conveyor belt-like efficiency, reflecting how routine such surgical procedures have become. The increased demand and complexity of the surgical workload, coupled with technological innovation, have combined to reduce the inpatient stay to 5–6 days (Dunstan & Riddle 1997, Woodman 1999). This has increased the pressure for nurses to provide quality care in a stressful, dynamic environment. This chapter will discuss the preparation of patients for cardiac surgery, together with an exploration of the morbidity and mortality associated with the various techniques. Risk stratification will be explored in addition to an overview of the surgical techniques commonly used. Importantly, the principles of cardiopulmonary bypass (CPB) will be examined and how this may affect postoperative nursing care. The effects of this device have led to the emergence of minimally invasive procedures to facilitate cardiac surgery, without the use of bypass techniques.

The two most common cardiac surgical procedures performed in the United Kingdom (UK) are coronary artery bypass grafting and valve repair or replacement. The nursing care for both will be discussed in depth and where there are differences between them, these will be identified. Finally, the reader is encouraged to explore the more recent developments and future trends in cardiac surgery, as outlined in Chapter 29.

CORONARY ARTERY BYPASS GRAFTING (CABG)

CABG surgery utilizes a section of vein or artery to bypass a blockage in a native coronary vessel and is the most common cardiac surgical procedure carried out today. The amount of CABG surgery has increased steadily in the past 15 years and now over 28 000 operations are carried out each year in the United Kingdom (BHF 2000). This figure is set to increase due to the rising numbers of people with cardiovascular diseases, coupled with an ageing population.

The main indications for CABG surgery are to relieve the symptoms of angina pectoris and to augment left ventricular function by improving coronary blood flow. CABG is more effective than percutaneous transvenous coronary angioplasty (PTCA) in those with extensive, multivessel disease (NHSCRD 1997). CABG should also be performed for stenoses in the left main stem (the primary section of the left coronary artery, emerging from the aorta, before it undergoes any anatomical division), due to the high risk of extensive infarction associated with attempted angioplasty in this major vessel. An investigation into the clinical outcomes of PTCA versus CABG for patients with multivessel disease found that those who had been randomized to PTCA required more medication, had more clinically significant angina and required significantly more interventions after a year than those who had undergone surgical revascularization (CABRI 1995).

Mortality

CABG surgery is a palliative, not a curative intervention. It does not increase longevity, as the underlying disease process of atherosclerosis is still present. Mortality rates for this form of surgery have increased in the last 10 years, reflecting the increased severity of disease and the length of time waiting for the operation. The observed mortality in a British cohort of patients undergoing CABG was noted to be 3.7% (65 of 1774) (Bridgewater et al 1998). CABG has higher initial risks of myocardial infarction (MI) and death than medical treatment of angina. A retrospective analysis of patients who had undergone CABG in Scotland noted that 10 years after surgery, 26% had died from cardiac causes, whilst 40% of the survivors had developed angina or required further interventions for cardiac symptoms (Bathgate & Irving 1997). Paradoxically, increased survival is only found in a specific subgroup of patients with advanced coronary artery disease. The very severity of their disease suggests that they should have a very high surgical mortality but they are more likely to die if they are not operated on. Their annual mortality rate is 2% if treated medically and this is reduced by surgery.

Research has also suggested that there is an unequal access to revascularization services. Women and those of Asian origin have been noted as having lower referral rates for hospital investigations and are often referred later than men (Lear et al 1994, Petticrew et al 1993). Surgical revascularization rates are lower for those in deprived areas, despite the higher incidence of coronary heart disease (CHD) seen in those from lower socio-economic groups (Ben-Shlomo & Chaturvedi 1995). These groups have high rates of morbidity and mortality from CHD and such inequalities need to be taken into account in the provision of equitable, target-effective services.

VALVE SURGERY

Valve surgery involves either surgical repair to a native valve or, more commonly, replacement of a diseased valve with either a mechanical or tissue prosthesis. Between the beginning of 1986 and the end of 1997, a total of 58 195 patients in the UK underwent first-time valve replacement surgery (Edwards & Taylor 1999).

The decision to replace a valve should be based on clinical and echocardiography findings. Valve dysfunction itself can be related to:

- congenital defects, such as a congenital bicuspid valve; infection, for example rheumatic heart fever and infective endocarditis. This can cause scarring and fusing of valve leaflets
- mechanical problems due to chamber enlargement, for example mitral regurgitation seen in left ventricular (LV) dilatation
- CHD causing damage to papillary muscles
- valve calcification which may be seen in older patients
- a congenital condition such as the Marfan syndrome, causing dilatation of the aortic root which houses the aortic valve (see Chapter 17).

Surgical technique

Valve surgery requires the use of cardiopulmonary bypass. If the patient requires the replacement of one valve, the procedure is generally quicker than for CABG surgery. However, if more than one valve is replaced with additional requirement for CABG, then the procedure will inevitably be longer.

Mortality

The mortality rate for valve replacement tends to be higher than for CABG. In specific terms, in the UK the 30-day mortality fell from 6.9% in 1986 to 3.8% in 1995, increasing again to 6.7% in the 2 years to 1997 (Edwards & Taylor 1999). A number of factors contribute to this. As highlighted, valve surgery is more complex. It may involve multiple valve replacements and combined valve and CABG. The underlying left ventricular function is often poorer in valve disease, due to the long-term insidious progress of valvular disorders. Whilst such figures are not overly high, they do give cause for concern and efforts should be made to identify patients at increased risk and ensure they are prepared adequately for surgery and are haemodynamically optimized where appropriate (Rooney 1996). Actuarial survival at 1, 5 and 10 years in the UK was 89.5%, 78.5% and 61.8% respectively between 1986 and the end of 1997 (Edwards & Taylor 1999). It is important, however, to remember factors such as advancing age, particularly when considering the long-term survival figures.

The most common indication for valve replacement, notably in the elderly, is calcific aortic stenosis, which accounts for approximately 60–70% of valve surgery (Prêtre & Turina 2000). The majority of individuals with aortic calcification usually have moderate to good left ventricular function and normal coronary arteries. The postoperative mortality rate for this procedure is 5–10% for patients over 80 years and 2–3% for younger patients. If CABG is to be carried out in conjunction with valve replacement, then mortality rises to 15–20%, reflecting underlying impaired cardiac function. Long-term survival rates are 95% at 1 year following surgery and 70% at 5 years (Prêtre & Turina 2000). Interestingly, aortic valve insufficiency is rare in elderly patients and only represents between 3–5% of the valve surgery work (Prêtre & Turina 2000). It should be undertaken when the patient has echocardiographic signs of declining ventricular function or has an ascending aorta dilated to more than 6 cm diameter or has developed clinical symptoms. Chronic mitral valve insufficiency is also a common reason for valve surgery, accounting for 30–35% of the valvular surgery caseload (Prêtre & Turina 2000).

Valve repair may be carried out by resecting the prolapsing leaflets, with excellent clinical results, and should be considered in older patients who have improved long-term outcomes following valve repair, rather than with replacement. The survival rates 1 year after repair are 90% for such patients, compared to 80% for replacement. This figure reduces to 64% 3 years after surgery (Prêtre & Turina 2000). Treatment of mitral stenosis accounts for only 1% of valve surgery and has a higher mortality in older patients (Prêtre & Turina 2000). Valve repair generally refers to the mitral valve. Aortic valve repair, rather than replacement, is extremely rare in adults.

Valve replacement in infective endocarditis

In cases of infective endocarditis, valve replacement should not be undertaken until the patient has responded to antibiotic or antiviral therapy. Emergency valve replacement should only be considered if there is significant disruption to the valve apparatus, compromising the haemodynamic function, or when the infection is clearly resistant to medical therapy (Spyrou et al 1997). The presence of an aortic valve ring abscess is usually regarded as an indication for early aortic valve replacement, because it has been thought to be an independent marker of a poor long-term outcome, although this has recently been challenged (Danchin et al 1999).

Valve surgery in the Marfan syndrome

This will entail replacement of the aortic root and valve with a composite graft (prosthetic valve and Dacron aortic root graft) due to dilatation and the subsequent risk of rupture and death. The point at which this should be performed is controversial. Gott et al (1999) advise replacement before the diameter of the aortic root exceeds 5.5–6.0 cm. However, as Chapter 17 and indeed the British Heart Foundation clinical guide (Child & Briggs 2001) highlight, replacement recommendations can vary between diameters of 5, 5.5 and 6 cm, depending on the chosen author.

RISK STRATIFICATION FOR CARDIAC SURGERY

Attempts have been made to undertake risk stratification of patients to try and reduce surgery-related mortality. The very nature of such surgery puts cardiac patients into a high-risk group. In addition, the compromised cardiac function that such patients already exhibit causes them to be at a higher risk of complications and further morbidity.

The challenge for risk stratification is to develop an objective scoring system which can be applied to all individuals undergoing cardiac surgery, whatever type it may be. One study gathered data from 3500 cardiac surgical patients, identifying 14 risk factors that could be scored to categorize each individual patient's risk. Essentially this was the probability of mortality within 30 days of surgery (Parsonnet et al 1989). Each risk factor was weighted and added up to an individual patient's total score. This allowed the individual to be placed in one of five groups of increasing risk (see Box 22.1). This is known as the Parsonnet score (Parsonnet et al 1989).

Box 22.1 Parsonnet's additive model of risk stratification (after Parsonnet et al 1989, Poloniecki et al 1998)

Risk factor and assigned weighting (%)
- Female gender: 1
- Weight ≥1.5 times ideal: 3
- Diabetes: 3
- Hypertension (systolic >140 mmHg): 3

Ejection fraction
- >50%: 0
- 30–49%: 2
- <30%: 4

Age
- 70–74: 7
- 75–79: 12
- ≥80: 20

Redo operation
- First: 5
- Second: 10
- Left ventricular aneurysm: 5
- Emergency surgery due to complications of percutaneous transluminal coronary angioplasty (PTCA) or angiography: 10
- Dialysis dependent: 10
- Catastrophic state, e.g. cardiogenic shock: 30
- Heart transplantation: 15
- Congenital heart disease: 5

Valve surgery:
- Mitral (pulmonary artery systolic pressure <60 mmHg): 5
- Mitral (pulmonary artery systolic pressure ≥60 mmHg): 8
- Aortic (gradient ≤120 mmHg): 5
- Aortic (gradient >120 mmHg): 7
- Coronary artery bypass grafting (CABG) at time of valve surgery: 2

Factors that need to be taken into consideration in a scoring system include older patients, who tend to be sicker and have multivessel disease. They also often have co-existent valvular disease and other co-morbid conditions (Vaska 1997a). Women have been identified as less likely to undergo cardiac investigations than men (Petticrew et al 1993) and have worse mortality after surgery because they tend to be sicker than their male counterparts. They are also significantly older, have smaller coronary arteries, a higher incidence of restenosis and are more likely to have diabetes mellitus than men. The factors which have been shown to increase postoperative length of stay include mitral valve, chronic pulmonary and cerebrovascular disease and atrial fibrillation (Johnson & McMahan 1997, Rosen et al 1999). Therefore, whilst an older patient with impaired left ventricular (LV) function is at increased risk, the severity of that risk can be estimated by knowing the actual age and LV function.

Each patient can have their scores added and the total will place them in one of the following categories:

- good risk   0–4%
- fair risk   5–9%
- poor risk   10–14%
- high risk   15–19%
- extremely high risk ≥20%

(after Parsonnet et al 1989).

Whilst this model is useful for stratifying those at increased risk of surgical morbidity, LV ejection fraction appears to be a more sensitive predictor of long-term surgical outcomes. A 5-year clinical follow-up of surgical patients found that those who had poorer underlying LV function preoperatively were more likely to have activity limitation 5 years after surgery (Caine et al 1999). Another study found that those who had experienced poor LV function preoperatively did not survive the 10 years after surgery (Bathgate & Irving 1997). More recently, the EuroSCORE has been developed. This was based upon analysis of risk factors and mortality for 19 030 consecutive adult patients undergoing cardiac surgery with CPB across Europe (Roques et al 1999). Three groups of risk factors have subsequently been identified in patient-, cardiac- and operation-related categories (Nashef et al 1999).

Waiting for surgery

For many patients there is a period of waiting for surgery after they have been informed it is required. This period may be several weeks, but for the majority will be several months and is inevitably a time of great anxiety for both the patient and their loved ones. Some will be living with severe symptoms, which may become more limiting during the waiting period. This actual period of waiting has been identified as the most stressful part of the surgical experience for both patients and their partners (Lindsay et al 1997).

Patients require information about lifestyle changes and the surgery itself, whilst partners are concerned about their abilities to meet the patient's emotional and physical needs after discharge. Partners have also been found to have significantly higher anxiety scores during the pre-operative period (Lindsay et al 1997). An optimistic outlook has a positive effect on how individuals cope with illness. Such individuals are thought to use more active coping strategies to achieve positive outcomes (King et al 1998).

Many centres run pre-operative nurse-led clinics for prospective patients to try and address some of these anxieties. Such clinics usually invite the patient and their partner to attend 2–3 weeks before their surgery is scheduled. Lepczyk et al (1990) provided pre-operative education to 72 patients undergoing coronary artery bypass surgery, with no previous cardiac surgery. In two groups, education was provided as an outpatient 2–7 days before surgery or on the afternoon of admission. The timings were close and the first group's range of 2–7 days pre-surgery was wide. Yet it was noted that knowledge was retained to a far better degree in the pre-admission group, although anxiety was moderate in both groups at the start of teaching and did not alter significantly in either (Lepczyk et al 1990). Anxiety was defined as the individual's inability to specify the source of threat or the object that is threatened. As surgery is clearly the threat, the authors concluded that fear may have been a more appropriate variable to analyse. In terms of a cost-effective pragmatic approach, it would still seem logical to provide teaching as a larger pre-operative group than on a one-to-one basis just prior to surgery. In addition, techniques such as breathing exercises could be practised at home prior to admission. If information is given too close to the time of surgery, the patient may be too distracted and will not fully comprehend the information.

The content of such clinics has also traditionally focused on orientating the patient to the hospital environment and their likely progress. Patients are shown around the ward areas and will often have some of their baseline investigations performed. As highlighted, factors such as atrial fibrillation and pulmonary complications have been found to be common factors responsible for prolonging the postoperative hospital stay and identifying potential at-risk patients should be a core component of the pre-operative nursing assessment (Johnson & McMahan 1997). However, it is important to remember that while this may be a good use of such time from a clinical viewpoint, it may only serve to heighten patients' anxieties about their forthcoming surgery.

PHYSICAL PREPARATION OF THE PATIENT

Patients are usually admitted 24 hours before surgery and will be seen by various members of the multidisciplinary team, such as the recovery nurse, surgeon, anaesthetist and physiotherapist (see Box 22.2). Certain necessary investigations may have been incorporated into the pre-operative clinic, therefore in some areas the patient may be admitted on the day of surgery.

A number of medications may need to be stopped several days prior to surgery, to minimize counterproductive effects in the immediate postoperative period (Box 22.3). The patient will also need to be

---

Box 22.2 Guide to assessment to be performed on admission for cardiac surgery

- Nursing assessment/social history
  Does the patient live alone or have a carer or partner who will assist once they return home to convalesce?
  Are there any areas that could hinder discharge, i.e. lack of transport, compliance with treatment?
  Does the patient/carer have any questions/anxieties about their admission?
  Do they know what their surgery will involve?
  Do they want to know what their surgery will involve?

- Symptom/medical history
  What symptoms does the patient have?
  Do the symptoms limit their activity in any way?
  What are the patient's risk factors for cardiovascular disease?
  Does the patient have any other co-morbid conditions, i.e. diabetes mellitus, a pressure sore?
  What is their current medication?
  Do they understand and comply with medication?
  Are there any known allergies?
  What is the patient's Parsonnet score?

- Baseline clinical observations: ECG, height, weight, temperature, blood pressure, pulse

- The anaesthetist's assessment will assess the patient's fitness to undergo a general anaesthetic and identify any potential problems, i.e. chest deformities, cigarette/cigar/pipe-smoking history, presence of respiratory conditions

- Assessment and consenting by the surgical team or surgeon. The patient will be clerked and an assessment will ensure that they are fit for the surgery in question. The patient must be able to give an informed consent regarding surgery

- Physiotherapy assessment. The patient will be introduced to appropriate mobility and deep-breathing exercises for use postoperatively.

- Common baseline investigations: full blood count (FBC), erythrocyte sedimentation rate (ESR), blood group and crossmatching for possible perioperative and postoperative transfusion. This possibility should be discussed with the patient. Clotting screen (for those taking anticoagulation medications), urea and electrolytes, chest X-ray (to identify the heart size and any respiratory disease and to be used as a baseline for postoperative assessment), ECG, echocardiogram (used to assess certain valve patients)

---

informed that their medication will be changed postoperatively; for example, anti-anginal treatments may be discontinued postoperatively after CABG surgery, while the anticoagulant warfarin may be

---

Box 22.3 Medications stopped before cardiac surgery

- Digoxin: to reduce postoperative arrhythmias and potential bradycardias. The effects of digoxin may fluctuate with alteration in the patient's potassium levels that may occur postoperatively
- Diuretics: to reduce postoperative arrhythmias and to facilitate a more accurate control of postoperative fluid balance
- Aspirin: to reduce tendency for postoperative bleeding
- Long-acting β-blockers: to minimize postoperative bradycardia and reduced cardiac contractility
- Warfarin converted to heparin 2–3 days pre-operatively: to allow a more precise management of the coagulation studies and to enable more prompt reversal of heparin's anticoagulation effects if required

---

commenced after valve replacement with a mechanical prosthesis.

On the day of surgery the patient may be required to remove any chest and leg hair (the latter for CABG patients only, to allow removal of the required vein). This has traditionally been undertaken to reduce the possibility of postoperative infection but removal of chest hair with razors can actually break the skin and act as a portal for infection. If hair removal is required, a depilatory cream should be used or electric hair clippers, to avoid skin trauma. The patient may be asked to shower, using a surgical soap to remove surface commensals and reduce the risk of postoperative infection. He or she should have nothing orally (nil-by-mouth) for 4–6 hours pre-operatively to reduce the risk of pulmonary aspiration during anaesthesia. A premedication will be administered 1–2 hours before surgery. Premedications are usually sedatives with analgesic and amnesic qualities, such as lorazepam or papaveretum.

ANAESTHESIA

Induction

Once the patient is in the anaesthetic room, they will be attached to an electrocardiogram (ECG) monitor and pulse oximetry. It is vitally important to monitor the patient during induction to quickly identify any adverse reactions to the anaesthetic and invasive procedures. The patient will usually be given an anaesthetic induction agent to reduce discomfort and prevent inappropriate movement. At this point a number of intravenous cannulae will be inserted. These are generally as follows:

- peripheral cannulae: for administration of medications/fluids
- arterial cannula: radial artery (but can be femoral) for arterial blood pressure monitoring and to allow arterial blood gas samples to be taken
- central venous cannula: internal jugular, for right atrial/central venous pressure monitoring and fluid/medication administration.

The patient will then be intubated and mechanically ventilated. A self-retaining urinary catheter will also be inserted. Intravenous antibiotics such as benzylpenicillin or cefuroxime are administered as prophylaxis to infection at this point and continued for a short period postoperatively. A gas mix of oxygen and air is used to mechanically ventilate the patient, rather than nitrous oxide which is a cardiac depressant (Rooney 1996). In the operating theatre, the patient will be attached to ECG monitoring, with the need to assess the ST segment to identify depression which signifies ischaemia. This will be the familiar 3-lead system placed on the chest, rather than 12-lead monitoring, and offers the opportunity to view a variety of leads during surgery. It is important to note that ECG monitoring will remain in place continuously until the patient is handed to the recovery or intensive care nursing staff, who will attach the patient to their own equipment. If a new monitor is required at any point, the rhythm remains monitored until the leads of the new equipment are attached and ready for use.

Both the arterial blood pressure and right atrial (central venous) filling pressure will be transduced for constant monitoring throughout surgery. Temperature probes will be placed in the nasopharynx to approximate the core temperature and a peripheral probe may be placed on the foot. If the patient's right heart dynamics are affected by a condition that will not accurately reflect their left heart function, such as with valvular disease, a pulmonary artery (PA) flotation catheter or direct left atrial line may be used instead (see Chapter 5).

Maintenance

Maintenance of anaesthesia will be achieved with intravenous opioids such as fentanyl and a benzodiazepine and inhaled volatile agents, for example isoflurane. Volatile agents can be titrated more effectively than intravenous opioids to maintain anaesthesia and control factors such as hypertension (Staples & Ramsay 1997). Fentanyl replaced morphine as the opioid of choice in cardiac surgery in the 1970s. Use of high-dose fentanyl (50–100 µg/kg/h) can delay extubation, whilst lower doses (5–10 µg/kg/h) allow extubation to occur within 1–2 hours of surgery. However, alfentanil is an alternative drug of choice.

Propofol is another commonly used intravenous anaesthetic agent (Covington 1998). It is short-acting and its mild myocardial depressant and vasodilator actions are well tolerated. Its hypotensive effects are avoided if it is given as an infusion. Propofol is now also commonly used postoperatively as a sedative until the patient is ready for extubation. The advantage is that its metabolism is rapid and extensive and awakening usually occurs some 10–20 minutes after the infusion has been discontinued (Covington 1998).

THE ROLE AND EFFECTS OF CARDIOPULMONARY BYPASS

William Harvey first described the circulation of blood in 1628 but it was to be another 250 years before the concept of circulatory support would have any influence on the treatment of cardiovascular disease. In 1812 Le Gallios wrote: 'If one could substitute for the heart a kind of injection of arterial blood, either naturally or artificially made, one would succeed easily in maintaining alive indefinitely any part of the body whatsoever' (cited by Westaby 2000, p. 2151). This potential, though somewhat gruesome, was demonstrated in 1850 by Brown Sequard who successfully perfused the head of a decapitated dog for 15 minutes by injecting oxygenated blood into the right and left common carotid and vertebral arteries. It was to be another 49 years before defibrillation was first demonstrated by Provost and Batelli on an animal and a further 48 years before it was successfully demonstrated on a human patient, in 1947. Defibrillation is commonly an integral part of the heart's 'recovery' phase on rewarming and weaning from bypass. The potential for perfusion was clearly a significant innovation but was useless without the facility to restore a life-supporting rhythm.

There are few reports of cardiovascular operations before 1900. Weil and Delorme proposed the removal of scar tissue from around the heart as a treatment for constrictive pericarditis as early as 1890 but this relatively simple procedure was not clinically demonstrated until 1920 (Westaby 2000). In 1925 Sir Henry Souttar described the relief of rheumatic mitral stenosis by introducing a finger through the left atrial appendage to widen the opening. The 19-year-old patient survived and had good relief of symptoms. Similar procedures undertaken to relieve aortic stenosis did not fare so well. Souttar wrote: 'The problem is to a large extent mechanical and as such should already be within the scope of surgery … In view of the extreme danger to the brain from even the shortest interruption to its blood supply, any manipulations which are carried out must therefore be executed in the full flow of the bloodstream and they must therefore not perceptively interfere with the contractions of the heart'.

The ingenuity of such pioneers as Blalock, Taussig, Brock and Tubbs pushed back the boundaries of cardiac surgery as we have come to know it. By 1948 Holmes Sellors and then Brock had performed a pulmonary valvotomy for stenosis using a transventricular approach (Westaby 2000). Subsequently a number of 'blind' procedures were developed in an attempt to close atrial and ventricular septal defects. As these procedures increased in their complexity, so did the obvious need for such repairs and modifications to be made under direct vision.

The aim was to facilitate intracardiac surgery under direct vision on a heart which was not required to support the patient's circulation. There were three significant techniques which became the forerunners to cardiopulmonary bypass (CPB) as we know it today. Bigelow demonstrated the principles of moderate hypothermia and temporary circulatory arrest in 1950. Systemic topical cooling of the body to 32°C in conjunction with venous outflow occlusion by temporarily clamping the superior and inferior vena cavae gave the surgeon 8–10 minutes in which to close an atrial or ventricular septal defect before irreversible brain damage occurred (Westaby 2000). The first clinical success employing this principle was described by Lewis in 1952.

It is now universally accepted that the single most important development in cardiac surgery has been the application and refinement of extracorporeal cardiopulmonary bypass. It was first used in 1953, on an 18-year-old woman for repair of an atrial septal defect (Westaby 2000). It has dramatically improved the ability to provide definitive surgical interventions for a host of cardiac defects.

Further surgical milestones were reached with the advent of cardioplegia (from the Latin meaning 'still heart'). For the first time, prolonged interruption of normal circulation but with protection of the myocardial muscle ('myocardial protection') became possible. This provided a decompressed, non-contracting and bloodless field in which to operate. Cardiopulmonary bypass is an incredibly sophisticated form of life support. It temporarily performs the functions of the heart (circulation of the blood) and the lungs (gas exchange) during open heart surgery. During CPB, the patient's condition on the heart–lung bypass machine or 'pump' is controlled and maintained by a highly trained perfusionist. In collaboration with the anaesthetist and surgeon, the perfusionist monitors the patient's haemodynamic and metabolic parameters, making adjustments accordingly. Naturally, vigilance and training are of paramount importance as the 'pump' provides total cardiopulmonary support for the patient. Should a malfunction or complication occur, the result could be catastrophic.

CPB is also known as an extracorporeal circulation because, via a number of silicone cannulae, blood is drained from the venous system into the heart–lung circuit outside the patient's body. As blood is pumped through the circuit it is oxygenated, has drugs and anaesthetic agents added and is warmed or cooled according to requirements. It is then filtered to remove any impurities and microscopic air bubbles before being transfused, via an arterial pump, back into the patient's circulation via the aorta (Fig. 22.1).

Circuit design

Advances in materials and design have allowed the CPB circuit to be safe and flexible enough to meet individual patient requirements. The development of disposable oxygenators in the late 1960s allowed perfusion to become practical and economically viable. These bubble oxygenators, whilst effective at the time, have been superseded by membrane oxygenators that allow for increased safety, less blood trauma and better control of blood gas exchange. The circuit itself consists of several components which can be combined in an integrated unit or mounted individually on the heart–lung machine and connected by tubing.

Venous reservoir

Due to the difference in height between the patient and the venous reservoir, venous blood will siphon out of the patient, via a length of PVC tubing into the entry port of the venous reservoir. As its name suggests, the venous reservoir acts as a storage area for blood draining from the heart before it is pumped from the reservoir into the oxygenator. The level of blood in the reservoir will give a good indication of the rate of drainage and of the patient's fluid volume needs. Some form of level detection will also be placed on the reservoir, which, when connected to the safety systems of the heart–lung machine, will either slow down or stop the pump, thus preventing air from being entrained into the circuit.

The reservoir also has two separate filtration systems built into it. One, for the venous blood, commonly has a pore size of 100 microns (red blood cells are about 7 microns). This will filter out any air, which

can be entrained down the venous line, and any debris such as blood clots or tissue. The other filtering system, which has a separate fluid pathway from that of the venous blood, is designed to filter the blood returning from the low-pressure cardiotomy suction. This will be of a much lower volume but will have a higher debris content. The pore size of this filter is about 25 microns. Once this blood has been filtered, it will be allowed to return to the venous blood in the main storage area of the reservoir.

The blood pump

The heart provides the energy required to push blood around the systemic and pulmonary circulation. Whilst on CPB this energy requirement is provided by the pump. In most instances this will be in the form of a roller pump.

A length of silicon tubing is squeezed between two rollers, adjusted so that they are just occlusive. The revolutions per minute of the pump will be directly proportional to the flow of blood. This type of pump is unfortunately also one of the main sources of trauma to the red cells, especially if set to be overocclusive. The squeezing effect of the rollers has a crushing effect, whilst the constant flexing of the tubing produces silicon debris which is carried away with the blood.

Another form of pump which is less commonly used is the non-occlusive or constrained vortex pump. In this type, centrifugal energy is imparted to the blood by the use of rapidly spinning cones or a small vaned turbine. These pumps are much less traumatic to the blood but are more expensive and therefore used mainly for longterm support such as extracorporeal membrane oxygenation (ECMO) or LV assist devices (LVAD). Whichever pump is used, it will be placed between the venous reservoir and the oxygenator and will be controlled by the safety systems on the heart–lung machine such as level and air detection devices.

Oxygenators

Whilst on CPB, blood is diverted away from the lungs and their function as a gas exchange device will be taken over by the oxygenator. It is designed to oxygenate the blood, remove carbon dioxide and control the temperature of the blood. The most common type of oxygenator in use today is the hollow fibre oxygenator. It is designed so that a large number of very fine, hollow fibres are bundled together and the total surface area available for gas transfer will be between 1.6 and 2 square metres (adult). The blood and gas

arterial line filter

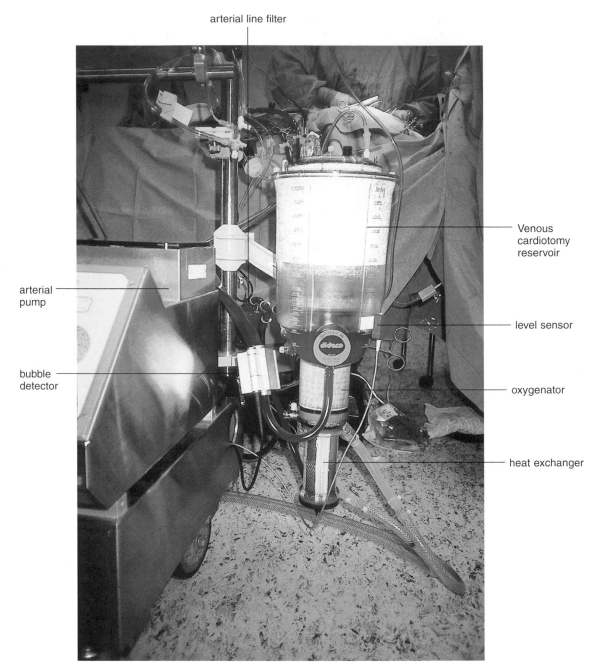

Venous
cardiotomy
reservoir

arterial
pump

level sensor

bubble
detector

oxygenator

heat exchanger

Figure 22.1 The cardiopulmonary bypass circuit.

follow two totally independent pathways, the gas flowing through the centre of the fibres and the blood passing over the outside. The fibres are permeable to oxygen and carbon dioxide.

Gas transfer occurs due to the concentration gradients that exist across the membrane. Blood entering the oxygenator (venous) is low in oxygen and high in carbon dioxide, while the gas is high in oxygen and carries no carbon dioxide. Oxygen therefore moves down the concentration gradient from the gas to the blood, whilst carbon dioxide moves in the opposite direction.

Oxygenation is controlled simply by altering the oxygen concentration of the gas going into the oxygenator (FiO_2) and carbon dioxide levels are controlled by altering the gas flow. A high gas flow will 'blow off' more carbon dioxide, whilst a low gas flow increases the retention of carbon dioxide in the body. Integral to the oxygenator is the heat exchanger, usually made of stainless steel, aluminum or polypropylene. The blood and water are completely separated from each other by this material. By accurately controlling the temperature of the water and blood, the patient temperature can be regulated.

Anticoagulation

The internal surface area of the CPB circuit will vary depending on the components used but in an adult circuit, will amount to approximately 1.5–2.5 square metres. The hollow fibres in the oxygenator will make up the majority of this area. Circulating blood will see this as a foreign surface and will initiate the clotting mechanism. This occurs via two pathways: the intrinsic, which is initiated by contact with foreign surfaces, and the extrinsic, which relies on tissue injury. These both combine with factor X to form the common pathway. In the common pathway the presence of prothrombinase and Ca^{2+} allows the conversion of prothrombin to thrombin. This in turn converts to fibrin, which, by trapping the circulating platelets, forms a clot.

The formation of clots during CPB is a potentially disastrous state and must be prevented. Heparin, which is extracted from animal lung tissue and intestinal mucosa, acts by combining with antithrombin III, increasing its effectiveness in the prevention of thrombin formation. Heparin dosage is calculated such that the activated clotting time (ACT) on bypass is at least four times the baseline value (which is normally 90–120 seconds). This dosage is usually between 2.5 and 3.5 mg/kg.

The heparin is administered just prior to cannulation and a sample is drawn to measure the ACT to verify adequate heparinization. Once the ACT is greater than 450 seconds, it is safe to commence bypass. ACTs are measured at regular intervals throughout the bypass to monitor the anticoagulation status. This is important as heparin is consumed during bypass and inadequate heparin levels can lead to the consumption of clotting factors at a subclinical level. This can in turn lead to an increase in postoperative blood loss. Other factors that alter the clotting time and need to be taken into consideration are temperature and the dilution of the blood by the fluid used to prime the circuit (pump prime).

Activated clotting times are also prolonged by aprotinin (Trasylol). Trasylol is an inhibitor of proteolytic enzymes and has been shown to have an important role in the protection of clotting mechanisms. Significant reductions in postoperative blood loss have been shown when Trasylol has been used (Bidstrup et al 1993). It is therefore indicated for patients at high risk of major blood loss during and following cardiac surgery.

Following the termination of CPB and once all surgical bleeding has been controlled, the aortic cannula is removed and the heparin is reversed with intravenous protamine. The precise mechanism of this antidote to heparin is not yet fully understood. However, 1 mg of protamine will reverse 80–100 units of heparin. Once again, an ACT is measured to confirm that clotting times have returned to normal pre-operative values. The accurate control of anticoagulation will play an important part in postoperative recovery, the length of time spent in the intensive care unit and the amount of blood products used. The reduction in both platelet count and activity that is associated with CPB can also lead to clotting problems, as can aspirin if it has been taken for a prolonged period pre-operatively. Protamine, which is obtained from salmon sperm, can also induce adverse reactions which may include hypotension, bradycardia and circulatory collapse. The incidence of these is reduced if protamine is administered slowly (Bell & Diffee 1991).

Myocardial preservation

One of the main requirements during open heart surgery is for a still, bloodless heart, hence the need for CPB. To prevent the flow of blood into the heart via the coronary arteries, a clamp is placed across the aorta between the heart and the aortic cannula, carrying blood back into the systemic circulation from the heart–lung machine. This is obviously only possible once full bypass has been established. It is of the utmost importance that the myocardium is protected from ischaemia during this period and several methods of myocardial preservation can be employed.

Crossclamp and fibrillation

This technique is only suitable for coronary artery grafting because it relies on short periods of ischaemia whilst the distal anastomosis of the vessel being grafted is carried out. The heart is then reperfused whilst the proximal anastomosis is attached to the aorta. The heart is protected during these short periods whilst the crossclamp is in place (no coronary flow) by several factors. The time period is relatively short at 6–15 minutes and if it is found that the anastomosis will take longer than anticipated, the heart can be reperfused briefly. The reduction in body temperature usually employed whilst on bypass, generally to about 32°C, offers protection to the heart by reducing myocardial oxygen demand.

The heart is electively put into ventricular fibrillation (VF) by using a low-voltage alternating current and this also has the effect of reducing myocardial oxygen demands. Once the anastomosis has been completed the crossclamp is removed and the heart restarted with a direct current (DC) shock via the internal defibrillator paddles. The heart can recover whilst the proximal anastomosis takes place and the process can then be repeated, depending on the number of grafts being placed.

Cardioplegia

There are many different ways of delivering and many different types of cardioplegic solutions. A few of the more common ones are listed here. Cardioplegia solutions offer myocardial preservation by using high doses of potassium to prevent the cardiac impulse from commencing, thus putting the heart into electromechanical arrest. The potassium levels required to achieve this are typically 15–30 mmol/l. The cardioplegia is then infused, under pressure, directly into the aorta, once it has been crossclamped. This can be via either a large-bore needle or, if the aorta is being opened, directly into the left and right coronary ostia. Whatever technique is used to deliver the cardioplegia, a repeat dosage may be given at appropriate intervals, thus maintaining myocardial protection.

Cold crystalloid cardioplegia

This can be made by adding one ampoule of cardioplegic infusion, such as St Thomas's cardioplegia (magnesium chloride 16 mmol, potassium chloride 16 mmol and procaine hydrochloride 1 mmol) to 1 litre of cold (4°C) Ringer's solution. The high potassium levels combined with the low temperatures will bring on rapid ventricular standstill. Using this technique, the myocardial oxygen consumption is reduced to such low levels that the heart is protected for about 60 minutes.

Cold blood cardioplegia

Whilst cold crystalloid cardioplegia is a simple technique, it has the disadvantage of not supplying any form of energy to the myocardium. Mixing blood with the cardioplegic solution (usually in the ratio of 4:1 or 1:1 blood to cardioplegia) has the advantage of using the blood as an energy scource. The technique is more complicated as it involves the use of a pump which takes oxygenated blood from the oxygenator and mixes it with cardioplegic solution, before passing it through a heat exchanger. The ratio of blood to cardioplegia is also governed by the size of the tubing. The temperature can be controlled independently by adjusting the water temperature passing through the heat exchanger and this would typically be in the range of 6–10°C. As well as arresting the heart with high levels of potassium, energy stores in the myocardium are replenished by the blood substrate. Repeat dosages can be given accurately due to the use of a pump.

Cardiopulmonary bypass and the links to nursing care

The inflammatory response to CPB

The exposure of blood to a large, foreign surface area and the mechanical shear forces generated by the pumps, tubing, oxygenators and cannulae present a gross insult to the body's immune and inflammatory response systems. Recently, improvements in the design of oxygenators, pumps and arterial filters and the use of biocompatible materials have led to a reduction in inflammatory responses, but it is still an important factor that needs to be taken into consideration when nursing a post-bypass patient.

Pulmonary effects

Lung damage is possibly the most commonly seen postoperative complication of CPB. Bypassing the flow of blood through the lungs in itself produces very abnormal physiological conditions. Activation of the complement anaphylatoxins C3a and C5a will lead to the activation of leucocytes. The release of oxygen free radicals and proteolytic enzymes caused by this will in turn increase vascular permeability.

This increase in capillary leakage, along with changes in the oncotic pressure of the blood caused by the haemodilution associated with CPB, can lead to intra-alveolar and interstitial oedema (the 'pump lung' syndrome). During the period of CPB the lungs will be deflated and this can lead to atelectasis (collapse of the lung, the alveolar walls sticking together). This will not be helped by conditions such as chronic bronchitis, obesity or pulmonary oedema. The perfusionist can try to reduce these effects by using pump-priming solutions that have a high oncotic value such as Gelofusine or HAES-steril. Thus, the mean oncotic pressure whilst going on to bypass does not change dramatically. The lungs are very effective as filters and will trap any particulate debris produced by the pump. The use of arterial line filters is designed to remove both this debris and the activated leucocytes.

Haemotological effects

Exposure of the blood to foreign surfaces and the dilution caused by the priming solutions all have an adverse effect on the blood. Blood components are damaged due to shear stresses from the CPB pump. Common complications include:

- a reduced haematocrit (HCT) – the amount of packed red cells in the total blood volume, sometimes known as the packed cell volume (PCV) – and haemoglobin levels
- decreased leucocyte and platelet counts
- plasma protein denaturation (creating a structural change).

These changes manifest themselves in the postoperative phase by:

- reduced phagocytic activity
- a low platelet count, until approximately 3 days postoperatively
- anaemia, which can take several weeks to correct.

Haemostasis is also disrupted due to the anticoagulation required to achieve successful bypass. As highlighted, this is reversed at the end of CPB with protamine sulphate (in a ratio of 1.3 mg:1 mg heparin). This binds with the heparin to neutralize its anticoagulant effect (Salipante 1998). However, rewarming can lead to a release of heparin which was previously sequestered in the tissues and this heparin rebound is a common cause of postoperative bleeding (Cooley 1995). The dose of protamine will vary depending on the patient's body mass and the patient will need to be observed by nursing staff for signs of an anaphylactic reaction to this drug, such as a profound blood pressure drop (Bell & Diffee 1991). If hypothermia has been used for cardioprotection, this will decrease platelet function and will also reduce the efficacy of protamine, which is most effective in normothermic patients (Earp & Mallia 1997).

Inevitably, changes in and the reduction of clotting factors, coupled with inaccurate control of anticoagulation, can lead to postoperative bleeding. This may require the use of large quantities of blood products or a return to theatre for further exploration to stem any bleeding points. In addition, the reduction in platelet count and activity associated with bypass may necessitate the postoperative administration of pooled platelets.

Neurological effects

Neurological sequelae to bypass are not uncommon and are well documented (Carrascal et al 1999, Hogue et al 1999, Lindsay 1999). A 50-year-old man has a 0.7% chance of suffering a cerebrovascular accident (CVA/stroke) during bypass (Glenville 1999). In the older population, Akins et al (1997) reviewed the effects of cardiac operations in patients aged 80 years or more over a 10-year period. Clearly CVA was of major concern, with a figure of 7.9% for those undergoing CABG surgery and 10.8% for aortic valve replacement (Akins et al 1997). Hogue et al (1999) examined data for 2972 CABG and valve surgery patients. The CVAs experienced were divided into early onset, when detected immediately after surgery, and 'delayed' if occurring after an initially uneventful neurological recovery. The patients were all 65 years and older; 1.6% suffered a CVA, with 65% of these being delayed.

It is important for a neurological examination to be performed following cardiac surgery. This will initially be by the intensive care unit (ICU) or recovery nurse, who will ask the waking patient to move all four limbs and squeeze their hand. Alternatively, the patient may be asked to follow a simple command such as opening their eyes or sticking out their tongue. Moving all four limbs does, however, show whether there are any residual weaknesses. The pupils are also examined for appropriate and equal size and reaction to light. Any concerns at this point are reported and usually monitored, with a more formal neurological assessment requested by the surgical or anaesthetic team if deficits such as limb weakness, a lack of orientation to time and place or unconsciousness remain after the first 24–48 hours, when sedation has been discontinued.

Risk factors for neurological sequelae include (after Ommen et al 1997):

- a history of neurological deficit
- a history of cardiac failure
- mitral regurgitation
- carotid artery bruits
- postoperative atrial arrhythmias.

Whilst in many cases neurological changes are subtle and not lasting in their effect, a small percentage of patients will present with more serious, longer lasting damage. This is usually embolic in origin. Any embolus caught in the brain, such as air, clot, atheroma or calcific debris, will produce local areas of ischaemia. The most common source of emboli is cannulation of the aorta and its repeated crossclamping. Prevention of these events by the perfusionist will involve the application of many techniques. These can include arterial filtration, careful control of temperature gradients within the system to prevent gases coming out of solution and careful selection of the appropriate equipment. Prevention of low flow rates and hypotension along with close control of blood gases will also protect the patient. It is also of prime importance that the surgeons are especially careful to remove surgical air from the heart before removing the aortic crossclamp.

In examining the risk factors as predictors of CVA, a prior neurological event, aortic atherosclerosis and the duration of CPB were independently associated with early neurological events (Hogue et al 1999). Delayed CVAs have been associated with diabetes, aortic atherosclerosis and the combination of low cardiac output and atrial fibrillation. In Hogue et al's study, female patients had a 6.9-fold increase in the risk of early CVA and a 1.7% increased risk of delayed CVA (Hogue et al 1999).

Post-pump delirium (PPD) or psychosis

Generally, altered neurological function is not uncommon postoperatively, but this may be more subtle, such as memory loss and mild personality changes (Glenville 1999). Presentation can, however, be more severe, from disorientation through to overt psychosis. This tends to be termed 'post-pump delirium' (Tucker 1993). The exact cause remains unclear but research has again correlated certain factors such as increasing age, type of operation and notably valve surgery, where emboli can be introduced into the circulation. There is a general recognition that the risk of neurological complications rises sharply with CPB times in excess of 3 hours.

PPD covers a range of symptoms from feelings of apathy to severe clinical psychosis requiring psychiatric intervention. It can be life threatening if the patient tries to remove intravenous lines or chest drains or extubate themselves, which many do. Incidence is noted as wide, varying from 11% to 57% of those undergoing CPB (Adams 1991), while prevalence is constant at 32% (Segatore et al 1998). However, despite its prevalence it can often be underdiagnosed.

The actual aetiology of PPD is unclear (see Box 22.4) but the hallmarks are abnormalities of attention, short-term memory deficits and inability to integrate and respond to incoming sensory stimulation (Segatore et al 1998). The care environment can also lead to development of PPD; ITUs are traditionally noisy environments, full of alien sounds and it can be difficult to differentiate between night and day and the semiconscious patient is easily disorientated. The typical post-operative care area is far from relaxing and can often contribute to the PPD. The constant sounds of equipment and staff and lack of obvious day/night cycles, coupled with use of sedatives and the patient's immobilized state will all lead to some degree of sensory disturbance. This can be minimized by talking to the patient by name and using touch where appropriate to communicate and grouping together activities so that the patient gets some rest. If the patient has any hearing aids or glasses these should be used to improve their sensory input.

It is vital that any delusions expressed by the patient are not reinforced by staff as this can prolong the deluded state. Sleep deprivation can also lead to PPD. Sleep patterns are influenced more by the actual recovery from surgery than the hospital environment, with those patients who sleep during the day having poorer quality night-time sleep (Knapp-Spooner & Yarcheski 1992), which could predispose to their developing symptoms of PPD.

It is important that PPD is diagnosed quickly and that any causative factors, such as infection, are identified and treated, and supportive measures should be instigated to protect the affected patient. Fifty percent of affected individuals will have either a metabolic or structural cause (Segatore et al 1998), although for the remainder it may be idiopathic. The clinical course is variable; PPD often emerges within 48 hours of surgery and may last between 2 and 5 days, resolving fairly rapidly within days or a few weeks, depending on the causal factor (Tucker 1993). Chemical sedatives such as haloperidol, propofol or diazepam may be required, along with measures to try and orientate the patient to time and place. It must be remembered that some patients will be extremely agitated and may become aggressive or violent and sedation and restraint will be necessary to protect them, other patients and staff.

Renal effects

There is a significant decrease in renal blood flow at the commencement of CPB, but urine output increases with the duration of bypass. Excretion of large volumes of dilute urine is seen in the first several hours after surgery, as the body attempts to correct the excess fluid needed to maintain the extracorporeal circuit. Patients will require close monitoring and intravenous supplementation of their potassium levels due to this profound diuresis. In those with pre-existing renal impairment, the insult of CPB can cause the development of acute renal failure (ARF) (Glenville 1999). The incidence of ARF requiring dialysis is relatively low, but still accounts for 1.5% of patients undergoing cardiac

> **Box 22.4** Factors that influence the development of post-pump delirium (PPD)
>
> *Pre-operative*
> - Increasing age of patient – most powerful predictor of PPD
> - Poor pre-operative cardiac status – if the patient has a low cardiac output then there may be an underlying poor cerebral perfusion
> - Co-morbidity
> - Hypoxia and sepsis
>
> *Surgery*
> - Poor postoperative cardiac status
> - Valvular surgery – greater risk from micro-emboli from valve lesions
> - Duration of time on CPB circuit – risk increases sharply when bypass time exceeds 2–3 hours
>
> *Postoperative*
> - Lack of normal sensory/tactile stimulation
> - Loss of sleep–wake cycles
> - Unfamiliar noises and surroundings
> - Loudness of surroundings
> - Anxiety
> - Infection
> - Medication
> - Sleep deprivation

surgery with CPB (Conlon et al 1999). The main problem of renal failure requiring dialysis is that it does increase mortality. Conlon et al (1999) analysed data for 2843 consecutive patients undergoing cardiac surgery with CPB. In the 2672 who underwent CABG, 0.7% developed renal failure that required some form of dialysis. The mortality in this group was 28%. The variables independently associated with dialysable renal failure included an elevated pre-operative creatinine level, the duration of CPB, the presence of diabetes, reduced cardiac ejection fraction and increased age.

Weaning from CPB

The weaning process from CPB commences once the patient has reached a normal temperature and when all anastomoses are completed and not bleeding. The desired temperature is generally 38°C via the nasopharyngeal probe. If the patient is to be fast tracked (see Chapter 29) the temperature may be taken to a slightly higher level than usual to reduce events such as shivering on return to the recovery/ICU area. Rewarming of the patient is accomplished slowly to allow the body to adjust to the increased metabolic rate accompanying the temperature rise. Spontaneous defibrillation of the heart can be facilitated by circulation of warm blood (Bell & Diffee 1991), although internal defibrillation may be required. Box 22.6 provides the general parameters for weaning from CPB.

Problems with weaning from CPB

CPB usually causes a reduction in cardiac contractility, manifested by a reduced cardiac output. This progresses during the postoperative period, reaching a nadir at 6 hours, will usually resolve within 24 hours (Staples & Ramsay 1997) and is more common in those with pre-existing poor LV function. Inotropes, such as intravenous dobutamine or adrenaline (epinephrine), or an assist device, such as the intra-aortic balloon pump (IABP, see Chapter 5), may be required if the patient cannot be weaned successfully.

The phenomenon of 'myocardial stunning' (see Box 22.7) occurs in 10% of post-CPB cases and is identified by decreased LV ejection fraction. It is more common in women over 70 and those undergoing urgent CABG surgery (Walton & Westrope 1996).

Low output states may be related to reperfusion injury after temporary ischaemia, as a consequence of inadequate myocardial protection during surgery. There is no predetermined point at which irreversible damage takes place but it will occur in the subendocardial cells, which are more sensitive to hypoxia, before the epicardial cells. It will also occur more quickly in hypertrophied or ischaemic hearts, due to the imbalance between myocardial oxygen supply and demand. It has been estimated that safe ischaemic time in surgery is in the region of 20 minutes (Brzozowski 1995). The potential for minimising myocardial injury during surgery is enhanced by the use of warm blood cardioplegia. This facilitates a more frequent early return to sinus rhythm after aortic crossclamping and a decrease in the amount of creatine kinase (CK) production, indicating reduced cell damage (Brzozowski 1995).

SURGICAL TECHNIQUES
Coronary artery bypass grafting

Both venous conduits and, more recently, arterial conduits are used for coronary artery bypass surgery (see Box 22.8). Direct aortocoronary artery bypass grafting commenced in 1967 with reversed saphenous vein grafts, which became an increasingly popular method due to the ease of anastomosis. Not all patients will have suitable veins, for example if they have varicosity. In this situation alternative conduits will be used such as cephalic or even synthetic veins. Due to an ageing population and more repeat ('redo') procedures, there remains an interest in finding alternative conduits to the saphenous veins and internal mammary arteries most commonly used in the UK. One possibility is to use the radial artery as an alternative conduit (Wolff et al 1997).

Box 22.5 A summary of the physiological effects of cardiopulmonary bypass (CPB)

Effects	Causes	Effects	Causes
Pulmonary		*Haematological*	
Atelectasis	lungs deflated on CPB	Haemolysis	erythrocyte damage
Pump lung	alterations in blood flow altered capillary permeability reduced colloid osmotic pressure	Low haemoglobin	haemodilution erythrocyte damage
		Coagulopathy/bleeding	inadequate heparin reversal
Cardiovascular			protein denaturation – consumption of clotting factors
Labile blood pressure:			
hypotension	hypovolaemia 3rd spacing bleeding reduced myocardial contractility		platelet damage
		Fluid imbalance	
		Volume depletion	fluid shifts to interstitium due to:
hypertension	raised systemic vascular resistance (SVR) due to hypothermia, increased catecholamines		low colloid osmotic pressure increased vascular permeability release of vasoactive substances
Depressed myocardial contractility: myocardial infarction (MI) myocardial stunning			haemodilution vasodilation (rewarming) blood loss diuresis
arrhythmias	inadequate myocardial protection acid–base imbalance electrolyte imbalance hypothermia handling of heart	*Urea and electrolyte (U&E) imbalance* Hyperglycaemia	haemodilution increased circulating catecholamines insulin secretion reduced alteration in glucose transport
Neurological			
Behavioural changes	embolisation, prolonged CPB time	Hypokalaemia	profound diuresis
cerebrovascular accident (CVA/stroke)	inadequate perfusion embolisation	Renal dysfunction	damage to erythrocytes

Surgery involves suturing the proximal end of a graft onto the ascending aorta. The distal end is then attached to the diseased vessel, distal to the occlusion or stenosis (Fig. 22.2). Arterial grafts are now becoming more common, as they are more resistant to atherosclerosis compared to venous grafts (Wolff et al 1997). They may respond to the demands on the coronary arterial circulation better than vein grafts, as they are naturally part of a high-pressure system. As arterial grafting offers better long-term revascularization than venous grafting and confers better myocardial protection, this may ultimately lead to a reduction in the amount of re-operations for occluded grafts. Graft occlusion occurs within a year of surgery in 15–20% of saphenous vein grafts and 10% of IMA grafts (Vaca et al 1997).

Box 22.6 Parameters for weaning from CPB

- Narrow complex QRS/stable rhythm
- Ventricles pink and showing uniform contraction
- Systolic blood pressure >80–100 mmHg
- Adequate filling pressures:
  Central venous pressure (CVP):   5–10 mmHg
  Pulmonary artery (PA) diastolic: 5–15 mmHg

Box 22.7 Signs of myocardial stunning (Walton & Westrope 1996)

- Significantly increased heart rate and low blood pressure
- Transient Q-waves
- Ventricular arrhythmias, i.e. ventricular fibrillation and tachycardia, idioventricular rhythms and ectopics
- Tachypnoea
- Decreased arterial oxygen saturations
- Sweating

Box 22.8   Vessels used in coronary artery bypass surgery

Venous
Saphenous
Cephalic (very rare)
Umbilical (very rare)

Arterial
Internal mammary arteries (IMAs) (aka internal thoracic arteries)
Gastro-epiploic
Inferior epigastric
Radial (increasing use)

Synthetic
e.g. Gortex (rare)

Box 22.9   Patency rates for grafts (*Cameron et al 1996, Dietl et al 1993)

- Internal mammary artery: 90–95% patent at 10 years
- Saphenous vein: 50% patent at 10 years
- Right internal thoracic artery: 85% patent at 17 years*
- Left internal thoracic artery: 92% patent at 17 years*
- Gastro-epiploic artery: 95% patent at 4 years
- Inferior epigastric artery: 80% patent at 1 year

Commonly used arterial grafts are the right or left internal mammary artery (IMA), also known as the internal thoracic artery, which supplies the anterior chest wall. IMA grafts are left attached to their native blood supply at the proximal end and the distal end is dissected away from the chest wall and used to bypass the occluded coronary vessel. This is usually the left anterior descending (LAD) artery. Its use is associated with excellent long-term patency, improved survival and fewer myocardial infarctions (Cameron et al 1996, Loop 1996, Pym et al 1997). Long-term results with saphenous veins show that they develop progressive atherosclerosis over a 5–10-year period, which does not appear to occur to the same degree in IMA grafts (Dietl et al 1993; see Box 22.9).

Arteries are living vessels and can dilate in response to increased myocardial blood flow demand and vasodilator drugs. However, they can also spasm and respond to vasoconstricting medication. The right

gastro-epiploic and radial arteries are prone to constrict more strongly as they are quite muscular (Pym et al 1997), although pre-operative calcium channel blockers may prevent this. The right gastro-epiploic artery (RGEA) can be used to revascularize the posterior wall of the heart which cannot be reached by the use of an IMA. The radial artery was first used in 1971 and abandoned because of poor short-term patency (Pym et al 1995), which may have been due to poor harvesting technique, causing spasm and intimal hyperplasia. Care must be taken to avoid arterial stabs or peripheral cannulation in the donor arm site. If the radial artery is to be considered, there are a number of questions that the patient must be asked (Wolff et al 1997).

- Are there any mobility problems with the arm?
- Is there a history of poor circulation or Raynaud's syndrome?
- Has there been any past surgery to the arms?
- Are there any renal problems? (The patient may require dialysis in the future and formation of a fistula.)

Postoperative arterial graft spasm can be prevented by avoiding trauma to the vessel wall during harvesting and in some centres pretreatment with the aforementioned intraluminal agents such as vasodilators and calcium channel blockers is routine (Pym et al 1995). Low-dose glyceryl trinitrate (GTN) infusion is sometimes used in the immediate postoperative period (up to 24 hours), although there is no evidence to support this practice. Due to extensive dissection, those undergoing total arterial revascularization have the potential for increased bleeding. If the RGEA has been used, there can be extensive bleeding into the abdominal cavity and the nurse will need to observe for signs of distension, guarding and tenderness, together with altered haemodynamics such as a lowering blood pressure (BP) and central venous pressure (CVP), together with a rising heart rate.

Minimally invasive cardiac surgery and minimally invasive direct coronary artery bypass (MIDCAB) are

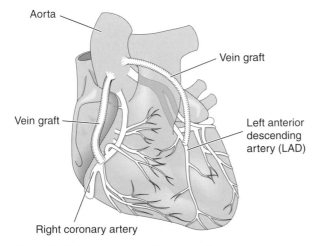

Figure 22.2 Coronary artery bypass grafts.

new and exciting developments in cardiac surgery (Mizell et al 1997). These techniques, avoiding the effects of the bypass machine, will impact on postoperative nursing care and are discussed in detail in the latter section of Chapter 29.

Valve surgery

Preparation for valve replacement surgery is almost identical to that of CABG surgery. The choice of prosthesis will influence the care that the patient will receive. Prosthetic valves are available in two forms (see Fig. 22.3):

- mechanical
- tissue: animal grafts or human cadaveric homografts.

The patient's lifestyle must be taken into account when discussing choice of prosthesis. Tissue valves

tend to wear out and require replacement within 5–8 years. However, they are often used for younger women who may be considering childbearing, as a repeat operation could be performed at a later date, while the teratogenic effects of warfarin are avoided. Elderly patients are also often offered tissue valves, to avoid possible long-term clinical problems of the required anticoagulation for mechanical valves. In addition, some individuals will be concerned about the detrimental effects of warfarin therapy and will also choose a tissue valve over a mechanical one.

However, in some cases, a mechanical valve may be the only real option, for example if the patient has a history of wearing out tissue valves and consequently has undergone multiple sternotomies, which increases the potential for complications. Many patients with valvular dysfunction will have been prescribed anticoagulant therapy prior to surgery due to impaired LV

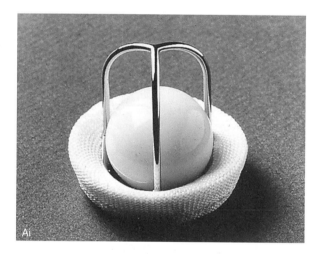

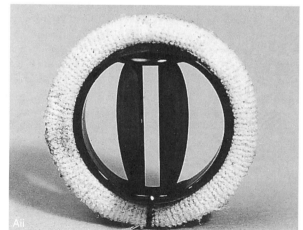

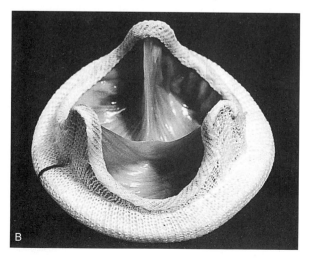

Figure 22.3 A: Prosthetic mechanical heart valves. (i) Starr-Edwards caged ball valve. (ii) St Jude Medical bileaflet valve. B: Tissue heart valve: Carpentier-Edwards porcine bioprosthetic valve. (Reproduced with permission from Julian DG, Camm AJ, Fox KM, Hau RJC, Poole-Wilson PA 1996 Diseases of the heart, 2nd edn. WB Saunders, London.)

function or atrial arrhythmias. Such patients will need to be admitted to hospital several days prior to surgery, so that warfarin can be discontinued and intravenous heparin commenced. The latter allows a much better immediate control and manipulation of coagulation studies for surgery.

In valve replacement surgery, the patient is placed on CPB, the diseased valve is completely excised and the replacement prosthesis sewn in. Due to the length of time this takes, patients are generally kept profoundly hypothermic (28°C). Consequently, they may spend longer in the recovery area whilst the sequelae of a longer CPB time are corrected. Valve patients are prone to bradyarrhythmias and atrioventricular (AV) nodal blocks in the immediate postoperative period, due to the proximity of the valvular tissue to the conducting tissue, particularly the AV node. Valve patients may have epicardial pacing wires sutured in place before the chest is closed and a suitable temporary pacing box should be kept nearby in case they develop an arrhythmia. They will also need to maintain a lower systolic blood pressure than graft surgery patients in the immediate postoperative period, to avoid putting undue pressure on the suture line around the valve. This may be achieved with cautious intravenous filling and the use of intravenous vasodilatory agents such as GTN.

Cardiac transplantation

This surgical procedure involves excising the patient's own diseased heart and replacing it with a heart from a cadaveric donor. This is known as orthotopic cardiac transplantation. The donor heart has to be the right size and be tissue typed to match the recipient. Transplantation is discussed in detail in the following chapter, but management will primarily differ from routine cardiac surgery in the following four areas: preventing infection, immunosuppression regimens, the risk and management of rejection and psychological support for the patient and carers related to receiving a new heart.

POSTOPERATIVE CARE FOR CARDIAC SURGERY

Transfer to the recovery area

Cardiac surgery patients are usually cared for in an intensive care or high-dependency environment for the first 12–24 hours after surgery. This enables close monitoring of their physical condition and allows for correction of the physical sequelae of CPB. Care will involve the following.

- Monitoring and optimizing the cardiovascular system. This occurs through the nurse manipulating the haemodynamic status against agreed parameters. It is achieved through a careful balance of observing the patient and their recorded pressures, such as the central venous and mean arterial pressures, and utilizing intravenous fluids and possibly vasodilatory drugs such as GTN and inotropic agents to augment the values. Chapter 18 explores in detail the skills of manipulating haemodynamics.
- Correcting the effects of anaesthesia and CPB.
- Maintaining the comfort of the patient by assessing for pain, type and required interventions, and attending to basic nursing needs. Initially, the patient is likely to have an infusion of analgesia. A catheter to monitor urinary output will prevent the need for the patient to consciously pass urine.
- Monitoring, controlling and correcting any bleeding.
- Correcting the patient's temperature.
- Monitoring and correcting cardiac arrhythmias.
- Observing for the signs of cardiac tamponade.
- Care and explanation to patient and family/carers.

Such acute care environments may be part of a general recovery or ICU, although some centres will have a dedicated cardiothoracic recovery or intensive care area. With the advent of surgical 'fast tracking' (see Chapter 29), such patients may spend a shorter amount of time in the recovery area or be admitted to a cardiac high-dependency unit (HDU) instead.

Once the patient has been rewarmed in theatre and the incisions are being sutured, the recovery area will be notified of the patient's imminent arrival. As the patient is transferred, the nurse will need to know the following.

- What operation the patient has had.
- If CABG, how many grafts were used, which vessels have been grafted and what type of grafts were used.
- If valve surgery, the location and type of prosthesis used, for example mechanical or tissue, location and number of pacing wires.
- Drains: the number of drains and where they are positioned. If opened, was the pleural cavity suctioned prior to the final positioning of the drain(s)? This has implications when the patient is sat upright or repositioned. If excessive drainage occurs this may indicate new bleeding, if the cavity had previously been suctioned. The colour and consistency should also be noted, to assess for fresh bleeding.
- The occurrence of any peri-operative complications, such as arrhythmias, labile blood pressure or problems weaning from CPB.

- Relevant medical history, such as asthma, smoking, hypertension, diabetes.
- Pre-operative arterial blood gases, if available.
- The presence of any infusions, such as GTN, sedatives, analgesia or inotropes.
- The presence of any assist devices, for example an IABP.

Such knowledge will assist in informing the nurse of the severity of the patient's condition and likely complications. It will also indicate the skill mix needed to care for the patient and possible additional preparations required, such as the ventilator model if weaning is anticipated as a problem and a pressure-relieving mattress if a longer stay in the unit is anticipated. The safety of the recovery environment must be ensured before the patient is admitted from the operating theatre. The bed space equipment must be configured to receive the patient, so that they can be attached to a ventilator immediately if necessary and their vital signs can be monitored with minimal delay.

Prior to surgery a pre-operative visit will allow the nursing team to know if the patient has any pre-existing respiratory problems (which may influence the mechanical ventilatory support), the nutritional status of the patient, whether they appeared anxious or frightened and their skin condition. A patient who was anxious preoperatively may need extra reassurance to enable them to comply with postoperative care, such as deep-breathing exercises following extubation. It is always sensible for the nurse who conducted the preoperative visit to be present when the patient returns from theatre, not only for the above reasons but to offer an element of familiarity to both patient and family or carers.

All alarm settings on the monitoring devices, such as ventilators, ECG monitors and blood pressure tranducers, need to be set for each individual patient and the alarms must be audible. This is to ensure the nurse is informed at an early stage should the patient's physiological parameters deviate from the acceptable levels. It must be emphasized that this is not a substitution for effective nursing observation and care of the patient. There should also be a thoracotomy tray/tolley nearby in case an emergency chest opening is required. This is usually when rapidly developing cardiac tamponade occurs although this is a relatively rare complication.

The first 12 hours

The care of the patient in the first 12 hours is largely focused on correcting the altered physiological processes that have occurred due to surgery and the effects of cardiopulmonary bypass (see Box 22.5). A partly preprinted prescription chart to cover the initial postoperative period is frequently used. This is because postoperative care will follow a fairly predictable pathway. Indeed, integrated care pathways (ICPs) have been particularly useful in the care of post-cardiac surgery patients (see Chapter 30). The prescription chart contains desired haemodynamic parameters for the patient's physiological observations. It will also detail what medications or intravenous fluids should be administered to achieve these parameters and thus optimize tissue perfusion during this critical period.

A printed example signed by the anaesthetist or surgeon may state:

Maintain systolic blood pressure between 90–110 mmHg.

If BP is >110 mmHg give GTN (1 mg/ml) between 1–15 ml/hour as required.

This all emphasizes the skill needed by nursing staff to manipulate and optimize the haemodynamic status of the patient. Additionally, this period can be very frightening for the patient and they may easily become disorientated which can lead to psychological disturbances. It is vital to talk to the patient and explain all actions and interventions and it is important that family members or carers are kept informed and encouraged to visit. They will not be used to the intensive care environment and will need a great deal of support at this stressful time.

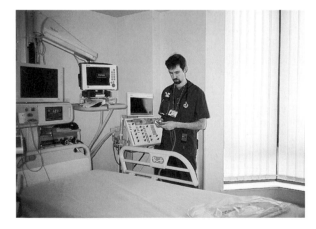

Figure 22.4 A bedspace being prepared for a patient's return from cardiac surgery. Note the nurse checking the emergency respiratory equipment in case the mechanical ventilator fails or the patient suffers severe respiratory compromise.

Until the advent of 'fast-track' surgical care, patients were routinely ventilated for perhaps 8–10 hours postoperatively, which would allow them to recover from the anaesthetic, whilst other sequelae of CPB were corrected. With the advent of fast tracking, early extubation against agreed criteria has become a more familiar practice (Edwards & Hess 1996). Therefore, many patients will be admitted to the recovery unit/ICU/HDU for a shorter period of ventilation or may even be self-ventilating on arrival. Some, however, will still be intubated, whilst others may be using a face mask over the endotracheal (ET) tube. Changes in respiratory management and shorter acting sedatives have revolutionized the recovery phase of such patients and made available valuable intensive care resources. Longer intubation times (>6 hours) are generally found in older patients and those with haemodynamic instability.

Caring for the ventilated patient

Mechanical ventilation applies positive pressure to force air into the lungs. In spontaneous breathing, air is drawn into the lungs by a negative intrathoracic pressure. This occurs via an increase in the thoracic cavity size created by movement of the respiratory muscles. This application of intrathoracic pressure by mechanical ventilation can cause major physiological changes which can have a profound effect on the cardiac surgical patient (Box 22.10).

To assist in minimizing these, any hypovolaemia must be corrected. Cardiac patients often require higher than normal filling pressures, due to their underlying LV dysfunction. This is linked to the physical principle of Starling's Law of the heart, whereby the more a myocardial fibre is stretched prior to its release, the greater the force of contraction and cardiac output. This stretch is achieved through increasing the preload with intravenous filling. However, the law is not linear and careful monitoring of the filling pressures (CVP and left atrial or pulmonary artery occlusion pressures if present) will guide these skills of optimization. There is a clear need to be aware of the degree of LV dysfunction present. Those patients with poor LV function (that is, an ejection fraction <30%) will quickly develop left-sided heart failure if fluid overloaded. It is important to remember that the absolute value of the CVP is not as important as its response to a fluid challenge (Hinds & Watson 1996). A rapidly rising CVP indicates that the limit of Starling's Law has been reached and the effects of heart failure may rapidly ensue. Filling pressures will also be artificially elevated due to mechanical ventilation and the

pressure exerted on the great veins, therefore these are best read at the end of the inspiratory phase.

The use of continuous positive airway pressure (CPAP) in a self-ventilating patient will also decrease the cardiac output by maintaining an elevated intrathoracic pressure throughout the whole respiratory cycle. This will result in a restriction of the venous return. CPAP (or positive end-expiratory pressure (PEEP), when mechanically ventilated) is indicated to normalize the patient's functional residual capacity and re-expand collapsed alveoli after CPB. Essentially, it prevents all the air leaving the lungs at the end of expiration to a set pressure. A high CPAP value may be regarded as 15 cmH$_2$O, a lower value perhaps 5 cmH$_2$O. Use of the former would be considered unusual due to the adverse effects on the cardiac output. The presence of a median sternotomy often results in restrictive pulmonary dysfunction and atelectasis in post-cardiac surgery patients which has been demonstrated on more than 60% of postoperative chest X-rays (Romand & Donald 1995). This will correct itself in 4–5 days after surgery, through the use of PEEP/CPAP (Romand & Donald 1995).

The following will need to be assessed on arrival in the recovery or acute unit and at hourly intervals whilst the patient remains mechanically ventilated.

- Respiratory rate (mechanical ventilation will normally be set at approximately 10–12 breaths per minute).
- Tidal volume (the amount of gas required for each breath). Low tidal volume, protective ventilation is now generally favoured. Much has been learnt from

---

Box 22.10 Physical changes due to mechanical ventilation (after Robb 1997)

Cardiac
- Reduced venous return
- Reduced cardiac output
- Reduced renal perfusion
- Reduced hepatic perfusion
- Reduced cerebral perfusion
- Arrhythmias common

Respiratory
- Decreased lung compliance
- Increased ventilator/perfusion ratio
- Barotrauma
- Oxygen toxicity
- Respiratory alkalosis

Other
- Increased airways disturbances
- Gastrointestinal disturbances
- Malnutrition
- Infection

the management of acute respiratory distress syndrome (ARDS) regarding possible damage to the lungs and a triggering of a pulmonary immune response through aggressive ventilation (Hirvela 2000). Tidal volumes tend to be more commonly set at 6–8 ml/kg.

• Minute volume (this is the tidal volume × the respiratory rate).

• Airway pressures (ideally these should be maintained at <30 cmH$_2$O. Higher airway pressures can occur with pre-existing lung disease and the anaesthetist or an experienced ICU nurse should be notified. High airway pressures can be damaging to the lungs and result in a possible pulmonary immune response or barotrauma. It is important to note that pain, endotracheal secretions, restlessness and fear can result in the patient 'fighting the ventilator' and raising the airway pressures. The underlying cause needs to be addressed.

• Oxygen–haemoglobin saturation (this will be monitored continually through pulse oximetry and intermittently through arterial blood gas analysis).

• Arterial blood gases (on arrival and some 15–20 minutes after changes to the ventilator settings).

• Auscultation of air entry (to ensure adequate mechanical ventilation of both lungs, to assess for bronchospasm and secretions).

Oxygen saturation of haemoglobin (SpO$_2$) can be measured non-invasively by use of a peripheral saturation probe (pulse oximetry), fixed to the finger or earlobe. Whilst pulse oximetry is used frequently in the postoperative setting, findings should be interpreted with caution in the hypothermic, haemodiluted patient. Such patients will be peripherally vasoconstricted and have dilutional anaemia, which will make any readings potentially less accurate. There is a tendency to take frequent arterial blood gas (ABG) measurements in the initial postoperative period which can mask changing trends. Monitoring of arterial oxygen saturations and end-tidal carbon dioxide levels, if the equipment is available, should reduce the need to take overly frequent ABGs (Staples & Ramsay 1997). Pulse oximetry and respiratory rate monitoring may also assist during the ventilation weaning process and reduce the number of ABGs taken (Noll & Byers 1995)

Suctioning

The patient will require endotracheal suctioning, as their gag reflex may be absent due to the use of muscle relaxants peri-operatively and sedation. It will also be reduced when awake, due to the endotracheal (ET) tube sitting in the trachea. It is of value for the nurse to be aware of pre-existing lung conditions or if the patient smokes, because both can result in a need for regular auscultation, suctioning and physiotherapy. Suctioning should only be performed when secretions can be detected on auscultation of the lung fields, to avoid undue respiratory trauma and peaking of the haemodynamic pressures. In addition, suctioning can be very distressing for the patient and has been shown to have the following detrimental effects (Puntillo 1990, Stone et al 1991):

• An increased blood pressure and heart rate. This can cause ischaemia and place haemodynamic pressure on the anastomoses
• Arrhythmias
• Pain and fear
• Hypoxia, due to air being rapidly drawn from the lungs
• A possible increase in the need for sedation, which will delay weaning from the ventilator

Indications for weaning from the ventilator

Whilst prolonged ventilation times have been used to achieve haemodynamic stability, development of 'fast-track' protocols has shown this to be unnecessary (Doering et al 1998). Criteria for early weaning and extubation will differ slightly from unit to unit. However, Keresztes & Kuruzar (1996) provide a useful example.

• Moderate to good LV function
• Age <70
• Uncomplicated and short CPB time
• Uncomplicated surgical course
• Limited co-morbidity

The above criteria demonstrate how subjectivity and individual clinical judgement will still play an active role. In addition, before extubating, the following criteria need to be met as recommended by Dunstan & Riddle (1997).

• Haemodynamic stability
• Normothermic
• Stable coagulation studies
• The patient is awake and can co-operate with commands
• Adequate analgesia has been administered
• Clear air entry and chest sounds on auscultation
• Acceptable wound drainage (<50 ml every 2 hours)
• The patient has undertaken a trial off the ventilator and maintained normal oxygen saturations. This may not occur in some units, if the patient appears

haemodynamically stable, with acceptable arterial blood gases on mechanical ventilation.

Acceptable weaning parameters:

- respiratory rate <25 bpm
- negative inspiratory force < -20 cmH$_2$O (in reality, this is rarely measured)
- acceptable arterial blood gas limits, for example:
  PaCO$_2$ < 6–7 kPa (30–55 mmHg)
  PaO$_2$ >10 kPa (> 70 mmHg) on a fraction inspired oxygen (FiO$_2$) of <40%
  SpO$_2$ >95%.

Further criteria for extubation can be found in Box 29.1.

The patient must obviously be able to protect their own airway and have a gag reflex present.

A negative pre-operative attitude to surgery, the patient's age and early haemodynamic instability are powerful predictors of delayed extubation (Doering 1997, Doering et al 1998, Ingersoll & Grippi 1991). After extubation, the patient must be observed for signs of stridor (noisy respirations, due to partial obstruction of the larynx or trachea), be sat upright but comfortably and be encouraged with deep-breathing exercises to clear any retained sputum, decreasing the risk of atelectasis. An ABG should be performed 30 minutes after extubation to assess progress. Ideally, oral fluids should be withheld for a short period in case re-intubation is required. However, most patients request a drink almost immediately and skills of clinical judgement are called upon in this situation. Wet mouth swabs may be of use. Some patients may ultimately require re-intubation due to cardiovascular instability, excessive bleeding or worsening respiratory function.

Common respiratory problems

Pulmonary complications account for 24% of deaths occurring within 6 days of surgery (Brooks-Brunn 1995). Diaphragmatic problems are common, related to phrenic nerve injury, due to cold cardioplegia, stretching or interrupted blood supply to the nerve.

Atelectasis (closure or collapse of the alveoli) occurs in 90% of cardiac surgery patients (Brooks-Brunn 1995). It can be undetectable or have overt clinical signs. It often responds to deep-breathing exercises or changing position and usually resolves within 24–48 hours.

Signs of atelectasis include:

- decreased breath sounds over the affected area (on auscultation)
- crackles (on auscultation)
- cough and sputum production

- X-ray findings.

Risk factors for atelectasis include (Brooks-Brunn 1995):

- increasing age
- obesity
- chronic lung disease
- smoking history
- poor pre-operative pulmonary education
- location of incision
- inadequate analgesia.

Pneumonia may develop if atelectasis persists as production of surfactant is altered, affecting lung expansion and enhancing bacterial growth. The incidence in cardiac surgery is highly variable and is in the region of 20–95% (Brooks-Brunn 1995). Respiratory complications can be minimized by a thorough respiratory assessment to identify those at risk and, when detected, institution of appropriate therapies. These include changing position, placing the patient in an upright position to facilitate chest expansion, encouraging deep breathing and expectorating, early mobilization and the utilization of the advice and skills of the physiotherapist.

Postoperative pain

Pain varies greatly in the postoperative patient and it is important to distinguish between incisional pain and ischaemic pain. Postoperative pain in the cardiac surgery patient is multidimensional and is related to:

- the location and type of surgical incisions
- intra-operative manipulation
- possible ischaemia
- the presence of invasive lines such as a urinary catheter, IV lines and an endotracheal (ET) tube
- chest drains
- the patient's norms: psychological, social, cultural and individual.

Median sternotomy pain is usually located along the incision site and may radiate into the subclavicular area and varies from dull, throbbing sensations to sharp constant pain. Coughing and deep breathing may exacerbate the discomfort experienced by the patient and is more intense in the first 3 days after surgery. Adequate pain relief depends on the individual's perception of pain rather than on the precise nature of the surgery (Hancock 1996). Patients who have undergone IMA grafting complain of chest discomfort over the harvest sites and sometimes numbness which may persist for several months after surgery (Holl 1995). Long-term discomfort persisting for 12–18 months has also been reported (Rowe & King 1998). Other symptoms include severe tenderness to palpation over the sternal areas, which may be related to damage to anterior branches of the intercostal nerves during harvesting (Pym et al 1995).

Physical signs indicative of pain, such as raised BP and tachycardia, may be masked due to the use of vasoactive drugs such as GTN and sodium nitroprusside (SNP) or use of β-blockers pre-operatively. Sedation may also inhibit the patient's ability to communicate any pain, as does the presence of an ET tube, which renders the patient unable to speak. Current management of pain in the immediate postoperative phase focuses on a combination of opioids, non-opiate analgesics and non-steroidal anti-inflammatory drugs (NSAIDs). NSAIDs must be used with caution as their inhibition of prostaglandin synthesis can affect renal function adversely and their inhibition of platelet aggregation can affect haemostasis (Hancock 1996). Morphine is the most commonly used analgesic and has been shown to be most effective when used in combination with non-opioid analgesics (Hancock 1996). Non-opioid analgesics include medication such as paracetamol. Opiates can be administered intravenously by bolus or infusion. Infusion avoids the peaks and troughs seen with bolus administration and minimizes any haemodynamic changes.

A descriptive study of patients recovering from CABG surgery in intensive care found that patients exhibited considerable pain which was not always relieved, due to nurses' underestimation of pain (Ferguson et al 1997). This study also identified a worrying practice of reduced analgesia administration over time with a corresponding increase in pain intensity.

The following recommendations were made:

- Standardized, regular, systematic assessment of pain is required
- Analgesia prescriptions should allow for a variation in dosage and agents to meet individual patients' needs
- Improved communication between health professionals is required for effective pain management

An investigation of the relationships between patient desire for control and the amount of analgesic administered in recovery/ITU after extubation found that desire for control, the patient's age and anxiety were predictors of the amount of analgesic administered. Less analgesia was administered as desire for control and age increased, while as anxiety increased, so did analgesia administration (Holl 1995). Nurses

need to keep patients informed and to include them in decisions about their analgesia, to promote a sense of control in postoperative care.

Temperature changes

All patients will undergo a period of rewarming before being weaned from CPB, but it is not uncommon to find that many patients are still very cold on admission to the postoperative unit. The aforementioned process will only return 65% of the patient's heat loss (Phillips & Skov 1988), but the degree of temperature drop will have been determined by the methods used for myocardial protection. Core temperature is elevated at the end of surgery to approximately 38°C but when CPB is discontinued, it can drop by 2–5°C. This is known as the 'afterdrop' phenomenon (Howell et al 1992). Afterdrop results when cold, stagnant blood is shunted to the body's core. Peripheral vasculature will remain constricted for 30–40 minutes after bypass ceases, so large areas of the body are unable to receive rewarmed blood. Afterdrop is usually noticed once the patient has been moved into the postoperative area and their temperature is being monitored once again.

Patients administered warm blood cardioplegia will not have undergone systemic hypothermia and are less likely to suffer from a drop in temperature. Those most at risk for postoperative hypothermia tend to be older and to have had long CPB times. Thus, patients undergoing complex procedures such as valve replacements or aortic arch surgery will be at higher risk than those undergoing CABG surgery.

The body's thermoregulatory mechanisms begin to respond during rewarming and as the effects of the anaesthetic and muscle relaxants diminish, the body's primary defence against cold – shivering – will occur (Holtzclaw 1986). This is undesirable, because it will increase the body's metabolic rate, oxygen consumption, carbon dioxide production and myocardial work (Phillips 1997). The body is unable to meet these increased needs due to reduced cardiac contractility and a reduced oxygen-carrying capacity, as a consequence of surgery (Earp & Mallia 1997, Holtzclaw 1986). Shivering will generate heat, but the body is unable to retain this and the use of any vasodilators in this period, such as GTN, will hasten heat loss. Heat conservation measures such as the use of extra blankets and head coverings should be considered for all postoperative patients. However, the use of two types of head coverings in a sample of 81 patients did not reveal any benefits over a control group in enhancing the rewarming process (Howell et al 1992). Interestingly, within this study, despite the groupings, patients who reached normothermia within 5 hours did tend to have experienced warmer core temperatures peri-operatively, were warmer on admission to the postoperative area, were generally younger and had shorter CPB times (Howell et al 1992).

Other causes of a failure to rewarm despite adequate filling should also be considered. These could include bleeding or myocardial dysfunction. A degree of caution needs to be exercised regarding the speed with which rewarming takes place. If too rapid, the cardiovascular system will be stressed by a sudden increase in the metabolic rate and oxygen consumption. This can lead to a 'rewarming acidosis' by causing the constricted peripheral vasculature to open and load the circulation with accumulated metabolites (Holtzclaw 1986).

Slow uniform rewarming is less likely to produce these dramatic effects, by avoiding the creation of steep temperature gradients. In general, on arrival in the postoperative area, the patient should be covered with blankets to conserve heat, while temperature probes should be attached to a peripheral site such as the foot and to a site approximating the core, usually the subaxilla. As the patient begins to warm, peripheral vasodilatation will occur and this may cause the blood pressure to drop dramatically. The skill of the nurse in carefully manipulating the intravenous fluids will be needed to maintain the haemodynamic status within the desired parameters.

Altered haemodynamics

A labile blood pressure, altered cardiac output and arrhythmias are all common in the immediate postoperative period and require intervention. Arterial blood pressure and right atrial (central venous) pressure are monitored continuously via transducers, so that any changes can be detected quickly. Multichannel ECG monitoring is utilized to improve rhythm recognition and detect any ischaemic changes.

Labile blood pressure

On arrival from theatre the patient's blood pressure is often high (>120 mmHg systolic) and this may require the use of vasodilators such as GTN or SNP to reduce it to acceptable limits. This may be as low as 90 mmHg in valve replacements and <120 mmHg in CABG surgery, to avoid physical stress to the suture line.

An elevated BP can be due to a number of causes:

- vasoconstriction due to hypothermia
- the release of sequestered adrenaline (epinephrine) on rewarming, occurring due to the physiological stress response

- pain
- agitation.

As previously highlighted, it is not uncommon for CABG patients to be prescribed a low-dose GTN infusion (1–2 mg/h), in order to prevent graft spasm if arterial grafts have been used, although there is no evidence to support its use. If the blood pressure is higher than the desired parameters, then GTN (1–15 mg/h) can be used as a first-line treatment. If this is unsuccessful then an arterio-venodilator such as SNP can be used and in severe cases, an α-adrenoceptor blocker such as phentolamine. Caution must be exercised with these drugs as the blood pressure response can be profound. The patient must also be observed for rewarming via the aforementioned monitored core and peripheral temperatures, but this will be together with the feel of the skin, because peripheral vessel dilatation can cause a rapid and sudden drop in blood pressure. Infusions may then need to be reduced or discontinued.

Rhythm disturbances

Alterations in heart rate and rhythm are common as a result of hypothermia and altered potassium concentrations, due to haemodilution. Common rhythm disturbances include atrial arrhythmias such as atrial fibrillation and AV nodal blocks (especially in those who have undergone valve surgery) and ventricular ectopy.

Patients with a history of such arrhythmias are at increased risk of developing these postoperatively. However, increased age is most strongly associated with arrhythmogenesis in this context. This is due to age-related cardiac changes, such as dilatation, muscle atrophy and impaired conduction (Ommen et al 1997). The cause of these postoperative arrhythmias include:

- pericardial inflammation/effusion
- excess catecholamine production and release
- autonomic imbalance (an imbalance between sympathetic and parasympathetic nervous stimulation)

Atrial arrhythmias

Atrial arrhythmias occur in 11–40% of CABG patients and over 50% of valve patients postoperatively (Ommen et al 1997). They are most frequent in the first 2–3 days postoperatively and are usually transient but reoccur in a significant number of patients. The most common arrhythmias seen in this period are:

- atrial fibrillation
- atrial flutter
- atrial tachycardia

Box 22.11   Arrhythmia management in the surgical setting (Ommen et al 1997)

Method	Indications
Digoxin	Frequently used as prophylaxis, but there is no evidence that it reduces the incidence of postoperative atrial fibrillation. It is indicated in those with left ventricular dysfunction and atrial tachyarrhythmias, and is used to control the ventricular rate; although benefits are limited when there are excess catecholamines.
β-blockers	Have a protective effect, decreasing the incidence of arrhythmias in the postoperative period. However, those β-blocked pre-operatively who have their medication withdrawn after surgery, have a high incidence of tachyarrhythmia.
Calcium channel blockers	Verapamil may control the ventricular rate; diltiazem is tolerated by those with poor left ventricular function but it can cause hypotension.
Amiodarone	Oral amiodarone given for 7 days preoperatively significantly reduces the incidence of postoperative atrial fibrillation (Daoud et al 1997). Intravenous administration is no more effective than digoxin in cardioverting the arrhythmia to sinus rhythm (Ommen et al 1997).
Epicardial pacing	Indicated in symptomatic bradycardias.
Electrical cardioversion	Early cardioversion may be necessary in individuals with haemodynamic compromise, although the factors that contribute to arrhythmia formation after surgery, i.e. inflammation, will still persist. Therefore the arrhythmia may reoccur. Atrial stunning sometimes occurs and the lack of contractility can lead to thrombus development (Ommen et al 1997).

Some patients may experience no symptoms, whilst others may report feelings of dizziness, light-headedness or palpitations. They may also have signs of haemodynamic compromise, due to a loss of atrioventricular synchrony, leading to reduced ventricular filling. Reduced diastolic filling times occur in fast ventricular rates.

Other potential complications include (Ellis 1998):

- thrombo-embolization
- compromised cardiac function
- longer hospital stay
- increased incidence of ventricular arrhythmias.

Arrhythmia management. A variety of medications may be used, although many of the research findings are conflicting, especially regarding the use of β-blockers and calcium antagonists. Prophylaxis should not be undertaken routinely, but could be considered in those at high risk of developing arrhythmias after surgery. As most atrial arrhythmias are due to surgical manipulation, anti-arrhythmic management must be reviewed and possibly discontinued before discharge. The aim of treatment is the restoration of sinus rhythm while ensuring a reduction in the ventricular rate and possible anticoagulation. Electrical cardioversion should be considered after 24 hours, if sinus rhythm has not returned. Box 22.11 provides a review of suggested management options for arrhythmias occurring following cardiac surgery.

Epicardial pacing

Epicardial pacing wires are used routinely in valve surgery. Such patients are at increased risk of transient AV block due to the proximity of the AV node and His bundle to the operative site. The pacing wires are made of Teflon-insulated stainless steel and the uninsulated tip is attached to the epicardial surface by the surgeon before the chest is closed. Generally two wires are attached on the right atrium and brought out of the chest wall in the right subcostal area. Two are attached on the right ventricular wall and brought out at the left subcostal area (Manion 1993). These can be used to speed up symptomatic bradycardias and to achieve AV synchrony should the patient develop a symptomatic AV conduction block. The wires are not attached to a pacing source unless the patient's condition warrants it. Any patient with pacing wires should have a temporary pacing box immediately available.

Atrial pacing is not indicated for the patient who develops atrial fibrillation. However, such patients may ocassionally require ventricular pacing if the rhythm develops with a slow ventricular response rate or, indeed, they may require anti-arrhythmic medication. Care should be exercised when handling epicardial wires to avoid 'microshock'. This is a potentially lethal situation which may arise from handling the pacing wires without gloves. This can ultimately cause an electric current to be passed directly along the wire to the heart (Lynn-McHale et al 1991). Wearing latex gloves when handling the pacing wires minimizes this risk by increasing the electrical resistance between the nurse and patient. The wires are also a potential source of infection as they are directly attached to the epicardial surface of the heart. The insertion site should be inspected daily for any signs of infection and be dressed with sterile gauze.

Removal of pacing wires occurs on postoperative days 3–5. They are removed by applying gentle traction until they slide out. If resistance is encountered, the wires should be cut close to the skin, allowing the insertion site to close over the wire. If the patient is anticoagulated, ensure that measurements such as the international normalised ratio (INR) are within an acceptable therapeutic range before wire removal. Warfarin is commonly used to prevent blood clot development around mechanical valves. The usual target INR value is 3.5, with a measurement within 0.5 regarded as acceptable (BNF 2001).

Risks have been reported during the removal of epicardial pacing wires. Carroll et al (1998) studied 145 patients who had right ventricular epicardial pacing wires placed during cardiac surgery. During wire removal 66% of patients experienced one or more premature ventricular contractions (PVC – ventricular ectopic), while 7% developed non-sustained ventricular tachycardia (VT). Interestingly, those who had undergone repeat cardiac surgery had significantly more non-sustained VT than did all other patients. Unsurprisingly, the conclusion drawn was the need for ECG monitoring *during* epicardial wire removal. All patients should be observed following pacing wire removal, for any adverse signs such as the development of cardiac tamponade or arrhythmias. The number of patients who subsequently require permanent pacing systems following cardiac surgery remains low. Del Rizzo et al (1996), in a study of 3493 consecutive patients, reported only 45 (1.3%) requiring a permanent system following surgery, while Gordon et al (1998) recorded a higher figure of 2.4% (255 patients amongst 10 421).

Postoperative low cardiac output

A low cardiac output state occurs frequently after cardiac surgery and is associated with a greater risk of death (Ellis 1997). This occurs more frequently in older patients with poor left ventricular function. Low output states are characterized by:

- the clinical signs of impaired cardiac function, in the presence of normal or high filling pressures
- a systolic blood pressure <90 mmHg

- mean arterial pressure <65 mmHg
- right atrial (central venous) pressure >10 mmHg
- tachycardia
- minimal wound drainage
- peripheral vasoconstriction
- decreased urine production
- failure to warm.

Other factors that can contribute to postoperative low cardiac output include:

- pre-operative myocardial dysfunction
- anaesthesia
- physiological responses to CPB
- electrolyte disturbances
- hypothermia
- coronary artery spasm and decreased coronary perfusion.

Cardiopulmonary bypass usually results in some degree of cardiac dysfunction (Staples & Ramsay 1997) and is more common in those with poor left ventricular function. Positive inotropes, such as adrenaline (epinephrine), can be used to augment the cardiac output until the heart has had time to recover. An often overlooked cause of myocardial dysfunction is perioperative myocardial infarction. All patients should have an ECG performed after admission to recovery. The presence of new, pathological Q-waves in two or more contiguous leads is the most accurate indicator of a peri-operative infarction. Cardiac enzyme analysis is not useful in this setting, as levels will be high due to cell damage from surgery. The troponin biochemical cardiac markers may be of some value (see Box 9.1).

Fluid management

Cardiac surgery involves major blood loss and relocation of plasma volume into the interstitium due to 'third spacing' (Ley et al 1990), exacerbated by the profound diuresis that occurs. Patients in the immediate postoperative phase have a severely depleted intravascular volume and exhibit varying degrees of hypovolaemia. Effective fluid management and the manipulation of haemodynamics will be guided by trends in a number of parameters, including the right atrial (central venous) pressure and haematocrit.

The nurse is also presented with several questions, including:

- how much fluid should be replaced?
- what form should fluid replacement take – crystalloid, colloid or blood?

There are a variety of products available for fluid replacement:

- blood and blood products
- crystalloids – balanced salt solutions
- colloids – balanced salt solutions that contain oncotically active particles, such as albumin.

Evidence regarding which is the best to use is conflicting. Blood is the optimal replacement fluid in severe blood loss, because it increases oxygen delivery and exerts oncotic pressure, so is less likely to cause further interstitial oedema, in comparison to crystalloids (Kavanagh et al 1995). However, it does carry a risk of infection and potential crossmatching errors. In the setting of normal haemoglobin levels, colloids are more effective at treating hypovolaemia than crystalloids. The body's response to stress is to retain increased amounts of sodium and water, thus negating the use for more of the same. Patients receiving colloids require less fluid replacement, gain less weight (so require less subsequent diuretic use) and have an improved haemodynamic status compared to crystalloids (Ley et al 1990).

Modified gelatins such as Gelofusine and Haemaccel are also used for intravascular resuscitation but they too carry a risk of allergic reactions, although this is seen less with Gelofusine (Kavanagh et al 1995). Haemaccel contains large amounts of calcium and should be avoided in hypercalcaemic patients and should not be given in the same giving set as blood, because calcium can cause the blood to clot.

Blood transfusion

CPB will result in the patient's blood becoming haemodiluted. Coupled with any damage to blood cells, this will always result in a lowered haemoglobin. Patients may require transfusing with up to six units of banked blood during and after surgery to correct their hypovolaemia and dilutional anaemia. It must be said that, generally, the decision to transfuse blood is now initiated cautiously. Such transfusions carry a number of risks, including infection and allergic reactions, which can increase morbidity. Peri-operative transfusion with packed red cells contributes to the systemic inflammatory response syndrome (SIRS) that can be seen postoperatively, by directly releasing bio-active substances into the circulation and enhancing the response of those already present (Fransen et al 1999).

Postoperatively, aside from any respiratory pathology, the patient remains well oxygenated at lowered haemoglobin levels and hence this is usually left to rectify itself over the coming days. The surgeon will provide instructions for the cardiac ITU nurse regarding when to transfuse blood and when to maintain colloid infusion. This will vary but usually blood is transfused

when the haemoglobin drops below 9 mg/dl. Some surgeons will use the level of the HCT or packed cell volume (PCV) to dictate transfusion. As haemoglobin is carried on red blood cells these measurements indicate the volume of red blood cells in the blood. An HCT/PCV below approximately 25% may indicate the need to transfuse, but again preferences will vary.

Autotransfusion is the collection and re-infusion of the patient's own blood which is salvaged intra-operatively and it has been in use since 1978. After surgery, the cardiotomy reservoir from the CPB circuit is attached to the mediastinal drains and this is then re-infused into the patient via a pump. Blood collected in this way can be transfused up to 6 hours after surgery, after which it must be discontinued and banked blood or other colloids used to limit any risk of infection (Ley 1996). A given amount of blood is therefore autotransfused each hour and it is recommended that 50 ml be left in the reservoir to avoid air entry.

Mediastinal blood differs from banked blood in the following ways (Goodnough et al 1999, Ley 1996).

- It is more dilute.
- HCT levels are lower than those found in banked blood, between 20–25% versus 35–42%.
- It is partially haemolysed, so there is platelet dysfunction.
- It is depleted of clotting factors and fibrinogen.
- It contains high proportions of cytokines.

Replacement of clotting factors and platelets may be required should the patient bleed excessively, although autotransfusion itself has not been implicated as a risk factor for bleeding. Whilst this procedure is almost universal, it cannot be used in those who have severe sepsis, blood coagulopathies, renal failure or chest malignancy (Ley 1996). Evidence to support its use is conflicting; several studies show a clear benefit, whilst others demonstrate a lack of efficacy (Goodnough et al 1999).

The patient will pass large volumes of dilute urine in the first 2–6 hours after surgery and will excrete large amounts of potassium. Urea and electrolyte levels will need to be assessed frequently as the patient may require regular potassium supplementation (for example, 20 mmol in at least 100 ml of fluid delivered via a central line, over perhaps 30–60 minutes) to maintain a serum potassium between 4 and 4.5 mmol/l. Supplements should be added to the crystalloid maintenance fluid, which is usually administered at 1 ml/kg/h. This is decreased once the patient is taking oral fluids.

A strict fluid balance chart needs to be maintained for the first 24 hours after surgery. Following this, daily weights can be used to assess any fluid gain. It is not uncommon to find a weight gain of 5 kg due to haemodilution in surgery and this can be treated by a short course of diuretics.

Late postoperative anaemia

Low haematocrit and haemoglobin levels *may* actually decrease again by the time of discharge, where Hb levels of 8–9 g/dl are not uncommon. It is important that this is corrected as it may cause fatigue and lethargy, limiting the patient's recovery. Patients have been shown to tolerate haemoglobin levels as low as 7 g/dl but this may vary with each individual in the context of compromised cardiac function (Crosby et al 1994).

Treatment of late postoperative anaemia varies. It may be left to correct itself or a transfusion may be given if there are very low Hb levels (for example, <7g/dl). Oral iron supplements may also be prescribed. However, in a study of 121 patients with a mean Hb level of 9.5 g/dl at 6 days after CABG, two regimens of iron supplement did not increase either the Hb or haematocrit above the control or placebo groups, at a mean of 59 days later (Crosby et al 1994).

Cardiac tamponade

Clearly one of the indications for maintaining close observation of the patient following cardiac surgery, at least in the initial postoperative period, is the danger of cardiac tamponade. This is a relatively rare occurrence and is defined as the accumulation of blood or serous fluid around the heart, usually in the pericardial sac. Progressively the blood constricts the pumping action of the heart and leads to haemodynamic collapse. In the first few hours following surgery this can occur rapidly and may lead to the chest being re-opened by the surgical team, on the unit, with no time to return to theatre. However, if a return to theatre can be achieved, this is more desirable as both equipment and trained staff are more easily available. Cardiac tamponade can occur in the later ward area but tends to be a slower accumulation of fluid. The condition emphasizes the need to observe recorded haemodynamic trends, as these most clearly identify the emerging problem.

The CVP will initially rise as pressure constricts the heart. The blood pressure will begin to drop, creating the so-called 'cross of danger'. The patient will become increasingly tachycardic but be aware of those who may be demonstrating the rate-slowing effects of β-blockers. In addition, many patients will initially be tachycardic on return from theatre, due to the physiological stress response and a need to maintain an adequate cardiac output. Pulsus paradoxus, an inspiratory decline in blood pressure of >10 mmHg, may noted on the arterial trace. Hinds & Watson (1996) warn that right heart tamponade, which may be due to loculated blood following cardiac surgery, is generally not associated with pulsus paradoxus. It is always useful at this stage to obtain a clotting screen to measure factors such as the ACT to assess the patient's propensity to bleed. Drainage from the chest drains may slow or stop but this is not always the case. It is not a priority to take a 12-lead ECG but if this is done, it will be seen that the amplitude of the complexes is much reduced. If awake, the patient can become increasingly restless.

Cardiac tamponade is a surgical emergency. The chest is usually re-opened to evacuate the blood and stem any bleeding. Within the initial 24–48 hours following surgery, aspiration via a wide-bore needle through the chest wall is usually not initiated, because the surgeon will need to remove clotted blood and locate and stem the bleeding site.

Management of postoperative bleeding

Haemostatic medication

Medication may be required to reduce blood loss and drugs commonly used to achieve haemostasis include:

- tranexamic acid
- desmopressin
- aprotinin
- aminocaproic acid (rarely used in the UK).

Antifibrinolytic drugs, such as tranexamic acid, are commonly used to treat blood loss in cardiac surgery. Tranexamic acid binds reversibly to plasminogen, blocking its activation and transformation into plasmin which enhances clot formation (Mannucci 1998). Desmopressin increases plasma concentrations of factor VIII and Von Willebrand's factor. Administering desmopressin during chest closure has been shown to reduce total blood loss and postoperative transfusion requirements, although only by a small amount. Consequently desmopressin is not recommended to reduce blood loss following cardiac surgery (Mannucci 1998).

Aprotinin inhibits kallikrein, so indirectly inhibits the formation of activated factor XII. It inhibits initiation of coagulation and fibrinolysis, but does not affect platelet function. It is effective in surgery where the patient has been taking aspirin, has infective endocarditis or is undergoing cardiac transplantation (Mannucci 1998). Prophylactic use of aminocaproic acid also results in a significant decrease in postoperative blood loss in CABG patients (Adamson et al 1994).

Overall, aprotinin is the most effective in reducing blood loss, followed by tranexamic acid, then aminocaproic acid. Aprotinin should also be given prophylactically to those who:

- are undergoing 'redo' surgery
- have haemostatic disorders
- have sepsis
- are taking antiplatelet agents
- are expected to require banked blood transfusions
- refuse transfusions for spiritual or other reasons

A clotting screen should also be obtained and the patient administered blood and clotting factors, such as fresh frozen plasma (FFP) and platelets if indicated. This is why it is important for the nurse to always know the amount of blood available within the blood fridge for transfusion. Administering a small amount of PEEP through the ventilator, if not resulting in an adverse effect on the cardiac output, may reduce bleeding by increasing the intrathoracic pressure through the whole respiratory cycle. It may be decided to administer further protamine, depending on the results of the clotting screen. If the blood loss is excessive, i.e. >500 ml in the first hour, then the patient will need to return to theatre for exploration and resuturing.

Wound drainage

Chest drains facilitate drainage of blood and serous fluid from the operating site, to reduce the risk of infection and clot formation. A closed underwater seal system is used to reduce infection risk and drains are attached to the external chest wall by a purse-string suture. Mediastinal tubes are used most frequently and pleural drains are used if the pleural space has been entered, for example if the patient has had a mammary artery graft. Mediastinal drainage is accomplished by use of one or two tubes. The drains are attached to low-pressure suction on admission to the recovery/ITU area (approximately $^-$15–20 cmH$_2$O/$^-$2 kPa), to promote drainage and reduce clot formation, which can lead to cardiac tamponade, and to prevent accumulation of blood, fluid and air in the mediastinal space in the pericardium (Calhoun Thomson et al 1997).

Stripping or milking of chest drain tubes is **not** recommended as this can increase negative intrathoracic pressure greatly, putting a strain on the anastomoses. This may then dislodge delicate clots around the suture lines and cause bleeding. Pressures between –100 cmH$_2$O and –400 cmH$_2$O have been reported during this practice (Duncan & Erickson 1982). Routine manipulation of chest tubes has been shown to be unnecessary in the first 8 postoperative hours and the

visible presence of clot in the chest tubes does not cause a lack of patency (Pierce et al 1991). A review of chest drain management found very few randomized controlled trials regarding chest drain management but found that there was no difference in occlusion rates if drains were milked or not (Godden & Hiley 1998).

Drainage should not be in excess of 200 ml in the first 2 hours. Excess drainage can indicate bleeding related to the surgery or inadequate reversal of anticoagulation and it may also occur if the patient's position is altered, although this is usually only transient.

The large blood losses seen in cardiac surgery are related to the (after Mannucci 1998):

- size of the surgical wound
- exposure of blood to artificial surfaces in the CPB circuit
- mechanical injury to platelets and coagulation factors
- hyperfibrinolysis during and after CPB.

Removal of chest drains.

Chest drains normally remain in place for 24 hours after surgery. They can cause the patient a great deal of discomfort as the drainage tubes can inhibit chest expansion, which could prevent the patient from breathing effectively or removing trapped secretions. Effective analgesia is paramount whilst the drains are in place and it is also necessary to ensure the patient has adequate analgesia before the drains are removed. Surgeon preference does vary, but generally drainage should be less than 100 ml in the previous 4 hours prior to removal. Two people will be required to remove the drains, one to pull the drain out and the other to tie off the purse-string suture.

To remove the chest drains, explain the procedure carefully to the patient to reduce anxiety and ensure compliance. It will be sore as they are pulled out and it is best to be honest. A small dose of intramuscular analgesia may be offered prior to removal to reduce soreness following the procedure.

- Disconnect suction from the drains and clamp the tubes near their origin so that they can be disconnected to aid manipulation
- Ask the patient to sit upright
- Cut the suture securing the tube to the chest wall and identify the purse-string suture
- Ask the patient to breathe in and hold their breath whilst the tubing is being removed (although there exists no evidence as to why this occurs (Godden & Hiley 1998))
- Remove the tube swiftly
- The assistant then pulls the purse-string tight and ties it off

- Order a post-removal chest X-ray to observe for possible pneumothorax.

Removal of the drains is painful for the patient, with 45% citing this as the worst memory of their recovery stay (Ferguson et al 1997). Patients have also reported feeling burning sensations, a feeling of pulling at removal and chest soreness after the procedure (Gift et al 1991). Removal of the chest drains is obviously more comfortable for the patient and enables them to move and breathe with less discomfort. The nurse should observe the patient for any signs of bleeding, infection or reduced breath sounds.

Leg pain after CABG

In patients who have had saphenous vein grafts, pain is common once mobilization has started, along with dependent oedema and numbness along the harvest site. Complications associated with use of the saphenous vein include delayed healing and may be related to poor harvesting technique. Use of pressure support stockings has been shown to reduce limb oedema in the first postoperative 5 days, although this was influenced by concomitant use of diuretics (Liehr et al 1992). This oedema can increase tension along the suture line and compromise the circulation, creating discomfort for the patient (Liehr et al 1992).

Wound infection

Sternal wound infection

The cause of wound infection is multifactorial and will depend on local and systemic factors, such as bacterial infection and sternal devascularization. Stasis in the sternal region limits fluid exchange and nutrient exchange, so oxygenation is reduced to the local area (Seyfer et al 1988). Bilateral and single mammary artery usage in CABG have been associated with a higher incidence of sternal wound infection, due to the fact that the internal mammary arteries supply the sternum with blood (Hussey & Leeper 1998).

Importantly, the likelihood of sternal wound infection is six times higher for patients who receive mechanical ventilation for longer than 48 hours. There are several reasons for this. A longer period ventilated means a prolonged stay in the ICU, exposing the patient to bacteria, while sputum and droplets when suctioning and disconnecting the ET tube can contaminate the sternal area. It is therefore strongly advisable, in the initial few days, to leave the sternal wound dressing intact and untouched, unless there are concerns regarding sternal stability or infection or the dressing becomes

saturated. Sternal wound infections can be potentially life threatening and will require aggressive treatment with antibiotic therapy. In severe cases, surgical debridement may be necessary.

Sternal wound dehiscence

Dehiscence refers to the breakdown of a surgical wound. Dehiscence of the sternal wound is a major cause of morbidity and mortality. Mortality ranges from 27% to 71% (Kuo & Butchart 1995). Again, devascularization of the sternum, which occurs as a result of using IMA grafts, is a factor in impaired sternal healing. The aim of sternal closure is to achieve maximal sternal stability. Kuo & Butchart (1995) use the example of closure of the sternum with interrupted horizontal stainless steel wires (no. 5 gauge) yielding a dehiscence incidence of only 1.6%, with infection associated in 41% of cases. Women have more sternal wound dehiscence due to the tension on the incision from breast tissue (Vaska 1997a). The occurrence of dehiscence is generally diagnosed by:

- pain
- discharge
- clicking sternum
- pyrexia
- a raised white cell count

Box 22.12 Risk factors for mediastinitis (Marggraf et al 1999)

Predisposing factors
- Diabetes mellitus
- Impaired cardiac function
- Malnutrition
- Extreme old age
- Male sex
- Smoking
- Steroid or immunosuppresive treatment
- Lengthy hospitalization:
  - increased risk due to longer exposure to hospital bacteria
- Obesity:
  - blood supply is compromised

Operative factors
- Use of bilateral mammary artery grafts:
  - reduces blood supply to the chest wall by up to 90%
  - main cause of impaired healing
- Prolonged surgical time
- Non-pulsatile CPB
- Frequent use of electrocautery
- Use of bone wax on sternum
- Large peri-operative blood loss

Mediastinitis

Mediastinitis is an acute or chronic inflammation of the mediastinum (Marggraf et al 1999), associated with retrosternal spread of infection to the heart, grafts, prosthetic material and sutures. It can also spread to the chest wall. It is rare and occurs in 0.4–5.0% of cardiac surgery but carries a mortality rate of 27% (Gallo & Todd 1990). It usually appears between 4 days to 4 weeks after surgery (see Box 22.12). It develops from sternal infections, where a small infected area becomes necrotic, develops inflammation and is followed by mediastinitis.

General deterioration in the patient's condition or the onset of sternal instability may be the only preceding signs. Other signs include:

- persistent fever
- elevated white cell count
- local erythema (redness of the skin)
- local tenderness
- purulent drainage from sternal wound site.

Those who recover from mediastinitis have been shown to have a significantly shorter life expectancy than those who do not develop the condition (Marggraf et al 1999).

Blood cultures should be taken if any infection is suspected. Staphylococcal organisms are found in 70% of wound cultures, whilst 40% have mixed infections. Fungi and Gram-negative organisms are rare (Marggraf et al 1999). Treatment ranges from aggressive antibiotic therapy to surgical debridement. High-dose vitamin C should also be given to promote effective wound healing. The incidence of dehiscence is eight times more common in those with decreased vitamin C levels (Young 1988). Broad-spectrum antibiotics, such as cephalosporins and vancomycin, should be commenced once cultures have been taken, with therapy being based on the results.

Some patients may require surgical treatment to remove infected tissue and foreign objects such as sternal wires, pacing wires and heavy sutures, to accomplish sternal closure. A closed irrigation system should be inserted after debridement to limit bacterial growth and remove all purulent material. It is not clear what the optimum composition of irrigation solutions should be but iodine, antibiotics and saline solutions are commonly used. If debridement and irrigation do not lead to healing, then it may be necessary to remove all or part of the sternum and repair the area with a muscle flap, commonly the omentum or a pectoralis major flap (Hussey & Leeper 1998).

Postpericardiotomy syndrome (PPS)

PPS is a delayed pericardial reaction after surgery characterized by fever, chest pain and a friction rub. It is a late complication of cardiac surgery and occurs in 10–50% of all cardiac surgery patients (Dziadulewicz & Shannon-Stone 1995). However, it has also been implicated in cardiac tamponade, although it is usually a benign condition and self-limiting. The aetiology is unclear but an auto-immune reaction is suspected, with the initial event being a myocardial injury causing the damaged tissue and blood within the pericardium to trigger the release of cardiac antigens, leading to an inflammatory reaction (Dziadulewicz & Shannon-Stone 1995). Its incidence is dramatically reduced with age and it has also been described as having seasonal variation, with the highest incidence occurring between May and July (Dziadulewicz & Shannon-Stone 1995).

Effective treatment is usually with NSAIDs, such as indometacin and ibuprofen. Indometacin has been implicated as causing coronary vasoconstriction whereas ibuprofen is a coronary artery vasodilator. Pain is often described as sharp, shooting or stabbing. Dull, deep pain may occur due to extension to the pericardial sac. Location of the pain is precordial or retrosternal with radiation to the left shoulder, which is not seen with other forms of pericardial disease (Kronick-Mest 1989). Pain can be accentuated with respiratory movement. Friction rubs occur and are described as scratching, grating or crunching and represent the roughened layers of the pericardial membrane (Kronick-Mest 1989).

Continued postoperative care

The patient will be transferred back to the ward area usually 24 hours after surgery (unless a fast-track candidate). All intravenous lines and the urinary catheter will be removed by 48 hours after surgery and the focus of nursing care here is to mobilize the patient and try and return them to maximal, normal functioning. Routinely the sternum is closed with surgical-grade steel wire and the muscle and skin with absorbable sutures. Skin clips are generally not used because of the length of time that would be required to remove them in an emergency if the chest had to be re-opened. For the leg wound, an absorbable suture, skin clips or an interrupted silk or nylon suture will be used. Surgeon protocol will vary regarding management of the wound, but generally nursing staff remove the dressing at approximately 3 days, unless there are concerns regarding the wound area or the dressing has become soiled. Some surgeons ask for a plastic sealant spray to be applied to the area, some do not. The patient will continue to be asked to support the chest wound, usually with a cushion or rolled towel, when coughing.

There are a wide range of physiological and psychological complaints that can occur postoperatively such as weakness, fatigue, pain from the donor limb, sternal discomfort, lack of concentration, poor sleep, appetite disturbances and emotional lability. Persistent gastro-intestinal (GI) complaints have been reported by some, with the most frequent being poor appetite, lack of taste and nausea (Beekmann-Ball & Grap 1992). It is important that patients and their carers are told that these are very common after surgery and will resolve in time.

Frequent problems encountered by patients in the first 8 weeks after surgery were examined by Tack & Gilliss (1990). Nursing diagnosis was used to categorize the experiences. These included pain, ineffective coping, sleep pattern disturbance, altered nutrition and activity intolerance (Tack & Gilliss 1990). This can be coupled with a general lack of information prior to discharge regarding diet, exercise, return to driving and medication (Goodman 1997). Patients have also been shown to exhibit a range of psychological states ranging from apathy, depression and mood swings to more positive states such as euphoria at being alive and the lack of pre-operative symptoms (Goodman 1997). Depression is common after cardiac surgery and is more common in men than women (Rankin 1990, Vaska 1997b).

Patients require ongoing support following discharge to help them adjust and recover (Tack & Gilliss 1990). Expectations of self-efficacy in patients recovering from cardiac surgery can be influenced by inpatient education and enhanced by outpatient telephone contact after discharge and may be influenced by cardiac functional class after surgery (Gortner & Jenkins 1990). The use of an audiotape explaining expected physical symptoms and their management has been noted to provide a positive effect on patients' physical functioning at 1 month after surgery (Moore 1996). The tape can be given to the patient before discharge and taken home.

After-discharge care can be delivered in a variety of ways. Patients will be invited to attend cardiac rehabilitation groups, but these are not always accessed for a variety of reasons. As cardiac surgery is performed in regional centres rather than district hospitals, the patient may not be able to attend, quite simply due to distance. Other services have been developed in recent years to bridge this gap in the form of cardiac liaison nurses (see Chapter 31), some of whom act as a link between the surgical centre and the patient at home. Others will aim to bridge the gap between primary and secondary care. The emerging cardiac nurse-led clinics offer the opportunity for patients to further understand their disease process, additional treatment options available and how they can adapt their lifestyle to improve their health. The clinics also offer a valuable opportunity to monitor the subsequent effects of surgical and medical management and to adjust medications within agreed protocols (patient group directions).

CASE STUDIES

When caring for the postoperative patient nurses may be faced with a bewildering array of physiological assessment data to interpret. They need to be able to identify the causes of any abnormal observations and know what action to take. The following scenarios aim to clarify some of the problems nurses may face and identify the most appropriate treatment.

Case study 22.1

Mrs Khan is a 72-year-old woman recovering from aortic valve replacement. This was a tissue valve plus internal mammary artery (IMA) graft to the left anterior descending artery. She has two drains in place, one mediastinal and one in the left pleural space. She is being mechanically ventilated. Her recorded clinical observations are:

- heart rate 126 bpm
- rhythm: atrial fibrillation (AF) (long standing)
- blood pressure (BP) 78/47 mmHg
- mean arterial pressure (MAP) 42 mmHg
- right atrial/central venous pressure 14 mmHg
- respiratory rate 12 breaths per minute
- lung auscultation: widespread crackles at the bases
- oxygen saturations via pulse oximetry: 87%
- FiO_2 0.5 (50%)
- urine output 14 ml/h (patient weight: 50 kg)

- temperature 34.8°C
- chest drainage <50 ml in the past 2 hours
- haemoglobin 8.7 g/dl.

Clinical discussion
In this example, Mrs Khan appears to show signs of poor cardiac function: very low BP and MAP, raised right atrial/central venous pressure and a tachyarrhythmia. She also has signs of impaired respiratory function: a low peripheral oxygen saturation, despite a high fraction of inspired oxygen. Abnormal breath sounds can be heard.

The nurse needs to identify the causes of these problems and plan the possible interventions. A low blood pressure can be caused by a number of conditions:

- bleeding
- underfilling of intravenous fluid

Case study 22.1 *continued*

- impaired myocardial contractility
- arrhythmia(s)
- the transducer level above the patient's mid-axilla point (or where the unit regards the zero point).

Mrs Khan is experiencing AF, which will reduce her cardiac output by up to 30%, due to the loss of AV synchrony. Although her arrhythmia is long standing, her ventricular rate is fast. This rate may be contributing to her low BP, reducing the diastolic filling time even further. However, it could also be a sign that her body's compensatory mechanisms are trying to maintain an adequate BP.

Her right atrial pressure (RAP) is higher than normal and coupled with the minimal wound drainage and adequate haemoglobin levels, rules out bleeding and underfilling as a cause of her low BP. Impaired myocardial contractility is the likely cause of Mrs Khan's

low BP in this example. Other evidence to support this are her reduced urine output and low core temperature, which reflect reduced renal and peripheral perfusion. The low oxygen saturation and abnormal breath sounds are likely to be due to pulmonary oedema as a result of impaired cardiac pumping.

Mrs Khan's filling pressures (RAP/CVP) are already at an unacceptably high level, therefore intravenous fluids would be inappropriate and would quickly induce further cardiac failure. Inotropic therapy is now required to augment the cardiac output and improve the blood pressure and myocardial contractility. She may also require nitrate therapy to dilate her peripherally, to reduce the venous return. This would allow her heart to pump less blood more effectively and also reduce her pulmonary congestion. However, the recorded BP must be monitored carefully, to prevent an undue drop.

Case study 22.2

Mr Butt is a 41-year-old man recovering from bilateral IMA grafting. He has three chest drains in place: one mediastinal and one in each pleural space. He is self-ventilating. His clinical observations are:

- heart rate 114 bpm
- rhythm: sinus tachycardia
- blood pressure 81/40 mmHg
- mean arterial pressure 54 mmHg
- right atrial/central venous pressure 1 mmHg
- respiratory rate: 16 breaths per minute
- lung auscultation: slight crackles at both bases
- oxygen saturation via pulse oximetry: 97%
- FiO_2 0.4 (40%)
- urine output 15 ml/h (patient weight: 74 kg)
- temperature 35.7°C

- chest drainage <30 ml in past hour
- haemoglobin 6.4 g/dl.

Clinical discussion
Mr Butt has a low BP and inadequate MAP, as evidenced by his reduced urine output, the cause of which needs to be identified. He is tachycardic and this could be either a cause (reduced diastolic filling time) or a response (a compensatory rate increase). His wound drainage is acceptable but his RAP is lower than normal, suggesting that he is underfilled. He appears to need filling because he has no other signs of cardiac dysfunction and his respiratory observations are also satisfactory. A decision needs to be made regarding whether to use colloid or blood. A look at his haemoglobin reveals an Hb level of 6.4 g/dl and so he should be given a unit of blood and then his clinical status re-assessed.

CONCLUSION

This chapter has reviewed the most common types of cardiac surgery occurring in the United Kingdom, with the associated care and the factors which may complicate recovery. Cardiac surgery is an area of increasing technological change, which presents challenges to all nurses working within this area. The numbers of individuals awaiting surgery is at present still rising and there is a challenge to be met in patients who have complex problems and are sicker than those presenting in the past. Newer surgical techniques, which are discussed throughout this textbook, offer hope to these patients with chronic and acute heart failure. The challenge for nursing is the need to continue to develop new and innovative ways of meeting the requirements, both physical and psychological, of cardiac surgical patients and their loved ones.

REFERENCES

Adams S 1991 Causes of PPD. Nursing 4(26): 9–12
Adamson R, Daily P, Dans N et al 1994 Effect of prophylactic epsilon-aminocaproic acid on blood loss and transfusion requirements in patients undergoing first-time coronary artery bypass grafting. A randomized, prospective, double-blind study. Journal of Thoracic and Cardiovascular Surgery 108(1): 99–106

Akins CW, Daggett WM, Vlahakes GJ et al 1997 Cardiac operations in patients 80 years and older. Annals of Thoracic Surgery 64: 606–614
Bathgate A, Irving J 1997 Ten year follow up of patients referred for coronary artery bypass grafting from a single district general hospital. Heart 78: 584–586

Beekmann-Ball G, Grap M 1992 Postoperative GI symptoms in cardiac surgery patients. Critical Care Nurse 12(1): 56–62

Bell P, Diffee G Jr 1991 Cardiopulmonary bypass. Association of Operating Room Nurses Journal 53(6): 1480–1496

Ben-Shlomo Y, Chaturvedi N 1995 Assessing equity in health care provision in the UK: does where you live affect your chances of getting a coronary artery bypass graft? Journal of Epidemiology and Community Health 49: 200–204.

BHF 2000 Coronary heart disease statistics database: annual compendium. British Heart Foundation, London

Bidstrup BP, Harrison J, Royston D, Taylor KM, Treasure T 1993 Aprotinin therapy in cardiac operations: a report on use in 41 cardiac centres in the United Kingdom. Annals of Thoracic Surgery 55(4): 971–976

BNF 2001 The British National Formulary, 41st edn. British Medical Association and the Royal Pharmaceutical Society of Great Britain, London

Bridgewater B, Neve H, Moat N, Hooper T, Jones M 1998 Predicting operative risk for coronary artery surgery in the United Kingdom: a comparison of various risk prediction algorithms. Heart 79(4): 350–355

Brooks-Brunn J 1995 Postoperative atelectasis and pneumonia. Heart and Lung 24(2): 94–115

Brzozowski L 1995 Myocardial protection during cardiac surgery. American Association of Critical-Care Nurses (AACN) Clinical Issues 6(3): 398–403

CABRI Trial Participants 1995 First year results of CABRI (Coronary Angioplasty versus Bypass Revascularisation Investigation). Lancet 346: 1179–1189

Caine N, Sharples LD, Wallwork J 1999 Prospective study of health related quality of life before and after coronary artery bypass grafting: outcome at five years. Heart 81(4): 347–351

Calhoun Thomson S, Wells S, Maxwell M 1997 Chest tube removal after cardiac surgery. Critical Care Nurse 17(1): 34–38

Cameron A, Davies K, Green G, Schaff H 1996 Coronary bypass surgery with internal-thoracic-artery grafts – effects on survival over a 15-year period. New England Journal of Medicine 334: 216–219

Carrascal Y, Guerrero AL, Maroto LC et al 1999 Neurological complications after cardiopulmonary bypass: an update. European Neurology 41(3): 128–134

Carroll KC, Reeves LM, Anderson G et al 1998 Risks associated with removal of ventricular epicardial pacing wires after cardiac surgery. American Journal of Critical Care 7(6): 444–449

Child AH, Briggs M 2001 The Marfan syndrome: a clinical guide. British Heart Foundation, London

Conlon PJ, Stafford-Smith M, White WD et al 1999 Acute renal failure following cardiac surgery. Nephrology, Dialysis, Transplantation 14(5): 1158–1162

Cooley D 1995 Conservation of blood during cardiovascular surgery. American Journal of Surgery 170 (suppl): 53–59

Covington H 1998 Use of propofol for sedation in the ICU. Critical Care Nurse 18(4): 34–39

Crosby L, Palarski VA, Cottington E, Cmolik B 1994 Iron supplementation for acute blood loss after coronary artery bypass surgery: a randomized, placebo-controlled study. Heart and Lung 23(6): 493–499

Danchin N, Retournay G, Stchepinsky O et al 1999 Comparison of long term outcome in patients with or without aortic ring abscess treated surgically for aortic valve infective endocarditis. Heart 81: 177–181

Daoud E, Strickberger S, Man K et al 1997 Preoperative amiodarone as prophylaxis against atrial fibrillation after heart surgery. New England Journal of Medicine 337(25): 1785–1791

Del Rizzo DF, Nishimura S, Lau C, Sever J, Goldman BS 1996 Cardiac pacing following surgery for acquired heart disease. Journal of Cardiac Surgery 11(5): 332–340

Dietl C, Madigan N, Menapace F et al 1993 Results of coronary artery bypass grafting using multiple arterial conduits. Journal of Cardiovascular Surgery 34: 513–516

Doering L 1997 Relationship of age, sex and procedure type to extubation outcome after heart surgery. Heart and Lung 26: 439–447

Doering L, Imperial-Perez F, Monsein S, Esmailian F 1998 Preoperative predictors of early and delayed extubation after coronary artery bypass surgery. American Journal of Critical Care 7(1): 37–44

Duncan C, Erickson R 1982 Pressures associated with chest tube stripping. Heart and Lung 11: 166–171

Dunstan J, Riddle M 1997 Rapid recovery management. The effects on the patient who has undergone heart surgery. Heart and Lung 26(4): 289–298

Dziadulewicz L, Shannon-Stone M 1995 Postpericardiotomy syndrome: a complication of cardiac surgery. American Association of Critical-Care Nurses (AACN) Clinical Issues 6(3): 464–470

Earp J, Mallia G 1997 Myocardial protection for cardiac surgery: the nursing perspective. American Association of Critical-Care Nurses (AACN) Clinical Issues 8(1): 20–32

Edwards D, Hess L 1996 Aggressive weaning in cardiac surgical patients. Dimensions of Critical Care Nursing 15(4): 181–186

Edwards MB, Taylor KM 1999 A profile of valve replacement surgery in the UK (1986–1997): a study from the UK Heart Valve Registry. Journal of Heart Valve Disease 8(6): 697–701

Ellis M 1997 Low cardiac output following cardiac surgery: critical thinking steps. Dimensions of Critical Care Nursing 16(1): 48–55

Ellis M 1998 Atrial fibrillation following cardiac surgery. Dimensions of Critical Care Nursing 17(5): 226–239

Ferguson J, Gilroy D, Puntillo K 1997 Dimensions of pain and analgesic administration associated with coronary artery bypass grafting in an Australian intensive care unit. Journal of Advanced Nursing 26: 1065–1072

Fransen E, Maessen J, Dentener M, Buurman W 1999 Impact of blood transfusions on inflammatory mediator release in patients undergoing cardiac surgery. Chest 116(5): 1233–1239

Gallo J, Todd B 1990 Mediastinitis after cardiac surgery. Critical Care Nurse 10(6): 64–68

Gift A, Spearing Bolgiano C, Cunningham J 1991 Sensations during chest drain removal. Heart and Lung 20: 131–137

Glenville B 1999 Minimally invasive cardiac surgery (editorial). British Medical Journal 319: 135–136

Godden J, Hiley C 1998 Managing the patient with a chest drain: a review. Nursing Standard 12(32): 35–39

Goodman H 1997 Patients' perceptions of their education needs in the first six weeks following discharge after cardiac surgery. Journal of Advanced Nursing 25: 1241–1251

Goodnough L, Brecher M, Kantner M, Aubuchon J 1999 Transfusion medicine. Part II Blood conservation. New England Journal of Medicine 340(7): 525–533

Gordon RS, Ivanov J, Cohen G, Ralph-Edwards AL 1998 Permanent cardiac pacing after a cardiac operation: predicting the use of permanent pacemakers. Annals of Thoracic Surgery 66(5): 1698–1704

Gortner S, Jenkins L 1990 Self-efficacy and activity level following cardiac surgery. Journal of Advanced Nursing 15: 1132–1138

Gott V, Greene P, Alejo D et al 1999 Replacement of the aortic root in patients with Marfan's syndrome. New England Journal of Medicine 340: 1307–1313

Hancock H 1996 The complexity of pain assessment and management in the first 24 hours after cardiac surgery: implications for nurses Part 1. Intensive and Critical Care Nursing 12: 295–302

Hinds CJ, Watson D 1996 Intensive care: a concise textbook, 2nd edn. WB Saunders, London

Hirvela ER 2000 Advances in the management of acute respiratory distress syndrome: protective ventilation. Archives of Surgery 135(2): 126–135

Hogue CW Jr, Murphy SF, Schechtman KB, Davila-Roman VG 1999 Risk factors for early or delayed stroke after cardiac surgery. Circulation 100(6): 642–647

Holl R 1995 Surgical cardiac patient characteristics and the amount of analgesics administered in the intensive care unit after extubation. Intensive and Critical Care Nursing 11: 192–197

Holtzclaw B 1986 Postoperative shivering after cardiac surgery: a review. Heart and Lung 15(3): 292–300

Howell RD, MacRae LD, Sanjines S, Burke J, De Stefano P 1992 Effects of two types of head coverings in the rewarming of patients after coronary artery bypass graft surgery. Heart and Lung 21(1): 1–5

Hussey LC, Leeper B 1998 Sternal wound infection: a case study of a devastating postoperative complication. Critical Care Nurse 18(1): 31–39

Ingersoll G, Grippi M 1991 Preoperative pulmonary status and postoperative extubation outcome of patients undergoing elective cardiac surgery. Heart and Lung 20(2): 137–143

Johnson L, McMahan M 1997 Postoperative factors contributing to prolonged length of stay in cardiac surgery patients. Dimensions of Critical Care Nursing 16(5): 243–250

Kavanagh R, Radhakrishnan D, Park G 1995 Crystalloids and colloids in the critically ill patient. Care of the Critically Ill 11(3): 114–119

Keresztes P, Kuruzar L 1996 Very early extubation: extubating in the OR following coronary artery bypass. Dimensions of Critical Care Nursing 15(4): 198–204

King K, Rowe M, Kimble L, Zerwic J 1998 Optimism, coping and long-term recovery from coronary artery surgery in women. Research in Nursing and Health 21: 15–26

Knapp-Spooner C, Yarcheski A 1992 Sleep patterns and stress in patients having coronary bypass. Heart and Lung 21(4): 342–349

Kuo J, Butchart E 1995 Sternal wound dehiscence. Care of the Critically Ill 11(6): 238–244

Kronick-Mest C 1989 Postpericardiotomy syndrome: etiology, manifestations and interventions. Heart and Lung 18(2): 192–197

Lear J, Lawrence I, Burden A et al 1994 A comparison of stress test referral rates and outcome between Asians and Europeans. Journal of Research into Social Medicine 87: 661–662

Lepczyk M, Raleigh EH, Rowley C 1990 Timing of preoperative patient teaching. Journal of Advanced Nursing 15: 300–306

Ley S 1996 Intraoperative and postoperative blood salvage. American Association of Critical-Care Nurses (AACN) Clinical Issues 7(2): 238–248

Ley S, Miller K, Skov P, Preisig P 1990 Crystalloid versus colloid fluid therapy after cardiac surgery. Heart and Lung 19(1): 31–40

Liehr P, Todd B, Rossi M, Culligan M 1992 Effect of venous support on edema and leg pain after coronary artery bypass graft surgery. Heart and Lung 21: 6–11

Lindsay M 1999 Cerebral vascular accident after cardiac surgery: its impact on nursing care. Progress in Cardiovascular Nursing 14(2): 47–52

Lindsay P, Sherrard H, Bickerton L, Doucette P, Harkness C, Morin J 1997 Educational and support needs of patients and their families awaiting cardiac surgery. Heart and Lung 26(6): 458–465

Loop FD 1996 Internal-thoracic-artery grafts: biologically better coronary arteries (editorial). New England Journal of Medicine 334(4): 263–265

Lynn-McHale D, Riggs K, Thurman L 1991 Epicardial pacing after cardiac surgery. Critical Care Nurse 11(8): 62–77

Magnusson L, Zemgulis V, Wicky S, Tyden H, Thelin S, Hedenstierna G 1997 Atelectasis is a major cause of hypoxia and shunt after cardiopulmonary bypass: an experimental study. Anesthesiology 87(5): 1153–1163

Manion P 1993 Temporary epicardial pacing in the post-operative cardiac surgery patient. Critical Care Nurse 13(2): 30–37

Mannucci P 1998 Hemostatic drugs. New England Journal of Medicine 339: 245–253

Marggraf G, Splittgerber F, Knox M, Reidemeister J 1999 Mediastinitis after cardiac surgery – epidemiology and current treatment. European Journal of Surgery 584 (suppl): 12–16

Mizell JL, Maglish BL, Matheny RG 1997 Minimally invasive direct coronary artery bypass graft surgery. Introduction for critical care nurses. Critical Care Nurse 17(3): 46–55

Moore S 1996 The effects of a discharge information intervention on recovery outcomes following coronary artery bypass surgery. International Journal of Nursing Studies 33(2): 181–189

Nashef SA, Roques F, Michel P, Gauducheau E, Lemeshow S, Salamon R 1999 European system for cardiac operative risk evaluation (EuroSCORE). European Journal of Cardiothoracic Surgery 16(1): 9–13

NHS Centre for Reviews and Dissemination (NHSCRD) 1997 Management of stable angina. Effective Health Care 3(5): 1–8

Noll M, Byers J 1995 Usefulness of measures of SVO2, SPO2, vital signs and derived dual oximetry parameters as indicators of arterial blood gas variables during weaning of cardiac surgery patients from mechanical ventilation. Heart and Lung 24: 220–227

Ommen S, Odell J, Stanton M 1997 Atrial arrhythmias after cardiothoracic surgery. New England Journal of Medicine 336(20): 1429–1434

Parsonnet V, Dean D, Bernstein A 1989 A method of uniform stratification of risk for evaluating the results of surgery in acquired adult heart disease. Circulation 79 (suppl): 3–12

Petticrew M, McKee M, Jones J 1993 Coronary artery surgery: are women discriminated against? British Medical Journal 306: 1164–1166

Phillips R 1997 Alterations in cardiac effort and oxygenation during shivering after cardiac surgery. Seminars in Perioperative Nursing 6(3): 176–184

Phillips R, Skov P 1988 Rewarming and cardiac surgery: a review. Heart and Lung 17(5): 511–520

Pierce J, Piazza D, Naftel D 1991 Effects of two chest tube clearance protocols on drainage in patients after myocardial revascularization surgery. Heart and Lung 20: 125–130

Poloniecki J, Valencia O, Littlejohns P 1998 Cumulative risk adjusted mortality chart for detecting changes in death rate: observational study of heart surgery. British Medical Journal 316: 1697–1700

Prêtre R, Turina M 2000 Valve disease. Cardiac surgery in the octogenarian. Heart 83(1): 116–121

Puntillo K 1990 Pain experiences of intensive care unit patients. Heart and Lung 19: 526–534

Pym J, Brown P, Pearson M, Parker J 1995 Right gastroepiploic to coronary bypass – the first decade of use. Circulation 92: II-45–II-49

Pym J, Luffman B, Parry M 1997 Total arterial revascularization of the heart: intentional or inevitable. American Association of Critical-Care Nurses (AACN) Clinical Issues 8(1): 9

Rankin S 1990 Differences in recovery from cardiac surgery: a profile of male and female patients. Heart and Lung 19: 481–485

Robb J 1997 Physiological changes that occur with positive pressure ventilation: part one. Intensive and Critical Care Nursing 13: 293–307

Romand JA, Donald F 1995 Physiological effects of continuous positive airway pressure (CPAP) ventilation in the critically ill. Care of the Critically Ill 11(6): 239–243

Rooney P 1996 Anaesthesia for cardiac surgery. British Journal of Theatre Nursing 6(6): 9–12

Roques F, Nashef SA, Michel P et al 1999 Risk factors and outcome in European cardiac surgery: analysis of the EuroSCORE multinational database of 19030 patients. European Journal of Cardiothoracic Surgery 15(6): 816–822

Rosen A, Humphries J, Muhlbaier L et al 1999 Effect of clinical factors on length of stay after coronary artery bypass surgery: results of the Cooperative Cardiovascular Project. American Heart Journal 138(1 part 1): 69–77

Rowe M, King K 1998 Long-term chest wall discomfort in women after coronary artery bypass grafting. Heart and Lung 27(3): 184–188

Salipante D 1998 Refusal of blood by a critically ill patient: a healthcare challenge. Critical Care Nurse 18(2): 68–76

Segatore M, Dutkiewicz M, Adams D 1998 The delirious cardiac surgical patient: theoretical aspects and principles of management. Journal of Cardiovascular Nursing 12(4): 32–48

Seyfer A, Shriver C, Miller T, Graeber G 1988 Sternal blood flow after median sternotomy and mobilization of the internal mammary arteries. Surgery 104: 899–904

Spyrou N, Anderson M, Foale R 1997 Listeria endocarditis: current management and patient outcome – world literature review. Heart 77(4): 380–383

Staples J, Ramsay J 1997 Advances in anesthesia for cardiac surgery: an overview for the 1990's. American Association of Critical-Care Nurses (AACN) Clinical Issues 8(1): 41–49

Stone K, Talaganis S, Preusser B, Gonyon D 1991 Effect of lung hyperinflation and endotracheal suctioning on heart rate and rhythm in patients after coronary artery bypass graft surgery. Heart and Lung 20: 443–450

Tack B, Gilliss C 1990 Nurse-monitored cardiac recovery: a description of the first 8 weeks. Heart and Lung 19 (5 part 1): 491–499

Tucker LA 1993 Post-pump delirium. Intensive and Critical Care Nursing 9(4): 269–273

Vaca K, Daake C, Lambrechts D 1997 Nursing care of patients undergoing thorascopic minimally invasive bypass grafting. American Journal of Critical Care 6(4): 281–286

Vaska P 1997a Cardiac surgery in special populations, part 2: women, pregnant patients and Jehovah's Witnesses. American Association of Critical-Care Nurses (AACN) Clinical Issues 8(1): 59–66

Vaska P 1997b Cardiac surgery in special populations, part 1: octogenarians, patients with neuropsychiatric disorders, and Blacks. American Association of Critical-Care Nurses (AACN) Clinical Issues 8(1): 50–58

Walton J, Westrope P 1996 Stunned myocardium: theoretical mechanisms of injury. Critical Care Nurse 16(2): 23–28

Westaby S 2000 Development of surgery of the heart and great vessels. In: Morris PJ, Wood WC (eds) Oxford textbook of surgery, vol 2, section 40.1. Oxford University Press, Oxford, pp. 2151–2159

Wolff C, Scott C, Banks T 1997 The radial artery: an exciting conduit in coronary artery bypass surgery. Critical Care Nurse 17(5): 34–39

Woodman R 1999 Cardiac surgery audit raises concern over equity of access. British Medical Journal 319: 277

Young M 1988 Malnutrition and wound healing. Heart and Lung 17(1): 60–67

23

Cardiac transplantation

*Wendy Cox**

Cardiac transplantation has developed rapidly during the last two decades in the United Kingdom (UK), establishing itself as a highly effective procedure for the management of severe refractory cardiac failure (De Maria et al 1996). Transplantation is largely confined to the Western world due to both cost and the cultural acceptance of brainstem death and transplant surgery (Shaw et al 1991). In 1990 approximately 3500 cardiac transplants were performed during the year worldwide (Large 1995) but due to limited donor organ supply, this figure is unlikely to increase. In the UK in 1997–8, 270 cardiac transplants occurred (BHF 2000).

This chapter explores the expanding scope of cardiac transplantation, examining the preparation for transplant with the need for planned and considered support for the patient and their loved ones. The issue of rejection, which many patients fear, is discussed in detail, together with the current drug regimens designed to reduce the risk and deal with its occurrence. The specific nursing care necessary in the immediate postoperative period is explored.

Cardiac transplantation offers a relatively low risk of death to the patient, with figures of 10–20% in the first year (Hosenpud et al 1997). It is also estimated that it offers a greater than 50% chance of surviving 11 years post transplantation and once the first year has passed there is a constant annual mortality of 4% (Hosenpud et al 1997). The current level of success is primarily attributed to advances in immunosuppressant therapy, antimicrobial agents, methods of detecting rejection and organ procurement and preservation (Muirhead 1992).

*Case study contributions from Sherrie Panther, Senior Sister, and Sheilagh Vidler, former Senior Nurse Manager, Transplant Unit, Harefield Hospital, Middlesex.

METHODS OF CARDIAC TRANSPLANTATION

There are two main surgical procedures in cardiac transplantation, both performed via a medial sternotomy.

Orthotopic transplantation

This more familiar surgical technique for cardiac transplantation was introduced by Shumway & Lower in 1964. The recipient's heart is removed and the donor heart is implanted. This will involve anastomosis of the donor atria to remnants of the recipient's atria (Fig. 23.1). More recently a new surgical technique has been introduced within some centres (Trento et al 1996). This new 'bicaval' technique for cardiac transplantation involves total excision of the heart with no recipient atria remaining. It has yet to be adopted generally, but it is hoped that the technique will help to reduce arrhythmia problems in the postoperative period.

Heterotopic transplantation

With this technique, a small donor heart is placed in the right side of the chest alongside the patient's own heart. This allows the optimum use of organs, as it utilizes a heart that would perhaps not otherwise be used if there were no suitable paediatric recipient. It can also be a life-saving opportunity in the critically ill patient (Cowell et al 1994) (Fig. 23.2). The transplanted heart functions in a similar fashion to a ventricular assist device, for the recipient's failing heart.

Indications for using this approach over the more traditional orthotopic approach include:

- elevated pulmonary vascular resistance
- a great degree of mismatch between donor and recipient body size, i.e. a 20% variant
- where there is a possibility of a useful recovery of the recipient's own heart. This usually involves simultaneous coronary artery bypass grafting. Contra-indications to heterotopic cardiac transplantation include intractable angina and persistent cardiac arrhythmias.

Due to the advent of increasingly successful means of bridging to transplantation, both with inotropes and mechanical assist devices, as well as the success of the domino procedure, heterotopic transplantation is now rarely performed.

Domino procedure

A high pulmonary vascular resistance (PVR) is an absolute contra-indication to orthotopic cardiac transplantation. This is because it would normally lead to acute right ventricular failure after transplantation, due to the transplanted heart being unable to cope with the high back pressure. In a patient with borderline PVR it is possible to use a heart with a hypertrophied right ventricle. This usually comes from a patient with cystic fibrosis who is receiving a

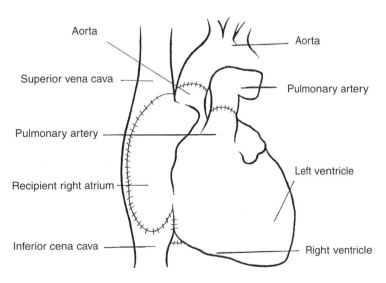

Figure 23.1 Orthotopic transplant.

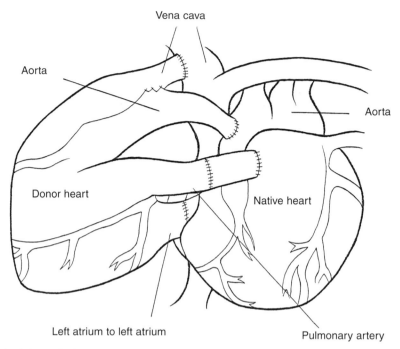

Figure 23.2 Heterotopic transplant.

heart–lung transplantation and where the right side of the heart has become accustomed to a greater workload, pumping blood into less compliant lungs. This is known as the domino procedure.

THE TRANSPLANT ASSESSMENT

Cardiac conditions requiring transplantation

The predominant indications for adult cardiac transplantation are cardiomyopathy and coronary artery disease. Each represents approximately equal numbers and together they account for the vast majority of cases. The percentage for each of these two diagnoses has varied from year to year, with cardiomyopathy representing the majority of cases in earlier years and coronary artery disease emerging in the late 1980s and early 1990s when the age criteria for transplantation were being expanded (Hosenpud et al 1997).

The indications for adult cardiac transplantation are:

- coronary artery disease
- cardiomyopathy

- valvular heart disease
- congenital heart disease
- retransplantation.

Details of all the above conditions may be found elsewhere in this book.

Congenital heart disease is the most common indication for paediatric cardiac transplantation and accounts for more than 75% of transplants in children less than 1 year old (Hosenpud et al 1997).

Assessment procedure and selection criteria

The aims of assessment for cardiac transplantation can be divided into three areas.

Clinical suitability for transplantation

Patients referred for cardiac transplantation are in end-stage cardiac failure, which can no longer be effectively treated either medically or surgically. The assessment procedure is vital to assess the patient's clinical suitability. The patient must be ill enough to require the transplant but be otherwise healthy enough to have a positive outcome (Allum 1998). The clinical assessment is essentially a series of tests (Box 23.1), following which the physicians and surgeons will discuss with the transplant team both the results and the patient's overall suitability (see Case study 23.2).

To inform the patient and family about transplantation and the associated risks and benefits

Transplant patients will have to offer informed consent to their operation, as with all forms of surgery and procedures. In order for this to be achieved, the benefits and risks of transplantation should be explained in detail, in simple language that the patient and family are able to understand (Thiroux 1995). The information given to patients in the assessment phase is summarized in Box 23.2. A senior member of the nursing/co-ordinating team will normally provide this information, with any additional information in writing.

To assess the support and psychological needs of the patient and family

Assessment for transplantation brings to the fore many suppressed feelings and emotions for patients and their family (Allum 1998). Patients who proceed through the process of transplantation are taken through an incredible series of events that begin with the proposal of the procedure and continue long after the operation. This process is accompanied by physical and psychological perils that require ongoing assessment and intervention.

Transplant nurses must not underestimate the stressors experienced during all stages of the process. The patient's ability to cope with the stressors that follow the transplant is an important factor in achieving the optimum quality of life. As well as medical problems, transplant patients may experience difficulties with body image, role change, family and marital stress, employment and financial issues as well as coping with a range of emotions (Kaba & Shanley 1997).

Implications for both the waiting period and post-transplantation lifestyle are therefore profound (Finkelmeier 1995). The commitment to undergo cardiac transplantation is a major undertaking that involves not only the recipient but also the entire family/carer support system. It is essential that the potential recipients realize that post transplantation they are still vulnerable to health problems and a new set can replace the old ones. It has also been suggested that the presence of a well-informed, supportive, caring partner throughout the transplant process correlates with the best outcome from surgery (Bunzel & Wollenek 1994).

It must also be remembered that whilst most patients are eager to be accepted onto the waiting list, some may actually decline. Some patients feel that they would rather continue as they are than take the risks associated with transplantation.

Box 23.3 indicates the general and specific cardiac criteria for transplantation, as well as the contra-indications.

THE PERIOD OF WAITING

Patients and families frequently report that the wait for the transplant is their worst time. It has been suggested that anxiety and depression are common

---

Box 23.1 Evaluation for transplant assessment

- Chest X-ray
- Echocardiogram
- Renal function – 24-hour urine (creatinine clearance and protein excretion)
- Respiratory function test
- Angiogram (including pulmonary vascular resistance (PVR) measurement)
- Infection screen – midstream urine (MSU), nose and throat swab
- Dental examination
- Height
- Weight
- Virology screen – HIV, hepatitis B and C, cytomegalovirus, toxoplasmosis
- Blood group and tissue typing
- Blood for haematological and biochemical assessment
- 24-hour ECG tape
- HLA/panel reactive antibody screening
- Auto-immune screen (cardiomyopathy patients only)

Box 23.2 Summary of information given to patients suitable for cardiac transplantation

- Benefits and risks of transplantation
- Lifestyle/rehabilitation implications
- The waiting period
- Postoperative care
- Complications
- Rejection and infection
- Medications action and side-effects
- Outpatient care
- Advised to make a will
- Contact numbers
- Support group information

> **Box 23.3** General criteria and contra-indications for cardiac transplantation
>
> | *General criteria* | *Contra-indications* |
> |---|---|
> | End-stage cardiac disease | Active infection |
> | New York Heart Association (NYHA) class III–IV | Irreversible renal/hepatic dysfunction |
> | Age <60 | High-dose steroid therapy |
> | | Ongoing drug or alcohol addiction |
> | | Smoking |
> | | High pulmonary vascular resistance (PVR) |
> | | Malignancy |

symptoms during this waiting period (Muirhead et al 1992). The euphoria of being accepted onto the transplant waiting list is often superseded by the realization of an uncertain future and the continuing deterioration in their medical condition.

Patients can wait from days to years for a cardiac transplant and they are at the end stage of their disease. It is estimated that at least one-third of patients will die whilst waiting for transplant. It is this uncertainty that can make the waiting period such a stressful one and fear of death is the overwhelming factor for many (Porter et al 1991).

Nurses often say that they feel awkward and inadequate when dealing with patients in this waiting period. Transplant support groups can provide valuable contact with other people waiting for transplant and most transplant centres run such groups, facilitated by specialist nurses. The groups provide a forum for discussing fears and anxieties in a sensitive and supportive setting. However, the groups can cause anxieties. Patients who attend may die before they receive their transplant, causing understandable concern to the others. There is also a national Transplant Support Network, whose aim is to introduce any patient, carer or family member to others who have been through a similar experience. It has been set up to complement and extend the support already provided by professional staff.

It should also be recognized that whilst every effort is made to allow patients to remain at home whilst waiting, sometimes they will require hospitalization to stabilize their condition. Occasionally patients require intensive support with the use of inotropes, intra-aortic balloon pumps or even ventricular assist devices. Caring for hospitalized pretransplant patients presents enormous challenges to nurses, both with the intensive nursing involved and with the psychological care of the patient and their family in such an uncertain time.

THE ROLE OF THE TRANSPLANT CO-ORDINATOR

Donor transplant co-ordinators are employed in every region of the UK to educate nurses and other health professionals as well as the public. All transplant co-ordinators liaise with the UK Transplant Support Service Authority (UKTSSA), based in Bristol, which runs a round-the-clock organ-matching and allocation service. Computerized data on all donors and clinical information about every patient waiting for a transplant are stored there. It is this service which contacts the recipient transplant co-ordinator at the transplant centre with details of a potential cardiac donor. Details about size, blood group and cytomegalovirus (CMV) status (antibodies formed by previous exposure to the CMV virus) are then matched with patients on the waiting list. All patients are ranked according to urgency. Transplants are not performed on a first-come first-served basis. Ultimately the transplant surgeon decides which patient is to receive the organ.

The recipient transplant co-ordinator is responsible for contacting the recipient, informing them of the offer and advising them to come to the hospital immediately. They are also responsible for organizing the organ retrieval team and co-ordinating the services at the transplant centre, such as theatre and pathology. The shorter the time between explant and implant, the more successful the transplant result. The ideal ischaemic time (the time from clamping of the aorta in donor hospital to unclamping in the recipient) should be no more than 4 hours with a cardiac transplant.

The transplant recipient, wishing to thank the donor family, often contacts the co-ordinator after the transplant. In such circumstances co-ordinators usually advise the recipients to contact the family by letter and can help with the wording. The letter will then be sent to the donor co-ordinator, who can forward it to the donor family. It has been well documented that families of organ donors gain comfort from the knowledge that their loved one's death has helped others (Snell 1997).

PRE-OPERATIVE PREPARATION

The patient is admitted for transplant preparation. Time is usually limited, as the organ retrieval team will already have been mobilized. Much of the recipient care is similar to that for any pre-operative cardiac patient (see Chapter 22). However, there are some important additions. These include infection screening and immunosuppression, both pre- and peri-operatively. The immunosuppression is calculated according to specific blood results and body weight.

POSTOPERATIVE PHASE

The immediate care following cardiac transplantation is undertaken in the intensive care unit (ICU) and is similar to that for other patients having undergone cardiac surgery (Kirk et al 1993) (see Chapter 22). Bleeding is likely because of pre-operative coagulopathy due to liver congestion and the effects of cardiopulmonary bypass. Pre-operative anticoagulant therapy and adhesion from previous surgery (for example, coronary artery bypass grafts) can also increase the risk of bleeding. Occasionally patients return to theatre for exploration of continual bleeding and require multiple transfusions with blood and blood products.

Renal function is often abnormal due to prolonged poor cardiac output and is exacerbated by cardiopulmonary bypass and the immunosuppressent ciclosporin, which is nephrotoxic. Despite current thinking, dopamine is usually given at a low dose to improve or sustain renal function, through dilatation of the vasculature in the kidney. Careful assessment of fluid balance is imperative. Haemofiltration is occasionally required in the initial postoperative phase.

Hyperkalaemia (high serum potassium) is poorly tolerated following cardiac transplantation. This is believed to be due to myocardial stunning and the effects of cardioplegia, the solution used to arrest the heart during transportation and surgery. Ciclosporin can induce hyperkalaemia, especially when serum levels are high or there is a degree of renal impairment. Potassium supplements are not routinely administered with diuretics.

As highlighted, care of a patient following cardiac transplantation is essentially the same as with more familiar open heart surgery. Many cardiac nurses frequently expect to be nursing transplant patients in isolation. However, protective isolation procedures have not been shown to have an impact on reducing the incidence of infection after heart transplantation (Wagoner 1997). Reverse barrier nursing is therefore no longer routinely performed. However, there are unique problems associated with the prevention, detection and treatment of rejection and infection.

Before discussing these in detail, the altered physiology and pharmacological responses of the transplanted heart will be addressed.

ALTERED PHYSIOLOGY

The orthotopic surgical procedure results in complete denervation of the nervous system of the transplanted heart, thereby depriving the heart of the important neural regulating mechanisms. Following the abolition of the usually dominant inhibitory vagal influences, the resting heart rate of the transplanted organ is generally higher than normal. The loss of vagal tone also alters the body's response to neurally mediated factors such as the Valsalva manoeuvre, carotid sinus massage, body position changes or neurally mediated drugs (Muirhead 1992), such as atropine.

The primary haemodynamic mechanisms of the transplanted heart are different from those of a normally innervated heart. The loss of direct stimulation requires a dependence on other mechanisms to support the circulation. The transplanted heart relies on preload augmentation for optimal contractility. It is also dependent on the effects of circulating catecholamines to maintain cardiac output by increasing heart rate and contractility. However, the maximum response to catecholamine receptor site stimulation in the denervated heart is less than the response produced by direct neural stimulation combined with catecholamine receptor effects in the innervated heart.

Postoperative myocardial function may be compromised as a result of factors such as surgical manipulation and the ischaemic time. Denervation does not allow the heart to compensate fully for acute changes in function. Myocardial dysfunction may respond to inotropic support until the transplanted heart recovers. The drug of choice tends to be isoprenaline as it is a pure β-agonist that will directly stimulate the β adrenergic receptors of the transplanted heart.

Stimulation of the β-sites results in an increase in heart rate and contractility and therefore an increase in cardiac output. Occasionally an intra-aortic balloon pump (IABP) or a ventricular assist device may be required during the initial postoperative phase.

The need for continued chronotropic support (stimulating the heart rate) after the patient has been weaned off the isoprenaline may be met by pacing the heart via epicardial wires. These wires pose an infection risk and cease to be effective in the long term. In this situation, a temporary wire or permanent system may be utilized.

ELECTROPHYSIOLOGY OF THE TRANSPLANTED HEART

Following surgery, the native sino-atrial (SA) node remains attached to the donor heart. It remains innervated and maintains its inherent automaticity. The electrical impulse produced by the native SA node is evident on the ECG as an extra P-wave (Fig. 23.3). This impulse will depolarize the native atrial remnant but will not cross the atrial suture line and is not responsible for the depolarization of the donor heart. The donor heart's SA node maintains its property of automaticity and is able to initiate a sinus impulse spontaneously. This sinus impulse is then conducted throughout the donor heart and depolarizes the myocardium, resulting in mechanical contraction. The donor heart's atrial contraction will produce a P-wave on the ECG that is related to the QRS complex.

Although it is generally accepted that the transplanted heart remains denervated, evidence suggests the possibility of partial reinnervation (Fitzpatrick et al 1993). Major electrophysiologic characteristics of the transplanted heart have significant implications for nursing practice. The loss of the aforementioned vagal influence results in an increased resting heart rate that is believed to be the heart's true intrinsic rate (Thompson 1995). The normal heart rate for the cardiac transplant recipient is 90–110 bpm (Kirk et al 1993). Thus tachycardia of the donor heart within this range is expected and does not indicate decreased cardiac output or myocardial dysfunction.

Psychological stress has been shown to produce a cardiovascular response in transplanted hearts (Thompson 1995). Thus the nurse should be aware that psychological stressors can produce a potentially detrimental cardiovascular response.

Arrhythmias

Arrhythmias are common in the immediate postoperative period due to the handling of the donor heart and oedema of the suture line (Williams & Sandiford-Guttenbeil 1991). The loss of vagal tone and myocardial catecholamine stores, along with what is known as the denervation supersensitivity phenomenon,

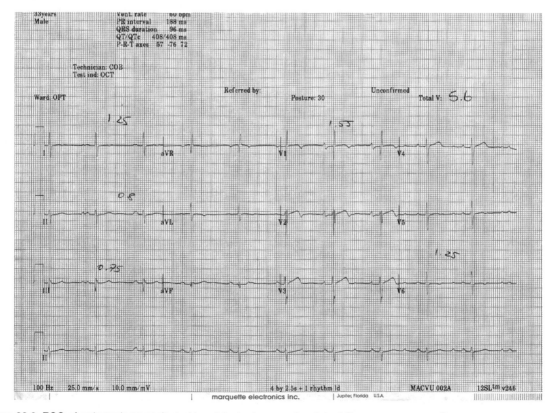

Figure 23.3 ECG of orthotopic transplanted heart (note donor and recipient P-waves are present).

increases the arrhythmogenic potential of the transplanted heart (Kirk et al 1993). Rejection episodes commonly manifest as arrhythmias, especially atrial in nature. When this occurs, treatment according to the antirejection protocol (see later) usually results in resolution of the rhythm disturbance.

Pharmacological agents effective in treating atrial arrhythmias, if rejection has been excluded, include procainamide and verapamil, as they exert their antiarrhythmic properties through a direct action on the myocardium.

Intravenous administration of digoxin to control a rapid ventricular rate will be ineffective in the denervated heart. The electrophysiologic effect of digoxin is to increase the refractory period of the SA node, thus decreasing conduction through the node. However, this effect is mediated through the parasympathetic nervous system and therefore has no immediate effect on the transplanted heart (Thompson 1995). Likewise, the loss of vagal tone influence in the heart makes atropine ineffective, as it inhibits parasympathetic stimulation, decreasing vagal tone and thus increasing heart rate. As highlighted, isoprenaline or pacing is the treatment of choice for bradycardia in the transplanted heart. It is essential that the nurse is aware of this in an emergency situation.

RESPONSE TO EXERCISE

The patient's response to exercise is affected by denervation. Normally any increase in oxygen demand is met by an immediate increase in heart rate. However, this action is a result of direct innervation and therefore does not occur in the transplanted heart, where all the nerves have been cut. The heart rate will gradually increase in response to circulating catecholamines, although it will never reach the peak rate seen in the normally innervated heart.

The reduced peak heart rate might be expected to be a limiting factor for cardiac output and exercise capacity after transplantation. However, the exercise capacity and peak heart rate of heart transplant recipients have been found to be similar to those of patients recovering from coronary artery bypass surgery and to those of patients undergoing medical therapy for heart failure (Banner 1992). At higher work loads, the stroke volume appears to plateau and this, combined with the blunted heart rate response, results in cardiac output falling below that of normal subjects (Banner 1992). Heart rate will also gradually decrease as a result of metabolism of catecholamines. Despite the lack of an immediate heart rate response, cardiac output can still increase rapidly due to an

enhanced Frank–Starling response (Starling's Law of the heart), increasing the stroke volume (Verani et al 1994) (see Chapter 18). Cardiac output and work capacity increase as a result of preload augmentation with intravenous fluids, to increase contractile force and thus maintain adequate tissue perfusion and oxygenation.

Contractility may also be enhanced owing to sensitivity to catecholamines and intrinsic contractile reserves (Thompson 1995). Administration of β-blockers accentuates the impairment in ventricular performance. Their use appears to be detrimental in the response to exercise, because ventricular performance during exercise increases principally through stimulation of the myocardial β-adrenergic receptors through circulating catecholamines (Verani et al 1994). The transplant patient should be encouraged to participate in regular exercise. The nurse's role involves recognizing the denervated heart's gradual response to exercise and emphasizing warm-up and cool-down exercises.

Many of the common complications after heart transplantation, such as infection, rejection, hypertension and hyperlipidaemia, have their greatest incidence during the first few months after transplantation, with a marked decrease in morbidity rates and complications after the first year (Brann et al 1998). Long-term clinical follow-up of the patient focuses on early diagnosis and treatment of complications and monitoring of immunosuppressive therapy. The following sections will deal with the important issues of rejection and infection. Rehabilitation/education are highlighted towards the end of the chapter and although all are separate issues it must be remembered that they are very much interdependent.

REJECTION

The success of transplantation is dependent on suppressing the recipient's immune system to minimize the risk of rejection. Yet there is still a need to maintain an adequate immune system to cope with infection.

The major histocompatibility complex (MHC) is the strongest immunological barrier to successful transplantation. It consists of a collection of polymorphic genes whose products are expressed at the cell surface. These antigens are important in the recognition of self and foreign antigens by lymphocytes. In humans, the genes are located on the short arm of chromosome 6 and are known as human leucocyte antigen (HLA) and labelled HLA A, B, C and DR. Since one copy of chromosome 6 is inherited from each parent, there is a one in four chance of siblings sharing identical HLA antigens (Dannie 1993). HLA/panel reactive antibody levels are determined during the assessment phase and if noted to be high, prospective crossmatching is performed between donor and recipient.

Rejection occurs because there are foreign antigens on and within the transplanted organ. An antigen is a foreign protein. A transplanted organ is recognized by the immune system as foreign because of antigens on the organ (Jackson 1991). Both antibody-mediated and T cell-mediated reactions are involved in graft rejection. Antibodies are directed against blood group antigens. These bind to graft tissue and cause complement-mediated lysis of the cells or they can direct cytotoxic macrophages or lymphocytes to attack the graft. Cell-mediated graft rejection is directed by CD4+ T-cells, which can activate macrophages at the graft site. Some may also be cytotoxic to graft cells (Brostoff & Male 1994).

To minimize the risk of graft rejection, immunosuppression is used. However, it is less effective after the initial lymphocyte response to an antigenic stimulus because this initial immune response triggers lymphocytic proliferation through the immune cascade system. In addition, activated T-cells release lymphokines critical to the events of rejection and are difficult to suppress. Therefore immunosuppression is best administered before the antigenic stimulus, that is, peri-operatively (Dannie 1993).

There are three distinct types of cardiac allograft rejection, hyperacute, acute and chronic, with distinct immunology. Each will be briefly discussed here with the nursing implications addressed.

Hyperacute rejection

Hyperacute rejection is defined as an immediate complication following cardiac transplantation, resulting in rejection and failure of the allografted organ within 24 hours (Rose 1993). It is understood to be due to pre-formed antibodies in the recipient, possibly due to previous transplantation, previous blood transfusions or pregnancy (Brostoff & Male 1994). All transplant assessment patients are screened for antibodies. Hyperacute rejection will present as failure of the graft when the patient is in theatre or the intensive care unit (Rose 1993). Prospective crossmatching (pre-operative crossmatching between donor and recipient) could help to avoid hyperacute rejection but due to the short ischaemic time required (less than 4 hours) this is not always possible, although attempts are being made to achieve this.

Acute rejection

Acute rejection remains the most important problem in the first 6 months after cardiac transplantation (Parameshwar 1996). Acute rejection is mediated by activated T-cells (CD4+) which have recognized differences in the HLA antigens. The activated T-cells then infiltrate the allograft. There is also some evidence to suggest that antibodies to the donor heart are made during acute rejection episodes. Antibodies and complement are believed to cause tissue damage and can be identified in biopsies of rejecting grafts (Rose 1993) (Plate 23.1).

Signs and symptoms of acute rejection

The clinical picture of acute rejection is unpredictable and will vary from the complete absence of symptoms to a patient presenting in acute heart failure. Symptoms may include fatigue, dyspnoea, weight gain, fluid retention and low-grade pyrexia. The electrocardiogram (ECG) may show a decrease in voltage (leads I, II, III, V1 and V6) and poor R-wave progression. Atrial arrhythmias are common. The echocardiogram may show poor ventricular wall motion and pericardial effusion. The ejection fraction (the fraction of blood in the ventricle ejected during systole) will also be reduced. There may be the presence of a third heart sound. An elevation of the jugular venous pressure can occur and sometimes a slight increase in the cardiothoracic ratio on chest X-ray will be noted.

Careful observation of the patient in the initial postoperative phase is a vital nursing role in order to detect the onset of acute rejection as early as possible. The patient will have temperature, apex pulse and blood pressure recorded 4 hourly and be maintained on strict fluid balance and daily weight. Gradually the patient will be educated to ensure that he or she is familiar with the symptoms of rejection for careful observation when at home. The medical team can therefore be alerted of any problems at the earliest opportunity.

Diagnosis

The most specific method for diagnosing acute rejection in the heart is by endomyocardial biopsy (Why 1991). Biopsies are performed with vascular access, usually via the right internal jugular vein. At least four sites in the right ventricle are biopsied to reduce the chance of a sampling error (Parameshwar 1996). Complications are rare and the biopsy can be performed as an outpatient procedure.

When such surveillance biopsies are performed, histological rejection is often seen in patients who are clinically well. Most transplant centres carry out routine surveillance biopsies in the first 12 months after transplantation. Initially they are performed weekly, then fortnightly, monthly and finally every 2–3 months depending on rejection episodes. The need for biopsies is assessed for each individual patient and they are generally only performed after the first year if clinically indicated. Patients who are treated for an episode of acute rejection are re-biopsied a week later to establish the adequacy of treatment.

Successful management of rejection requires prompt diagnosis and aggressive treatment in the transplant recipient (Muirhead 1992). Rejection episodes are expected and most patients will experience at least one within the first 3 months after transplantation. This is normally during the postoperative stay (Vlahakes et al 1994). It is important that the patient realizes this as it can come as a huge disappointment in a recovery with few apparent complications. It is essential that the transplant nurse reassures the patient that rejection episodes can normally be treated with a course of intravenous steroids and that the heart will not suddenly stop working because they are rejecting.

Treatment of rejection is normally based on the results of the biopsy. In cases where the patient is haemodynamically compromised, treatment will have to commence before the results of the biopsy are available.

In treatment, four factors have to be considered.

- Level of background immunosuppression, especially ciclosporin level and renal function.
- The patient's clinical and haemodynamic state.
- Histological grade of biopsy (see Box 23.4).
- The patient's previous history of rejection.

Immunosuppression

Transplant immunosuppression has three components:

- Initial or so-called induction therapy.
- Maintenance immunosuppression.
- Treatment of acute rejection episodes.

Induction immunosuppression. Patients will normally receive a premedication of ciclosporin and azathioprine, calculated according to the patient's weight and renal function. Some centres use azathioprine only and introduce ciclosporin gradually post-operatively, in order to preserve kidney function. It is

---

Box 23.4	Classification of cardiac biopsy grading for rejection (reproduced from Billingham et al 1990 with permission from Elsevier Science)

Grade	Nomenclature
0	No rejection
1	A = Focal infiltrate without necrosis
	B = Diffuse but sparse infiltrate without necrosis
2	One focus only with aggressive infiltration and/or myocyte damage
3	A = Multifocal aggressive infiltrates and/or myocyte damage
	B = Diffuse inflammatory process with necrosis
4	Diffuse aggressive polymorphous +/– infiltrate, +/– oedema, +/– haemorrhage, +/– vasculitis, with necrosis

---

usual to give antithymocyte globulin and steroids peri-operatively, with gradual introduction of ciclosporin from 2 days post transplant. The exact regimen varies from centre to centre.

Maintenance immunosuppression.

Ciclosporin. Ciclosporin (cyclosporin) is a fungal metabolite which works selectively on lymphocytes. It prevents activation of killer T-lymphocytes and inhibits interleukin-II production. It is therefore effective against the cell-mediated immune response present in acute rejection. Its discovery revolutionized transplantation but it is extremely nephrotoxic and its use must be monitored carefully by trained transplant physicians.

It is available in intravenous, liquid and capsule form and is administered by continuous intravenous infusion or orally twice a day. Dosage is calculated by measuring trough blood levels and serum creatinine levels (White-Williams 1993). In the initial postoperative phase the aim is to achieve a trough ciclosporin level above 300 ng/ml as soon as possible. This is providing that renal function is adequate. The optimum trough level can be reduced gradually after 3 months, to 100–200 ng/ml at 1 year post transplantation, when the risk of acute cell-mediated rejection has lessened.

Ciclosporin doses should be taken 12 hours apart and patients must be warned not to take the drug prior to their blood being taken for levels, as it is essential to obtain a trough level. Most patients take capsules but all must be informed not to take the dose with grapefruit juice as this can enhance absorption and so increase blood levels.

Ciclosporin has numerous side-effects:

- Nephrotoxicity
- Hepatotoxicity

- Increased risk of infection
- Hypertension
- Hirsutism (excess growth of hair)
- Hypercalaemia
- Hypomagnesaemia
- Muscle weakness/tremors/headaches
- Lymphoma
- Gingival hyperplasia (overgrowth of the gums)
- Thrombocytopenia

As the levels are reduced, the side-effects lessen but they are still unpleasant for the patient who will need support and encouragement.

Ciclosporin interacts with many drugs including anti-epileptics such as phenytoin and phenobarbital, both of which reduce plasma levels. It also interacts with oral contraceptives which raise levels of ciclosporin, so transplant recipients of child-bearing age must be offered contraceptive advice. All patients taking ciclosporin are told to check with the transplant centre before taking any drug prescribed by physicians, other than those with transplant experience. More recently, Neoral, a micro-emulsion ciclosporin formulation, has been developed to enhance the oral absorption of ciclosporin.

Azathioprine (Imuran). Azathioprine inhibits purine (protein) metabolism and suppresses the proliferation of rapidly dividing cells (White-Williams 1993). It is used in conjunction with other immunosuppressive agents as it is not very effective on its own. It is absorbed rapidly from the gastro-intestinal tract, the dose being 2 mg/kg daily. It is normally given orally at night.

Azathioprine may need to be reduced or discontinued if there is bone marrow suppression. Normally the white cell count is the most sensitive indicator of this occurrence. The drug is normally stopped if the white cell count falls below 4.0×10^9. Thrombocytopenia is also a problem but is uncommon without white cell suppression. Liver function tests are often abnormal after surgery and azathioprine should be discontinued if the patient is clinically jaundiced.

Azathioprine has a variety of side-effects:

- Hepatitis
- Alopecia
- Rash
- Anaemia
- Leucopenia
- Thrombocytopenia
- Increased risk of infection
- Nausea
- Fever

- Rash
- Increased tendency for gout

An important drug interaction that patients must be aware of is that of azathioprine and allopurinol. This combination can cause dangerous bone marrow suppression as allopurinol inhibits the metabolism of azathioprine. If allopurinol must be given, azathioprine dosage must be reduced to one quarter of the above and there must be careful monitoring of the full blood count.

Corticosteroids. Corticosteroids have a diverse effect on the immune system. They directly inhibit antigen-driven T-cell proliferation through their ability to block interleukin-I. Interleukin-II plays an important part in T-cell activation but it is dependent on interleukin-I, so indirectly, corticosteroids block its release. Corticosteroids also have generalized anti-inflammatory effects and their ability to prevent fever in sepsis almost certainly derives from the blocking of interleukin-I release. This is especially hazardous when assessing postoperative patients who are taking corticosteroids as they could have an infection or be rejecting, both of which may present with pyrexias, but the signs would be masked.

Corticosteroids are given to maintain immunosuppression when ciclosporin levels are lowered, as part of triple therapy. This is used in patients prone to recurrent rejection, following a rejection episode or to help clear 'persistent' rejection.

Corticosteroids have numerous side-effects:

- Weight gain
- Increased appetite
- Mood swings
- Salt and fluid retention
- Glucose intolerance
- Acne
- Fragile skin/poor wound healing
- Ulcers
- Cushingoid syndrome
- Osteoporosis
- Bruising

The impact of taking corticosteroids on the body image and emotional state requires a high level of support and empathy (Allum 1998). Prolonged use is therefore undesirable and the aim is to taper off the dose so that the majority of patients are not taking the drug at 1 year post transplantation (Parameshwar 1996).

FK506. FK506 (tacrolimus) acts in a similar way to ciclosporin by selectively inhibiting the early phase of T-cell activation and thus cytokine activation. It is used for rescue therapy in persistent rejection and has been shown to decrease the frequency of such episodes (Rinaldi et al 1997). However, it is not a standard immunosuppressive agent for cardiac transplantation. It is more potent than ciclosporin, yet does not appear to cause some of the cosmetic side-effects (hirsutism, gum hyperplasia). Hypertension may also be less common than with ciclosporin.

FK506 side-effects include:

- nephrotoxicity
- diabetes mellitus
- peripheral neuropathy
- tremor
- headache
- hypertension
- hyperkalaemia
- leg cramps
- malaise
- peripheral oedema
- cardiogenic shock.

Mycophenolate mofetil. Mycophenolate mofetil (MMF) acts by inhibiting the de novo purine metabolism in lymphocytes (T- and B-cells) leading to the depletion of immunocompetent cells (Renlund et al 1996). MMF tends to be used as maintenance immunosuppression.

MMF's main side-effects are:

- bone marrow suppression
- diarrhoea
- gastro-intestinal symptoms.

Cyclophosphamide. Cyclophosphamide can be used for a variety of reasons. It tends to be used for prophylaxis of rejection in patients with a positive HLA crossmatch. It can also be used to treat antibody-mediated rejection and is sometimes used in conjunction with plasmapheresis. It is useful as a substitute for azathioprine in hepatic dysfunction. The dose is calculated according to the patient's weight.

Cyclophosphamide's common side-effects include:

- nausea and vomiting
- bone marrow suppression
- alopecia
- hepatic disturbance.

There is also a possible increased malignancy risk with long-term use.

Treatment of acute rejection episodes.
Treatment of rejection is according to the histological grade of rejection (see Box 23.4).

Polyclonal antibodies. Antithymocyte globulin (ATG) is a polyclonal animal-derived antibody to human lymphocytes which makes them susceptible to phagocytosis (ingestion by phagocyte cells). It is used in induction therapy when ciclosporin cannot be used, when there is a rejection episode unresponsive to methylprednisolone, a rejection episode where ciclosporin cannot be given and finally in cases of severe rejection where steroids alone are inadequate. Rabbit (RATG)- and horse (HATG)-derived globulins are most commonly used.

Severe anaphylactic reactions can occur, so a test dose must always be given. If no reaction occurs, administration is commenced after an antihistamine and paracetomol have been administered to minimize any reaction. The drug is infused via a central line over several hours, with careful observation of the haemodynamic vital signs. Its effectiveness is monitored by T-cell levels. The normal dose is once a day for 3 days. The main side-effects are fever, cytopenia, thrombocytopenia and serum sickness.

Monoclonal antibodies (OKT3). OKT3 is produced from mice by cloning hybrid cells that produce a supply of specific antibodies. It is used for rejection that has not responded to steroids or ATG. It is a potent immunosuppressant that rapidly blocks the function of T-lymphocytes. It is administered intravenously as a bolus injection once a day for 10–14 days. Premedication with intravenous methylprednisolone, Piriton and oral paracetamol is administered to minimize side-effects. However, severe reactions can still occur and these include convulsions, haemodynamic response, intestinal complications, first-dose 'cytokine release phenomenon', pulmonary oedema and viral infections (Wagner et al 1994). It is a very expensive treatment with only moderate results, so its use is limited (Wagner et al 1994).

Total lymphoid irradiation. Total lymphoid irradiation (TLI) has been shown to be effective in the management of recurrent cellular rejection (Hunt et al 1991). Allograft dysfunction develops in a proportion of heart transplant recipients without a cellular infiltrate in endomyocardial biopsies and with normal coronary angiography. The mechanism for this remains unclear. It has been suggested that TLI could also be beneficial to this group of patients (Madden et al 1996).

Acute rejection is uncommon after the first year. The three most important long-term complications in cardiac transplant recipients are coronary artery disease, malignancy and renal disease due to ciclosporin-induced nephrotoxicity (Parameshwar 1996).

Chronic rejection

Long-term results of heart transplantation are strongly influenced by graft failure resulting from chronic transplant dysfunction, also known as chronic rejection. Survival beyond the first year post transplantation is essentially dictated by the development of transplant coronary artery disease (TCAD) (Large 1995). Indeed, it may emerge in some individuals as early as 6 months after transplantation (Hary et al 1992).

This chronic process is characterized by concentric narrowing of arterioles; that is, intimal thickening with proliferation of smooth muscle cells. Another feature is the irregular thickening of the donor coronary artery wall that affects the entire length of the vessel, including the small branches. It stops at the junction between donor and recipient tissue (Billingham 1994). The pathogenic mechanism that triggers and maintains the process is the subject of many studies. Both antibody and cell-mediated immunity may be involved (Tullius & Tilney 1995).

It has been proposed that potential non-immunologic risk factors for the development of TCAD include:

- prolonged ischaemic time (above 4 hours)
- reperfusion injury
- ciclosporin dosage
- transplant size
- lipid abnormalities
- age and gender of donor.

Potential immunologic contributors are believed to be:

- HLA incompatibility
- cytomegalovirus (CMV) infection
- panel reactive antibody
- number and intensity of acute rejection episodes (after Tullius & Tilney 1995).

Another possible explanation could be that during transplantation, ischaemic and reperfusion damage cause injury to the endothelium of the transplanted heart. As a result of the non-specific injury, activation of complement and coagulation cascades takes place. The damaged endothelium releases various cytokines and growth factors. In turn, smooth muscle cell proliferation is stimulated, contributing to the intimal thickening (Raisanen-Sokolowski & Hayry 1996).

One of the most striking features of TCAD is that the myocardium can maintain adequate function and be free of a cellular infiltrate while simultaneously harbouring advanced coronary obstructive lesions (Rose 1996). Consequently most patients with TCAD are asymptomatic until late in the course of the disease (see Case study 23.1). Annual coronary angiography is therefore part of the follow-up in most centres. Despite denervation, angina does occur in some of these patients (Parameshwar 1996).

Treatment is hampered by the diffuse nature of the disease. Coronary artery bypass surgery and angioplasty are possible and are generally performed if the lesions are proximal. The only definitive treatment is retransplantation but the shortage of donors and a prognosis worse than that of first-time transplantation limit the applicability (Parameshwar 1996).

INFECTION

Infection is a potential complication of immunosuppressant drug therapy and continues to be a significant cause of morbidity and mortality in transplant patients (Vlahakes et al 1994). Infection represents a major cause of hospital re-admission after cardiac transplantation and remains a leading primary cause of death during the first year after surgery (Smart et al 1996).

Early infections occur within the first month of transplant and are usually dominated by nosocomial organisms such as *Staphylococcus aureus*, *Pseudomonas aeruginosa*, enterococci and other Gram-negative organisms (Gentry 1993). The types of infection most often seen are pneumonia, urinary tract infection, wound infection and catheter-related bacteraemia (Wagoner 1997). Patients are screened pre-operatively to allow antibiotic therapy to commence quickly. Prophylactic antibiotic cover is routinely given in most centres, although it is under constant review as it increases the risk of infection, with multiple antibiotic-resistant organisms and fungal infections.

Normally central lines, temporary pacing wires and similar devices should be changed electively at least once a week. Only tunnelled and long lines are suitable for long-term use. The nurse has an important role in preventing the spread of nosocomial infection by maintaining and promoting excellent handwashing techniques and in following strict asepsis for dressing changes. The nurse should also monitor patients for signs and symptoms of infection (pyrexia may be absent due to the effects of immunosuppression).

Late infection usually occurs between the first month and the first year after transplantation. This is because immunosuppression is at its highest during this time. In immunocompromised patients certain infections which, with a normal immune system, would be harmless act as pathogens; these infections are known as 'opportunistic'. Patients are particularly susceptible to opportunistic infections during treatment for acute rejection, as extra immunosuppression is administered. As previously stated, acute rejection is also more likely to occur within the first year.

Viral opportunistic infections

Cytomegalovirus (CMV)

CMV infection occurs either because of re-activation or transmission with the allograft. CMV is a significant cause of morbidity and mortality after heart transplantation (Wagoner 1997). CMV infection is usually seen in the first 6 months after transplantation but can cause recurrent infection and long-term debility. It has also been linked with transplant coronary artery disease (Tullius & Tilney 1995).

CMV infection commonly presents after immunosuppression has been augmented for a period of acute rejection (see Case study 23.2). Patients will generally present with pyrexia and malaise or with evidence of involvement of specific organ systems (pneumonia, colitis, encephalitis and, rarely, myocarditis). The patient can be almost asymptomatic or extremely unwell, requiring intensive support. Diagnosis is made by analysis of viral cultures by a laboratory familiar with isolation of the virus.

Treatment is normally with a 14-day course of ganciclovir, administered intravenously via a central line. It is almost exclusively excreted in an unchanged form in the urine, so the dose is modified in renal impairment. It is also known to cause granulocytopenia and thrombocytopenia but it must be remembered that bone marrow suppression is also a manifestation of CMV infection.

Treatment with ganciclovir has been shown to shorten the clinical course of the disease and decreases morbidity.

Herpes simplex

Herpes simplex infection is common in the first 3 months post transplantation. Prophylactic treatment with aciclovir is very effective (Parameshwar 1996).

Fungal opportunistic infections

Oropharyngeal infection with candida is common in patients on high doses of corticosteroids and can usually be prevented with oral nystatin. Resistant or severe infections respond to a short course of fluconazole.

Aspergillus

Aspergillus infection is relatively rare but it causes serious invasive disease and has a high mortality (Wagoner 1997). Outbreaks of aspergillus are associated with poor ventilation, building work and spore-contaminated air conditioning systems (Gentry 1993). Infection usually follows a period of increased immunosuppression and notably treatment with ATG. The lung is the most common site of infection and diagnosis is made by lung biopsy. Nebulized amphotericin is the drug of choice for treatment for invasive aspergillosis. Liposomal amphotericin can be given for severe infection but is nephrotoxic so must be used with caution.

Pneumocystis carinii pneumonia

This is a protozoan infection. It is a rare but serious complication. Diagnosis is by transbronchial biopsy. It is almost never seen when low doses of co-trimoxazole are used as prophylaxis. The length of time it is used as prophylaxis varies centre by centre but always covers the crucial first 3 months post transplantation.

Toxoplasmosis

Toxoplasma can cause myocarditis. It is usually transmitted with the allograft, in patients who have not developed antibodies to the agent. Pyrimethamine is used in some centres and co-trimoxazole may also be effective. Both are used as prophylactics. Transplant patients should be advised to wear gloves when gardening and handling cat litter, as Toxoplasma is found in cat faeces.

All transplant patients are advised about the signs and symptoms of infection and are told that prophylactic antibiotics are required prior to dental or surgical procedures. Advice with regard to travelling abroad is offered, including the avoidance of all live vaccines, such as the combined mumps-measles-rubella vaccine or the Sabin oral polio vaccine. They are also advised to initially avoid crowds and coming into contact with people known to have infections, such as coughs and colds.

MALIGNANCY

The administration of cytotoxic agents, either for immunosuppression or for chemotherapy, is associated with an increased incidence of malignancy. Malignancy is one of the recognized side-effects of long-term immunosuppression (Wagoner 1997). Malignant cutaneous tumour is the most common and is associated with the use of azathioprine where the metabolite causes enhanced photosensitivity, which is believed to contribute to the growth of a tumour.

Post-transplant lymphoproliferative disease is a form of lymphoma that has occurred with the advent of ciclosporin (Sullivan et al 1984). This tumour usually develops at 12–18 months post transplant. It occurs most often in the bowel, has diffuse involvement of nodal and extranodal tissue and its prognosis varies (Wagoner 1997). Often it is of B-cell origin and may be induced by the Epstein–Barr virus (Sullivan et al 1984). Treatment varies but usually consists of high-dose intravenous aciclovir, because of its effect on Epstein–Barr virus replication.

HYPERLIPIDAEMIA

Hyperlipidaemia is a common problem after heart transplantation. Elevated cholesterol levels have been reported as early as 3 weeks after transplantation and usually they have become raised in the first 6–18 months. Hypercholesterolaemia is associated with increased concentrations of low-density lipoproteins (Wagoner 1997), which are known to precipitate atheroma formation. Several factors have been associated with the development of hyperlipidaemia after transplantation (Kubo et al 1992). These include a prior history of ischaemic heart disease, pre-existing lipid abnormalities and cumulative dosage of corticosteroids and ciclosporin.

The treatment of hyperlipidaemia post transplantation includes weight loss, exercise, a low-fat diet and the reduction of corticosteroids and ciclosporin. Lipid-lowering agents have been reported by several centres as an effective therapy (Ballantyne et al 1992).

REPRODUCTIVE HEALTH

In spite of the fact that parenting and child bearing become considerations in females of child-bearing age (Wagoner 1997), most centres have discouraged pregnancy after cardiac transplantation. The most frequent maternal complications have been found to be hypertension, premature labour and pre-eclampsia. The most frequent neonatal complications have been found to be prematurity and low birth weight (Wagoner et al 1993). There have been no reports of fetal abnormalities. Paternity after organ transplantation is more common and is considered safer (Wagoner 1997).

Male and female recipients should consider the possibility that the child may lose a parent from complications of transplantation or may have to deal with prolonged illness in that parent. Thus, counselling with an honest prognosis of heart transplantation is an essential nursing role when caring for a cardiac transplant patient who is considering parenthood. It is usually the nursing team in the transplant follow-up clinics who become involved in this aspect of care.

QUALITY OF LIFE

The majority of patients say that they had not anticipated the enormous impact that the transplant would have on their lives (Iliffe & Swan 1993). The aim of transplantation is to improve quality of life and increase survival (Madden & Hodson 1996). Health and functional ability are believed to be the main factors that affect this quality (Grady & Jalowiec 1995). It is important to achieve optimum exercise capacity and functional status through progressive exercise training and rehabilitation. Most transplant centres have a rehabilitation programme. Patients are normally enrolled onto a structured exercise regime that they are encouraged to continue at home following discharge. Their exercise capacity is formally examined at 6-monthly intervals, through use of a treadmill.

In general, social, sexual and psychiatric adjustment have shown to be improved after heart transplantation (Mai et al 1990). Indeed, in one study over 80% of heart transplant recipients reported no limitations in activity (Brann et al 1998). Long-term survival for heart transplant recipients is mainly dependent on adopting certain lifestyle behaviours, such as a lifelong regimen of immunosuppressive therapy, dietary control, exercise regulation and taking precautions to prevent infection. It is a vital nursing role when caring for patients after a heart transplant to commence education regarding the above issues as soon as possible after their return from the intensive care unit. Involvement of the family or carers is positively encouraged.

Stressors for recipients after transplant include fear of organ rejection and death, body image change, mood swings, depression, the financial burden, lifestyle changes and side-effects of immunosuppression (Hwang 1996, Mai et al 1990). It appears that while life is not perfect, patients are willing to accept the problems as a trade-off for being alive. Most heart transplant recipients perceive symptoms such as rejection as having a relatively small impact on their quality of life (Mai et al 1990). This perception is primarily due to the recipient's attempt to adapt to symptoms, alter their lifestyle and 'redesign their dream' (Hwang 1996).

Many heart transplant recipients return to work and see employment as having a positive effect on their quality of life. Some, however, just want to enjoy life (Bellchambers 1993). Brann demonstrated that only slightly more than one-third of the heart transplant recipients they studied had returned to employment at 1 year post transplantation (Brann et al 1998). It must be remembered that some employment might not be suitable for recipients and some employers might show reluctance in employing them. Nurses have a role in counselling patients and encouraging them to develop skills to find suitable employment.

THE FUTURE

It could be said that cardiac transplantation is a victim of its own success. The major problems to be overcome are organ rejection and availability of donors. As the demand for organs continues to grow, the gap between supply and demand will become even more significant. The death rates from cerebrovascular (CVA) and road traffic accidents continue to fall, so consequently do donor rates (Parrott 1996). Across the UK and Europe there is a steady state or fall in organ donor rates, while demand and waiting lists rise.

In some countries, including some states in America, all families are asked to agree to the donation of organs and tissues from their deceased relatives. Hospital staff are required to ask the family whether or not the person concerned carried any kind of donor card. This is known as 'required request'. Alternatively, in some countries, including Austria, Belgium and France, hospitals will automatically remove organs and tissues unless they know that the patient, when alive, was not in favour of organ donation. This is known as 'presumed consent'. In this country there are no plans to change from the current system of 'opting in' but it is hoped that initiatives such as the Organ Donor Registry will improve donation rates by raising awareness.

Against this background, it should come as no surprise that the attention of researchers has focused on the possibility of animal-to-human transplantation (xenotransplantation). Xenografts trigger an immune response that is even stronger than that produced in response to allografts. However, the degree of response partly depends on the phylogenetic (relative genetic) distance between the source animal and the recipient. In this respect, the immunological and genetic problems are less with so-called concordant xenografts; that is, anthropoids/apes to man. However, dwindling numbers already threaten most if not all of the ape species. They are also slow to breed and have small

---

Case study 23.1

Andrew Black is a 50-year-old physics teacher transplanted 7 years ago for ischaemic heart disease. His only recent admission to hospital had been for his annual 'MOT' angiogram, which showed slight narrowing in the circumflex coronary artery.

Andrew presented at clinic because he had noticed a decrease in his exercise tolerance. He and his wife were keen walkers. He was now unable to walk half a mile without becoming breathless and complained of 'angina-type pain' across his chest, which spread down his left arm.

On examination his jugular venous pressure (JVP) was not elevated. Elevation may have indicated fluid retention due to heart failure. Heart sounds were also normal. Ischaemic changes were noted on the 12-lead ECG and there was a reduction in cardiac function on the echocardiogram. Biochemical cardiac markers were normal.

Andrew was admitted to the ward to undergo a repeat coronary angiogram. This confirmed increased narrowing in the circumflex artery. After discussion with Andrew, the cardiologist performed an angioplasty and insertion of stent. Andrew had an uneventful recovery following this and was discharged the next day, for review in a month. He was also referred to the lipid clinic (as his cholesterol was 9.7 mmol) and to the dietitian. He was advised to resume his exercise regime as before, because he was now symptom free.

---

numbers of offspring. For all these reasons, apes are unlikely ever to be used for transplants.

The research is now focusing on a more distant species, the pig. However, this would be a discordant xenograft, which is likely to trigger a strong immediate immune response. This would subsequently result in hyperacute rejection, acute vascular thrombosis and activation of naturally occurring xeno-antibodies. Efforts to frustrate this immune response are underway. Strategies being pursued include human gene insertion to modify the source animals, gene knockout to modify the source animal, antibody masking and modification of the host through bone marrow chimerism (in which bone marrow from the donor is transplanted along with the organ) (Klotzko 1998). Even if all the problems with rejection were surmounted, society and doctors will still have to come to terms with the ethical issues, although the Transplantation Society has officially endorsed the concept.

CONCLUSION

This chapter has reviewed the indications for nursing care and issues of immunosuppression and rejection

Case study 23.2

Alex Carey was 27 years old when he was referred to the transplant centre. He was born with tetralogy of Fallot and had corrective surgery as a child. He had been well until 18 months ago since when he had developed exertional dyspnoea, being unable to walk more than 50 metres on the flat. He was accompanied to the transplant ward by his mother. Alex's father died one year ago.

On admission he was noted to be in atrial fibrillation, with a ventricular rate of 120 bpm, his blood pressure was 100/65 mmHg and oxygen saturations 92% via oximetry. His medications included amiodarone 200 mg once a day (od), warfarin 1–2 mg od, bumetamide 3 mg od and isosorbide mononitrate 20 mg od.

Alex underwent left and right heart catheterisation to assess his cardiac function, coronary arteries and pulmonary pressures. An echocardiogram, electrocardiogram (ECG), chest X-ray, respiratory function tests (to investigate the exertional dyspnoea) and 24-hour ambulatory ECG recording were all performed. Blood was taken to determine blood group, tissue type, hepatitis B and C status, cytomegalovirus (CMV) status, HLA/panel reactive antibody levels, biochemistry, liver function and full blood count. A 24-hour urine collection for protein excretion and creatinine clearance was completed.

The transplant social worker, psychologist and transplant co-ordinator saw Alex and his mother. An experienced transplant nurse provided pre- and post-transplant information in both written and verbal form, to allow both son and mother time to ask questions and to assimilate the information given.

Alex was an inpatient for 3 days during which time his mother was noted to be extremely anxious, requiring constant reassurance about the assessment process from the nursing staff. The nurses noted that Alex appeared very withdrawn. His mother was his constant companion so the nurses found it difficult to talk to him on his own, to determine how he felt about the possibility of a transplant.

When the tests were all completed, the results were reviewed by the transplant team, which included the consultant surgeon and cardiologist, social worker, transplant psychologist, junior doctors and nursing team involved in his care. Alex was considered suitable for transplantation and graded as urgent. His blood group was A positive and he was CMV negative. Alex was issued with a pager and he and his mother went home to await the transplant call.

Alex received a call for a possible transplant 7 months later. He arrived on the transplant ward at 21.30 hrs accompanied by his mother. He was prepared for surgery by the nursing team and transferred to theatre at 22.30 hrs. He arrived in the intensive care unit (ICU) at 05.00 hrs the next morning, following an orthotopic cardiac transplant. The donor was a 27-year-old female who had suffered a subarachnoid haemorrhage. The donor was blood group A positive and CMV negative.

On arrival in the ICU Alex had a central venous line and was receiving the following infusions: dopamine at 5 μg/kg/min (renal dose) and RATG 100 mg/250 ml. He was atrially paced via temporary epicardial pacing wires at a fixed rate of 100 bpm. Pericardial and mediastinal drains were in place, on negative 5 cm suction and a urinary catheter had been passed to assess his renal function. He was mechanically ventilated via an endotracheal tube. Alex's blood pressure on arrival was 100/40 mmHg and the CVP was 7 cmH$_2$O. As Alex warmed up the drainage from the pericardial drains increased for a couple of hours but required no intervention. He received a total of six units of whole blood peri- and postoperatively.

He was transferred to the ward after 24 hours with the infused dopamine at 5 μg/kg/min, fixed atrial pacing at a rate of 100 bpm, 35% oxygen and he was fully awake and orientated.

Alex had an uneventful recovery and was discharged home after 3 weeks. When he attended his first outpatient appointment he complained of feeling generally unwell and 'full of cold'. He was pyrexial at 37.6°C. On examination a third heart sound was evident and mild peripheral oedema was noted. The 12-lead ECG showed a drop in voltage and his ejection fraction was decreased on the echocardiogram. Alex underwent a cardiac biopsy and was admitted to the transplant ward to await the result. He was now afraid about what would happen if he were rejecting. The nursing and medical staff reassured him that it was perfectly normal to reject and that treatment was usually quite simple.

Alex's renal and hepatic functions were unchanged. The biopsy result indicated 1B rejection (see Box 23.4). He commenced a course of methylprednisolone, 1 g a day for 3 days. The steroids made him feel very 'high' and he complained of having trouble sleeping due to his mind racing. A repeat biopsy the following week indicated no rejection.

Alex continued to feel unwell. He developed a persistent temperature and a troublesome unproductive cough. Oxygen saturations dropped to 91% and he became dyspnoeic on minimal exertion. The CMV titre was raised and a transbronchial biopsy confirmed that he had developed CMV pneumonitis. A central line was sited and ganciclovir 300 mg bd intravenously was commenced, for 14 days. White cell screens were regularly performed and renal function was monitored throughout the treatment.

Alex felt his breathing had improved after 5 days of treatment and he became apyrexial. After a 14-day course of ganciclovir, the CMV titre was negative and repeat cardiac biopsy showed no rejection. He was discharged home, to be reviewed again in a week.

---

associated with cardiac transplantation. Careful co-ordination of all involved services is of vital importance to reduce the ischaemic time and offer the greatest chance of transplant success. Importantly, support for the patient, family and carers, particularly during the waiting period, is a necessary and required skill for both the nursing and all the health-care team. The rate of change and development in transplantation is so rapid that the issues of drug-free tolerance, genetic manipulation of the immune system and xenotransplantation are now within our grasp. It is entirely possible that the hypotheses of transplanted organ tolerance and effective immunosuppression of concordant and discordant xenografts may be possible in the near future (Parrott 1996).

Transplantation is an exciting and evolving field which presents many challenges to nurses. It has come a long way in the past two decades but still has a long way to go.

REFERENCES

Allum L 1998 Transplantation. In: Shuldham C (ed) Cardiorespiratory nursing. Stanley Thornes, Cheltenham, pp. 489–515

Ballantyne CM, Radovancevic B, Farmer JA et al 1992 Hyperlipidemia after heart transplantation: report of a six year experience, with treatment recommendations. Journal of the American College of Cardiology 19(6): 1315–1321

Banner NR 1992 Exercise physiology and rehabilitation after heart transplantation. Journal of Heart and Lung Transplantation 11(4 part 2): S237–S240

Bellchambers J 1993 Employing transplant recipients: a pilot study. Nursing Standard 7(32): 28–31

BHF 2000 British Heart Foundation coronary heart disease statistics database: annual compendium. BHF, London

Billingham ME 1994 Pathology and aetiology of chronic rejection of the heart. Clinical Transplantation 8(3 part 2): 289–292

Billingham ME, Cary NR, Hammond ME et al 1990 A working formulation for the standardization of nomenclature in the diagnosis of heart and lung rejection: Heart Rejection Study Group of the International Society for Heart Transplantation. Journal of Heart Transplantation 9(6): 587–593

Brann WM, Bennett LE, Keck BM, Hosenpud JD 1998 Morbidity, functional status and immunosuppressive therapy after heart transplantation: an analysis of the Joint International Society for Heart and Lung Transplantation/United Network for Organ Sharing Thoracic Registry. Journal of Heart and Lung Transplantation 17(4): 374–382

Brostoff J, Male D 1994 Clinical immunology: an illustrated outline. Mosby, Boston, pp. 100–106

Bunzel B, Wollenek G 1994 Heart transplantation: are there psychosocial predictors for clinical success after surgery? Journal of Thoracic and Cardiovascular Surgery 42(2): 103–107

Cowell R, Morris-Thurgood J, Coghlan J et al 1994 Post operative haemodynamic improvement with paced linkage of the donor and recipient heart following heterotopic cardiac transplantation. Clinical Cardiology 17(10): 542–546

Dannie E 1993 Immunosuppressive agents. Nursing Times 89(4): 34–38

De Maria R, Minoli L, Parolini M et al 1996 Prognostic determinants of six month morbidity and mortality in heart transplant recipients. The Italian Study Group on Infection in Heart Transplantation. Journal of Heart and Lung Transplantation 15(2): 124–135

Finkelmeier BA 1995 Heart, lung and heart–lung transplantation. In: Finkelmeier BA (ed) Cardiothoracic surgical nursing. JB Lippincott, Philadelphia, pp. 329–337

Fitzpatrick AP, Banner N, Cheng A, Yacoub M, Sutton R 1993 Vasovagal reactions may occur after orthotopic heart transplantation. Journal of the American College of Cardiology 21(5): 132–137

Gentry LO 1993 Cardiac transplantation and related infections. Seminars in Respiratory Infection 8(3): 199–206

Grady KL, Jalowiec A 1995 Review of the quality of life after transplantation. In: Williams BAH, Grady KL, Sandiford-Guttenbeil DM (eds) Organ transplantation: a manual for nurses. Springer, New York, pp. 329–344

Hary P, Neunauder S, Yilmaz J et al 1992 Cellular and molecular mechanism in allograft arteriosclerosis. Transplantation Proceedings 24: 2359–2361

Hosenpud JD, Bennett LE, Keck BM, Fiol B, Novick RJ 1997 The Registry of the International Society for Heart and Lung Transplantation: fourteenth official report 1997. Journal of Heart and Lung Transplantation 16(7): 691–712

Hunt SA, Strober S, Hoppe RT, Stinson EB 1991 Total lymphoid irradiation for treatment of intractable cardiac allograft rejection. Journal of Heart and Lung Transplantation 10(2): 211–216

Hwang HF 1996 Patient and family adjustment to heart transplantation. Progress in Cardiovascular Nursing 11(2): 16–39

Iliffe J, Swan P 1993 Heart and heart lung transplantation. In: Tschudin V (ed) Ethics: aspects of nursing care. Scutari Press, London, pp. 56–71

Jackson SA 1991 The immune system: basic concepts for understanding transplantation. Critical Care Nursing Quarterly 13(4): 83–88

Kaba E, Shanley E 1997 Identification of coping strategies used by heart transplant recipients. British Journal of Nursing 6(15): 858–862

Kirk AJ, Richens D, Dark JH 1993 A manual of cardiopulmonary transplantation. Edward Arnold, London

Klotzko AJ 1998 The beast inside. Nursing Times 94(31): 51–52

Kubo SH, Peters JR, Knutson KR et al 1992 Factors influencing the development of hypercholesterolemia after heart transplantation. American Journal of Cardiology 70(4): 520–526

Large SR 1995 Cardiac transplantation – the next decade. British Journal of Hospital Medicine 53(9): 440–447

Madden BP, Hodson ME 1996 Rehabilitation considerations for the transplant patient. In: Bach JR (ed) Pulmonary rehabilitation. The obstructive and paralytic conditions. Hanley and Belfus, Philadelphia, pp. 193–202

Madden BP, Backhouse L, McClosky D, Reynolds L, Tait D, Murday A 1996 Total lymphoid irradiation as rescue therapy after heart transplantation. Journal of Heart and Lung Transplantation 15(3): 234–238

Mai FM, McKenzie FN, Kostuk WJ 1990 Psychosocial adjustment and quality of life following heart transplantation. Canadian Journal of Psychiatry 35(3): 223–227

Muirhead J 1992. Heart and heart–lung transplantation. Critical Care Nursing Clinics of North America 4(1): 97–109

Muirhead J, Meyerowitz BE, Leedham B, Eastburn TE, Merrill WH, Frist WH 1992 Quality of life and coping in patients awaiting heart transplantation. Journal of Heart and Lung Transplantation 11(2 part 1): 265–271

Parameshwar J 1996 Follow-up after cardiac transplantation. British Journal of Hospital Medicine 56(7): 350–354

Parrott NR 1996 Transplantation: where are we now? International Journal of Intensive Care 3(4): 126–133

Porter JL, Bailey C, Bennen G et al 1991 Stress during the waiting period: a review of pre transplant fears. Critical Care Nursing Quarterly 13(4): 25–31

Raisanen-Sokolowski A, Hayry P 1996 Chronic allograft arteriosclerosis: contributing factors and molecular mechanisms in the light of experimental studies. Transplant Immunology 4(2): 91–98

Renlund DG, Gopinathan SK, Kfoury AG, Taylor DO 1996 Mycophenolate mofetil (MMF) in heart transplantation: rejection, prevention and treatment. Clinical Transplantation 10: 136–139

Rinaldi M, Pellegrini C, Matinelli L et al 1997 FK506 effectiveness in reducing acute rejection after heart transplantation: a prospective randomised trial. Journal of Heart and Lung Transplantation 16(10): 1001–1010

Rose M 1993 Antibody-mediated rejection following cardiac transplantation. Transplantation Reviews 7(3): 140–152

Rose M 1996 Role of antibody and indirect antigen presentation in transplant-associated coronary artery vasculopathy. Journal of Heart and Lung Transplantation 15(4): 342–349

Shaw LR, Miller JD, Slutsky AS et al 1991 Ethics of lung transplantation with live donors. Lancet 338: 678–681

Shumway N, Lower R 1964 Special problems in transplantation of the heart. Annals of the New York Academy of Sciences 120: 773–777

Smart FW, Naftel DC, Costanzo MR et al 1996 Risk factors for early, cumulative and fatal infections after heart transplantation: a multiinstitutional study. Journal of Heart and Lung Transplantation 15: 329–341

Snell J 1997 Life from death. Nursing Times 93(27): 30–31

Sullivan JL, Medveczky P, Forman SJ, Baker SM, Monroe JE, Mulder C 1984 Epstein–Barr virus induced lymphoproliferation: implications for antiviral chemotherapy. New England Journal of Medicine 311(18): 1163–1167

Thiroux J 1995 Ethics: theory and practice, 5th edn. Prentice Hall, Englewood Cliffs, New Jersey, pp. 379–382

Thompson CJ 1995 Denervation of the transplanted heart: nursing implications for patient care. Critical Care Nursing Quarterly 17(4): 1–14

Trento A, Czer LSC, Blanche C 1996 Surgical technique for cardiac transplantation. Seminars in Thoracic and Cardiovascular Surgery 8(2): 126–132

Tullius SG, Tilney NL 1995 Both alloantigen-dependent and independent factors influence chronic allograft rejection. Transplantation 59(3): 313–318

Verani MS, Nishimura S, Mahamarian JJ, Hays JT, Young JB 1994 Cardiac function after orthotopic heart transplantation: response to postural changes, exercise and beta-adrenergic blockade. Journal of Heart and Lung Transplantation 13(2): 181–193

Vlahakes GJ, Lemmer JH, Behnendt DM, Austen WG 1994 Transplantation. Handbook of Patient Care in Cardiac Surgery. Little, Brown, Boston, pp. 229–261

Wagner FM, Reichenspurner H, Uberfuhr P et al 1994 How successful is OKT3 rescue therapy for steroid-resistant acute rejection episodes after heart transplantation? Journal of Heart and Lung Transplantation 13(3): 438–442

Wagoner LE 1997 Management of the cardiac transplant recipient: roles of the transplant cardiologist and primary care physician. American Journal of Medical Sciences 314(3): 173–184

Wagoner LE, Taylor DO, Olsen SL et al 1993 Immunosuppressive therapy, management and outcome of heart transplant recipients during pregnancy. Journal of Heart and Lung Transplantation 12(6 part 1): 993–999

White-Williams C 1993 Immunosuppressive therapy following cardiac transplantation. Critical Care Nursing Quarterly 16(2): 1–10

Why H 1991 Endomyocardial biopsy technique. Nursing Standard 6(5): 49–50

Williams BA, Sandiford-Guttenbeil DM 1991 Heart and heart–lung transplantation. In: Williams BAH, Grady KL, Sandiford-Guttenbeil DM (eds) Organ transplantation: a manual for nurses. Springer, New York, pp. 129–164

24

Cardiopulmonary resuscitation in adults

Tom Quinn
Richard Hatchett

Cardiopulmonary arrest is the cessation of an effective circulation and respiratory effort. This is generally regarded as the ultimate medical emergency. The term 'cardiac arrest' is frequently used to indicate the same condition but technically this is the absence of an effective circulation only. In considering resuscitation skills, it is important to remember that the body does not store oxygen and therefore the brain will die within minutes if an effective circulation is not initiated by definitive treatments such as defibrillation or maintained by basic life support (BLS).

The majority of cardiac arrests occur in the community setting, with four-fifths of these resulting from coronary heart disease (Kuisma & Alaspaa 1997). Three-quarters of fatal coronary events occur in the home (Norris 1998). The major non-cardiac causes of cardiac arrest as identified within the literature (Kuisma & Alaspaa 1997, Silfvast 1991) are shown in Box 24.1.

True survival rates from prehospital cardiac arrest are difficult to ascertain because of methodological differences in collecting and reporting patient data. Reported survival in the United Kingdom (UK) ranges from 1.9% to 18.4% (NHS Executive 1996). In a Scottish series of 1476 patients resuscitated from cardiac arrest

---

Box 24.1   The major non-cardiac causes of cardiac arrest

- Non-traumatic bleeding
- Pulmonary embolism
- Dissecting aortic aneurysm with cardiac tamponade
- Intracerebral haemorrhage
- Intoxication
- Trauma
- Asthma
- Near drowning
- Malignancy
- Choking
- Hanging

by ambulance personnel, approximately 40% of patients who had a spontaneous circulation on reaching hospital were discharged home without major neurological deficit (Cobbe et al 1996). It has been suggested that, given the circumstances required for resuscitation to be successful, it is remarkable that anyone survives at all (Weaver 1991).

The outlook for patients who suffer cardiac arrest while in hospital differs from that of patients requiring resuscitation in the community but a successful outcome remains the exception. A survey of resuscitation attempts in British hospitals reported survival rates of around 15%. Patients who arrested in specialized units (coronary care or accident and emergency) were more likely to survive than those in general wards (Tunstall-Pedoe et al 1992). However, in the latter report baseline characteristics and details of the type of arrest were not given.

CARDIAC ARREST: DEFINITION AND DIAGNOSIS

Cardiac arrest will be defined for the purposes of this chapter as a loss of consciousness with absence of circulation, accompanied by absent or gasping respiration. These characteristics are, of course, features of death itself and cardiopulmonary resuscitation (CPR) is not appropriate in many cases, for example in terminal illness or where resuscitation attempts would be futile. These issues will be considered later.

It is important to note that in the setting of a witnessed cardiac arrest, patients may continue to make some spontaneous respiratory effort for a few minutes, although this is likely to present as agonal gasping. A classic study by Bayes de Luna et al (1989) of ambulatory electrocardiogram (ECG) monitoring reported that about three-quarters of patients developed ventricular fibrillation (VF) at the time of collapse. Several authorities have identified key factors which influence the chances of a successful outcome following cardiac

arrest. The arrest must be witnessed, bystander BLS commenced within 4 minutes, defibrillation (for VF or pulseless ventricular tachycardia (VT)) attempted within 8 minutes and advanced life support (including drugs and endotracheal intubation) administered as soon as possible. Together, these components describe a sequence of events known as the 'chain of survival' (Cummins et al 1991) (Fig. 24.1).

It is important that resuscitation is attempted as soon as possible following cardiac arrest, as indicated in the 'chain of survival' concept described above. Resuscitation initiated by a bystander helps to maintain cardiac arrest patients in a treatable rhythm and triples the chance of survival (Herlitz et al 1994). Unless a greater proportion of patients with cardiac arrest receive resuscitation from bystanders, the benefits of equipping ambulance personnel and hospital departments with specialized equipment and training will have little impact on survival (Fitzpatrick et al 1992). Efforts to ensure that every citizen can perform 'perfect' resuscitation are unrealistic but having some lifesaving skills, and using them to the best of one's capability, is certainly better than doing nothing at all (Wills 1997).

BASIC LIFE SUPPORT

Basic life support (BLS) is the term used to describe the measures used to maintain a clear airway and support patients' breathing and circulation, without the use of equipment (European Resuscitation Council 1998a, Nolan & Gwinnutt 1998a) apart from a simple protective device such as a plastic shield used for aesthetic purposes. The key steps encompassed within the term BLS include ensuring personal safety of the rescuer, patient assessment, summoning skilled help at the earliest opportunity, airway maintenance, expired air ventilation and chest compressions (European Resuscitation Council 1998a, Nolan & Gwinnutt 1998a). In those circumstances where additional

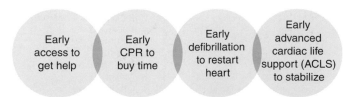

Figure 24.1 The 'chain of survival' (after Cummins et al 1991).

equipment, for example oropharyngeal airways or a pocket mask, is used by the rescuer, this is conventionally termed 'BLS with airway adjuncts'. Early defibrillation, using an automated external defibrillator (AED) when individuals are required to provide emergency aid as part of their job, is gaining acceptance within the health professions (Bossaert et al 1998, Kaye et al 1995, Quinn 1998). This will be discussed later in this chapter. If a defibrillator is available and the rescuer is competent in use of the device, then clearly this should take priority over all other activity once cardiac arrest is confirmed.

The objective of BLS is the maintenance of cerebral and coronary perfusion by artificial ventilation and circulation pending the application of definitive treatment such as the aforementioned defibrillation. It is very unlikely that a patient who sustains cardiac arrest will regain spontaneous circulation following the application of BLS measures alone. There have been reports of spontaneous termination of ventricular fibrillation (Mustafa et al 1998, Van Hemel & Kingma 1993) but such an occurrence is thought to be extremely rare and the overwhelming majority of patients in cardiac arrest will require resuscitation. BLS should be considered as a holding measure to 'buy time' rather than an attempt to restart the heart,

maintaining oxygenation of the brain and heart until defibrillation or other measures are available. Considerable emphasis is therefore given to the importance of summoning appropriate skilled help and equipment as soon as the initial assessment reveals absence of breathing.

In the hospital setting, this will usually be a call for the cardiac arrest team and in the community, use of the universal emergency numbers (999 or 112) to summon an ambulance. The single most important determinant of survival from adult cardiac arrest is the time elapsing from the patient collapsing to the delivery of defibrillation (Cobbe et al 1991). There is therefore considerable emphasis in the literature, in public education campaigns and in formal BLS courses on the importance of making this call at the earliest opportunity.

The recommended sequence of action for adult BLS is summarized in Figure 24.2. BLS is essentially a series of psychomotor skills. It has been known since research in the 1980s that the skills of BLS require physical practice, not just the learning of theory, and are most appropriately taught and refreshed under the supervision of a skilled trainer such as a resuscitation training officer. The following guidance, unless stated to the contrary, applies to the single-handed rescuer

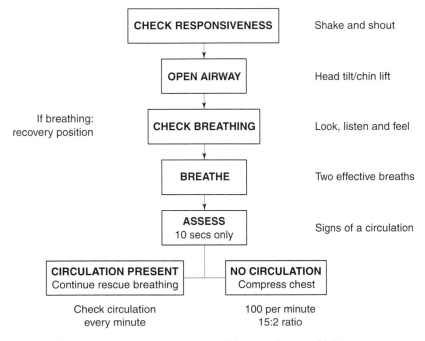

Figure 24.2 Cardiopulmonary basic life support algorithm. (Reproduced with permission from the Resuscitation Council (UK).)

confronted by a collapsed adult. Resuscitation of babies and young children and the management of cardiac arrest in special circumstances such as pregnancy, drowning and hypothermia are not covered in this chapter.

Safety of the rescuer is paramount

There is a saying well known to those in emergency services that 'two casualties are not better than one'. The rescuer's first duty is to ensure their own safety, whatever the setting: the potential hazards in the community are limitless and may include speeding road traffic, electrical cables and wires, noxious substances and falling masonry, as well as distressed, drunken or aggressive onlookers. In the hospital setting (arguably a more controlled environment), hazards such as electrocution, slippery floors and spilled water from a bedside locker should not be overlooked. The appropriate management of relatives, friends and persons close to the patient in cardiac arrest, who may wish to be present at the bedside during a resuscitation attempt, will be discussed later.

Patient assessment and recognition of cardiac arrest

The patient's level of responsiveness is assessed using the 'shake and shout' manoeuvre. The patient who responds to these simple stimuli is unlikely to be experiencing a cardiac arrest and should be assessed further to determine the appropriate management. Faced with an unresponsive adult, the rescuer should shout for help from bystanders or colleagues. The patient's airway should be opened to ensure the flaccid tongue is not preventing breathing. The head-

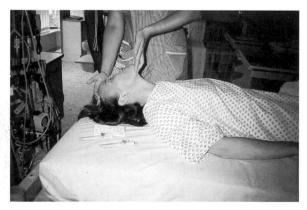

Figure 24.3 The head-tilt, chin-lift manoeuvre to open the airway.

tilt, chin-lift manoeuvre is used to achieve this (Fig. 24.3). This manoeuvre should be avoided if at all possible where there is a history of neck or head injury, for example in the setting of a road accident, fall or diving accident. With the airway open, the rescuer should look, listen and feel for breathing (more than the occasional gasp) for 10 seconds. In the patient who is breathing spontaneously a circulation check should be made (see below). If this is also present they should be placed in the recovery position (see below) while help is summoned. The patient is continually re-assessed for signs of deterioration.

The call for help is crucial

Different actions are required depending upon the circumstances of the collapse. In an adult who is unresponsive and not breathing and where there is no suspicion of trauma or drowning, the most likely cause of the arrest is presumed to be ventricular fibrillation and an immediate call for an emergency ambulance (in the community) or the cardiac arrest team (in hospital) is required. There is now an absolute imperative to get a defibrillator to the patient as rapidly as possible. In situations where the loss of consciousness is associated with trauma or drowning or the patient is an infant or child, then BLS should be administered for about 1 minute before help is summoned. This is because reversal of hypoxia is considered the main priority in such cases.

Rescue breathing

Once the diagnosis of cardiac arrest has been made and appropriate help summoned, either personally (leaving the patient initially, if alone) or delegated to a colleague or bystander, the rescuer should immediately commence BLS. Two *effective* breaths, which make the patient's chest rise and fall, are recommended. Up to five attempts are allowed to achieve this before moving on to the next steps. The patient should be turned on to their back and any visible obstruction removed from the mouth. Dentures, unless very loose, are generally left in place. Expired air ventilation is commenced by pinching the patient's nose and creating a good seal of the rescuer's lips around the patient's mouth. A steady blow is made into the mouth for 1.5–2 seconds.

Volumes of expired air in the region of 400–600 ml should be sufficient to make the chest rise and fall. The rescuer should remove their mouth from the patient's after each breath to facilitate expiration and to avoid contact with regurgitated matter. If the chest fails to rise and fall with each breath, the airway should be reassessed and the head-tilt chin-lift checked for adequacy. Failure to achieve effective breaths after five attempts should not impede rapid progress to the next steps outlined below.

Assessing the circulation

After two adequate rescue breaths have been achieved (or after five attempts, even if they have not) the victim is assessed for signs of a circulation. There have been reports of difficulties with palpating for the carotid pulse (Eberle et al 1996, Flesche et al 1994). The guidelines therefore now recommend that the rescuer check for any movement, including swallowing or breathing, and assess the patient's colour as guides to the adequacy of circulation, if there is any doubt regarding the presence of a carotid pulse. Non-health-care rescuers are generally advised not to attempt the carotid pulse check, for the above reason. This assessment should take no more than 10 seconds. If there is confidence that a circulation is present, then rescue breathing should be continued if the patient is not breathing. The recommendation is that 10 breaths are given (taking about 1 minute to achieve this) and the circulation re-assessed. This sequence continues until help arrives, the patient recovers or the rescuer becomes exhausted. Should the patient appear to recover, re-assessment of vital signs is required.

Chest compressions

In the absence of a circulation or where there is any doubt and in the absence of a defibrillator, the rescuer should commence chest compressions at a rate of about 100/minute, alternating with rescue breaths in a ratio of 15:2 (compressions:breaths). The patient's chest should be exposed and the lower half of the sternum located. Using index and middle fingers, the rescuer should identify the lower rib margin and, keeping the fingers together, slide them upwards to the point where the ribs meet the sternum. With the middle finger on this point, the rescuer places the index finger on the sternum and slides the heel of their other hand down the sternum until it reaches the index finger of the first. This should be the lower half of the sternum. The heel of one hand is placed over the other, with fingers interlocked. With the rescuer now placed vertically above the patient's chest and with arms straight, the sternum is pressed upon to depress it 4–5 cm (about one-third of the chest depth), then released without losing contact between rescuer's hands and patient's chest (Fig. 24.5). This is repeated about 100 times per minute, with compression and release taking an equal amount of time. After 15 compressions, two rescue breaths are given as described above. The sequence of alternating compressions to rescue breaths is continued with a ratio of 15:2. Resuscitation efforts are continued until qualified help and/or equipment arrives, the patient appears to recover or the rescuer becomes exhausted.

The recovery position

The unconscious patient is at risk of airway contamination from regurgitated stomach contents or debris in the mouth or upper airway, including loose dentures,

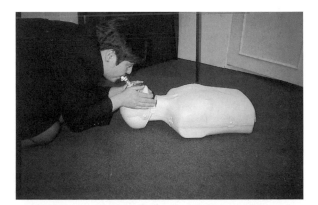

Figure 24.4 Using the pocket mask at the top of the patient. The airway is opened and a good seal can occur between rescuer and casualty to provide ventilation. Saliva or vomit does not touch the rescuer and a view of the chest rising can be seen more easily. NB: The risk of infection, particularly serious infection such as hepatitis B or HIV, is remote. No cases of AIDS have ever been reported from mouth-to-mouth resuscitation (Handley 1999).

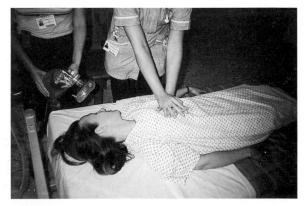

Figure 24.5 The hand position for effective chest compressions in resuscitation.

and from mechanical obstruction arising from the tongue falling back. In the absence of contra-indications such as suspected head and/or neck trauma, the safest place for the unconscious patient is on their side, facilitating drainage of stomach contents and reducing the risk of obstruction. The European Resuscitation Council (1998a) recommend the following position.

Having removed any objects such as spectacles or keys which might injure the patient from their pockets, the rescuer kneels beside the patient and opens the airway using the head-tilt chin-lift manoeuvre. The patient's arm nearest to the rescuer is placed out at a right angle to their body, the elbow bent and palm uppermost. The far arm is brought across the chest, the back of the hand held against the nearest cheek. The far leg is grasped just above the knee by the rescuer's free hand and pulled up with the foot remaining on the ground. The rescuer pulls on this leg to roll the victim, on their side, towards the rescuer. The upper leg is adjusted to ensure that both the hip and knee are bent at right angles. The head is tilted back to assist in airway maintenance, with the hand under the patient's cheek adjusted as necessary. The patient must be regularly re-assessed to ensure adequate breathing and circulation (Fig. 24.6).

Two-rescuer resuscitation

Where there are sufficiently skilled personnel available, two-person BLS may be administered with each sharing the task but at the same ratio of 15 compressions to two rescue breaths. The first priority in such circumstances, however, remains the prompt call for an ambulance or the cardiac arrest team. It is useful for the rescuer administering chest compressions to count 'one, two, three ...' so that the person responsible for rescue breathing is ready to proceed without delay. Good team-work can reduce the effects of fatigue by swapping tasks or resting while the other person continues the BLS.

Choking

A partial or complete obstruction of the airway is terrifying for any person and can be fatal. The person will often be able to clear an obstruction merely by coughing. The choking person often grips his throat with his hand in the so-called 'international distress sign'. In cases of partial obstruction, the person may be distressed and coughing and there may be an associated inspiratory wheeze. If airway obstruction is complete the victim loses the ability to speak, breathe or cough and rapidly loses consciousness. Death is inevitable without rapid action by rescuers.

The conscious person who appears to be choking should be encouraged to cough, because in some cases this may be all that is required to relieve the obstruction. If the person is deteriorating (for example, they stop coughing or breathing or lose consciousness) the situation is potentially grave. Obvious debris should be removed from the mouth and back slaps should be administered. Lean the person well forward and administer up to five sharp slaps between the shoulder blades with the heel of one hand (Fig. 24.7). If the person is lying down, kneel beside them and give up to five sharp slaps as described above.

If back slaps do not relieve the obstruction, abdominal thrusts are indicated (Fig. 24.8). Standing behind the person, the rescuer places a clenched fist between the umbilicus and xiphisternum. With this fist grasped by the rescuer's other hand, the rescuer pulls sharply inwards and upwards. If the person is on the ground, the rescuer should kneel astride them, placing them on

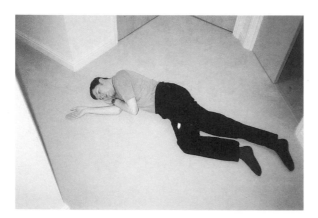

Figure 24.6 A person in the recovery position.

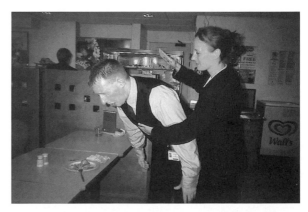

Figure 24.7 Back slaps administered to a choking person.

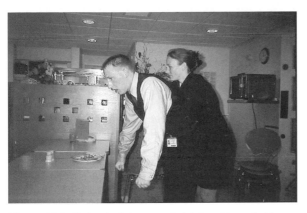

Figure 24.8 Abdominal thrusts administered to a choking person.

their back. Abdominal thrusts should be administered in this position, while taking care to avoid pressure on the person's chest and rechecking the mouth after every five slaps or thrusts.

Should the person with airway obstruction become unconscious the sequence for basic life support described above should be instituted. Rescue breaths should be attempted alternately with back slaps and abdominal thrusts.

THE ADVANCED LIFE SUPPORT ALGORITHM

The key aspects of cardiopulmonary resuscitation in adults are summarized in the advanced life support

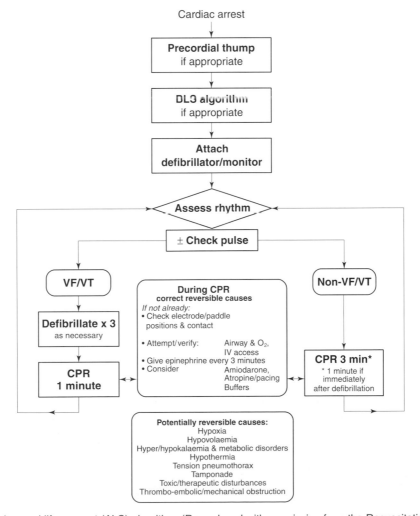

Figure 24.9 The advanced life support (ALS) algorithm. (Reproduced with permission from the Resuscitation Council (UK).)

(ALS) algorithm (Fig. 24.9). The algorithm, it should be remembered, is not the complete guideline to resuscitation but merely a graphic summary and it is recommended that readers obtain further information and advice from their resuscitation training officer or equivalent expert. Current guidelines may be found in Resuscitation Council (UK) (2000).

It is the ECG manifestation of cardiac arrest that gives rescuers a guide to the appropriate treatment and, in some cases, the prognosis of the patient. The ECG manifestations in cardiac arrest can be divided into two pathways. These are rhythms amenable to defibrillation – ventricular fibrillation (VF) and pulseless ventricular tachycardia (VT) – and a pathway where defibrillation is not used – asystole and electromechanical dissociation (EMD). EMD can be defined as the features of cardiac arrest despite normal (or near normal) electrical excitation (Colquhoun & Camm 1999). Basically, a rhythm appears that would normally offer a pulse but in EMD it does not. The principles of management for these two pathways are summarized in Figure 24.9.

Defibrillation

The importance of early defibrillation cannot be stressed enough. Current guidelines reflect advances in defibrillator technology made over recent years. Automated external defibrillators (AEDs) have been developed to remove the difficulties of cardiac rhythm analysis from the less experienced rescuer, using specialized software designed to discriminate cardiac arrest rhythms where a shock is indicated from those in which a shock is not indicated, with a high degree of accuracy. Thus, AEDs provide a means of delivering defibrillation, where appropriate, to victims of cardiac arrest without the need to await the arrival of a cardiac arrest team. AEDs have been successfully deployed by ambulance services (Cobbe et al 1991), St John Ambulance volunteers (Walters et al 1994), nursing students (McKee et al 1994), police officers (Haynes et al 1991) and even airline cabin crew (O'Rourke et al 1997).

An important aspect of current resuscitation guidelines is that they are designed to include the management of cardiac arrest using AEDs as well as the traditional manual defibrillators which many nurses will already be familiar with. It is strongly recommended that all registered nurses be trained in, and authorized to use, AEDs, whatever the setting (Quinn 1998). This life-saving skill would seem to fall into the category of a 'logical and desirable' development in nursing practice as discussed in the UKCC document

The scope of professional practice (UKCC 1992). Survival from cardiac arrest in the community and hospital settings alike remains the exception, not the norm, so patients' chances of a successful resuscitation are likely to be increased with the widespread availability of early defibrillation by so-called 'first responders', including nurses using AEDs (Bossaert et al 1998, Quinn 1998). The only interventions shown unequivocally to be of value in improving long-term outcomes from adult cardiac arrest are BLS and early defibrillation. Current guidelines therefore place considerable emphasis on these aspects of resuscitation.

Advanced airway care

The European Resuscitation Council have published specific guidance on airway management techniques (Baskett et al 1996). Endotracheal intubation remains the 'gold standard' for securing the airway, with laryngeal mask airways (LMA) gaining prominence as a more accessible technique for less experienced personnel. The latter is a curved tube terminating in a spoon-shaped rubber mask with an inflatable rim. It is held like a pen, the curve following the roof of the mouth and passed blindly into the hypopharynx. This isolates and seals the laryngeal inlet, with remarkable reliability up to inflation pressures of 25 cmH$_2$O (Simons 1999). It is an excellent and highly recommended device for the cardiac arrest trolley or cupboard, administering a high percentage of oxygen yet, particularly for nursing staff who are not intubating routinely, it is a technique that is easy to master and practise.

The bag-valve device can be tricky to use for smaller and less experienced hands. It may be more effective for one nurse to hold the mask in place with two hands and hold the airway open while a colleague uses their hands to squeeze the bag. A reservoir bag added to the end of the self-inflating system will allow oxygen to be drawn into the system as opposed to *air* and oxygen. This will offer a much high percentage of oxygen for resuscitation (Simons 1999) (Fig. 24.10).

Drugs

In terms of drugs and their administration during resuscitation, the intravenous route remains the preferred option for most cases. Drug absorption by the endobronchial route is less reliable and therefore the use of the central venous route represents the 'gold standard'. Accessibility does, however, depend upon available skills and equipment. Direct intracardiac injection, while popular in previous years, is not supported by current opinion. While animal-based exper-

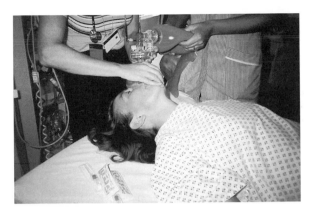

Figure 24.10 Two nurses using the bag-valve device. NB: Note the reservoir bag at the end of the device to increase the percentage of oxygen delivered.

imental studies have demonstrated improvements in myocardial and cerebral blood flow following administration of adrenaline (epinephrine), this has not been shown to improve survival in humans, irrespective of the dose administered (Woodhouse et al 1995). Adrenaline (epinephrine) should be administered with caution to patients whose arrest is associated with solvent abuse, cocaine and similar agents (Lange et al 1989). Evidence to support the use of other medication remains limited and the recommendations on drug administration tend to be based on tradition rather than 'hard' evidence. The main therapeutic options are summarized in Figure 24.9.

GUIDELINES ARE NOT PROTOCOLS

The current resuscitation guidelines may appear less prescriptive than the 'resuscitation protocols' of the past. This is a reflection of the need for patient care to be applied to individuals on the basis of the presenting circumstances and the available expertise. Words and flow charts must be interpreted with common sense and an appreciation of their intent (Nolan & Gwinnutt 1998b). Local policies will continue to codify the responsibilities of nurses and others employed within a particular setting, with less emphasis than in the past on drug administration and more on proven treatments such as defibrillation (Quinn 1998).

AFTER THE EVENT: POSTRESUSCITATION CARE

Resuscitation efforts do not cease when the patient regains a spontaneous circulation. To optimize the chances of a return to pre-arrest health status, it is nec-

essary to re-assess the patient's condition and to correct life-threatening conditions that may have caused the arrest in the first place, for example by administering a thrombolytic agent to a patient with acute myocardial infarction. Attention is required to the simple 'ABCs' of resuscitation: the airway must be patent and breathing supported if necessary. Supplementary oxygenation is mandatory and correction of haemodynamic, biochemical and other physiological variables may be required. Many patients will merely require ECG monitoring on a coronary care unit but for some more detailed monitoring and support, including mechanical ventilation, will be necessary. Outcome following resuscitation may be influenced by the place of care in the hours following a return of circulation, irrespective of age (Premachandran et al 1997).

LEGAL AND ETHICAL ISSUES

It is hardly surprising that cardiopulmonary resuscitation raises a number of legal and ethical issues, since by definition decision making in this area of professional practice is unparalleled by any other. Deciding whether or not a patient should be subjected to the indignity and frank brutality of a resuscitation attempt is fraught with difficulty. Involving patients in decisions about their care is morally, legally and clinically desirable (Florin 1994), although doctors and patients have not always agreed on this sensitive issue (Morgan et al 1994). Most patients want to discuss their resuscitation status (Hill et al 1994, Morgan et al 1994) but not all patients want to have to make the final decision (Liddle et al 1993).

Each case requires clinicians and patient together to weigh up the likely chances of a successful outcome and of the impact on dignity and quality of life of the individual concerned. Discussion of cardiopulmonary resuscitation may not be appropriate for all patients, however, but should be sensitively addressed in, for example, cases where the patient is at risk of cardiac or respiratory failure or is terminally ill. Efforts to develop guidelines based on prediction of mortality following resuscitation have been reported by several authors (Beuret et al 1993, Dautzenberg et al 1993, Schultz et al 1996).

In legal terms, failure to attempt resuscitation when there is a recognized professional duty to act to save life may result in criminal proceedings (Doyal & Wilsher 1993). This is particularly the case where there is evidence that the patient might have survived had resuscitation been provided. This may, for example, be in a previously healthy individual struck down by an episode of ventricular fibrillation, although survival even with prompt defibrillation is not guaranteed in this group. Registered nurses have a professional duty to act at all times in the best interests of the patient and this would include the collapsed person in the street as well as the patient on the ward.

In their discussion of proposals for formal guidelines, Doyal & Wilsher (1993) suggest three instances where non-resuscitation is acceptable. First, where a competent patient, having been informed of the probable consequences of resuscitation, indicates that they do not wish to be subjected to this treatment and, in effect, issues an 'advance directive'. Second, where the patient is not legally competent to give or refuse consent to treatment, the responsible clinician judges that resuscitation would not be in the patient's best interests. Finally, in those cases where the likelihood of a successful outcome approaches zero, irrespective of the patient's competence to consent. This latter scenario would include those patients in the prehospital setting who are 'found dead', where no BLS has been attempted prior to the arrival of ambulance personnel. This would also include a situation where time had elapsed from the onset of cardiac arrest (if known) and the arrival of professional help had been prolonged. It may also be where the ECG rhythm demonstrates asystole despite a period of BLS and in those patients who are found to be in a state of decomposition, demonstrate signs of rigor mortis or decapitation (Marsden et al 1995).

Resuscitating elderly patients raises many questions. While outcomes are less favourable when compared with younger patients, this is not necessarily the case when the older patient is in otherwise good health and the presenting rhythm is ventricular fibrillation or ventricular tachycardia (Tresch 1991). Yet more than a quarter of senior doctors have indicated that they would not resuscitate healthy patients over the age of 70 (Hill et al 1994). In one series, geriatricians were more likely to recommend resuscitation for elderly patients than were general physicians (Davies et al 1993).

The overall responsibility for decisions regarding CPR and 'do not attempt resuscitation' (DNAR) orders lies with the consultant concerned (BMA/RCN 2001). He or she should be prepared to discuss the issue with all members of the health-care team involved in the patient's care. A DNAR decision should be dated and recorded in the patient's notes, with the reason for the order. The primary nurse or senior member of the nursing team should record it in the nursing notes, and inform other members of the team. Communication of decisions to the patient and people close to the patient is part of this process. Unless the patient refuses, decisions should also be communicated to the patient's family and others close to them (BMA/RCN 2001).

Marsden et al (1995) have designed a useful algorithm for ambulance staff faced with the issues of whether to resuscitate that may be of use to some nursing staff. It certainly stimulates discussion. It does err on the side of caution, advising 1 minute's worth of CPR even if there is no evidence of cardiopulmonary resuscitation in the previous 15 minutes (Marsden et al 1995). The AED has been highlighted as useful here, because it can be used throughout the resuscitation attempt to assess whether there is an arrhythmia amenable to defibrillation. After the final minute's worth of CPR, if the AED again finds no shockable rhythm and a flat line persists on the ECG screen for over 10 seconds, it is advised that resuscitation attempts are stopped (Marsden et al 1995). This is a difficult situation for both ambulance and nursing staff, as they are not permitted to diagnose death, and one which community and hospital health care teams need to discuss.

RELATIVES AND RESUSCITATION

There has been considerable interest in the need to support relatives and loved ones both during and after and indeed in anticipation of resuscitation. Sigsbee & Geden (1990) studied the anxiety levels of cardiac patients' family members and their ability to learn how to perform basic life support. When anxiety was measured through use of the State Anxiety Inventory, anxiety levels had declined 2 months after completion of the training programme. McLauchlan et al (1992) trained a group of patients with recurrent VT in the skills of BLS, together with a friend or family member. This was prompted by doctors' perceptions that anxiety would be increased by such training. Measured anxiety levels had in fact lowered 3 months after training in both groups.

Dracup et al (1997), in the largest published series, studied patient–family pairs randomized to undergo training in BLS, BLS with risk factor modification, BLS with social support intervention or 'usual care'. BLS training was, however, restricted to family members only. Patients whose family members learned BLS with the social support intervention reported better psychosocial adjustment with less anxiety and hostility than patients in the other groups. Control patients reported better psychosocial adjustment and less emotional distress than patients in the BLS-only and BLS-risk factor modification groups. The authors concluded that there was a need to tailor family BLS training so that instruction does not result in negative psychosocial states in patients. In terms of skill retention, Moser et al (1990) found that this was poor at 7 months following training and indeed may start to wane as little as 2 weeks after initial training in family members and the lay public, as well as nurses, physicians and emergency medical technicians (Moser & Coleman 1992).

The presence of family members during the resuscitation of a loved one has raised much debate since it emerged as an issue in the early 1990s. The American nursing press appeared to lead the way with a debate occurring over several weeks in the *Journal of Emergency Nursing* in 1991 (Martin 1991). Subsequently, the emergency department at the Foote Hospital in Michigan reported a positive 9-year experience of allowing relatives to witness resuscitation attempts, while being supported by a member of the professional team (Hansen & Strawser 1992). This was usually a religious minister. The hospital had questioned whether it was ethical to prevent relatives being with a loved one at what might be the end of the patient's life.

The issue does seem to raise several points. Healthcare professionals may run the risk of deciding whether individuals can cope with a resuscitation situation without actually asking them. There is also the possibility of generalizing to all relatives from a small number of negative experiences where relatives did become distressed at witnessing the scene. The Foote Hospital experienced no relative interference in resuscitation attempts and the small number who became hysterical or fainted were quickly escorted from the room.

The *British Medical Journal* undertook the debate in 1994, with a personal account from Sarah Adams of being present at resuscitation attempts on her brother at an equestrian event (Adams et al 1994). The subsequent letters demonstrated mixed feelings. There was concern that the often necessarily light-hearted comments used by staff as a coping mechanism would be upsetting to relatives (Schilling 1994), while Crisci (1994), describing experiences in southern Italy, believed that relatives can be hostile and even assaulting when they believe events are going wrong. By 1996 the Resuscitation Council were recommending that relatives should be allowed to witness resuscitation and that they be supported by appropriately trained medical staff (Resuscitation Council 1996). The primary issue appears to be considering and enquiring about the needs of relatives at this unhappy time. Staff should not leave relatives alone in the resuscitation room but explain what is occurring *before* entering the event, as well as after. The debate has inevitably occurred in paediatric nursing (Goldstein et al 1997), where the important issue is raised of not making parents feel uncomfortable if they in fact wish to leave.

TEACHING BASIC AND ADVANCED LIFE SUPPORT SKILLS

There is currently a clear emphasis in the UK to move away from ringfencing the skills of basic life support for health-care professionals alone. Quite simply, the 'chain of survival' needs to be strengthened at each link. The British Heart Foundation has made great strides with its Heart Start programme which teaches BLS to the lay public. Its success is that it encourages members of the public to set up their own support groups to learn and teach the skills. This is augmented by a regular magazine and certification to encourage nationwide support and a sharing of initiatives. The programme has more recently advanced into teaching school children; which unlike other European countries is a relatively new initiative in the UK.

The government White Paper *Saving lives: our healthier nation* (Department of Health 1999) pledged implementation and training for placing (automated external) defibrillators in public places, reinforcing the 'chain of survival' and the need to initiate early definitive treatment. Such moves require a shift from who should and should not be allowed to perform BLS and advanced life support (ALS) to what the patient needs to survive a cardiopulmonary arrest. The days when only the doctor was allowed to defibrillate must be relegated to the past and an appropriate assessment system for a wide range of personnel needs to take its place. *The scope of professional practice* (UKCC 1992) asks nursing staff to reflect on the skills necessary to provide appropriate care to the patient and resuscitation must surely come into this domain.

The UK Resuscitation Council provides and supports ALS courses nationally, lasting a minimum of 2 days, which teach and assess a variety of skills including airway management, defibrillation and leading a team through an arrest. Individual hospital policies would then be adhered to by the practitioner, following completion. The Crown Report (1998) signalled support for multidisciplinary protocols for administering medications and this leads the way for nursing staff to administer first-line resuscitation drugs in line with the hospital policy and ALS algorithm.

The valued role of the resuscitation officer or trainer can offer innovative in-house programmes to augment formal teaching. Records can be maintained on courses staff have attended and their learning needs. Those who arrive at work having already completed a reputable ALS course can be assessed on the hospital equipment to ensure orientation and safety. Mock arrests will also allow staff to practise skills regularly. Studies in the 1980s demonstrated how poor the skills of resuscitation were in hospital staff (Skinner 1985, Wynne 1987). They also demonstrated that confidence may remain as competence declines. Regular teaching seemed the ideal and logical answer but there is still debate regarding the best way to teach the skills to encourage retention. It is clear that the ability to perform the skills wanes quickly and after a year candidates may be back to the level of competency similar to that before the training (Wynne et al 1999). Certainly, in BLS there is a need for 6-monthly to yearly practical updates. It is likely that this may also be required as frequently in the more complex skills of ALS but logistics and cost may militate against this.

CONCLUSION

The management of cardiopulmonary arrest presents professional, ethical, legal and practical challenges for the nurse. Recently published guidelines have been simplified to reduce the requirement for complex decision making during a resuscitation attempt. The emphasis given to BLS and defibrillation reflects the strong evidence base for these interventions compared to other techniques and medications. Skills should be regularly updated under the supervision of a resuscitation training officer or similar skilled individual. Defibrillation is a time-dependent, life-saving technique which, with the advent of AEDs, is within the scope of every nurse's responsibility.

REFERENCES

Adams S, Whitlock M, Higgs R, Bloomfield P, Baskett PJF 1994 Should relatives be allowed to watch resuscitation? British Medical Journal 308: 1687–1689

Baskett PJF, Bossaert L, Carli P et al 1996 Guidelines for the advanced management of the airway and ventilation during resuscitation. A statement by the Airway and Ventilation Management Working Group of the European Resuscitation Council. Resuscitation 31(3): 201–230

Bayes de Luna A, Coumel P, Leclercq JF 1989 Ambulatory sudden cardiac death: mechanisms of production of fatal arrhythmia on the basis of data from 157 cases. American Heart Journal 117(1): 151–159

Beuret P, Feihl F, Vogt P, Perret A, Romand J, Perret C 1993 Cardiac arrest: prognostic factors and outcome at one year. Resuscitation 25(2): 171–179

BMA/RCN 2001 Decisions relating to cardiopulmonary resuscitation: a joint statement from the British Medical Association, the Resuscitation Council (UK) and the Royal College of Nursing, London.

Bossaert L, Handley A, Marsden A et al 1998 European Resuscitation Council guidelines for the use of automated external defibrillators by EMS providers and first responders. Resuscitation 37(2): 91–94

Cobbe SM, Redmond MJ, Watson JM, Hollingworth J, Carrington DJ 1991 'Heartstart Scotland': initial experience of a national scheme for out of hospital defibrillation. British Medical Journal 302(6791): 1517–1520

Cobbe SM, Dalziel K, Ford I, Marsden AK 1996 Survival of 1476 patients initially resuscitated from out of hospital cardiac arrest. British Medical Journal 312(7047): 1633–1637

Colquhoun M, Camm JA 1999 Asystole and electromechnical dissociation. In: Colquhoun MC, Handley AJ, Evans TR (eds) ABC of resuscitation. BMJ Books, London, pp. 11–13

Crisci C 1994 Should relatives watch resuscitation? Local factors may influence decision (letter). British Medical Journal 309: 406

Crown Report 1998 A report on the supply and administration of medicines under group protocols. Department of Health, London.

Cummins RO, Ornato JP, Thies WH, Pepe PE 1991 Improving survival from sudden cardiac arrest: the 'chain of survival' concept. A statement for health professionals from the Advanced Cardiac Life Support Subcommittee and Emergency Cardiac Care Committee, American Heart Association. Circulation 83(5): 1832–1847

Dautzenberg PL, Broekman TC, Hooyer C, Schonwetter RS, Duursma SA 1993 Patient related predictors of cardiopulmonary resuscitation of hospitalized patients. Age and Ageing 22(6): 464–475

Davies KN, King D, Silas JH 1993 Professional attitudes to cardiopulmonary resuscitation in departments of geriatric and general medicine. Journal of the Royal College of Physicians of London 27(2): 127–130

Department of Health 1999 Saving lives: our healthier nation. Stationery Office, London

Doyal L, Wilsher D 1993 Withholding cardiopulmonary resuscitation: proposals for formal guidelines. British Medical Journal 306(6892): 1593–1596

Dracup K, Moser DK, Taylor SE, Guzy PM 1997 The psychological consequences of cardiopulmonary resuscitation training for family members of patients at risk of sudden death. American Journal of Public Health 87(9): 1434–1439

Eberle B, Dick WF, Schneider T, Wisser G, Doetsch S, Tzanova I 1996 Checking the carotid pulse check: diagnostic accuracy of first responders in patients with and without a pulse. Resuscitation 33(2): 107–116

European Resuscitation Council 1998a The 1998 European Resuscitation Council guidelines for adult single rescuer basic life support. Resuscitation 37(2): 67–80

European Resuscitation Council 1998b The 1998 European Resuscitation Council guidelines for adult advanced life support. Resuscitation 37(2): 81–90

Fitzpatrick B, Watt GCW, Tunstall-Pedoe H 1992 Potential impact of emergency intervention on sudden deaths from coronary heart disease in Glasgow. British Heart Journal 67(3): 250–254

Flesche CW, Breuer S, Mandel LP, Breivik H, Tarnow J 1994 The ability of health professionals to check the carotid pulse. Circulation 90 (suppl 1): 288

Florin D 1994 Decisions about cardiopulmonary resuscitation. British Medical Journal 308(6945): 1653–1654

Goldstein A, Berry K, Callaghan A 1997 Resuscitation witnessed by relatives (letter). British Medical Journal 314: 144

Handley AJ 1999 Basic life support. In: Colquhoun MC, Handley AJ, Evans TR (eds) ABC of resuscitation. BMJ Books, London, pp. 1–4

Hansen C, Strawser D 1992 Family presence during cardiopulmonary resuscitation: Foote Hospital emergency department's nine-year perspective. Journal of Emergency Nursing 18: 104–106

Haynes BE, Mendoza A, McNeil M, Schroeder J, Smiley DR 1991 A statewide early defibrillation initiative including laypersons and outcome reporting. Journal of the American Medical Association 266(4): 545–547

Herlitz J, Ekstrom L, Wennerblom B, Axelsson A, Bang A, Holmberg S 1994 Effect of bystander initiated cardiopulmonary resuscitation on ventricular fibrillation and survival after witnessed cardiac arrest outside hospital. British Heart Journal 72(5): 408–412

Hill ME, McQuillan G, Forsyth M, Heath DA 1994 Cardiopulmonary resuscitation: who makes the decision? British Medical Journal 308: 1677

Kaye W, Mancini ME, Giuliano KK et al 1995 Strengthening the in-hospital chain of survival with rapid defibrillation by first responders using automated external defibrillators: training and retention issues. Annals of Emergency Medicine 25(2): 163–168

Kuisma M, Alaspaa A 1997 Out-of-hospital cardiac arrests of non-cardiac origin. Epidemiology and outcome. European Heart Journal 18(7): 1122–1128

Lange RA, Cigarroa RG, Yancy CW et al 1989 Cocaine-induced coronary artery vasoconstriction. New England Journal of Medicine 321(23): 1557–1562

Liddle J, Gilleard C, Neil A 1993 Elderly patients' and their relatives' views on CPR. Lancet 342(8878): 1055

Marsden AK, Ng GA, Dalziel K, Cobbe SM 1995 When is it futile for ambulance personnel to initiate cardiopulmonary resuscitation? British Medical Journal 311: 49–51

Martin J 1991 Rethinking traditional thoughts. Journal of Emergency Nursing 17: 67–68

McKee DR, Wynne G, Evans TR 1994 Student nurses can defibrillate within 90 seconds. An evaluation of a training programme for third year student nurse in the use of an automatic external defibrillator. Resuscitation 27(1): 35–37

McLauchlan CA, Ward A, Murphy NM, Griffith MJ, Skinner DV, Camm AJ 1992 Resuscitation training for cardiac patients and their relatives – its effect on anxiety. Resuscitation 24(1): 7–11

Morgan R, King D, Prajapati C, Rowe J 1994 Views of elderly patients and their relatives on cardiopulmonary resuscitation. British Medical Journal 308(6945): 1677–1678

Moser DK, Coleman S 1992 Recommendations for improving cardiopulmonary resuscitation skills retention. Heart and Lung 21(4): 372–380

Moser DK, Dracup K, Guzy PM, Taylor SE, Breu C 1990 Cardiopulmonary resuscitation skills retention in family members of cardiac patients. American Journal of Emergency Medicine 8(6): 498–503

Mustafa MUA, Baker CSR, Stephens JD 1998 Spontaneously terminating ventricular fibrillation and asystole induced by silent ischaemia causing recurrent syncope. Heart 80(1): 86–88

NHS Executive 1996 Review of ambulance performance standards. Final report of steering committee. NHS Executive, London

Nolan J, Gwinnutt C 1998a The 1998 European Resuscitation Council guidelines for adult single rescuer basic life support. British Medical Journal 316: 1870–1876

Nolan J, Gwinnutt C 1998b The 1998 European Resuscitation Council guidelines for adult advanced life support. British Medical Journal 316: 1863–1869

Norris RM 1998 Fatality outside hospital from acute coronary events in three British health districts, 1994–5. United Kingdom Heart Attack Study Collaborative Group. British Medical Journal 316(7137): 1065–1070

O'Rourke MF, Donaldson E, Geddes JS 1997 An airline cardiac arrest program. Circulation 96(9): 2849–285

Quinn T 1998 Cardiopulmonary resuscitation: new European guidelines. British Journal of Nursing 7(18): 1070–1077

Resuscitation Council (UK) 1996 Should relatives witness resuscitation? Report from a project team of the Resuscitation Council (UK). Resuscitation Council, London

Resuscitation Council (UK) 2000 Resuscitation Council guidelines. Resuscitation Council, London

Schilling RJ 1994 Should relatives watch resuscitation? No room for spectators. British Medical Journal 309: 406

Schultz SC, Cullinane DC, Pasquale MD, Magnant C, Evans SRT 1996 Predicting in-hospital mortality during cardiopulmonary resuscitation. Resuscitation 33(1): 13–17

Sigsbee M, Geden EA 1990 Effects of anxiety on family members of patients with cardiac disease learning cardiopulmonary resuscitation. Heart and Lung 19(6): 662–665

Silfvast T 1991 Cause of death in unsuccessful prehospital resuscitation. Journal of Internal Medicine 229: 331–335

Simons R 1999 The airway at risk. In: Colquhoun MC, Handley AJ, Evans TR (eds) ABC of resuscitation. BMJ Books, London, pp. 19–24

Skinner D 1985 CPR skills of preregistration house officers. British Medical Journal 290: 1549

Tresch DO 1991 CPR in the elderly: when should it be performed? Geriatrics 46(12): 47–56

Tunstall-Pedoe H, Bailey L, Chamberlain DA, Marsden A, Ward M, Zideman DA 1992 Survey of 3765 cardiopulmonary resuscitations in British hospitals (the BRESUS study). British Medical Journal 304(6838): 1347–1351

UKCC 1992 The scope of professional practice. UKCC, London

Van Hemel NM, Kingma JH 1993 A patient in whom self-terminating ventricular fibrillation was a manifestation of myocardial reperfusion. British Heart Journal 69(6): 568–571

Walters G, Glucksman E, Evans TR 1994 Training St. John Ambulance volunteers to use an automated external defibrillator. Resuscitation 27(1): 39–45

Weaver WD 1991 Resuscitation outside the hospital – what's lacking? New England Journal of Medicine 325(20): 1437–1439

Wills A 1997 Having some lifesaving skills must be better than having none. British Medical Journal 314(7075): 222

Woodhouse SP, Cox S, Boyd P, Case C, Weber M 1995 High dose and standard dose adrenaline do not alter survival compared with placebo in cardiac arrest. Resuscitation 30(3): 243–249

Wynne GA 1987 Inability of trained nurses to perform basic life support. British Medical Journal 294: 1198

Wynne GA, Gwinnutt C, Bingham B, Van Someren V, Colquhoun M, Handley AJ 1999 Teaching resuscitation. In: Colquhoun MC, Handley AJ, Evans TR (eds) ABC of resuscitation. BMJ Books, London, pp. 54–60

25

Management and support of patients with internal cardioverter defibrillators

Jayne James

The development of the internal cardioverter defibrillator (ICD) has provided considerable advances in survival rates for patients experiencing sudden cardiac events. However, its use may have wider consequences for individuals and their families or carers living with this device, both physically, socially and psychologically (Cooper et al 1986). Many patients and their families find discharge home a difficult time in adjusting to the new device. This chapter discusses the role and functioning of the ICD and focuses upon strategies of support that nurses may provide themselves or facilitate through other health-care professionals. In addition, within the community, families of ICD patients often witness the device administering a shock. Not surprisingly, stress-related problems have been described arising from this responsibility. It is therefore suggested that a more family-centred approach is needed to enable the role that relatives and carers play to be recognized and supported.

It should always be remembered that patients receiving this device have a complex and life-threatening illness, which will require innovative nursing strategies to enable individuals and their families or carers to obtain maximum quality of life. Whilst some care strategies are suggested here, it is vital that current nursing practice is continuously evaluated and developed for the benefit of this unique group of patients.

THE DEVELOPMENT OF THE ICD

Patients who are likely to receive this device include those who have survived a sudden cardiac death (SCD) event or patients considered at risk of a SCD, for example following extensive myocardial infarctions (Knight et al 1997). SCD essentially means the occurrence of death within 1 hour following cardiac symptoms (Mason & McPherson 1992). Traditionally, patients experiencing life-threatening arrhythmias prior to the development of the ICD were offered a variety of anti-arrhythmic drug therapies. More recently, use of this treatment alone has been questioned due to serious side-effects and poor patient tolerance (Singh et al 1995). A number of studies have identified marked improvements in survival rates for patients receiving the ICD device when compared to drug therapy alone (Bremner et al 1993, Nichols & Wolverton 1991).

Bremner et al (1993) studied a group of 381 patients receiving an ICD and reported survival rates of 99%, 97% and 96% at 1, 2 and 3 years after implantation. More recently, the Multicenter Automatic Defibrillator Implantation Trial (MADIT) (Moss et al 1996) and the Antiarrhythmic Versus Implantable Defibrillator Trial (AVID) (AVID Investigators 1997) established significant improvements in survival rates with the use of ICD therapy when, again, it was compared to drug therapy alone.

The ICD was developed by Miroswki in the United States and was first implanted into a human in 1980 (Mirowski 1984). American literature still continues to dominate this field of enquiry. The device first consisted of a 'shock box concept' but now offers a multiprogrammable tiered therapy, with further improvements still expected (Nichols & Collins 1995). It has been estimated that in total 75 000 patients have already received this device worldwide (Schuster et al 1998). Within the UK 400–500 devices are presently being implanted per year and it is estimated that already a total of 2000 patients benefit from the ICD (British Pacing and Electrophysiology Group 1999).

It is envisaged that use of this device will expand considerably (Kalbfleisch et al 1989, Page 1994, Teplitz 1991), with predictions suggesting a further 30 000 ICDs will be implanted annually worldwide by the middle of the millennium (Rehak 1995). Arising from this expansion, ICD patients needing treatment are likely to receive care in a variety of settings, not only in specialist areas. Nurses, whether in the hospital or community, will need knowledge of the specific needs of ICD patients and their families to promote confidence in the care they provide.

DEVICE FUNCTION

The present-day ICD system is battery operated, able to monitor heart rate and rhythm and record action taken (Collins 1994). It is capable of providing anti-tachycardia pacing (fast pacing), pacing for bradycardia (slow pacing), burst pacing for ventricular tachycardia and cardioversion or defibrillation shocks. Arrhythymias such as ventricular tachycardia (VT) and ventricular fibrillation (VF) are treated by administering varying joules of shocks (Teplitz 1991). Each device is individually programmed but can take as little as 10 seconds to recognize the arrhythmia and 4 seconds to deliver the shock (CPI 1998a). The device's ability to react quickly to an arrhythmic event means that some patients may receive little or no warning of a shock (James 1997a). Devices can give up to five consecutive shocks to correct the arrhythmia (Currier & Packa 1992) and the amount of joules delivered may increase during this period (Reid 1993). The intensity of the internal shock, whilst requiring less energy, has the same effect as external defibrillation because it is delivered directly to the source (James & Tagney 1998). As there are a variety of models currently available, specific technical details are not given here but can be obtained from the manufacturers' manuals.

The device can be programmed to administer treatment in a variety of ways, with most patients given tiered therapy (Kruse 1998). Tiered therapy consists of various options of treatment. First, as VT starts, this triggers and administers a series of fast pacing impulses. The rhythm is then assessed and if normal rhythm has not returned, pacing impulses will be given again. If the programmed number of impulses fails to stop or slow the VT, the device moves to the next tier of treatment which is cardioversion. This will be delivered in gradual incremental levels of higher intensity. Finally, if this still fails or the patient deteriorates into VF, defibrillation will be administered. These three options may take over 2 minutes (Kruse 1998). The battery enables anything from 4 to 9 years of monitoring and treatment. Timing of the battery replacement depends on usage and the age of the device (Kruse 1998, Teplitz 1991).

Future improvements likely to be seen include increased life of the device, continued reduction in size and improvements to the leads, batteries and its capacitors. It is envisaged that this will result in less complex follow-up procedures and these should be possible over the telephone (Morris et al 1999).

DEVICE COMPOSITION

The device consists of a pulse generator which is surgically implanted either into the abdomen, submammary or subcutaneously via a clavicular incision (Fig. 25.1). The subclavian vein is accessed to enable the lead system to be positioned. Two sensing electrodes are then threaded through this vessel until the base of the right ventricle is reached. They are then left lying on the endocardial surface of the heart (Collins 1994).

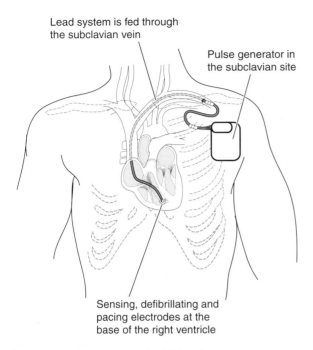

Lead system is fed through the subclavian vein

Pulse generator in the subclavian site

Sensing, defibrillating and pacing electrodes at the base of the right ventricle

Figure 25.1 Placement of the ICD device.

The lead wire is attached to the pulse generator at the site chosen for its insertion. Whilst original models were bulky, weighing 200 g (Nathan & Barnett 1997), current models are continually reducing in size. Some now weigh as little as 78 g (CPI 1998a).

De-activation of the device can be instigated by application of a magnet. The actual process of this varies dependent on the device. For example, some models require the magnet to be held over the area and de-activation occurs immediately, whilst other models require you to wait 30 seconds until a bleeping sound stops (Kruse 1998). Nurses caring for ICD patients need to know the specific manufacturer's protocol for the models used in their unit. De-activation of the device may be necessary if it malfunctions or during resuscitation when external defibrillation may be deemed necessary (Collins 1994).

SELECTION OF PATIENTS FOR AN ICD

Likely candidates for the ICD are patients who have experienced at least one sudden cardiac death event (Morris et al 1999). At least 90% of SCD events can be attributed to coronary artery disease (Bolles & Funk 1995). In particular, these events are mainly due to ventricular arrhythmias (Mason & McPherson 1992). Approximately 29% of those experiencing SCD survive

the initial cardiac arrest (Bolles & Funk 1995) and of these survivors, between 10% and 30% are likely to have another SCD event within a year (Myerberg et al 1984). This rises to 50% by 5 years (Cobb et al 1992).

There is increasing prophylactic use of this device for patients who are considered at risk of a SCD event but who may not have had an episode of ventricular tachyarrhythmia. This, for example, could be patients who have experienced extensive myocardial infarctions (Block & Breithardt 1999, Knight et al 1997). In addition, patients with cardiomyopathy or heart failure who may be at risk of ventricular tachyarrhythmias may be candidates for this device (James & Tagney 1998). Patients receiving the ICD often have a poor left ventricular ejection fraction, often as low as 35% (Moss et al 1996), and some patients may already have received coronary artery bypass grafting (Bolles & Funk 1995).

In addition to the medical rationale for patient selection, there also appears to be a gender difference in patients likely to receive this device, with available research indicating that mainly male patients receive the ICD (AVID Investigators 1997, Bremner et al 1993, Moss et al 1996). Despite the low rate of device implantation in women, statistics confirm the far slower general reduction in deaths from heart disease when compared to men (BHF 2000; see also Chapter 2). This present gender imbalance could be attributed to the fact that women are less likely to be referred for cardiac investigations which would identify them as likely candidates for the ICD. Further investigation is needed with regard to identifying gender imbalances in patient selection and to making sure that processes are in place to ensure that all patients who would benefit from this device are given the opportunity.

THE PERIOD LEADING TO IMPLANTATION

In many instances, prior to the decision to implant the device patients have often experienced lengthy periods of hospitalization. This may be related to recovery and treatment of SCD events. In addition, a series of drug 'cocktails' are likely to have been tried in the first instance (Teplitz 1991). Extensive diagnostic tests to ascertain the suitability of the device for individual patients will include electrophysiology studies (EPS), coronary angiography and echocardiography. During these tests patients may learn for the first time the poor state of their heart. Not surprisingly, patients and families have described this period as a time of crisis (Dougherty 1994, Pycha et al 1986).

Preparation for implantation

Nurses caring for patients awaiting an ICD implantation need to consider not only the specific preparation but also the preceding events that patients and families or carers may have experienced. This is important, particularly when planning clinical nursing strategies to facilitate maximal quality of life on return home. For example, a number of SCD events may have resulted in some memory impairment (Dougherty 1997), therefore use of repetition, audiovisual aids and other techniques may be needed to ensure understanding (Mason & McPherson 1992).

Patients with an ICD have described concerns arising from health-care professionals' lack of knowledge about the device (Dougherty 1997). To be told 'You're at the forefront of technology' (Reid 1993) may not instill confidence in your care. It is essential therefore that nurses preparing patients and their families are conversant with the physical, psychological and emotional problems which may occur following the implantation of the ICD (James 1997b).

IMPLANTATION OF THE DEVICE

The device is usually implanted in specialist units, to ensure relevant expertise and suitable management in case of surgical emergencies such as vessel perforation (Collins 1994). Implantation of the device is a straightforward procedure usually performed under local anaesthetic with the patient heavily sedated. During the procedure the device function is checked by precipitating a shock from the device in a controlled clinical environment. Due to the amnesiac effects of sedation, patients may or may not remember this happening.

IMMEDIATE POST-IMPLANTATION CARE

On return to the ward, the patient's heart rate and rhythm will be closely monitored. Patients will be continuously monitored via an ECG for episodes of VT or VF and for inappropriate shocks (Kruse 1998). The EPS department should be immediately informed of any such events. If sustained postoperative arrhythmias do occur and the device appears to be unable to correct these, standard resuscitation procedures should be followed (James & Tagney 1998). If external defibrillation is deemed necessary, paddle position will depend on the positioning of the generator. For example, anterior/posterior positioning may be used to avoid external defibrillation over the device site (Collins 1994).

> **Box 25.1** Complications associated with ICD implantation
>
> - Lead dislodgement, failure and fractures
> - Inappropriate shocks
> - Subcutaneous migration of the device
> - Major vessel or cardiac perforation
> - Serious wound infections (this may lead to device removal)

Patients will initially remain on bedrest. Care will include management of pain and wound site observation (Moser et al 1993). Given the serious nature of postoperative wound infections, prophylactic antibiotics are routinely administered (Kennergren 1996). Patients usually begin to mobilize the following day and may resume normal activities within 2–4 weeks (Nathan & Barnett 1997). Physical complications arising from this procedure are not frequent but Box 25.1 lists some complications which should be monitored for in the immediate postoperative period and subsequently following discharge.

In addition to these physical aspects of care, it is vital that patients and their families/carers are able to talk about their feelings surrounding the device from the outset. Patients may be anxious at the anticipation of their first shock (Molchany & Peterson 1994) and if they do receive a shock whilst in hospital, may need to talk through this experience (Teplitz et al 1990).

PREPARATION FOR DISCHARGE

In comparison to lengthy periods of hospitalization prior to the fitting of the device, discharge home following implantation (providing recovery is uneventful) is usually within 48 hours (CPI 1998b). This abrupt end to what for many was a lengthy and often intensive period of care can leave patients and families/carers feeling vulnerable and isolated from support. As discharge is a time when emotions are often heightened it is not surprising that patients and families/carers have described initial problems in adjusting to living with this device, particularly during the first few months following implantation (Dougherty 1995). This indicates the need for strategies to be developed which provide continued support and education within the community setting. This should enable patients and their families or carers to fully understand and adjust to living with the ICD.

As those close to the patient are likely to be providing the majority of support when home, it is essential that they are included in preparation for discharge (James 1997a).

Patients commonly feel very anxious around discharge. However, levels of anxiety generally do reduce over time (Dougherty 1995). High anxiety levels on discharge may affect patients' ability to understand and retain information given. Some patients have difficulty understanding that the device will not prevent the arrhythmias occurring but will provide immediate treatment via shock delivery when they do occur (Anderson & Camm 1993). It is essential that this is fully understood to ensure that patients are expecting the device to administer a shock. In addition, repeated cardiac arrests may have further diminished patients' ability to retain information (Dougherty 1997). Despite these problems, patients and carers receive most of their information before discharge. Whilst written sources are available to take home, they largely deal with safety aspects of the care, giving limited attention to possible feelings and emotions. Time is needed for patients and families to talk through how they are feeling and continued support needs to be available following discharge home.

Within inpatient care there is very limited time available for the preparation of living with this device (James 1997a). Notably there is little time for preparation for situations in which the shocks may occur, for example during stressful situations (Reid 1993). Suggestions to improve this have included role play, repetition of information, family involvement and video-taped information (James 1997b). Role playing with patients and families could possibly assist in demonstrating ways in which they may deal with certain situations (Nichols & Wolverton 1991). It is vital that clinical nursing practice strategies such as these are evaluated to ensure they are meeting patients' and carers' needs.

Case study 25.1 outlines a possible situation which could be role played. Box 25.2 summarizes possible points for discussion.

Safety advice given to patients on discharge

An important part of the nurse's role in preparing patients and their families/carers for discharge is providing information aimed at ensuring safety factors

---

Case study 25.1

Brian, who has recently had an ICD implanted, decides to accompany his wife on her weekly supermarket visit. The visit goes without incident until they visit the crowded coffee shop. While they are sitting drinking their tea, Brian says he's feeling increasingly light-headed and thinks he might be about to receive a shock. An assistant comes over and offers to ring for an ambulance.

Box 25.2 Points for discussion (Case study 25.1)

- Avoidance of patient injury by:
  - encouraging patient to lie down (if time)
  - making some space on the floor, removal of furniture.
- Coping with onlookers.
- Patient assessment including monitoring the pulse rate and checking the patient's recovery after the shock.
- Remember the patient may receive more than one shock and may lose consciousness.
- Role of relative in patient support. Reminder that they can touch their loved one without fear of injury during a shock.
- Assessing whether an ambulance is necessary.
- Organizing the patient to go home or to hospital if necessary.
- Obtaining advice from the regional centre at a later point.
- Encouraging those involved to discuss concerns and worries regarding this experience.

Box 25.3 ICD patient advice

- Check wound site daily for signs of infection, such as soreness, exudate or fever.
- Keep incision site dry until healed (Kruse 1998).
- Avoid excess arm movements to the affected arm for the first 6 weeks.
- Wear MedicAlert bracelet with details of the ICD (Knight et al 1997).
- Carry an ICD identification card, including model number and personnel to contact in case of an emergency (Moser et al 1993).
- Record the date, time and nature of an event requiring a shock (Kruse 1998).
- Ring the regional centre for advice initially after each shock and when worried or concerned.
- Avoid strong magnetic fields as they can cause device malfunction. The pulse generator should be at least 12" away from magnetic fields, for example security wands in airports or cellular phones (CPI 1998b).
- Avoid caffeinated drinks such as coffee, as they may precipitate arrhythmias (Kruse 1998).
- Magnetic resonance imaging is contra-indicated.
- Initially patients are unable to drive for 6 months (DVLC 1998). Reinstatement of a driving licence is then individually assessed (Gold & Oliver 1990).
- Women should be individually counselled regarding the possibility of becoming pregnant and the implications of this for their own and their baby's health.

are adhered to. Box 25.3 summarizes the advice patients currently receive.

PREPARING PATIENTS AND THEIR FAMILIES/CARERS FOR AN ICD SHOCK

Nurses can play a key role in the preparation and support of both patients and families/carers for the delivery of the shock. This should include preparation for what may happen and enabling patients and others to understand and come to terms with the experience afterwards (James 1997a). Patients should be informed that they could be either conscious or become unconscious during a shock and that they may receive little or no warning of this ICD activation (James 1997a). Information is given that they may receive up to five consecutive shocks to correct the arrhythymia. In addition, it is advisable that they sit or lie down if there is warning of an impending shock (Medtronic 1998). In addition, certain precautions are advised to avoid injury when the ICD is activated; for example, climbing ladders should be avoided and swimming should be within their depth and accompanied by someone else.

Family/carer preparation

As highlighted, due to time constraints discharge preparation concentrates on safety aspects related to the device, with little opportunity given for discussion of family or carer needs. Despite this omission, once home, patients look mainly to their family or carers for support (Kuiper & Nyamathi 1991) and it is usually these people who will be present during the delivery of a shock. This can be a distressing experience and therefore it is essential that they are equally well prepared.

Carers should be re-assured that they will not experience adverse effects if touching the patient during a shock; they may, however, expect to feel a mild tingling sensation and will probably feel the patient jolt (Knight et al 1997).

If patients are admitted to hospital for other treatments, it is important that both their own and their families'/carers' wishes are respected if a shock from the device is anticipated. Within the hospital setting, patients' and significant others' preferences are being increasingly sought regarding whether they wish to remain during patient resuscitation (Williams 1996). In ICD patient care, this is also a vital issue. When a shock does occur, it is important that mechanisms that patients and families or carers have developed to cope are continued and supported.

FOLLOW-UP CARE

Attendance at follow-up clinics is necessary to enable the number and types of events to be monitored. It also allows physiologic assessment, device evaluation and adjustment and modifications to drug regimens to be continued (Bremner et al 1993). In addition, battery replacement will be necessary as power depletes and this occurrence can be carefully monitored during the clinic time. Surgical replacement of the battery is required but this does not usually mean lead replacement and is completed under local anaesthetic.

The health-care professionals offering follow-up care do vary. Some clinics in America will have nurse specialists (De Borde et al 1991), whilst others will have limited nursing participation. It appears that due to time factors, there may be little opportunity during these visits for patients and others to discuss how they may be coping with the device. It therefore appears essential that alternative support is provided for the needs of ICD patients in addition to the physical functioning of the device (James 1997a).

Presently there appear to be few rehabilitation programmes available. For patients to regain previous fitness levels it is important that they are aware of the pulse rates which have been set to trigger pacing and defibrillation (Kruse 1998). Individual programmes are suggested which enable patients to avoid misconceptions such as fears of triggering a shock from the device which may inhibit them returning to a safe level of fitness.

COMMON PATIENT ADJUSTMENT PROBLEMS ASSOCIATED WITH ICD IMPLANTATION

Whilst it is essential that nurses caring for ICD patients develop practice to ensure safe and competent physical care, in addition they will need to understand the feelings and emotions that may be evoked by living with this device. This knowledge will help nurses to ensure that care is not only technically correct but meaningful and relevant to patients and their families.

Fears about the device function

As patients are reliant on this device, unsurprisingly many fears relate to the device efficiency. Patients worry about the possibility of device malfunction and battery failure and that the battery will eventually need replacement (Cooper et al 1986).

Unpredictability of the device

Many patients have a problem in coming to terms with the unpredictability of the device, as there may be little warning of an impending shock (Dunbar et al 1993). This may leave patients feeling a loss of control over their lives and a reluctance to rejoin previous social groups due to the risk of shock delivery and their friends' subsequent reactions (Molchany & Peterson 1994). Some patients, in an attempt to try to gain some control, may blame the shock on an unrelated incident. They may then stop activities they enjoy in their attempts to reduce the number of shocks they receive (Dunbar et al 1993). Without correct advice and support, patients may find themselves doing less and less in their misguided attempt to reduce the frequency of shocks.

Worries about health-care professionals' lack of knowledge

Outside regional centres of expertise little may be known about the function or impact this device may have on patients' and families'/carers' lives. Lack of confidence in health-care professionals' abilities and knowledge has led some patients and families to limit how far they will travel. Some patients will be unwilling to travel too far from their regional centre (James 1997b) and this may restrict holidays and other pursuits. One ICD patient described how a paramedic refused to connect him to an ECG monitor 'for fear of him blowing up their machine' (Veseth-Rogers 1990, p. 17).

Emotional needs

The life-threatening nature of the ICD patient's condition leads some to see an association between the shock delivery and a close call with death (Dunbar et al 1993). Arising from this, patients often describe the need to talk about their feelings and may relive the shock many times over in their attempts to come to terms with what has happened (Sneed & Finch 1992). Despite this need to talk, patients often feel unable to burden those close with their feelings (Teplitz et al 1990). Nurses may be ideally placed to fulfil this role or could be instrumental in liaison with other health-care professionals such as counselling services to ensure these needs are fully addressed. Whilst support groups may be available in some areas (Teplitz et al 1990), their effectiveness to provide emotional support needs to be carefully evaluated. Often the patient and partner attend together but neither may feel able to

discuss certain issues honestly for fear of upsetting the other. In addition, some may feel inhibited about discussing personal issues within this forum. It is essential that patients and significant others are individually assessed, as there will be individuals who may benefit from confidential support and discussion.

Anger and anxiety

Feelings of anger and anxiety have been described by many ICD patients. These emotions are often heightened around the time of discharge but again, tend to reduce over time (Dougherty 1995). Interestingly, levels of both these emotions appear closely correlated to the number of shocks received; the greater the number of shocks, the higher the incidence of emotional problems (Luderitz et al 1994). Other emotions include depression, which can occur in as many as 50% of patients (Kuiper & Nyamathi 1991, Morris et al 1999).

Changes in the perception of body image can be a problem, particularly in patients with older, more bulky devices. Abdominal insertion may mean changes in clothing style, as restrictive garments may hamper the functioning of the device (Pycha et al 1990). It is vital that the reasons why patients experience these extreme emotions are explored to enable coping strategies to be developed.

Changes in sexual activity

Patients are advised that they are unlikely to receive a shock during sexual activity and if this does occur, their partner will not be harmed (De Borde et al 1991). Despite this re-assurance, patients' sexual activity is often reduced following ICD implantation (Luderitz et al 1994). A combination of factors may contribute to this including declining self-esteem, body image change and role alteration within the family (Sneed & Finch 1992). In addition, this may be partly attributed to health-care professionals' omission in not addressing this issue specifically when preparing patients for life at home (Albarran & Bridger 1997). It is suggested that continued follow-up within the community may assist patients and their families/carers to feel able to address such intimate topics.

FAMILY/CARER EXPERIENCES OF SUPPORTING ICD PATIENTS

As highlighted above, the family or carers frequently provide the main support for ICD patients on discharge. Recovery and adjustment are therefore influenced by and affected by those close (James 1997a). The degree to which they cope will determine how well the patient adjusts to living with this device. Despite this fact, the effects on the family and carers are often underestimated or overlooked (James 1997b). It is vital that those who are providing this support have their needs and problems understood and strategies of support offered. NB: Within this section, the term 'family' will be used to refer to both family or carers who may be involved in ICD patients' lives when discharged.

Family needs

Families of ICD patients need to discuss their feelings both in terms of their concerns for the loved one but also the effect this treatment option may have on them and the family's functioning. Despite this need, families and carers have described being unable to express their emotions for fear of precipitating patient anxiety, possibly leading to arrhythmias and shock treatment (Simons et al 1992). Supporting a loved one who collapses, receives a shock and may even lose consciousness is an enormous responsibility, yet it is assumed that the family will take on this responsibility and that they will be fully capable. However, many describe feeling very frightened and apprehensive at this prospect (Dunbar et al 1993). In addition, it appears friends may feel unable to cope with the responsibility of taking an ICD patient out. Therefore, unlike other recoveries, families of ICD patients may at this time feel isolated from their own support mechanisms (James 1997b). Nurses can provide support during this time and assist in allaying fears of those close.

Feelings of family members

Stress-related problems are common in family members and carers. These include insomnia (Nichols & Wolverton 1991), anxiety, frustration and despair (Pycha et al 1990). There is worry about the ability to cope should a shock occur (James 1997a) and some have described feeling helpless and uncertain as to what to do (Dunbar et al 1993).

In addition to the concerns for their partner, families and carers worry about the implications for themselves, such as increased patient dependency (Kuiper & Nyamathi 1991). Some patients may feel frightened to be alone in case of a shock. Therefore, whilst those close may crave personal space, they also feel guilty if they are not present when a shock occurs (Dunbar et al 1993). Sometimes those close try to protect the patient

from emotional upsets such as family arguments but this can lead to concealed resentment and anger (Simons et al 1992). Not surprisingly, higher levels of psychological problems are reported in families where the device is activated than in those who have not experienced a shock (Dougherty 1997).

Family assessment

Families and carers may face additional potential problems, because some centres teach cardiopulmonary resuscitation (CPR) in case of device malfunction (Kruse 1998). Arguably, families should be assessed to ascertain their ability to cope with this role and their feelings surrounding this added responsibility (Sirovatka 1993).

Family dynamics

Due to the patient's increased dependence on those close, role reversal may occur once the patient is discharged (Teplitz et al 1990). This may give rise to areas of conflict. Some patients may not be able to return to work and this may again affect the family functioning. Prohibition from driving following device implantation may be only for 6 months but it could be indefinite, dependent on the incidence of shocks (DVLC 1998). Patients and their families have reported enormous repercussions from this, including resentment of wives about having to drive and husbands becoming critical of their spouse's driving. Driving prohibition can be such an issue that some patients have described driving despite medical advice to the contrary (Craney & Powers 1995, Sneed & Finch 1992). The use of taxis or friends may ease the strain on both patients and their families, while nurses can provide a key role in assisting patients and families to make such choices as they adjust to living with this device.

At present, most investigations of ICD patients' adjustment to the device consist of male samples. Little is known about particular issues related to female patients and their families' needs (James 1997b). Currently, there is limited information available on the experiences of female ICD patients becoming pregnant. This information is vital as the device is increasingly used and it is likely that more younger women will be receiving ICDs. Issues for male caregivers and female ICD patients, such as child-rearing concerns, need further investigation and the development of supportive strategies. More discussion regarding women's issues and ICDs can be found in James et al (1999).

KEY RECOMMENDATIONS FOR CLINICAL NURSING PRACTICE

- Further research is needed to evaluate existing clinical nursing practice. Patients' and families'/carers' perceptions of their experiences need to be investigated and can then form a basis of care.

- Continued education is needed to enable nurses caring for ICD patients to formulate meaningful care which meets patients' and family needs. This will also enable patients to have confidence in the care they receive.

- Greater patient and family preparation is needed for the experiences likely to be encountered. This will include possible role and lifestyle changes.

- A shift in nursing approach is needed from the physical aspects of care towards a more holistic model which recognizes and deals with associated psychological and emotional effects of these treatments. Nurses are ideally placed to provide this.

- Strategies are required to enable patients and families to talk about and understand their ICD experiences. This will enable adjustment to living with the ICD.

- A shift in emphasis towards a family-centred approach, which recognizes this resource as part of patient recovery, as well as the needs of the family and carers themselves.

- Clinical nursing practice strategies within the community need to be developed, particularly aimed at continued patient and family support at home, to enable greater quality of life for both. This needs to become holistic and patient centred to enable appropriate and necessary support mechanisms to become more accessible to patients and their families.

IMPLICATIONS FOR CLINICAL NURSING PRACTICE

As nurses are increasingly faced with medical technological advances such as the ICD, it is vital that continued professional development is undertaken to enable patients and families to have confidence in the care they receive. Whilst it is essential that physical aspects of nursing care are fully addressed, nurses will need to ensure that they do not lose sight of the context in which these episodes occur. Care needs to be formulated beyond the tasks developed by technology (Mackellaig 1995). The therapeutic value of the nurse/patient/family/carer relationship needs to be recognized and developed to enable patients and carers to return to their maximal quality of life.

More recently, the National Institute for Clinical Excellence (NICE) has produced guidance on the use of ICDs (NICE 2000). These recognise both the relatively low use of the device in the UK compared to other countries such as the United States and Germany, and the regional variations in its use. Importantly, guidance includes those patient groups for whom the ICD should routinely be considered. These include those suffering cardiac arrest due to either VT or VF, and those with spontaneous VT causing syncope or significant haemodynamic compromise. The use of the ICD is divided into secondary and primary prevention categories. The potential for adverse psychological impact through the implantation of the device is recognised, with a call for adequately funded and staffed support services. Finally, and as a closing point, nurses caring for ICD patients will need:

the ability to be simultaneously the technically competent nurse, and the personally involved humanistic practitioner. It is about being able to share a world of meaning with the patient and family. It is about exhibiting a concerned attitude for the welfare of the patient and the family. (Walters 1995, p. 1002)

REFERENCES

Albarran J, Bridger S 1997 Problems with providing education on resuming sexual activity after myocardial infarction: developing written information for patients. Intensive and Critical Care Nursing 13(1): 2–11

Anderson M, Camm J 1993 Legal and ethical aspects of driving and working in patients with an implantable cardioverter defibrillator. American Heart Journal 127(4:2): 1185–1193

AVID Investigators 1997 The Antiarrhythmics Versus Implantable Defibrillators. A comparison of antiarrhythmic-drug therapy with implantable defibrillators in patients resuscitated from near-fatal ventricular arrhythmias. New England Journal of Medicine 337: 1576–1583

BHF 2000 British Heart Foundation coronary heart disease statistics database: annual compendium. BHF, London

Block M, Breithardt G 1999 The implantable cardioverter defibrillator and primary prevention of sudden death: the multicenter automatic defibrillator implantation trial and coronary artery bypass graft (CABG)-patch trial. American Journal of Cardiology 83(5B): 74D–78D

Bolles M, Funk M 1995 Quality of life in younger persons with an implantable cardioverter defibrillator. Dimensions of Critical Care Nursing 14(2): 100–110

Bremner S, McCauley K, Axtell K 1993 A follow-up study of patients with implantable cardioverter defibrillators. Journal of Cardiovascular Nursing 7(3): 40–51

British Pacing and Electrophysiology Group 1999 National pacemaker database. BPEG, London

CPI 1998a Physician's system manual. Guidant Corporation, St Paul, Minnesota

CPI 1998b Therapy in action. AICD patient handbook. Guidant Corporation, St Paul, Minnesota

Cobb L, Weaver W, Fahrenbruch C, Hallstrom A, Copass M 1992 Community based interventions for sudden cardiac death: impact, limitations, and changes. Circulation 85(11): 98–102

Collins M 1994 When your patient has an implantable cardiovertor defibrillator. Australian Journal of Nursing March 1: 34–39

Cooper D, Luceri R, Thurer R, Myerburg R 1986 The impact of the automatic implantable cardioverter defibrillator in quality of life. Clinical Progress in Electrophysiology and Pacing 4(4): 306–309

Craney J, Powers M 1995 Factors related to driving in persons with an implantable cardioverter defribrillator. Progress in Cardiovascular Nursing 10(3): 12–17

Currier D, Packa D 1992 The patient with an implantable cardiac defibrillator: a case study. Focus on Critical Care 19(2): 150–154

De Borde R, Aarons D, Biggs M 1991 The automated implantable cardioverter. Clinical Issues in Critical Care Nursing 2(1): 170–177

Dougherty C 1994 Longitudinal recovery following sudden cardiac arrest: survivors and their families. American Journal of Critical Care 3: 145–154

Dougherty C 1995 Psychological reactions and family adjustment in shock versus no shock groups after implantation of internal cardioverter defibrillator. Heart and Lung 24(4): 281–291

Dougherty C 1997 Family-focused interventions for survivors of sudden cardiac arrest. Journal of Cardiovascular Nursing 12(1): 45–58

Driving Vehicle Licensing Centre (DVLC) 1998 The at-a-glance guide to the current medical standards of fitness to drive. Crown Publications, Swansea

Dunbar S, Warner C, Purcell J 1993 Internal cardioverter defibrillator device discharge: experiences of patients and family members. Heart and Lung 22(6): 494–501

Gold R, Oliver M 1990 Fitness to drive: updated guidance on cardiac conditions in holders of ordinary driving licenses. Health Trends 22: 31–32

James J 1997a The psychological and emotional impact of living with an automatic internal cardioverter defibrillator (AICD): how can nurses help? Intensive and Critical Care Nursing 13(6): 316–323

James J 1997b Living on the edge – patients with an automatic internal cardioverter defibrillator (AICD): implications for nursing practice. Nursing in Critical Care 2(4): 163–167

James J, Tagney J 1998 Caring for patients with an ICD. Nursing Times 94(48): 50–51

James J, Albarran J, Tagney J 1999 Going home: the lived experiences of women following ICD implantation. Advancing Clinical Nursing 3: 169–178

Kalbfleisch K, Lehmann M, Steinman R et al 1989 Re-employment following implantation of the automatic cardioverter defibrillator. American Journal of Cardiology 64: 199–202

Kennergren C 1996 Impact of implant techniques on complications with current implantable cardioverter-defibrillator systems. American Journal of Cardiology 78(5a): 15–19

Knight L, Livingston N, Gawlinski A 1997 Caring for patients with third-generation implantable cardioverter defibrillators: from decision to implant to patient's return home. Critical Care Nurse 17(5): 46–63

Kruse L 1998 Keeping pace with implanted defibrillators. Registered Nurse 61(8): 30–35

Kuiper R, Nyamathi A 1991 Stressors and coping strategies of patients with automatic implantable cardioverter defibrillators. Journal of Cardiovascular Nursing 5(3): 65–76

Luderitz B, Jung W, Deister A, Manz M 1994 Patient acceptance of implantable cardioverter defibrillator devices: changing attitudes. American Heart Journal 4(2): 1179–1184

Mackellaig J 1995 Has technology dimmed our view of t he best care for our patients? Care of the Critically Ill 11: 92

Mason P, McPherson C 1992 Implantable cardioverter defibrillator: a review. Heart and Lung 21: 141–147

Medtronic 1998 On a safe course … life with the PCD. Medtronic, Switzerland

Mirowski M 1984 The implantable cardioverter-defibrillator – an update. Journal of Cardiovascular Medicine 9: 191–199

Molchany C, Peterson K 1994 The psychosocial effects of support group intervention on AICD recipients and their significant others. Progress in Cardiovascular Nursing 9(2): 23–29

Morris M, Kenknight B, Warren J, Douglas J 1999 A preview of inplantable cardioverter defibrillator systems in the next millennium: an integrative cardiac rhythm management approach. American Journal of Cardiology 83(5B): 44D–48D

Moser S, Crawford D, Thomas A 1993 Updated guidelines for patients with automatic implantable cardioverter defibrillators. Critical Care Nurse 13(2): 62–71

Moss A, Jackson W, Cannon D et al 1996 Improved survival with an implanted defibrillator in patients with coronary disease at high risk for ventricular arrhythmia. New England Journal of Medicine 335(26): 1933–1940

Myerberg R, Kessler K, Estes D 1984 Long term survival after pre-hospital cardiac arrest: analysis of outcome during an eight year study. Circulation 70: 538–546

Nathan A, Barnett M 1997 Implantable cardioverter defibrillators: a patient booklet. British Heart Foundation, London

NICE 2000 NICE guidance on technologies for specialist cardiac services. The National Institute for Clinical Excellence, London

Nichols K, Collins J 1995 Update on inplantable cardioverter defibrillators: knowing the differences in devices and their impact on patient care. AACN (American Association of Critical-Care Nurses) Clinical Issues 6(1): 31–34, 160–162

Nichols S, Wolverton C 1991 Outcome criteria for patients with implantable cardioverter defibrillators. Dimensions in Critical Care Nursing 10(5): 294–304

Page P 1994 Ethical and cost benefit issues of research involving patients with an implantable defibrillator. Canadian Journal of Cardiology 10(3): 339–341

Pycha C, Gulledge A, Hutzler J, Kadria N, Maloney J 1986 Psychological responses to the implantable defibrillator: preliminary observations. Psychosomatic Medicine 27(12): 841–845

Pycha C, Calabrese J, Gulledge D, Maloney J 1990 Patient and spouse acceptance and adaptation to implantable defibrillators. Cleveland Clinic Journal of Medicine 57: 441–444

Rehak M 1995 Research corner. Quality of life perceptions of implanted cardioverter-defibrillator patients. Prairie Rose 63(1): 6–7

Reid S 1993 After VT: living with a AICD implant. Australian Nurses Journal 22(9): 9–13

Schuster P, Philips S, Dillon D, Tomich P 1998 The psychosocial and physiological experiences of patients with an implantable cardioverter defibrillator. Rehabilitation Nursing 23(1): 30–37

Simons L Cunningham S, Catanzaro M 1992 Emotional responses and experiences of wives of men who survive a sudden cardiac death event. Cardiovascular Nursing 28(3): 17–21

Singh S, Fletcher R, Fisher SG et al 1995 Amiodarone in patients with CHF and asymptomatic ventricular arrhythmia. New England Journal of Medicine 333(2): 77–82

Sirovatka B 1993 The implantable cardioverter defibrillator: patient and family education. Dimensions of Critical Care 12(6): 328–334

Sneed N, Finch N 1992 Experiences of patients and significant others with automatic implantable cardioverter defibrillators after discharge from the hospital. Progress in Cardiovascular Nursing 7(3): 20–24

Teplitz L 1991 Nursing diagnosis of automatic implantable cardioverter defibrillator patients. Dimensions of Critical Care Nursing 10: 199–201

Teplitz L, Egenes K, Brask L 1990 Life after sudden death: the development of a support group for automatic implantable cardioverter-defibrillator patients. Journal of Cardiovascular Nursing 4(2): 20–32

Veseth-Rogers J 1990 A practical approach to teaching the automatic implantable cardioverter defibrillator patient. Journal of Cardiovascular Nursing 4(2): 7–19

Walters J 1995 A hermeneutic study of the experiences of relatives of critically ill patients. Journal of Advanced Nursing 22: 998–1005

Williams K 1996 Relatives want to witness resuscitation. Nursing Standard 11(2): 7

FURTHER READING

James J 1999 Caring for patients with an automatic internal cardioverter defibrillator: seeking a balance between technological and patient and family-centred care – implications for practice. Coronary Health Care 3(1): 25–31

26

Transmyocardial revascularization: the rebirth of an old idea

Mary Ibbotson

End-stage coronary heart disease is a manifestation of chronic ischaemic heart disease. It is characterized by a reduction in left ventricular function and intractable, untreatable angina pectoris. As this book has demonstrated, not only is coronary disease a major cause of death in the Western world, it is also a leading cause of severe disability for millions of people. The characteristic symptoms of angina, dyspnoea and fatigue degrade the quality of life for sufferers. Physical activity is limited, independence is reduced and self-esteem is lost. This results in frequent hospital admissions and death may eventually occur from recurrent infarctions or pump failure. The implications for loss of income, dependence on family and the state, as well as the demand on health resources, are huge. Thus any intervention that may alleviate these burdens attracts serious consideration.

Despite advances made in coronary revascularization, there is a small but significant number of patients for whom conventional treatments are not suitable or appropriate. Transmyocardial revascularization (TMR), a more recent form of cardiac laser surgery, provides a chance for such patients who have few other options. Although the mechanism of TMR is not fully understood, clinical benefits have been demonstrated. These include a reduction in angina, an improvement in myocardial perfusion and a decrease in hospital re-admission rate (Horvath et al 1996). Thus renewed interest has arisen in this method of indirect revascularization which was abandoned 30 years ago due to the success of coronary artery bypass grafting (CABG).

DESCRIPTION

Using a laser, channels are created from the epicardial surface of the left ventricle to its cavity in an attempt to improve the perfusion and hence oxygenation of the ischaemic myocardium (Fig. 26.1). It is thought that although the epicardial surface rapidly seals, the majority of the channels remain patent through to the

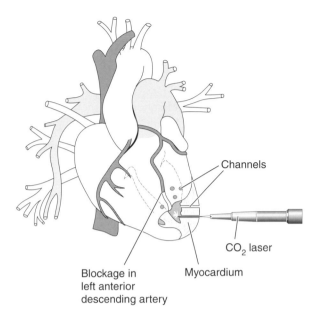

Figure 26.1 Transmyocardial revascularization.

ventricle, allowing oxygen-rich blood to perfuse directly into the myocardium. However, it is possible that these channels close so there may be an alternative mechanism to explain the observed benefit of TMR. It may be that the laser channels connect to intramyocardial vessels or that new vessel growth, 'angioneogenesis', is induced or a combination of both mechanisms. The advantage of this revolutionary treatment is that it can be performed on the beating heart without the use of cardiopulmonary bypass.

THEORETICAL CONCEPT

During the process of evolution, the human heart has advanced further than the heart of a reptile, which has underdeveloped coronaries but extensive radial flaps into the ventricle. This rudimentary circulation is also seen in the developing human embryo. Oxygen diffuses through these flaps to supply energy to the myocardium. The adult human heart has residual flaps or 'sinusoids' and it is possible that these could transport oxygenated blood to the ischaemic myocardium if they were linked to the laser channels created by TMR.

HISTORICAL BACKGROUND

At the beginning of the 20th century coronary heart disease was treated extracardially using techniques to reduce the heart's activity in order to decrease its oxygen demand. As surgeons found access to the

myocardium, indirect revascularization techniques were developed with variable success.

In 1933 Wearn et al discovered channels naturally occurring between the left ventricular cavity and the coronary arteries. These tiny channels, the aforementioned sinusoids, run a meandering course between the muscular fibres of the myocardium, anastomosing with each other and with capillaries. In 1935 Beck grafted muscle or mediastinal fat to the surface of the heart to demonstrate the ability of the myocardium to source a new blood supply. In 1954, the 'Vineberg procedure', in which the internal mammary artery was implanted into the left ventricular wall, appeared to give the most long-term benefit and is still occasionally used today, although scarring often closes up the tunnels created. In 1957 Massimo & Boffi implanted plastic tubes with side-wall holes to allow blood flow into the myocardial sinusoids. Sen et al (1965), followed by White & Hershey (1968), made puncture holes through the myocardium to allow blood to flow from the left ventricle, although Pifarre et al (1969) argued that these mechanical holes closed within 6 weeks due to fibrosis.

Research into methods of indirect revascularization was curtailed with the advent of the CABG operation. With the advantage of extracorporeal circulation and myocardial protection of the non-beating heart, CABG became the gold standard for treating coronary heart disease.

Despite this change of interest, in 1971 Mirhoseini pioneered the first successful attempt to create artificial transmyocardial channels using a carbon dioxide (CO_2) laser in the canine model (Fisher 1998). Having perforated the myocardium with channels and then ligated the left anterior descending coronary artery, he proved that the channels remained open with no scarring after sacrifice of the dogs at up to 5 months. From 1983, Mirhoseini operated on patients with end-stage coronary heart disease (CHD), using TMR as an adjunct to CABG on vessels that were not graftable. Sustained improvement in cardiac function occurred along with increased perfusion as shown by scintigraphy scanning. One patient who died 4 years postoperatively from unrelated causes underwent post mortem. Patent channels were found over the entire length except for the outer 2 mm of the heart's surface, with development of normal endothelial linings (Mirhoseini et al 1990).

In 1990 the first patient to undergo sole TMR with a beating heart was operated on by Crew and Fisher at Seton Medical Center in California (Fisher 1998). They had commissioned a prototype CO_2 laser from a Massachusetts company called Laser Engineering, who subsequently set up a daughter company, PLC Systems, to develop the Heart Laser. PLC was given permission by the Food and Drug Administration (FDA) in America to commence clinical trials on TMR which took place between 1990 and 1996. The results, as discussed later, showed an improvement in myocardial ischaemia, angina and quality of life for the patient after TMR. The FDA advisory panel finally granted approval for its use in the spring of 1998. There are now several other companies producing lasers for TMR and the field has opened wide for its future use.

RATIONALE

Today cardiologists have become more aggressive with drug therapies and interventions such as thrombolysis and percutaneous transluminal coronary angioplasty (PTCA) together with stenting. These, along with CABG, form the current basic strategies for cardiac revascularization and have had a significant effect on survival. Thus, an ageing population is returning for surgery with an increasingly complex disease. Although the risk of further surgery is raised for these patients, with the development of new technology, intervention may be justified if it provides additional years of quality life.

There is, however, no definitive cure for progressive coronary heart disease. Angioplastied vessels or bypass grafts occlude with time, angina returns and re-operation may be indicated. Less graft material is available with each operation. Disease may be distal to the point of previous interventions. There is a certain threshold beyond which PTCA or bypass surgery is contra-indicated.

Koerner et al (1998) argue that transplantation is the only option for end-stage CHD with a justifiable 5-year survival prognosis. However, strict inclusion criteria, due to the imbalance between the number of patients referred and availability of donor organs, mean that transplantation is not a realistic option for many sufferers. In addition, in contrast to the severe coronary insufficiency of patients awaiting transplant, most patients being considered for TMR have only slightly to moderately impaired left ventricular function, suggesting preservation of a relatively large amount of viable myocardium (Schoebel et al 1997).

Klein et al (1998) contend that there is a need to focus not only on the proximal lesions of coronary arteries but also on the distal lesions of the smallest vessels for the patient with end-stage coronary heart disease. These culprit lesions, not amenable to conventional treatment, may benefit from revascularization of the surrounding area, resulting in the relief of anginal symptoms.

Hence indirect revascularization has experienced a renaissance from the pre-bypass era but it has only been made possible through laser technology. Where previous techniques failed, the laser may well provide the answer for revascularization with more long-term channel patency.

SCIENTIFIC EVIDENCE

There is now an increasing amount of literature on TMR, not only on the efficacy of the procedure but also on its mechanism. Conflicting data have provided a great deal of controversy on the subject and to date, there is no scientifically valid answer to the mechanism of action.

To summarize the many different theories, Grundfest et al (1998) describe six hypotheses for TMR.

1. Channels endothelialize, stay open and allow blood flow from the ventricle to the myocardium.
2. Channels close but connections form with the coronary vasculature. Cellular injury stimulates the release of growth factors which cause angioneogenesis.
3. Channels close and produce small scars. This improves the compliance of the ventricle, as a reduction in viable myocardium means a reduction in oxygen requirements.
4. Channels and surrounding damaged areas cause denervation of the myocardium. This has the effect of masking anginal symptoms, although ischaemia is still present.
5. Channels alter the conduction characteristics of the myocardium, improving its contractility.
6. Channels bear no relationship to clinical improvement; this is a response to other factors such as optimization of drug regimens, diet, rest, exercise and psychological status, i.e. the placebo effect.

Some of these hypotheses will now be discussed in the light of recent evidence on TMR.

Evidence of patent channels after TMR was originally reported by Mirhoseini & Cayton (1981) and supported by several others in both the clinical and laboratory settings. Conversely, researchers have also demonstrated closed channels or no improvement in regional blood flow in the myocardium (Gassler et al 1997, Krabatsch et al 1998). March (1997) observed patent channels visible shortly after operation but stated that the vascularity of channels diminished with time, as scar tissue was identified within the laser tracts when specimens were examined after 2 years. This could account for the deterioration of some patients with time after TMR. Muller et al (1998) cite a study by Krabatsch which found that after 1 year more than 70% of TMR patients reported a recurrence of their original disease. Recent reports are now questioning the validity of this simple original theory and are concentrating on laser-induced angioneogenesis.

Chronic ischaemia appears to be a key factor for the success of TMR. In this situation collaterals are usually extensively developed, which may provide the link with laser channels. In support of this, Frazier & Kadipasaoglu (1996) point out that patients with occluded grafts but established collaterals fair better after TMR than those with patent grafts but poor distal run-off. Heusch & Schulz (1998) believe that many patients who are suitable for TMR have hibernating myocardium. This is defined as a state of chronic reduction of contractile function which is fully reversible upon reperfusion (Rahimtoola 1985). This manifestation of prolonged ischaemia is best identified by positron emission tomography (PET) scanning, which will be described later.

Ischaemia is a powerful promoter of angioneogenesis (Schoebel et al 1997). The cellular injury caused by TMR may stimulate new vessel growth, which would explain the gradual improvement observed after TMR. For example, Horvath et al (1994) described no improvement in myocardial perfusion in patients at 3 months postoperatively but significant improvement by 6 months. In theory, angioneogenesis should be evidenced by increased perfusion of the myocardium yet radionuclide scans have not always demonstrated a positive change. Kadipasaoglu & Frazier (1999) point out that this may be because of the subtle nature of the changes or because of the limitations of the specificity of available diagnostic methods. PET scanning is the best method but its high cost means that it is not available in most units. Several studies have failed to show an increase in myocardial perfusion but this has not correlated with the observed clinical improvement (Horvath et al 1997, Milano et al 1998, Vincent et al 1997). Therefore one must question whether TMR does affect myocardial perfusion to the same degree as observed clinical benefit.

It is possible that TMR denervates the myocardium, whether or not it is in conjunction with the process of angioneogenesis, which could contribute to the reduction of angina seen clinically (Al-Sheikh et al 1999, Stundt & Kwong 1999). If denervation does occur, the patient would feel less angina and could therefore work through their pain, so that their perfusion would increase through the development of collaterals. However, the clinical studies that have shown an improvement in myocardial perfusion (Cooley et al 1996, Donovan et al 1997, Frazier et al 1995, Horvath et al 1996, Lansing et al 1996) suggest that the mechanism of TMR does more than simply reduce anginal symptoms. Similarly, one would expect to see a corresponding rise in myocardial infarction and sudden death if denervation were the only explanation and yet this has not occurred (Roethy et al 1999).

It could be argued that the improvement in angina class is too subjective, especially in the absence of unequivocal objective data. However, if the clinical benefit is due to a placebo effect, one would expect it to decline after the first few months. Instead, improvement has been reported to increase for up to 2 years (Horvath et al 1996). However, not all studies have been as positive. Nagele et al (1998) found a declining trend in patients' symptoms after 6 months post-TMR. Schofield et al (1999) demonstrated little improvement in cardiovascular performance following TMR.

There is confusion due to the fact that the mechanism of TMR is not yet fully understood but perhaps a combination of mechanisms is responsible for the observed clinical improvements. As with many innovations, there is a lot more hyperbole than hard data, which makes objective analysis difficult. In addition, in contrast to the clinical setting of chronic ischaemia, many experiments performed in the laboratory induce acute ischaemia. This may explain the differences seen between human and animal responses to TMR and highlights the difficulty of analysing such conflicting data.

Large trials have been sanctioned by the FDA in America. The phase I study in 1990 on 15 patients demonstrated that TMR with the CO_2 laser was safe for human use. The phase II study was carried out on 200 non-randomized patients between 1992 and 1995. This showed a reduction of angina class, perfusion defects and re-admission rate and a mortality of 9%. Age and poor ventricular function pre-operatively were identified as predictors of poor outcome. Phase III began in 1995 to randomize patients to either TMR or medical management. It demonstrated a significant improvement in myocardial perfusion, unstable angina, myocardial infarction and mortality in the TMR group. Thus recruitment was halted after almost 200 patients and those that were in the medical management group were given the opportunity to 'cross over' to the TMR group. The FDA withheld approval in 1997 because of concern about the high mortality in the crossover group, as well as insufficient follow-up data. It was argued, however, that those in the crossover group were more unstable because of failure of medical treatment. Nevertheless, the FDA panel recommended conditional approval in April 1998 after further data were presented on 1-year follow-up of all groups. This has given American centres official approval to offer TMR as a treatment and many other centres around the world are now following suit.

However, since then, Schofield et al (1999) have published findings on their British study of nearly 200 patients randomized to either TMR or medical therapy, with less positive results than their American counterparts. They claimed that the outcomes from TMR were neither significant nor clinically important and, moreover, that the TMR patients had a higher mortality than those managed medically. Although a moderate improvement in angina status was reported, with a minimal improvement in exercise tolerance, hospital re-admission rate and nitrate use, it was argued that it could not be justified against the poor survival rate and cost to the health system. Results of perfusion scans and measurements of left ventricular function were disappointing.

The British study has stimulated further controversy amongst scientists and clinicians. In current research there is emphasis on combining two modalities, TMR and CABG, to create the 'hybrid' procedure. This is indicated by the presence of suitable vessels to bypass along with regions of ischaemic myocardium devoid of target or bypassable vessels.

Misfeld et al (1998) compared sole TMR surgery versus TMR and single graft surgery. They believed that the immediate angina relief seen in both groups could not be explained by angioneogenesis but could be due to denervation of the lasered myocardium. In those patients with the graft, enhanced myocardial protection may have been given during the early postoperative phase. This group had a better peri-operative course, therefore the graft may well have been protective initially but there was no difference in clinical outcome in the long term. They concluded that grafting should be attempted if at all possible in addition to TMR. Trehan et al (1996) reported on a large series of patients in India who underwent TMR and CABG, with good results. He maintained that it was difficult to achieve complete revascularization with bypass alone, due to the widespread presence of diffuse disease and the small physical size of Asian hearts.

Lastly, Morgan & Camponella (1998) examined the effect of TMR as an adjunct to CABG, having postulated that up to 20% of patients referred for CABG are not suitable for complete revascularization. They recorded an improvement in angina class and concluded that TMR as an adjunct to CABG provided the surgeon with an additional tool to improve the outcome for this group of patients. Thus the use of a combination of direct and indirect revascularization, the so-called 'hybrid' operation of TMR and CABG, appears to be a promising way forward to achieve optimum revascularization.

An area which is attracting more recent interest is percutaneous (trans) myocardial revascularization (PMR/PTMR). This procedure involves endocardial lasering of the myocardium by the cardiologist in the catheter laboratory (Kantor et al 1999). The proposed mechanism of action is the promotion of angioneogenesis which is identical to TMR. PTMR is performed by a percutaneous approach via the femoral artery, from which the catheter is guided into the left ventricle under fluoroscopic screening. A fibre-optic laser is used with a series of short pulses to create approximately 30 channels of partial-wall thickness. The epicardial surface of the myocardium is not broken so there should be less risk of tamponade than with TMR. In addition, both a general anaesthetic and thoracotomy are avoided, which may reduce postoperative complications and length of hospital stay. However, problems can occur with excessive tissue trauma and conduction abnormalities. Initial results suggest that PTMR is safe and effective (Whitlow 1999), but further evidence is necessary in the form of large randomized trials.

THE LASER

There are three types of laser associated with TMR.

1. Carbon dioxide (CO_2) infrared laser
2. Holmium:yttrium-aluminium-garnet (YAG) infrared laser
3. Excimer ultraviolet laser

The goal of all these lasers is to maximize therapeutic benefit while minimizing myocardial tissue damage (Lee & Rosengart 1999). Each laser has its advantages and disadvantages, as follows.

Most experience of TMR has been gained with the CO_2 laser. The advantages are that it uses a high-energy source with a short time on, each channel can be drilled in one pulse, it has rapid tissue absorption and vaporization and creates channels which have smooth walls. This laser is capable of a highly focused beam, producing minimal structural tissue trauma. The disadvantages of the CO_2 laser are that it is an expensive, large machine with a restrictive articulated arm. It requires a full ventricle to absorb the laser beam, there is a risk of damaging other structures due to the high energy of its beam and its relative long pulse duration causes substantial thermal injury.

The second laser, the holmium:YAG, is small and easy to operate and its tissue-tearing properties may actually encourage new vessel growth. The fibre-optic delivery allows accurate control, which means that it can also be used for PTMR. The disadvantages are that each channel requires several shots (about 30 compared with one shot of the CO_2 laser). The firing is not synchronized with the cardiac cycle, which may induce arrhythmias, and its tissue tearing may actually encourage clot formation rather than angioneogenesis. It is not such an effective tissue ablator as the other two lasers because it has a tendency to cause mini-explosions, resulting in greater thermal and structural injury.

Finally the excimer laser is the most recent addition to TMR. It is also small, with fibre-optic delivery, but is more flexible than the holmium:YAG, as it has a range of energies and repetition rates. It causes less thermal damage than the other lasers due to its short pulse duration. However, its disadvantages are that multiple pulses are necessary to create each channel (200 for every single firing with the CO_2 laser), it is not synchronized with the cardiac cycle and its non-uniform beam profile creates irregular channels.

Thus it can be seen that each laser varies in power, pulse length, repetition rate and beam quality and that no one laser is ideal. As with any new technology, there is continual evolution and change. One common feature, however, is that they all cause shock waves and thermal injury, although it is not clear how significant these effects are.

Muller et al (1998) believe that the most important result of inducing a shock wave is the 'enervation' of hibernating myocardium by restimulating vasomotor activity. Therefore, the more advanced the ischaemia, the more difficult it is to retrieve hibernating myocardium effectively. This may explain the different responses to TMR. The researchers also discuss the effect of thermal injury. The laser produces burn scars to the tissue which result in hypoxia and necrosis. This in turn stimulates the growth of new vessels, angioneogenesis. The effect takes time and may account for the delayed benefit of TMR. However, it is not yet known how thick the band of necrosis should be in order to provide the optimum environment for angioneogenesis.

Verdaasdonk et al (1998) have studied the effect of each laser on tissue. The vapour exploding from the laser seeks the path of least resistance. With a fibre-optic laser the opening to the surface is occluded, therefore the channel wall is ruptured, leaving an irregularly shaped hole whereas with a CO_2 laser, the vapour escapes straight through the end of the channel into the ventricle, leaving the channel walls smooth and unscarred. However, the shape of the channel created may not have any bearing on the clinical outcome, as results have been comparable regardless of which laser is used. Until the physiology of TMR is understood, it is not clear which types of channel have the best potential to induce reperfusion of the myocardium. Moreover, it cannot be demonstrated whether one laser is more effective than another until the significance of their characteristics is recognized. In the meantime, further research is necessary to compare their function in the clinical setting.

PATIENT ASSESSMENT

After TMR it is hoped that the patient will be able to return to a more active lifestyle and experience a better quality of life. However, it is important to educate the patient and their families about the likely outcome from TMR. As with any intervention, benefit cannot be guaranteed. Improvement of symptoms, if at all, may not occur for several months. The patient is likely to experience angina initially as they still have the same underlying heart disease as before surgery. Angioneogenesis may take up to a year to occur so any benefit will probably be gradual.

There are important ethical issues to be considered concerning informed consent. Some patients are in a vulnerable position, as they are desperate for a treatment for their symptoms. Because TMR is such a novel procedure, it attracts attention from patients who are looking for an answer to their problem. The media also sometimes encourage a belief that new is always better. Hence health-care professionals must emphasize the possibility of an unsuccessful outcome, associated with a potentially high-risk operation. The current mortality at 1 year post TMR is approximately 10% (Burns et al 1999) which is higher than many conventional cardiac interventions. Having discussed the individual's risk assessment for TMR, they should be given time to consider their options and an opportunity to return for further consultation. There is rarely only one path to follow; the surgeon and cardiologist usually discuss various options between them and advise the patient accordingly.

March (1997) states that careful patient selection is paramount for TMR. In the FDA study described earlier, patients with unstable angina had a worse outcome than those with stable angina. Thus, he argues that a stable pattern of angina is the best setting for TMR and that acute myocardial ischaemia will be further aggravated by TMR. He advocates stabilization of the patient by drug therapy and intra-aortic balloon pump (IABP) in order to optimize their cardiovascular status prior to TMR. This is supported by Frazier & Kadipasaoglu (1996) who maintain that the pre-operative presence of congestive heart failure, unstable angina or malignant arrhythmia is a strong predictor of poor postoperative outcome following TMR. In addition, Nagele et al (1998) found that patients with a low ejection fraction had a worse outcome and that the highest risk was in the early postoperative period. It was thought that the laser treatment compromised left ventricular function, either because of myocardial oedema or infarctions in adjacent tissue. However, left ventricular ejection fraction is also the strongest predictor of survival for conventional revascularization.

The assessment for TMR is likely to proceed along the following course:

1. Referral to surgeon by cardiologist, following coronary angiography. This is to demonstrate the anatomy and disease process of the coronary arteries as well as left ventricular wall motion.
2. Consultation with surgeon. This will involve a physical examination and past medical history; assessment of angina (see Canadian Cardiovascular Society Classification table: Box 26.3), individual risk stratification; elimination from conventional surgery; explanation of procedure, risks and benefits; discussion of available options and preferences of patient; plan of action.
3. Discussion with nurse specialist, who will become the contact source in order to arrange tests, offer support, reinforce verbal information and provide additional written information.
4. Myocardial scintigraphy, to demonstrate myocardial perfusion at cellular level (see Box 26.1).
5. Multiple gated acquisition (MUGA) scan to assess ventricular function. Injection of a radio-isotope is given intravenously to act as a marker for scanning the heart. A series of image frames are taken of the cardiac cycle to represent ventricular performance. The left ventricular ejection fraction can then be calculated as an exact percentage value.
6. Echocardiogram: to assess ventricular size and function, including movement of each wall, using ultrasound technology.
7. Exercise tolerance test: to assess exercise capacity on a treadmill whilst monitoring for the onset of ischaemic changes.

Box 26.1   Myocardial scintigraphy by perfusion scanning

Underperfused but viable regions of the heart can be determined in the nuclear medicine department using different techniques of scanning and radio-active tracers. These perfusion markers accumulate in the myocardium after intravenous injection and their uptake can be recorded and interpreted. Using single photon emission tomography (SPET) and 201-thallium as the tracer, a comparison can be made between the regional distribution of perfusion at stress with that at rest. The patient's myocardium is stressed either physically or pharmacologically and then scanned immediately while the tracer is still highly accumulated. The tracer will flow more easily through healthy vessels than diseased ones, therefore greater uptake will be seen in the non-ischaemic areas.

After 3–5 hours the scan is repeated to show the redistribution at rest. Reversible ischaemia can be demonstrated if the deficit shown at stress improves at rest. If the deficit fails to improve at rest, then it is said to be 'fixed' and is likely to be the result of previous damage such as a myocardial infarction. This permanent scarring is unlikely to respond to revascularization attempts. However, due to limited resolution of this type of scanning, it is not always clear if the reduced tracer uptake is due to necrotic or hibernating myocardium. As the latter may respond to TMR, it is worth investigating the *metabolism* of the myocardium.

18-F-Flurodeoxyglucose (FDG) is often used as the tracer to determine carbohydrate metabolism and myocardial viability. A positron emission tomograph (PET) scan records the tracer uptake and quantitative information is derived. PET scans are considered to be the gold standard for assessing myocardial viability but not all nuclear medicine centres are able to afford this service.

In both SPET and PET scans, data can be projected onto a colour three-dimensional image of the heart in order to demonstrate tracer distribution. Three orientations are shown: short axis, vertical long axis and horizontal long axis. Thus all myocardial regions can be identified.

---

8. Routine pre-operative diagnostic tests: electrocardiogram (ECG), chest X-ray, bloods (such as full blood count, urea and electrolyte levels).

SURGICAL PROCEDURE

The patient is anaesthetized as for general cardiac surgery. This includes intubation with a single-lumen endotracheal tube, peripheral arterial and venous cannulation, quadruple lumen central catheterization, attachment to pulse oximetry as well as core and peripheral temperature probes, and urinary catheterization. In addition, a pulmonary artery (PA) catheter is

Box 26.2 Generally accepted criteria for TMR

Inclusion criteria
- Severe coronary artery disease
- Severe angina (Canadian Cardiovascular Society Classification III or IV) on maximum anti-anginal therapy
- Coronary vasculature not suitable for conventional therapy (CABG, PTCA)
- Moderate to good left ventricle (ejection fraction >35%)
- Evidence of reversible or hibernating myocardium

Exclusion criteria
- Unable to tolerate anaesthesia
- Poor left ventricle (ejection fraction <35%)
- Severe chronic obstructive pulmonary disease
- Unstable angina or myocardial infarction within last 2 weeks
- Irreversible ischaemia or fixed defects shown on perfusion scan

inserted for measurement of cardiac output, pulmonary artery pressures and systemic and pulmonary vascular resistances. A transoesophageal echocardiogram (TOE) probe is inserted into the patient's oesophagus and positioned to visualize the left ventricular (LV) cavity and mitral valve apparatus. ECG electrodes are linked to the laser device.

The patient is placed in the right lateral position and a left anterolateral thoracotomy is made (6–10 cm long) in the fifth intercostal space. The pericardium is

Box 26.3 Canadian Cardiovascular Society classification of angina pectoris (reproduced with permission from Campeau 1976)

Class I	Ordinary physical activity does not cause angina, such as walking and climbing stairs. Angina with strenuous, rapid or prolonged exertion at work or recreation.
Class II	Slight limitations of ordinary activity, such as walking or climbing stairs rapidly; walking uphill; walking/stair climbing after meals/in cold/wind/under emotional stress; only during the first few hours after awakening; walking more than two blocks on the level; climbing more than one flight of ordinary stairs at a normal pace and in normal conditions.
Class III	Marked limitation of ordinary physical activity, such as walking one or two blocks on the level or climbing one flight of stairs in normal conditions and at normal pace. Comfortable at rest.
Class IV	Inability to carry out any physical activity without discomfort. Anginal symptoms may be present at rest.

opened and the epicardial surface of the myocardium is exposed. The operator places the laser handpiece on the heart and fires the laser by activating a foot pedal. The laser is synchronized to fire on the R-wave of ECG, just after ventricular systole, when the ventricle is refilling with blood. Channels are created at approximately 1 cm^2 intervals over the ischaemic area. After four shots the surgeon applies digital compression over the holes for approximately 1 minute by which time bleeding has usually stopped. It is rarely necessary for sutures to be required. The handpiece is cleaned and four more shots are made and this is continued until the surgeon is satisfied that sufficient channels have been made. The number of channels created depends on the extent of ischaemia and the size of the heart, but is usually in the region of 30–40. However, Lansing (1999) maintains that better results are achieved if the entire left ventricle is lasered, regardless of the area of ischaemia, in order to promote an angioneogenic response.

Successful penetration of the ventricular wall is confirmed by visualization of laser vaporization by TOE, with the blood-filled cavity of the left ventricle absorbing the laser energy. By firing the laser in diastole in synchronization with the ECG, the risks of damaging intraventricular structures or inducing arrhythmias are minimized.

Wound closure occurs in routine fashion, leaving a single mediastinal drain and a pleural drain. The patient is transferred from the operating theatre to the intensive care unit.

If TMR is combined with CABG as the hybrid procedure, the grafts are usually sewn on first to bypass any suitable vessels, followed by lasering to the remaining ischaemic areas. This aims to achieve maximum revascularization. The incision may be a sternotomy rather than a thoracotomy and the heart and lung bypass machine may be used initially for grafting. This would then be weaned off in the usual fashion with reversal of heparinization before lasering could begin.

POSTOPERATIVE CARE

The care of the patient post TMR follows the same principles as for any cardiac surgery. Management of adequate oxygenation, cardiac function, haemodynamic status, sedation and pain are fundamental. However, it is important to remember that the patient has the same coronary artery disease as he or she had pre-operatively. The procedure may actually cause an acute deterioration in left ventricular function due to the added trauma of lasering, therefore the patient has to be managed with caution. Whilst each patient has to be treated individually, there are some common factors associated with TMR.

Maintaining adequate cardiac output

Low cardiac output is the primary concern and could be due to myocardial ischaemia, oedema, wall rigidity, bleeding or arrhythmias. On arrival from theatre the patient will have the pulmonary artery catheter in situ, in order to continuously measure arterial and mixed venous oxygenation. The patient's cardiac index should be continuously monitored, with the aim of maintaining it above 2 l/min/m². Any deterioration of left ventricular function may be shown by a fall in blood pressure, urinary and/or cardiac output or by an elevation of left atrial pressure. This should be treated early by low-dose inotropic support such as dobutamine which should increase myocardial contractility. There should also be a low threshold for use of an intra-aortic balloon pump to support left ventricular function. Low-dose dopamine may be commenced to increase blood flow to the renal and mesenteric vessels. These measures should help to prevent severe ischaemia in these end-stage cardiac disease, and thus vulnerable, patients.

Maintaining adequate oxygenation

The patient will be intubated and mechanically ventilated. Continuous pulse oximetry is monitored and arterial blood gases are taken regularly to assess oxygenation levels. The patient usually begins to wake from 2 hours onwards following the procedure. Extubation occurs when the patient is warm, alert and haemodynamically stable within acceptable parameters. Oxygen therapy continues after extubation via mask or nasal cannulae. The arterial catheter is removed soon after extubation.

Maintaining haemodynamic status

The crystalloid overload and constricted circulation normally associated with cardiopulmonary bypass will not apply here. The patient's stiff ventricle with reduced function warrants caution with intravenous crystalloid and colloid replacement. Fluid replacement is guided primarily by haemodynamic parameters (such as the central venous pressure: CVP) and response to fluid filling, electrolyte levels and lung sounds. Blood loss should be measured in the chest drains, although it is usually minimal with TMR. The chest drains should also be checked for patency and air leaks. They are normally removed when blood loss is less than 100 ml over 8 hours, usually on the second postoperative day.

Preventing arrhythmias

The patient's ECG is monitored continuously and serum potassium levels should be checked hourly. Ventricular arrhythmia in the early postoperative phase may occur due to ischaemia, irritability of the ventricle after lasering, damage to conduction pathways by the laser or electrolyte imbalance. It is commonly treated by a Class III anti-arrhythmic drug such as amiodarone intravenously. In addition, oxygenation should be optimized, electrolyte levels corrected and ischaemia minimized by an intravenous nitrate infusion.

Managing pain

Pain can be managed using opiates initially, either by intravenous patient-controlled analgesia (PCA) or by epidural infusion. The advantage of PCA is that patients are more in control of their analgesia requirements once they are awake. Effective pain management is essential in order to maintain haemodynamic status, relieve anxiety and, most importantly, to minimize myocardial oxygen demand.

INTERMEDIATE CARE

The patient will usually be in intensive care for about 2 days, depending on their individual condition. Each unit has its own protocol but general criteria for transfer out of the intensive care unit (ITU) are when the patient is awake and co-operative, extubated, well saturated and haemodynamically stable. The TMR patient is managed slowly because of their haemodynamic unpredictability and chronic disease process. When they are ready they may be moved into an intermediate unit, where they should continue to be monitored due to the risk of late arrhythmias. Intravenous therapy will be titrated down and stopped. Oxygen therapy will cease when no longer deemed necessary from recorded data and patient observation. Mobilization and independence will be gradually increased.

The patient is recommended on their pre-operative anti-anginal medication, subject to their heart rate and blood pressure being within a normal range, with the aim of continuing this for at least 6 months. This allows time for potential angioneogenesis to occur whilst the patient is supported by adequate medication and this can be titrated down at a later stage.

The patient will be anticoagulated with intravenous or subcutaneous heparin which may be followed by oral warfarin. Heparin is discontinued once the patient is mobile and warfarin has reached a therapeutic level (international normalised ratio (INR): 2–3).

Anticoagulation with warfarin may be maintained for 3–6 months, to reduce the possibility of the channels re-occluding. Aspirin is then commenced indefinitely. If amiodarone has been prescribed for arrhythmias, the patient may be maintained on a low oral dose for 6 weeks.

The thoracotomy wound should continue to be assessed for signs of infection. This may manifest itself as purulent wound drainage, inflammation, fever or raised white blood cell count. Treatment would include antibiotic therapy and wound cleaning and dressing with the appropriate agents.

Analgesia is normally continued for several weeks after surgery as a thoracotomy tends to be painful due to the disturbance of thoracic nerves and muscles as well as ribs, particularly on movement. However, exercise should not be avoided for this reason as the stiffness will become worse. Relaxation techniques may help to relieve pain and stiffness.

AFTER HOSPITAL DISCHARGE

The total length of hospital stay is currently approximately 7 days but this obviously depends on the individual's recovery. As for any cardiac surgery, the patient may feel anxious on returning home after discharge from the controlled, safe environment of hospital. This is particularly evident with patients who have had TMR, as outside knowledge of this relatively new procedure is limited. Patients may feel isolated and vulnerable in the community and they may continue to rely on hospital staff for support and advice. Links should be forged between hospital and community health-care professionals.

Patients may be followed up at more frequent intervals than for most cardiac operations, for example at 3, 6 and 12 months postoperatively and annually thereafter. It is useful to monitor their response to TMR in relation to their angina status, functional ability and perfusion changes. For this purpose, an exercise test, echocardiogram, radionuclide scan and physical examination may be performed. It is also an opportunity for health-care professionals and patient to exchange information and give each other feedback on progress. Much can be learnt from the patient's experience.

Carlson (1997) describes how patients are partners in the recovery process and that active participation in their own care is necessary to prevent complications and promote the healing process. The role of the TMR liaison nurse or rehabilitation nurse is important to provide support and health education to enable the patient to undertake this part in their recovery.

As highlighted after TMR it is hoped that the patient will be able to return to a more active lifestyle and experience a better quality of life than before. However, it is important to remind the patient and their family about the delay in improvement of symptoms and that, at worst, benefit may not be seen. The patient is likely to experience angina initially as they still have the same underlying heart disease. They will need regular review of their medication to control any symptoms but it is hoped that their drug regimen can gradually be reduced. The patient may also continue to experience socio-economic problems, such as housing, employment or benefit difficulties, due to the chronic nature of their condition and delay in clinical benefit. Communication between hospital and employer or social services is often necessary to educate people about TMR.

It could be argued that TMR is only a palliative treatment, involving symptom control for end-stage cardiac patients, and nothing more. It remains to be seen if consistent evidence emerges in the future demonstrating an additional reduction in morbidity and mortality.

Discharge advice

- Gradual increase of activity as tolerated. Eventual aim to increase exercise to achieve 20 minutes brisk walking every day. Encourage attendance at cardiac rehabilitation programme.
- Wound care: observe for signs of infection (swelling, pain, redness, oozing) and seek medical advice. Sutures are usually dissolvable.
- Medication: anticoagulation, anti-anginal, antihyperlipidaemia, analgesia therapies. Ensure knowledge of medication regimens, side-effects and necessary blood tests.
- General advice: no heavy lifting or driving for one month, continue deep breathing and coughing exercises, resume sexual activity as desired.
- Angina: take glyceryl trinitrate spray or tablets if chest pain occurs, and rest. Seek medical advice if not effective.

FUTURE DIRECTIONS

TMR has its place in the armoury of cardiac interventions. This method of indirect revascularization has attracted renewed interest as a treatment option for end-stage coronary artery disease. Furthermore, it has been demonstrated to be clinically effective. There is a strong link between the stimulation of coronary microcirculation and improvement in myocardial perfusion. However, further rigorous experimental and clinical evaluation is necessary. The mechanism of action, at present largely based on assumptions, needs to be determined in order to predict benefit to patients. Nevertheless, in the same way as penicillin was used for 20 years before its mechanism of action was fully understood, TMR should continue to be developed as a therapeutic treatment for the end-stage coronary artery disease patient.

Medical science should attempt to understand how a therapy works, but the attempt should not jeopardize the pursuit of a beneficial therapy. (Frazier & Kadipasaoglu 1996)

Future research will concentrate on the properties of different lasers. The optimum shape, size and number of channels made by the laser need to be evaluated. Channel patency remains a controversial subject and its significance in the long term must be addressed.

The use of TMR as an adjunct to CABG is developing as a means of achieving complete revascularization. Clinical trials are currently under way to determine the effect on morbidity and mortality. Minimally invasive coronary surgery with TMR is also being investigated.

Percutaneous transmyocardial revascularization (PTMR), involving endocardial lasering of the myocardium by the cardiologist in the catheter laboratory, is generating considerable interest. It remains to be seen if clinical trial results are comparable to TMR.

Potentially PTMR could be used in conjunction with PTCA.

Finally the injection of vascular endothelial growth factors is being investigated as a means of enhancing myocardial perfusion by therapeutic angioneogenesis. Endothelial cells are activated to give rise to new vessel growth in an ischaemic area. Delivery of growth factors may be via coronary artery catheters, intrapericardial implantation or direct myocardial injection (Lee & Rosengart 1999). It is possible that this could be applied in combination with TMR to augment each effect.

Patient selection for TMR is undoubtedly a key factor. Although the relatively high mortality with TMR is a cause for caution, it has to be remembered that the patients concerned are in a high-risk group. The reduction of symptoms and an improved quality of life are arguably sufficient endpoints. It is not foreseen that TMR will ever be used as a front-line treatment or as a replacement for CABG. However, the technology of the laser has broadened the choices for the patient with refractory angina.

An attempt has been made here to represent the current level of understanding on TMR but, as with any pioneering technology, advances are continuously being made. New findings are emerging in the literature at a rapid rate which stimulate new controversies and hypotheses daily. Thus it is unavoidable that areas of this chapter will be outdated and superseded by new theories by the time of publication. However, it is hoped that this chapter has provided a basis for what is proving to be an exciting concept in the treatment of coronary artery disease.

REFERENCES

Al-Sheikh T, Allen K, Straka S et al 1999 Cardiac sympathetic denervation after transmyocardial laser revascularization. Circulation 100(2): 135–140

Beck C 1935 The development of a new blood supply to the heart by operation. Annals of Surgery 102(5): 801–813

Burns S, Caine N, Schofield P, Sharples L, Tait S, Wallwork J 1999 The transmyocardial laser revascularization international registry report. European Heart Journal 20: 31–37

Campeau L 1976 Grading of angina pectoris. Circulation 54(3): 522–523

Carlson P 1997 Patient care and expectations for recovery after transmyocardial laser revascularization. American Association of Critical-Care Nurses (AACN) Clinical Issues 8(1): 33–40

Cooley D, Frazier O, Kadipasaoglu K et al 1996 Transmyocardial laser revascularization: clinical experience with twelve-month follow-up. Journal of Thoracic and Cardiovascular Surgery 111(4): 791–799

Donovan C, Clements F, Coleman R, Landolfo K, Lowe J, Ryan T 1997 Improvement in inducible ischaemia during

dobutamine stress echocardiography after transmyocardial laser revascularization in patients with refractory angina pectoris. Journal of the American College of Cardiology 30(3): 607–612

Fisher J 1998 The history of transmyocardial revascularization. In: Klein M, Gams E, Schulte H (eds) TMLR: management of coronary artery diseases. Springer, Berlin, p. 111

Frazier O, Kadipasaoglu K 1996 Invited commentary. In: Burkhoff D, Fisher PE, Apfelbaum M, Kohmoto T, De Rosa CM, Smith C 1996 Histologic appearance of transmyocardial laser channels after four and a half weeks. Annals of Thoracic Surgery 61(5): 1532–1535

Frazier O, Cooley DA, Kadipasaoglu KA et al 1995 Myocardial revascularization with laser: preliminary findings. Circulation 92 (9 suppl 1): ii, 58–65

Gassler N, Helmchen U, Stubbe H, Wintzer H, Wullbrand A 1997 Transmyocardial laser revascularization: histological features in human nonresponder myocardium. Circulation 95(2): 371–375

Grundfest W, Papaiannou T, Shi W et al 1998 Basic science consideration in TMR: in vitro and in vivo studies. In:

Klein M, Gams E, Schulte H (eds) TMLR: management of coronary artery diseases. Springer, Berlin, p. 131

Heusch G, Schulz R 1998 Hibernating myocardium: a review. In: Klein M, Gams E, Schulte H (eds) TMLR: management of coronary artery diseases. Springer, Berlin, p. 11

Horvath KA, Cohn LH, Mannting F 1994 Improved myocardial perfusion and relief of angina after transmyocardial laser revascularization (abstract). Circulation 90 (suppl 1): 640

Horvath KA, Cohn LH, Cummings N, Mannting F, Shernan S 1996 Transmyocardial laser revascularization: operative techniques and clinical results at two years. Journal of Thoracic and Cardiovascular Surgery 111(5): 1047–1053

Horvath KA, Cohn LH, Cooley DA et al 1997 Transmyocardial laser revascularization: results of a multicenter trial with TLR used as sole therapy for end-stage coronary artery disease. Journal of Thoracic and Cardiovascular Surgery 113(4): 645–653

Kantor B, McKenna CJ, Caccitolo JA et al 1999 Transmyocardial and percutaneous myocardial revascularization: current and future role in the treatment of coronary artery disease. Mayo Clinic Proceedings 74(6): 585–592

Kadipasaoglu K, Frazier O 1999 Transmyocardial laser revascularization: effect of laser parameters on tissue ablation and cardiac perfusion. Seminars in Thoracic and Cardiovascular Surgery 11(1): 4–11

Klein M, Dauben H, Gams E, Schulte H 1998 Transmyocardial laser revascularisation: clinical observations concerning the use of an excimer laser system. In: Klein M, Gams E, Schulte H (eds) TMLR: management of coronary artery diseases. Springer, Berlin, p. 201

Koerner M, Koerfer R, Tenderich G 1998 Borderline indications for heart transplantation and alternative measures. In: Klein M, Gams E, Schulte H (eds) TMLR: management of coronary artery diseases. Springer, Berlin, p. 99

Krabatsch T, Hetzer R, Lieback E, Schaper F, Tambeur L 1998 Transmyocardial laser revascularisation in the treatment of severe diffuse coronary artery disease. In: Klein M, Gams E, Schulte H (eds) TMLR: management of coronary artery diseases. Springer, Berlin, p. 177

Lansing A 1999 Transmyocardial laser revascularisation. Lancet 353: 1704–1707

Lansing A, Singh S, Lash JA 1996 Transmyocardial revascularization for intractable angina. Journal of the Kentucky Medical Association 94(10): 432–436

Lee L, Rosengart T 1999 Transmyocardial laser revascularization and angioneogenesis: the potential for therapeutic benefit. Seminars in Thoracic and Cardiovascular Surgery 11(1): 29–35

March R 1997 Transmyocardial laser revascularization: current experience and future direction. Journal of Clinical Laser Medicine and Surgery 15(6): 301–306

Massimo C, Boffi L 1957 Myocardial revascularization by a new method of carrying blood directly from the left ventricular cavity into the coronary circulation. Journal of Thoracic Surgery 34: 257–264

Milano A, Pratali S, De Carlo M, Pietrabissa A, Bortolotti U 1998 Transmyocardial holmium laser revascularization: feasibility of a thoracoscopic approach. European Journal of Cardio-thoracic Surgery 14 (suppl 1): S105–110

Mirhoseini M, Cayton MM 1981 Revascularization of the heart by laser. Journal of Microsurgery 2(4): 253–260

Mirhoseini M, Shelgikar S, Cayton M 1990 Clinical and histological evaluation of laser myocardial revascularization. Journal of Clinical Laser Medicine and Surgery 8(3): 73–77

Misfeld M, Fuhrmeyer F, Kraatz E, Schmidtke C, Sievers H 1998 TMLR with and without additional single grafting: differences in postoperative outcome? In: Klein M, Gams E, Schulte H (eds) TMLR: management of coronary artery diseases. Springer, Berlin, p. 241

Morgan I, Camponella C 1998 Transmyocardial laser revascularisation in Edinburgh. British Journal of Theatre Nursing 7(12): 4–9

Muller G, Dorschel K, Schaldach B 1998 Transmyocardial laser revascularisation: a matter of the right wavelength? In: Klein M, Gams E, Schulte H (eds) TMLR: management of coronary artery diseases. Springer, Berlin, p. 123

Nagele H, Stubbe HM, Nienaber C, Rodiger W 1998 Results of transmyocardial laser revascularization in non-revascularizable coronary artery disease after three years follow up. European Heart Journal 19(10): 1525–1530

Pifarre R, Jasuja L, Lynch R, Neville W 1969 Myocardial revascularization by transmyocardial acupuncture: a physiological impossibility. Journal of Thoracic and Cardiovascular Surgery 58(3): 424–431

Rahimtoola S 1985 A perspective on the three large multicentre randomized clinical trials of coronary bypass surgery for chronic stable angina. Circulation 72 (6 part 2): 123–135

Roethy W, Burkhoff D, Yamamoto N 1999 An examination of potential mechanisms underlying transmyocardial laser revascularization induced increases in myocardial blood flow. Seminars in Thoracic and Cardiovascular Surgery 11(1): 29–35

Schoebel F, Frazier O, Jessurun G et al 1997 Refractory angina pectoris in end-stage coronary artery disease: evolving therapeutic concepts. American Heart Journal 134(4): 587–602

Schofield P, Sharples L, Caine N et al 1999 Transmyocardial laser revascularisation in patients with refractory angina: a randomised controlled trial. Lancet 353: 519–524

Sen P, Kinare S, Parulkar G, Udwadia T 1965 Transmyocardial acupuncture: a new approach to myocardial revascularization. Journal of Thoracic and Cardiovascular Surgery 50: 181–189

Stundt T, Kwong K 1999 Clinical experience with the holmium:YAG laser for transmyocardial laser revascularization and myocardial denervation as a mechanism. Seminars in Thoracic and Cardiovascular Surgery 11(1): 19–23

Trehan N, Kohli VM, Mishra M, Mishra A, Jangid DR, Bapna R 1996 Transmyocardial laser revascularization as an adjunct to CABG. Indian Heart Journal 48(4): 381–388

Verdaasdonk R, Beek J, Grundeman P, Sachinopoulou A 1998 Working mechanism of pulsed CO_2, holmium and excimer laser system with regard to transmyocardial revascularisation (TMR): in vivo implications. In: Klein M, Gams E, Schulte H (eds) TMLR: management of coronary artery diseases. Springer, Berlin, p. 143

Vincent JG, Bardos P, Kruse J, Maass D 1997 End stage coronary disease treated with the transmyocardial CO_2 laser revascularisation: a chance for the 'inoperable' patient. European Journal of Cardiothoracic Surgery 11(5): 888–894

Vineberg A 1954 Clinical and experimental studies in the treatment of coronary artery insufficiency by internal mammary implant. Journal of the International College of Surgeons 22(5): 513–518

Wearn J, Klumpp T, Mettier S, Zschiesche L 1933 The nature of the vascular communications between the coronary arteries and the chambers of the heart. American Heart Journal 9: 143–164

White M, Hershey JE 1968 Multiple transmyocardial puncture revascularization in refractory ventricular fibrillation due to myocardial ischaemia. Annals of Thoracic Surgery 6(6): 557–563

Whitlow P 1999 Percutaneous transmyocardial revascularization versus medical therapy in patients with refractory angina. American College of Cardiology ACCIS meeting, March

27

Complementary therapies for cardiac health

Carol L Cox

The role of cardiac health promotion has changed substantially over the past decade. It has extended its importance for people with coronary artery disease and for those with critical cardiac dysfunction who require high dependency and intensive care. Previously the emphasis on cardiac health promotion concentrated mainly on modifying risk factors by educating people about healthy lifestyles (Jowett & Thompson 1989). Healthy lifestyle issues addressed traditional Western perspectives such as exercise in moderation, maintaining a healthy diet, getting plenty of rest and cessation of smoking. More recently a multifactorial approach to promoting cardiac health has been assumed (Alspach 1991, Hudak & Gallo 1994) which involves some modification of or major changes in lifestyle (Alspach 1991). European Atherosclerosis Society 1987, Health Education Council 1984, Hudak & Gallo 1994).

Traditional approaches are intended to reduce the risk of myocardial infarction and are frequently regarded by patients as a hardship which compromises their lifestyle. Therefore people are shifting towards the use of complementary therapies as a way of support in promoting their health (Bryne 2001, Mackereth 1998). Western medicine, according to Sasaki (1992), provides many remedies for the problems and diseases people encounter in their lives but by concentrating on illness and failing to address the essence of health, modern medicine falls short of many people's needs. Many complementary therapies are identified as systems of medicine, for example, acupuncture, homeopathy and herbalism. This is in contrast to treatments such as iridology, which is a diagnostic tool, or massage and aromatherapy, which are therapeutic interventions (Rankin-Box 1991). Complementary therapies can be defined as therapies which build upon the therapeutic relationship and address the physical, emotional, mental, psychological and spiritual dimensions of a person's condition (McMahon & Pearson 1991).

This chapter provides a discussion and overview of the various complementary therapies that may be incorporated into the care of the patient experiencing cardiac disease. Analysis is provided as to their perceived benefit to the well-being of the patient.

The British Medical Association (BMA) suggested in 1993 that approximately 180 different types of complementary therapies were practised by the public in the United Kingdom (UK) (Bryne 2001). An increase in the use of complementary therapies throughout the UK has meant that cardiac health promotion has begun to embrace not only traditional Western views but also complementary therapies which are derived, in the main, from Eastern perspectives about the promotion of health and the development of a sense of well-being. In 1993, Cameron-Blackie identified that the MORI poll of 1989 demonstrated that three out of four people surveyed thought complementary therapies should be available through the National Health Service (NHS). In addition, a survey conducted by the National Association of Health Authorities and Trusts (NAHAT) in 1992 indicated that the majority of purchasers of health care were in favour of some or all complementary therapies being available on the NHS (Cameron-Blackie 1993). There is a growing awareness amongst the public of the limitations of orthodox medical care and the side-effects of treatment (Leddy & Pepper 1993) which has led to the recent trend of people integrating complementary therapies with conventional/traditional medicine. It is postulated that this leads to a holistic approach to care.

With the increase in popularity of integrating complementary therapies with traditional medicine, it is important to consider ways in which complementary/integrative therapies can be used to promote cardiac health. In order to inform the reader, this chapter begins with a brief review of the history of orthodox medicine. Recent progress in therapeutics and the growing integration of complementary therapies into cardiac health care are considered and the empowerment of patient – the patient in control – in terms of cardiac health promotion is discussed. There is a focus on prevention and healing rather than cure. Following this, a review of therapies integrated with orthodox medicine and their associated benefits is outlined so that consideration can be given to how these are used in promoting health and a sense of well-being.

There are many types of complementary therapies which could be included in this chapter. However, some of these therapies, such as iridology, macrobiotics, naturopathy and spiritual healing, have not demonstrated clinical effectiveness through research.

Only those therapies which have been demonstrated clinically to be of benefit to patients in promoting cardiac health are addressed. A recommendation is made that the therapies addressed in this chapter should be used in conjunction with traditional Western medicine. Integration of therapies leads to a less fragmented way of promoting cardiac health. Inherent in this is the intention for people to be more motivated about promoting their own cardiac health and feeling better.

HISTORICAL OVERVIEW OF ORTHODOX MEDICINE

Hippocrates is considered to be the father of modern medicine. He established the beginnings of a sound body of scientific knowledge and a code of conduct which has been passed on for generations in traditional, orthodox medicine. The Hippocratic oath articulates the ethical principles which guide doctors. Hippocrates emphasized a holistic approach to healing and a scientific evaluation to treatment.

During the Renaissance, or Age of Discovery, Andreas Vesalius produced the first accurate anatomical representation of the body and in the 17th century William Harvey described human circulation (Cumston 1996). Antonji Van Leeuwenhoek invented the light microscope and discovered micro-organisms and cellular structures. In the late 18th century Edward Jenner developed the principle of vaccination (Longmate 1970). Following on from this, in the 19th century, Louis Pasteur conducted his work and developed the germ theory of disease (Cumston 1996). This contributed substantially to medicine's understanding of illness transmission and the prevention and containment of epidemics.

The age of invention followed. By 1860 the thermometer, stethoscope, ophthalmoscope and laryngoscope were in use. This was followed with the introduction of the gastroscope, cystoscope and sphygmomanometer by 1883. During this period, Crawford Long demonstrated general anaesthesia in 1842 using ether and in 1895 Wilhelm Roentgen took the first X-rays of the body (Longmate 1970). Ten years later radiological evidence of kidney function was made evident by the use of radio-opaque contrast medium. In the early 20th century inroads into the prevention of cholera, diphtheria and typhoid were made via the principle of immunization. Antiseptic surgical techniques developed by Joseph Lister made operative procedures safer and at the beginning of the Second World War the pharmaceutical revolution began (Webster 1981). Of major importance during this time was the discovery of penicillin by Sir Alexander Fleming, Ernest Boris Chain and Sir Howard Walter Florey (Longmate 1970). Its widespread use reduced mortality from infections such as septicaemia, osteomyelitis, meningitis and pneumonia. Tuberculosis was all but extinguished with the introduction of BCG vaccination and the development of streptomycin. Increasingly the focus became centred on cure. As more sophisticated drug therapy evolved, many diseases were cured quickly whereas 50 years earlier they would have resulted in death. Insulin was an effective treatment in diabetes and cortisone facilitated impressive results in organ transplantation.

In the mid 20th century cardiac surgery edged forward, introducing the cardiopulmonary bypass (CPB) machine and an ability to keep patients alive beyond previous scientific imagination. Congenital heart disease could be treated and in 1967 Christian Barnard made history with the first heart transplantation. Although Dr Barnard's patient lived only for 18 days, heart transplantation is now commonplace (see Chapter 23).

Other scientific breakthroughs in orthodox medicine continued. Lithotripsy has meant shattering kidney stones without the need for painful surgery. In vitro fertilization techniques have produced opportunities for medically induced conception amongst infertile couples. Genetic and physiologic problems, like spina bifida and other disorders, in the unborn and developing fetus are being detected. Surgeons operate on fetuses whilst they are in the womb.

Acquired immune deficiency syndrome (AIDS) is now considered to be pandemic. By 1990 the United States (US) Department of Health and Human Services Seventh Report (1990) indicated that approximately 1–1.5 million people were considered to be infected with the human immunovirus (HIV) in the United States alone. Within the last few years HIV and AIDS drug treatment has been revolutionized. Where there was little hope of long-term survival, people affected by conditions like HIV and cancer have been able to resume a normal working life. Magnificent contributions to orthodox medicine have been made over the past 100 years. Randomized controlled trials have been carefully organized to eliminate misleading results and methods of evaluation of treatment have improved. These trials have shown the medical profession how to treat disease effectively.

All of the aforementioned medical achievements are important and critical to health but through its evolution traditional medicine has become more and more particularistic in its approach to treatment. The human being is regarded as discrete parts and separate in mind and body (Leddy & Pepper 1993). Despite the considerable breakthroughs in traditional approaches to medical care and its many triumphs, especially those demonstrated through randomized controlled trials, an increasing number of people are becoming aware of its drawbacks and limitations. People are coming to regard traditional medicine with scepticism and intolerance, particularly when the system fails them, and are turning to complementary therapies for support (Bryne 2001, Mackereth 1998). It appears science alone is not enough to satisfy all the needs of today's patients (Chopra 1991, 1993). In this era of evidence-based medicine, health care and nursing, a paradoxical issue arises regarding therapies which people want yet which followers of traditional approaches would argue hold little evidence of efficacy, primarily in relation to the absence of randomized controlled trials. People are seeking more than what can be provided through the dispensing of a prescription or surgery. People are seeking a holistic approach to their care.

RECENT PROGRESS IN THERAPEUTICS AND THE GROWING INTEGRATION OF COMPLEMENTARY THERAPIES INTO CARDIAC HEALTH CARE

Over the past decade health-care providers, in particular general practitioners (GPs), have recognized that complementary therapies are beneficial and are integrating acupuncture, homeopathy, massage and other therapies in order to provide a more holistic approach to their patients' care. In conjunction with this, programmes of health education and promotion which include the use of complementary therapies are being adopted by practice nurses, health visitors and district nurses who are linked to practices through primary care groups. The aim of promoting holistic health has led to the integration and provision of complementary therapies within the NHS. Nurses in the hospital setting, in particular in intensive care and coronary care, are using aromatherapy to promote rest (Price 1998, Price & Price 1995, Stevensen 1994, 2001) and various forms of massage to reduce anxiety, promote sleep and provide comfort (Cox & Hayes 1997, 1998, Richards 1998).

It has been recognized that many conditions cannot be cured through orthodox medicine. This recognition is fuelling the integration of complementary therapies into the provision of care as these are viewed as gentler, safer and more natural ways of promoting health and healing when cure cannot be achieved. Complementary therapies are considered to have less risk of causing harm to people who use them. Unlike traditional approaches in which synthetic, refined medicines are prescribed by doctors, the treatments employed by complementary therapists are generally derived from natural sources. Many doctors who embrace holistic perspectives find the integration of natural products into their armament of treatment modalities compelling.

A number of medical products which are traditionally prescribed to patients, for example digoxin, have toxic side-effects. Complementary therapies, by and large, involve treatments that are externally applied to the patient and where substances are taken internally, these are natural products which have been diluted to such a degree they are regarded as non-toxic.

EMPOWERMENT OF PATIENTS: THE PATIENT IN CONTROL

According to Park (1992), everything a person does can be done in a way that promotes healthy functioning or it can be done in such a way that it becomes harmful. Discovery through health education and health promotion activities empowers people to take control of their own health. Taking control leads to prevention of ill health and healing of the self. Cardiac health promotion activities are targeted towards healing rather than cure in cardiovascular disease and particularly so after myocardial infarction.

When promoting cardiac health, the complementary therapist adopts the perspective that patients are in control of their treatment. The therapist listens to what patients have to say about their symptoms and is receptive to what patients perceive to be the cause. Patients often feel the therapist is on their side and therefore lifestyle recommendations are more likely to be taken on board. Complementary therapists adopt the lifestyle they recommend to their patients. A major advantage of adopting a complementary approach to care is that it is holistic. In practice, complementary therapists enquire in more depth into the patient's lifestyle, relationships and occupational issues than traditional health-care practitioners, whilst addressing the patient's fears and anxieties. Therefore patients feel valued and a more positive mindset to promote their own health is established. Acutely ill patients and the dying express feelings of hope and are less anxious as some forms of complementary therapies relieve suffering and discomfort (Cox & Hayes 1998).

Complementary therapists postulate that health is more than freedom from disease. Health is associated with the balance of the patient's spiritual, emotional and physical being. Illness may be prevented by maintaining equilibrium. When patients become knowledgeable about how to manage their own health

through the integration of complementary therapies, the symptoms associated with ill health are less likely to emerge or become established.

REVIEW OF THERAPIES INTEGRATED WITH ORTHODOX MEDICINE AND ASSOCIATED BENEFITS

Acupuncture

The word acupuncture is derived from the Latin *acus* (needle) and *punctura* (puncture). Acupuncture is an ancient Chinese treatment rooted in Confucian and Taoist philosophy which was refined over 2000 years ago. Daoist and Taoist philosophy deal with lifestyle and behaviour and encourage moderation, harmony and balance in all things. The actual origin of acupuncture is not known but excavations in China have revealed stone needles dating back to 3000 BC. In the second century BC it was the dominant therapeutic technique in China (Unschuld 1985), working from the outside of the body inward. As time passed, the primary theories associated with acupuncture became related to concepts of energy flowing in meridian systems. Acupuncture forms a large part of traditional Chinese medicine and within the last three decades there has been an increased acceptance and incorporation of acupuncture within traditional Western medicine. The British Medical Association recognizes acupuncture as a discrete clinical discipline (BMA 1993).

Acupuncture involves the insertion of fine sterile needles into specific points on the body. According to Downey (2001), central to the theory associated with acupuncture is the concept of the human body as self-healing and self-rectifying. The body is a dynamic whole, a network of inter-relating and interacting energies which through even distribution and flow maintains health (Firebrace & Hill 1988). Conventionally trained health-care providers postulate that acupuncture works within the nervous system by releasing endorphins, which are naturally produced opiates. These practitioners also postulate that acupuncture is associated with the gate theory of pain, which was described by Melzack & Wall in 1965, in which physiological gates along the spinal cord open or close in relation to transmission of pain along nerve fibres.

Acupuncture acts by stimulating other nerve fibres, thus blocking the transmission of pain signals to the brain. As a complementary therapy, it has been shown to be effective in the treatment of many forms of pain and disorders including postoperative pain management, in conjunction with physiotherapy, pain relief in induction of labour, control of vomiting following chemotherapy and myocardial infarction, emotional distress and in the control of withdrawal symptoms associated with alcohol and drug abuse. It is administered in a number of different health-care settings including GP surgeries, in hospital acute care wards, outpatient clinics, occupational health centres, sports medicine facilities and obstetrical wards as well as in drug rehabilitation and mental health centres.

Practitioners who perform acupuncture undergo specialized training and take care to ensure that the whole person is treated rather than providing acupuncture for symptomatic relief alone (Downey 2001). An acupuncturist attempts to promote health by helping the patient to live according to the philosophies of Dao and Tao which are associated with avoiding excess and extremes. Thus working to excess, consuming excessive amounts of alcohol, overanxiety and promiscuity are discouraged.

Alexander technique

The Alexander technique is a form of experiential learning and practice for people who want to change something about themselves (Park 1992). The technique was developed by an Australian, Frederick Matthias Alexander, at the beginning of the 20th century. Frederick was an extremely difficult child who did not respond well to formal education. He suffered from respiratory problems which made it difficult for him to attend school regularly. Subsequently, Frederick was able to indulge his love of the country. He had a passion for horses and spent most of his time observing their movements. Therefore he developed keen skills in observation of movement. In his teenage years, he developed a tremendous love for the theatre and music and eventually he became an actor. However, he experienced a problem with his breathing and voice each time he performed on stage. Intrigued by this, he undertook self-examination, for approximately 10 years, to discern the cause. Through the use of mirrors he was able to watch his movements when he spoke and decided it was his posture that was affecting his breathing and speaking voice. Over time he discovered that the relationship between his head, neck and spine was the key to how the rest of his body functioned. He termed this the 'primary control' and postulated that when it was in balance and harmony, it had an invigorating effect on his entire body. Other actors noticed that Frederick's breathing and voice improved and wanted to learn his technique. Thus the Alexander technique evolved. Key to the practice is the understanding that changing is an art and cannot be rushed or forced. According to Park, Frederick indicated that the change involves carrying out an activity 'against the habit of life' (Park 1992).

Practising the Alexander technique involves a series of practical experiments and observational exercises. The exercises are not fitness or stretching exercises but rather opportunities to explore in detail aspects of yourself and to consider aspects of which you may have been previously unaware. Each exercise is carried out slowly and purposefully whilst paying attention to the process of how you are doing the exercise. The purpose of the exercises is to develop self-awareness. For people who use this form of experiential learning and practice in cardiac health promotion, a sense of well-being and self-control is experienced.

Aromatherapy

It has been estimated that over 40 000 years ago Australian aborigines were using plant extracts to promote health and a sense of well-being. Many of the plant extracts the aborigines used to treat illnesses are still in use today. Blackwell (1991) and Stevenson (2001) suggest that the Australian tea tree, *Maleleuca alternifolia*, which has antibacterial and antifungal properties, was used by the aborigines and it is used in aromatherapy today. Six thousand years ago the Egyptian doctor Imhotep used aromatherapy to facilitate breathing and to stimulate the skin in massage. Essential oils derived from plants have been used by the Hebrews, Greeks and Romans. It is also known that Hippocrates recommended a daily bath scented with oils.

Avicenna, an Arab scholar, is attributed with undertaking the first distillation of essential oils in the 10th century AD. However, Williams (1989) indicates that archaeological evidence suggests that the use of essential oils in the Indus Valley civilization occurred 5000 years earlier. Therapeutic use of essential oils is attributed to RM Gattefosse, a French chemist, who lived in the early 20th century. Gattefosse used lavender oil after severely burning his hand in a laboratory accident. He found that his hand healed quickly and did not scar. Gattefosse published the findings of his research in a text entitled *Aromatherapie* in 1931.

Aromatherapy has been identified as having a distinct therapeutic effect in reducing or alleviating symptoms of distress, thus aiding the person to move towards responsibility for managing their own health and wellness (Price & Price 1995). It is the fastest growing of all complementary therapies and is used by many nurses and midwives to promote rest, sleep, comfort and reduce anxiety in critical care, acute care labour and delivery suites and the hospice environment (Cannard 1994, Price 1998, Stevensen 1994). It has been shown to be an effective treatment when used by patients experiencing side-effects from chemotherapy and radiotherapy.

Art, music, poetry and dance therapy

From the beginning of time, human beings have engaged in self-expression through forms of art, music, writing and dance. The Hippocratic model of 2000 years ago held that 'there is one flow; one common breathing; all things are in sympathy' (Graham 1991). Twenty thousand years ago the Shaman healers used dance, drawing and story telling as a means to promote health and well-being. Shamans were considered to be holistic practitioners who attempted to harmonize the individual and environment. Drawing, listening to music, writing poetry and dancing are considered gentle, non-invasive forms of caring for the self that instil feelings of relaxation and calmness. In instances where tension and anxiety are experienced over long periods of time, this can have a depressing effect on the immune system, leading to ill health and disease (Ryman 1994).

Art therapy, music therapy, dance therapy and reading poetry are activities which provide a form of pleasure which reduces feelings of anxiety and are often prescribed when people experience depression. In the coronary care setting, music has been shown to reduce anxiety and effect a happier emotional state (Bolwerk 1990, Davis-Rollans & Cunningham 1987). In the book *Soulskin*, Krysl stated 'Everything is in resonance. Each note of the scale resonates with the atomic number of one of the elements, with a colour of the spectrum, and with the placement of the planets around the sun. Your body has its note. If you are ill, this note can make you well. If in pain, this note diminishes that pain' (Krysl 1996). In terms of cardiac health promotion, people have indicated that following myocardial infarction, these therapies have helped them change their lifestyle and gain a sense of well-being.

Chinese herbal medicine/herbal medicine

Herbal treatments have been at the centre of medicine throughout history. Recorded practice associated with the use of herbal medicines dates back to at least the first century BC in Greece and Egypt and the first Western recording of 455 plants used for medicinal purposes was recorded by Theophrastus in the third century BC (Griggs 1981). Chinese herbal medicine has been practised for at least 5000 years. Unlike acupuncture, which works from the outside into the body, herbal treatment is posited to work from inside the body outwards. In 1500 BC the Chinese Emperor Yen compiled a text on herbal medicine and in 200 AD this text was condensed into a medical text which listed over 350 herbs. This established the basis of Chinese pharmacology. In the 16th century the general catalogue of herbs entitled *Li Shi Zheng's Beng Cao Ganu Mu* was written. Chinese herbal medicine is well established and represents one of the fastest growing complementary therapies in the United Kingdom.

Chinese herbal medicine and herbal medicine in general employ the properties of a variety of herbs to promote health and prevent illness as well as to treat disease. Herbal treatments are prescribed for physical, mental and emotional problems and may be used alone or in conjunction with other complementary therapies. Herbal medicine is considered to be a gentle form of treatment and is postulated to restore balance and harmony to the physical, mental and emotional forces in a person's body. In terms of Chinese medicine, most of the herbs used are exported from China and Taiwan and are dispensed in the United Kingdom from Chinese pharmacies.

The World Health Organization has acknowledged the importance of herbal medicine in terms of treating health problems (World Health Organization 1978). The role of the professional herbalist was identified in the 1968 Medicines Act in the United Kingdom. This act makes provision for herbal medicines that cannot be sold over the counter to be prescribed by a professional herbalist. In the UK the National Institute of Medical Herbalists, founded in 1864, regulates standards of practice and training in herbal medicine.

Herbal treatments are based on the premise that the 'vital force' or 'life energy', which is known as *Chi* or *Ki* in Chinese medicine, must be in balance and unrestricted in the human body. When this vital force is in balance and circulating freely, optimal well-being occurs. Any imbalance or disharmony will result in ill health or disease. In terms of Chinese medicine, there are two opposing forces within chi known as the Yin and Yang. When there is an imbalance between the Yin and Yang or when the energy flow becomes restricted, balance is lost and disease or illness will occur. Chi flows through meridians (channels) in the body and any interruption to this energy flow can cause problems to develop in organs which correspond with the meridians. The Chinese herbalist attempts to determine where energy blockages or imbalances occur and then attempts to restore the energy balance through the use of specific herbs.

In terms of integrative therapy within traditional medicine, herbal medicine has a variety of applications. It is considered to be a gentle and highly effective system of health care. Therapeutic effectiveness has been found in treating cardiovascular problems, migraine headaches, inflammation and various skin conditions (Busby 2001). In terms of cardiac health promotion in particular, the gentle actions of herbal treatment have been shown to promote rest, enhance immunity, act as vasodilators, anti-inflammatory and antifungal agents as well as expectorants and mild diuretics (Weiss 1988, Williams & Home 1995).

Homeopathy

The name homeopathy is derived from the Greek words *homios* meaning 'like' and *pathos* meaning 'suffering'. Homeopathic medicine is produced from natural sources such as plants, metals, minerals, poisonous venoms, insect stings and bacteria. For example, the extract from the common annual belladonna (deadly nightshade) plant, which is found in waste places, quarries and on wooded hills throughout central and southern Europe, is used to lessen irritability and treat pain. As a drug, belladonna has been found in small doses to allay cardiac palpitations and when used as a plaster applied to the epigastric region, it relieves discomfort. Belladonna has also been found to be a powerful antispasmodic in treating intestinal colic (Fox 1993).

The principles of homeopathy were known during the time of Hippocrates and are considered to have originated in the fifth century BC. Approximately 200 years ago, the German doctor and chemist Samuel Hahnemann (1755–1843) established the modern principles of homeopathy. Hahnemann was concerned that surgical procedures were barbaric and that medicines were given without any sound rationale for their use. He criticized the side-effects of many medicines and began experimenting with animal, mineral and vegetable products on human volunteers. Hahnemann developed a taxonomy for each of the products he investigated which was published as the Law of Similars in 1796 (Haehl 1985). Central to homeopathy is the view that each person is unique and reacts differently to the same disorder. Hahnemann proposed three essential principles which form the basis of homeopathy today. First, if large doses of a product promote symptoms in a healthy person, then much smaller doses could cure people who have similar symptoms of disease. Second, the 'minimum dose' principle was theorized which states that the greater the dilution of a curative product, the more effective it becomes. This theory is known as 'potentization'. Third, the principle of 'whole-person prescribing' was established which means taking into consideration the person's personality, mood, temperament, physical and emotional health and living conditions. Therefore, although two people may have the same disorder, they may be treated with a different homeopathic medicine.

Homeopathy is a holistic approach to promoting health. Treating like with like stimulates the body to heal itself. Hahnemann referred to this healing as the 'vital force' which, through the aid of homeopathic medicines, assisted the body in recovering from illness and achieving perfect health. Homeopathic medicines are prepared and dispensed in four basic forms depending on the type of prescription: powders, granules, tablets and liquids. The original substance is diluted many times in a water and alcohol base. With each dilution, the liquid is shaken vigorously, a process known as 'succussion'. Homeopaths postulate that this gives the final medicine its power to heal. Dilutions of the substance may be in decimal (1/10th) or centesimal (1/100th) forms. The number of stages in dilution determines the potency of the final product.

The principles of homeopathy are similar to the principles of immunization, whereby the introduction of a small amount of the substance into the body stimulates the immune system so that when the body is confronted with a disease, health can be maintained. The essential tenet of homeopathic treatment is to tailor the specific treatment to the individual person. Many GPs are trained in the use of homeopathy and prescribe it in conjunction with conventional medicines to promote cardiac health. For example, homeopathic medicine is often prescribed to aid in the cessation of smoking. The demand for homeopathic treatment is growing and it is one of the increasing number of integrative therapies available through the NHS.

Massage and touch

The word massage is derived from Arabic, Greek, Hindi and French words which describe forms of touch, pressing and shampooing (Horrigan 2001). It is a systematic manipulation of the soft tissues of the body. Regardless of the individual touch technique that has been developed by the massage therapist, manipulations will be gliding, kneading, percussing, compressing, shaking or vibrating.

In an ancient Chinese book titled *The Cong-Fou of the Tao-Tse*, the techniques of modern massage were described. Approximately 100 years ago a French translation of the text appeared and the French brought Chinese massage to the Western world. Although there are now many forms of massage, such as the Swedish movements of massage which were systematized by Per Henrik Ling, a Swedish gymnast, in the early 19th century, the French terminology for massage strokes is used. Strokes that glide are termed *effleurage*; those that knead are termed *petrissage*; those that strike are termed *tapotement*; those that compress are termed *friction* and those that shake or vibrate are termed *vibration*.

According to Tappan (1988), massage probably began as soon as the cave dwellers rubbed their bruises. Therapeutic massage undoubtedly developed from local folk medicine and although the origin of Chinese medicine is lost in antiquity, it appears massage has always been an essential aspect. Documents in the British Museum indicate massage was performed in China around 3000 BC (Horrigan 2001). It has been found useful and integral to the healing process and is frequently prescribed for its psychological, physiological, mechanical and reflex effects. Hippocrates learned the art of massage and prescribed it for his patients in 400 BC and Asclepiades, who was an eminent Greek doctor, abandoned the use of all other medicines in favour of massage, which he claimed effected cure by restoring the nutritive fluids of the tissues to their natural, free movement. He discovered that sleep could be induced by gentle stroking.

During the First and Second World Wars massage was used extensively to promote physical and emotional rehabilitation in battle-worn soldiers. Massage therapy has been embraced by the caring professions and in particular by nurses. In the primary and secondary care sectors, massage is used extensively in areas such as pain clinics, cancer wards, hospices, care of the elderly units and physiotherapy departments.

Massage has been shown to be effective in promoting sleep and recovery in critically ill patients (Richards 1998). The effects of massage and associated therapeutic touch have been shown to reduce anxiety, promote comfort and rest in the intensive care environment (Cox & Hayes 1997, 1998). Through massage, aspects of sleep deprivation can be ameliorated (Bonnet 1994).

Meditation

Meditation is considered to be a hard discipline akin to a good programme of physical exercise (Leshan 1995). It has been practised for over 2000 years in Asia and is documented as a part of the monastic life found in Buddhist monasteries. Maharishi Mahesh Yogi developed transcendental meditation in the early 1960s and it was enthusiastically embraced by the flower children who said it brought about a sense of peace and feelings of well-being. The Friends of the Western Buddhist Order established a slightly different form of meditation in Britain in 1967 and consequently a large number of British people practise meditation for about 20 minutes once or twice each day. Meditation involves sitting quietly and sweeping away all thoughts from the conscious mind. This frees the unconscious mind to do its work. Many GPs prescribe its use, particularly as a means of reducing anxiety and stress. The British Association for the Medical Application of Transcendental Meditation boasts a membership of over 700 GPs and hospital doctors.

Leshan (1995) indicates that people meditate to find or recover something of themselves that they have lost. It is used as a means of achieving spiritual awareness and fulfilment, as well as reducing or alleviating inner turmoil and feelings of stress. Through its use a deep sense of relaxation occurs. Meditation is designed to improve physical, psychological and spiritual well-being by accessing more of an individual's human potential. It is said to bring the person closer to the self and reality.

There are many forms of meditation. Probably the most popular is transcendental meditation (TM) which is frequently prescribed to reduce stress levels. In order to practise TM the person sits quietly and repeats a personally significant word or 'mantra' in their head. The critical element of TM is that the 'mantra' or word should either be nonsensical, such as 'la di', or of a positive nature, such as 'peace'.

Buddhist meditation encompasses specific breathing techniques associated with the abolition of negative feelings. Whilst employing these techniques, the person focuses on positive, constructive thoughts which are designed to alter attitudes about the self. This form of meditation is postulated to bring about a greater sense of self-worth and spiritual contentment.

Mantra meditation is a technique centred on repeating a basic word or sound. The mind drifts without direction. In that a basic word or sound is repeated, mantra meditation is similar to TM. The word or sound should have no meaning whatsoever and, as in Buddhist meditation, is intended to free the unconscious mind to do its work. This form of meditation is postulated to produce feelings of tranquillity and serenity.

There are contra-indications to meditation. People who are suffering from depression or have epilepsy or organic psychiatric disorders such as schizophrenia should not meditate unless this has been approved by their doctor. Meditation brings about deep states of relaxation. An increase in α-wave activity, which is normally associated with rest, has been implicated in inducing focal seizures.

In terms of promoting cardiac health, people who meditate indicate they sleep better and experience less anxiety. Many people recovering from myocardial infarction have used meditation as a means to reduce their smoking and drinking habits. Research associated with TM suggests people who suffer from anxiety, sleeplessness, migraine, tension headache, irritable bowel syndrome, stomach ulcers, asthma and high blood pressure may benefit (Jones 1998).

Osteopathy

Osteopathy is derived from the Greek words *osteo* meaning 'bone' and *pathos*, meaning 'disease or suffering'. It involves the physical manipulation of the musculoskeletal system to diagnose problems, alleviate pain, enhance mobility and improve general health. It is based on the principle that 'structure governs function'. The bones, ligaments, joints and muscles of the body influence function and through manipulation, re-alignment occurs which improves function not only in terms of the musculoskeletal system but the rest of the body as well, including its internal organs.

Osteopathic medicine was developed over 100 years ago by an American, Andrew Taylor Still, in the 1870s. Still was an engineer who became a surgeon. However, after working in the army he became disillusioned with traditional medicine due to its brutality and lack of compassion. His engineering background led him to believe that for normal function to occur a sound structure was required. The fundamental principle that 'structure governs function' was born and this remains the foundation of today's osteopathy. When the integrity of a structure is maintained health is promoted. When re-alignment is implemented, the body's self-healing mechanisms can work effectively.

The first school of osteopathic medicine was established by Still in Kriksville, Missouri, in 1892. In 1917, one of Still's students established the British School of Osteopathy. Today over 5 million people seek treatment from osteopaths (Jones 1998). In 1993 it became the first complementary therapy regulated by law in Britain.

Osteopathic treatment centres on the spine. Still postulated that the spine was the most important part of the body as it houses that part of the nervous system, the spinal cord, which governs movement and bodily function. Misalignment of the bones, ligaments and joints associated with the spine and the muscles surrounding them has an effect on the functioning of the body.

In terms of promoting and maintaining health, osteopathy involves manipulative techniques to correct problems. Treatments vary from simple massage in order to relax muscle tension, stretching which improves joint mobility and gentle manipulation to high-velocity thrusts which force bones into alignment. All the techniques used are standard and well established. Many people indicate that osteopathy improves their range of motion, helps them to relax and brings about dramatic results in terms of range of neck and spinal movement, the reduction of sciatic discomfort and relief of low back pain. Osteopathy is considered particularly useful in treating sports injuries, migraine and tension headaches, dizziness and many forms of arthritic discomfort.

Reflexology

Reflexology stems from an understanding of the reflex action of the nervous system. Reflexology is a treatment which involves the application of varying degrees of pressure to focal points on the hands and feet in order to facilitate healing from within. Essentially, the purpose of reflexology is to promote health and a sense of well-being. Approximately 5000 years ago in China and India, as well as amongst the American Indians, various forms of pressure to the feet and hands were used in the treatments of pain and illnesses (Goodwin 1994).

At the end of the 19th century, Dr William Fitzgerald, an American ear, nose and throat specialist at Boston General Hospital, discovered that pressure applied to specific points on the hand and foot could cause partial anaesthesia in areas of the ear, nose and throat. Using this technique he performed minor surgical procedures without the aid of conventional anaesthetics. In 1913 Dr Fitzgerald began to map the zones of the hands and feet and in 1917, in collaboration with a colleague, Dr Edwin Bowers, he published a text describing 'zone therapy'. Fitzgerald postulated there were 10 longitudinal zones running through the body which were related to specific organs. These were reflected on the hands and feet. With controlled pressure, Fitzgerald suggested a response could be produced elsewhere in the body. According to Fitzgerald, reflexology stimulates not only a particular organ associated with the pressure point but also the inter-relationship between organs and other body systems. Shortly thereafter in 1920, Dr Joseph Riley further developed the technique and published the book *Zone therapy simplified* in which specific horizontal zones of the feet are associated with zone pathways. In the 1960s Doreen Bailey visited America and met Dr Riley's research assistant, Eunice Ingham, who had been refining Riley's technique. Bailey introduced the practice to the UK and established the Bailey's School of Reflexology in 1968.

The theory associated with reflexology suggests that every part of the body is connected by pathways which terminate in the soles of the feet, palms of the hands and ears, tongue and head (Ashkenazi 1993, Booth 1994). Reflexologists believe that the feet are the windows of the body and that they can detect problems in the body by palpating small sand-like grains on the soles of the feet. They indicate that these grains are crystalline deposits of calcium located at the end of nerves in the feet. The areas of the soles of the feet in which they feel the minute grains are related to weak or overactive areas in the body. They claim they can bring about healing by using their thumbs and fingers to rebalance the flow of energy in the zones.

Although there is scepticism as to whether energy can be rebalanced by applying pressure to the foot, many people have indicated they benefit from the therapy. Reflexology is postulated to promote relaxation and is prescribed for people suffering with chronic diseases like arthritis, anxiety-related problems and stress-related disorders. According to the Association of Reflexologists, reflexology is designed to boost energy levels and enhance emotional and spiritual well-being.

Shiatsu

Shiatsu is a Japanese word which means 'finger pressure'. It developed from early forms of massage, called *anma*, in Japan, which employ rubbing, stroking, squeezing, tapping, pushing and pulling to influence the muscle tissue and circulatory systems of the body. In contrast to many forms of massage, Shiatsu uses few techniques. It involves the use of gentle manipulation and hand pressure to bring health and vitality into a person's life. To the casual observer it may appear little is happening in terms of physical activity but through the simple uncomplicated rotation of a limb or the light pressure of the hand or thumb, it is postulated much is happening internally to the body's energy (Lundberg 1992).

The practice of Shiatsu was developed in the early part of the 20th century by Tamai Tempaka who was a Japanese medical practitioner. Tempaka incorporated Western medical knowledge of anatomy and physiology with gentle manipulation, stretches and pressure to form the practice of Shiatsu. In 1964 Shiatsu was officially recognized as a formal therapy by the Japanese government. This recognition distinguished it from the older form of traditional massage, anma. Shiatsu was introduced to the UK about 25 years ago and the Shiatsu Society was founded in 1981.

Central to the principles of Shiatsu is the 2000-year-old philosophy of traditional Chinese medicine which states that energy is manifested from the universe in the forces of Yin and Yang, the positive and negative aspects of *Chi* or *Ki* which flows within the body, forming a matrix that links the vital organs with all other parts of the body. Chi supports the body and all its functions. In Chinese treatments the emphasis is on restoring harmony to the Chi in the body. Chi is considered the primary substance of the universe and arises from the interaction of Yin and Yang.

Shiatsu is commonly used as a treatment for stress-related disorders and for treating back and neck problems. Although there is little scientific evidence that quantifies its benefits, one Chinese study found it effective in treating chronic low back pain and promoting sleep and a double blind trial published in the *Journal of the Royal Society of Medicine* indicated that Shiatsu improved morning sickness in women attending the Royal Maternity Hospital in Belfast (Jones 1998).

Tai Chi

In China, people of all ages begin the day by performing traditional Chinese exercises in parks, woods or wherever they live. A common sight is tai chi chuan which is an exquisite slow exercise, a soft martial art that develops and relaxes the whole body (Lam 1991). Tai chi originated in the Sung Dynasty of the 12th century. It was developed by a Taoist monk Chang San Feng, who was a soldier, spiritualist and martial arts expert. According to legend, Chang San Feng observed a duel between a snake and crane. During the duel the snake mesmerized the crane by its artful speed and grace. Chang San Feng was so impressed with the agility of the snake that he developed a system of non-combative martial art exercises that integrated the snake-like movements with relaxation techniques, breathing exercises and meditation. Tai Chi is frequently referred to as a moving meditation. Tai Chi has grown in popularity since the early 1970s. It is widely practised in the UK and is regarded as a beautiful and soothing antidote to the stresses and strains of modern life. Although there are many forms of Tai Chi, all forms are designed to aid the flow of vital energy in the body. This helps to establish balance. When practised regularly, Tai Chi improves posture, suppleness and respiratory functioning. It stimulates the circulatory and lymphatic systems and promotes relaxation of the nervous and musculoskeletal systems.

Yoga

In 8000 BC the yoga cult in India used respiratory exercises for religious and healing purposes. The word yoga was derived from the Sanskrit word for 'union' which means promoting union between the mind and body. Like Tai Chi, yoga is considered a moving meditation. Although the origins of yoga are unknown, the practice as known today probably began about 5000 years ago. It was brought to the UK in the Victorian era and has become increasingly popular since its introduction.

Yoga is an exercise system that enhances the psyche (mind) and soma (body). The postures adopted in yoga increase suppleness and strength whilst inducing relaxation. In practice, yoga alleviates stress and counters negative emotions. It induces an inner calm through concentration on postures (exercises) and breathing. This is postulated to enhance digestion, relieve tension, reduce feelings of anxiety and bring about spiritual well-being. Yoga is frequently prescribed as a treatment for back pain and depression.

Breathing is central to the philosophy of yoga. Therapeutic effects occur through correct breathing. Anxiety, tension and stress manifest themselves in disorders such as indigestion, irritable bowel syndrome and headache. Through breathing exercises which use all of the lung and respiratory muscles in expanding the chest, oxygenation of the blood is improved, the involuntary nervous system is stimulated and energy and vitality are enhanced.

There is considerable evidence that yoga is a valuable form of complementary therapy. In 1985, the *British Medical Journal* indicated that regular practice of yoga by asthmatic patients reduced the number of attacks they experienced and also reduced the dosage of medication required to manage their symptoms (Jones 1998). Yoga has been used in NHS hospitals and hospices for treating the terminally ill as well as treating myalgic encephalomyelitis and emphysema. In terms of cardiac health promotion, yoga has been shown to be effective in reducing anxiety and other stress-related conditions such as palpitations and high blood pressure. Balance and harmony are induced through yoga and this promotes a healthy lifestyle.

CONCLUSION

Complementary therapies can be used to promote cardiac health in a variety of ways when integrated with traditional Western approaches to care. Recent progress in therapeutics and the growing integration of complementary therapies provide a holistic approach to cardiac health promotion. The empowerment of patients is central to a focus on prevention and healing rather than cure.

It is recommended that the therapies addressed in this chapter should be used in conjunction with traditional Western medicine. Integration of these therapies leads to a less fragmented way of promoting cardiac health so that people become more motivated about promoting their own cardiac health and feeling better.

REFERENCES

Alspach J 1991 Core curriculum for critical care nursing, American Association of Critical Care Nurses, 4th edn. WB Saunders, London

Ashkenazi R 1993 Multidimensional reflexology. International Journal of Alternative and Complementary Medicine 11(6): 8–12

Blackwell A 1991 Tea tree oil and anaerobic (bacterial) vaginosis. Lancet 337: 300

Bolwerk C 1990 Effects of relaxing music on state anxiety in myocardial infarction patients. Critical Care Nursing Quarterly 13: 63–72

Bonnet M 1994 Sleep deprivation. In: Kryger N, Roth T, Dement W (eds) Principles and practice of sleep medicine, 2nd edn. WB Saunders, Philadelphia, pp. 50–67

Booth B 1994 Reflexology. Nursing Times 5: 38–40

British Medical Association 1993 Complementary medicine: new approaches to good practice. Oxford University Press, Oxford

Bryne C 2001 Choosing a therapy. In: Rankin-Box D (ed) The nurses' handbook of complementary therapies, 2nd edn. Baillière Tindall, London and the Royal College of Nursing, London, pp. 9–14

Busby H 2001 Herbal medicine. In: Rankin-Box D (ed) The nurses' handbook of complementary therapies, 2nd edn. Baillière Tindall, London and the Royal College of Nursing, London, pp. 179–184

Cameron-Blackie G 1993 Complementary therapies in the NHS. National Association of Health Authorities and Trusts, Birmingham

Cannard G 1994 On the scent of a good night's sleep. Trial project. Midland Health Board News January: 3

Chopra D 1991 Unconditional life. Bantam Books, London

Chopra D 1993 Ageless body, timeless mind. Harmony Books, New York

Cox C, Hayes J 1997 Reducing anxiety: the employment of therapeutic touch as a nursing intervention. Complementary Therapies in Nursing and Midwifery 3(6): 162–167

Cox C, Hayes J 1998 Experiences of administering and receiving therapeutic touch in intensive care. Complementary Therapies in Nursing and Midwifery 4(5): 128–133

Cumston CG 1996 History of medicine. Routledge, London

Davis-Rollans D, Cunningham S 1987 Physiologic responses of coronary care patients to selected music. Heart and Lung 16: 370–378

Downey S 2001 Acupuncture. In: Rankin-Box D (ed) The nurses' handbook of complementary therapies, 2nd edn. Baillière Tindall, London and the Royal College of Nursing, London, pp. 121–128

European Atherosclerosis Society 1987 Strategies for the prevention of coronary heart disease: a policy statement of the European Atherosclerosis Society. European Heart Journal 8: 77–88

Firebrace P, Hill S 1988 New ways to health – a guide to acupuncture. Hamlyn, London

Fox A 1993 General practice management of gastrointestinal problems assisted by Vegatest techniques. British Homeopathic Journal 82: 87–91

Goodwin H 1994 Reflex zone therapy. In: Rankin-Box D (ed) Complementary health therapies: a guide for nurses and the caring professions. Chapman and Hall, London, pp. 59–84

Graham H 1991 The return of the shaman: the emergence of a biophysical approach to health and healing. Complementary Medical Research 5(3): 165–171

Griggs B 1981 Green pharmacy: a history of herbal medicine. Jill Norman and Hobhouse, London

Haehl R 1985 Samuel Hahnemann, his life and work, volumes 1 and 2. B. Jain, New Delhi

Health Education Council 1984 Coronary heart disease prevention: plans for action. Pitman, London

Horrigan C 2001 Massage. In: Rankin-Box D (ed) The nurses' handbook of complementary therapies, 2nd edn. Baillière Tindall, London and the Royal College of Nursing, London, pp. 215–221.

Hudak C, Gallo B 1994 Critical care nursing; a holistic approach, 6th edn. Lippincott, Philadelphia

Jones H 1998 Doctor, what's the alternative? Hodder and Stoughton, London

Jowett NI, Thompson DR 1989 Comprehensive coronary care. Scutari Press, Middlesex

Krysl M 1996 Sound healer. In: Krysl M (ed) Soulskin. National League for Nursing, New York, p. 47

Lam Kam Chuen 1991 The way of energy. Gaia Books, London

Leddy S, Pepper J 1993 Conceptual bases of professional nursing, 3rd edn. JB Lippincott, Philadelphia

Leshan L 1995 How to meditate. Thorsons, London

Longmate N 1970 Alive and well: medicine and public health 1830 to the present day. Penguin, Harmondsworth

Lundberg P 1992 Shiatsu. Gaia Books, London

Mackereth P 1998 Body, relationship and sacred space. Complementary Therapies in Nursing and Midwifery 4(5): 125–127

McMahon R, Pearson A 1991 Nursing as therapy. Chapman and Hall, London

Park G 1992 The art of changing. Ashgrove Press, Bath

Price L, Price S 1995 Aromatherapy for health professionals. Churchill Livingstone, Edinburgh

Price S 1998 Using essential oils in professional practice. Complementary Therapies in Nursing and Midwifery 4(5): 144–147

Rankin-Box D 1991 Proceed with caution. Nursing Times 87: 34–36

Richards K 1998 Effect of a back massage and relaxation intervention on sleep in critically ill patients. American Journal of Critical Care 7(4): 288–299

Ryman L 1994 Relaxation and visualisation. In: Wells R, Tschudin V (eds) Wells' supportive therapies in health care. Baillière Tindall, London, pp. 67–86

Sasaki P 1992 Foreword. In: Lundberg P Shiatsu. Gaia Books, London, pp. 6–7

Stevensen C 1994 The psychophysiological effects of aromatherapy following cardiac surgery. Complementary Therapies in Medicine 2: 27–35

Stevensen C 2001 Aromatherapy. In: Rankin-Box D (ed) The nurses' handbook of complementary therapies, 2nd edn. Baillière Tindall, London and the Royal College of Nursing, London, pp. 129–137

Tappan F 1988 Healing massage techniques. Holistic, classic, and emerging methods. Appleton and Lange, Norwalk

Unschuld P 1985 Medicine in China: a history of ideas. University of California Press, Berkeley

US Department of Health and Human Services 1990 Seventh Report to the President and Congress on the Status of Health Personnel in the United States. US Department of Commerce National Technical Information Service, Springfield, Virginia

Webster C 1981 Biology, medicine and society 1840–1940. Cambridge University Press, London

Weiss R 1988 Herbal medicine. Beaconsfield Press, Beaconsfield

Williams D 1989 Lecture notes on essential oils. Eve Taylor, London

Williams L, Home V 1995 A comparative study of some essential oils for potential use in topical applications for the treatment of the yeast Candida albicans. Australian Journal of Medical Herbalism 7(3): 57–62

World Health Organization 1978 The promotion and development of traditional medicine. WHO technical report series no. 662. WHO, Geneva

Professional issues in cardiac care

This section emphasizes the changing role of nurses and nursing in cardiac care. The large variety of ethical issues and debates related to cardiac care offers a reflection on many of the complex situations that nurses can become involved in. The emergence in recent years of critical pathways (integrated care pathways) and their contribution to cardiac care, the growth of early extubation protocols, minimally invasive surgery and what the future may offer the cardiac patient, their loved ones and the nursing profession are explored in detail.

28

Ethical issues in cardiac care

Graham Rumbold

This chapter begins by addressing the question of why do nurses in general, and cardiac nurses in particular, need to study ethics. In answering this question the nature of ethics will be explored. It will then progress to discuss some key ethical theories – *deontology* and *utilitarianism* – and principles – *beneficence and non-maleficence*. This will be followed by a discussion of issues and dilemmas which are pertinent to cardiac nursing: cardiopulmonary resuscitation, organ transplantation and cessation of treatment. The chapter concludes with suggestions for further reading on both the topics discussed within it and other aspects of ethics pertinent to nursing.

WHY STUDY ETHICS?

In order to answer this question, one needs first to understand something of the nature of ethics. Ethics is a branch of philosophy and 'is concerned with human actions and their effects and the value of those actions' (Rumbold 1999). Unlike many of the sciences, it is not a precise discipline. While it seeks to find answers, on one level, to questions such as 'What is right? What is good?' and at another level to resolve practical dilemmas such as whether to carry out a particular treatment or not, it can seldom provide a definitive answer. What it seeks to do is provide a means of formulating answers to questions and so guide actions. However, as will be seen, in many situations different people might arrive at differing answers and so take different actions which are neither necessarily correct or incorrect. The important thing is to justify the decisions and actions on the basis of sound ethical reasoning.

It [ethics] provides a framework for dealing with issues, problems and dilemmas. An understanding of ethical or moral theories helps a person to decide on an appropriate line of action although it will not necessarily provide them with an answer. (Rumbold 1999)

So, why do nurses and other health-care workers need to study ethics? The answer to this question has to some extent already been answered but there are a number of specific reasons. Two of these are particularly relevant in the context of cardiac care. First, nurses in the course of their day-to-day work face a number of problems that have an ethical dimension. Sometimes the ethical nature of the problem is fairly obvious, such as whether to tell a patient that their condition is terminal or having to respond to a suggestion that a patient not be resuscitated. On other occasions the ethical dimension may be less explicit, the decision may appear to be essentially a clinical one and yet will be influenced by the ethical beliefs and values of the actors.

Second, and this is particularly the case in cardiac care, recent years have seen advances in medical knowledge and technology, which have created new ethical questions. Organ transplants, the use of life support machines such as mechanical ventilation, cryogenics and genetic engineering all pose questions, the answers to which cannot be found in traditional moral codes. Even cardiopulmonary resuscitation, which today is taken as an almost routine procedure, is a comparatively recent technique and still causes ethical debate.

ETHICAL THEORIES AND PRINCIPLES

An understanding of ethical theories provides a framework to guide ethical decision making, while ethical principles can provide a rationale for choices. Here two theories are discussed: deontology and utilitarianism. The reason for selecting these, rather than others, is that they have been major influences, at least in Western philosophy, in recent times. Furthermore, as will be seen, they have each influenced thinking within health care. Two principles are then explored: beneficence and non-maleficence. These two principles have been central to medical ethics since the time of Hippocrates and still underpin much thinking in medical, if not nursing, ethics.

Deontology

Deontology is derived from the Greek word *deon* meaning duty. While the notion of duty-based ethics can be traced back to the Stoic philosophers (about 300 BC), the greatest impetus to this way of thinking came from the 18th-century German philosopher Immanuel Kant. Kant argued that it was the intention rather than the consequences of an act that determines whether the act is morally right. The good intention is

to do one's moral duty. He argued that for a moral principle to be binding on one as a duty, it must be universal, unconditional and imperative. This he called the *categorical imperative* and stated it as follows:

Act only on the maxim through which you can at the same time will that it should become a universal law.

Thus, Kant argued, to determine whether a maxim, or principle, was a moral law, one asked the question 'What if the antithesis were adopted as a law?'. Kant applied this test to two examples, promise keeping and truth telling. What if we adopted the principle that we should make promises which we had no intention of keeping? Kant argued that this would be self-contradictory and therefore could never become a universalized law, for if we made promises which we never intended keeping then there would be no point in making promises. The whole point of making a promise is the implication that it will be kept. Therefore, if there is a law it should be (a) only make promises which one intends to keep and (b) keep them. Kant applied a similar argument to truth telling and concluded that there was no justification for telling an untruth and that there is a moral duty to tell the truth. What he said was that in every utterance one should be truthful. This implies that while one should never tell an untruth, it is acceptable to withhold the truth – to say nothing.

This clearly has implications for health professionals. If we are to apply Kant's rule in the situation where a patient is suffering from a terminal condition and asks to be told their prognosis, then we are bound to tell them the truth. To say 'we don't know' when we do is to tell an untruth and in such a situation to make no reply is not a feasible option.

A second and particularly pertinent principle derived by Kant was what he described as *respect for persons*. Kant argued that people should always be treated as ends in themselves and never as means. This is clearly consistent, as we shall see later, with beneficence and non-maleficence and also with the concept of respecting autonomy. Kant argues that respect for autonomy is a universal law and is supported both by the categorical imperative and the concept of respect for persons. However, he argued that respect for the autonomy of one individual had to be seen within the context of respect for the autonomy of others (Rumbold 1999).

Thus, if we are to apply Kant's thinking within the health-care setting, there are two important implications. First, that every patient should be treated as a person in their own right and that whatever is done to them must be for their benefit and not to benefit others. To carry out any form of experimentation on a patient unless the intention were to benefit them would, according to Kant's reasoning, be unjustified. There may also be benefits for others and this would be acceptable but if the benefit were *only* for others then there would be no justification. It also calls into question the use of placebos, especially when the patient is unaware that they are being given a placebo, for to do so is to deceive the patient and thus not treat them with the respect due to an autonomous being. Second, one might be justified in not acceding to the request of one patient if in so doing the autonomy of other patients is impinged. It is implicit in the concept of respecting autonomy that *all* should respect the autonomy of others. The patient has a duty to respect the autonomy of other patients, just as much as the health professional has a duty to respect the autonomy of patients.

Utilitarianism

Utilitarianism is some times referred to as consequentialism, for what is seen as morally justifying any action or non-action are the outcomes. It is the consequence or end which determines the rightness or wrongness of actions and not necessarily the act in itself. This is clearly in contradiction to deontological theories which would argue, for example, that to tell the truth is right and to tell an untruth is wrong, whatever the end result. Consequentialists would argue that there may be occasions when not telling the truth is justified if the end result is for the good.

The two best-known proponents of this line of thinking were Jeremy Bentham (1748–1832) and John Stuart Mill (1806–73). 'Although they put forward different accounts, they agree on the fundamental point that what has ultimate value is happiness. Good outcomes are those that yield happiness' (Singleton & McLaren 1995). And, as Mill himself wrote:

The creed which accepts as the foundation of morals, Utility, or the Greatest Happiness Principle, holds that actions are right in proportion as they tend to produce happiness, wrong as they tend to produce the reverse of happiness. By happiness is intended pleasure, and the absence of pain; and by unhappiness, pain, and the privation of pleasure. (cited in Warnock 1962, p. 257)

Where Bentham and Mill differed was over how pleasure or happiness can be measured. Bentham held that all pleasures can be quantified and argued that the morally good act was that which produces the greatest happiness for the greatest number of people. Mill, while accepting the basic principles of Bentham's theory, rejected the idea that all pleasures can be measured quantitatively and argued that pleasures differ qualitatively.

Pleasures that befit rational human beings rather than those held in common with lesser animals have greater value. He also placed more emphasis on the social character of happiness than did Bentham. The goal of moral actions is the greatest happiness of all members of society. (Rumbold 1999).

It is important to note that neither Bentham nor Mill says that it is the happiness of the individual which morally justifies an action but that of either the majority or all. Thus, in any situation it is the consequences for the *greater number*, rather than the individuals involved, that have to be considered.

The philosophy of Bentham and Mill is often referred to as *hedonistic consequentialism* because of the emphasis placed on achieving happiness or pleasure and avoiding pain. There are two further refinements of consequentialist or utilitarian ethics: *act utilitarianism* and *rule utilitarianism*. The former, as the name suggests, places emphasis on the act itself and argues that an act can be morally justified if it results in a good consequence. Thus, just as Bentham and Mill, act utilitarians would seek to determine the most appropriate action in each situation. They might thus determine that the same act is morally good in one situation but morally wrong in another. Rule utilitarians, similarly to deontologists, argue that there are moral rules and that these are determined by the extent to which generally applying the rule would result in the greatest good. Thus rule utilitarians would argue, for example, that truth telling is a moral rule on the basis that if it were generally adopted the overall result would be for the good. Whereas act utilitarians might argue that in some situations to tell an untruth might be justified if the intended consequences were good.

In the case of the terminally ill patient who asks to know their prognosis, rule utilitarians would agree with deontologists and say that the patient should be told the truth, even though in that particular situation the consequence may not necessarily be good; the patient may become very depressed and give up all hope. Whereas act utilitarians might argue that if there is a strong likelihood of a bad consequence, the nurse would be justified in telling an untruth.

While utilitarianism, and hedonistic or act utilitarianism in particular, has some attractions, it does have its problems. The attraction is that it enables one to judge each situation on its own merits and try to determine the best course of action. There are, however, some flaws in the argument. Utilitarians base their argument on a number of suppositions. First, they presuppose that everyone knows what happiness is and that everyone understands it in the same way. Second, it presupposes that everyone becomes happy in the same way. Third, if as utilitarians claim, everyone can estimate what actions promote happiness, then it leaves each individual free to set their own criterion of morality. The result would be chaos, which of course rule utilitarianism seeks to overcome.

The questions which can be argued, and utilitarians have failed to answer satisfactorily are 'How can we know what happiness is?' and 'How can we determine the best way of achieving it?'. Nevertheless, in some situations the notion of the greatest good or happiness for the greatest number can be a useful guide to decision making. (Rumbold 1999)

Certainly, it can provide a useful guide when determining how best to allocate limited resources, whether this be at a national level, where the government has to determine which health needs have the greater priority, or at ward level, where a nurse may have to balance the needs of an individual patient with those of all the patients in the ward.

Deontological theories and rule utilitarianism are equally not without their difficulties. On the one hand, ethical decision making appears simpler in as much as, if one knows the rule, one simply applies it whatever the consequences. And, in so doing, it may feel justified. On the other hand, one might feel very uncomfortable with the consequences of one's actions and might even feel that they are sufficiently harmful to make one question the morality of the act and even of the rule itself. For, as health professionals, we have an inherent desire to act always in a way which will benefit the patient and not cause harm.

Beneficence and non-maleficence

The principles of beneficence and non-maleficence are essential elements of medical ethics, at least within the Western world. They have their foundations within the teachings of Hippocrates and are integral to the Hippocratic oath. The oath in its original form stated:

I will follow that system of regimen which, according to my ability and judgement, I consider for the benefit of my patients, and abstain from whatever is deleterious and mischievous.

And, as Hippocrates stated elsewhere: 'As to diseases, make a habit of two things – to help, or at least to do no harm'.

Put simply, the principle of beneficence is a moral injunction to always do good. More specifically, within the health-care setting, it implies only acting in a way which will benefit the patient.

Beneficence is traditionally seen as residing at the foundation of health care and refers specifically to the principle that the goal of actions in relation to patients ought to be to promote health, to relieve from unnecessary pain and suffering and to prolong life. (Beauchamp & Childress 1983)

The principle of non-maleficence is linked to that of beneficence, meaning to not inflict harm. 'It can be argued that the principle of non-maleficence is not a principle in its own right, but merely an idea encompassed by the principle of beneficence' (Rumbold 1999). Or the two might be seen as opposite ends of a continuum (Singleton & McLaren 1995). However, there may be situations, as has been argued by Gillon (1986), where the principle of non-maleficence takes precedence over that of beneficence. There may be occasions where, for example, the risk of harm from a medical intervention outweighs the potential benefits. In more general terms, many (Gillon 1986, Glover 1977) argue that the principle of non-maleficence is more widely binding than that of beneficence in as much as, while we do not have a duty to do good for everyone, we do have a duty to not harm anyone. Mill, on the other hand, when defining his principle of utility, defined happiness as pleasure *and* the absence of pain, thereby equating doing good, that is causing pleasure, with not doing harm, that is preventing pain.

The principles of beneficence and non-maleficence are clearly entwined in the Hippocratic oath:

I will use treatment to help the sick according to my ability and judgement, but I will never use it to injure or wrong them.

And similarly, the United Kingdom Central Council (UKCC) *Code of professional conduct* (1992) states that in the exercise of accountability a registered nurse, midwife or health visitor must:

1. act always in such a manner as to promote and safeguard the interests and well being of patients and clients
2. ensure that no action or omission on your part … is detrimental to the interests, condition or safety of patients and clients.

While it can be argued that to not do harm is to benefit someone, it does not, as has already been suggested, follow that in doing something which is beneficial we can necessarily avoid doing harm. The debate is further confounded by the fact that increasingly patients are submitted to medical interventions which, while not actually causing them harm, do not benefit them either – interventions which are *futile*; 'particularly in the context of critically ill, dying patients, the provision of care that cannot reverse their decline might well be described as a futile effort' (Zucker & Zucker 1997). The medical futility debate is one which has gained momentum in recent years, not least in the area of intensive or high-dependency care. The increasing use of medical technology and life-sustaining interventions which have often been shown not to give any lasting benefit has caused many to question the basis of universally employing such procedures.

Summary

Before moving on to discuss issues in cardiac nursing, it would seem useful to summarize the key points which have arisen in the foregoing discussion. Two major ethical theories have been discussed – deontology and utilitarianism – both of which provide frameworks for ethical decision making. While each will approach ethical decision making from a different philosophical stance, there are some points of agreement, not least regarding the principle that one should do good. The differences are about how one determines what is good and whose good is paramount. Deontologists claim that the answer to the first question is determined by moral law, while utilitarians argue that it is the consequences of actions that determine their rightness or wrongness. In answer to the second question, deontologists, such as Kant in particular, would argue that it is the good of the individual that is paramount, while utilitarians would argue that it is the good of the greater number that needs to be considered.

However, as we have seen, the principles of beneficence and non-maleficence are compatible with both schools of thought. Kant emphasizes this in his principle of respect for persons and Mill's definition of utility clearly supports these principles. The key principles, then, which should underpin ethical decision making in health care are beneficence, non-maleficence and respect for the individual. One of the as yet unanswered questions is who decides? Who decides what will benefit the patient or which treatments may be futile or even harmful? We shall address these questions as we explore some specific issues.

CARDIOPULMONARY RESUSCITATION

The issues related to decisions as to whether or not a patient or groups of patients should be eligible for resuscitation have already been touched upon briefly in Chapter 24. Here the debate is expanded and will focus on two related issues: (a) the futility debate in respect of cardiopulmonary resuscitation (CPR) and who should be involved in the decision-making process.

The problem of medical futility involves two questions.

1. Are there medical interventions administered to a specific patient with a particular disease that we can label *futile* or *useless*, because we are sufficiently confident that they will not be beneficial?
2. If so, are physicians entitled, or indeed obligated, to refuse to provide those interventions to the patient in question even if the treatment is requested or demanded by the patient or appropriate surrogate? (Brody 1997)

These are by no means easy questions to answer but the health professions cannot escape them. First, health care is an expensive enterprise and in many countries dependent upon public funds so the justification for spending funds on interventions which have little or no cost benefit has to be addressed. Second, we need to address the question as to what extent specific interventions are beneficial to the individual patient.

It has become standard practice in hospitals and emergency care settings to attempt CPR if a patient suffers a cardiopulmonary arrest. In order to answer the question of how appropriate the widespread use of this procedure is, we need to briefly set it within historical context. CPR came to the fore in the 1960s with the introduction of coronary care units (CCUs). These units, equipped with monitors and staffed by specialist trained personnel, enabled instantaneous notification of the onset of potentially fatal arrhythmias. It also meant that within seconds of an arrest, resuscitation could be attempted.

The success of CPR led to a phenomenon fairly typical of American medicine – the uncritical use of technology that has proved beneficial to a small number of patients for treating other patients who have not been shown to benefit. CPR soon became the standard reaction to any patient in any US health care setting who suffered a cardiac arrest. (Brody 1997)

CPR is an expensive procedure. It requires the use of considerable resources, both human and material. The question is, are we justified in using these resources in situations where the known success rate is noticeably small? The utilitarian response to this question is 'no' for two reasons. First, employing these resources for such a small number of people deprives many others of access to health-care resources given that the total resource is limited. Second, while, when successful, it may bring happiness and relief of pain to a few, the majority for whom it is not successful gain no benefit. As Tom Quinn has already pointed out in Chapter 24, the procedure itself subjects the patient to 'indignity and frank brutality', so in itself it causes pain. It also causes considerable distress to the patient's relatives. There would seem little justification in performing CPR other than in cases where the success rate is known to be perhaps 50% or more, which for the most part means those patient groups for whom it was originally designed.

Recognition of the fact that in some cases CPR may be futile has led to the use of 'do not attempt resuscitation' (DNAR) orders. While, in the light of the argument above, the use of such orders may be justified, there are also dangers involved. The utilization of guidelines based on relatively arbitrary selected criteria, for example age, may mean that many are deprived of resuscitation when the likelihood of success of the procedure may be as great as for those for whom it is automatically performed. As Quinn (Chapter 24) points out, research (Tresch 1991) has shown that for some elderly patients CPR has a success rate close to that of younger patients. And, more crucially, when they meet the diagnostic criteria, they may have a considerably greater likelihood of success than when the procedure is performed on less healthy younger patients.

The question that has to be addressed is who makes the decision? Who should decide whether an individual patient, or specific groups of patients, should be deemed suitable for resuscitation? The debate has tended to focus on decisions *not to resuscitate* (see Chapter 24) and very seldom on the decision *to resuscitate*. The assumption is made that all patients who suffer a cardiac arrest should be resuscitated unless there is reason not to. The decision to resuscitate or not is generally made by the physician and it is only in the latter situation that any discussion is likely to take place with either other health professionals involved or with the patient and their family. There is an assumption that people want to be resuscitated and therefore the question is only addressed if there is felt to be reason for not doing so. Yet, should not patients have the right to be involved in either decision? Bandman & Bandman (1990) argue that it should not be the health professional who decides but the patient: 'Playing God by deciding who has the required quality of life and who therefore lives or dies also reveals a serious moral pitfall of arbitrarily abrogating the equal rights of individuals to decide whether to

live or die'. The point is that there may be patients who, although they meet the medical criteria for resuscitation, would choose not to be resuscitated. Yet, the only occasions when, if at all, the question is discussed with patients is when there are reasons for not resuscitating. The doctrine of respect for persons would suggest that with this procedure, as with any other treatment, the patient has the right to consent. The more recent guidelines from the British Medical Association and the Royal College of · Nursing (BMA/RCN 2001) have addressed some of these issues and should be consulted in this debate.

ORGAN TRANSPLANTATION

The transplantation of major human organs, such as heart and lung(s), has become almost routine and few now remember the debates that occurred in the early years. Initially much of the debate centred around the rightness or wrongness of the procedure per se. Then, with the high rate of failure, questions of futility were raised. Today, with a much higher success rate for heart/lung transplants in the majority of cases, the issue of futility is seldom raised, although there are situations where the appropriateness of the procedure is questionable. Consider Case study 28.1.

This case raises a number of questions. Should he have been allowed a third transplant? Should he even have been given the second one when other needy candidates did not have even one? Given that there was no reason not to give him the first transplant, he met all the criteria and was assessed as a suitable candidate and there was no reason to expect that the procedure would not be successful. It could be argued that the staff were then obligated to offer a second transplant when the first failed. Having accepted the patient for treatment they then had an obligation to prevent his death. They had removed his own heart and therefore, it could be argued, had an obligation to

---

Case study 28.1

A 45-year-old man, married with two children, was assessed as a suitable candidate for a heart transplant, meeting all the criteria. A suitable match was found and the surgery performed. Initially he made a satisfactory recovery, but then 6 months later his new heart began to fail. He was then placed back on the waiting list for a further transplant. Three months later another heart became available and the man underwent a second transplant operation. Again the heart failed and he subsequently died. In the meantime, however, the suggestion was made that he be offered a third transplant.

repair the damage that was done. But was their obligation to this man greater than that to others on the waiting list? In giving this man a second transplant and in considering offering him a third, they were denying other patients a chance.

It could be argued that it would be medically futile to undertake a third transplant, given that two had already failed. It might be argued that it was futile to undertake even a second. The application of the principle of non-maleficence does hold some weight, in as much as the staff had an obligation to prevent harm to this man. However, they also have an obligation to prevent harm to all other patients on their waiting list, since they have already accepted them for the transplant programme. It could be argued that in undertaking a second and certainly a third transplant, they might be actually causing more harm than good to this man and his family. The mental anguish caused by waiting for a suitable donor, coupled with the uncertainty of a successful outcome following a first failure, could outweigh the potential benefit. The case also raises issues about justice. The question is, is it fairer to offer one person more than one opportunity for treatment if in so doing others are denied any opportunity?

The case study raises the issue of justice at the micro level, while the implementation of transplant programmes raises the issue of justice at the macro level. Transplant surgery is expensive. It ties up a lot of resources, both human and material. The question is therefore posed as to whether, given that health-care resources are limited, it is just to allocate so much resource which benefits a few, rather than spreading that resource wider and benefiting far more. Would it be more just to abandon transplant surgery and devote the freed-up resources to, for example, hip replacements? Space does not permit extensive discussion of the principle of justice and the reader is referred to suggestions for further reading at the end of this chapter. However, we need to acknowledge that injustice in health care is inevitable if resourcing is insufficient to meet all needs. There are bound to be winners and losers (Rumbold 1999).

The ideal solution to the dilemma posed would be to so increase resources that all those who need a heart transplant and all those who need hip replacements would be able to obtain them at the point at which their need was identified. The reality is that this is not, and is highly unlikely to be, a possibility. This being the case, how do we answer the question? One might expect the utilitarian response to be that the resources should be allocated to those requiring hip replacements rather than those requiring heart transplants, on the basis that this would bring greater happiness for a

greater number. However, the argument is not that simple. For when we talk of the greater number we are referring to the greater number within society as a whole. Patients requiring heart transplants are often of a younger age group than those requiring hip replacements. The former, if successfully treated, will be enabled to return to the workforce and therefore contribute to the wealth of society. The latter, being elderly, will, despite their increased mobility, nevertheless remain if not dependent financially on the state, at least not able to make an economic contribution, having already ceased to be economically active.

Therefore, it can be argued that in treating patients who require heart transplants rather than those requiring hip replacements, greater good is achieved for the greater number. A counter argument is that the longer hip replacements are delayed, the greater the demand for care those people will place upon society, thus causing a greater burden rather than greater benefit for the greater number. This discussion illustrates to some extent an inherent weakness in utilitarianism. It is not always obvious who is 'the greater number'. And, of course, it also fails to address the needs of the individual.

Kant argued that people should be treated as ends in themselves and not as means. Deciding to treat a particular group of individuals, for example those requiring transplants, on the basis of the extent to which a greater number will benefit is to treat those individuals as means to an end. If people are to be treated as ends in themselves, each individual should be assessed and treated on the basis of their need and not on the extent to which their treatment will benefit others. Furthermore, deontologists would argue that the injunction to save life takes priority over that to improve health. Therefore, given that we possess the knowledge and skill to do so, performing transplant surgery takes priority over hip replacements.

The foregoing discussion illustrates that there are often no clearcut answers to ethical questions. In this particular case, transplants versus hip replacements, it is possible to put forward a reasoned argument on both sides. And this is what is important; that in making ethical decisions one is able to present a logical, reasoned argument to support one's position. A further issue related to organ transplant is that of consent – consent of the donor. 'The patient's right to respect requires free and fully informed consent from the donor or nearest of kin, as with any other intrusion into the body' (Bandman & Bandman 1990). The donor or, as is more frequently the case with heart transplantation, the nearest of kin has the same rights as anyone else to sufficient information in order to consent.

The person from whom consent is obtained has a right to know exactly what the procedure entails and the purposes for which the organ(s) will be used; that is, is it to save life or to enhance the quality of life of another, or will the organ(s) be placed in a bank for use on a future occasion? (Rumbold 1999)

Recent cases in the United Kingdom (UK) have highlighted the anguish caused to relatives when they have discovered that organs from a deceased family member, usually children and young infants, have been retained without their knowledge or consent following post-mortem examination. There can be no moral justification for such practices for they fail to respect either the deceased or their families as persons.

There is also the question as to who should give consent. Obviously, in the case of living donors consent is obtained from the donor themselves but this clearly cannot apply in the case of major organ transplants such as heart or liver or for that matter more minor organs such as corneas. In these instances consent (at present in the UK) must be obtained from the nearest of kin. Thus, while a patient may carry a donor card and may have made their wishes clearly known to health-care staff, their wishes can be overridden by the relatives at the time of death. The UKCC (1987), in its elaboration of Clause 9(2), states: 'The death of a patient/client does not absolve the practitioner from this obligation'. The obligation referred to is to prevent the release of confidential information; however, there are equally sound moral reasons for applying this principle to respecting the patient's wishes.

The requirement to obtain consent from relatives at the time of death creates a number of problems. First, staff may feel reluctant to raise the issue for fear of causing additional stress to the family. Second, the family may feel under pressure to consent. Third, because of the emotional stress they are already experiencing the family may not be capable of giving *informed* consent, which requires that a person fully understands the nature of the decision they are being asked to make. Nurses in such a situation perhaps have a role to play as both patient's and relative's advocate. If they are aware of what the patient's wishes were, they can make this known. And, 'as relatives' advocate in ensuring that their rights to considerate care and to give informed consent – and also their interests – are respected' (Rumbold 1999).

CESSATION OF TREATMENT

So far we have been concerned with decisions about whether or not to treat, be it CPR or transplantation.

The more difficult decision that often has to be made is when to discontinue treatment. The case study discussed above touched on this issue, though there the question was more strictly about whether to repeat treatment. In the discussion about CPR the issues about who should decide who should or should not be resuscitated were addressed. However, there is also the question as to when to stop the procedure and who should make that decision.

To my knowledge, all of the discussion about unilateral decision making, value judgments, and futility relates to the decision whether or not to start CPR. I am aware of no serious policy consideration ever being given to demanding the consent of the patient or family as to when to stop CPR. In principle, however, these two decisions seem equally value laden. (Brody 1997)

Part of Brody's concern is about the timing of the decision. Who decides when to stop and who can say that judgement is accurate? Would another 5 minutes have produced a successful outcome? Clearly one can never know and there has to come a point at which the procedure is terminated. More importantly, the issue Brody raises is who makes the decision. Clearly, in this situation it cannot be the patient, who is unconscious. But is there a case for involving the relatives?

While an immediate response might be 'yes', there are practicalities which have to be considered. The decision has to be made quickly, not least because treatment has to continue while the decision is being made. If relatives are to be involved in the decision-making process they would need time in order to absorb and understand the information on which to make the decision, and time is limited. Also, because of their emotional state they may not be capable of making a rational decision. It does therefore seem that while ideally one would want to involve the relatives, it is in reality not a feasible idea. However, there are other situations in which either the patient or relative can, and should, be involved in the decision to discontinue treatment.

The cessation of the employment of extraordinary means to prolong the life of the body when there is irrefutable evidence that biological death is imminent is the decision of the patient and/or family. (American Medical Association 1974)

Case study 28.2 is drawn from the author's own experience when working on night duty in a CCU. Although the final outcome was for the good, there are questions raised by this case. First, if he had not been a hospital employee, it is doubtful that so many attempts to resuscitate would have been carried out, which raises the question of equity. Second, at no time

Case study 28.2

George, aged 56 years, was employed as a hospital porter. During the night while he and a colleague were pushing the mortuary trolley across the road (the hospital was sited on either side of a main road) he arrested. He was rushed into CCU where he was successfully resuscitated. During the course of the night he arrested a further five times and each time was successfully resuscitated. Eventually after 2 months he returned to work.

was he asked if, should he arrest again, he wished to be resuscitated, yet there were several opportunities to do so since he regained a fully conscious state after each attempt. As he was a bachelor and had no immediate relatives living in the vicinity there was no one else who could be consulted. The decision on each occasion was made by the physician alone.

This raises a further point, that when a decision is made to continue or discontinue treatment it should not rest solely with one health professional, nor even with that one professional and the patient and/or family. The area in which the question of cessation of treatment most frequently occurs is that of patients on life-support machines such as mechanical ventilators, in particular those in a persistent vegetative state (PVS).

In the case of the PVS patient, the determination of irreversibility can only be made by doctors ... the determination of continued treatment as futile and thus optional, should be a shared judgement. (Mitchell et al 1993)

The decision then should involve not just the doctor and the patient's relatives but also other health-care professionals, in particular the nurses. Often, because the nurses are more closely involved with both patient and relatives, they are likely to have a greater knowledge and understanding of their wishes and values. The decision to discontinue treatment is never a purely clinical one, it is equally an ethical one and 'Expertise in clinical diagnosis does not automatically confer expertise in ethical decision-making' (Singleton & McLaren 1995).

To not involve the patient's relatives in the decision making is to not respect them as persons. And to not take into account the known values and wishes of the patient, even though they are no longer able to articulate them, is to fail to respect them as a person. On the other hand, utilitarians would argue that there is no doubt about the decision. If the clinical evidence is that the patient's condition is irreversible, then to continue treatment, thus tying up valuable resources, is not justified.

Of course, it is not only in life-threatening situations, such as those so far discussed, that the issue of discontinuing treatment arises. Patients have the same right to discontinue treatment as they do to decide whether or not to accept it in the first place. Earlier, following discussion of the principles of beneficence and non-maleficence, the question posed was 'who decides what is in the patient's best interests?'. Traditionally it has been the physician who has decided. However, today, with greater emphasis being placed on patients' rights and in particular their right to autonomy, there is a greater recognition that they should be involved in the decision-making process. To respect patients as persons implies respecting their autonomy. Kant argues that respect for autonomy is a universal law, and is supported by both the categorical imperative and the concept of respect for persons. Utilitarians, such as Mill, also support the principle of respect for autonomy, on the basis that such respect would maximize human happiness. 'If individuals are allowed the freedom to act autonomously they will be happier, and the sum total of happiness will be increased' (Rumbold 1999). However, neither Kant nor the utilitarians would argue that autonomy is absolute. The exercise of autonomy has to be tempered by respect for others and one can only exercise one's autonomy to the extent that it does not impinge upon the rights and freedom of others.

But what is meant by autonomy? Autonomy can be defined as 'the capacity to think, decide, and act on the basis of such thought and decision freely and independently and without let or hindrance' (Gillon 1986). However, 'Autonomy does not mean freedom to do as one wants or to act in accordance with one's desires. It embodies the notions of freedom and liberty, but only within the constraints of reason' (Rumbold 1999).

Thus, in order to decide and act autonomously, the patient requires sufficient information on which to make a reasoned decision. And respect for autonomy implies that the patient, having received and understood the relevant information and made their decision, has the right to expect that health professionals will respect that decision. The health professional may not agree with the decision; they may consider it ill advised or even absurd, in which case they should try to explore more fully with the patient the rationale behind the decision, but at the end of the day they have to respect that the patient has the right to decide for themselves and act upon their decision. Once that decision has been made and, however reluctantly, complied with, the health professional is then absolved of the moral responsibility for the outcome. However, they would, particularly if discontinuation of treatment may lead to a deterioration in the patient's condition, even death, be advised to obtain a signed statement from the patient that it is their free and uncoerced decision.

It is also worth noting that if a patient declines to undergo treatment which was the reason for their admission to hospital in the first place and they do not require any other treatment or there is no alternative treatment which they may find more acceptable, then they are in essence in breach of contract. For in agreeing to come into hospital in the first place, they have entered into a contract which implies that (a) they have the right to receive appropriate care and (b) they will accept that care. If they then refuse to accept that care or its continuation, they become in effect trespassers and should be required to sign a self-discharge form and leave the hospital. If they refuse to do so, the hospital authorities can require that they be removed. This may appear rather harsh but rights imply duties and freedom implies responsibility. Thus in exercising their autonomy they must be prepared to accept the consequence of their actions.

CONCLUSION

This chapter began by exploring two ethical theories – deontology and utilitarianism – and two principles –

beneficence and non-maleficence. In the second half of the chapter specific issues were explored – cardiopulmonary resuscitation, organ transplantation and cessation of treatment. The discussion of these specific issues drew upon the theories and principles covered in the first part. In addition, in discussing the final issue, a third principle – respect for autonomy – was introduced as a logical development of the earlier theories and principles, in particular as being implicit within the concept of respect for persons.

The discussion of the specific issues has demonstrated how the major theories and principles can provide a basis on which to make ethical decisions. However, as has been illustrated, conclusions reached by differing theoretical approaches do not always converge. This serves to illustrate the complexity of ethical decision making and demonstrates that, as was suggested in the opening paragraphs of the chapter, there are not always clearcut answers. There may be more than one justifiable answer to any question and the one is not necessarily more 'right' than the other. While we might have a 'gut feeling' that a particular action is right or wrong, we do need, particularly within the context of professional practice, to be able to provide a reasoned argument to support that feeling. It is hoped that this chapter has provided some assistance to enable the reader to do this.

REFERENCES

American Medical Association 1974 Cited in: Rumbold G 1999 Ethics in nursing practice, 3rd edn. Baillière Tindall, Edinburgh, p. 98

Bandman EL, Bandman B 1990 Nursing ethics through the life span, 2nd edn. Prentice Hall, Englewood Cliffs, NJ

Beauchamp TL, Childress JF 1983 Principles of biomedical ethics, 2nd edn. Oxford University Press, New York

BMA/RCN 2001 Decisions relating to cardiopulmonary resuscitation. A joint statement from the British Medical Association, the Resuscitation Council (UK) and the Royal College of Nursing, London

Brody H 1997 Medical futility: a useful concept? In: Zucker MB, Zucker HD (eds) Medical futility and the evaluation of life-sustaining interventions. Cambridge University Press, Cambridge, pp. 1–4

Gillon R 1986 Philosophical medical ethics. John Wiley, Chichester

Glover J 1977 Causing death and saving lives. Penguin Books, London

Mitchell KR, Kerridge IH, Lovat TJ 1993 Medical futility, treatment withdrawal and the persistent vegetative state. Journal of Medical Ethics 19(2): 71–76

Rumbold G 1999 Ethics in nursing practice, 3rd edn. Baillière Tindall, Edinburgh

Singleton J, McLaren S 1995 Ethical foundations of health care. Mosby, London

Tresch D 1991 CPR in the elderly: when should it be performed? Geriatrics 46(12): 47–56

UKCC 1987 Confidentiality: an elaboration of Clause 9 of the second edition of the UKCC's code of professional conduct for the nurse, midwife and health visitor. UKCC, London

UKCC 1992 Code of professional conduct for the nurse, midwife and health visitor, 3rd edn. UKCC, London

Warnock M (ed) 1962 Utilitarianism. Fontana Library, Glasgow

Zucker MB, Zucker HD (eds) 1997 Medical futility and the evaluation of life-sustaining interventions. Cambridge University Press, Cambridge

FURTHER READING

On deontology and utilitarianism

Fromer MJ 1981 Ethical issues in health care. CV Mosby, St Louis
See references to 'utilitarianism' and 'natural law'
Husted GL, Husted JH 1991 Ethical decision making in nursing. CV Mosby, St Louis
See Chapter 5 – Theories and standards
Paton HJ (ed) 1948 The moral law. Hutchinson University Library, London
Includes translation of Kant's work
Warnock M (ed) 1962 Utilitarianism. Fontana Library, Glasgow

On autonomy

Husted GL, Husted JH 1991 Ethical decision making in nursing. CV Mosby, St Louis
See references to autonomy
Rumbold G 1999 Ethics in nursing practice, 3rd edn. Baillière Tindall, Edinburgh
See Chapter 14 – Beneficence, non-maleficence and autonomy

On beneficence and non-maleficence

Rumbold G 1999 Ethics in nursing practice, 3rd edn. Baillière Tindall, Edinburgh
See Chapter 14 – Beneficence, non-maleficence and autonomy
Singleton J, Mclaren S 1995 Ethical foundations of health care. Mosby, London
See Chapter 5 – The principles of beneficence and non-maleficence

On futility

Schneiderman LJ, Jecker NS 1995 Wrong medicine: doctors, patients and futile treatment. Johns Hopkins University Press, Baltimore
Zucker MB, Zucker HD 1997 Medical futility and the evaluation of life-sustaining interventions. Cambridge University Press, Cambridge

On justice

Benjamin M, Curtis J 1992 Ethics in nursing, 3rd edn. Oxford University Press, New York
See Chapter 7 – Cost containment, justice and rationing
Singleton J, McLaren S 1995 Ethical foundations of health care. Mosby, London
See Chapter 5 – The principle of justice
Rumbold G 1999 Ethics in nursing practice, 3rd edn. Baillière Tindall, Edinburgh

General nursing and medical ethics (in addition to titles already listed)

Bandman EL, Bandman B 1990 Nursing ethics through the life span, 2nd edn. Prentice Hall, Englewood Cliffs, NJ
Beauchamp TL, Childress JF 1983 Principles of biomedical ethics, 2nd edn. Oxford University Press, New York
Seedhouse D 1988 Ethics – the heart of health care. John Wiley, Chichester
Varga AC 1980 The main issues in bioethics. Paulist Press, New York
Veatch RM 1981 A theory of medical ethics. Basic Books, New York

29

Fast tracking and new revascularization techniques

Ann-Marie Openshaw
Moira Durbridge

The advances in cardiac surgical and cardiopulmonary bypass techniques, together with shorter acting and more appropriate sedatives, have allowed a critical review of the management of post operative cardiac patients. This chapter explores these issues, together with a review of the emergence of early extubation (fast-track) protocols and the development of high-dependency (HDU) nursing. The latter section of the chapter offers a review of the more recent developments in cardiac surgery and possible future directions. This provides an indication of how nursing care will need to adapt to meet the ever-changing trends.

The demand for cardiac surgery has increased dramatically since the 1980s and while coronary heart disease (CHD) continues to be prevalent in Western society, the need for this specialty will continue to escalate. Data have demonstrated that there was a twofold increase in coronary artery bypass graft (CABG) surgery in the 10 years to 1999, with approximately 28 000 such operations now occurring each year in the United Kingdom (UK) (BHF 2000). In addition, cardiac surgery is performed for other reasons besides myocardial revascularization. This includes valve replacement, correction of congenital abnormalities and transplantation, but it is the demand for CABG that is placing the most strain on cardiac unit resources.

Due to the nature of cardiac surgery, the cost implications are a major issue for the government and more acutely for the individual budget holders and trusts that contract for this specialized surgery. The cost is influenced by the duration of hospitalization, the severity of illness pre-operatively and the complexity and intensity of care provided postoperatively (Parsonnet et al 1989).

Until the advent of 'fast-track' care in the late 1980s, postoperative cardiac patients were cared for exclusively in an intensive care unit (ICU) where they received elective mechanical ventilation overnight and close haemodynamic monitoring for 24–48 hours. Over the last few years, this approach has been under review by many cardiac centres, due mainly to advances in medical, surgical and anaesthetic techniques. Such a review has opened treatment to patients with increased severity of coronary heart disease, patients who are older and those who have previously undergone extensive medical therapy. This includes patients who have undergone previous angioplasty/stent or revascularization (Cheng et al 1996).

By the 1980s, the burden on the system had become so great that problems arose, such as:

- intensive care beds becoming blocked by sick cardiac patients
- operations being cancelled
- the length of stay in hospital increasing
- a lack of funds to meet the increasing costs.

Therefore, by the 1980s, in addition to clinical advances and review, there arose a need to streamline and evaluate the care for patients undergoing cardiac surgery, while still preserving quality of care and positive outcomes (Maxam-Moore & Goedecke 1996).

'Fast-track' care, which is also known as early extubation or rapid recovery, is the method that many cardiothoracic centres throughout the world have adopted to meet this need. The growth of the specialized recovery units and/or high-dependency units (HDUs) appears to be following this hand in hand.

The remainder of this section will examine the changing needs of the cardiac patient. This will include more recent myocardial revascularization techniques, the concept and definition of early extubation protocols and the advantages and disadvantages of this process of care. The all-important selection criteria will be explored, in relation to cost, the nurse's role and the managerial issues of the emerging HDUs. The aim is to provide an overview of the available literature and to demonstrate that, currently, early extubation protocols offer the most appropriate way forward in the management of cardiac patients.

The need for early extubation protocols has been brought to the fore by several specific factors. These include the pressure on hospital trusts to reduce waiting list times to meet government targets, emphasized by documents such as The Patient's Charter (Department of Health (DoH) 1992, 1996), together with the recognition that sicker patients were blocking intensive care unit beds. In the latter case this will inevitably mean a higher incidence of cancellations, leading to an increase in the average length of stay in hospital generally.

Aps (1995) defines fast tracking as 'the specific intra-operative management leading to an improved postoperative condition, with a consequent reduction in both the need for cardiorespiratory support and formal ICU facilities'. This definition is important because it incorporates some of the aspects of total fast-track management vital to a successful patient outcome, notably the intra-operative management. It does not aim to negate the value of postoperative nursing care but emphasizes how events during surgery can affect the fast-track management. It also places emphasis upon the role of the anaesthetist in taking specific management measures in theatre to promote early extubation. This may be actively waking the patient or taking steps such as the implementation of aggressive fluid management strategies. The latter may involve, for example, applying a filter to the bypass circuit to correct the positive fluid balance the patient will have acquired due to the use of an extracorporeal bypass circuit.

Short-acting sedatives such as propofol can be viewed in two ways. Their properties may facilitate a move to the ICU/recovery area while still sedated, with the knowledge that the nursing team can actively wake and extubate the patient when certain parameters are met. However, on arrival, such an approach may be affected by the skill of the nurse, the workload of the unit or clinical problems that may start emerging to prevent earlier extubation. A more aggressive approach by the anesthetist, utilizing the properties of the short-acting sedatives, may have achieved extubation at an earlier stage. Some anaesthetists may wish to leave the patient intubated for a short time to reduce the incidence of potential myocardial ischaemia. Therefore the definition can also be seen as limited, in that it does not include other important issues such as:

- pre-operative assessment
- the length of operation time
- rewarming and the maintenance of haemodynamic stability.
- the control of pain and sedation
- weaning from the ventilator

All of these factors play an important role in the successful early extubation of a patient following cardiac surgery and all need to be discussed individually.

WEANING FROM THE VENTILATOR AND EARLY EXTUBATION

One of the crucial factors that effective fast-track management centres upon is the early extubation of selected patients and their subsequent care in a designated cardiac recovery unit or a specialized HDU. This may follow rapid transfer from an ICU rather than receiving elective and sometimes prolonged ventilation.

Early extubation was defined by Higgins (1992), as well as other authors, as extubation within 8 hours of the patient's arrival from the operating theatre. In some centres this figure may now be nearer to 6 hours or less but again, may be dictated by skill mix and staff availability. In reality, early extubation will also encompass any patients who are not ventilated routinely overnight but who are cared for in the ICU environment (Davies 1997). This can become necessary if there are bed shortages on the recovery or HDU or if the hospital does not contain the latter facility. If the patient is suitable for early extubation but has to be cared for in an ICU overnight, then the management should not differ from that of patients who are transferred to a step-down unit. The use of integrated care pathways is of great value in monitoring and applying the necessary standard of care in situations like this.

Aps et al (1986) have always advised caution about the term 'early', stating that it can be misleading, implying that extubation is performed before normal criteria for extubation are met. This obviously is not the case and must be stressed to the patient and loved ones, if they are informed that they have been preselected for early extubation.

The move towards early extubation would seem to contradict the traditional view that the myocardium could be vulnerable to ischaemia if the patient is awake. Results from the numerous studies carried out on early versus late extubation show that it is safe to practise early extubation on the majority of patients. These studies report that patients extubated within 6 hours or less have fewer days in intensive care, earlier mobilization and similar morbidity, haemodynamic patterns, re-intubation rates and require less postoperative sedation compared with patients extubated the next day. Studies have also concluded that early extubation may be beneficial in terms of cardiac function (Cheng et al 1996, Quasha et al 1980, Westaby et al 1993).

Discontinuation of positive pressure ventilation results in improved cardiac filling and cardiac output due to the elimination of increased intrathoracic pressure. Higgins (1992) has suggested that endotracheal intubation contributes to morbidity which increases with the length of time a patient is intubated. This may, for example, be from the concomitant development of chest infection.

Increasingly over the last few years, the role of extubation has become nurse led. This move was aided by the UKCC document *The scope of professional practice* in 1992. This altered the interpretation of nurses' roles and emphasized individual professional accountability in clinical decision making (Bowler &

Mallik 1998). This is primarily through a reflection on what the patient or client group requires, with a removal of the terms 'extended' or 'expanding' roles which appear, through an almost hierarchical system, to limit rather than appropriately expand practice.

Traditionally, all patients were weaned from the ventilator and extubated by an anaesthetist but now most centres and their medical staff back the practice of nurses taking the lead in the weaning and subsequent extubation. Elmquist (1992) supports this role, stating that the ability to make the crucial decision to extubate is an essential skill of any nurse caring for a postoperative patient. She also highlights that this skill results from knowledge and good assessment techniques, together with extensive practice and experience. Nurses generally work in collaboration with the anaesthetist and physiotherapist as well as following their local extubation policy. Each centre's extubation guidelines will differ slightly from the next, so a general example is shown in Box 29.1.

Box 29.1 illustrates how clinical judgement plays an important role in assessing factors such as 'acceptable haemodynamics'. Such a criterion may be broken into more specific outcomes but patients are dynamic beings and may require differing goals, depending on their underlying clinical condition. It is here that guidance, education and support from more experienced colleagues can assist junior staff to understand what constitutes an acceptable clinical picture for extubation. In the classroom setting, case studies are a valuable method to explore patient parameters in a holistic fashion and learn how a variety of interdependent factors can lead to a decision to extubate.

Maxam-Moore & Goedecke (1996) offered an alternative algorithm to guide nursing staff and anaesthetists through the multiple steps and decision-making points on the way towards safe and timely extubation (see appendix). The overall outcome is obviously to have a fit patient who is haemodynamically stable enough to be transferred to a high-dependency (step-down) unit as soon as possible following cardiac surgery.

Box 29.1 Example of criteria for extubation

- Awake and co-operative
- Able to protect airway (cough and gag reflex)
- Respiratory rate 10–25 breaths/min
- Tidal volume >5 ml/kg (if measured, this is not always the case)
- PaO_2 >10 kPa on FiO_2 of 40%, $PaCO_2$ <7 kPa
- Minimal blood loss (<100 ml/h)
- Acceptable haemodynamics and electrocardiogram (ECG)

On a general level, when the patient has regained consciousness, obeyed commands such as squeezing the nurse's hand, moved all limbs appropriately and has met agreed haemodynamic parameters, mechanical ventilation is weaned off. In addition, the patient will have to be centrally warm and demonstrate minimal drainage from intercostal drains. If the patient's arterial blood gas analysis is satisfactory, the endotracheal tube is removed and supplemented with humidified oxygen. If the arterial blood gases remain satisfactory and there have been no other changes in the condition, then the patient is deemed ready to be transferred to the HDU where they usually would stay until the following morning.

PRE-OPERATIVE ASSESSMENT

Cardiac surgery using cardiopulmonary bypass induces profound physiological and psychological changes and therefore carries an increased risk of morbidity and mortality (see Chapter 22). The mortality rates in England have risen over the last decade from approximately 1% to 3%. This is mainly due to the referred patients being increasingly older and/or more debilitated. With the cost of medical treatment increasing and inevitable economic contraction, increasing morbidity as well as mortality rates have become a very significant issue. Predicting the length of stay pre-operatively remains invaluable in controlling expenditure and using resources efficiently and effectively. As well as cost implications, Tuman et al (1992) state that morbidity is an important indicator of the quality of care and quality of life for patients postoperatively. Inevitably the ability to predict morbidity is an important issue when considering which patients may be suitable for fast-track care.

Many papers have studied risk stratification and all have strived to develop a model that cardiothoracic centres can use to uniformly predict morbidity and complication rates postoperatively. Risk assessment methods devised in the past have either been too complicated for everyday practical use or have not been adaptable in the cardiac field. The Acute Physiological and Chronic Health Evaluation (APACHE), for example, requires postoperative variables such as blood pressure and temperature to be included, which excludes its use as a pre-operative indicator.

A variety of risk factors have been identified in various reports on this subject but not all have been uniformly included, so it seems unlikely that individual centres would agree with one another on which formulae to use. For example, when considering gender, there seems to be a difference of opinion regarding its importance as a predictive variable. Parsonnet et al, in their 1989 study, included this variable, stating that females have a higher operative mortality than males, perhaps due to their smaller artery size. In a 1992 study, Higgins excluded gender from the criteria, arguing that smaller body size and/or coronary artery size cannot be linked to gender alone.

Repeat or 'redo' cardiac surgery, which is usually performed after a period of time when symptoms have reoccurred, is another important factor due to the large number of patients in this category. The Parsonnet scoring system, as well as other studies such as Tuman et al (1992), do include this as a risk, primarily because of the advanced nature of disease that these patients present with, plus the potential for technical problems such as bleeding to occur.

In current practice, it seems that the Parsonnet scoring system is widely used as a baseline indicator of operative risk, essentially the probability of mortality within 30 days of surgery, because the indicators used are simple and universally available. However, although the Parsonnet score is a fairly reliable assessment of pre-operative morbidity and mortality, it does not always predict initial postoperative recovery. Many centres therefore use additional criteria to identify suitable patients for fast-track management, with such selection criteria being over-ridden to exclude or include patients at the discretion of the surgeon or anaesthetist. This obviously would take into account any peri-operative variables such as length of time on bypass or excessive bleeding. Increasingly the EuroSCORE is being utilised within cardiac centres in the UK (Roques et al 1999) (see Chapter 22). In general, however, a patient who scores a Parsonnet higher than 10 is often deemed unsuitable to be fast tracked but, as practice shows, not all patients follow the rule and some patients with higher Parsonnet scores fast track very successfully. Box 29.2 provides an example of the Parsonnet scoring system. The associated categories of increasing risk created from the weighting are: good (0–4%), fair (5–9%), poor (10–14%), high (15–19%) and extremely high risk (≥20%).

SEDATION AND ANALGESIA CONTROL

Another factor that has to be considered pre-operatively is the type of premedication used. Most of the literature agrees that the types of premedication and anaesthesia chosen are highly significant in the subsequent ability to rapidly wean the patient from mechanical ventilation and to extubate early. High-dose opioid analgesia was generally thought of as inappropriate by Aps et al (1986) and the routine

---

Box 29.2 Parsonnet's additive model of risk stratification (after Parsonnet et al 1989, Poloniecki et al 1998)

Risk factor and assigned weighting (%)
- Female gender: 1
- Weight ≥1.5 times ideal: 3
- Diabetes: 3
- Hypertension (systolic >140 mmHg): 3

Ejection fraction
- >50%: 0
- 30–49%: 2
- <30%: 4

Age
- 70–74: 7
- 75–79: 12
- ≥80: 20

Redo operation
- First: 5
- Second: 10
- Left ventricular aneurysm: 5
- Emergency surgery due to complications of percutaneous transluminal coronary angioplasty (PTCA) or angiography: 10
- Dialysis dependent: 10
- Catastrophic state, e.g. cardiogenic shock: 30
- Heart transplantation: 15
- Congenital heart disease: 5

Valve surgery
- Mitral (pulmonary artery systolic pressure <60 mmHg): 5
- Mitral (pulmonary artery systolic pressure ≥60 mmHg): 8
- Aortic (gradient ≤120 mmHg): 5
- Aortic (gradient >120 mmHg): 7
- Coronary artrey bypass grafting at time of valve surgery: 2

---

addition of a benzodiazepine to an Omnopon and scopolamine premedication was abandoned following their study at St Thomas' Hospital in London. Authors such as Maxam-Moore & Goedecke (1996) generally agree and have incorporated anaesthesia management into their early extubation protocols.

The traditional approach to anaesthesia has been to administer high-dose opioids in conjunction with a benzodiazepine such as midazolam to control sedation and prevent wakening during surgery. Inhaled agents such as isoflurane are now more commonly used as well as propofol. Propofol is a non-opioid sedative hypnotic (Maresch 1997) which is quick acting and has a very short half-life, allowing it to be titrated as necessary but to be eliminated rapidly following termination of the infusion or after bolus use. Postoperatively, if propofol is used, care must be taken not to wean the infusion too quickly as the patient may become very anxious and agitated on waking, particularly if still mechanically ventilated.

Propofol can induce hypotension, bradycardia and a reduction in myocardial contractility but this is no more than with other anaesthetics. When compared to midazolam, propofol provides the aforementioned faster wake-up time and better control of the depth of sedation (Sherry 1997) which is imperative for early extubation. Despite propofol's expense, it is ultimately more cost effective for this group of patients due to the reduced time they spend in the ICU environment.

Pain management is imperative for any postoperative patient but following cardiac surgery, the natural physiological stress response to pain and anxiety can be extremely detrimental to recovery. Catecholamines are produced which cause tachycardia, hypertension and increased contractility which together increase myocardial oxygen requirements. As well as these haemodynamic effects, the patient is less likely to breathe deeply and cough which predisposes them to atelectasis and secretion retention. This in turn may result in respiratory infection and hypoxia and can prolong the length of stay in hospital.

High-dose opioids cannot be given in fast-track management due to their profound respiratory depressant properties but this does not mean that low-dose infusions of opioid analgesia are excluded. Chong et al (1992) highlighted that the appropriate use of analgesics such as morphine does not prevent early extubation. Low-dose opioid infusions as well as bolus therapy can be used safely and effectively. Devices facilitating patient-controlled analgesia (PCA) have also been shown to be useful following cardiac surgery, as it enables the patient to control their own pain, enhancing comfort and reducing dependence on the nurse (Hancock 1996).

LENGTH OF OPERATION TIME

Developing techniques in cardiac surgery have led to an appreciable reduction in aortic crossclamp, cardiopulmonary bypass and total operating time. However, there are some who argue that this should not necessarily result in rapid recovery. In the early 1990s, Siliciano (1992) favoured prolonged intubation and mechanical ventilation, arguing that patients were now sicker pre-operatively and should be cared for more conservatively. Verrier et al (1995) also favoured more prolonged ventilation as they believed that the stress of being wakened early and extubated causes increased myocardial ischaemia. There are various studies in progress exploring this argument but there is currently no definitive research to deter centres from fast tracking patients.

REWARMING AND HAEMODYNAMIC STABILITY

During cardiac surgery, patients are maintained in a hypothermic state to protect the vital organs of heart, brain and lungs from hypoxia. Since hypothermia was first introduced into clinical practice by Bigelow and colleagues in 1950 (Youhana 1995), it has been the cornerstone of myocardial protection for most cardiac operations. Although hypothermia plays a crucial role in organ preservation, it can induce cardiac arrhythmias and platelet dysfunction and may interfere with drug and anaesthetic elimination. In the first few hours following surgery, it can also cause intense shivering which dramatically increases myocardial oxygen demand and the potential for ischaemia (Giuffre et al 1994).

Traditionally, the temperature of the patient was brought down below 30°C and topical hypothermia such as crushed ice placed around the heart was common. The belief was that the colder the heart, the less likely there was to be ischaemic injury perioperatively. Mild hypothermia of 30–32°C is now advocated. Consequently if patients are not as cold at the end of surgery, then rewarming is easier and less time consuming, therefore allowing extubation to occur at an earlier stage (Seifert 1998). Leslie & Sessler (1998) suggest that a mild hypothermia of approximately 34°C enables the optimal balance between the risks and benefits for fast-track patients.

Core rewarming is usually initiated whilst bypass is still in progress and most centres aim to achieve a core temperature of 38°C prior to the patient coming off bypass. During the first few hours postoperatively, however, this warm blood circulates to the peripheries and peripheral vasodilatation occurs. This in turn brings about rapid shifts of cold peripheral blood back to the body's centre which results in an 'afterdrop' of the patient's core temperature. This afterdrop scenario is not as apparent if the patient's core temperature was only reduced to 32°C.

In the past, peripheral rewarming in the cardiac ICU was brought about by radiant heat lamps or warmed blankets, but forced warm air devices are now more commonly used. This means that rewarming is extremely efficient but should not be carried out too quickly and needs to be closely monitored. Subsequent vasodilatation can lead to critical hypotension if not managed correctly. Once the patient achieves a satisfactory core temperature and meets the other necessary criteria for extubation, then the recovery can proceed according to preset guidelines or via an integrated care pathway (ICP) if these are used.

MULTIDISCIPLINARY POLICIES AND PROTOCOLS

The advanced nature of rapid weaning and early extubation has meant that cardiac surgery patients are now being managed very differently. Specialized cardiac recovery and HDUs are now common and nursing staff in these areas, as well as in ICUs, have developed their skills and expertise to take on the management of fast-track patients safely and effectively.

In many areas the nurses tend to take the lead in the bedside management of patients postoperatively with parameters such as blood pressure, central venous pressure (CVP) and urine output being set by the medical staff or by the interdisciplinary team within an ICP. The medical staff generally prescribe a range of medications and intravenous fluids which are administered at the discretion of the nurse in conjunction with their observations and clinical assessment of the patient.

HDUs are generally classed as intermediate care facilities, providing care for patients in between ICU or cardiac recovery and the ward area. Many definitions of HDUs exist but the Association of Anaesthetists of Great Britain and Ireland (1991) classes them as being 'an area for patients who require more intensive observation than can be provided on a general ward. It would not normally include patients requiring mechanical ventilation but could manage those receiving invasive monitoring'. This definition is still valuable and very much used (Brooks 2000).

HDUs vary in their function, especially regarding patient criteria for admission and nursing skill mix, but nearly all cardiac HDUs invasively monitor their patients.

A variety of issues must be raised when examining their use:

- The nurse:patient ratio
- Patient admission and discharge criteria
- The skill mix, experience and knowledge of the nursing staff
- What medical and other support teams will be needed and the speed of access
- Environment and geographical location in relation to the ICU/recovery unit, theatres and the ward area

In recent years, nurses have expanded their scope of practice enormously. Edwards & Hess (1996) believe that the fast-track approach has forced nurses to re-evaluate their approach to the care of cardiac surgical patients. Nurses are now more skilled than ever and incorporate many expanded roles into their routine day, including extubation, arterial blood gas analysis, advanced life support and the ability to monitor and record cardiac output studies as appropriate (Anderson & O'Brien 1995). In the realm of the ICU and HDU, nurses need to be autonomous practitioners with the experience and knowledge to make informed decisions based on their clinical observations and assessment skills and in line with agreed protocols.

According to Batey & Lewis (1982) autonomy is the freedom to make discretionary and binding decisions consistent with one's scope of practice and freedom to act on those decisions. Many critical care units work within a philosophy that advocates a high level of autonomy for their nurses. This is extremely important to the well-being of patients, as it is the nursing team who are with the patient for the majority of their recovery. To work within a culture of nurse autonomy, nurse managers of any cardiac postoperative care facility must ensure that both medical and paramedical staff are confident about and recognise the level of skill and experience of nursing staff.

Agreement should be reached regarding the postoperative guidelines or ICPs that are being used. Without multidisciplinary collaboration, the overall standard of care given to any patient can never reach an optimum level. This multidisciplinary team should obviously include doctors and other specialists such as anaesthetists and physiotherapists, with any new practice issues discussed prior to implementation. Conflict, however, does often arise when many different specialists are involved in the recovery of a patient.

Management regimes will vary from centre to centre but it is important for the nursing staff to know who to seek advice from if the need arises. For example, do the surgeons or the anaesthetists provide medical support for the unit? Protocols and policies must be available that allow any nurse to make an informed decision regarding which course of action to take if required in a clinical situation.

The location of the unit is very important when setting these protocols. Logistically, it is obviously better if the postoperative care facilities such as ICU and HDU are near to theatres and each other. If working relationships between the different areas a patient has to move between are good, then seamless care for the patient will become more of a reality. Before a HDU is set up, it is necessary to consider both the case load and the potential demand. This will allow the correct number of beds to be opened to meet

the requirements. Aps et al (1986) highlighted that the demands for open heart surgery, especially coronary artery bypass surgery, tend to exceed the postoperative facilities available and this remains true today. Fortunately, the number of HDUs or equivalent areas has increased since the 1980s but postoperative care facilities still need to be addressed in some centres.

If a HDU is available to complement an ICU, it offers a number of advantages to the hospital.

- A potential reduction in the pressure on ICU beds
- A reduction in the number of cancelled elective surgery cases
- A reduction in the number of unscheduled transfers to other ICUs
- A reduced number of premature discharges from ICU

All HDUs are more cost effective if they have an even number of beds as the usual nurse:patient ratio is 2:1. The financial benefits or drawbacks of a HDU have to be weighed against what the outcome for the patient would be using existing postoperative facilities, usually the ICU and the ward. If there is no HDU, the other options are to keep patients in the ICU longer than necessary or to care for them on a cardiac ward using an individual specialist nurse (specialing). This remains an extremely poor utilization of resources (Edbrooke 1996).

It is important to note that the emphasis of care in the HDU is placed on positive rehabilitation rather than the invasive medical technology required in the ICU. This leads to a calmer, more relaxed environment for patients and their family and friends. With highly trained and skilled nurses overseeing the patient's return to normality, the quality of care and support offered in HDUs provides a confidence boost for patients during a difficult time in their recovery. It is very important that nurses working in HDUs or similar environments maintain their development of new skills, ideas and research and keep up to date with current trends. The field of cardiac surgery is constantly changing and we need to keep abreast of any new changes in practice, as highlighted below, and how the postoperative facilities must accommodate such work.

In view of the Calman Report (1993), it is anticipated that nurse-led units will become more common with specialist critical care nurse practitioners or similar roles becoming more commonplace. The emergence and growth of high-dependency nursing continues to offer a challenging role to the cardiac nurse. In conjunction with this is the refining and development of new cardiac surgical techniques. HDUs do, however, remain the focus of much controversy. For some, they provide a means of increasing throughput without compromising intensive care resources. For others, they merely transfer the problem of blocked beds and staff shortages from one area to another. HDUs may have a valuable place within the cardiac arena but they are certainly not a panacea. It seems that the debate and interest in these issues are set to continue.

The final section of the chapter examines the continuing areas of development and reflects on the future direction of cardiac surgery.

THE EMERGENCE OF NEW MYOCARDIAL REVASCULARIZATION TECHNIQUES

Historical perspectives

Prior to the inception of cardiopulmonary bypass, coronary surgery was performed by various surgeons on the beating heart (Kolessov 1967, Murray et al 1954, Sabiston 1974). The successful development of an extracorporeal circulation circuit offered a solution to the problems encountered by the early cardiac surgeons. These were primarily arterial pressure changes when manipulating the beating heart, difficulties with accurate anastomosis suturing due to coronary wall motion and obscured vision as a result of collateral blood flow (Borst et al 1997).

Coronary artery bypass graft (CABG) surgery conducted via a median sternotomy with cardiopulmonary bypass (CPB) has been the traditional method of revascularizing the myocardium for more than 30 years. This technique provides the surgeon with a bloodless target area, the ability to manipulate the heart to expose all coronary branches and a motionless surgical field (Borst et al 1997). It also enables the cardiac surgeon to operate with greater precision and with adequate visualization of the whole operative area. However, conventional CABG with cardioplegic arrest is not without risks and side-effects. Mortality and morbidity associated with CABG are primarily attributed to:

- the cardiopulmonary bypass
- the median sternotomy
- aortic crossclamping
- global cardiac arrest
- hypothermia (after Mizell et al 1997).

The deleterious effects of CPB are well documented (Acuff et al 1996, Buffolo et al 1996, Wilcock et al 1997) and are outlined in Chapter 22. These include a significant risk of brain injury, principally cerebrovascular accident (CVA/stroke) and neuropsychological

deficit (Wilcock et al 1997). Some authors have calculated the morbidity related to such adverse cerebral outcomes at 6.1% (Roach et al 1996). The current trend to operate on an increasingly ageing client group is likely to exacerbate the problem further. Other reported complications include bleeding, fluid retention, renal ischaemia, impaired lung function, myocardial ischaemia and coagulopathy (Edmunds 1995).

Borst et al (1997) attribute any temporary depression in myocardial contractility to cardioplegic cardiac arrest and cite the whole-body inflammatory reaction that can be triggered as another objection to cardiopulmonary bypass. Many authors believe that the avoidance of CPB is the most effective and important means of decreasing the systemic inflammatory response following cardiac surgery (Butler et al 1993, Edmunds 1995). These concerns, together with the development of newer operative techniques such as thoracoscopic surgery, improved pharmacology and the development of dedicated instrumentation, have led many cardiac surgeons to explore less invasive methods of myocardial revascularization.

Terminology

With the advent of various, more recent techniques and the continual evolution of aspects of the MIDCAB procedure, the terminology may seem confusing. Generally, MIDCAB stands for minimally invasive direct coronary artery bypass, but different surgeons and centres use the term MIDCAB to describe different procedures. In some centres, 'minimally invasive' is used to describe operations via limited access (such as the LAST – left anterior small thoracotomy – procedure; McAlpine 1997), while other surgeons refer to the term as meaning beating heart surgery (but with a median sternotomy). Off-pump or beating heart surgery applies to any cardiac operation which does not use cardiopulmonary bypass. An off-pump procedure may therefore be a MIDCAB operation, a LAST procedure or a beating heart minimally invasive port access valve operation. Not surprisingly, the literature contains a host of acronyms and abbreviations. The most common are shown in Box 29.3.

Of these acronyms/abbreviations, all but the last group are myocardial revascularization techniques and similar developments are being accomplished within the cardiology sphere. Many of the techniques described are still evolving. In addition, new innovations, surgical instrumentation and operative techniques continue to be developed. Minimally invasive cardiac surgery is no longer revolutionary but it is being expanded, modified and perfected. As new

---

Box 29.3 Common terminology for cardiac surgical techniques

CABG	• Coronary artery bypass grafting/grafts • Traditional method of revascularizing the myocardium, since the development of cardiopulmonary bypass and associated machinery • Complete revascularization can be performed. The heart is arrested using warm or cold blood, antegrade or retrograde crystalloid cardioplegia. Aortic crossclamping is applied	Beating heart surgery	• CPB is avoided • The heart is not arrested; surgery is conducted on the beating heart • Numerous myocardial stabilization devices have been tried • Often referred to as off-pump surgery
OBCAB	• Off-pump coronary artery bypass surgery. This is probably the most common term used to describe any beating heart surgery	LAST procedure	• Left anterior small thoracotomy • Refers to single-vessel grafting: left internal mammary artery to left anterior descending coronary artery • Sometimes referred to as keyhole surgery • Sometimes referred to as thoracoscopic surgery • The procedure is performed without the use of cardiopulmonary bypass or cardioplegia
MIDCAB	• Minimally invasive direct coronary artery bypass surgery • May also be referred to as minimally invasive direct vision coronary surgery • Sometimes called reduced or limited access cardiac surgery • Usually involves beating heart surgery • May refer to mini-thoracotomy approach or median sternotomy • Rarely refers to video-assisted surgery or heart port	Heart port	• Thoracoscopic procedure • No direct visualization of the heart • Three small incisions made • Sometimes referred to as port access • Often used for closure of atrial septal defects in children
		Minimally invasive valvular surgery	• Avoids use of median sternotomy • At present, length of stay only marginally decreased • Small incisions rather than full sternotomy used

---

developments pervade the cardiac arena, the treatment options for coronary artery disease continue to increase and the decision as to the most suitable procedure for the patient becomes more complex. The relative advantages and disadvantages of these newer cardiac surgical procedures will now be discussed.

MINIMALLY INVASIVE DIRECT CORONARY ARTERY BYPASS SURGERY

The MIDCAB procedure is an accepted, more recent revascularization technique, although it is not without its critics and continues to be veiled in some controversy (Treasure 1997). The procedure has been suggested as beneficial in the following areas. It offers selected patients a less invasive surgical approach, milder pericardial adhesions, fewer difficulties with mobilization, improved healing of the incision site, faster rehabilitation and improved cosmetic appearance of the wound (Mizell et al 1997). However, research must continue to be ongoing. Not least, some centres have reported cost savings relating to MIDCAB work versus traditional CABG surgery. The

demerits of the MIDCAB operation are poorer visualization of the operative area, technically the procedure is more demanding and the long-term results have yet to be scrutinized. Another disadvantage is that most usually, only two coronary arteries may be bypassed using this technique.

From a patient perspective, the immediate benefits of MIDCAB are clear. Mortality and morbidity are reduced (Robinson et al 1995), early postoperative recovery is enhanced (Vitello-Cicciu et al 1998) and hospitalization time is reduced (Westaby 1995). For many patients, the appeal of earlier return to work and fewer neuropsychological effects prompts them to opt for this procedure, if they meet the appropriate patient selection criteria. Arguably, the greatest benefits are those gained by avoiding the pernicious effects of cardiopulmonary bypass. Due to the elimination of extracorporeal support, reduced heparinization and no aortic crossclamping, the incidence of myocardial infarction, cerebrovascular accident, respiratory and renal failure and bleeding are all reduced (Benetti et al 1991).

As a consequence, transfusion of blood products, infusions of inotropic agents and the length of time ventilated, intubated and spent in a critical care environment are all reduced. Treasure (1997) suggests that if the need for blood transfusion is completely eliminated, the likelihood of other systems functioning better is increased.

Further advantages are afforded in the reduced incidence of post-pump/postcardiotomy delirium. The use of the cardiopulmonary bypass machine is unfortunately associated with a significant risk of brain injury (Wilcock et al 1997). While only 2% of patients suffer a CVA, a much larger group will suffer neuropsychological damage. This is most usually a diffuse encephalopathy of which the aetiology is uncertain; global hypoperfusion or micro-embolism during the procedure are the most likely culprits. The presentation of neuropsychological damage following cardiac surgery can vary from mild irritability or slight confusion to a violent psychosis.

From a nursing perspective, the dependency of patients with post-pump delirium can be substantial, requiring significant extra resources in nursing time. From the patient's or a relative's/carer's point of view, experiencing or witnessing symptoms such as confusion, poor memory, mood swings, impaired cognitive ability, visual disturbances or acute paranoia can be extremely distressing. Any measures to reduce the cerebral abnormalities, therefore, are likely to be welcomed by nurses, patients and relatives/carers alike.

The two main sources of the aforementioned emboli are the cardiopulmonary bypass circuit and the aorta. Within the CPB circuit emboli are formed when blood comes into contact with a foreign surface, such as the tubing, oxygenator and the heat exchanger. This activates platelets and the intrinsic blood coagulation pathway, leading to the formation of platelet aggregation and thrombus emboli respectively. The second common source of emboli is atheroma dislodged from the ascending aorta during aortic cannulation, cross-clamping and unclamping (Wilcock et al 1997). As neither cardiopulmonary bypass nor aortic cross-clamping is required for the MIDCAB procedure, emboli formation in this way should be eliminated and therefore the incidence of neuropsychological deficit as well as CVA should be significantly reduced. A note of caution is the inability to perform complete revascularization and the long-term consequences of this have yet to be realised.

Patient selection for MIDCAB

Essentially, the criteria for selecting patients for the MIDCAB procedure are largely dependent on the institution in which they are treated. The patient's risk profile is a key feature. Most institutions would consider the following.

- Number and territory of blocked arteries
- Co-morbidities
- Risk stratification (i.e. Parsonnet's Predicted Operative Mortality Scale)
- General health status
- Surgeon's preference
- Patient preference

A significant calcified aorta is considered by many surgeons as a good indication for MIDCAB, to reduce the incidence of embolic events.

Some patients who are unsuitable for traditional revascularization techniques and in whom interventional cardiological procedures are not feasible may be considered for MIDCAB surgery (Mizell et al 1997). These may include elderly patients (older than 70 years), patients with acute or end-stage renal failure requiring renal replacement therapy, patients with chronic airways limitation, other systems failure or even patients with a treatable carcinoma (Benetti et al 1991, Buffolo et al 1996, Calafiore et al 1996). Patients requiring re-operation who are of advanced years may be more readily considered for the MIDCAB procedure than for traditional revascularization. As the current trend for re-operations and an increasingly elderly cardiac surgical population is likely to continue, the impact and value of MIDCAB and beating heart surgery cannot be overstated (Foster et al 1984, Hannan et al 1990). Several UK centres are also undertaking combined procedures (MIDCAB with PTCA).

Patients who are excluded from minimally invasive and beating heart programmes are those with disease of the left main stem and patients with valvular heart disease concomitant with coronary artery disease (Buffolo et al 1996). At present, the ability to perform safe and timely surgery in this group, without the use of cardiopulmonary bypass, is still not available.

Care needs of MIDCAB patients

Both the peri-operative and postoperative care needs of patients have been revolutionized with the introduction of MIDCAB surgery. Historically, a cardiac intensive care unit bed had been an absolute prerequisite for patients undergoing cardiac surgery. Further to this, routine patients had frequently required intubation for perhaps 8–10 hours and hospitalization for up to 7 days. In recent years this has been changing (see above) but now the MIDCAB patient can be extubated even earlier, in the operating room or within 3 hours of surgery (Vitello-Cicciu et al 1998). They rarely require full cardiac intensive care facilities and they may be discharged home as early as the second or third postoperative day. For many patients, these advantages alone present a compelling argument for continued studies into minimally invasive cardiac surgery. Some UK centres provide comprehensive cardiac surgical outreach services for patients discharged from the third postoperative day (e.g. the University Hospitals of Leicester NHS Trust). This is likely to be an expanding area in the future, as the focus of inpatient to outpatient care continues to subtly change.

The management and care of MIDCAB and beating heart patients are relatively straightforward and simple, certainly in terms of respiratory, critical care, fluid and electrolyte and neurological management. The whole process of recovery is accelerated such that a 'routine' beating heart or MIDCAB patient may be out of bed and eating on the evening of surgery and be free of every line, tube, cannula and drain and be ambulant on day 1 postoperatively. The ability to expedite a patient's progress has been further enhanced by the introduction and development of ICPs, cardiac surgical HDUs and, not least, the expertise of cardiac and critical care practitioners, both medical and nursing.

From a psychological perspective, the negative effects of a prolonged period in an ICU can be avoided and several UK cardiac centres report successfully 'fast tracking' patients to high-dependency areas or even directly back to cardiac surgical wards. Patients selected for beating heart or MIDCAB procedures may be suitable for same-day admission programmes, allowing them to be admitted to hospital only 4–5 hours prior to their operation. These patients would have received pre-operative education and information, together with all routine investigations on an outpatient basis a week or two before surgery. Thus it may be that a patient who can access a same-day admission programme, who has beating heart surgery, an unremarkable postoperative recovery and who can be discharged home with outreach facilities could be in hospital for only 72 hours.

THE LAST PROCEDURE

Although Kolessov originally pioneered the LAST technique in 1967, it has only recently been revisited as a revascularization option for patients with coronary artery disease. Since 1994, some surgeons have selected the LAST procedure as the operation of choice for patients requiring single bypass grafting.

In this procedure, the left internal thoracic (mammary) artery (LIMA) is grafted to the left anterior descending artery (LAD) via a left anterior small thoracotomy. As with MIDCAB, the LAST procedure is performed on the beating heart without the use of cardiopulmonary bypass. Rather than the usual median sternotomy, a small (5–10 cm) incision is made in the anterior portion of the fourth or fifth intercostal space.

According to Weinschelbaum et al (1998a), the primary indications for the LAST operation are:

- total occlusion of a branch of the LAD coronary artery, not suitable for PTCA
- severe obstruction of a LAD unsuitable for stenting
- presence of multiple risk factors precluding conventional CABG with cardiopulmonary bypass
- re-operation for a single bypass graft to the LAD
- combined strategy in two or three vessel disease with MIDCAB to the LAD and PTCA to the other vessels
- LIMA to LAD grafting in patients undergoing valve procedures (two simultaneous mini-thoracotomies with cardiopulmonary bypass).

While the LAD is the primary vessel grafted via a small anterior thoracotomy, some surgeons have reported approaching the right coronary artery in the same manner (Cohen & Glenville 1997). Other authors have demonstrated that a variety of conduits can be used for this procedure including the gastro-epiploic artery and the inferior epigastric artery, as well as radial arteries (Acar et al 1992, Buche et al 1992, Suma et al 1993). Suma and associates (1995) believe that the LAST procedure is also valuable for coronary artery redo operations, to avoid injury to the patent old graft and the myocardium, at risk from sternal re-entry.

Although the LAST procedure appeared a promising technique, some surgeons have been disappointed with results. Graft failure seems the primary concern, which (like most of the newer minimally invasive procedures) may be related to the steep learning curve involved with this operation. Calafiore et al (1996) have still asserted that for patients with single LAD disease, the LAST procedure is a good operation which provides acceptable results. Some surgeons believe that many of the early failures can be attributed to technical flaws that were and will be overcome with experience (Weinschelbaum et al 1998a). Again, as knowledge, skill, expertise and instrumentation continue to improve in this area, the results too should be more encouraging.

MINIMALLY INVASIVE VALVE OPERATIONS

Minimally invasive procedures are now extending into all areas of cardiac surgery, including valve operations. Currently the clinical experience and consequently the literature are limited for this procedure, although Cosgrove et al (1998), Mohr et al (1998) and Weinschelbaum et al (1998b) have all presented some encouraging results. The optimum incision site remains an area of debate with some surgeons using an 8 cm parasternal incision over the third and fourth costal cartilages, some preferring a mini-sternotomy extended into the fourth interspace on the right, with yet others opting for the port access endovascular cardiopulmonary bypass system (EndoCPB, Heartport Inc, Redwood City, CA). There are clearly real and potential advantages and disadvantages associated with each.

The port access system is a closed endovascular system that allows for cardioplegic arrest, aortic crossclamping and decompression. The latter is the venting of blood from the left side of the heart and draining it back to the CPB machine under low-grade suction, utilizing an overflow cannula (Schwartz et al 1996, Stevens et al 1996). This video-assisted technique enables mitral valve replacement and complex repair through a right lateral mini-thoracotomy with an incision site of usually less than 4 cm. Valve repair operations are possible due to the three-dimensional view produced by the stereoscope that provides clear visualization of all the relevant valve structures. However, some serious complications have been reported with this approach, most notably aortic dissections (Mohr et al 1998, Reitz 1997).

The parasternal incision is beneficial in that the small incision site causes less peri-operative and post-operative bleeding. In addition, fewer respiratory complications are experienced and hence an early extubation time is achieved, due to less discomfort from the smaller wound (Cosgrove et al 1998). Cosgrove et al further suggest that this approach is advantageous in as much as the pericardium is not opened over the left ventricular outflow tract, making re-operation safer and easier. Conversely, critics of this incision believe that the negative features of possible instability of the anterior part of the chest wall, the higher incidence of bradycardias and arrhythmias postoperatively (due to the proximity to the sino-atrial node) and the 'sacrifice' of an internal thoracic (mammary) artery are too great. The use of mini-sternotomy enables preservation of the internal thoracic artery, reduces postoperative arrhythmias, yet maintains many of the benefits of a small incision.

Another reported problem is postoperative confusion. According to Baldwin (1998), the incidence of neurological complications associated with this operation is considerable and well documented on the Internet. Unlike beating heart or MIDCAB procedures, aortic crossclamping and cardiopulmonary bypass are not eliminated with this technique, so one may advocate that the only discernible benefits of minimally invasive valve surgery are those associated with the avoidance of a full sternotomy.

While some authors argue that minimally invasive valvular surgery is a useful procedure which is effective in reducing surgical trauma and cost, it should be noted that patients requiring re-operations, those in New York Heart Association (NYHA) class IV and patients with severe left ventricular dysfunction have a higher hospital mortality (Cosgrove et al 1998, Weinschelbaum et al 1998b).

VENTRICULAR SEPTAL DEFECT CLOSURE USING MINIMALLY INVASIVE SURGICAL TECHNIQUES

Lin and colleagues (1998), among others, have reported successfully performing ventricular septal defect (VSD) closure using minimally invasive cardiac techniques in paediatric cases. Lin et al's experience demonstrated that the closure of VSDs could be undertaken safely using video-assisted endoscopic techniques under femoral–femoral cardiopulmonary bypass. As with other minimally invasive procedures, reduced discomfort, excellent cosmetic healing, reduced complications and quick functional recuperation were the attractive features of the procedure, again allowing for early discharge. Reduced drainage in the first 24 hours following surgery and the avoidance of a sternotomy are particularly desirable benefits for paediatric patients.

COST

In today's health-care climate, cost issues are a real and vital consideration. Safe, effective alternatives to traditional myocardial revascularization with economic benefits are constantly being sought. Indeed, the development of beating heart and minimally invasive programmes in South America was entirely cost driven (Benetti et al 1991, Buffolo et al 1996).

Cost containment is achieved through:

- reduced operating theatre time
- reduced critical care (ICU) time
- reduced hospitalization

- reduced use of disposables (cannulae, oxygenators, cardioplegic sets, etc.)
- less use of blood products
- less pharmacology (after Westaby 1991, 1995).

The treatment modalities available for coronary artery disease are numerous and include not only surgical options but also a growing number of interventional cardiological procedures. The risk/benefit/cost equation of each procedure should be calculated so that the most appropriate treatment can be offered to each patient at the lowest cost.

INSTRUMENTATION

As minimally invasive and beating heart surgery has developed, so too has the necessary instrumentation. Numerous apparatus, devices and appliances have been produced for virtually each stage of the procedure. These include:

- coronary stabilization devices
- percutaneous femoral–femoral bypass
- Hemopump® device (dlp, a division of Medtronic, Grand Rapids, MI)
- new myocardial protection techniques (intracoronary shunts)
- suckers and blowers to improve visualization of the operative field
- visual enhancement systems.

Blowers that instil air to disperse blood from the operative field are essential in improving visualization. These instruments are improving continually, enabling safer, quicker operations with fewer complications.

Coronary stabilization devices

The development of mechanical immobilization devices to locally reduce coronary motion has been a significant step in recent beating heart surgery programmes. Numerous devices have appeared on the market which allow the surgeon to perform microsurgery without contending with the normal beating heart movement. The aim of the device is to provide an area of akinisia without significantly affecting normal physiology. Coronary stabilization devices enable the surgeon to operate via a conventional sternotomy while providing good visualization, effective vessel stabilization and easy access to arteries. The Octopus Tissue Stabilizer and the CTS Access Ultima System are two stabilization devices in frequent use currently in the UK.

Visual enhancement systems

More recent devices which gently blow blood away from the target site to allow better anastomotic visualization, such as the Visu-Flow (Research Medical, Midvale, UT), are improving performance within the minimally invasive cardiac field.

ANAESTHETIC CONSIDERATIONS OF OFF-PUMP SURGERY

Off-pump cardiac surgery presents challenges not only for cardiac surgeons and cardiac nurses but also for cardiac anesthetists. The patient's haemodynamic status may change by manipulation of the heart to access the anastomosis site and by the movement of stabilizing devices. Anaesthetic interventions such as the administration of low-dose inotropes, infusions and intravenous fluids can correct these difficulties (Nierich et al 1999).

The use of high thoracic epidural anesthesia (TEA) has allowed many centres to extubate patients earlier, compared with standard opioid anaesthetics, with few reported complications. Advances in pharmacology together with refinements in anaesthesia are likely to contribute to the use and development of off-pump surgery. According to Nierich (1999), anaesthetic management during off-pump surgery for CABG is focused on the following.

- Providing a maximum of cardiac protection, by the use of a cardiac protective anaesthetic technique
- Providing safe induction and maintenance of general anesthesia
- Maintaining haemodynamic stability through the use of adequate monitoring and pharmacological support
- Enabling surgical exposure within the limits of haemodynamic and cardiac stability
- Enabling early postoperative recovery and mobility
- Providing excellent postoperative analgesia (after Nierich 1999)

The use of TEA is growing in popularity among cardiac anesthetists (Nierich 1999). The beneficial cardiac effects of TEA are:

- reduction of myocardial oxygen consumption (by reducing respiratory and cardiac effort)
- vasodilatation of epicardial coronary arteries
- vasodilatation of internal thoracic arteries
- increase of collateral blood flow during myocardial ischaemia.

There remains some controversy with respect to the significance of early extubation post cardiac surgery. Most studies seem to suggest that there is no positive effect on cognitive function with early extubation, although some believe that it has no deleterious effects either and can facilitate patient care in the postoperative period (Dumas et al 1999).

MINIMALLY INVASIVE SAPHENOUS VEIN HARVESTING

Developments and technology have not only progressed to enable minimally invasive procedures within the sternum, but 'keyhole' surgery as a whole has developed by leaps and bounds in virtually every surgical sphere. It is not surprising, therefore, that newer techniques have emerged to enable surgeons to remove the entire saphenous vein through two small incisions. De Laria et al (1981) comment that harvesting the entire saphenous vein leaves the patient with the longest incision used for any operation. This is not without significance when considering leg wound complications, postoperative pain and discomfort and when attempting to provide early rehabilitation and early discharge programmes. Although major leg wound infections are thankfully low (1–2%), minor complications such as incisional pain, limb swelling and delayed healing are common (Utley et al 1989).

Nurses caring for patients post CABG surgery will often find that leg wound pain or oozing leg wounds are a more frequent problem than sternal infections or discomfort. Certain patients may have an elevated risk for developing leg wound problems. These include diabetic and obese patients, as well as patients on steroid medication and those with peripheral vascular disease. Finding methods to limit these risks and to reduce complications is a welcome development for both patients and clinicians.

During the video-endoscopic vein harvesting procedure the surgeon inserts endoscopic surgical instruments, including a miniature camera, through a small incision in order to remove the vein. The surgeon is then able to view the inside of the leg on a television monitor during the surgery, without having to expose the full length of the vein. Data provided by Allen (1998) demonstrated a statistically significant drop in leg wound complications with endoscopic as opposed to traditional vein harvesting (19% with the latter, 4% with the former). As numerous manufacturers continue to design new systems for endoscopic vein harvesting, it is a technique that is likely to increase and develop further, especially as early results seem promising.

COMPUTER-ASSISTED CARDIAC SURGERY

Looking to the future, it seems clear that new systems and new technologies will continue to influence the progression of cardiac surgical procedures. The latest in this line of innovative equipment are computer-assisted devices which enable the surgeon to sit at a console which affords a clear three-dimensional view of the surgical field. By operating the control levers, the surgeon's movements are transmitted to the instruments within the heart (Linden 1999). Carpentier et al (1999) have described their experience of using this computer-assisted system for both coronary artery surgery and valve repair. Patients undergoing valve repair had one 5 cm incision, while those for coronary artery surgery received three 1 cm ports. Early indications seem to suggest that patients progress well (all patients in Carpentier's study were discharged home with no significant co-morbidities), although as with most of the other more recent procedures, the long-term results will need to be evaluated.

CONSENT

The issue of obtaining informed consent remains a topical and pertinent one. Clinical governance, national directives and guidelines and the trust's own policies encourage the building of a partnership between health-care professionals and patients. An important aspect of this partnership is the obtaining of informed consent. Increasingly, there is an expectation that clinicians should provide patients with appropriate, current information and literature and relevant details relating to the risks and benefits of the procedure. It is therefore incumbent on clinicians to explain to patients selected as suitable for minimally invasive cardiac operations the specific risks and benefits and also any alternative treatment options. This should include the implications of treatment including pre-, peri- and postoperative effects and consequences. Information should also include the benefits and risks of non-intervention. Some suggest that each surgeon should be able to provide patients with their own mortality figures related to each procedure.

CONCLUSION

The proliferation of various minimally invasive procedures in recent years has urged many surgeons to consider their use (Jansen et al 1998, Subramanian et al 1997, Weinschelbaum et al 1998a). However, indiscriminate use of these techniques remains inadvisable, until the long-term statistics can be evaluated. Indeed, the old surgical maxim 'big mistakes through little holes' should always be borne in mind. In 1998 the Society of Thoracic Surgeons/American Association for Thoracic Surgery's Committee on New Technology produced a policy statement regarding minimally invasive coronary artery bypass surgery. This statement suggested that the newer technologies and hybrid procedures were likely to continue and advised that as this occurs, 'It is incumbent on practitioners to appropriately educate themselves as well as to document and disseminate new information'. The same committee further produced *Course guidelines for minimally invasive cardiac surgery* which provided advice concerning programme cost and funding, programme content, faculty and director and credentialling. The very publication of these papers demonstrates some concern that these more recent techniques should be carefully monitored and evaluated. The considerable benefits should be judiciously weighed against the results over time, so that the long-term patency of the grafts is not sacrificed for a shorter, fashionable operation. The gold standard of outcomes remains CABG on bypass.

Buffolo et al (1996) presented results that suggest that all types of arterial conduits may be used for coronary artery bypass on the beating heart and provided data with an acceptable mortality of 2.5%. They further suggest that the results demonstrate that serious complications were lower than those in patients undergoing CABG with cardiopulmonary bypass and that the patency rate was not discernibly different. In the future, more combined procedures such as MIDCAB with PTCA or intracoronary artery stenting are likely to be performed. Dual-modality options are likely to become available for patients with improved operative techniques, advanced PTCA technology and increased quality of radiological services.

As the landscape of cardiac surgery continues to change and various new surgical treatment modalities are developed for myocardial revascularization, the chief considerations should be the quality of the procedure, the risks of the procedure and the probable long-term benefits. Undoubtedly, the skill and the experience of the operator together with the age and clinical condition of the patient will also be determining factors in the type of operation selected. Although there are likely to remain sceptics of the minimally invasive cardiac operation, it is perhaps a measure of its value that more than 40 years after it was first attempted, surgeons the world over continue to try to perfect this technique. Many cardiac surgeons, both in the United Kingdom and abroad, feel that greater research in the form of randomized, prospective studies is needed to further advocate this approach.

As with any new, technically complex procedure, the learning curve for these operations needs consideration. The pre-, peri- and postoperative management of patients is different for minimally invasive and beating heart cases, often requiring additional skills from the health-care professionals caring for them. While many clinicians will embrace these changes and learn the new skills, others may not have the desire, the opportunity or the ability to alter their current practice. What is certain is that techniques designed to reduce both the physiological and psychological trauma to patients and to improve vessel access and visualization for the surgeon will continue to influence the cardiac surgical field.

APPENDIX: EXTUBATION ALGORITHM (after Maxam-Moore & Goedecke 1996)

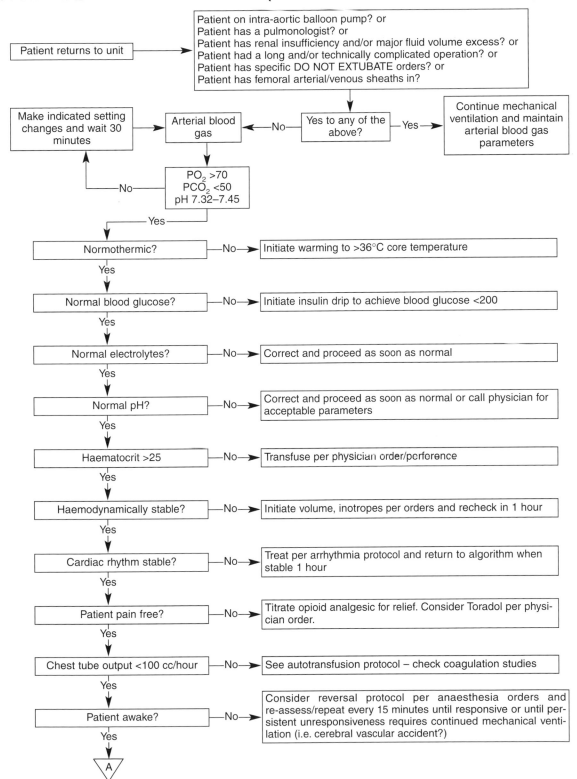

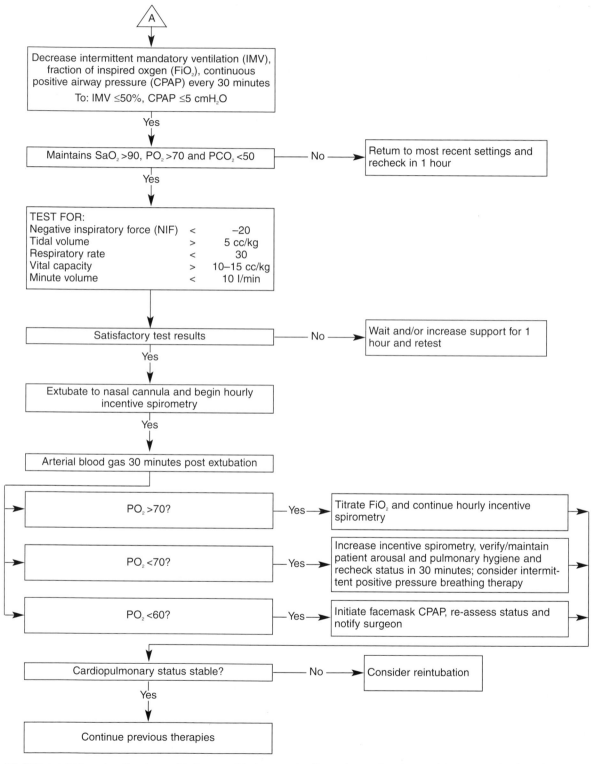

NB: This extubation algorithm is provided as a guide to promote discussion and an appropriate progression in patient care. Terminology and measurement criteria will differ between units as the multidisciplinary team plan care together.

REFERENCES

Acar C, Jebara VA, Portoghese M et al 1992 Revival of the radial artery for coronary artery bypass grafting. Annals of Thoracic Surgery 54(4): 652–659

Acuff TE, Landreneau RJ, Griffiths BP, Mack MJ 1996 Minimally invasive coronary artery bypass grafting. Annals of Thoracic Surgery 61(1): 135–137

Allen KB 1998 Endoscopic versus traditional saphenous vein harvesting: a prospective randomized trial. Presented at the 34th Annual Meeting of the Society of Thoracic Surgeons Meeting, New Orleans, January 24–28

Anderson J, O'Brien M 1995 Challenge for the future; the nurse's role in weaning patients from mechanical ventilation. Intensive and Critical Care Nursing 1: 2–5

Aps C 1995 Fast tracking in cardiac surgery. British Journal of Hospital Medicine 54(4): 139–142

Aps C, Hutter JA, Williams BT 1986 Anaesthetic management and post operative care of cardiac surgical patients in a general recovery ward. Anaesthesia 41(5): 533–537

Association of Anaesthetists 1991 The high-dependency unit – acute care in the future? AAGBI, London

Baldwin J 1998 Surgery for acquired heart disease: editorial re minimally invasive port-access mitral valve surgery. Journal of Thoracic and Cardiovascular Surgery 115(3): 563–564

Batey MV, Lewis FM 1982 Clarifying autonomy and accountability in nursing service. Part 1. Journal of Nursing Administration 12(9): 13–18

Benetti FJ, Naselli G, Wood M, Geffner L 1991 Direct myocardial revascularisation without extracorporeal circulation. Experience in 700 patients. Chest 100(2): 312–316

BHF 2000 The British Heart Foundation coronary heart disease statistics database: annual compendium. British Heart Foundation, London

Borst C, Santamore WP, Smedira NG, Bradee JJ 1997 Minimally invasive coronary artery bypass grafting: on the beating heart and via limited access. Annals of Thoracic Surgery 63(6 suppl): S1–S5

Bowler S, Mallik M 1998 Role extension or expansion: a qualitative investigation of the perceptions of senior medical and nursing staff in an adult intensive care unit. Intensive and Critical Care Nursing 14(1): 11–20

Brooks N 2000 Quality of life and the high-dependency unit. Intensive and Critical Care Nursing 16: 18–32

Buche M, Schoevaerdts JC, Louagie Y et al 1992 Use of the inferior epigastric artery for coronary bypass. Journal of Thoracic and Cardiovascular Surgery 103(4): 665–670

Buffolo E, De Andrade CS, Branco JN, Teles CA, Aguiar LF, Gomes WJ 1996 Coronary artery bypass grafting without cardiopulmonary bypass. Annals of Thoracic Surgery 61(1): 63–66

Butler J, Rocker GM, Westaby S 1993 Inflammatory response to cardiopulmonary bypass. Annals of Thoracic Surgery 55(2): 552–559

Calafiore AM, Giammarco GD, Teodori G et al 1996 Left anterior descending coronary artery grafting via left anterior small thoracotomy without cardiopulmonary bypass. Annals of Thoracic Surgery 61(6): 1658–1663

Calafiore AM, Giammarco GD, Teodori G et al 1998 Surgery for acquired heart disease: midterm results after minimally invasive coronary surgery. Journal of Thoracic and Cardiovascular Surgery 115(4): 763–771

Calman KC 1993 Hospital doctors: training for the future. Report of the Working Group on Specialist Medical Training (the Calman Report). Department of Health, London

Carpentier A, Loulmet D, Aupede B et al 1999 Computer assisted cardiac surgery. Lancet 353: 379–380

Cheng DCH, Carroll J, David T et al 1996 Early tracheal extubation after coronary artery bypass graft surgery reduces costs and improves resource use. A prospective randomized controlled trial. Anaesthesiology 85(6): 1300–1310

Chong JL, Pillai R, Fisher A, Grebenik C, Sinclair M, Westaby S 1992 Cardiac surgery moving away from intensive care. British Heart Journal 68(4): 430–433

Cohen A, Glenville B 1997 Keyhole coronary bypass surgery. British Journal of Hospital Medicine 57(7): 326–329

Cosgrove DM 3rd, Sabik JF, Navia JL 1998 Minimally invasive valve operations. Annals of Thoracic Surgery 65(6): 1535–1538

Davies N 1997 Nurse-initiated extubation following cardiac surgery. Intensive and Critical Care Nursing 13(1): 77–79

De Laria GA, Hunter JA, Goldin MD, Serry C, Javid H, Najafi H 1981 Leg wound complications associated with coronary revascularisation. Journal of Thoracic and Cardiovascular Surgery 81(3): 403–407

Department of Health 1992 The patient's charter. HMSO, London

Department of Health 1996 The patient's charter and you: a charter for England. Department of Health, London

Dumas A, Dupuis GH, Searle N, Cartier R 1999 Early versus late extubation after coronary artery bypass grafting: effects on cognitive function. Journal of Cardiothoracic and Vascular Anaesthesia 13(2): 130–135

Edbrooke DL 1996 High dependency – so much promise, so little progress. Care of the Critically Ill 12(3): 80–81

Edmunds LH Jr 1995 Why cardiopulmonary bypass makes patients sick: strategies to control the blood–synthetic surface interface. Advances in Cardiac Surgery 6: 131–167

Edwards D, Hess L 1996 Aggressive weaning in cardiac surgical patients. Dimensions of Critical Care Nursing 15(4): 181–186

Elmquist L 1992 Decision making for extubation of the post anaesthetic patient. Critical Care Nurse Quarterly 15(1): 82–86

Foster ED, Fisher LD, Kaiser GC, Myers WO 1984 Comparison of operative mortality and morbidity for initial and repeat coronary artery bypass grafting: the Coronary Artery Surgery Study (CASS) Registry Experience. Annals of Thoracic Surgery 38(6): 563–570

Giuffre M, Heidenreich T, Pruitt L 1994 Rewarming cardiac surgery patients: radiant heat versus forced warm air. Nursing Research 43(3): 174–178

Hancock H 1996 The complexity of pain assessment and management in the first 24 hours post cardiac surgery: implications for nurses. Intensive and Critical Care Nursing 12(5): 295–302

Hannan EL, Kilburn H Jr, O'Donnell JF, Lukacik G, Shields EP 1990 Adult open heart surgery in New York State. An analysis of risk factors and hospital mortality rates. Journal of the American Medical Association 264(21): 2768–2774

Higgins TL 1992 Early endotracheal extubation is preferable to late extubation in patients following coronary artery surgery. Journal of Cardiothoracic and Vascular Anaesthesia 6(4): 488–493

Jansen EW, Borst C, Lahpor JR 1998 Coronary artery bypass grafting without cardiopulmonary bypass using the Octopus method: results in the first one hundred patients. Journal of Thoracic and Cardiovascular Surgery 116(1): 60–67

Kolessov VI 1967 Mammary artery–coronary artery anastomosis as method of treatment for angina pectoris. Journal of Thoracic and Cardiovascular Surgery 54(4): 535–544

Leslie K, Sessler DI 1998 The implications of hypothermia for early tracheal extubation following cardiac surgery. Journal of Cardiothoracic and Vascular Anaesthesia 12 (6 suppl 2): 30–34

Lin P, Chang CH, Chu JJ 1998 Minimally invasive cardiac surgical techniques in the closure of ventricular septal defect: an alternative approach. Annals of Thoracic Surgery 65(1): 165–169

Linden B 1999 Computer assisted cardiac surgery. Cardiac Care Update 6(3): 6

Maresch KJ 1997 Propofol: improving patient outcome. Dimensions of Critical Care Nursing 16(2): 58–60

Maxam-Moore VA, Goedecke RS 1996 The development of an early extubation algorithm for patients after cardiac surgery. Heart and Lung 25(1): 61–68

McAlpine L 1997 The left anterior small thoracotomy technique: a new approach for coronary artery bypass grafting. Critical Care Nurse 17(5): 40–45

Mizell J, Maglish B, Matheny R 1997 Minimally invasive direct coronary artery bypass graft surgery: introduction for critical care nurses. Critical Care Nurse 17(3): 46–55

Mohr FW, Falk V, Diegeler A, Walther T, Van Son JA, Autschbach R 1998 Minimally invasive port-access mitral valve surgery. Journal of Thoracic and Cardiovascular Surgery 115(3): 567–574

Murray G, Porcheron R, Hilario J, Roschlau W 1954 Anastomosis of a systemic artery to the coronary. Canadian Medical Association Journal 71: 594–597

Nierich AP 1999 Anaesthesia in beating heart CABG surgery. Medtronic, Grand Rapids, MI, pp. 46–49

Nierich AP, Diephuis J, Jansen EW et al 1999 Embracing the heart: perioperative management of patients undergoing off-pump coronary artery bypass grafting using the Octopus tissue stabilizer. Journal of Cardiothoracic and Vascular Anaesthesia 13(2): 123–129

Parsonnet V, Dean D, Bernstein AD 1989 A method of uniform stratification of risk for evaluating the results of surgery in acquired adult heart disease. Circulation 79 (suppl 1): 3–12

Poloniecki J, Valencia O, Littlejohns P 1998 Cumulative risk adjusted mortality chart for detecting changes in death rate: observational study of heart surgery. British Medical Journal 316: 1697–1700

Quasha AL, Loeber N, Feeley TW, Ullyot DJ, Roizen MF 1980 Postoperative respiratory care: a controlled trial of early and late extubation following coronary artery bypass grafting. Anaesthesiology 52(2): 135–141

Reitz B 1997 Minimally invasive cardiac surgery. Presentation at the World Congress on Minimally Invasive Cardiac Surgery, Paris, May

Roach GW, Kanchuger M, Mangano CM 1996 Adverse cerebral outcomes after coronary bypass surgery. New England Journal of Medicine 335(25): 1857–1863

Robinson MC, Gross DR, Zeman W, Stedje-Larsen E 1995 Minimally invasive coronary artery bypass grafting: a new method using an anterior mediastinotomy. Journal of Cardiac Surgery 10(5): 529–536

Roques F, Nashef SA, Michel P et al 1999 Risk factors and outcome in European cardiac surgery: analysis of the EuroSCORE multinational database of 19 030 patients. European Journal of Cardiothoracic Surgery 15(6): 816–822

Sabiston DC Jr 1974 The coronary circulation. Johns Hopkins Medical Journal 134(6): 314–329

Schwartz DS, Ribakove GH, Grossi EA 1996 Minimally invasive cardiopulmonary bypass with cardioplegic arrest: a closed chest technique with equivalent myocardial protection. Journal of Thoracic and Cardiovascular Surgery 111(3): 556–566

Seifert PC 1998 Advances in myocardial protection. Journal of Cardiovascular Nursing 12(3): 29–38

Sherry KM 1997 The use of propofol for ICU sedation in patients following cardiac surgery. British Journal of Intensive Care 7(3): 91–94

Siliciano D 1992 Early extubation is not preferable to late extubation in patients undergoing coronary artery bypass surgery. Journal of Cardiothoracic and Vascular Anaesthesia 6(4): 494–498

Stevens JH, Burdon TA, Peters WS 1996 Port access coronary artery bypass grafting. A proposed surgical method. Journal of Thoracic and Cardiovascular Surgery 111(3): 567–573

Subramanian VA, McCabe JC, Geller CM 1997 Minimally invasive direct coronary artery bypass grafting: two year clinical experience. Annals of Thoracic Surgery 64(6): 1648–1653

Suma H, Wanibuchi Y, Terada Y, Fukuda S, Takayama T, Fututa S 1993 The right gastroepiploic artery graft: clinical and angiographic mid term results in 200 patients. Journal of Thoracic and Cardiovascular Surgery 105(4): 615–622

Suma H, Kigawa I, Horii T, Tanaka J, Fukuda S, Wanibuchi Y 1995 Coronary artery reoperation through the left thoracotomy with hypothermic circulatory arrest. Annals of Thoracic Surgery 60: 1063–1066

Treasure T 1997 Minimal access surgery. Heart 77: 304–306

Tuman KJ, McCarthy RJ, March RJ, Najafi H, Ivankovich AD 1992 Morbidity and duration of ICU stay after cardiac surgery. A model for preoperative risk assessment. Chest 102(1): 36–44

UKCC 1992 The scope of professional practice. UKCC, London

Utley JR, Thomason ME, Wallace DJ et al 1989 Preoperative correlates of impaired wound healing after saphenous vein excision. Journal of Thoracic and Cardiovascular Surgery 98(1): 147–149

Verrier ED, Wright IH, Cochran RP, Spiess BD 1995 Changes in the cardiovascular surgical approach to achieve early extubation. Journal of Cardiothoracic and Vascular Anaesthesia 9(5) (suppl 1): 10–15

Vitello-Cicciu J, Fitzgerald C, Whalen D 1998 On the horizon: minimally invasive cardiac surgery. Journal of Cardiovascular Nursing 12(3): 1–16

Weinschelbaum E, Rodriguez C, Cabello ML et al 1998a Left anterior descending coronary artery bypass grafting through minimal thoracotomy. Annals of Thoracic Surgery 66(3): 1008–1011

Weinschelbaum E, Stutzbach P, Machain A et al 1998b Valve operations through a minimally invasive approach. Annals of Thoracic Surgery 66(3): 1106–1109

Westaby S 1991 Cutting costs in cardiac surgery. Time to break the mould. Surgery 86: 2040–2055

Westaby S 1995 Coronary surgery without cardiopulmonary bypass. British Heart Journal 73(3): 203–205

Westaby S, Pillai R, Parry DA et al 1993 Does modern cardiac surgery require conventional intensive care? European Journal of Cardiothoracic Surgery 7(6): 313–318

Wilcock D, Cherryman GR, Keal R, Spyt TJ, Jarvis M 1997 Cerebral consequences of cardiopulmonary bypass: demonstration with diffusion weighted, susceptibility and FLAIR magnetic resonance imaging. Protocol. University Department of Radiology, Leicester Royal Infirmary and Department of Radiology and Department of Cardiac Surgery, Leicester General Hospital (unpublished research proposal)

Youhana AY 1995 Warm blood cardioplegia. British Heart Journal 73(3): 206–207

30

Critical pathways: aiming for seamless care

Myrna Scott

The care of patients following cardiac surgery has undergone significant changes in recent years, notably with the advent of new surgical techniques, high-dependency units (HDUs) and early extubation (fast-tracking) programmes. Today during one admission, patient care will be provided at a much faster pace by multidisciplinary teams in four to five distinct units, in addition to other departmental involvement. The over-riding issue has therefore become the need to deliver seamless, co-ordinated and collaborative care in order to meet these changing needs. Delivery of care is also influenced by financial constraints, the pressure from waiting lists and increased consumer awareness and expectations.

As a result, pre-existing models of nursing may not offer the flexibility to address the requirements of current cardiac practice. Managed care, the overall concept behind critical/integrated care pathways, has emerged from the literature as a potential method of organizing multidisciplinary care to meet these changeable demands (Henry & Duffy 1995, Redick et al 1994, Scott 1996). However, it still remains important to explore the utility and effectiveness of this new export from the United States (US) in fully addressing such management and clinical issues before adopting the process.

This chapter is based on a selective review of managed care literature and the findings of my own research, originally completed as part of a Masters degree in nursing at King's College, London (Scott 1996). This action research project implemented and evaluated a managed care programme for cardiac surgical fast-track patients in the intensive care unit (ICU) and has formed the basis for ongoing work and evaluation. The study was undertaken at St Bartholomew's Hospital, London, and the ICU is named with staff permission. The concept of managed care will be explored and clarified and the driving forces behind its introduction in the US and Britain will be discussed.

Much of the literature portrays the introduction of both managed care and critical pathways as a pain-free process. This chapter aims to provide an honest account, highlighted by my own experiences, of the challenges and practicalities of introducing such a new initiative into the clinical area. The focus will be on the difficulties with developing multidisciplinary collaboration, creating the pathway itself, maintaining momentum and auditing. The benefits and disadvantages of practising managed care will also be discussed in relation to recent results from the ICU in the original study and from new literature. More recently, authors have called for published evaluation and appraisal tools for the implementation of critical pathways. The current lack has led to variable forms of evaluation (Johnson & Smith 2000).

The importance of nurse-led innovations which illuminate the implicit work of nursing and the requirement for nursing research which provides the foundation for such work is emphasized throughout. Changes in nurses' roles and practice which were stimulated both by the research innovation and managed care will be examined, together with recommendations for future practice.

CONFUSION OVER CONCEPTS AND DEFINITIONS OF MANAGED CARE?

Terms such as managed care, case or care management and continuing care co-ordination have been used interchangeably in the literature (Girard 1994, Kelly 1992). This is complicated by the use of 'managed care' in the US to refer to the overall managerial and financial insurance system used in many states to provide health care (Gross 1995). However, managed care and case management are the two essential and most commonly used concepts. The two are intrinsically linked, sharing a similar historical background which has led to confusion over definitions and use in practice (Goodwin 1994). Similarly, there are many different names for critical pathways, such as care or structured pathways, care maps, anticipated recovery paths, integrated care pathways (ICPs), multidisciplinary care plans and clinical algorithms or guidelines. To simplify, the terms managed care and critical pathway will be used throughout this chapter.

WHAT IS MANAGED CARE?

Managed care is a system of organizing unit-based care and promoting multidisciplinary communication and co-ordination. This occurs throughout a specific period of illness so that identified clinical outcomes are achieved within a set time frame (Cohen & Cesta 1997, Zander 1990). This adapted definition was used in my own study to foster the ICU philosophies of teamwork yet maintain individual responsibility for care. Unlike case management, managed care enables members of staff with different competencies to use the system and provide consistent levels of care (Zander 1991).

In reviewing the literature, Scully & Nichols (1990) identified certain key managed care characteristics. These included: the identification of at-risk populations, matching of services to need, cost control, advocacy, co-ordination of hospital and community care, problem solving, quality management and multidisciplinary involvement. These principles were adapted to the inpatient acute setting and subsequently developed into a separate nursing care model which was used in the study. This can be incorporated into team, primary or alternative nursing systems to promote advanced practice (Hampton 1993, Micheels et al 1995, Mosher et al 1992, Van Buskirk & Vanderbilt 1995, Zander 1987, 1991).

WHAT IS CASE MANAGEMENT?

Case management is based around an entire stay in hospital rather than one episode of illness in one unit. A single case manager co-ordinates and evaluates care from admission to discharge (Leclair 1991). Case managers can practise as clinical nurse specialists, autonomous unit-based primary nurses or patient services managers (O'Malley 1992, Zander 1988). The model has been criticized for duplicating care and costs by overlapping roles and increasing stress due to large workloads (Jones 1995). However, it has been advocated for the care of complicated, long-term patients, such as chronically ill ventilated patients (Burns et al 1997).

WHAT IS A CRITICAL PATHWAY?

The critical (or integrated care) pathway is the tool of managed care which facilitates delivery and audit of patient care (Figs 30.1–30.3). The pathway, printed on paper or via the computer screen, is used at the bedside to guide multidisciplinary care giving and to enable practitioners to record and evaluate patient problems and outcomes. The critical pathway is a blank template on which the multidisciplinary team have described standardized patterns of care and key interventions by all disciplines, which need to be carried out sequentially for the patient's specific condition. This ensures that care is delivered within a set time frame and expected outcomes are achieved with efficient use of resources (Cohen & Cesta 1997, Del Tongo-Armanasco et al 1989, Mosher et al 1992, Zander 1990). The pathways are based on evidenced-based practice, recent research and bench marking. The latter is a method of comparing current practice processes and outcomes against recognized best practice leaders (Capuano et al 1999). They can also be used as best practice tools for audit and training as they incorporate existing standards and help develop new ones (Roebuck 1998). Pathways utilize key components of the nursing process and are thus easily extrapolated into practice (Girard 1994). The design and development of pathways along with their benefits and disadvantages will be discussed later.

WHAT ARE CRITICAL PATHWAY VARIANCES?

The Care Map (™, owned by the Center for Case Management Inc, South Natick, Massachusetts) was introduced in 1991 as an extension to the original critical pathway. Unlike traditional care plans, it included a patient outcome index with indicators for measuring quality against a time frame (Zander 1992). Today's pathways also contain an inbuilt quality audit to monitor variances (Fig. 30.3).

Variances include patient outcomes, 'critical events' (such as extubation) or care which are not achieved or differ from those expected and ultimately hinder or facilitate a patient's progress along the predicted pathway (Hampton 1993, Zander 1991). Variances are often categorized according to the cause of the problem or improvement: patient or family (e.g. postoperative bleeding), care giver or clinician (e.g. shortage of nurses), hospital, system or community services (e.g. shortage of ward beds) (Zander 1991). Recording of variances on a specific variance sheet in the pathway supplants the traditional nursing kardex. Ideally, variances are recorded as they actually occur along with the action taken to correct the variance and keep the patient on the pathway. Patient outcomes are evaluated continuously during admission until resolution. The practicalities of collecting and auditing these variances will be discussed later.

WHAT FACTORS DROVE THE INTRODUCTION OF MANAGED CARE IN THE UNITED KINGDOM?

As with the majority of innovations in health care, the issue of cost is both a primary driving and controlling force. Case management, first used in the 19th century,

was adopted in the 1960s by American and British community workers to co-ordinate services and resources (Bergen 1992, Jones 1995). It was introduced to the acute sector in the 1980s by American nurse administrators to strategically address spiralling health costs while maintaining quality (Micheels et al 1995, Zander 1988) and to advance professional status and primary nursing (Ethridge & Lamb 1989, Kramer 1990, Zander 1987). Managed care structured the use, cost, quality and effectiveness of health services at the patient–provider level as control shifted to purchasers of care. By 1990 it had been adopted by over 50% of American hospitals (Light 1994) which invested heavily in the race to introduce pathways for many patient groups. However, early enthusiasm dwindled with the realization that managed care was not the panacea for all financial difficulties (Gearner Thompson 1994, Yandell 1995).

In the United Kingdom (UK), managed care was recognized as a means to increase accountability for resources at a clinical level. It has, however, been primarily adopted to address policy issues and cultural changes in health care such as fragmentation of care, primary and consumer-led services (Benton 1995, Cameron 1994, DoH 1989) and evidence-based care (Deighan & Hitch 1995, Fawcett-Hensey 1995, Tingle 1996). In my research study, managed care was promoted as a quality initiative to address problems such as co-ordination of fast tracking. Cost was never a motivating factor or measured, as it was believed that outcome-focused care would ultimately and positively affect expenditure.

REVIEW OF THE LITERATURE ON MANAGED CARE

The literature review is essential to explore the meaning and utility of managed care and to justify its use within the UK health service. The review provided much evidence to support the safe use of managed care but large gaps were identified in the body of knowledge which my own research and more recent studies have addressed.

In my own study the selective review of mainly American literature included general and critical care studies ranging from psychogeriatrics to intensive care. They were divided into two broad categories: anecdotal descriptive studies of the development and qualitative benefits of the system and quantitative studies on outcomes. Managed care and case management were promoted as systems capable of positively influencing many quality indicators. These included: improved communication and co-ordination of resources which reduced lengths of stay (Flynn &

Last / First Name: **Patient, Any**
Hospital Number: **12345678**   Date of Birth: **01/02/34**

Barts and The London NHS

NHS Trust

ITU ADMISSION BOOK NUMBER:		DATE:	__/__/20__		
FIRST HOUR FOLLOWING OPERATION (ITU)			V or n/a	Time Shift	Initials
TRANSFER	• Pre-transfer: check all safety equipment on bed & area & set up morphine. • **Handover from anaesthetist – patient Hx, op, complications, RS & CVS parameters.** • **Pre-transfer check of vital signs, pacing wires, lines & infusions, drains, IABP, name band, ICP pack, notes, CXRs & transfusion form.** • Transfer with anaesthetist, ITU nurse and CTT (cardiothoracic team). • **GRADE OF INTUBATION: 1 / 2 / 3 / 4** • **REVERSAL AGENTS POST-OP: YES/NO (IF No d/w ITU SPR)**	N A N MDT A A/N		
ADMISSION	<u>OUTCOME: WAKING & WEANING ASSESSMENT AT END OF HOUR 1</u>			
Respiratory monitoring	• Attach patient to ventilator: SIMV, pressure support 8 cmH₂O & PEEP 5 cmH₂O (as per weaning algorithm) unless respiratory problem/anaesthetic request. If self-ventilating: use T-Piece/mask & specs (SBH) or mask only (LCH). Report to nurse. • Check & record ventilator settings/alarms, air entry, ET cuff pressure. • Check ABG and SaO₂ & adjust settings using FiO₂ protocol/NIC/SPR. <u>AIMS: VENTILATED PO₂ >10 kPa, PCO₂ 4.5–6 kPa, SaO₂ >95%.</u> <u>EXTUBATED: PO₂ >10 kPa, PCO₂ <7 kPa, SaO₂ >95% (extubation criteria).</u>	A N N		
Cardiac monitoring	• Establish cardiac monitoring, alarms, axilla & peripheral temps, warm using blankets or assess need for Bair Hugger per consultant preference. • Record chest drainage & attach drains to suction (–5 kPa)(SBH) or 30–50 cmH₂O (LCH) / autotransfusion (–10 kPa). • Sit patient at 45° to aid drainage & ventilation, if awake sit bolt upright. • Establish IV access and infusions per prescription. • Establish baseline observations: every 15mins (plus drains) for 1 hour; 30mins for 2 hours according to stability, then hourly. <u>AIMS FOR: HR, Rhythm, K⁺, Pacing, BP, MAP, CVP, LA, PAOP, CI, SVRI, SVO₂ & IABP scripted on fluid chart according to pre- & intra-operative condition.</u>	N D		
HR/Pacing	• Titrate infusions (inc K⁺, Mg²⁺) &/or pacing to achieve HR & rhythm aims. • Care & safety of pacing wires: check & record threshold once per shift.	N		
Colloid	• Assess need for colloid &/or blood/blood products according to: Hb </=8.5g/dl (LCH), overall blood loss (Mr Wood) or </=25% (other consultants), Hb, INR, platelets, perfusion and aims for CVP/LA/PAOP & urine output & review effects.	N		
Vasoactive Infusions	• Titrate inotropes or vasodilators to achieve target BP, MAP, CI, SVRI when CVP/LA/PAOP optimised – review with NIC/CTT if ineffective.	N		
CO Studies	• Perform cardiac calculations (CO measurement protocol) with supervision if required.	N		
IABP	• Check & hourly recording of IABP settings, peripheral perfusion & pedal pulses. • Observe insertion site: change dressing PRN according to Unit protocol.	N		
Drains	<u>OUTCOME:</u> BLEEDING <200mls/hr: if bleeding, report to NIC/CTT, record blood loss volumes as variances & treat according to consultant preferences.	N		
Fluid Management	<u>OUTCOMES: ADEQUATE URINE OUTPUT (>0.5mls/kg/hr)</u> <u>POTASSIUM 4.5–5mmols/l with supplements PRN</u>	N		
Sedation & Pain Control	<u>OUTCOME: CNS INTACT & PAIN FREE/CONTROLLED</u> • Check pupils on admission and hourly until awake. • On waking assess ability to obey commands and move all limbs equally: report any deficits in **endarterectomy** patients immediately to NIC & CTT. • Commence sedation/pain score on admission (SBH). • **Establish morphine infusion / PCA (SBH) within 15mins of admission.** • Give paracetamol PR 6 hourly as prescribed (check consent signed). • If severe pain (>2) give bolus dose morphine 3–5mg & assess. • **Assess need for sedation – if required use boluses of propofol and ONLY use infusion if excessively agitated or unstable.** • **Reassess sedation level & requirements after 1ˢᵗ hour or earlier in readiness for weaning.**	N		
Blood Sugar	• Check BM stix on admission & 4 hourly – establish insulin sliding scale as per diabetic chart if patient diabetic or if BM >15mmol/l if not diabetic.	N		
General	• Check & record pedal pulses 6 hourly (IABP check hourly). • Check chest & leg wounds and record drainage from any leg drains. • Aspirate NG tube 6 hourly.	N		
Clinical Tests	• **ECG within first hour** • Bloods for ABG & BM. • **Script fluid chart: colloid, 5% dextrose (SBH) / D/Saline (LCH), morphine, propofol, paracetamol PR, antibiotics and PRN drugs (KCl, furosemide, anti-emetics according to protocol).** • Script GTN to a maximum of 10mg/hr (SBH) or 20mg/hr (LCH) then add SNP. • Liase with nurse and script CVS parameters. • Start GRASP.	N N D D D N		

Figure 30.1 Hours 0–1 of the critical pathway for cardiac surgery at St Bartholomew's Hospital ICU. (Reproduced with kind permission from St Bartholomew's Hospital: Barts and the London NHS Trust.) NB: This is provided as an example in the development of a critical pathway. It is recognised that practice has and will advance in areas such as extubation (such as moving beyond T-piece weaning for the majority of patients). Abbreviations are explained to all new staff as part of the orientation to the pathway.

Last / First Name: **Patient, Any**
Hospital Number: **12345678**   Date of Birth: **01/02/34**

Barts and The London **NHS**
NHS Trust

ITU ADMISSION BOOK NUMBER:		DATE:	__/__/20__		
HOURS 2–6 (covers all care for first 24 hours if required) FOLLOWING OPERATION (ITU) UNTIL TRANSFER TO CHDU			V or n/a	Time Shift	Initials
RESPIRATORY WEANING	OUTCOME: APPROPRIATE EXTUBATION				
Establish adequate breathing on Water's Bag	▪ Manipulate respiratory support to achieve set aims: ABGs, SaO₂ & RR. ▪ **CONSULT WEANING ALGORITHM (SBH)**, changing FiO₂ protocol & NIC/SPR as required. ▪ **If CVS stable & acceptable bleeding, sit patient upright and wake every 15mins to trial on Water's Bag; transfer to T-piece if RR 10–25, TV >5ml/kg, SaO₂ >95% – start 15 min observations.** ▪ Pre-oxygenate (avoid excessive bagging) and suction if required.	N		
On T-Piece	▪ **Check ABG in 20mins to ensure patient meeting set aims.** ▪ **Active management: reassess continually & encourage deep breathing, wean FiO₂ to 0.4 with SaO₂ >95%.** ▪ **If on T-Piece >1 hour add CPAP +5cm: reassess continually for extubation.**	N		
Extubation Criteria (Unit Protocol)	▪ Awake, orientated, co-operative, equal limb movements. ▪ Able to protect airway (cough & gag reflex present). ▪ Respiratory rate **10–25** breaths/min. ▪ Tidal volume >5ml/kg (if measured). ▪ PaO2 >10kPa on FiO₂ of 0.4, PaCO₂ <7kPa. ▪ Acceptable haemodynamics, EGG and blood loss <100mls/ hr. ▪ **If criteria achieved check with NIC/SPR and extubate according to unit protocol.**	N		
Post Extubation Management and Education	▪ Establish on 6l via humidified mask plus 4l via nasal specs (SBH) ▪ **Wean FiO₂ according to ABG (1/2 hour post extubation) & SaO₂.** ▪ Encourage deep breathing & coughing 1/2 hourly, reinforce use of PCA and support of chest wound, consider treatment by physiotherapist, if available. ▪ NBM for 1 hour then re-establish oral medications.	N		
CARDIOVASCULAR & DRAIN MANAGEMENT	▪ Aim to achieve set parameters in first 4 hours by titration of vasodilators/ inotropes, colloid, IABP, pacing and maintenance of potassium levels. ▪ **Report a colloid balance of +ve 2 litres to SHO (CXR may be ordered).** ▪ Report & record volume of any bleeding >100mls/hr to NIC & CT SHO. Request FBC & clotting.	N		
MANAGEMENT OF PAIN & SEDATION & PATIENT EDUCATION	OUTCOME: AWAKE, ORIENTATED, PAIN FREE/ CONTROLLED ▪ **Aim to stop use of propofol and actively wake & assess patient using voice control and analgesia.** ▪ Assess pain & sedation levels using score: titrate analgesia (0–3 mg/hr) to achieve pain level 0–1. Change from continuous to PCA in hours 1–4 (SBH). ▪ Assess understanding of PCA & sedation score and re-educate/reinforce. ▪ Explain weaning process and plan of care to the patient & relatives.	N		
FLUID MANAGEMENT	▪ Monitor urine output hourly – if inadequate consider a fluid challenge/ furosemide bolus and reassess checking with NIC/CT SHO. ▪ Continue crystalloid maintenance at 1 ml/kg/hr (inclusive of drugs) and reduce when oral fluids (2l restriction) tolerated; light diet if tolerated. ▪ Aim to keep K⁺ 4.5–5 mmols/l ▪ Educate patient about potential nausea and use of anti-emetics.	N		
PRESSURE AREA CARE MOBILISATION EYE & MOUTH CARE	▪ **Aim to roll off canvas and assess pressure areas using Waterlow score within 4 hours: SCORE_____ STAGE_____** OUTCOME: APPROPRIATE MOBILISATION educate patient about pressure area care: if intubated roll 2–4 hourly with limb exercises; if extubated encourage limb exercises & consider leg dangling over edge of bed. ▪ Eye & mouth care as per Unit Standards. ▪ Replace glasses/hearing aid/dentures ASAP.	N		
CARE OF NEXT OF KIN	▪ Aware of operation and progress along critical pathway. ▪ Orientated to ITU/CRU/CHDU & visiting policies. ▪ **First contact details checked on Patient Information Section.** ▪ Aware of transfer process to CHDU & patient's goals for next 24 hours. INQUIRIES:	N		
DISCHARGE & TRANSFER CRITERIA	OUTCOME: APPROPRIATE DISCHARGE TO CHDU or CHDU ICP or ITU ICP HOURS 24–48 POST-OP as appropriate TO CHDU: Extubated >1 hour, no deterioration in extubation criteria & blood loss <50 ml/hr: check ABG/BM pre-transfer. ▪ When criteria met patient assessed by NIC & CHDU contacted re transfer. ▪ GRASP & variance record completed & filed in ITU. ICP Pack, Notes, CXRs, ECGs & transfusion forms sent with patient to CHDU. TO CHDU ICP: achievement of ICP set outcomes but lack of CHDU bed TO ITU ICP HOURS 24–48: patient not achieving ICP outcomes and requiring continued ITU care to resolve ongoing variances	N		
	Signature and Initials		**Status / Agency**		
Day Nurse					
Night Nurse					
Day Nurse					
Doctor					

Figure 30.2 Hours 2–6 of the critical pathway. (Reproduced with kind permission from St Bartholomew's Hospital: Barts and the London NHS Trust.)

Last / First Name:		Barts and The London **NHS**
Hospital Number:	Date of Birth:	NHS Trust **Cardiac Intensive Care Unit**

Date Time	Code	VARIATION	ACTION	EVALUATION	Signature Designation

PATIENT
1. PAIN
2. BLEEDING
3. ARRHTHMIAS
4. CEREBRAL PROBLEM
5. PRIMARY RESPIRATORY PROBLEM
6. SLOW RESPIRATORY WEANING
7. CARDIOVASCULAR INSTABILITY
8. INADEQUATE URINE OUTPUT
9. NAUSEA & VOMITING
10. PYREXIA
11. OTHER

MULTIDISCIPLINARY TEAM
12. NURSE AVAILABILITY
13. DOCTOR AVAILABILITY
14. PHYSIO AVAILABILITY
15. OTHER

HOSPITAL / SYSTEM
16. CHDU
17. EQUIPMENT AVAILABILITY
18. OTHER

ADMISSION BOOK NO:

TIME OF ARRIVAL	
F_iO_2 ON ARRIVAL	
TIME OF EXTUBATION	
F_iO_2 AT EXTUBATION	
TYPE/TOTAL AMOUNT OF ANALGESIA BY EXTUBATION	
TYPE/TOTAL AMOUNT OF SEDATION BY EXTUBATION	
TOTAL BLOOD LOSS AT EXTUBATION	
DATE/TIME OF DISCHARGE	

WHITE COPY: Notes   PINK COPY: Central Audit   YELLOW COPY: Local Audit

Figure 30.3 The variance audit sheet of the critical pathway. (Reproduced with kind permission from St Bartholomew's Hospital: Barts and the London NHS Trust.)

Kilgallen 1993, Shiell et al 1993, Wigfied & Boon 1996), identification of problems at an earlier stage, improved documentation (Miller et al 1995) and continuity of care, increased positive feedback from patients (Johnson 1995, Riches et al 1994), promotion of standardized research-based care and heightened autonomy and education for nurses (Marr & Reid 1992). The quantitative studies reported trends towards shorter lengths of stay, cost savings, fewer complications and shorter consultation times (Bultema et al 1996, Dukes Crawley & Till 1995, Farley 1995, Luther & Crofts 1997, Rudy et al 1995, Zander 1988).

Although the literature advocated the adoption of managed care, closer examination of the studies suggested mixed and slightly ambiguous findings. They appeared to use a paucity of formal evaluation tools, making them difficult to compare. Managed care was often inadequately described, presenting the critical pathway as a separate entity. There was little discussion of effects on staff, existing philosophies and models of care or multidisciplinary collaboration. The few disadvantages cited included a tendency towards task orientation and lack of individuality (Laxade & Hale 1995a,b).

Review of the studies using managed care for cardiac surgery

The studies related to cardiac surgery use a variety of terms to describe the accelerated process of recovery after surgery: early extubation, fast tracking and rapid recovery (see Chapter 29). In the study the term 'fast tracking' was used to encompass the changes to intra-operative anaesthesia, postoperative sedation and analgesia which facilitated the aim of safely extubating all patients within 6 hours of surgery and covered the whole recovery process in ITU until discharge to the cardiac high dependency unit (CHDU) (Aps 1992, Higgins 1995).

The majority of studies reviewed describe either isolated early extubation protocols (Anderson & O'Brien 1995, Blondin et al 1996, Edwards & Hess 1996, Keresztes & Kuruzar 1996, Maxam-Moore & Goedecke 1996) or the development of cardiac recovery units in the UK (Aps 1995, Howard 1995, Massey & Meggit 1994, Packham 1990). Hampton (1993) and Ley (1995) briefly and anecdotally described the potential benefits of pathways for cardiac patients. A small number of studies combined managed care with cardiac fast tracking (Henry & Duffy 1995, Redick et al 1994, Riches et al 1994, Schriefer 1994, 1995) of which only one was British. Riches et al (1994) outlined the implementation of pathways in a London trust using a co-

ordinator whose role remained unclear. They highlighted the importance of multidisciplinary teamwork and a bottom-up approach to facilitate changes in practice and attitudes. Improved communication was also reported and positive feedback from patients with use of the pathway. Only Redick et al (1994) and Henry & Duffy (1995) described the use of managed care in any great detail. Redick et al (1994) did not describe the managed care model used but suggested that pathways could aid the planning of staffing requirements and identification of research questions. These studies, although innovative, lacked any systematic evaluation of the difficulties associated with implementing changes and there was little discussion of the disadvantages of managed care for cardiac patients themselves.

A few American studies did recognize that staff have to change their attitudes and practice for early extubation programmes to succeed. Blondin et al (1996), Keresztes & Kuruzar (1996) and Maxam-Moore & Goedecke (1996) described early extubation programmes without managed care. Blondin et al's (1996) study alluded to the concerns of practitioners managing fast-track patients including a 'fear of weaning too fast' and a lack of the necessary 'assertive extubation thought process', but these issues were not examined in any depth. Keresztes & Kuruzar (1996) describe a case where a patient was unexpectedly extubated in theatre and transferred to ICU. They emphasized that early extubation requires not only protocol and system changes but improved communication, staff education and evaluation of outcomes. They described the need to change nursing priorities towards airway management and control of sedation and analgesia in addition to teamwork and patient education. Importantly, they discussed the ethical considerations related to the nurses' concerns over the practice of early extubation and patient safety. Only Henry & Duffy's (1995) study combined early extubation with managed care and they directly identified the need to change practices, perceptions and attitudes when introducing these systems. However, whilst their study used a multidisciplinary, problem-solving approach with in-service education to tackle the difficulties of introducing fast tracking, it was unfortunately not systematically evaluated.

OUTLINE OF THE CURRENT ACTION RESEARCH STUDY

The study addressed changes to cardiac services caused by formation of a trust. At St Bartholomew's Hospital an integral cardiac recovery unit (CRU) was developed within the ICU along with an adjacent CHDU. Although the ICU had pre-existing protocols for extubation and discharge, the fast-track programme was introduced before a nursing strategy was developed to address the needs of these new patients. The need to change clinical practice and attitudes along with education to facilitate fast tracking was largely unrecognized. The study sought to inject nursing input to the pre-existing fast-track programme by implementing and systematically evaluating managed care.

The research originally took place between September 1995 and August 1996. An action research approach was used to facilitate a bottom-up, participatory process 'with' and 'for' practitioners rather than 'on' them (Reason 1988, Reason & Rowan 1981). This collaborative form of research encouraged participants to reflect on their practices and become involved in research in their own environment (Carr & Kemmis 1986). My joint practitioner–researcher role allowed me to drive nursing inquiry and practice to facilitate change within a multidisciplinary framework. However, full involvement was difficult for new staff and not desired by some members of the cardiothoracic team. I regarded the ICU nurses as the key to successful fast tracking and action research enabled their contribution to practice to be acknowledged and nurtured.

The five overlapping phases of the eclectic approach to research (Hart & Bond 1995, Holter & Schwartz-Barcott 1993, Meyer 1995, Webb 1989) and the research methods used are highlighted in Figure 30.4. This gives some insight into the essence and scale of the project. The process of developing the managed care system is outlined in Figure 30.5.

The research explored the issues surrounding the initial changes in cardiac services before introducing more change in the form of managed care. The research had five aims:

- to examine practitioners' perceptions of the changes in cardiac services
- to implement and evaluate a managed care programme for cardiac fast-track patients in ICU
- to examine practitioners' perceptions of using managed care and fast tracking in the reality of practice
- to explore patients' and relatives' experiences of the transfer process between clinical areas
- to examine my own perceptions of the changes and my role as action researcher.

The action research approach allowed a complementary combination of quantitative and qualitative methods of data collection to be used as outlined in Figure 30.4.

It is vitally important to pilot the pathway before implementation to identify problems and areas in need of revision. Piloting can also demonstrate the effectiveness of the pathway on outcomes and thus sustain practitioner involvement in the project (Cardozo et al 1998, Farley 1995, Lutjens 1995). The methods of data analysis allowed me to preserve, interpret and present the essence of such a huge quantity of data. This made the findings accessible, a prerequisite to establish the rigor and credibility of the qualitative research approach (Guba & Lincoln 1985, Meyer 1995).

Data analysis produced findings relating to four areas of concern: health practitioners' perceptions of fast tracking; practitioners' experiences of the whole process of change including managed care; the utility of the critical pathway; and patients' and relatives' perceptions of transfer. Some of these findings, including interview excerpts and case studies from the study, will be used along with recent literature to highlight the challenges of introducing managed care in practice.

THE CHALLENGES OF INTRODUCING MANAGED CARE

Figure 30.5 summarizes the key issues in planning and developing the introduction of managed care. Many of these apply universally to project development but each clinical area will have its own unique characteristics and politics to be accommodated. The most important and recurring elements of successful change are involvement, information, education and feedback for participants.

PLANNING FOR MANAGED CARE
Key change agents

The role of the change agent/researcher–practitioner was paramount in producing a planned and long-lasting change. The change agent needs to develop and nurture the culture of change (Doran et al 1998). The issue of using change agents from inside or outside the area is debatable. Doran et al (1998) suggested that doctors should lead the change process but the success of this nurse-led project challenges this view. However, doctors in the multidisciplinary team are essential to lead other doctors through the process, particularly when fundamental practices have to be changed, such as anaesthetic techniques to facilitate early extubation (Doran et al 1998). As a sister on the ICU, I found that familiarity allowed trust to develop

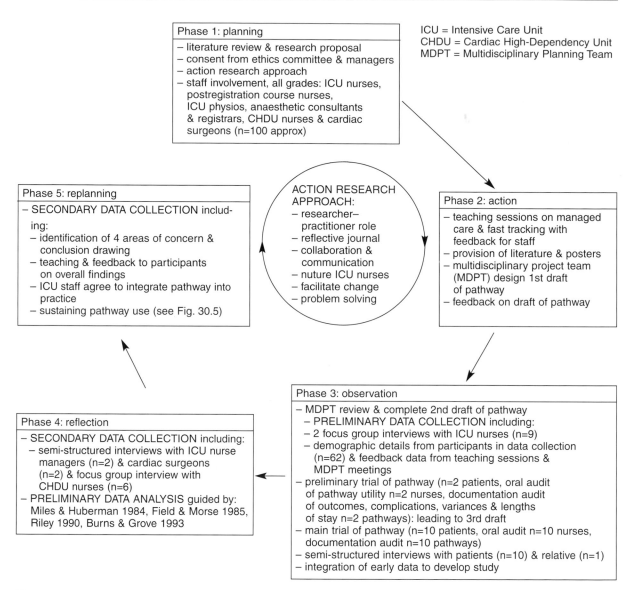

Figure 30.4 Summary of the research approach and methodology for implementing critical pathways.

and encouraged participation. This will also increase the clinical credibility of the research (MacGuire 1990).

Regardless of their discipline, change agents need to be knowledgeable and confident but should avoid casting themselves as experts, producing a hierarchical relationship with staff. The whole process is a learning experience, drawing out the tacit knowledge of practitioners in addition to creating new knowledge (Hunt 1987, Nolan & Grant 1993). Staff can feel threatened by the introduction of unplanned change and irritated by unexplained new procedures and documentation. Making the reasons for change explicit and discussing

the management of change in teaching sessions can ease the process (Haffer 1986, McGovern & Rodgers 1986).

Implementation of the pathway in practice is time consuming. I monitored all patients in the study from their pre-operative day, during their admission to ICU and until discharge home. Close observation of the ICU recovery period, in conjunction with the nurse in charge, was essential to ensure that the patients who had consented to participate in the trial were cared for safely, as emphasized by Keresztes & Kuruzar (1996). It was important that the ICU practitioners were sup-

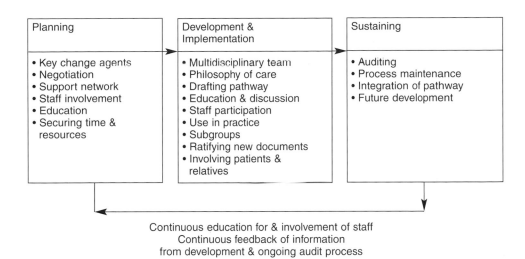

Figure 30.5 Key elements in planning, developing, implementing and sustaining the process of managed care.

ported while gaining experience in fast tracking (Capuano et al 1999) and using the new documentation. My role enabled me to promote more proactive, outcome-focused care and to address emergent issues as they actually occurred. Priority should be given to providing a team of change agents with common goals and full-time commitment to facilitate the process.

Negotiation and support

Negotiation with all levels of staff, particularly key members of each multidisciplinary group, is imperative to give people time to respond to proposals in order to gain support at local and regional levels for the introduction of change. Recent literature highlights the importance of multidisciplinary work to implement pathways successfully (Newman 1995, Roebuck 1998), with support from medical staff a prerequisite (Cardozo et al 1998). In the study, not all individuals were interested in managed care, but it is worthwhile investing some time with uninterested staff to discuss any concerns and ensure they understand the documentation. Regional resources include audit teams, research and development nurses, cardiac health promotion nurses, course tutors and managed care co-ordinators. The *Directory of UK NHS trusts using care pathways* (Royal College of Nursing Institute 1998) and nursing Internet sites are also useful.

Communication and collaboration

The ICU has been promoted as a key area for collaboration (Mechanic & Aiken 1982). However, as in other collaboration projects (Baggs et al 1992, Johnson 1992, Lorentzon 1995), nurses and doctors in the study had different perceptions about the degree of partnership and input required to facilitate it. Obstacles to communication existed between all groups of practitioners in the study, exacerbated by differing philosophies of care and power struggles over patient management. These were manifested as disparities in the degree of trust, level of understanding and respect for each other's practices and views. In particular, the ICU nurses questioned the CHDU nurses' capability to care for fast-track patients despite the CHDU nurses' previous experiences, as highlighted in these excerpts from separate focus group interviews.

My only concerns about fast tracking post-extubation and going round to the ward [CHDU] is the level of the nurses' knowledge and the care ... often post-extubation patients can be quite sick. (Senior ICU nurse)

...I went back [to CHDU] a couple of hours later just to check what those gases were so that I could fill out my form and they hadn't been done and I was thinking 'Oh dear!' and they [the patient] were fine. I think maybe we worry too much. (Senior ICU nurse)

...what sometimes is amusing, is sometimes there can be a very junior nurse looking after the patient in ICU who has probably not had a tenth of the ICU experience some of us have had and then saying 'Well, are you all right taking the patient?'. But that's part of it and that's accepted. (CHDU nurse)

However, the excerpts below demonstrate that the senior ICU nurses initially experienced difficulty in changing their practices and attitudes, as suggested by Henry & Duffy (1995) and Keresztes & Kuruzar (1996). They were educationally and psychologically unprepared to withdraw their care at an earlier stage in fast-track patients' recovery.

They [junior ICU nurses] are wondering where their responsibility for the patient ends ... they don't feel as if they've finished the job. (Senior ICU nurse)

I find it very odd taking a patient over [to CHDU] with all the drips and drains in and handing over. I still find that strange even now. (Senior ICU nurse)

Interactive multidisciplinary groups can be used to enable practitioners to challenge each other's attitudes and actions in a controlled environment. This can increase awareness of roles, knowledge, values, conflicts and the nurses' input to care. Multidisciplinary problem-solving groups and equality in information giving, education, involvement and support will also promote collaboration and communication.

Education, feedback systems and discussion

Education is probably the most important element in implementing and sustaining managed care. At St Bartholomew's ICU, education and discussion occur through various group and bedside teaching sessions which currently focus on variance management. Written information, including orientation packages for nurses and doctors, flyers and posters supplement the process (Doran et al 1998). Updating practitioners with feedback on the progress of pathway development and audit results is imperative to ensure that they understand the implications for practice and feel involved.

Involvement and ownership

All the strategies used during the planning stage will promote a sense of involvement and ownership in managed care. During the study, the experience of practitioners who used the pathway on a daily basis, especially those involved in practice groups, was utilized by encouraging problem solving to review practice protocols and redraft the pathway. A sense of ownership will give practitioners control over the direction of the care process and particularly over fast tracking.

Securing time and financial resources

The scale of financial and organizational commitment described in the American literature can be daunting.

However, the same results can be produced in the UK using local resources as long as time is secured for project work. Initial negotiations with managers should address this issue as implementation is very time consuming, particularly auditing and education. Funding bodies such as hospital or unit trustees can be approached to cover development costs, such as the printing of pathways and teaching materials. In addition, a research grant to fund a study can be sought from health service bodies such as the King's Fund.

DEVELOPMENT AND IMPLEMENTATION OF THE CRITICAL PATHWAY

Building the multidisciplinary managed care team

Recent articles have stressed the need for careful team selection and collaboration to help drive the development process (Cardozo et al 1998, Doran et al 1998). It was a challenge to bring together key members of different disciplines involved with cardiac patients and encourage them, despite local politics and power struggles, to work together. Practitioners were invited to join the project team on the strength of their commitment to practice, experience (juniors and seniors) and potential ability to collaborate. The team comprised the ICU senior nurse, a senior and junior sister, the ICU physiotherapist, an ICU anaesthetic consultant, a cardiothoracic senior registrar and senior house officer and myself. Meetings allowed long-standing clinical issues, such as weaning criteria and consultants' preferences for the haematocrits (HCT level), to be discussed and incorporated into the pathway. Importantly, the collaboration of the project team became central to the success of the study.

Developing a common philosophy of care

A joint philosophy of cardiac care is essential for fast tracking to succeed (Riches et al 1994, Scott 1996). Although the team agreed on the goals of managed care and fast tracking and formulated a basic philosophy, the various disciplines involved in the study exhibited different knowledge and beliefs. Practitioners often manifested their lack of understanding of the process by creating their own agendas for fast tracking which were reflected in the disparate approach to postoperative care. It is important to assess practitioners' understanding of managed care and the needs of specific groups of patients during the development stage.

The study helped to clarify understanding of fast tracking and a philosophy was drafted following a project review in September 1997. The philosophy advocated that the ICU, in promoting 'recovery from cardiac surgery', aimed to admit all cardiac patients for individualized, co-ordinated and safe extubation using managed care. In addition, the ICU anaesthetic, consultant–ICU, nurse-led service would promote nursing autonomy and practice.

Critical pathways: making the implicit ... explicit

The principal attribute of a critical pathway is simply making the implicit or hidden processes of care, particularly everyday nursing care, more explicit. The total process of care delivered by all disciplines can then be scrutinized, evaluated and understood. The study was the first to suggest that pathways and variance analysis play an important part in highlighting the effort involved by practitioners, particularly nurses, in ensuring safe patient progress and achievement of outcomes.

Designing the critical pathway

Designing the critical pathway is time consuming but crucial in making the care process explicit. The change

agent needs to maintain momentum to ensure the pathway is designed within a strict time frame. Design was guided by Cohen & Cesta's (1997) framework and adapted with examples from other units (Fig. 30.6).

The basic layout of the pathway was based, with permission, on a neurosurgical pathway used at a sister hospital (Luther 1995, Luther & Crofts 1997) and adapted to the needs of the ICU. Utilizing pre-existing frameworks can save time in the development stage (Zevola et al 1997). To reduce duplication, the ICU at St Bartholomew's now uses the admission sheet compiled in the pre-admission clinic or ward, and after 48 hours a more detailed ICU sheet is compiled.

In making care explicit, the project team identified the total process of care involved for fast-track patients. The pathway charted all identified specialist care required during ICU, incorporating unit standards and protocols, which must be carried out sequentially within the first 6 hours of admission for fast-track patients. However, the pathway covers care required for the first 24 hours in the ICU.

The pathway was divided into two time periods: hours 0–1 (Fig. 30.1) and hours 2–6 (Fig. 30.2). However, the second time period actually covers all care required by the patient if they have to remain in the ICU for up to 24 hours, such as postextubation

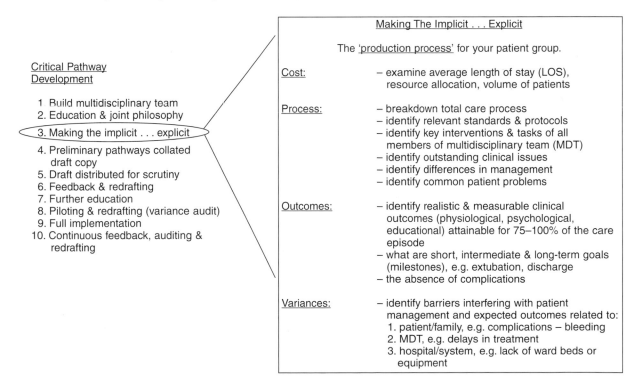

Figure 30.6 A framework for the multidisciplinary design of the critical pathway.

management and pressure area care. The first period covers all interventions required to admit the patient from theatre and settle them into the ICU. The emphasis in the first hour is patient safety, monitoring and administration of analgesia. By the end of the first hour the nurse can evaluate the patient for readiness to fast track: wake, wean and extubate.

Edwards & Hess (1996) reported that fast-track weaning protocols increase nurses' decision-making capabilities and responsibility for extubation. The additional use of a pathway increases nurses' control over the whole process of care in the ICU. The set time periods introduced the idea of time managed, active and outcome-focused care, providing sound guidelines to assist clinical decision making. They also highlight the potential for complications and the need for continual assessment of the patient's individual progress. The pivotal change associated with fast tracking is the emphasis on practitioners to proactively manage and wean patients.

In addition, the pathway was designed as a teaching tool to meet the needs of all levels of ICU staff, including agency nurses. Inclusion of weaning, extubation and discharge criteria on the pathway increased its utility as a bedside guide. Compared to other pathways, it is very detailed and perhaps prescriptive. However, nurses in the study stated that it 'jogs the memory' and acts as an 'aide-mémoire', particularly for junior nurses and for those who fast track more than one patient per shift. This level of detail is useful for complicated but less commonly seen conditions such as diabetic ketoacidosis (Van Buskirk & Vanderbilt 1995). Hassaballa et al (1998) described a scheme to ensure pathways are used by practitioners by inserting them into inpatient notes on admission.

Use in practice

The pathway was created for use at the beside to guide care through each time period. Each stage of the pathway is completed as care, outcomes or variances occur rather than in retrospect at the end of the shift. This provides a more accurate picture of the changing clinical situation and encourages use of the nursing process and clinical decision-making skills to assess needs, identify potential problems and take action.

The pathway integrates existing pressure area assessment, patient information and discharge sheets to aid auditing, reduce writing and save paper. Written guidelines to accompany the pathway are included in bedside folders. These document the answers to common queries such as what to do when a patient deteriorates. In this case, all patients who return to theatre for bleed-

ing continue to be cared for using the pathway on re-admission to the ICU. Patients who require ICU care for more than 48 hours are transferred to a general care plan which covers the needs of long-term cardiac patients and is compatible with the pathway.

Ratification of the new critical pathway

Like any new clinical document, the completed pathway needs to be scrutinized and ratified by senior nurses and consultants before use in practice (Cardozo et al 1998, Keresztes & Kuruzar 1996). Clinical accuracy and safety can be assessed using individual trust protocols and guidelines from professional bodies such as the Royal College of Nursing.

Involvement of patients and relatives/carers

Moyer (1994) reported that relatives of standard cardiac patients were confused about transfers and the length of ICU stay despite pre-operative teaching. These findings were supported in relation to fast tracking in the study. A simplified version of the pathway can be used as a teaching aid for patients and relatives (Doran et al 1998, Ley 1995, Zevola et al 1997). It can be used as a guide to progress with the understanding that individual recovery may differ slightly from the pathway and other patients. The pathway can also be used, where appropriate, to inform patients who are concerned over their incomplete memories of the ICU (Scott 1996). Recent literature advocates increased patient and family involvement to promote recovery supported by home care pathways, home care nursing teams and telephone support links after discharge (Capuano et al 1999, Doran et al 1998, Riddle et al 1996). These initiatives promote fast tracking as a more seamless process for both patients and relatives/carers.

Sustaining the momentum of managed care

Recent longitudinal studies recognize that to sustain momentum the most important factors are continued audit, review of guidelines and feedback of progress to practitioners (Capuano et al 1999, Riddle et al 1996). In fact, the ICU currently uses the tenth draft of the pathway following audits and protocol reviews. The pathway should be treated as a 'living document', developing and changing in conjunction with practitioners' experience, knowledge and research. Integral to the design process is reviewing, updating and integrating existing models of care, clinical standards and documentation to address the need for evidence-based care. Discussion of strategies to maintain momentum will focus on the importance and challenges of auditing variances, updating standards and further developing the pathway.

Why is the auditing of variances important?

Auditing provides an ongoing focus for the development of managed care. It systematically and tangibly demonstrates the utility of the pathway in clinical practice, providing information on common patient problems, delivery of care and outcomes. Variance tracking also reveals data on staffing issues, skill mix and bed availability which can affect discharge and safety of the environment (Redick et al 1994, Scott 1996).

Exception reporting, such as variance monitoring, is relatively new in the UK. If combined with continuous quality improvement, it can be used by the multidisciplinary team to identify and solve the causes of variances. This can lead to the verification of practice and, if required, the redrafting of clinical protocols and pathways and formulation of research and education strategies (Coffey et al 1995, Eisenberg & Redick 1998, Redick et al 1994, Schriefer 1995, Scott 1996, Shulkin & Harris 1996, Zevola et al 1997).

What are the challenges of variance tracking and audit?

Despite the importance of auditing there is little published literature on how to undertake the process. The few centres with long-term experience have reported that variance management can be time consuming and inaccurate if incorrectly performed (Yandell 1995). The major issue in variance management is use of terminology and the biggest challenges are the practicalities of variance data collection and analysis. With little advice available, most units will have to devise their own methods of audit according to resources and needs. Help can be obtained from hospital audit teams and research staff and the process is facilitated by the use of computerized documentation. The following section provides guidelines on initiating the process.

Terminology

The early literature on variance tracking categorized variances as 'negative' or 'positive' which can have contradictory connotations for practitioners. Supposedly 'negative' variances, such as slow to wean, can imply that staff have 'failed' if patients 'deviate' from the pathway's set outcomes. Equally, it is important to recognize and record 'positive' variances such as patients who achieve set outcomes and are discharged early. This 'negative' and 'positive' terminology can be avoided by constructively presenting results which demonstrate the effort and difficulties involved in fast tracking patients and which themselves encourage discussion and quality initiatives.

Collection of variance data

The biggest difficulty is the collection of variance sheets when the patient is discharged. The study ICU has a duplicate variance sheet which staff remove and deposit in a specific tray for the audit team. The original copies of the pathway and variance sheet transfer with the patient to CHDU. Collected variance sheets are then compared with the admission book to detect missing ones. Monitoring the compliance rate in completing and collecting variance sheets alerts the audit team to the need for reminders.

Analysis of variance data

Initial auditing has been limited due to the volume of data. Current audit at the ICU in the study has involved monitoring of the monthly number of patients on the pathway, the nursing compliance in completing and collecting pathways and the number and type of variances recorded. From this they have calculated the number of patients experiencing each type of variance as shown on the bar chart in Figure 30.7. The pie chart (Fig. 30.8) demonstrates in more detail which variances occurred first during the initial 6 hours of admission (Byers, Cahill, personal communication).

The most frequent variances are postoperative bleeding, slow respiratory weaning and cardiovascular instability. Bleeding is the primary variance. Of note are the number of patients with no variances and the number of CHDU variances due to lack of beds for patient transfer. After the study the categories of variances were clarified. 'Primary respiratory problem', such as chronic obstructive pulmonary disease (COPD) or asthma, was added to differentiate these patients from those with no history of pulmonary disease but who were identified as a 'slow respiratory wean' due to other causes such as sedation. Variances which are not used, such as the multidisciplinary team category, may be due to a lack of understanding, requiring teaching or the removal of redundant variances from the pathway.

Developing the audit process in the future

The emerging issue for the ICU is how to move the audit process forward, specifically in tackling the root

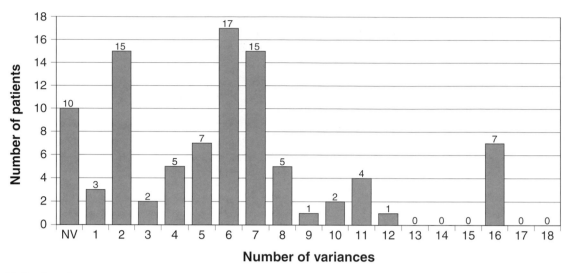

Patient variances

NV	No variances	5	Primary respiratory problem	10	Pyrexia	14	Physio' availability
1	Pain	6	Slow respiratory weaning	11	Other	15	Other
2	Bleeding	7	Cardiovascular instability	**Multidisciplinary team**		**Hospital/system**	
3	Arrhythmias	8	Inadequate urine output	12	Nurse availability	16	CHDU (no bed)
4	Cerebral problem	9	Nausea and vomiting	13	Doctor availability	17	Equipment availability
						18	Other

Total number of patients: 66
13 variance sheets missing – 80% nursing compliance in completion of variance sheets
74% of patients were discharged from ITU within 24 hours
23% (15 patients) **'fast tracked' within 6 hours of admission**

Figure 30.7 An example of the number of patients in 1 month experiencing each type of variance. (Reproduced with kind permission of Heather Byers, Senior Sister, ICU, St Batholomew's Hospital, London)

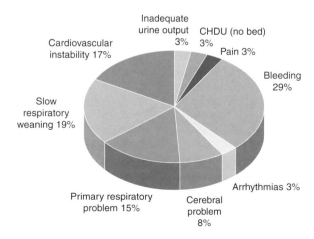

Figure 30.8 The distribution of the first variance to be reported within the first 6 hours post surgery in 1 month. The variance 'CHDU' indicates that the cardiac high-dependency unit was unable to take the patient due to a lack of a bed or staff at that time. (Reproduced with kind permission of Heather Byers, Senior Sister, ICU, St Batholomew's Hospital, London)

causes of variances and ultimately refining the pathway. With the primary and most frequently occurring variances identified, the next stage is determining whether the variances precipitate or are related to each other, causing a cascade effect resulting in patients not meeting their expected outcomes.

Current investigation of a possible link between the three main variances centres on whether postoperative patients bleed and become cardiovascularly unstable which in turn slows their respiratory weaning. This has prompted a review of the bleeding protocol. The ICU staff anecdotally noted that although a large number of patients bled, this did not seem to slow their progress. Indeed, the audit results for 1 month showed that 30% of patients had bleeding as a variance but 74% of the total were still discharged within 24 hours. The audit team attributed the high numbers of bleeding variances to the low volume of blood measured per hour (over 100 ml) which is used to define bleeding according to the protocol. It was possible that this amount of post operative bleeding was normal and did not impact on the patients' progress.

A literature review and telephone survey of other cardiac ICUs revealed little data to guide the protocol. Therefore, in conjunction with the cardiac surgeons, the acceptable volumes of post operative bleeding were changed to <200 ml for the first post operative hour, followed by <100 ml for the second hour before treatment is required. Due to the range of clinical experience on the ICU, the limit was increased cautiously to ensure that bleeding was still reported early. The pathway has now been altered along with teaching for staff. A recent audit has demonstrated that those patients who are identified as having a bleeding variance are actually those who require medical or surgical intervention and are therefore 'true bleeders'. The audit has shown that the new protocol has reduced the number of bleeding variances without adversely affecting patient care or prompt treatment of bleeding (Yorke, personal communication). Future projects include developing a treatment protocol for bleeding, taking into account consultant preferences. By examining the availability of doctors to institute the protocol it may eventually be deemed appropriate for the ICU nurses to initiate treatment (Boley, personal communication). Finally, it is imperative to concentrate on clarifying the causes of one variance at a time as this may rectify others.

When variance management becomes established the frequency of auditing can be reduced. This may be, for example, from monthly to quarterly using a smaller sample group of patients. Yandell (1995) reported that some hospitals have completely stopped auditing as they felt their pathways were fully developed but this may stop new clinical problems from being detected.

Using the audit process to develop clinical practice

The pathway can also be developed by commissioning subgroups to tackle variances and changes to standards arising from the audit. For example, Capuano et al (1999) instituted an oxygen-weaning protocol to supplement their pathway. Other adjuncts include nurse-driven protocols allowing nurses to independently discharge patients (Doran et al 1998) and extubate and remove pulmonary artery catheters to expedite discharge (Zevola & Maier 1999).

Multidisciplinary atrial fibrillation protocols appear to reduce the incidence of arrhythmias (Dunstan & Riddle 1997, Riddle et al 1996) and ensure they are treated more promptly (Doran et al 1998). Other protocols promote postoperative activity to facilitate rehabilitation (Capuano et al 1999, Riddle et al 1996) and facilitate prophylaxis of gastro-intestinal problems such as poor appetite and nausea (Riddle et al 1996). Importantly, Capuano et al (1999) stressed the need for medical staff to support nurses in initiating new protocols such as early ambulation which can be stressful for both staff and patients. The American literature reports efforts to reduce the quantity of routine laboratory tests and X-rays to reduce costs without affecting quality (Capuano et al 1999, Riddle et al 1996).

What are the benefits and difficulties of using critical pathways?

Some of the advantages and disadvantages of the system have already been discussed. However, it is important to summarize the main benefits and difficulties or, more positively, what has been learnt from using it in practice.

Unlike the literature, the study made no huge claims of improving communication and collaboration as these variables are infinitely hard to measure. Long-term change is difficult to achieve with ever-changing staff and the influence of local politics. However, the project team was perceived as bridging the gap between the ICU and cardiac teams. Importantly, senior management recognized the need to involve staff in new developments.

Importantly for myself, the study had some positive effects on nursing practice. The pathway has been well supported and is currently completely integrated into daily practice by users who find it flexible to the needs of patients, particularly those who were slow to wean. Use of the critical pathway has made nursing care more explicit, highlighting the implicit work of the ICU nurses. The pathway has supported clinical practice while the nurses developed the skills and knowledge of early extubation and fast tracking. It has increased nursing input and control over the process, reducing the risk of maverick treatments by new staff, and has promoted fast tracking as an ICU anaesthetic, consultant–ICU, nurse-led service. The study also facilitated a degree of empowerment, although this is also hard to measure, by encouraging education, self-reflection, discussion and the use of inherent skills and knowledge. There was also the encouragement of long-term nursing innovation through continuation of the audit process.

Coffey et al (1995) and Yandell (1995) caution against attributing too many advantages to pathways as any improvements in quality indicators may be due to a short-term 'Hawthorne effect' (providing the results desired by the research) and the subjective benefits of improved teamwork and shared objectives. Burns et al (1997) and Cardozo et al (1998) suggested that pathways were only tools and only as good as the design and the users, requiring expert clinicians to implement them.

Roebuck (1998) suggested that the degree of change required, including the adoption of a care system incorporating a new nursing perspective, documentation and multidisciplinary teamwork, can be regarded as a disadvantage to using the system.

Pathways have been criticized for being rigid and not individualized, with early literature suggesting that a pathway will only cater for 70–75% of the patient group (Laxade & Hale 1995a). However, the study and the literature have demonstrated that they can be individualized by users (Gearner Thompson 1994, Luther 1995) through acting on variance information (Van Buskirk & Vanderbilt 1995), producing separate or mini-pathways for individual problems and incorporating more flexible time frames for outcomes (Laxade & Hale 1995a).

Pathways have also been described as task orientated (Laxade & Hale 1995a). They are clearly a learning tool and guide for inexperienced nurses and these features actually suit cardiac care which can be quite routine. Without the pathway, if certain key interventions are not carried out by practitioners, problems may not be identified at an early stage and outcomes not achieved. The focus on time management inherent in pathways allows practitioners to spend more time with patients actively waking, weaning and support-

ing them at the bedside. As a result the patients are actively but appropriately moved forward in terms of outcomes. Roebuck (1998) reported that the use of evidence-based pathways and identification of variances for cardiology patients has maintained individualized patient care. The reduction in documentation has allowed nurses to spend more time with patients, resulting in a 90% reduction in complaints.

THE DIFFICULTIES OF OUTCOME-FOCUSED CARE FOR NURSING PRACTICE

Only a handful of authors, such as Jones (1995), Keresztes & Kuruzar (1996) and the current study, have clearly identified potential risks posed by the practices of managed care and fast tracking for nurses. The ICU nurses, including myself, expressed concerns over potential pressure on staff, particularly from the cardiac team, as they tried to achieve the set outcomes.

The nurses expressed feelings of stress, guilt and blame. They were anxious about being criticized or 'found out' if their patient 'failed' to fast track, as demonstrated in these excerpts from a focus group with senior ICU nurses.

The idea of fast tracking is really good but there are elements of stress as well … a lot of medical staff hover around wondering why you haven't managed to get them on the T-piece or extubate, as if it's your fault. (Senior ICU nurse)

… it's far more upsetting for everyone when the people they're supposed to be fast tracking go wrong… (Senior ICU nurse)

The study identified 'calculated risk taking' as a feature of fast tracking with some nurses enjoying the extra pressure and autonomy associated with it. This has to be balanced by clinical judgement and confidence and supported by the pathway and clinical guidelines. The difficulties inherent in managed care need to be addressed during system development. Doran et al (1998) acknowledged the need for organizations to nurture the culture of change so that associated risk taking is supported.

FUTURE CHALLENGES

The future of critical pathways will be directed by the changing needs of patients, including the chronically critically ill and those undergoing new procedures.

Yandell (1995) cautioned against the overuse of pathways and uncertainty initially surrounded their appropriateness for medical and ICU patients whose conditions can be unpredictable (Johnson 1995, Ritter et al 1992). However, with moves toward the integration of standards and clinical guidelines it was inevitable that pathways would be introduced for some critical care groups (Deighan & Hitch 1995, Tingle 1996).

The multidisciplinary project team were more flexible than many units at the time in their inclusion criteria. The only exclusions from the pathway are the small percentage of patients post transmyocardial revascularization (TMR) and a separate pathway is being planned for them in the future. The pathway has now been extended to cover the first 48 hours in the ICU and to include those admitted with an intra-aortic balloon pump (IABP), as suggested by Capuano et al (1999), and those with pulmonary artery (PA) flotation catheters and inotropes. It is also part of an ICP package for the whole stay in hospital.

More recently, pathways have been devised for a wider range of less predictable critical care groups, including trauma patients (Latini 1996, Latini & Foote 1992), patients requiring long-term ventilation (Burns et al 1997), the chronically critically ill (Rudy et al 1995) and organ donors (Holmquist et al 1999). This has encouraged ICU nurses in my trust to develop a pathway for patients with cervical spine injuries. The Heart Hospital in London has included a column headed 'process note' in its pathways. This allows staff, if they wish, to write a *brief* note for a patient who has achieved an outcome but where it may have been difficult with regards to clinical skills, stressful for staff and/or patient or additional staff support was required. The observation charts provide further valuable data. This is a useful example of how a pathway has been adapted to more fully reflect patient care (Hatchett, Gardner, personal communication).

Miller et al (1999) have extended this work to high-risk cardiac patients whose risk for operative morbidity and mortality increases in line with their level of postoperative complications, lengths of ICU stay and requirement for nursing resources. They suggested that these patients, identified using pre-operative risk classification models (Parsonnet et al 1996), can be cared for using 'risk-specific clinical pathways'. These incorporate 'risk-specific treatment plans' to address postoperative complications particular to this group, such as arrhythmias and respiratory insufficiency. The use of risk stratification to select patients for particular pathways may give more accurate information on true variances and therefore the resources required for high-risk patients.

Finally, in the future an increasing number of patients will undergo new cardiac surgical revascularization procedures. These include minimally invasive direct coronary artery bypass surgery (MIDCAB), which avoids the need for cardiopulmonary bypass (Koncsol et al 1999) (see Chapter 29) and trans/percutaneous myocardial revascularization (TMR/PMR). These more recent techniques have their own complications and outcomes which need to be included in pathways.

Case study 30.1

Bob Miller, a 65-year-old man underwent three coronary artery bypass grafts (CABG) and a left internal mammary artery graft (LIMA) with no intra-operative complications. He was admitted to the intensive care unit at 11.30 hours. One variance was recorded: code 4 – cerebral problem – manifested as severe agitation on waking immediately on admission to the ICU. The nurse prioritized her care around assessing readiness to wean and controlling his agitation with some first-hour outcomes, such as the 12-lead ECG, not being achieved. Guidelines in the pathway for administration of analgesia and controlled doses of propofol, along with continuous assessment of sedation and pain levels, allowed the nurse at the bedside to wean Bob while sedated rather than fully resedate and reventilate him. Subsequently, he woke up appropriately and was extubated after 3 hours 10 minutes. He was then discharged to the CHDU after 4 hours 45 minutes. The pathway acted as a reminder to the nurse to ensure that the ECG was performed when appropriate.

Case study 30.2

Jim Weaver, a 62-year-old man, was admitted to the ICU at 16.30 hours following two CABGs and a LIMA graft. No intra-operative complications were recorded but he was administered midazolam in theatre. Seven variances were recorded. Code 1 – 'pain' manifested as a pain-free (recorded as 0 or no pain on the pain score) but overdrowsy patient (recorded as 2 on the score or requiring stimulation to wake) resulting in the PCA being restricted. Code 2 – 'bleeding' manifested as bleeding more than 200 ml in the first hour. Code 5 – 'slow respiratory wean' with Jim requiring respiratory stimulants and a nasal airway until more awake. Code 6 – 'cardiovascular instability' manifested as hypertension requiring glyceryl trinitrate (GTN) and sodium nitroprusside (SNP) infusions. Code 7 – 'other' manifested as nausea. Code 8 – 'nurse availability' recorded as the cardiac recovery unit being short staffed and Jim was not rolled off the canvas within 4 hours of admission. Despite these variances, he was extubated in 4 hours 15 minutes. The focus on active patient management in the pathway encouraged practitioners to continually wake, support and wean him. After early extubation Jim stayed in the cardiac recovery unit (CRU) overnight due to bed shortages (Code 16 – 'CHDU'). Early the next morning the ICU nurses discharged him to CHDU using the discharge criteria on the pathway.

Case study 30.3

Richard Rollings, a 49-year-old man, was admitted to the ICU following one coronary bypass graft and a LIMA graft. Intra-operatively he bled, requiring clotting factors and a Trasylol infusion. He was admitted to ITU at 12 midday. Variances were recorded in order of occurrence. Code 2 – 'bleeding' manifested as blood loss of 400 ml and 200 ml for the first 2 hours of admission. Clotting was rechecked and as it was abnormal, Richard was treated with fresh frozen plasma and platelets and variance re-evaluated as bleeding of 150 ml for the first half of the third hour of admission. Richard was treated with protamine and tranexamic acid, Trasylol continued. Code 7 – 'cardiovascular instability' manifested as hypotension, blood pressure 80/55 mmHg, sinus tachycardia with a rate of 122 bpm, low central venous pressure 2–4 mmHg and requiring blood, blood products and Gelofusine to be transfused. Code 6 – 'slow respiratory wean' due to continued light sedation and ventilation because of bleeding and hypotension. The first-hour outcome of readiness for weaning was not achieved. Richard was transferred to theatre for re-sternotomy at 14.50 hours. He returned to the ICU at 16.00 hours following repair to a leak at the LIMA site and a 'generalized ooze'. He continued to have mild coagulopathy. Variances from the first admission were completed and Richard was restarted on the same pathway again to guide care and outcomes during his second admission. Good progress occurred following the second operation and he was weaned to extubation after 6 hours. Richard was discharged to CHDU the next morning.

CONCLUSION

Van Buskirk & Vanderbilt (1995, p. 66) stated that 'The science of Care Maps ™ is not finished: because of its evolving nature, it never will be'. The long-term success and ongoing development of the managed care project in this study support this view. However, the intensive care phase of the patient's treatment cannot exist in isolation from the rest of their care. The plethora and variety of studies reviewed highlight that managed care can be used at all stages of the cardiac patient's care. Therefore it is essential that managed care should be introduced within a total quality management framework which encompasses all aspects of patient care and all the services involved (Johnson 1995, Van Buskirk & Vanderbilt 1995). This process will promote seamless care from the pre-admission clinics to postdischarge care at home. Most importantly, this will promote multidisciplinary practice and the development of nurses' roles and practice in the move towards clinical effectiveness and shared governance. It is important that all groups keep talking to each other and sharing ideas of implementation. Such implementation does not have to be set in tablets of stone and how units have adapted the pathways to meet their patients' needs should be shared. This will increase the value of the tool and prevent it from becoming a mere paper exercise.

REFERENCES

Anderson J, O'Brien M 1995 Challenges for the future: the nurse's role in weaning patients from mechanical ventilation. Intensive and Critical Care Nursing 11(1): 2–5

Aps C 1995 Fast-tracking in cardiac surgery. British Journal of Hospital Medicine 54(4): 139–142

Baggs JG, Ryan SA, Phelps CE, Richeson JF, Johnson JE 1992 The association between interdisciplinary collaboration and patient outcomes in a medical intensive care unit. Heart and Lung 21(1): 18–24

Benton DC 1995 The role of managed care in overcoming fragmentation. Nursing Times 91(29): 25–27

Bergen A 1992 Case management in community care: concepts, practices and implications for nursing. Journal of Advanced Nursing 17: 1106–1113

Blondin J, Schriefer J, Shinozaki T et al 1996 The Quality Cup winner: Fletcher Allen Health Care's early extubation team. Quality Management in Health Care 4(2): 42–54

Bultema JK, Mailliard L, Getzfrid MK et al 1996 Geriatric patients with depression. Improving outcomes using a multidisciplinary clinical path model. Journal of Nursing Administration 26(1): 31–38

Burns N, Grove SK 1993 The practice of nursing research. Conduct, critique and utilization, 2nd edn. WB Saunders, Philadelphia

Burns SM, Daly B, Tice P 1997 Being led down the critical pathway: a perspective on the importance of care managers vs critical pathways for patients requiring prolonged mechanical ventilation. Critical Care Nurse 17(6): 70–75

Cameron F 1994 Models of specialist practice. In: Humphris D (ed) The clinical nurse specialist: issues in practice. Macmillan, Basingstoke, pp. 16–28

Capuano TA, Sullivan K, Rothenberger C et al 1999 A benchmark project to improve cost and quality outcomes for CABG patients. Dimensions of Critical Care Nursing 18(1): 36–43

Cardozo L, Aherns S, Steinberg J et al 1998 Implementing a clinical pathway for congestive heart failure: experiences at a teaching hospital. Quality Management in Health Care 7(1): 1–12

Carr W, Kemmis S 1986 Becoming critical: education, knowledge and action research. Falmer Press, London

Coffey RJ, Othman JE, Walters JI 1995 Extending the application of critical path methods. Quality Management in Health Care 3(2): 14–29

Cohen EL, Cesta TG 1997 Nursing case management: from concept to evaluation, 2nd edn. Mosby Year-Book, St Louis, pp. 12–16

Deighan M, Hitch S (eds) 1995 Clinical effectiveness from guidelines to cost-effective practice. Health Services Management Unit. Earlybrave Publications, Essex

Del Togno-Armanasco V, Olivas G, Harter S 1989 Developing an integrated nursing case management model. Nursing Management 20(10): 26–29

Department of Health 1989 Working for patients. HMSO, London

Doran KA, Henry SA, Anderson BJ 1998 Breakthrough change for adult cardiac surgery in a community-based cardiovascular program. Quality Management in Health Care 6(4): 29–36

Dukes Crawley W, Till AH 1995 Case management: more population based data. Clinical Nurse Specialist 9(2): 116–120

Dunstan JL, Riddle MM 1997 Rapid recovery management: the effects on the patient who has undergone heart surgery. Heart and Lung 26(4): 289–298

Edwards D, Hess L 1996 Aggressive weaning in cardiac surgical patients. Dimensions of Critical Care Nursing 15(4): 181–186

Eisenberg AA, Redick EL 1998 Transsphenoidal resection of pituitary adenoma: using a critical pathway. Dimensions of Critical Care Nursing 17(6): 306–312

Ethridge P, Lamb GS 1989 Professional nursing case management improves quality, access, and costs. Nursing Management 20(3): 30–35

Farley K 1995 The COPD critical pathway: a case study in progress. Quality Management in Health Care 3(2): 43–54

Fawcett-Hensey A 1995 Is managed care for nursing too? Journal of Nursing Management 3: 219–220

Field PA, Morse JM 1985 Nursing research: the application of qualitative approaches. Croom Helm, London

Flynn AM, Kilgallen ME 1993 Case management: a multidisciplinary approach to the evaluation of cost and quality standards. Journal of Nursing Care Quality 8(1): 58–66

Gearner Thompson D 1994 Critical pathways: good idea, right reason? Critical Care Nurse 14(6): 112

Girard N 1994 The case management model of patient care delivery. Association of Operating Room Nurses Journal (AORNJ) 60(3): 403–415

Goodwin DR 1994 Nursing case management activities. How they differ between employment settings. Journal of Nursing Administration 24(2): 29–34

Gross P 1995 Managed care: the perfect package. Health Service Journal 105: 20–23

Guba E, Lincoln Y 1985 Effective evaluation. Jossey-Bass, London

Haffer A 1986 Facilitating change: choosing the appropriate strategy. Journal of Nursing Administration 16: 18–22

Hampton DC 1993 Implementing a managed care framework through care maps. Journal of Nursing Administration 23(5): 21–27

Hart E, Bond M 1995 Action research for health and social care. A guide to practice. Open University Press, Buckingham

Hassaballa H, Payne J, McFolling S, Marder RJ 1998 Enhancing clinical pathway placement. Quality Management in Health Care 7(1): 13–17

Henry L, Duffy J 1995 A cardiovascular intensive care nursing staff response to managed care: a change in practice. Critical Care Nursing Quarterly 18(3): 28–35

Higgins TL 1992 Pro: early endotracheal extubation is preferable to late extubation in patients undergoing coronary artery surgery. Journal of Cardiothoracic and Vascular Anaesthesia 6(4): 488–493

Holmquist M, Chabalewski F, Blount T 1999 A critical pathway: guiding the care for organ donors. Critical Care Nurse 19(2): 84–98

Holter IM, Schwartz-Barcott D 1993 Action research: what is it? How has it been used and how can it be used in nursing? Journal of Advanced Nursing 18: 298–304

Howard C 1995 Fast-track care after cardiac surgery. British Journal of Nursing 4(19): 1112–1117

Hunt M 1987 The process of translating research findings into nursing practice. Journal of Advanced Nursing 12: 101–110

Johnson ND 1992 Collaboration – an environment for optimal outcome. Critical Care Nursing Quarterly 15(3): 37–43

Johnson S 1995 Pathway to the heart of care quality. Nursing Management 1(8): 26–27

Johnson S, Smith J 2000 Factors influencing the success of ICP projects. Professional Nurse 15(12): 776–779

Jones A 1995 An analysis of case management – the efficient utility of human resources, but to what end? Journal of Nursing Management 3: 143–149

Kelly KC 1992 Managing care: a search for role clarity. Journal of Nursing Administration. 22(3): 9–10

Keresztes PA, Kuruzar L 1996 Very early extubation: extubating in the OR following coronary artery bypass. Dimensions of Critical Care Nursing 14(4): 198–204

Koncsol K, De Voogd K, Hravnak M, Zenati M 1999 Minimally invasive coronary artery bypass grafting: a kinder cut. Dimensions of Critical Care Nursing 18(2): 21–23

Kramer M 1990 The magnet hospitals: excellence revisited. Journal of Nursing Administration 20: 35–44

Latini EE 1996 Trauma critical pathways: a care delivery system that works. Critical Care Nursing Quarterly 19(1): 83–87

Latini EE, Foote W 1992 Obtaining consistent quality patient care for the trauma patient by using a critical pathway. Critical Care Nursing Quarterly 15(3): 51–55

Laxade S, Hale CA 1995a Managed care 1: an opportunity for nursing. British Journal of Nursing 4(5): 290–294

Laxade S, Hale CA 1995b Managed care 2: an opportunity for nursing. British Journal of Nursing 4(6): 345–350

Leclair D 1991 Introducing and accounting for RN case management. Nursing Management 22(3): 44–49

Ley J 1995 Putting critical pathways on the map. Critical Care Nurse 15(3): 106–113

Light DW 1994 Managed care: false and real solutions. Lancet 344: 1197–1199

Lorentzon M 1995 Multidisciplinary collaboration: life line or drowning pool for nurse researchers? Journal of Advanced Nursing 22: 825–826

Luther T 1995 Report of a pilot managed care project in neurosciences. Royal Hospitals Trust, London

Luther T, Crofts L 1997 Managed care: integrated care pathways in neurosciences. Nursing Progress: Royal Hospitals NHS Trust Journal 1: 5–10

Lutjens LFJ 1995 Determinants of hospital length of stay. Journal of Nursing Administration 25(4): 14

MacGuire JM 1990 Putting nursing research findings into practice: research utilization as an aspect of the management of change. Journal of Advanced Nursing 15: 614–620

Marr JA, Reid B 1992 Implementing managed care and case management: the neuroscience experience. Journal of Neuroscience Nursing 24(5): 281–285

Massey D, Meggit G 1994 Recovery units: the future of postoperative cardiac care. Intensive and Critical Care Nursing 10: 71–74

Maxam-Moore VA, Goedecke RS 1996 The development of an early extubation algorithm for patients after cardiac surgery. Heart and Lung 25(1): 61–68

McGovern W, Rodgers JA 1986 Change theory. American Journal of Nursing 86: 566–567

Mechanic D, Aiken LH 1982 A cooperative agenda for medicine and nursing. New England Journal of Medicine 307: 747–750

Meyer JE 1995 Lay participation in care in a hospital setting: an action research study. Unpublished PhD thesis. University of London, London

Micheels TA, Wheeler LM, Hays BJ 1995 Linking quality and cost effectiveness: case management by an advanced practice nurse. Clinical Nurse Specialist 9(2): 107–111

Miles MB, Huberman A 1984 Qualitative data analysis. A source book of new methods. Sage, London

Miller J, Newton V, Havercroft J 1995 Nursing patients through 'pathways of care'. Professional Nurse 10(12): 759–762

Miller KH, Gatson Grindel C, Patsdaughter CA 1999 Risk classification, clinical outcomes, and the use of nursing resources for cardiac surgery patients. Dimensions of Critical Care Nursing 18(2): 44–49

Mosher C, Cronk P, Kidd A et al 1992 Upgrading practice with critical pathways. American Journal of Nursing 92(1): 41–44

Moyer JA 1994 Factors related to length of ICU stay for CABG patients. Dimensions of Critical Care Nursing 13(4): 194–200

Newman B 1995 Enhancing patient case management and critical pathways. Australian Journal of Advanced Nursing 13(1): 17–25

Nolan M, Grant G 1993 Action research and quality of care: a mechanism for agreeing basic values as a precursor to change. Journal of Advanced Nursing 18: 305–311

O'Malley J 1992 Future directions: managing the cost–quality paradigm. Critical Care Nursing Quarterly 15(3): 80–85

Packham R 1990 Making room for recovery. Nursing Times 86(40): 74–75

Parsonnet V, Bernstein AD, Gera M 1996 Clinical usefulness of risk stratified outcome analysis in cardiac surgery in New Jersey. Annals of Thoracic Surgery 61: S8–11

Reason P 1988 Human inquiry in action: developments in new paradigm research. Sage, London

Reason P, Rowan J 1981 Human inquiry: a sourcebook of new paradigm research. John Wiley, Chichester

Redick EL, Stroud AR, Kurack TB 1994 Expanding the use of critical pathways in critical care. Dimensions of Critical Care Nursing 13(6): 316–321

Riches T, Stead L, Espie C 1994 Introducing anticipated recovery pathways: a teaching hospital experience. International Journal of Health Care Quality Assurance 7(3): 21–24

Riddle MM, Dunstan JL, Castanis JL 1996 A rapid recovery program for cardiac surgery patients. American Journal of Critical Care 5(2): 152–159

Riley J 1990 Getting the most from your data. A handbook of practical ideas on how to analyse qualitative data. Technical and Educational Services, Bristol

Ritter J, Fralic MF, Tonges MC, McCormac M 1992 Redesigned nursing practice: a case management model for critical care. Nursing Clinics of North America 27(1): 119–128

Roebuck A 1998 Critical pathways: an aid to practice. Nursing Times 94(35): 50–51

Royal College of Nursing Institute 1998 Directory of UK NHS trusts using care pathways. RCN Institute, Oxford

Rudy EB, Daly BJ, Douglas S et al 1995 Patient outcomes for the chronically critically ill: special care unit versus intensive care unit. Nursing Research 44(6): 324–331

Schriefer J 1994 A winning combination – critical pathways and clinical algorithms. Quality Management in Health Care 2(1): 22

Schriefer J 1995 Managing critical pathway variances. Quality Management in Health Care 3(2): 30–42

Scott ML 1996 Evaluating the implementation of managed care for cardiac fast-track patients in an intensive therapy unit: an action research study. Unpublished MSc thesis. University of London, London

Scully G, Nichols S 1990 Case management: a compilation of definitions. Case Management October: 42–44

Shiell A, Kenny P, Farnworth MG 1993 The role of the clinical nurse co-ordinator in the provision of cost-effective orthopaedic services for elderly people. Journal of Advanced Nursing 18: 1424–1428

Shulkin DJ, Harris CM 1996 Coordinating initiatives in critical pathways and information systems. Quality Management in Health Care 4(2): 37–41

Tingle J 1996 Clinical guidelines: risk management and legal issues. British Journal of Nursing 5(5): 266–267

Van Buskirk MC, Vanderbilt D 1995 Evaluating patient care by the use of a diabetic ketoacidosis CareMap (TM) in an intensive care unit setting. Journal of Nursing Care Quality 9(3): 59–68

Webb C 1989 Action research: philosophy, methods and personal experiences. Journal of Advanced Nursing 14: 403–410

Wigfield A, Boon E 1996 Critical care pathway development: the way forward. British Journal of Nursing 5(12): 732–735

Yandell B 1995 Critical paths at Alliant Health System. Quality Management in Health Care 3(2): 55–64

Zander K 1987 Nursing case management: a classic. Definition 2(2): 1–3

Zander K 1988 Nursing case management: strategic management of cost and quality outcomes. Journal of Nursing Administration 18(5): 23–30

Zander K 1990 Managed care and nursing case management. In: Mayer GG, Madden MJ, Lawrenz E (eds) Patient care delivery models. Aspen Publishers, Rockville, MD, pp. 37–61

Zander K 1991 What's new in managed care and case management. The New Definition 6(2): 1–2

Zander K 1992 Quantifying, managing and improving quality: 1. How care maps link CQI to the patient. The New Definition 7(2): 1–3

Zevola DR, Maier B 1999 Improving the care of cardio-thoracic surgery patients through advanced nursing skills. Critical Care Nurse 19(1): 34–44

Zevola DR, Raffa M, Brown K et al 1997 Clinical pathways and coronary artery bypass surgery. Critical Care Nurse 17(6): 20–33

31

The future of cardiac nursing

Stuart Jones
Catherine Rimmer
Richard Hatchett

In looking to what the future may hold for cardiac nursing, one needs to take stock of where we are now and how we have arrived at this point. The previous chapters have addressed the amazing progress in the care of the cardiac patient over recent years. This includes the more invasive techniques now used by cardiologists, developments in technology and the refinements in surgery. The increased use of angioplasty and stenting, the development of internal cardioverter defibrillators (ICDs) for life-threatening arrhythmias and the utilization of surgical techniques performed without the clinical risk of the bypass machine are further examples. This latter development for coronary revascularization has, in some techniques, removed the need for a sternotomy, thereby reducing the physical limitations a patient experiences when recovering from surgery. It also aims to reduce the length of inpatient stay as compared to conventional bypass surgery (Shiono & Sezai 1998). The advent of early extubation protocols (fast tracking) and the development of high-dependency units (HDUs) have given an additional impetus to this progress.

These advances in medical and surgical procedures not only have great implications for nursing practice in the future but also carry notable significance for the patient and their significant others. Such changing care requirements require nurses in all areas of cardiac care to adapt their knowledge base and skills and inevitably their role. Indeed, from a nursing perspective, nurse-led clinics and the consultant nurse roles are both more recent examples of innovative methods of health-care provision that recognize a chronic, rather than a curable health experience. Such changes mean that nursing staff need to maintain a personal philosophy of updating in their practice and education.

Glen & Clark (1999) argue that modern nurse training has led to a perceived lack of skills and confidence. The ever-present practice/theory gap may have widened, a situation which can be addressed in part by utilizing structured in-house education to augment the services of the university system. To facilitate these learning needs within cardiac nursing, the role of the lecturer/practitioner or clinical facilitator could be envisaged. The role is a promising way forward and its development in cardiac nursing can provide both practical support and education for new and existing staff (Smith 1997). However, for this role to be a success, support is required from both service and education and the role has to be well defined to avoid work overload (Wright 1988).

Current nurse education aims to encourage and empower nurse students to take responsibility for their own learning, while the teacher has a duty to provide and facilitate appropriate learning and training activities, with feedback and support (McManus & Sieler 1998). This self-responsibility and facilitative approach are vital if learning is to be encouraged as an ongoing process. There is a recognized increased pressure for qualified nursing to be a graduate profession (Munro 1999) but it is essential that the learning activities are relevant to the work environment and tailored accordingly.

Parsons (1998) cited the level of education, meaning accessibility and appropriateness to role, as a measure of job satisfaction amongst nursing staff, along with task variety. One way to increase this element of variety would be to introduce rotation within the specialized area. This could include cardiac surgery, coronary care, cardiology and the angiography department. This may also empower staff to have a more informed approach to patient care through experiential learning. Perhaps the broader knowledge and experience developed on rotation will also assist nurses to use admission and discharge procedures as an initial impetus for health promotion. In addition, rotation and the achievement of objectives within those areas may fulfil expected role competencies or be used via appraisal as the move to the next nursing grade.

The shortening of inpatient stay will reduce the nurse's already limited time for psychological care of the patient and their family or carers. There is a danger of the two-way therapeutic relationship between patient and nurse being lost in the constant endeavour to increase patient throughput. In some hospitals cardiac liaison teams, who provide information, education and support both pre- and postoperatively, are countering this.

When considering the above points, it should be realized that in the future people suffering from heart disease will spend most of their time outside the hospital setting. Even following acute episodes of treatment, such as cardiac surgery, patients are being discharged much earlier. This, in addition to the need for more rehabilitation and health education, argues for more supportive services. It is imperative that greater links are forged between the hospital environment and the primary health-care setting, a situation which traditionally has not been the case. However, there are already some tenuous links via the aforementioned cardiac liaison teams that continue to monitor patients after their discharge.

One of the earliest of these liaison services designed for the support and care of cardiac surgery patients was set up at Manchester Royal Infirmary by Sister Anne Porter. This was initiated through recognition that the needs of patients and their families were not being met after discharge. The service has since provided information and support to patients from the time of being placed on the waiting list to pre-admission clinics, through the postoperative period and then postdischarge support, for as long as the patients require it. Many tertiary cardiac centres provide some level of cardiac liaison service although others, despite the research demonstrating the importance of information provision (Mitchell 1997, Speechley 1989, Teasdale 1995) and support, continue not to do so.

At the present time, the service primarily provided by cardiac liaison teams is in the form of pre-admission clinics. The aims of these clinics are fourfold.

• They provide information about the impending admission, in order to meet patient and carer psychological and physical needs. Mitchell (1997) believes that by offering preparatory information at a level that matches individual coping style, anxiety levels can be reduced. By reducing patient anxiety, a less expensive recovery has been demonstrated in certain forms of surgery (Hough et al 1991).

• They enquire into social circumstances, so enabling patients to begin making suitable provisions following discharge. It also allows staff time to start making appropriate requests to social services or health authorities regarding funding for care packages. In some teams, this assessment is also being carried out in the form of a questionnaire, which is sent out prior to the pre-admission clinic. Appropriate discharge planning is essential not only on humanitarian grounds but, as Alderman (1997) states, with proactive planning, patient throughput can be increased and the length of inpatient stay decreased.

• Appropriate pre-operative investigations can be undertaken at this clinic. Early identification of problematic results means there is opportunity to rectify them or to order other appropriate investigations and treatments, for example, carotid studies or dental checks. This will ensure patients are in an improved physical state of health prior to surgery. In addition, Worley (1986) claims that patients who attend a pre-admission clinic are likely to have fewer postoperative complications. Alternatively, if they are discovered not to be a suitable candidate for surgery at this time, there is opportunity to prepare another patient and valuable surgery time is not wasted (Livingstone et al 1993).

• Such clinics also provide an opportunity to begin identifying a patient's heart disease risk factors. Although this may not be the ideal place to address risk factors or commence health education, the situation may still lend itself to this. Within our own cardiac liaison team, we have learned never to assume that if a patient is a diabetic, taking antihypertensive or cholesterol-reducing medication, that they necessarily understand the implications for heart disease. Haddock & Burrows (1997) believe that even a 10-minute intervention in surgical pre-admission clinics may be a trigger for those with no intention to stop smoking to think about stopping and to work towards improving their health. Early identification of predisposing factors assists in tailoring postoperative advice to the individual's needs.

As this text has demonstrated, achieving a healthier lifestyle is a positive step in reducing morbidity and mortality from coronary heart disease. A study by Smith & Smith (1994) highlights the importance of lifestyles and behaviours being tackled as a whole, rather than as single behaviours, in order for health promotion activities to be effective. This must become an integral component of the service provided for cardiac patients and emphasized at primary, secondary and tertiary levels.

The desired general outcomes of the pre-admission clinics are that the patient and family are both physically and psychologically more appropriately prepared for the treatment and that medical, nursing and social interventions can be planned in advance. This may include recognizing the need to optimize medication before surgery through to preplanning social services for ultimate discharge. These preparations are significant influences in reduced hospital stays (Newton 1996, Worley 1986).

Cardiac liaison teams in many hospitals also provide the back-up or support services after discharge. The provision of individual information, advice and support is invaluable in decreasing patient anxiety (Huerta-Torres 1998), as patients can find surgery particularly stressful in a condensed hospital stay. The service utilizes qualified and experienced nurses to assess the physical and emotional capabilities of the patient and their carers, so that an informed decision can be made as to whether a patient is suitable for an early discharge. Patients who have been educated as to what to expect after discharge may find the transition between home and hospital a little easier (Huerta-Torres 1998). When giving advice and instructions for home, the inclusion of family members or carers is useful in clarifying misconceptions and assists in decreasing anxieties about managing at home following discharge.

Occasionally the views of the cardiac liaison nurse and those of the medical staff may differ, especially in regard to discharge. The patient may be medically fit for home yet the liaison nurse, with a much broader insight into how patients and families cope after discharge, together with a knowledge of the individual patient and their condition, may recognize problems. This may potentially necessitate an extended inpatient stay. The doctors' experience of the patient will mainly be in the context of their hospital stay and they may know little about the individual's family circumstances and potential problems. However, with the constraints and changes within modern health care, there has to be greater collaboration between nursing and medical staff in the future (Fagin 1992).

The discrepancies in authority between the multidisciplinary roles are beginning to be met by the formalization of treatment plans, such as critical/integrated care pathways. These provide a structured plan of treatment and set goals that a patient has to meet before discharge (see Chapter 30). Huerta-Torres (1998) claims that an advantage of this is that often when patients know they are progressing satisfactorily and according to plan, compliance with treatments and activities increases. The role of the cardiac liaison nurse is defined within this plan and a patient's discharge is conditional on their authority and satisfactory discharge arrangements.

One area where the use of critical pathways is particularly pertinent is in the increasing number of short-stay programmes that are developing. The programme involves selection criteria covering both medical and social factors, agreed by medical and nursing staff. Once on the programme, patients follow a pathway aimed at reducing hospital stay, targeting a discharge date of 3–4 days postoperatively.

This service provides community pre-admission education, as well as the option of initial regular home visits if appropriate. As it is reported that patient care and education is most fragmented when moving between the community, hospital and back to the community (Robinson & Hill 1999), their integration should assist in improving patient care. These pathways require input from the multidisciplinary team and so the decision to discharge a patient is very much a collaborative effort.

Several studies have examined early discharge programmes (Donald 1995, Hollingsworth et al 1993, Knowleden et al 1991) and one benefit they appear to demonstrate is an earlier recovery rate. Other potential benefits of shorter inpatient stay include a reduction in the incidence of hospital-acquired infection, shorter waiting lists and more efficient use of acute hospital beds (Clarke 1997).

It is imperative that patients who are selected for short-stay programmes but who then do not meet the requirements for discharge as planned are well supported and not made to feel as if they have failed. This task is often left to the nursing staff as they spend more time with the patients, and specifically to the cardiac liaison nurses, who will have been involved in the initial selection process and who maintain contact with the patient after discharge. However, there is undoubtedly an inequality in the services for patients simply because of the distance they live from the hospital. This inequality may affect whether they are invited to a pre-admission clinic or whether they have a home visit from the aforementioned support services. In some cases this has left liaison teams feeling unable to offer some patients any form of visit.

The cardiac liaison teams form part of the emerging nurse-led clinics that are growing within both cardiac and other specialties. Such clinics by definition facilitate increased nurse autonomy in practice, that is, away from direct medical dominance. The nurses do work as part of a multidisciplinary team but accept direct referrals and manage their own caseload of patients. They tend to operate in the community within general practitioner (GP) practices or as part of outpatient services reviewing, educating and adjusting medication with patients. The latter issue of adjusting medication has more recently been enhanced by the first report of the Crown Committee (Crown Report 1998). This Department of Health document called for nurses to adjust medication within multidisciplinary agreed protocols (patient group directions). In fact, it is formalizing what has been happening to a lesser or greater extent for many years.

More recently, the Crown Committee's second report discussed the issue of nurse prescribing, through independent and dependent prescribers (NHS Executive 1999). The former group would be responsible for assessing the patient's condition, devising a treatment plan and prescribing as part of that plan. The latter would encompass those prescribing for patients whose condition had been diagnosed by an independent pre-

scriber. The report was not restricted to nurses alone but also extended to other groups such as specialist physiotherapists and chiropodists. Within the nursing profession, specific groups were identified and included specialist diabetic and asthma nurses. Cardiac nurses were not included at that time. The government received the report favourably, with its suggestion of a new prescribers advisory committee where members of the particular groups could apply for the appropriate prescriber status. Such an advancement has huge implications for nurse education, if safe and appropriate practice is to be maintained.

More recently, consultation between various interested professional bodies and the Department of Health has occurred, regarding how nurse prescribing can be safely and effectively extended (Department of Health (DoH) 2000a). The Secretary of State Alan Milburn announced funding of £10 million between 2001 and 2004 to support education and training to this end. Certain groups of nurses will be able to prescribe to a revised nurses' formulary, following specialist education. Rather like the original formulary designed for practitioners such as district nurses and health visitors, the aim is to increase the services to patients rather than to enhance the professional status of any one occupation.

There is a growing but still relatively small amount of literature exploring the breadth of services that nurse-led clinics offer. This may include health promotion advice, monitoring and adjustment of drugs such as warfarin and quite simply explaining and offering psychological support. However, there has been limited exploration of the professional issues and the power balance between varying health-care disciplines and managers that have allowed the services to succeed. Other issues of importance include the current lack of specific education pathways for nurse-led practice because such developments must encompass the issue of public protection. A suggested educational pathway may incorporate a broad base including legal issues and divide into the various specific elements such as cardiac, diabetes, family planning, etc.

Many nurses do appear to be practising competently within nurse-led clinics so education planning within such a pathway must analyse how knowledge and skills have been acquired in the practice area. Assessment may include examination which takes a case study analytical approach, assessment within the clinics such as of physical examination, reflective diaries highlighting case histories and decisions taken, as well as the more familiar testing of specific pharmacological and physiological knowledge. Of concern in an era of nurse shortages is that many experienced cardiac nurses may be taken away from the bedside to run such clinics. In addition, the effects on other colleagues, such as the potential for deskilling junior doctors, may be an issue of concern. However, such a career pathway may keep skilled nurses in practice by maintaining motivation through the provision of a career pathway and further remuneration. Such nurses are then available to teach more junior staff and to hone their own skills.

In regard to wider issues, the National Service Framework for Coronary Heart Disease was released in March 2000 to much publicity (DoH 2000b). This was under the broad initiative of clinical governance and is based upon concerns regarding the need to improve and, importantly, standardize the quality of cardiac services available to the public. The framework sets out a 10-year programme designed to achieve the target of reducing heart disease and cerebral vascular accident by 40% by 2010 (Mayor 2000). Twelve standards were identified for the prevention, diagnosis and treatment of coronary heart disease. The National Institute for Clinical Excellence (NICE) is the specific body producing clinical guidance products, many of which focus upon the treatment of specific conditions. The aim is to bring together all the evidence relating to the various available treatment options. Such guidance can be regarded as a summation of the state of knowledge on a particular condition at a particular time (NHS Executive 2000).

The NICE also has the role of appraising existing interventions, as well as offering guidance on new treatments. In relation to the latter, the government stated that frequently there appeared differing judgements and interpretation regarding the significance of evidence, resulting in variations in access for patients. In relation to the existing interventions, the most significant are being appraised by the NICE, particularly where there appear to be wide differences in clinical practice or inappropriate use (NHS Executive 2000).

The government provided £50m in funding to launch the programme and specific targets were set including the 8-minute response time for ambulances in 75% of emergency calls. This is an attempt to reduce the still variable 'call to needle time' in thrombolysis therapy and the slow access to defibrillation. The increased numbers of defibrillators in public places highlighted in the previous White Paper *Our healthier nation* (DoH 1999) was reiterated in the framework. The aim, by April 2002, was to ensure that 75% of eligible patients received thrombolysis within 30 minutes of arrival at hospital. Some could have argued that this was still a long time but the framework had to take account of all the varying structures

in place that would require alteration or enhancement to meet the targets.

Clinical guidelines were also incorporated and included the clear push for the improved use of known effective medications following, for example, myocardial infarction and for patients with angina. In the former these were notably aspirin, β-blockers and statins. Although the framework has been a concerted effort to equalize good standards of practice and service across the country, an astute nurse or observer will note that, inevitably, the medical profession will always be somewhat resistant to any form of control regarding clinical decisions. However, the framework, although recommending drug dosages and treatments for particular cardiac events, does provide broad statements such as 'patients with acute myocardial infarction should usually receive the following, unless contra-indicated' (DoH 2000b, ch. 3). The framework is a positive development for nurses in that good practice guidelines can justify decisions and care delivered, particularly in the more autonomous nurse-led clinics. Guidelines do not, however, take the place of astute clinical judgement and good educational preparation. Ultimately, the framework will lead to adaptation of the cardiac nurse's role into various guises to implement and achieve the targets and this should make fuller and more satisfying use of current academic preparation.

The consultation document *The new NHS: modern, dependable* (NHS Executive 1998, p. 4) sets a specific target to provide 'fair access to health services in relation to people's needs, irrespective of geography, socio-economic group, ethnicity, age or sex'. In some areas of the country this is being partially tackled by consultants attending outreach clinics at smaller referring hospitals, who are also taking the initiative to establish their own cardiac liaison service. The development of these services has been achieved in response to the need for more locally based resources (NHS Executive 1998).

Another initiative which assists in providing equality for patients in requesting advice are telephone helplines. This is a service which will no doubt increase over the coming years (Williams et al 1995). Further evidence of the advantages of telephone helplines are highlighted by Keeling & Dennison (1995). Their study examined a follow-up nurse-initiated telephone service for post myocardial infarct (MI) patients, following predischarge contact. Benefits included occasion to reinforce health education, answer questions about physical problems, provide emotional and psychological care and opportunity to refer onto other appropriate agencies, such as social workers. Research into nurse-led telephone consultations in the primary care sector has shown them to be as effective as surgery/health centre consultations in meeting patients' and carers' needs (Marklund et al 1991). The helplines do, however, leave those with communication problems, for example those without a telephone, the deaf or some ethnic minorities, at a disadvantage (Payne 1998). It is believed that in health care 60% of information is given by visual clues, such as pallor, posture and demeanour (Crouch 1998), indicating that those monitoring the helplines will require special skills in order to provide a safe and effective service.

To reduce some of the limitations of telephone helplines, it could be envisaged that with the reforms in the way GPs purchase care, such as through primary care groups (PCGs), a specialist cardiac nursing support service could be established. On many occasions the specialist nurse post is initially funded by research charities, with this eventually being taken over by the employer once the role is established (Wilson-Barnett 1992). This is presently the case with the British Heart Foundation cardiac liaison nurse posts.

The UKCC consultation document *A higher level of practice* (UKCC 1998) states that there should be an increased emphasis on delivering care in the user's own locality and this can be fulfilled by specialist cardiac nurses attached to a GP's surgery. A system of community-orientated cardiac specialist nurses would also achieve some equity, so that no matter how far away from a specialist centre the patient lived, there would still be specialized knowledge at a local level. Essentially this is a further example of nurse-led practice and could reduce the pressure on the GP by potentially providing another source who could refer patients back to the hospital setting if necessary. 'Today the shift towards a primary care led NHS, and other health and social policy changes, plus technological advances and increases in scientific knowledge, demand that the professions develop in new ways' (UKCC 1997, p. 2).

Beyond this, health education could also be provided not only to the patient and their family or loved ones but in a wider context to the community as a whole. If initiatives are introduced at a local level, then hopefully messages regarding a healthier lifestyle will have a greater impact. Specialist nurses working in a local area would be much more aware of relevant issues relating to heart disease and may be able to help communities make changes earlier by planning or lobbying. They are also well placed to aid changes in health knowledge and behaviour, because in order to achieve significant health promotion outcomes, long-term planning and support is required (Robinson & Hill 1999). It is rarely possible to achieve this during hospitalization.

Inroads are being made into the reduction of heart disease (National Audit Office 1996), but it still remains the largest cause of premature death in this country (DoH 1999). Improvements in this area were highlighted as a key target for the government's health plans in *Saving lives: our healthier nation* (DoH 1999).

In Manchester, a scheme has been organized to follow up patients after a cardiac event. On discharge from hospital, information regarding the patient is sent to the GP. This includes risk factors for heart disease. These patients are then visited by the GP or district nurse and advice is offered not only to the patient but also to the family regarding healthy lifestyles. The aim is to set up a register of coronary heart disease patients and audit patient management, in order to improve primary and secondary prevention in this area.

Despite such incentives and the increasing number of treatments available for cardiac conditions, it is essential to remember that none of these presents a long-term cure and that cardiac disease is a chronic condition. In an ideal world, through long-term health education, people would examine their risk factors, modify their lifestyle and the number of patients requiring hospitalization would perhaps reduce. However, measures beyond health education will be required in order to make significant long-term impacts on the reduction of coronary heart disease.

This chapter would not be complete without reflecting on *The scope of professional practice*, the significant document released by the UKCC in 1992. It emphasized the need for individual practitioners to reflect on their own practice and knowledge base and to 'honestly acknowledge any limits of personal knowledge and skill and take steps to remedy any relevant deficits in order effectively and appropriately to meet the needs of patients and clients'. The scope reflected on the previous practice of demarcating specialist skills as 'extended roles', which appeared to limit rather than extend the parameters of practice. Appropriate education and assessment are always at the forefront of practice but the document allowed cardiac nurses, in particular, to reflect on the nursing service and highlight to managers that we could be more innovative and educate ourselves more appropriately to meet patient needs.

Beyond cardiac nursing itself, the early chapters within this book highlighted *The Black Report* released in 1980 (Townsend et al 1992). This commented on the differences in mortality and morbidity from all major disease between the social classes. Primarily, it demonstrated the poorer health experience of lower occupational class groups and that this applied at all stages of life. Such inequalities appeared to widen in the 1980s, demonstrated in the publication of *The health divide* in 1987, updated in 1992 (Townsend et al 1992), and more recently in *Saving lives: our healthier nation* (DoH 1999). It has also been recognized that inequalities in social environments lead to variations in health and life expectancy, again with those in the lower social classes faring worse (DoH 1995). Poverty can lead to difficulty in making the best decisions regarding health and Blackburn (1991) suggests that as well as the physical effects of poverty there are also the psychological effects, which can lead to health-damaging actions such as smoking. Despite a reduction in the overall number of people smoking and the evidence of its detriment to health (DoH 1998), certain groups continue to smoke and it is estimated to account for a fifth of all deaths in the UK (Poulter et al 1996).

Another area that can be affected by poverty is diet, with an agreement that the UK population has a generally unhealthy diet (Cadman & Wiles 1996). This includes too much fat, sugar and salt and insufficient amounts of fibre, vitamins and minerals. The growing fast food industry and the enormous amount of media advertising of these products do not assist people in this consumer age to eat more healthily (Hitchings & Moynihan 1998). The National Children's Home (1991) stated that a healthy diet costs 17% more than an unhealthy one and research shows that children's diets remain high in fat and sugar (Adamson et al 1992). This is particularly relevant when it is known that eating habits are formed in early life (Lamb & Sissons Joshi 1996).

In addition, while these risk factors are present, it is also unlikely that the incidence of diabetes will decrease, a recognized risk factor for heart disease (Poulter et al 1996). The government has now accepted the links between poverty and ill health (Inside Track 1999) and is beginning to address the issues surrounding this by the introduction of health action zones, to target local areas where inequalities in health are particularly pronounced. This encourages innovative approaches and has involved programmes to increase awareness of low-cost healthy food, resource centres for young mothers and healthy schools schemes (Inside Track 1999). In addition, for the first time in Britain, a minister specifically for public health is in post. In linking care provision to the community we serve, the launch of the NICE should also assist in standardizing practice throughout the country.

This chapter has attempted to demonstrate that health is a dynamic concept requiring many varied and innovative approaches if it is to be optimized. Yet as we are all aware, only when all risk areas are more fully addressed will future generations benefit, but for the foreseeable future heart disease is here to stay. At the grass-roots level, nurses involved in the care of the cardiac patient must ensure that they rise to the challenge of this innovative and holistic care. There is a need to keep pace with the technological advances and our increasing knowledge of the concepts of health and ill health. In the final link, as individuals and in our multidisciplinary care teams we need to review and adapt our practice accordingly. This is not only through an increasing knowledge base but through the evaluation of how varying disciplines can cross traditional barriers in care provision to speed service access, more adequately monitor treatments and provide full support and information. If nursing innovations are to survive and also be used to raise the professional status of nursing, then appropriate auditing must be instigated to show clearly our value in the health-care arena. In addition, evidence-based practice will augment this approach by demonstrating a structured and logical approach to health-care needs. The ultimate aim should not be an overwhelming protection of our knowledge or hierarchies but to meet the cardiac patient's, carer's and society's needs in an era of chronic ill health.

REFERENCES

Adamson AJ, Rugg-Gunn AJ, Appleton DR, Butler TJ, Hackett AF 1992 Dietary sources of energy, protein, unavailable carbohydrate and fat in 11–12 year-old English children in 1990 compared with results in 1980. Journal of Human Nutrition and Dietetics 5: 371–385

Alderman C 1997 Anticipating anxiety (interview with H Walsgrove). Nursing Standard 12(1): 22–23

Blackburn C 1991 Poverty and health, working with families. Open University Press, Buckingham

Cadman L, Wiles R 1996 Nutrition advice in primary care: evaluation of practice nurse nutrition training programmes. Journal of Human Nutrition and Dietetics 9(2): 147–156

Clarke A 1997 Benefits and drawbacks of hospital-at-home schemes. Professional Nurse 12(10): 734–736

Crouch R 1998 Between the lines. Nursing Standard 12(28): 22–23

Crown Report 1998 A report on the supply and administration of medicines under group protocols. Department of Health, London

Department of Health 1995 Variations in health: what can the Department of Health and the NHS do? Report of the Variations Sub-group of the Chief Medical Officer's Health of the Nation working group. HMSO, London

Department of Health 1998 Smoking kills. Executive summary. Stationery Office, London

Department of Health 1999 Saving lives: our healthier nation. Stationery Office, London

Department of Health 2000a Consultation on proposals to extend nurse prescribing. Department of Health, London

Department of Health 2000b National Service Framework for Coronary Heart Disease. Department of Health, London

Donald IP 1995 Gloucester hospital-at-home: a randomised control trial (research looking at the benefits of the scheme for elderly medical patients). Age and Ageing 24(5): 434–439

Fagin CM 1992 Collaboration between nurses and physicians no longer a choice. Academic Medicine 67(5): 295–303

Glen S, Clark A 1999 Nurse education: a skill mix for the future. Nurse Education Today 19(1): 12–19

Haddock J, Burrows C 1997 The role of the nurse in health promotion: an evaluation of a smoking cessation program in surgical pre-admission clinics. Journal of Advanced Nursing 26: 1098–1110

Hitchings E, Moynihan PJ 1998 The relationship between television food advertisements recalled and actual foods consumed by children. Journal of Human Nutrition and Dietetics 11(6): 511–517

Hollingsworth W, Todd C, Parker M, Roberts JA, Williams R 1993 Cost analysis of early discharge after hip fracture. British Medical Journal 307: 903–906

Hough D, Crosat S, Nye P 1991 Patient education for total hip replacements. Nursing Management 22(3): 80I–80P

Huerta-Torres V 1998 Preparing patients for early discharge after CABG. American Journal of Nursing 98(5): 49–51

Inside Track 1999 Unequal Britian. Inside Labour 1(2) (suppl): vi–vii

Keeling AW, Dennison PD 1995 Nurse-initiated telephone follow-up after acute myocardial infarction: a pilot study. Heart and Lung 24(1): 45–49

Knowleden J, Westlake L, Clarke S, Wright K 1991 Peterborough hospital at home: an evaluation. Journal of Public Health Medicine 13: 182–188

Lamb R, Sissons Joshi M 1996 The stage model and processes of change in dietary fat reduction. Journal of Human Nutrition and Dietetics 9(1): 43–53

Livingstone J, Harvey M, Kitchen N, Shah N, Westell C 1993 Role of pre-admission clinics in a general surgical unit: a six months audit. Annals of the Royal College of Surgeons of England 75: 211–212

Marklund B, Koritz P, Bjorkander E, Bengtsson C 1991 How well do nurse-run telephone consultations and consultations in the surgery agree? Experience in Swedish primary health care. British Journal of General Practice 41: 462–465

Mayor S 2000 Heart disease framework aims to cut deaths in England. British Medical Journal 320: 665

McManus E, Sieler P 1998 Freedom to enjoy learning in the 21st century; developing an active learning culture in nursing. Nursing Education Today 18: 322–328

Mitchell M 1997 Patients' perceptions of pre-operative preparation for day surgery. Journal of Advanced Nursing 2: 356–363

Munro R 1999 Growing demand for nurse degrees. Nursing Times 95(9): 9

National Audit Office 1996 Review of the implementation of health promotion policies. HMSO, London

National Children's Home 1991 Poverty and nutrition survey. National Children's Home, London

Newton V 1996 Care in pre-admission clinics. Nursing Times 92(1): 27–28

NHS Executive 1998 The new NHS: modern, dependable. A national framework for assessing performance. Consultation Document. Department of Health, London

NHS Executive 1999 The review of prescribing, supply and administration of medicines. NHS Executive, London

NHS Executive 2000 Faster access to modern treatment: how NICE appraisal will work. NHS Executive, London

Parsons LC 1998 Delegation skills and nurse job satisfaction. Nursing Economics 16(1): 18–26

Payne D 1998 Language barrier warning over NHS helpline. Nursing Times 94(5): 8

Poulter N, Sever P, Sever S 1996 Cardiovascular disease: practical issues for prevention, 2nd edn. Lynn Whitfield, Surrey

Robinson SE, Hill Y 1999 Our healthier hospital? The challenge for nursing. Journal of Nursing Management 7(1): 13–17

Shiono M, Sezai Y 1998 Less invasive coronary artery bypass without cardiopulmonary bypass. Artificial organs. Blackwell Science, Oxford, pp. 769–774

Smith AM, Smith C 1994 Dietary intake and lifestyle patterns: correlates with socio-economic, demographic and environmental factors. Journal of Human Nutrition and Dietetics 7(4): 283–294

Smith K 1997 Is there a role for the research practitioner? Managing clinical nursing. Churchill Livingstone, New York, pp. 33–38

Speechley V 1989 Patient teaching. Surgical Nurse 2(6): 20–22

Teasdale K 1995 Theoretical and practical consideration on the use of reassurance in the nursing management of anxious patients. Journal of Advanced Nursing 22(1): 79–86

Townsend P, Davidson N, Whitehead M (eds) 1992 Inequalities in health: the Black Report and the Health Divide. Penguin, Harmondsworth

UKCC 1992 The scope of professional practice. UKCC, London

UKCC 1997 Press statement: UKCC position on advanced practice. Advanced practice project: description and discussion. Annexe 1 to cc/97/06, p. 2. UKCC, London

UKCC 1998 Higher level of practice. Consultation document. UKCC, London

Williams S, Crouch R, Dale J 1995 Providing health-care advice by telephone. Professional Nurse 10(12): 750

Wilson-Barnett J 1992 Guest editorial. Specialist in nursing: effectiveness and maximisation of benefit. Journal of Advanced Nursing 21: 1–2

Worley B 1986 Pre-admission testing and teaching: more satisfaction at less cost. Nursing Management 17(12): 32–33

Wright S 1988 Joint appointments: handle with care. Nursing Times 84(1): 32–33

INDEX